THIRD EDITION

FOUNDATIONS OF NURSING IN THE COMMUNITY

Community-Oriented Practice

THIRD EDITION

FOUNDATIONS OF NURSING IN THE COMMUNITY

Community-Oriented Practice

MARCIA STANHOPE, RN, DSN, FAAN
The Good Samaritan Professor and Chair in
Community Health Nursing
College of Nursing
University of Kentucky
Lexington, Kentucky

JEANETTE LANCASTER, RN, PhD, FAAN
Visiting Professor, Department of Nursing Studies
The University of Hong Kong
Professor, University of Virginia
Formerly, Sadie Heath Cabaniss Professor and Dean
School of Nursing
University of Virginia
Charlottesville, Virginia

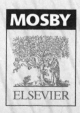

MOSBY

ELSEVIER

MOSBY
ELSEVIER

3251 Riverport Lane
St. Louis, Missouri 63043

Notice

Knowledge and best practice in this field are constantly changing. As new research and experience broaden our knowledge, changes in practice, treatment, and drug therapy may become necessary or appropriate. Readers are advised to check the most current information provided (i) on procedures featured or (ii) by the manufacturer of each product to be administered, to verify the recommended dose or formula, the method and duration of administration, and contraindications. It is the responsibility of the practitioner, relying on his or her own experience and knowledge of the patient, to make diagnoses, to determine dosages and the best treatment for each individual patient, and to take all appropriate safety precautions. To the fullest extent of the law, neither the Publisher nor the Authors assume any liability for any injury and/or damage to persons or property arising out of or related to any use of the material contained in this book.

The Publisher

Previous editions copyrighted 2002, 2006

Library of Congress Cataloging-in-Publication Data or Control Number

Stanhope, Marcia.
  Foundations of nursing in the community : community-oriented practice
/ Marcia Stanhope, Jeanette Lancaster. -- 3rd ed.
       p. ; cm.
  Includes bibliographical references and index.
  ISBN 978-0-323-06655-6 (pbk. : alk. paper)
  1. Community health nursing. I. Lancaster, Jeanette. II. Title.
  [DNLM: 1. Community Health Nursing. 2. Community Health Services.
WY 106 S786fa 2010]
  RT98.S78197 2010
  610.73'43--dc22
                        2009022207

Managing Editors: Linda Thomas and Nancy O'Brien
Developmental Editor: Carlie Bliss Irwin
Publishing Services Manager: Anne Altepeter
Senior Project Manager: Cheryl A. Abbott
Design Direction: Kimberly Denando

Printed in China

Last digit is the print number: 9   8   7   6   5   4   3   2   1

I would like to dedicate this edition to the memory of my brother Gerald who taught me much, through his life and struggles with his disabilities, about the importance of listening and taking action to promote his quality of life and the need for a responsive health care system.

Marcia Stanhope

About the Authors

Marcia Stanhope, RN, DSN, FAAN

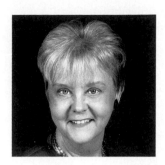

Marcia Stanhope is currently The Good Samaritan Professor and Chair in Community Health Nursing at the University of Kentucky College of Nursing in Lexington, Kentucky. She has practiced community and home health nursing, has served as an administrator and consultant in home health, and has been involved in the development of multiple nurse-managed centers. She has taught public and community health, primary care nursing, and administration courses. Dr. Stanhope formerly served as associate dean at the University of Kentucky College of Nursing, also directed the Division of Community Health Nursing and Administration, and co-directed the Doctorate of Nursing Practice program from its inception. She has been responsible for both undergraduate and graduate courses in public and community health nursing. She also has taught at the University of Virginia and the University of Alabama, Birmingham. Her presentations and publications have been in the areas of home health, community health and community-based nursing practice, primary care nursing, and nurse-managed centers with emphasis on vulnerable populations. Dr. Stanhope holds a diploma in nursing from the Good Samaritan Hospital in Lexington, Kentucky, and a bachelor of science in nursing from the University of Kentucky. She has a master's degree in public health nursing from Emory University in Atlanta and a doctorate of science in nursing from the University of Alabama, Birmingham. Dr. Stanhope is the co-author of four other Mosby/Elsevier publications: *Public Health Nursing* (also with Dr. Lancaster), *Handbook of Community-Based and Home Health Nursing Practice, Public and Community Health Nurse's Consultant,* and *Case Studies in Community Health Nursing Practice: A Problem-Based Learning Approach.* Dr. Stanhope received the 2000 Public Health Nursing Creative Achievement Award from the Public Health Nursing Section of the American Public Health Association. She was inducted into the University of Kentucky Distinguished Alumni Hall of Fame, May 2005, joining 257 other graduates of the University of Kentucky who have received this honor. Other honors include recognition as an Edgerunner by the American Academy of Nursing, October 2006, for her work with nurse-managed centers.

Jeanette Lancaster RN, PhD, FAAN

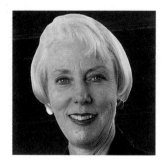

Jeanette Lancaster is currently a visiting professor in the Department of Nursing Studies at the University of Hong Kong. She served for 19 years as the Sadie Heath Cabaniss Professor of Nursing and Dean at the University of Virginia School of Nursing in Charlottesville, Virginia. Dr. Lancaster also served as president of the American Association of Colleges of Nursing. She has practiced psychiatric nursing and taught both psychiatric and community health nursing. She formerly directed the master's program in community health nursing at the University of Alabama, Birmingham, and served as dean of the School of Nursing at Wright State University in Dayton, Ohio. Her publications and presentations have been largely in the areas of community and public health nursing, leadership and change, and the significance of nurses to effective primary health care. Dr. Lancaster is a graduate of the University of Tennessee, Memphis, College of Nursing. She holds a master's degree in psychiatric nursing from Case Western Reserve University in Cleveland and a doctorate in public health from the University of Oklahoma. Dr. Lancaster is the author of another Mosby/Elsevier publication, *Nursing Issues in Leading and Managing Change,* and co-author (with Dr. Stanhope) of *Public Health Nursing.* She edits the interdisciplinary journal, *Family & Community Health.* She most recently has taught undergraduate and graduate courses in public health nursing and health promotion in the Department of Nursing Studies, Faculty of Medicine at the University of Hong Kong.

Contributors

We gratefully acknowledge the following individuals who wrote chapters for the seventh edition of *Public Health Nursing,* upon which the chapters in this book are based.

Brenda Afzal, MS, RN
Director of Health Programs
School of Nursing
665D SNB
University of Maryland
Baltimore, Maryland

Debra Gay Anderson, PhD, RNC
Associate Professor
College of Nursing
University of Kentucky
Lexington, Kentucky

Dyan A. Aretakis, MSN, FNP
Project Director
Teen Health Center
University of Virginia Health System
Charlottesville, Virginia

Edie Devers Barbero, PhD, RN
Assistant Professor
School of Nursing
University of Virginia
Charlottesville, Virginia

Linda K. Birenbaum, RN, PhD
Public Health Program Supervisor
Washington County Health and Human Services–Public
  Health
Hillsboro, Oregon

Christine Di Martile Bolla, RN, DNSc
Assistant Professor
Department of Nursing
Dominican University of California
San Rafael, California

Angeline Bushy, PhD, RN, FAAN
Professor and Bert Fish Memorial Eminent Scholar Chair
Daytona Campus Coordinator
School of Nursing
University of Central Florida
Daytona Beach, Florida

Jacquelyn C. Campbell, PhD, RN, FAAN
Anna D. Wolf Professor and Chair
School of Nursing
Johns Hopkins University
Baltimore, Maryland

Ann H. Cary, PhD, MPH, RN, A-CCC
Professor and Director
School of Nursing
Loyola University, New Orleans
New Orleans, Louisiana

Deborah C. Conway, MSN, RN
Assistant Professor
University of Virginia School of Nursing
Charlottesville, Virginia

Marcia K. Cowan, MSN, CPNP
Pediatric Nurse Practitioner
The Pediatric Center of Tullahoma, PC
Tullahoma, Tennessee

Cynthia E. Degazon, PhD, RN
Associate Professor
Hunter Bellevue School of Nursing
Hunter College of the City University of New York
New York, New York

Janna Dieckmann, PhD, RN
Assistant Professor
School of Nursing
University of North Carolina at Chapel Hill
Chapel Hill, North Carolina

Diane B. Downing, RN, MSN
Public Health Program Specialist
Arlington County Department of Human Services
Arlington, Virginia
Clinical Instructor
Georgetown University
School of Nursing and Health Studies
Washington, DC

James J. Fletcher, PhD
Retired, Associate Professor of Philosophy
Department of Philosophy and Religious Studies
George Mason University
Fairfax, Virginia

Kathleen Ryan Fletcher, RN, MSN, APRN-BC, CNP
Assistant Professor, School of Nursing
Director, Senior Services
University of Virginia Health System
Charlottesville, Virginia

Doris Glick, RN, PhD
Associate Professor
School of Nursing
University of Virginia
Charlottesville, Virginia

Jean Goeppinger, PhD, RN, FAAN
Professor
Schools of Nursing and Public Health
University of North Carolina at Chapel Hill
Chapel Hill, North Carolina

Monty Gross, PhD, RN, CNE
Associate Professor
Department of Nursing
James Madison University
Harrisonburg, Virginia

Cynthia Z. Gustafson, PhD, APRN-BC
Chair and Associate Professor
Department of Nursing
Director of the Parish Nurse Center
Carroll College
Helena, Montana

Patty J. Hale, RN, PhD, FNP, FAAN
Professor and Graduate Program Coordinator
Department of Nursing
James Madison University
Harrisonburg, Virginia

Susan B. Hassmiller, PhD, RN, FAAN
Senior Advisor for Nursing
The Robert Wood Johnson Foundation
Former Chair, Disaster Services
American Red Cross
Princeton, New Jersey

Diane C. Hatton, DNSc, RN
Professor
Community Health Nursing Concentration Chair
San Diego State University
San Diego, California

Bonnie Jerome-D'Emilia, PhD, RN
Professor
Department of Nursing
Rutgers Camden College of Arts and Sciences
Camden, New Jersey

Joanna Rowe Kaakinen, PhD, RN
Associate Professor
School of Nursing
University of Portland
Portland, Oregon

Lisa M. Kaiser, RN, MSN, PhD(c)
Associate Faculty
National University
LaJolla, California

Kären M. Landenburger, RN, PhD
Professor
Nursing Program
University of Washington, Tacoma
Tacoma, Washington

Susan C. Long-Marin, DVM, MPH
Epidemiology Manager
Mecklenburg County Health Department
Charlotte, North Carolina

Karen S. Martin, RN, MSN, FAAN
Health Care Consultant
Martin Associates
Omaha, Nebraska

Mary Lynn Mathre, RN, MSN, CARN, CLNC
President
Patients Out of Time
Sole Proprietor of Medical Legal Management
Howardsville, Virginia

Robert E. McKeown, PhD
Professor of Epidemiology, Department Chair
Arnold School of Public Health
University of South Carolina
Columbia, South Carolina

DeAnne K. Hilfinger Messias, RN, PhD, FAAN
Associate Professor
College of Nursing and Women's and Gender Studies Program
University of South Carolina
Columbia, South Carolina

Lillian H. Mood, RN, MPH, FAAN
Retired, State Director of Public Health Nursing, Assistant Commissioner, and Community Liaison for Environmental Quality Control
South Carolina Department of Health and Environmental Control
Chapin, South Carolina

Marie Napolitano, RN, PhD, FNP
Associate Professor
School of Nursing
University of Portland
Portland, Oregon

Lisa L. Onega, PhD, RN, FNP, GNP
Professor
Waldron College of Health and Human Services
Radford University
Radford, Virginia

Bonnie Rogers, DrPH, COHN-S, LNCC, FAAN
Director
North Carolina Occupational Safety and Health Education and Research Center
Director, Public Health/Occupational Health Nursing Programs
University of North Carolina
Chapel Hill, North Carolina

Barbara Sattler, RN, DrPH, FAAN
Professor, Family and Community Health
School of Nursing
University of Maryland
Baltimore, Maryland

Juliann G. Sebastian, ARNP, PhD, FAAN
Dean and Professor
College of Nursing
University of Missouri—St. Louis
St. Louis, Missouri

George F. Shuster, RN, DNSc
Associate Professor
College of Nursing
University of New Mexico
Albuquerque, New Mexico

Mary Cipriano Silva, RN, PhD, FAAN
Professor Emeritis
College of Nursing and Health Science
George Mason University
Fairfax, Virginia

Jeanne Merkle Sorrell, PhD, RN, FAAN
Professor
College of Nursing and Health Science
George Mason University
Fairfax, Virginia

Francisco S. Sy, MD, DrPH
Director
Division of Extramural Activities and Scientific Programs
National Center on Minority Health and Health Disparities
National Institutes of Health
Bethesda, Maryland

Anita Thompson-Heisterman, MSN, RN, CS, FNP
Assistant Professor
University of Virginia
School of Nursing
Charlottesville, Virginia

Heather Ward, MSN, ARNP
Master's Student
University of Kentucky
College of Nursing
Lexington, Kentucky

Carolyn A. Williams, RN, PhD, FAAN
Professor and Former Dean
College of Nursing
University of Kentucky
Lexington, Kentucky

Judith Lupo Wold, PhD, RN
Associate Professor Emeritus
School of Nursing
College of Health and Human Sciences
Georgia State University
Atlanta, Georgia

Janet T. Ihlenfeld, RN, PhD†

Ancillary Contributors

Virginia Nehring, PhD, RN
Professor Emeritus
Wright State University
College of Nursing and Health
Dayton, Ohio
Test Bank

Lisa Turner, RN, MSN
Associate Professor
University of Kentucky
School of Nursing
Lexington, Kentucky
PowerPoint Slides

Reviewers

Joanne Dalton, PhD, RN
Associate Professor of Nursing
Regis College
Weston, Massachusetts

Kathleen M. Lamaute, EdD, FNP, CNAA, BC, CNE
Associate Professor of Nursing
Molloy College
Rockville Centre, New York

Phyllis More, PhD, RN, BC
Professor of Nursing
Bloomfield College
Bloomfield, New Jersey

Beth Pritchett, APRN, BC
Associate Professor of Nursing
Bluefield State College
Bluefield, West Virginia

†We are indebted to Janet T. Ihlenfeld RN, PhD, who ably authored "The Nurse in the Schools" chapter in the seventh edition of *Public Health Nursing: Population-Centered Health Care in the Community.* Before her death, Dr. Ihlenfeld was a professor of nursing at D'Youville College where she taught both child health and community health nursing. Her knowledge and teaching experience made her an ideal author for the chapter on "The Nurse in the Schools."

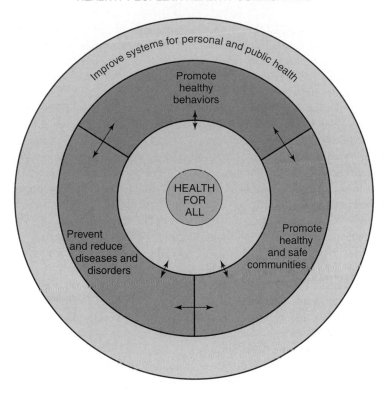

Community Nursing Definitions

Community-Oriented Nursing Practice is a philosophy of nursing service delivery that involves the generalist or specialist community-oriented nurse providing "health care" through community diagnosis and investigation of major health and environmental problems, health surveillance, and monitoring and evaluation of community and population health status for the purposes of preventing disease and disability and promoting, protecting, and maintaining "health" in order to create conditions in which people can be healthy.

Nursing Practice in the Community is the synthesis of nursing theory and public health theory applied to promoting, preserving, and maintaining the health of populations through the delivery of personal health care services to individuals, families, and groups. The focus of practice is health of individuals, families, and groups and the effect of their health status on the health of the community as a whole.

Community-Based Nursing Practice is a setting-specific practice whereby care is provided for "sick" individuals and families where they live, work, and go to school. The emphasis of practice is acute and chronic care and the provision of comprehensive, coordinated, and continuous services. Nurses who deliver community-based care are generalists or specialists in maternal-infant, pediatric, adult, or psychiatric-mental health nursing.

From *Healthy People 2010: Understanding and Improving Health,* March 2001.

Preface

As we look back at the preface to the second edition of this text, it is clear that many of the concerns at that time about health care still exist. In the United States, an increasing amount of money is spent annually on health care, yet nearly 46 million people lack health coverage. Of these, a large number are children and employed people. In a recent report entitled *2008 America's Health Rankings* (2008) many of the findings about the health of individuals and their communities are discouraging. What is most discouraging is that many of the most significant health maladies at present are both preventable and are public health concerns. Also, regrettably, health status indicators are not improving. The findings of this report, which assesses health status annually by individual states, were confirmed in the reflections of former Surgeon General Everett Koop in an editorial in the *American Journal of Public Health* in late 2006. He commented that in nearly 6 decades of public health work, he was "awed at what has been achieved and shocked at what has not" (Koop, 2006, p. 2090). He commented on the many medical miracles that have saved lives and led to longer lives but that have often failed to make those added years any freer of disability and discomfort. He went on to talk about preventable health problems, including obesity; orthopedic injury; unintentional pregnancies, many of which lead to abortions; and lack of adequate preparation to deal effectively with potential influenza pandemics, bioterrorism, or HIV/AIDS.

Further, health care around the world is vastly uneven. From the high performing countries in terms of health to the poor and disadvantaged countries in Africa and other nations, there are enormous differences in economic indicators and education, as well as in the quality of life for their citizens in regard to health. To illustrate, the United States currently is 28th in terms of health life expectancy with an average life expectancy of 69 years. Japan leads all countries with an average life expectancy of 75 years. Regrettably, among 18 other industrialized nations, the United States ranked last in death from treatable conditions before age 75. Between 2003 and 2008, the United States fell below Finland, Portugal, the United Kingdom, and Ireland on this health indicator (America's Health Ratings, 2008).

For several years, many of us in public health and public health nursing have believed that a number of national priorities are misaligned. In recent years we have spent more money on war than on dealing with poverty. We continue to reimburse more fully for complex reparative procedures than spend money on prevention, including health education and health promotion. Despite the fact that many people across the world know that lifestyle plays a large role in morbidity and mortality, only a portion of the people in each country "walk the talk" in terms of their own personal behavior. It is important to remember that numerous deaths each year are still attributed to tobacco, alcohol, and illicit drug use; diet and activity patterns; microbial agents; toxic agents;

firearms; sexual behavior; and motor vehicle accidents. Over the years the most significant improvements in the health of the population have come from advances in public health such as improvements in motor vehicle safety, food and water sanitation, food pasteurization and refrigeration, immunizations, workplace safety, and emphasis on personal lifestyle and environmental factors that affect health. Changes in the public health system are essential if the health of the people in the United States is to improve.

The need to focus attention on health promotion, lifestyle factors, and disease prevention led to the development of a healthy public policy in the United States. This policy was designed by a large number of people representing a wide range of groups interested in health. The policy is reflected in the document *Healthy People 2010,* which identifies a comprehensive set of national health-promotion and disease-prevention objectives. Despite the development of these guidelines for health and the acceptance of the goals and objectives set forth, health indicators are simply not measuring up to what the expectations were.

To develop healthy populations, individuals, families, and communities, there must be a commitment to health goals. In addition, society, through the development of health policy, must support better health care, the design of improved health education, the financing of strategies to alter health status, and the support of alliances and coalitions that truly and consistently work together to improve health care. Of most importance, healthy public policy must be evidence based and outcomes of the policies evaluated.

Our message to you our readers is to ask "How are you going to use the knowledge and skills that you have to make a difference in health care?" We ask you to remember that behind every public health decision, there is a political decision. This means that your role in health care is broad and includes care to individuals, families, communities, and the nation. In late 2008, Bill Foege, MD, MPH, former head of the Centers for Disease Control and Prevention and now with the Bill and Melinda Gates Foundation, offered these comments that have direct usefulness to students of public health nursing, "Leadership in the future will require knowing the rules of coalitions. Most coalitions (however) are formed around an idea. The best will be formed around an outcome" (American Academy of Nursing, 2008 meeting). His words emphasize that public health work is not the work of a soloist and that the work should focus on the outcome versus the process. We hope that this text will provide you with some of the tools to accomplish the goal Dr. Foege sets forth. It is our belief that nurses are the backbone of public health in both developed and developing countries.

This text focuses on the processes and practices for promoting health principally by the nurse, who is considered to be an ideal person to demonstrate and teach others how to promote health. To be effective, health promotion requires that people cease focusing on how to "fix" themselves and others only when they detect physical and emotional problems and that they instead assume personal responsibility for health promotion. Such a change in emphasis requires that health care providers incorporate health-promotion techniques into their practice.

Because people do not always know how to improve their health status, the challenge of nursing is to initiate change. Public health nursing focuses on the health of individuals, families, and groups to change the health of the population as a whole. The practice takes place in a variety of public and private settings and includes disease prevention, health promotion, health protection, education, maintenance, restoration, coordination, management, and evaluation of care of individuals, families, and populations, including communities.

To meet the demands of a constantly changing health care system, nurses must be visionary in designing their roles and identifying their practice areas. To do so effectively, nurses must understand concepts and theories of public health, the changing health care system, the actual and potential roles and responsibilities of nurses and other health care providers, the importance of a health-promotion and disease-prevention orientation, and the necessity to involve consumers in the planning, implementation, and evaluation of health care efforts.

This text was written to provide nursing students and practicing nurses with a comprehensive source book that provides a foundation for designing nursing strategies for individuals, families, and populations, including communities. The book integrates health-promotion and disease-prevention concepts into all aspects of practice.

■ REFERENCES

Koop CE: Health and health care for the 21st Century: for all the people, *Am J Public Health* 96(12):2090-2091, 2006.
America's Health Rankings: *2008 America's Health Rankings: a call to action for individuals and their communities,* Minnetonka, Minn, 2008, United Health Group, available at http://www.americashealthranking.org/2008/overview/html.

ORGANIZATION

The text is divided into seven sections:
* *Part I,* **Perspectives in Health Care Delivery and Nursing,** describes the historical and current status of the health care delivery system and nursing practice in the community.
* *Part II,* **Influences on Health Care Delivery and Nursing,** addresses specific issues and societal concerns that affect nursing practice in the community.
* *Part III,* **Conceptual Frameworks Applied to Nursing Practice in the Community,** provides conceptual models for nursing practice in the community; selected models from nursing and related sciences are also discussed.
* *Part IV,* **Issues and Approaches in Health Care Populations,** examines the management of health care and select community environments, as well as issues related to managing cases, programs, disasters, and groups.
* *Part V,* **Issues and Approaches in Family and Individual Health Care,** discusses risk factors and health problems for families and individuals throughout the life span.
* *Part VI,* **Vulnerability: Predisposing Factors,** covers specific health care needs and issues of populations at risk.
* *Part VII,* **Nursing Practice in the Community: Roles and Functions,** examines diversity in the role of nurses in the community and describes the rapidly changing roles, functions, and practice settings.

PEDAGOGY

Each chapter is organized for easy use by students and faculty. Chapters begin with a list of Additional Resources that directs students to chapter-related tools and resources contained in the Appendixes on the book's Evolve website, or when using Patty Hale's *Real World Community Health Nursing: An Interactive CD-ROM* with the textbook. Objectives guide student learning and assist faculty in knowing what students should gain from the content. The Chapter Outline alerts students to the structure and content of the chapter. Key Terms and their definitions are also provided at the beginning of the chapter to assist the student in understanding unfamiliar terminology. The key terms are in boldface within the text.

The following features are presented in most or all chapters:

BRIEFLY NOTED BOXES

Present notes to the student that may be a fact of interest, a special consideration for clinical practice, or a contemporary issue that stimulates debate and discussion.

HOW TO Boxes

Provide specific, application-oriented information.

Evidence-Based Practice

Illustrates the use and application of the latest research findings in public health, community health, and nursing.

Levels of Prevention Boxes

Apply primary, secondary, and tertiary prevention to the specific chapter content.

Healthy People 2010

Contains selected objectives from this landmark document that fit the specific chapter content. The new *Healthy People 2020* objectives are scheduled to be released in 2010 and will be added to the book's Evolve website as soon as they are available.

CASE STUDY

Real-life clinical situations help students develop their assessment and critical thinking skills.

CLINICAL APPLICATION

At the end of each chapter, these boxes provide the reader with an understanding of how to apply chapter content in the clinical setting through the presentation of a case situation with questions students will want to think about as they analyze the case.

REMEMBER THIS!

Provides a summary in list form of the most important points made in the chapter.

WHAT WOULD YOU DO?

Stimulates student learning by suggesting a variety of activities that encourage both independent and collaborative effort.

In the back of the book you will find additional important sources of information.

Numerous **Appendixes** provide additional resources and key information.

Answers to Clinical Application Questions provide answers for each Clinical Application question.

TEACHING AND LEARNING PACKAGE

A website, http://evolve.elsevier.com/stanhope/foundations, includes instructor and student materials.

For the instructor:
- Annotated Chapter Outlines
- Critical Thinking Activities
- Test Bank, with 800 questions
- Image Collection, with all illustrations from the book
- Learning Objectives
- Critical Analysis Questions and Answers
- PowerPoint slides

For the student:
- Quiz, containing NCLEX®-format study questions
- Case Studies, with Questions and Answers
- Community Assessment Applied
- Chapter-Specific WebLinks

Acknowledgments

We would like to thank our families, friends, and colleagues who supported us in the completion of the third edition. Special thanks go to our co-workers at the University of Kentucky College of Nursing and the University of Virginia School of Nursing who provided generous support and assistance. We especially thank Linda Thomas, Carlie Bliss Irwin, and Cheryl Abbott at Elsevier and the peer reviewers for their time and thoughtfulness in completing the revisions.

We would like to extend special thanks to the contributors of the seventh edition of Public Health Nursing *for their careful and thoughtful reviews and critique of the chapters of this book.*

Marcia Stanhope

Jeanette Lancaster

Contents

THIRD EDITION

FOUNDATIONS OF NURSING IN THE COMMUNITY

Community-Oriented Practice

PART I

Perspectives in Health Care Delivery and Nursing

Chapter 1

Community-Oriented Nursing and Community-Based Nursing

Carolyn A. Williams

ADDITIONAL RESOURCES

These related resources are found either in the appendix at the back of this book or on the book's website at http://evolve.elsevier.com/stanhope/foundations.

Appendix

• Appendix E.3: The Health Insurance Portability and Accountability Act (HIPAA)

Evolve Website

• Community Assessment Applied
• Case Study, with questions and answers
• Quiz review questions
• WebLinks, including link to *Healthy People 2010* website

Real World Community Health Nursing: An Interactive CD-ROM, second edition

If you are using this CD-ROM in your course, you will find the following activities related to this chapter:
• *Definitions and More* in **Public and Community Health: The Big Picture**
• *Can You Tell the Difference?* in **Public and Community Health: The Big Picture**
• *What Is Public Health Nursing?* in **Public and Community Health: The Big Picture**

OBJECTIVES

After reading this chapter, the student should be able to:

1. Describe the core functions of public health and the services generally provided by practitioners of public health.
2. Discuss the role of the public health nurse specialist and how the role influences nursing practice in the community.
3. Explain community-based nursing practice.
4. Describe community-oriented nursing practice.
5. Examine how community-based nursing practice differs from community-oriented nursing practice.

CHAPTER OUTLINE

WHAT IS PUBLIC HEALTH?
PUBLIC HEALTH CORE FUNCTIONS DEFINED
POPULATION-FOCUSED NURSING PRACTICE
PRACTICE FOCUSING ON INDIVIDUALS, FAMILIES, AND GROUPS

Community-Oriented Nursing
Community-Based Nursing
CHALLENGES FOR THE FUTURE

KEY TERMS

aggregate: a population group.

assessment: systematic data collection about a population. This includes monitoring the population's health status and providing information about the health of the community.

assurance: the public health role of making sure that essential community-oriented health services are available.

community: people and the relationships that emerge among them as they develop and use in common some agencies and institutions and share a physical environment.

community-based: occurs outside an institution. Services are provided to individuals and families in a community.

community-based nursing: the provision of acute care and care for chronic health problems to individuals and families in the community.

community health nursing: nursing practice in the community, with the primary focus on the health care of individuals, families, and groups in a community. The goal is to preserve, protect, promote, or maintain health.

community-oriented nursing: nursing that has as its primary focus the health care of either the community or a population of individuals, families, and groups.

community-oriented practice: broader in scope than community-based practice. A form of care in which the nurse provides health care after doing a community diagnosis to determine what conditions need to be altered so that individuals, families, and groups in the community to stay healthy.

policy development: providing leadership in developing policies that support the health of the population.

population: a collection of people who share one or more personal or environmental characteristics.

population-focused: emphasizes populations who live in a community.

population-focused practice: the core of public health, a practice that emphasizes health protection, health promotion, and disease prevention of a population.

primary health care services: both primary care and public health services that are designed to meet the basic needs of people in communities at an affordable cost.

public health: community efforts designed to prevent disease and promote health. It can be what members of society do collectively to ensure conditions that support health.

public health core functions: these include assessment, policy development, and assurance.

public health nursing: a specialty of nursing that synthesizes nursing, social, and public health sciences to provide care to populations.

secondary health care services: services designed to detect and treat disease in the early acute stage.

subpopulations: subsets of the population who share similar characteristics. For example, people older than 65 years who live in a residential home would be a subpopulation of a larger population of older persons in the community.

tertiary health care services: services designed to limit the progression of disease or disability.

Professional nurses must actively participate in developing cost-effective, high-quality, innovative, and useful ways to provide care to citizens. Because of the growing costs of hospital care, more services are being provided in **community-based** settings. Increasingly, nurses will engage in what is called **community-based nursing** (CBN). In CBN, the nurse focuses on "illness care" of individuals and families across the life span. The aim is to manage acute and chronic health conditions in the **community,** and the practice is family-centered illness care. While providing health care to individuals and families, the nurse maintains an appreciation for the values of the community. CBN is not a specialty in nursing but rather a philosophy that guides care in all nursing specialties.

In contrast, **community-oriented nursing** has as its primary focus the health care either of the community or populations as in **public health nursing** (PHN) or of individuals, families, and groups in a community; in the past and by some today this has been called **community health nursing.** In community-oriented community health nursing the goal is to preserve, protect, promote, or maintain health. The key difference between CBN and community-oriented nursing is that community-based nurses deal primarily with illness-oriented care whereas community-oriented nurses provide health care to promote quality of life. They both deal with individuals and families, and the community-oriented nurse also typically deals with groups in the community. Table 1-1 lists the similarities and differences between community-oriented nursing and CBN.

As mentioned, community-oriented nursing includes PHN. This is a specialty area whose primary focus is on the health care of communities and populations rather than on individuals, groups, and families. The goal of this specialty is to prevent disease and preserve, promote, restore, and protect health for the community and the population within it. The focus is on the public health ethic of "the greatest good for the greatest number." This specialty is built on the blending of nursing and the discipline of public health (American Nurses Association, 2007).

This chapter examines both CBN and community-oriented nursing. It describes the similarities and differences between these two areas of nursing and also discusses public health and the core functions and services that are included in public health practice. In addition, the essential services of public health nurses are discussed, since nurses working from both a CBN and a community-oriented community health nursing framework may use some of these skills. To work effectively in the community regardless of the focus, it

Table 1-1	**Select Examples of Similarities and Differences between Community-Oriented and Community-Based Nursing**	
	Community-Oriented Nursing	**Community-Based Nursing**
Philosophy	Primary focus is on "health care" of individuals, families, groups and the community, or populations	Focus is on "illness care" of individuals and families across the life span
Goal	Preserve, protect, promote, or maintain health and prevent disease	Manage acute or chronic conditions
Service Context	Personal health care Population health	Family-centered illness care
Community Type	Varied, usually local community	Human ecological
Client Characteristics	• Individuals at risk • Families at risk • Groups at risk • Communities • Usually healthy • Culturally diverse • Autonomous • Able to define their own problem • Primary decision maker	• Individuals • Families • Usually ill • Culturally diverse • Autonomous • Able to define their own problem • Involved in decision making
Practice Setting	• Community agencies • Home • Work • School • Playground • May be organization • May be government	• Community agencies • Home • Work • School
Interaction Patterns	• One-to-one • Groups • May be organized	• One-to-one
Type of Service	• Direct care of at-risk persons • Indirect (program management)	• Direct illness care
Emphasis on Levels of Prevention	• Primary • Secondary (screening) • Tertiary (maintenance and rehabilitation)	• Secondary • Tertiary • May be primary

Roles	***Client and Delivery Oriented: Individual, Family, Group, Population***
	• Caregiver
	• Social engineer
	• Educator
	• Counselor
	• Advocate
	• Case manager
	
	Group Oriented
	• Leader (personal health management)
	• Change agent (screening)
	• Community advocate/developer
	• Case finder
	• Community care agent
	  • Assessment
	  • Policy developer
	  • Assurance
	  • Enforcer of laws/compliance
		Client and Delivery Oriented: Individual, Family
		• Caregiver
		
		Group Oriented
		• Leader (disease management)
		• Change agent (managed-care services)

Priority of Nurse's Activities	• Case findings • Client education • Community education • Interdisciplinary practice • Case management (direct care) • Program planning and implementation • Individual, family, and population advocacy	• Case management (direct care) • Patient education • Individual and family advocacy • Interdisciplinary practice • Continuity of care provider

is useful to know exactly what public health is and how the functions of that discipline work to improve the health of people in their communities.

BRIEFLY NOTED

PHN, or community-oriented nursing and CBN practice are not all the same. The primary difference lies in the focus of public health nurses on populations and the health of the community versus a focus on illness care of individuals and families.

WHAT IS PUBLIC HEALTH?

Public health is a scientific discipline that includes the study of epidemiology, statistics, and assessment—including attention to behavioral, cultural, and economic factors—as well as program planning and policy development. In recent years, efforts in the United States to change the way in which health care is delivered have focused heavily on looking at ways to change the delivery of medical care and on health insurance. Limited attention has been focused on looking at the health of the population. Although people are excited when a new drug is discovered that cures a disease or when a new way to transplant organs is perfected, it is important to know about the significant gains in the health of populations that have come largely from public health accomplishments. For example, public health has influenced the safety and adequacy of food and water, sewage disposal, public safety from biological threats, and changes in personal behaviors such as smoking. The dramatic increase in life expectancy for Americans during the 1900s and 2000s, from less than 50 years in 1900 to more than 77 years in 2005, was the result primarily of improvements in sanitation, control of infectious diseases through immunizations, and other public health activities (U.S. Department of Health and Human Services, 2007). The population-focused preventive programs begun in the 1970s have led to changes in tobacco use, blood pressure control, dietary habits (except obesity), automobile safety restraint, and injury-control measures. These changes in health behavior have decreased deaths due to stroke, coronary heart disease, and cancer; as a result overall death rates have decreased by 45%. Yet chronic disease is on the increase because of the high prevalence of unhealthy lifestyles and behaviors (U.S. Department of Health and Human Services, 2007).

Another way of looking at the benefits of public health practice is to look at how early deaths can be prevented. The U.S. Public Health Service estimates that medical treatment can prevent only about 10% of all early deaths in the United States, whereas population-focused public health approaches could help prevent about 70% of early deaths in America through measures that influence the way people eat, drink, drive, engage in exercise, and treat the environment (U.S. Department of Health and Human Services, 2000). Public health practice provides many benefits, especially

considering the small portion of the health care budget in the United States that is used for this prevention and population-focused specialty. Some of this decline in the 1980s and 1990s occurred as public health agencies increasingly provided personal care services to people who were unable to obtain care elsewhere. Providing such care shifted resources and energy away from public health's traditional population-focused activities (Institute of Medicine, 2003). As overall health needs become the focus of care in the United States, a stronger commitment to population-focused services is emerging. In July 2008, The Trust for America's Health released a study that highlighted the effects of preventive services on improving lives and reducing costs as well as ways to change the health care system. The threats of bioterrorism, highlighted by the events of September 11, 2001, and the anthrax scares increase awareness for public safety. Important to the public health community is the emergence of modern-day epidemics and infectious diseases, such as the mosquito-borne West Nile virus and other causes of mortality, many of which affect the very young. Most of the causes are preventable (Baker and Koplan, 2002).

BRIEFLY NOTED

Because of the importance of influencing a population's health and providing a strong foundation for the health care system, the U.S. Public Health Service and other groups strongly advocate a renewed emphasis on the population-focused essential public health functions and services that have been most effective in improving the health of the entire population.

Public health is best described as what society collectively does to ensure that conditions exist in which people can be healthy (Institute of Medicine, 2003). Public health is a community-oriented, population-focused specialty area. The overall mission of public health is to organize community efforts that will use scientific and technical knowledge to prevent disease and promote health (Institute of Medicine, 2003). The three **public health core functions** are *assessment, policy development,* and *assurance.*

PUBLIC HEALTH CORE FUNCTIONS DEFINED

Figure 1-1 describes public health in America. These functions provide a framework for defining the services to be provided by the public health system. The core functions are defined as follows:
- **Assessment** is systematic data collection on the population, monitoring the population's health status, and making information available about the health of the community.
- **Policy development** refers to efforts to develop policies that support the health of the population, including using a scientific knowledge base to make policy decisions.

PUBLIC HEALTH IN AMERICA

Vision:
Healthy people in healthy communities

Mission:
Promote physical and mental health and
prevent disease, injury, and disability

Public health
• Prevents epidemics and the spread of disease
• Protects against environmental hazards
• Prevents injuries
• Promotes and encourages healthy behaviors
• Responds to disasters and assists communities in recovery
• Ensures the quality and accessibility of health services

Essential public health services by core function
Assessment
  1. Monitor health status to identify community health problems
  2. Diagnose and investigate health problems and health hazards in the community

Policy Development
  3. Inform, educate, and empower people about health issues
  4. Mobilize community partnerships to identify and solve health problems
  5. Develop policies and plans that support individual and community health efforts

Assurance
  6. Enforce laws and regulations that protect health and ensure safety
  7. Link people to needed personal health services and assure the provision of health
     care when otherwise unavailable.
  8. Ensure a competent public health and personal health care workforce
  9. Evaluate effectiveness, accessibility, and quality of personal and population-based
     health services

Serving All Functions
  10. Research for new insights and innovative solutions to health problems

FIGURE 1-1 Public health in America. (From U.S. Public Health Service: *The public health functions steering committee members*, Washington, DC, July 1995, Office of Disease Prevention and Health Promotion.)

• **Assurance** is making sure that essential community-oriented health services are available. These services might include providing essential personal health services for those who would otherwise not receive them. Assurance also includes making sure that a competent public health and personal health care workforce is available.

A working group within the U.S. Public Health Service developed the Health Services Pyramid (Figure 1-2). In this pyramid, population-focused public health programs with the goals of disease prevention, health protection, and health promotion provide a foundation for **primary, secondary, and tertiary health care services.** Each service level in the pyramid is important to the health of the population. The base of the pyramid shows the effective services that will support the top tiers and contribute to better health. All tiers of the pyramid need to be adequately financed (U.S. Public Health Service, 1994/2000). Since the pyramid was developed it has been used to show how health care services can be offered to specific population groups (Colorado Department of Public Health and Environment, 2008). In reality, health care in the United States has been organized with the pyramid upside down. That is, more attention, support, and

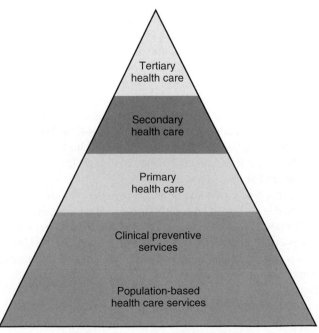

FIGURE 1-2 Health services pyramid.

HOW TO	Participate, as a Public Health Nurse, in the Essential Services of Public Health

1. Monitor health status to identify community health problems.
   - Participate in community assessment.
   - Identify subpopulations at risk for disease or disability.
   - Collect information on interventions to special populations.
   - Define and evaluate effective strategies and programs.
   - Identify potential environmental hazards.
2. Diagnose and investigate health problems and hazards in the community.
   - Understand and identify determinants of health and disease.
   - Apply knowledge about environmental influences of health.
   - Recognize multiple causes or factors of health and illness.
   - Participate in case identification and treatment of persons with communicable disease.
3. Inform, educate, and empower people about health issues.
   - Develop health and educational plans for individuals and families in multiple settings.
   - Develop and implement community-based health education.
   - Provide regular reports on the health status of special populations within clinic settings, community settings, and groups.
   - Advocate for and with underserved and disadvantaged populations.
   - Ensure health planning, which includes primary prevention and early intervention strategies.
   - Identify healthy population behaviors and maintain successful intervention strategies through reinforcement and continued funding.
4. Mobilize community partnerships to identify and solve health problems.
   - Interact regularly with many providers and services within each community.
   - Convene groups and providers who share common concerns and interests in special populations.
   - Provide leadership to prioritize community problems and develop interventions.
   - Explain the significance of health issues to the public and participate in developing plans of action.
5. Develop policies and plans that support individual and community health efforts.
   - Participate in community and family decision-making processes.
   - Provide information and advocacy for consideration of the interests of special groups in program development.
   - Develop programs and services to meet the needs of high-risk populations as well as broader community members.
   - Participate in disaster planning and mobilization of community resources in emergencies.
   - Advocate for appropriate funding for services.
6. Enforce laws and regulations that protect health and ensure safety.
   - Regulate and support safe care and treatment for dependent populations such as children and frail older adults.
   - Implement ordinances and laws that protect the environment.

   - Establish procedures and processes that ensure competent implementation of treatment schedules for diseases of public health importance.
   - Participate in the development of local regulations that protect communities and the environment from potential hazards and pollution.
7. Link people to needed personal health services and ensure the provision of health care that is otherwise unavailable.
   - Provide clinical preventive services to certain high-risk populations.
   - Establish programs and services to meet special needs.
   - Recommend clinical care and other services to clients and their families in clinics, homes, and the community.
   - Provide referrals through community links to needed care.
   - Participate in community provider coalitions and meetings to educate others and to identify service centers for community populations.
   - Provide clinical surveillance and identification of communicable disease.
8. Ensure a competent public health and personal health care workforce.
   - Participate in continuing education and preparation to ensure competence.
   - Define and support proper delegation to unlicensed assistive personnel in community settings.
   - Establish standards for performance.
   - Maintain client record systems and community documents.
   - Establish and maintain procedures and protocols for client care.
   - Participate in quality assurance activities such as record audits, agency evaluation, and clinical guidelines.
9. Evaluate the effectiveness, accessibility, and quality of personal and population-based health services.
   - Collect data and information related to community interventions.
   - Identify unserved and underserved populations within the community.
   - Review and analyze data on the health status of the community.
   - Participate with the community in the assessment of services and outcomes of care.
   - Identify and define enhanced services required to manage the health status of complex populations and special risk groups.
10. Research for new insights and innovative solutions to health problems.
   - Implement nontraditional interventions and approaches to effect change in special populations.
   - Participate in the collecting of information and data to improve the surveillance and understanding of special problems.
   - Develop collegial relationships with academic institutions to explore new interventions.
   - Participate in the early identification of factors that are detrimental to the community's health.
   - Formulate and use investigative tools to identify and impact care delivery and program planning.

From the Association of State and Territorial Directors of Nursing: *Public health nursing: a partner for healthy populations,* Washington, DC, 2000, ASTDN.

funding are given to tertiary and secondary care than to primary and preventive services including population-focused care. The "How To" box on p. 7 lists the essential public health services.

These services need to be implemented to support the base of the pyramid and to support the services offered through the top tiers of the pyramid. Together, all services at all levels will contribute to better health in America.

POPULATION-FOCUSED NURSING PRACTICE

PHN is a specialty with a distinct focus and scope of practice; it requires a special knowledge base. The role of the public health nurse has changed over the years in response to the following:
- Changes in health care
- Priorities for health care funding
- The needs of the population
- The educational preparation of nurses

As noted in Chapter 2, PHN began more than 100 years ago; early public health nurses provided direct care to people, most often in their homes. The Henry Street Settlement, established in New York City in the late 1800s by Lillian Wald, was an early model for PHN. At Henry Street Settlement the nurses took care of the sick in their homes and also looked at the overall population of low-income people in the community from which their home care patients came. The primary focus that has differentiated PHN from other specialties has been the emphasis on the population rather than on single individuals or families. Following the example of Lillian Wald, public health nurses have done the following:
- Looked at the community or population as a whole
- Raised questions about the overall health status and the factors associated with that status, including environmental factors such as physical, biological, social, economic, and cultural aspects

HOW TO   Distinguish the Specialty of Public Health Nursing

- *Population-focused:* Primary emphasis on populations that live in the community, as opposed to those that are institutionalized.
- *Community-oriented:*
  - Concern for the connection between the health status of the population and the environment in which the population lives (physical, biological, sociocultural).
  - An imperative to work with members of the community to carry out core public health functions.
- *Health and preventive focused:* Predominant emphasis on strategies for health promotion, health maintenance, and disease prevention, particularly primary and secondary prevention.
- *Interventions at the community and/or population level:* The use of political processes to affect public policy as a major intervention strategy for achieving goals.
- *Concern for the health of all members of the population or community, particularly vulnerable subpopulations.*

- Worked with the community to improve health status
- Provided health education to individuals, families, and groups to encourage healthier living

The primary goal of public health—the prevention of disease and disability—is achieved by ensuring that conditions exist in which people can remain healthy. The Policy Development process "How To" box describes ways to distinguish what actually makes up the specialty of PHN.

In 1981 the PHN section of the American Public Health Association (APHA) defined PHN and described how this role contributes to health care delivery. This statement was reaffirmed in 1996 (American Public Health Association, 1996). PHN is defined as a specialty that brings together knowledge from the public health sciences and nursing to improve the health of the community. It is defined by the Quad Council of Public Health Nursing Organizations as population-focused, community-oriented nursing practice. The goals of PHN are "the promotion of health, the prevention of disease and disability for all people through the creation of conditions in which people can be healthy" (American Nurses Association, 2007). Box 1-1 presents the process of PHN from the APHA definition.

Public health nurses, like others in public health, engage in assessment, policy development, and assurance activities. These functions are achieved when nurses work in partnerships with others, including nations, states, communities, organizations, groups, and individuals. Public health

▌ Evidence-Based Practice

This research used a participatory approach to explore environmental health (EH) concerns among Lac Courte Oreilles (LCO) Ojibwa Indians in Sawyer County, Wisconsin. The project focused on health promotion and community participation. Community participation was accomplished through a steering committee that consisted of the primary author and LCO College faculty and community members. The assessment method used was a self-administered survey mailed to LCO members in Sawyer County.

Concern for environmental issues was high in this tribal community, particularly because of what they would mean to future generations. Concern was higher among older members and tribal members living on rather than off the reservation. Local issues of concern included those related to the environment such as motorized water vehicles, effects from global warming, effects of aging septic systems on waterways, unsafe driving, and contaminated lakes/streams. Health concerns included diabetes, cancer, stress, obesity, and the use of drugs and alcohol. The LCO community can use survey results to inform further data needs and program development.

NURSE USE: The community was most interested in developing a program addressing drug and alcohol use. Community participation in the assessment would increase the possibility that a drug and alcohol program would be successful.

From Severtson C et al: A participatory assessment of environmental health concerns in an Ojibwa community, *Public Health Nurs* 19(1):47-58, 2002.

nurses carry out this mission by participating in the essential public health services described earlier in the chapter.

Although population-focused practice is the central feature of PHN, many of the skills and activities are used when community-oriented nurses and community-based nurses work in the community. For this reason, these practices are described in detail here. A **population** or **aggregate** is a collection of people who share one or more personal or environmental characteristics. Members of a community can be defined either in terms of geography (e.g., a county, a group of counties, a state) or a special interest (e.g., children attending a particular school). These members comprise a population. Generally, there are **subpopulations** within the larger population. Examples of a subpopulation within a population of a county are high-risk infants younger than 1 year old, unmarried pregnant adolescents, or individuals exposed to a particular event such as a chemical spill.

In **population-focused practice,** problems are defined (assessments/diagnoses) and solutions (interventions), such as policy development or providing a given preventive service, are implemented for or with a defined population or subpopulation as opposed to diagnoses, interventions, and treatment carried out at the individual level. This contrasts with basic professional education in nursing, medicine, and other clinical disciplines, which emphasizes developing competence in decision making at the level of the individual client by assessing health status, making management decisions (ideally with the client), and evaluating the effects of care. The ways in which nurses provide care to people with high blood pressure can demonstrate how population-focused practice differs from the clinical direct care practice so often used in nursing. Specifically, in a clinical direct care situation a nurse practicing in the community might decide that a person is hypertensive based on certain clinical signs. The nurse would evaluate different interventions to find the best one for this person and implement an intervention such as a change in diet. In contrast, a public health nurse engaged in population-focused practice would ask the following questions:

- What is the prevalence rate of hypertension among various age, race, and gender groups?
- Which subpopulations have the highest rates of untreated hypertension?
- What programs could reduce the problem of untreated hypertension and decrease the risk of further cardiovascular morbidity and mortality?

Public health nurses are typically concerned with more than one subpopulation, and they often deal with the health of the entire community. Assessment, one of the public health core functions, is a logical first step in examining a community setting to determine its health status.

The core public health function of assessment includes the following:

- Engaging in activities that involve the collection, analysis, and dissemination of information on both the health and health-relevant aspects of a community or a specific population.
- Questioning, for example, whether the health services of the community are available to the population and are adequate to address needs.
- Monitoring the health status of the community or population and the services provided over time.
- Evaluating the social, economic, environmental, and lifestyle characteristics and practices of a population as well as the health services and capacity available within the community to support good health for the population.

Listed in the "How To" box is a general set of questions that can be used or modified to gather assessment data.

Excellent examples of assessment at the national level are the U.S. Department of Health and Human Services' efforts

---

Box 1-1	**The Process of Public Health Nursing**

PHN is a systematic process of working with the client as partner that does the following:

- Assesses the health and health care needs of a population in collaboration with other disciplines to identify subpopulations (aggregates), families, and individuals at increased risk of illness, disability, or premature death.
- Develops and plans interventions to meet these needs. The plan includes resources available and those activities that contribute to health and its recovery and the prevention of illness, disability, and premature death.
- Implements the plan effectively, efficiently, and equitably.
- Evaluates progress to determine the extent to which these activities have influenced the health status outcomes of the population.
- Utilizes the results to influence and direct the delivery of care, the use of health resources, and the development of local, regional, state, and national health policy and research to promote health and prevent diseases.

Data from American Public Health Association: *The definition and role of public health nurses: a statement of the American Public Health Association's Public Health Nursing section,* Washington, DC, 1996, The Association; American Public Health Association: *The definition and role of public health nursing in the delivery of health care: a statement of the Public Health Nursing section,* Washington, DC, 1981, The Association; American Nurses Association: *Public health nursing: scope and standards of practice,* 2007, American Nurses Publishing.

HOW TO	**Assess: Assessment Questions to Ask**

- What are the major health problems in this community?
- Which population groups are at greatest risk?
- How are risks distributed geographically?
- What services are available?
- What services need to be provided but are unavailable?
- What is the level of quality of the available and needed services?
- What do citizens think their most pressing health needs are?
- Are the most pressing health needs considered to be the same by both providers and citizens?
- What is the history of agency collaboration and cooperation in this community?

Healthy People 2010

Overview and Goals

In 1979, the Surgeon General issued a report that began a 20-year focus on promoting health and preventing disease for all Americans. The report, entitled *Healthy People,* used morbidity rates to track the health of individuals through the five major life cycles of infancy, childhood, adolescence, adulthood, and older age.

In 1989, *Healthy People 2000* became a national effort of representatives from government agencies, academia, and health organizations. Their goal was to present a strategy for improving the health of the American people. Their objectives are being used by public and community health organizations to assess current health trends, health programs, and disease-prevention programs.

Throughout the 1990s, all states used *Healthy People 2000* objectives to identify emerging public health issues. The success of the program on a national level was accomplished through state and local efforts. Early in the 1990s, surveys from public health departments indicated that 8% of the national objectives had been met and progress on an additional 40% of the objectives was noted. In the mid-course review published in 1995, it was noted that significant progress had been made toward meeting 50% of the objectives.

Using the progress made in the past decade, the committee for *Healthy People 2010* proposed the following two goals:
• To increase years of healthy life
• To eliminate health disparities among different populations

They hope to reach these goals by measures such as promoting healthy behaviors, increasing access to quality health care, and strengthening community prevention.

The major premise of *Healthy People 2010* is that the health of the individual can rarely be separated from the health of the larger community. Therefore the vision for *Healthy People 2010* is "Healthy People in Healthy Communities."

Data from U.S. Department of Health and Human Services: *Healthy People 2000: national health promotion and disease prevention objectives,* DHHS Pub. No. 91-50212, Washington, DC, 1991, U.S. Government Printing Office; U.S. Department of Health and Human Services: *Healthy People 2010: understanding and improving health,* ed 2, Washington, DC, 2000, U.S. Government Printing Office; U.S. Department of Health, Education, and Welfare: *Healthy people: the surgeon general's report on health promotion and disease prevention,* DHEW Pub. No. 79-55071, Washington, DC, 1979, U.S. Government Printing Office.

to organize the goal-setting, data collection and analysis, and monitoring necessary to develop the series of publications describing the health status and health-related aspects of the U.S. population. These efforts began with *Healthy People* in 1980, and continued with *Promoting Health, Preventing Disease: 1990 Health Objectives for the Nation* and *Healthy People 2000,* and most recently *Healthy People 2010* (*Healthy People 2010* box) (U.S. Department of Health and Human Services, 2000).

In a local health department, public health nurses would participate in and provide leadership for assessing community needs, the health status of populations within the community, and environmental and behavioral risks. They also look at trends in the factors that determine health in the community, identify priority health needs, and determine the adequacy of existing community resources.

Policy development is a core function of public health and one of the core intervention strategies used by PHN specialists. Policy development relies heavily on planning and begins with the identified needs and priorities set by the people involved. It also includes building constituencies that can bring about policy changes. It is important to know what the powerful people in the community think about a specific public health concern. Health and human service providers as well as the people who will be served or affected must be included. PHN is a "with the people," not a "to the people" or "for the people," approach to planning. Historically, health care providers have been accused of providing care for or to people without actually involving the recipients in the decisions. The beneficiaries of services in public health need to be included from the very beginning in identifying the need, planning the intervention, and deciding on the format for the evaluation (Box 1-2).

Box 1-2   Policy Development Process

The policy development function:
• Is essentially a planning process that uses the assessment data to define health needs, set priorities, identify alternatives, outline a plan including the determination of available and needed resources, and determine who needs to be involved to ensure some measure of success.
• Serves as a resource and/or catalyst to help elected officials or heads of community organizations develop population-based health plans.
• Assists people who make policies to do so in such a way that the needs of many people or groups are met. It also advises these individuals and/or groups about which needs are most important and should be handled first.
• Consistently advocates for better health conditions for the population as a whole.

The third core public health function, *assurance,* focuses on the responsibility of public health agencies to be sure that activities are appropriately carried out to meet public health goals and plans. Not only does PHN include assessment or investigative functions, but the role also requires skill in collaboration, consultation, and cooperation. The assurance function makes sure that the activities designed during the policy development or planning phase are carried out. This is done through collaboration with people in a variety of health and human service organizations to promote, monitor, and improve both the availability and quality of providers and services. PHN is not a good field for people who like to work alone. Although there is considerable opportunity for autonomy in thinking and planning, effective and consistent collaboration is vital to success. Assurance does not always mean to provide something.

Rather, another agency may provide the needed service. Assurance means making certain that the services determined to be needed are provided by some agency within the community. Further, assurance includes assisting communities to implement and evaluate plans and projects. It includes maintaining the ability of both public health agencies and private providers to manage day-to-day operations as well as the capacity to respond to critical situations and emergencies.

In PHN, the nurse often reaches out to those who might benefit from a service or intervention. In other forms of nursing, the client is more likely to seek out and request assistance. As is discussed in later chapters, often the people or populations most in need of public health services are the least likely to ask for them. Examples include homeless, poor, and mentally ill people. The dominant needs of the population outweigh the expressed needs of one or a few people. Because resources are often limited, careful assessment to identify key needs is important.

However, the special contributions of public health nurse specialists include looking at the community or population as a whole, raising questions about its overall health status and factors associated with that status, including environmental factors (physical, biological, sociocultural), and working *with the community* to improve the population's health status.

PRACTICE FOCUSING ON INDIVIDUALS, FAMILIES, AND GROUPS

As mentioned, community-based nursing practice, with its focus on the provision or assurance of care to individuals and families in the community, is different from **community-oriented practice.** The latter is broader in scope and is a form of care in which the nurse provides health care after doing a community diagnosis to determine what conditions need to be altered for individuals, families, and groups in the community to stay healthy. Although it is hoped that all direct care providers contribute to the community's health in the broadest sense, not all are primarily concerned with the population focus, or the "big picture." All nurses in a given community, including those working in hospitals, physicians' offices, and health clinics, contribute positively to the health of the community. Examples of community settings for treating individuals include ambulatory surgery, outpatient clinics, physician and advanced-practice nursing offices and clinics, and employment and school sites, as well as preschool programs, housing projects, and migrant camps. These sites often provide individual-focused health care services. This contrasts to **population** (i.e., large group)-**focused** services. A specific example is the federally funded program for preschool children called *Head Start.* From a community-oriented nursing care perspective, nursing services could be provided to individual children by conducting developmental-level screening tests to evaluate each child's level of cognitive and psychomotor development in comparison

Evidence-Based Practice

The purpose of this study was to evaluate whether an 8-week support and education program could be beneficial for parents at high risk for experiencing parenting problems and for engaging in child abuse. The participants were parents of infants and toddlers, and the project was aimed at alleviating parental stress and improving parent-child interaction among parents who attended an inner-city clinic. Participants were 199 parents of children 1 through 36 months of age. Serious life stresses that defined at-risk parents included poverty, low social support, personal histories of childhood maltreatment, and substance abuse. Program effects were evaluated in terms of improvement in self-reported parenting stress and observed parent-child interaction. Positive effects were documented for the group as a whole and within each of three subgroups: two community samples and a group of mothers and children in a residential drug treatment program. Program attendance and the amount of gain in observed parenting skills were the factors related to a positive outcome.

NURSE USE: This program was offered in partnership with academic researchers and the public clinic. The nurses in this agency can ensure better outcomes in parenting by providing a long-term program for high-risk parents.

From Huebner C: Evaluation of a clinic-based parent education program to reduce the risk of infant and toddler maltreatment, *Public Health Nurs* 19(5):377-389, 2002.

with established standards for children of the same age. The community-based nurse may deliver illness care to the children in the school. In contrast, a public health or population-focused approach would look at the entire group of children being served by the program as well as the characteristics of the facilities and its programs to see if they are effective in achieving the goals of making the school population healthier.

COMMUNITY-ORIENTED NURSING

Most nurses practicing in the community and many staff public health nurses—both historically and at present—focus on providing direct care services, including health education, to persons or families outside of institutional settings, either in the home or in a clinic. Historically, the term *community health nurse* applied to all nurses who practiced in the community, regardless of whether they had preparation in PHN. Thus nurses providing secondary or tertiary care in a home, school, or clinic or any nurse who did not practice in an institutional setting could be considered a "community health nurse." To a large extent the development of what has been called *community health nursing* was influenced by the development within medicine of the specialty of community medicine. At that time both community medicine and community health nursing reached out to the community and began doing community assessments to determine more effectively the needs of the people. Thus disease prevention and health promotion could be targeted to specific needs in a given community. Specifically, the community health nurse operated from a health care focus that is based on an understanding of broader community needs.

The nurse is continually evaluating the community to see if changes are occurring that will influence the health of the people who live there. The case study on the Evolve website is an example of community-oriented nursing practice. Work through the case study and answer the questions for understanding this area of specialty.

The practice of community-oriented nursing involves health promotion, health maintenance, health education, management, coordination, and continuity of care in the management of the health care of individuals, families, and groups in a community. A holistic approach is used, and the goal of this care is to provide personal health services that promote and preserve the health of the community in which the clients live. This nurse uses both nursing and public health theory to guide practice.

Evidence that entry-level nurses are practicing effectively in the community includes the following (Turnock, 2006):

- Provides quality services that can control costs
- Focuses on disease prevention and health promotion
- Organizes services where people live, work, play, and learn
- Provides for referrals when clients need them
- Works in partnerships and with coalitions and other health care providers
- Works across the life span and with culturally diverse populations
- Works with at-risk populations to promote access to services
- Participates in epidemiologic investigations and disaster services
- Develops the community's capacity for health
- Works with policymakers for policy change
- Works to make the environment healthier

As can be seen, community-oriented nurses emphasize health protection, maintenance, and promotion and disease prevention, as well as self-reliance among clients. Regardless of whether the client is a person, a family, or a group, the goal is to promote health through education about prevailing health problems, proper nutrition, beneficial forms of exercise, and environmental factors such as safe food, water, air, and buildings. The nurse is likely to be involved in immunizing individuals as well as organizing the immunization programs for vaccinating the community for influenza, for example, and educating the community about the value of this service. Other individual and family services include provision of maternal and child health care, treatment of common communicable and infectious diseases and injuries, and provision of basic screening programs for problems such as lice, vision, hearing, and scoliosis.

Nurses have always been involved in providing family-centered care to individuals, families, and groups across the life span; however, they also work to identify high-risk groups in the community. Once such groups are identified, the nurse can work with others to develop appropriate policies and interventions to reduce risk and provide beneficial services. Both community-oriented nurses and

Levels of Prevention   Related to Public Health

PRIMARY PREVENTION
The public health nurse develops a health education program for a population of school-age children that teaches them about the effects of smoking on health.

SECONDARY PREVENTION
The public health nurse provides an influenza vaccination program in a community retirement village.

TERTIARY PREVENTION
The public health nurse provides a diabetes clinic for a defined population of adults in a low-income housing unit of the community.

community-based nurses must be aware of cultural diversity and provide care that is appropriate to the needs of the recipient. Likewise, both groups of nurses provide care in homes.

COMMUNITY-BASED NURSING

As mentioned, the goal of CBN is to manage acute or chronic conditions while promoting self-care among individuals and families (Oermann and Heinrich, 2003). In CBN the nursing care is family centered, which means that the nurse works to improve the competencies of families to enable them to take better care of themselves. The nurse pays particular attention to the uniqueness of each family and works to plan the most useful interventions. A "cookbook" approach cannot be used since no one nursing approach will fit each family or individual. Cultural diversity is taken into account as are the situations and stressors facing the person or the family at a given time. The nurse promotes client autonomy and helps clients learn to do as much as possible for themselves.

The nurse practicing CBN is more likely to give direct care to people than are nurses who practice from a community-oriented framework. The nurse assesses client needs and also the services that are available in order to plan the most appropriate course of action. Throughout care delivery, the nurse teaches and counsels clients so they can more fully develop their own ways of taking care of themselves. Box 1-3 provides definitions of each of the four key modes of nursing practice seen in the community.

CHALLENGES FOR THE FUTURE

Over the past few years, the places in which care is given have changed dramatically. In previous decades the majority of care was given in an inpatient setting. At present, the trend is to move more care into community settings and to reduce the number of hospital days for "sick" clients. There are a variety of reasons for the change. First, community care is often much less expensive than hospital care. Because the cost of health care in the United States has risen considerably over the past decade, there is a significant need to find new

Box 1-3	Definitions of the Four Key Nursing Modes in the Community

Community-Oriented Nursing Practice: a philosophy of nursing care delivery that involves generalist or specialist public health and community health nurses providing "health care" through community diagnosis and investigation of major health and environmental problems, health surveillance, monitoring, and evaluation of community and population health status, to prevent disease and disability, promoting, protecting, and maintaining "health" in order to create conditions in which people can be healthy.

Public Health Nursing Practice: the synthesis of nursing and public health theory applied to promoting and preserving the health of populations. Practice focuses on the community as a whole, and the effect of the community's health status (resources) on the health of individuals, families, and groups. The goal is to prevent disease and disability and promote and protect the health of the community as a whole.

Community Health Nursing Practice: the synthesis of nursing and public health theory to promote, preserve, and maintain the health of the population through the delivery of personal health services to individuals, families, and groups. The focus is on the health of individuals, families, and groups and how their health status affects the community as a whole.

Community-Based Nursing Practice: a setting-specific practice whereby care is provided for "sick" individuals and families where they live, work, and attend school. The emphasis is on acute and chronic care and the provision of comprehensive, coordinated, and continuous care. These nurses may be generalists or specialists in maternal-infant, pediatric, adult, or psychiatric mental health nursing.

F. *Staff nurses in a public health clinic or community health center*
G. *Director of nursing in a health department*
Choose three categories on the list above and interview at least one nurse in each category.
1. *Determine the scope of their practice.*
2. *Are they carrying out population-focused practice?*
3. *Could they?*
4. *How?*
5. *Ask them if they would change their role if this were possible.*
6. *Inquire whether they believe their role is either community-oriented nursing or CBN practice. Compare and contrast their answers with what you have learned about these roles.*
Answers are in the back of the book.

REMEMBER THIS!

- Public health is what members of a society do collectively to ensure that conditions exist in which people can be healthy.
- Assessment, policy development, and assurance are the core public health functions at all levels of government.
- Assessment refers to systematic data collection on the population, monitoring of the population's health status, and making information available on the health of the community.
- Policy development refers to the need to provide leadership in developing policies that support the health of the population, including use of the scientific knowledge base in decision making about policy.
- Assurance refers to the way public health practice makes sure that essential community-wide health services are available. This may include providing essential personal health services for those who would otherwise not receive them. Assurance also includes making sure that a competent public health and personal health care workforce is available.
- Setting is frequently viewed as the feature that distinguishes PHN from other specialties. A more useful approach is to use characteristics such as the following: a focus on populations who live in the community, an emphasis on prevention, concern for the interface between health status of the population and the environment (physical, biological, sociocultural), and the use of political processes to influence public policy to achieve one's goals.
- Specialization in PHN is seen as a subset of community-oriented nursing practice.
- Population-focused practice is the focus of specialization in PHN. The focus on populations in the community and the emphasis on health protection, health promotion, and disease prevention are the fundamental factors that distinguish PHN from other nursing specialties.
- Population is defined as a collection of individuals who share one or more personal or environmental characteristics. The term *population* may be used interchangeably with the term *aggregate*.

ways to deliver care that is accessible to the recipients, less expensive, and with adequate quality to meet client needs. Also, care in the community is usually more appealing to people who prefer to remain at home rather than be treated in a hospital. Currently, care is given in homes, schools, and at the work site, as well as in a variety of outpatient clinics. This trend is expected to grow, and it is expected that the role of the nurse in community settings will likewise grow and continue to change. There are many factors that will affect the changing role of the nurse in the community, such as the new and emerging infectious diseases, the need for emergency preparedness, the increases in chronic illness, and the continued reduction of numbers of days in the hospital for serious illnesses.

CLINICAL APPLICATION

Debate with classmates where and how PHN specialists practice and how their practice compares with what has been defined as CBN. Be specific about the differences.

Debate with classmates which of the nurses in the following categories are practicing population-focused nursing:
A. *School nursing*
B. *Staff nurses in home care*
C. *Director of nursing for a home care agency*
D. *Nurse practitioners in a health maintenance organization*
E. *Vice-president of nursing in a hospital*

WHAT WOULD YOU DO?

1. Define each of the following:
   a. The core functions of public health
   b. The specialist in PHN
   c. The nurse whose practice is community based
   d. The community-oriented nurse
2. Discuss with classmates examples in your community in which the CBN role is the ideal role to meet client needs. Also identify examples in which the most useful nursing role would be that of the community-oriented nurse. How can you justify your opinion if classmates disagree?
3. With three or four of your classmates, develop a plan for identifying two or three nurses in your community who are in an administrative role and discuss the following with them:
   a. How they define the populations they serve
   b. The strategies they use to monitor the population's health status
   c. The strategies they use to ensure that the populations are receiving basic needed services
   d. The initiatives they are taking to address problems

Can you compare and contrast their answers to what you have learned about roles in different settings?

■ REFERENCES

American Nurses Association: *Public health nursing: scope and standards of practice*, Washington, DC, 2007, American Nurses Publishing.

American Public Health Association: *The definition and role of public health nurses: a statement of the American Public Health Association's Public Health Nursing section*, Washington, DC, 1996, The Association.

American Public Health Association: *The definition and role of public health nursing in the delivery of health care: a statement of the Public Health Nursing section*, Washington, DC, 1981, The Association.

Baker EL, Koplan JP: Strengthening the nation's public infrastructure: historic challenge, unprecedented opportunity, *Health Aff* 21(6):15–27, 2002.

Colorado Department of Public Health and Environment: *MCH core public health services pyramid, 2008: health care program for children with special needs,* Denver, 2008, CDPH.

Institute of Medicine: *The future of the public's health: the 21st century,* Washington, DC, 2003, National Academy Press.

Oermann M, Henrich K: *Annual review of nursing education,* Vol 1, 2003, Springer.

Turnock B: *Public health: career choices that make a difference,* Boston, 2006, Jones and Bartlett.

U.S. Department of Health and Human Services: *Health U.S.: 2007,* Washington, DC, 2008, National Center for Statistics.

U.S. Department of Health and Human Services: *Healthy People 2010 objectives,* Washington, DC, 2000, U.S. Department of Health and Human Services.

U.S. Public Health Service: *The core functions project,* Washington, DC, 1994 (update 2000), Office of Disease Prevention and Health Promotion.

The History of Public and Community Health and Nursing

ADDITIONAL RESOURCES

These related resources are found either in the appendix at the back of this book or on the book's website at http://evolve.elsevier.com/stanhope/foundations.

Appendix

- Appendix E.3: The Health Insurance Portability and Accountability Act (HIPAA): What Does It Mean for Public Health Nurses

e Evolve Website

- Community Assessment Applied
- Quiz review questions

- WebLinks, including link to *Healthy People 2010* website

Real World Community Health Nursing: An Interactive CD-Rom, second edition

If you are using this CD-ROM in your course, you will find the following activities related to this chapter:

- *Stories of Public Health Nursing Leaders* in **Community/Public Health Nursing History**
- *What's My Line?* in **Community/Public Health Nursing History**

OBJECTIVES

After reading this chapter, the student should be able to:

1. Discuss historical events that have influenced how current health care is delivered in the community.
2. Relate the contributions of Florence Nightingale, Lillian Wald, and Mary Breckinridge to current public health and nursing.
3. Explain significant historical trends in the development of public health nursing.

4. Examine the ways in which nursing has been provided in the community, including settlement houses, visiting nurse associations, official health organizations, and schools.
5. Discuss the status of nursing in public health practice in the twenty-first century.

CHAPTER OUTLINE

EARLY PUBLIC HEALTH

PUBLIC HEALTH DURING AMERICA'S COLONIAL PERIOD AND THE NEW REPUBLIC

CONTINUED GROWTH IN PUBLIC HEALTH NURSING

PUBLIC HEALTH NURSING DURING THE EARLY TWENTIETH CENTURY

ECONOMIC DEPRESSION AND THE IMPACT ON PUBLIC HEALTH

FROM WORLD WAR II UNTIL THE 1970s

COMMUNITY AND PUBLIC HEALTH NURSING FROM THE 1970s TO THE PRESENT

Based on a chapter written by Janna Dieckmann for *Public Health Nursing,* 7th edition.

KEY TERMS

American Association of Colleges of Nursing (AACN): members are baccalaureate and higher degree nursing education programs. The association serves as the national voice for these programs.

American Nurses Association (ANA): a national association for registered nurses in the United States, founded in 1896 as the Nurses' Associated Alumnae of the United States and Canada.

American Public Health Association (APHA): national organization founded in 1872 to facilitate interdisciplinary efforts and promote public health.

American Red Cross: a national organization founded in 1881 through the efforts of Clara Barton that today seeks to reduce human suffering through health, safety, and disaster-relief programs in affiliation with the International Committee of the Red Cross.

Breckinridge, Mary: pioneering nurse who established the Frontier Nursing Service to deliver community health services to families in rural Kentucky.

district nursing: a system in public health nursing in which a nurse was assigned to a geographic district in a town to provide a variety of health services for its residents.

Frontier Nursing Service (FNS): provides community health services to rural families in Kentucky. Begun in 1925 by Mary Breckinridge when she developed outpost centers throughout the mountain areas in Kentucky to provide midwifery and nursing, medical, and dental care. A hospital was established and began operating in Hyden, Kentucky, in 1935.

instructive district nursing: an early term for visiting nursing. Begun in Boston, it emphasized health education and care to families.

Metropolitan Life Insurance Company: a life insurance company that provided home nursing services for its beneficiaries and their families from 1909 to 1952.

National League for Nursing (NLN): a national nursing organization that began as the American Society of Superintendents of Training Schools of Nursing and later the National League for Nursing Education. The NLN initially established nurse training standards and promoted collegial relations among nurses.

Nightingale, Florence: an English nurse who is credited with establishing nursing as a discipline.

official health agencies: agencies operated by state or local governments to provide a wide range of public health services, including community and public health nursing services.

Rathbone, William: a British philanthropist who founded the first district nursing association in Liverpool. With Florence Nightingale, he advocated for district nursing throughout England.

settlement houses: neighborhood centers providing social and health services.

Shattuck Report: the first attempt to describe a model approach to the organization of public health.

Social Security Act of 1935: enacted to protect the health of people and included funds for education and employment of public health nurses.

visiting nurse associations: agencies staffed by nurses who provide care for patients and families most often in the home.

visiting nurses: nurses who provide care wherever the client may be—at home, work, or school.

Wald, Lillian: the first public health nurse in the United States and an influential social reformer. She founded the Henry Street Settlement (later the Visiting Nurse Service of New York).

One of the best ways to make plans for today and tomorrow is to look at the past. What worked? What did not work? What past lessons about health care, nursing, and communities can be used to plan for the future? Learning about history helps people understand what has influenced developments in the past, as well as what is happening in the present. This is especially true in times of rapid changes in society. How have nurses developed into the professionals they are today and what have been their supports and obstacles?

For more than 120 years, nurses in the United States have responded effectively to public health problems. Public health emphasizes prevention; however, measuring the outcomes of preventive work has always been a challenge. In the short run, it has been easier to document the effectiveness of a treatment or intervention than to document prevention. Recent terrorism attacks and natural disasters such as massive hurricanes, fires, and mud slides, have renewed emphasis on public health to prevent disease, waste and chemical contamination, and assaults from humans and the environment.

Most current health threats caused by communicable diseases, the environment, pressures of a fast-paced life, chronic illness, and aging have been present over time. Fear of terrorist attacks and natural disasters have added to public health challenges, and this includes feelings of helplessness in preventing and defending against them. The specific ways in which these threats affect people have changed. Over the years, nurses practicing in the community have been flexible, creative, and able to work with people from many backgrounds and with varied skills. Although a select few historical figures are highlighted who have demonstrated unusual success, remember that many nurses have contributed to building organizations and providing services to improve the health of the public. Effective planning for the future is built upon learning from all of our predecessors.

Nursing leaders who have worked in the community have done so to improve the health status of individuals, families, and populations. They have spent time, energy, and effort working with high-risk or vulnerable groups. Part of the appeal of public health nursing has been its autonomy of practice and independence in problem solving and decision making, as well as the interdisciplinary nature of the specialty. Many of the varied and challenging nursing and public health roles can be traced to the late 1800s when public health efforts focused on environmental conditions such as sanitation, control of communicable diseases, education for health and prevention of disease and disability, and care of sick persons in their homes. This chapter describes the beginnings of public health, the role of nursing in the community, the contributions made by nurses to public health, and the influence of nurses on community health.

EARLY PUBLIC HEALTH

People in all cultures have been concerned with the events surrounding birth, death, and illness. They have tried to prevent, understand, and control disease. Their ability to preserve health and treat illness has depended on their knowledge of science, the use and availability of technologies, and the degree of social organization. For example, ancient Babylonians understood the need for hygiene and had some medical skills. They used medicine to treat sick people. The Egyptians in about 1000 BCE (before the Common Era) developed a variety of pharmaceutical preparations and constructed earth privies and public drainage systems. In England, the Elizabethan Poor Law of 1601 guaranteed medical care for poor, blind, and "lame" individuals. This minimal care was generally provided in almshouses supported by local government. The goal was to regulate the poor as well as to provide care during illness. Table 2-1 presents milestones of public health efforts that occurred during the seventeenth, eighteenth, and nineteenth centuries.

The Industrial Revolution in nineteenth-century Europe led to social changes while making great advances in transportation, communication, and other forms of technology. Previous care-giving structures, which relied on families, neighbors, and friends, became inadequate because of migration, urbanization, and increased demand. During this period, small numbers of Roman Catholic and Protestant religious women provided nursing care in institutions and sometimes in the home. Many lay women who performed nursing functions in almshouses and early hospitals in Great Britain were poorly educated and untrained. As the practice of medicine became more complex in the mid-1800s, hospital work required a more skilled caregiver. Physicians and community advocates wished to improve the quality of nursing services. Early experiments led to some improvement in care, but it was because of the efforts of Florence Nightingale that health care was revolutionized when she founded the discipline of nursing.

Table 2-1	Milestones in the History of Public Health—Public and Community Health Nursing: 1600-1865
Year	**Milestone**
1601	Elizabethan Poor Law written
1617	Sisterhood of the Dames de Charité organized in France by St. Vincent de Paul
1789	Baltimore Health Department established
1798	Marine Hospital Service established; later became Public Health Service
1812	Sisters of Mercy established in Dublin, where nuns visited the poor
1813	Ladies Benevolent Society of Charleston, South Carolina, founded
1836	Lutheran deaconesses provided home visits in Kaiserwerth, Germany
1851	Florence Nightingale visited Kaiserwerth, Germany, for 3 months of nurse training
1855	Quarantine Board established in New Orleans; beginning of tuberculosis campaign in the United States
1859	District nursing established in Liverpool by William Rathbone
1860	Florence Nightingale Training School for Nurses established at St. Thomas Hospital in London
1864	Beginning of Red Cross

PUBLIC HEALTH DURING AMERICA'S COLONIAL PERIOD AND THE NEW REPUBLIC

In the early years of America's settlement, as in Europe, the care of the sick was usually informal and was provided by the women of the household. These women not only provided care during sickness and childbirth but also grew or gathered healing herbs for use throughout the year. This traditional system became insufficient as the number of urban residents grew in the early 1800s.

British settlers in the New World influenced the American ideas of social welfare and care of the sick. Just as the American legal system is based on English common law, colonial Americans established systems of care for the sick, poor, aged, mentally ill, and dependent based on the model of the Elizabethan Poor Law. Early county or township government was responsible for the care of all dependent residents, and they were strict about caring only for their own residents. Those outside residents were returned to their home county for care. Few hospitals existed, and then only in the larger cities. Pennsylvania Hospital, the first hospital in the future United States, was founded in Philadelphia in 1751.

Early colonial public health efforts included the collection of birth and death statistics, improved sanitation, and control of the many communicable diseases brought in at the seaports. The colonists did not have a system to ensure that public health efforts were supported and enforced. Epidemics often occurred and strained the limited local organization for health during the seventeenth, eighteenth, and nineteenth centuries (Rosen, 1958).

After the American Revolution, the threat of disease, especially yellow fever, led to public interest in establishing government-sponsored, or official, boards of health. By 1800, with a population of 75,000, New York City had established a public health committee for monitoring water quality, sewer construction, drainage of marshes, planting of trees and vegetables, construction of a masonry wall along the waterfront, and burial of the dead (Rosen, 1958).

Industrialization with its growth of cities coupled with inadequate housing and sanitation led to epidemics of small-pox, yellow fever, cholera, typhoid, and typhus. Tuberculosis and malaria were always present, and infant mortality was about 200 per 1000 live births (Pickett and Hanlon, 1990). American hospitals in the early 1800s were generally unsanitary and staffed by poorly trained workers. Physicians had limited education, and medical care was scarce. Public dispensaries, similar to outpatient clinics, and private charitable efforts tried to provide some care for the poor. The federal government focused its early public health work on providing health care for merchant seamen and protecting seacoast cities from epidemics. At this time some agencies began to provide lay nursing care in homes including the Ladies' Benevolent Society of Charleston (Buhler-Wilkerson, 2001), South Carolina; lay nurses in Philadelphia; and visiting nurses in Cincinnati, Ohio (Rodabaugh and Rodabaugh, 1951). Although these programs provided useful services, they were not adopted elsewhere.

By the mid-nineteenth century, public health problems were more strongly associated with poor urban living conditions. The few urban boards of health focused on communicable disease and environmental health. In 1850 the Massachusetts Sanitary Commission published the **Shattuck Report,** which called for major improvements in state government action for public health. This landmark report recommended the following changes (Kalisch and Kalisch, 1995):

- Establishing a state health department and local health boards in every town
- Conducting sanitary surveys and collecting vital statistics
- Improving environmental sanitation
- Control of food, drug, and communicable diseases
- Providing well-child care and health education
- Controlling smoking and the use of alcohol
- Town planning
- Teaching preventive medicine in medical schools

It took 19 years for the first of these recommendations to be implemented in Massachusetts; other states later adopted some of these steps. The Shattuck Report is important because it was the first proposal for modern approach to public health organization. These recommendations remain important in the twenty-first century.

Florence Nightingale's vision of trained nurses and her model of nursing education influenced the development of professional nursing and, indirectly, public health nursing in the United States. In 1850 and 1851, Nightingale carefully studied nursing "system and method" by visiting Pastor Theodor Fliedner at his Kaiserwerth, Germany, School for Deaconesses. Her work with Pastor Fliedner and the Kaiserwerth Lutheran deaconesses, with their systems of **district nursing** later led her to promote nursing care for the sick in their homes.

During the Crimean War (1854-1856), the British military established hospitals for sick and wounded soldiers in Scutari in Asia Minor. The care of soldiers was poor, with cramped quarters, poor sanitation, lice and rats, not enough food, and inadequate medical supplies (Kalisch and Kalisch, 1995; Palmer, 1983). When the British public demanded improved conditions, **Florence Nightingale** asked to work in Scutari. Because of her wealth, social and political connections, and knowledge of hospitals, the British government sent her to Asia Minor with 40 ladies, 117 hired nurses, and 15 paid servants. In Scutari, Nightingale progressively improved the soldiers' health using a population-based approach that improved both environmental conditions and nursing care. Using simple epidemiology measures, she documented a decreased mortality rate from 415 per 1000 at the beginning of the war to 11.5 per 1000 at the end (Cohen, 1984; Palmer, 1983). Like Nightingale's efforts in Scutari, public health nurses today identify health care needs that affect the entire population. They then mobilize resources and organize themselves and the community to meet these needs.

After the Crimean War, Nightingale returned to England in 1856. Her fame was established. She organized hospital nursing practices and nursing education in hospitals to replace untrained lay nurses with Nightingale nurses. Nightingale thought that nursing should promote health and prevent illness, and she emphasized proper nutrition, rest, sanitation, and hygiene (Nightingale, 1894, 1946).

In 1859 British philanthropist **William Rathbone** founded the first district nursing association in Liverpool, England. Based on the success of these "friendly visitors" who provided care to needy people (Kalisch and Kalisch, 1995), Nightingale and Rathbone's support for nursing in the home led to the organization of district nursing in England (Nutting and Dock, 1935).

With growing urbanization in the United States during the Industrial Revolution, the number of jobs for women rapidly increased. Educated women became teachers, secretaries, or saleswomen, and less-educated women worked in factories. As it became more acceptable to work outside the home, women were more willing to become nurses. The first nursing schools based on the Nightingale model opened in the United States in the 1870s. The early graduate nurses worked as private duty nurses or were hospital administrators or instructors. The private duty nurses often lived with the families for whom they cared. Because it was expensive to hire private duty nurses, only the well-to-do could afford their services. Community nursing began in an effort to meet urban health care needs, especially for the disadvantaged, by providing visiting nurses. In 1877 in New York City, trained nurse Francis Root was hired by a New York mission to visit the sick poor. Her goal was to care for sick people in their homes.

Visiting nurses took care of several families in one day (rather than attending to only one patient or family as the private duty nurse did), which made their care more economical. The movement grew, and **visiting nurse associations** were established in Buffalo (1885), Philadelphia (1886), and Boston (1886). Wealthy people interested in charitable activities funded both settlement houses and visiting nurse associations.

BRIEFLY NOTED

Wealthy upper-class women, freed from some of the social restrictions that had previously limited their social life and contributions, began to do charitable work and created, supported, and supervised early visiting nurses.

Visiting nurses promoted prevention through home visits and well-baby clinics. They worked with physicians, gave selected treatments, kept temperature and pulse records, taught families how to care for the sick, and also taught personal and environmental prevention measures, such as hygiene and good nutrition (Figure 2-1). Many early visiting nurse agencies employed only one nurse, who was supervised by members of the agency board. Board members were wealthy or socially prominent women. These ladies were critically important to the success of visiting nursing through their efforts to open new agencies, to financially support existing agencies, and to make the services socially acceptable.

In 1886 in Boston, two women, to improve their chances of gaining financial support for their cause, coined the term **instructive district nursing** to emphasize the relationship of nursing to health education. Support for these nurses was also secured from the Women's Education Association, and the Boston Dispensary provided free outpatient medical care. In February 1886 the first district nurse was hired in

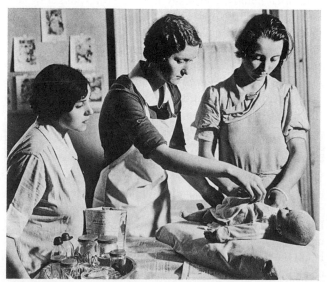

FIGURE 2-1 Public health nurse demonstrating well-child care during a home visit. (Courtesy Visiting Nurse Service of New York.)

Boston, and in 1888 the Instructive District Nursing Association was incorporated as an independent voluntary agency (Brainard, 1922).

Other nurses established **settlement houses** and neighborhood centers, which became hubs for health care and social welfare programs. For example, in 1893 trained nurses **Lillian Wald** and Mary Brewster began visiting the poor on New York's Lower East Side. They established a nurses' settlement that became the Henry Street Settlement and later the Visiting Nurse Service of New York City. By 1905 public health nurses had provided almost 48,000 visits to more than 5000 patients (Kalisch and Kalisch, 1995). Lillian Wald emerged as a prominent leader of public health nursing during these decades (Box 2-1 and Figure 2-2).

BRIEFLY NOTED

Lillian Wald demonstrated an exceptional ability to develop approaches and programs to solve the health care and social problems of her times. What can we learn from her and what can be applied to today's nursing practice?

The public wanted to limit disease among all classes of people, partly for religious reasons, partly as a form of charity, but also because the middle and upper classes were afraid of diseases that were prevalent in the large communities of European immigrants. During the 1890s in New York City, about 2,300,000 people were packed into 90,000 tenement houses. The environmental conditions of immigrants in tenement houses and sweatshops were familiar features of urban life across the northeastern United States and upper Midwest. From the beginning, community nursing practice included teaching and prevention (Figure 2-3). Community interventions led to improved sanitation, economic improvements, and better nutrition. These interventions were credited with reducing the incidence of acute communicable disease by 1910.

The **American Red Cross**, through its Rural Nursing Service (later the *Town and Country Nursing Service*), initiated home nursing care in areas outside larger cities. Lillian Wald obtained the initial donations to support this agency, which provided care to the sick, instruction in sanitation and hygiene in rural homes, and improved living conditions in villages and farms. These nurses dealt with diseases such as tuberculosis, pneumonia, and typhoid fever. By 1920 there were 1800 Red Cross Town and Country Nursing Services. This number eventually grew to almost 3000 programs in small towns and rural areas.

BRIEFLY NOTED

The emphasis of community nursing has varied and changed over time. In recent years federal and state financing have influenced the growth. Florence Nightingale and Lillian Wald were two amazing early leaders whose legacy continues to provide ideas for the present and the future.

Box 2-1   Lillian Wald: First Public Health Nurse in the United States

Public health nursing evolved in the United States in the late nineteenth and early twentieth centuries largely because of the pioneering work of Lillian Wald. Born on March 10, 1867, Lillian Wald decided to become a nurse after Vassar College refused to admit her at 16 years of age. She graduated in 1891 from the New York Hospital Training School for Nurses and spent the next year working at the New York Juvenile Asylum. To supplement what she thought had been inadequate training in the sciences, she enrolled in the Woman's Medical College in New York (Frachel, 1988).

Having grown up in a warm, nurturing family in Rochester, New York, her work in New York City introduced her to an entirely different side of life. In 1893, while conducting a class in home nursing for immigrant families on the Lower East Side of New York, Wald was asked by a small child to visit her sick mother. Wald found the mother in bed after childbirth, having hemorrhaged for 2 days. This home visit confirmed for Wald all of the injustices in society and the differences in health care for poor persons versus those persons able to pay (Frachel, 1988).

She believed poor people should have access to health care. With her friend Mary Brewster and the financial support of two wealthy laypeople, Mrs. Solomon Loeb and Joseph H. Schiff, she moved to the Lower East Side and occupied the top floor of a tenement house on Jefferson Street. This move eventually led to the establishment of the Henry Street Nurses Settlement. In the beginning, Wald and Brewster helped individual families. Wald believed that the nurse's visit should be friendly, more like a friend than someone paid to visit (Dolan, 1978).

Wald used epidemiological methods to campaign for health-promoting social policies to improve environmental and social conditions that affected health. Not only did she write *The House on Henry Street* to describe her own public health nursing work, but she also led in the development of payment by life insurance companies for nursing services (Frachel, 1988).

In 1909, along with Lee Frankel, Lillian Wald established the first public health nursing program for life insurance policy holders at the Metropolitan Life Insurance Company. She urged that nurses at agencies such as the Henry Street Settlement provide complex nursing care. Wald convinced the company that it would be more economical to use the services of public health nurses than to employ their own nurses. She also convinced them that services could be available to anyone desiring them, with fees graduated according to the ability to pay. This nursing service designed by Wald continued for 44 years and contributed several significant accomplishments to public health nursing, including the following (Frachel, 1988):

1. Providing home nursing care on a fee-for-service basis
2. Establishing an effective cost-accounting system for visiting nurses
3. Using advertisements in newspapers and on radio to recruit nurses
4. Reducing mortality from infectious diseases

Lillian Wald also believed that the nursing efforts at the Henry Street Settlement should be aligned with an official health agency. She therefore arranged for nurses to wear an insignia that indicated that they served under the auspices of the Board of Health. Also, she led the establishment of rural health nursing services through the Red Cross. Her other accomplishments included helping to establish the Children's Bureau and fighting in New York City for better tenement living conditions, city recreation centers, parks, pure food laws, graded classes for mentally handicapped children, and assistance to immigrants (Backer, 1993; Dock, 1922; Frachel, 1988; Zerwekh, 1992).

Data from Backer BA: Lillian Wald: Connecting caring with action, *Nurs Health Care* 14:122–128, 1993; Dock LL: The history of public health nursing, *Public Health Nurs* 14:522, 1922; Dolan J: *History of nursing,* ed 14, Philadelphia, 1978, Saunders; Frachel RR: A new profession: the evolution of public health nursing, *Public Health Nurs* 5(2):86–90, 1988; Zerwekh JV: Public health nursing legacy: historical practical wisdom, *Nurs Health Care* 13:84–91, 1992.

Occupational health nursing, which began as industrial nursing, grew out of early home visiting efforts. In 1895 Ada Mayo Stewart began to work with employees and families of the Vermont Marble Company. As a free service for the employees, Stewart provided obstetric care, sickness care, and some postsurgical care. Interestingly, she provided few services for work-related injuries (Kalisch and Kalisch, 1995).

School nursing was also an extension of home visiting. In New York City in 1902, more than 20% of children might be absent from school on a single day due to conditions such as pediculosis, ringworm, scabies, inflamed eyes, ear discharge, and infected wounds. School medical inspection began in 1897 and focused on excluding infectious children from school rather than on providing or obtaining medical treatment so they could return to school. Lillian Wald introduced the English practice of providing nurses for the schools. Lina Rogers, a Henry Street Settlement resident, became the first school nurse. She worked with the children in New York City schools and made home visits to teach parents and provide follow-up care to children absent from school. The new school nurses found that many children were absent because

they lacked shoes or adequate clothes. Many of the children were often hungry, and many took care of younger or sick children (Hawkins, Hayes, and Corliss, 1994). School nursing was a success, and New York City added more nurses. School nursing spread to several large cities across the country. The scope of school nursing is highly variable across the United States at present. In some areas, poor funding has led to unmanageably high nurse-student ratios.

CONTINUED GROWTH IN PUBLIC HEALTH NURSING

The *Visiting Nurse Quarterly*, begun in 1909 by the Cleveland Visiting Nurse Association, initiated a professional form of communication for clinical and organizational concerns. In the same year the University of Minnesota began the first university nursing program. In 1911 a joint committee of existing nursing organizations convened, under the leadership of Lillian Wald and Mary Gardner, to standardize nursing services outside the hospital. They recommended the formation of an organization to address public health nursing

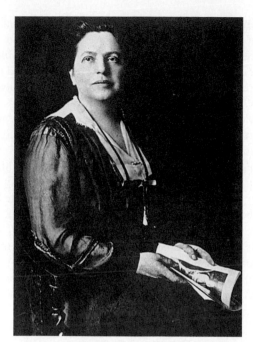

FIGURE 2-2 Lillian Wald. (Courtesy Visiting Nurse Service of New York.)

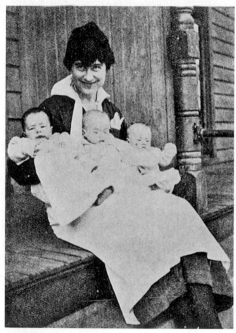

FIGURE 2-3 Teaching well-child care was a significant public health nursing role. (Courtesy Instructional Visiting Nurse Association of Richmond, Va.)

concerns. The committee invited 800 agencies involved in public health nursing to send delegates to an organizational meeting in Chicago in June 1912. After a heated debate on its name and purpose, the delegates established the National Organization for Public Health Nursing (NOPHN) and chose Lillian Wald as its first president (Dock, 1922). Unlike other professional nursing organizations, the NOPHN membership included both nurses and their lay supporters.

The NOPHN, which worked "to improve the educational and service standards of the public health nurse and promote public understanding of and respect for her work" (Rosen, 1958, p. 381), soon became the dominant force in public health nursing (Roberts, 1955).

BRIEFLY NOTED

Learning about the history of a practice agency, such as a visiting nurse association, can provide important perspectives on current agency values, decision-making structures, funding, clinical priorities and service areas, and obstacles to success.

At this time newly graduated nurses often were unprepared for home visiting. Nursing school courses were inadequate in teaching home care because these diploma schools of nursing emphasized hospital care of patients. Nurses working in the community needed additional education. In 1914 Mary Adelaide Nutting, working with the Henry Street Settlement, began the first postgraduate nursing course in public health nursing at Teachers College, New York City (Deloughery, 1977). The American Red Cross provided scholarships for graduates of nursing schools to attend the public health nursing course. In 1923 the Rockefeller Foundation endowed a School of Nursing at Yale University and Frances Payne Bolton, a U.S. Representative and wealthy Cleveland woman, endowed the School of Nursing at Western Reserve University.

Public health nurses were also active in the **American Public Health Association (APHA),** which was established in 1872 to facilitate interdisciplinary efforts and promote the "practical application of public hygiene" (Scutchfield and Keck, 1997, p. 12). The APHA focused on important public health issues, including sewage and garbage disposal, occupational injuries, and sexually transmitted diseases. In 1923 the Public Health Nursing Section was formed within APHA to provide a national forum for the discussion of strategy for public health nurses within the context of the larger public health organization. Public health organizations expanded to rural areas where they targeted epidemics and maternal–child health. To accomplish this, local health units, or official health agencies, were established, staffed primarily by public health nurses. These nurses became leaders on health care issues by collaborating with local officials, nurses, and other health care providers.

The experience of Orange County, California, during the 1920s and 1930s illustrates the growing importance of the nurse in the community. Based on the efforts of a private physician, social welfare agencies, and a Red Cross nurse, the county board created the public health nurse position in 1922. Presented with a shining new Model T car, sporting the bright orange seal of the county, the nurse began her work by dealing with the serious communicable disease problems of diphtheria and scarlet fever. Typhoid became epidemic when a drainage pipe overflowed into a well, infecting those who drank the water; also infected were those who drank raw milk from an infected dairy. Almost 3000 residents were immunized. At weekly well baby conferences, nurses taught mothers how to care for their infants and the infants were weighed and immunized.

PUBLIC HEALTH NURSING DURING THE EARLY TWENTIETH CENTURY

In 1918 during World War I, the Vassar Training Camp School for Nurses was started as a unique and patriotic aspect of nursing education. The American Red Cross and the Council of National Defense jointly supported this novel program, which proposed that nursing education be shortened from 3 to 2 years for college graduates. This school provided initial skills training for graduates from 435 colleges. Students completed nursing education at local hospital schools so that they could become Army Reserve officers to meet urgent wartime needs. The program ended when peace was declared (Buhler-Wilkerson, 1989; Kalisch and Kalisch, 1995).

The personnel needs of World War I in Europe depleted the ranks of public health nurses, yet the NOPHN identified a need for a second and third line of defense at home. There was a major patriotic duty for public health nurses to stay at home near the end of the war, and after the war the worldwide influenza epidemic swept the United States. The NOPHN and the American Red Cross formed a coalition to aid those with influenza. Houses, churches, and halls were turned into hospitals. Some nurse volunteers died of this disease. The NOPHN also loaned a nurse to the U.S. Public Health Service to establish a public health nursing program for military outposts, which was the first federal government sponsorship of nurses (Shyrock, 1959; Wilner, Walkey, and O'Neill, 1978).

Limited funds during the early twentieth century was the major obstacle to extending nursing services in the community. Most early visiting nurse associations relied on contributions from wealthy and middle-class supporters. Consistent with the goal of promoting economic independence, poor families were asked to pay a small fee for nursing services.

In 1909, with advocacy by Lillian Wald, the **Metropolitan Life Insurance Company** began a program using visiting nurse organizations to provide care for sick policyholders. By 1912, 589 Metropolitan nursing programs provided care through existing agencies or through visiting nurses hired directly by Metropolitan Life. By 1918 Metropolitan Life calculated an average decline of 7% in the mortality rate of policyholders and almost a 20% decline in the deaths of children younger than 3 years of age. The insurance company attributed this improvement, as well as reduced costs for the insurance company, to the work of visiting nurses.

Nurses also influenced public policy by advocating for the U.S. Children's Bureau and the Sheppard-Towner Program. Wald and other nursing leaders urged that the Children's Bureau be established to address national problems of maternal and child welfare. Beginning in 1912, Children's Bureau experts investigated the effects of income, housing, employment, and other factors on infant and maternal mortality. Their work led to federal child labor laws and the 1919 White House Conference on Child Health.

Problems of maternal and child morbidity and mortality spurred the Maternity and Infancy Act (often called the *Sheppard-Towner Act*) in 1921, which provided federal matching funds to establish maternal and child health divisions in state health departments. Education during home visits by public health nurses included promoting the health of mother and child, as well as encouraging prompt medical care during pregnancy. Although credited with saving many lives, the Sheppard-Towner Program ended in 1929 in response to concerns by the American Medical Association and others that the legislation gave too much power to the federal government and too closely resembled socialized medicine (Pickett and Hanlon, 1990).

BRIEFLY NOTED

Just as in the twentieth century, we still see lack of funds limiting the ability to offer important public health services.

Innovations in health care resulted both from changes in public support for nursing and from individual commitment and private financial support. In 1925 **Mary Breckinridge** established the **Frontier Nursing Service (FNS)**. This creative service was based on systems of care used in Scotland (Box 2-2 and Figure 2-4). Breckinridge introduced the first nurse-midwives into the United States. The pioneering spirit of the FNS influenced the development of public health programs to improve the health care of the rural and often inaccessible population in the Appalachian sections of southeastern Kentucky (Browne, 1966; Tirpak, 1975) (Figure 2-5). FNS nurses were trained in nursing, public health, and midwifery. Their work, in a 700-square mile area, led to reduced pregnancy complications for their patients and one-third fewer stillbirths and infant deaths (Kalisch and Kalisch, 1995). The FNS still provides comprehensive health and nursing services to the people of that area and supports the Frontier School of Midwifery and Family Nursing.

African-American nurses faced many kinds of challenges when trying to work in public health nursing. Jessie Sleet (Scales), a Canadian educated at Provident Hospital School of Nursing (Chicago), became the first black public health nurse when she was hired by the New York Charity Organization Society in 1900 (Buhler-Wilkerson, 2001; Hine, 1989; Thoms, 1929). In 1925, just 435 black public health nurses were employed across the United States, and in 1930, only six black nurses held supervisory positions in public health nursing organizations.

Nursing education was largely segregated until the 1960s. Even public health nursing certificate and graduate education

Box 2-2   Mary Breckinridge and the Frontier Nursing Service

Born in 1881 into the fifth generation of a well-to-do Kentucky family, Mary Breckinridge devoted her life to the establishment of the Frontier Nursing Service (FNS). Learning from her grandmother, who used a large part of her fortune to improve the education of southern children, Breckinridge later used money left to her by her grandmother to start the FNS (Browne, 1966).

Tutored in childhood and later attending private schools, Mary Breckinridge did not consider becoming a nurse until her husband died. She "yearned for adventure and struggled for the opportunity to 'do something useful'" (Hostutler et al., 2000). In 1907 she enrolled at St. Luke's Hospital School of Nursing in New York. She later married for a second time and had two children. Her second marriage ended after her daughter died at birth and her son died at age 4. From the time of her son's death in 1918, she devoted her energy to promoting the health care of disadvantaged women and children (Browne, 1966).

After World War I and work in postwar France, she returned to the United States passionate about helping the neglected children of rural America. To prepare herself for what would become her life's work, she studied for a year at Teacher's College, Columbia University, to learn more about public health nursing (Browne, 1966).

Early in 1925 she returned to Kentucky. She decided that the mountains of Kentucky were an excellent place to demonstrate the value of community health nursing to remote, disadvantaged families. She thought that if she could establish a nursing center in rural Kentucky, this effort could then be duplicated anywhere. The first health center was established in a five-room cabin in Hyden, Kentucky. Establishing the center took not only nursing skills but also the construction of the center and later the hospital and other buildings; it required extensive knowledge about developing a water supply, disposing of sewage, getting electric power, and securing a mountain area in which landslides occurred (Browne, 1966). Despite many obstacles inherent in building in the mountains, six outpost nursing centers were established between 1927 and 1930. The FNS hospital was built in Hyden, Kentucky, and physicians began entering service. Payment of fees ranged from labor and supplies to funds raised through annual family dues, philanthropy, and the fund-raising efforts of Mary Breckinridge (Holloway, 1975).

The FNS established medical, surgical, and dental clinics; provided nursing and midwifery services 24 hours a day; and served nearly 10,000 people spread over 700 square miles. Baseline data were obtained on infant and maternal mortality before beginning services. FNS services are especially remarkable considering the environmental conditions in which rural Kentuckians lived. Many homes had no heat, electricity, or running water. Often physicians were located more than 40 miles from their patients (Tirpak, 1975).

During the 1930s, nurses lived in one of the six outposts, from which they traveled to see patients; they often had to make their visits on horseback. Like her nurses, Mary Breckinridge traveled many miles through the mountains of Kentucky on her horse, Babette, providing food, supplies, and health care to mountain families (Browne, 1966).

Over the years, several hundred nurses have worked for the FNS. Although Mary Breckinridge died in 1965, the FNS has continued to grow and provide needed services to people in the mountains of Kentucky. This service continues today as a vital and creative way to deliver community health services to rural families.

Data from Browne H: A tribute to Mary Breckinridge, *Nurs Outlook* 14(5):54–55, 1966; Goan MB: *Mary Breckinridge: the frontier nursing service and rural health in Appalachia,* Chapel Hill, NC, 2008, The University of North Carolina Press; Holloway JB: Frontier Nursing Service 1925-1975, *J Ky Med Assoc* 73(9):491–492, 1975; Hostutler J et al: Nurses: then and now and models of practice, *Am J Nurs* 100(2):82–83, 2000; Tirpak H: The Frontier Nursing Service: fifty years in the mountains, *Nurs Outlook* 33:308–310, 1975.

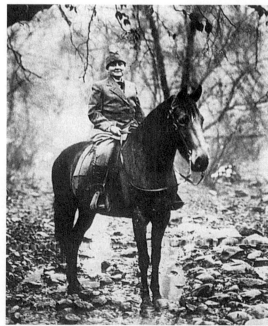

FIGURE 2-4 Mary Breckinridge, founder of the Frontier Nursing Service. (Courtesy Frontier Nursing Service of Wendover, Ky.)

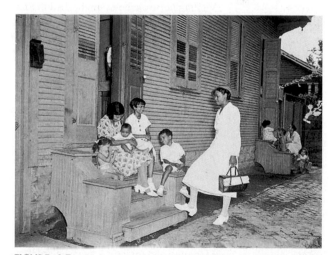

FIGURE 2-5 African-American nurse visiting a family on the doorstep of their home. (Courtesy New Orleans Public Library WPA Photograph Collection.)

was segregated in the South; study outside the South was difficult to afford, and study leaves from the workplace were seldom granted. To address this problem, a collaboration was established in 1936 between the United States Public Health Service and the Medical College of Virginia (Richmond).

These partners established a certificate program in public health nursing in which the federal government paid the nurses' tuition.

ECONOMIC DEPRESSION AND THE IMPACT ON PUBLIC HEALTH

During this period the tension between preventive care and care of the sick, and the related question of whether nursing interventions should be directed toward groups and communities or toward individuals and their families persisted. Although each nursing agency was unique and services varied from region to region, voluntary visiting nurse associations tended to emphasize care of the sick, and official public health agencies provided more preventive services. Not surprisingly, this splintering of services led to rivalry between "visiting," or community, and "public health" nurses and interfered with the development of comprehensive community nursing services (Roberts and Heinrich, 1985). For example, one household could receive services from several community nurses representing different agencies. Residents in the same home might have separate visits for a postpartum woman and new baby, for a child sick with scarlet fever, and

for an elderly bedridden person. This was confusing, costly and duplicated services.

The "combination service" merged sick care services and preventive services into one comprehensive agency by combining visiting nurse and official public health agencies. However, compared with visiting nurse organizations, public health nurses in **official health agencies** often had less control of the program because physicians and politicians determined services and the assignment of personnel. The "ideal program" of the combination agency was hard to administer, and many of the combination services implemented between 1930 and 1965 later reverted to their former, divided structures of visiting nurse agencies and official health departments.

The economic crisis of the 1930s Depression deeply influenced nursing. Not only were agencies and communities unable to meet the huge needs of the poor, but decreased funding for nursing services reduced the numbers of nurses in hospitals and in the community. The Federal Emergency Relief Administration (FERA) supported nurse employment through grants-in-aid for state programs of home medical care. FERA purchased nursing care from existing visiting nurse agencies, which supported nurses and prevented

Table 2-2   Milestones in the History of Community Health and Public Health Nursing: 1866-1945

Year	Milestone
1866	New York Metropolitan Board of Health established
1872	American Public Health Association established
1873	New York Training School opened at Bellevue Hospital, New York City, as first Nightingale-model nursing school in the United States
1877	Women's Board of the New York Mission hired Frances Root to visit the sick poor
1885	Visiting Nurse Association established in Buffalo
1886	Visiting nurse agencies established in Philadelphia and Boston
1893	Lillian Wald and Mary Brewster organized a visiting nursing service for the poor of New York, which later became the Henry Street Nurses Settlement; Society of Superintendents of Training Schools of Nurses in the United States and Canada was established (in 1912 it became known as the National League for Nursing Education)
1896	Associated Alumnae of Training Schools for Nurses established (in 1911 it became the American Nurses' Association)
1902	School nursing started in New York; Lina Rogers was the first school nurse
1903	First nurse practice acts
1909	Metropolitan Life Insurance Company initiated the first insurance reimbursement for nursing care
1910	Public health nursing program instituted at Teachers College, Columbia University, in New York
1912	National Organization for Public Health Nursing formed with Lillian Wald as the first president
1914	First undergraduate nursing education course in public health offered by Adelaide Nutting at Teacher's College
1918	Vassar Camp School for Nurses organized; U.S. Public Health Service (USPHS) established division of public health nursing to work in the war effort; worldwide influenza epidemic began
1919	Textbook, *Public Health Nursing*, written by Mary S. Gardner
1921	Maternity and Infancy Act (Sheppard-Towner Act)
1925	Frontier Nursing Service using nurse-midwives established
1934	Pearl McIver becomes the first nurse employed by USPHS
1935	Passage of the Social Security Act
1941	Beginning of World War II
1943	Passage of the Bolton-Bailey Act for nursing education, and Cadet Nurse Program established; Division of Nursing begun at USPHS; Lucille Petry appointed chief of the Cadet Nurse Corps
1944	First basic program in nursing accredited as including sufficient public health content

agency closure. More than 10,000 nurses were employed by the Civil Works Administration (CWA) programs and assigned to official health agencies. "While this facilitated rapid program expansion by recipient agencies and gave the nurses a taste of public health, the nurses' lack of field experience created major problems of training and supervision for the regular staff" (Roberts and Heinrich, 1985, p. 1162). Thus new graduates were inadequately prepared to work in public health and required considerable agency orientation and teaching (National Organization for Public Health Nursing, 1944).

Changes at the federal level affected the structure of community health resources and led to a "new era in public health nursing" (Roberts and Heinrich, 1985, p. 1162). In 1933 Pearl McIver became the first nurse employed by the U.S. Public Health Service to provide consultation services to state health departments. McIver was convinced that the strengths and ability of each state's director of public health nursing would determine the scope and quality of local health services. Together with Naomi Deutsch, director of nursing for the Federal Children's Bureau, and with the support of nursing organizations, McIver and her staff of nurse consultants influenced the direction of public health nursing. Between 1931 and 1938, more than 40% of the increase in public health nurse employment was at local health agencies. Even so, more than one-third of all counties in the nation lacked local public health nursing services.

The **Social Security Act of 1935** tried to overcome the national setbacks of the Depression. Title VI of this act provided funding to expand opportunities for health protection and promotion through education and employment of public health nurses. More than 1000 nurses completed educational programs in public health in 1936. Title VI also provided $8 million to assist states, counties, and medical districts to establish and maintain adequate health services, as well as $2 million for research and investigation of disease (Buhler-Wilkerson, 1985, 1989; Kalisch and Kalisch, 1995).

In the late 1930s and especially in the late 1940s, Congress supported categorical funding to provide federal money for priority diseases or groups rather than for a comprehensive community health program. In response, local health departments designed programs to fit the funding priorities. This included maternal and child health services and crippled children (1935), venereal disease control (1938), tuberculosis (1944), mental health (1947), industrial hygiene (1947), and dental health (1947) (Scutchfield and Keck, 1997). This pattern of funding continues in the twenty-first century.

World War II increased the need for nurses both for the war effort and at home. Many nurses joined the Army and Navy Nurse Corps. U.S. Representative Frances Payne Bolton of Ohio led Congress to pass the Bolton Act of 1943, which established the Cadet Nurses Corps. This legislation supported increased undergraduate and graduate enrollment in schools of nursing. Funding became more available to

educate nurses by providing financial support for them to go to school, with many focusing on public health.

Because of the number of nurses involved in the war, civilian hospitals and visiting nurse agencies shifted care to families and nonnursing personnel. "By the end of 1942, over 500,000 women had completed the American Red Cross home nursing course, and nearly 17,000 nurse's aides had been certified" (Roberts and Heinrich, 1985, p. 1165). By the end of 1946, more than 215,000 volunteer nurse's aides had received certificates. During this time community health nursing expanded its scope of practice. For example, more community health nurses practiced in rural areas and many official agencies began to provide bedside nursing care (Buhler-Wilkerson, 1985; Kalisch and Kalisch, 1995).

Following the War there was increased need for services from local health departments to respond to sudden increases in demand for care of emotional problems, accidents, alcoholism, and other responsibilities new to official health agencies. Changes in medical technology improved the ability to screen and treat infectious and communicable diseases (e.g., using antibiotics to treat rheumatic fever and venereal diseases). Job opportunities for public health nurses increased, and nurses were a major portion of health department staff. More than 20,000 nurses worked in health departments, visiting nurse associations, industry, and schools. Table 2-2 highlights significant milestones in community and public health nursing from the mid-1800s to the mid-1900s.

FROM WORLD WAR II UNTIL THE 1970s

By 1950, Americans were living longer and the leading causes of death had changed from infectious diseases to heart disease, cancer, and cerebrovascular disease. Nurses influenced the reduction of communicable diseases through their work with immunization campaigns, improved nutrition, and better hygiene and sanitation. The availability of more medications, better housing, and good emergency and critical care services also extended the lives of many people. The over-65-year-old population grew from 4.1% in 1900 to 9.2% of the total in 1950. Chronic illnesses and longer lives brought new health challenges including the need to provide long-term care and to treat chronic diseases.

During the 1930s and 1940s, more Americans chose to obtain care in hospitals, since this was where physicians worked and where technology was readily available to diagnose and treat illness. Health insurance programs now allowed middle-class people to get care in hospitals that had previously been available only to those who could afford to pay their own bills. In 1952, Metropolitan Life Insurance Company and John Hancock Life Insurance Company ended their support of visiting nurse services for their policyholders and the American Red Cross ended its programs of direct nursing service.

Nursing organizations also continued to change. The functions of the NOPHN, the National League for Nursing Education, and the Association of Collegiate Schools of Nursing were distributed to the new **National League**

Evidence-Based Practice

Nursing has a long and rich past, yet this is rarely conveyed to undergraduate nursing students; as a result, nurses devalue the achievements of earlier nurses. This chapter argues that studying the history of nursing has a number of benefits for undergraduate students as well as the profession at large. It provides students with a realistic understanding of nursing and what has influenced past developments to bring us to the present situation. As such, it provides students with the context of nursing practice and thus a firm foundation on which other nursing courses can build. Introducing students to the history of nursing introduces them to a heritage of working in the community as well as institutions; of working independently as well as interdependently; and of ongoing struggles to forge a professional status based on philanthropy, ethics, and later, education. Studying the history of nursing, especially at the beginning of the undergraduate program, allows students to understand what factors have influenced past events and how these factors continue to have an impact on nursing today and into the future.

In addition to the contextual benefits gleaned from the study of the history of nursing, fundamental critical thinking skills can be developed by encouraging students to question the evidence before them and to seek out influencing factors or the "bigger picture." Additional benefits include the ability to debunk some well-known nursing myths that have affected nursing over the years, the ability to explore gender roles in nursing and discuss how gender affects today's practice, and the ability to understand the unwritten rules of the clinical environment.

NURSE USE: The influence of nursing needs to be valued and understood within the context of the time it was being practiced, because students who have an appreciation of nursing's past have a better understanding of nursing and who nurses are. Through the history of nursing, students can better understand that they are entering a profession that has a rich and diverse past and that this can provide a firm platform upon which to base their other studies. By studying the history of nursing, they also develop their critical thinking skills, which allows them to question and evaluate information that is presented to them on a daily basis.

From Madsen W: Teaching history to nurses: will this make me a better nurse? *Nurs Educ Today* 28(5):524–529, July 2008.

for Nursing (NLN). The **American Nurses Association (ANA)** continued as the second national nursing organization. In 1948 the NLN adopted the recommendations of Esther Lucile Brown's study of nursing education, *Nursing for the Future*, and this considerably influenced how nurses were prepared. She recommended that basic nursing education be done in colleges and universities. In the 1950s, public health nursing became a required part of most baccalaureate nursing education programs. In 1952, nursing education programs began in junior and community colleges. Louise McManus, a director of the Division of Nursing Education at Teachers College, Columbia University, wanted to see if bedside nurses could be prepared in a 2-year program. The intent was to prepare nurses more quickly than in the past to ease the prevailing nursing shortage (Kalisch and Kalisch, 1995). This would also move more nursing education into American higher education. Mildred Montag, an assistant professor of nursing education at Teacher's College, became the project coordinator. In 1958, when the 5-year study was completed, this experiment was determined to be a success.

Currently, associate degree nursing (ADN) programs educate the largest percentage of nurses, although baccalaureate program rates are growing. Both health care and ADN education have changed. Both have moved away from a heavy focus on inpatient care to community-based care. Curricula in ADN programs often include content and clinical experiences in management, community health, home health, and gerontology. These clinical areas have typically been key components of baccalaureate education. The **American Association of Colleges of Nursing (AACN)** was founded in 1969 to respond to the need for an organization that would further nursing education in American universities and 4-year colleges, including establishing essentials of nursing education for baccalaureate and higher degree programs.

COMMUNITY AND PUBLIC HEALTH NURSING FROM THE 1970s TO THE PRESENT

During the 1970s, nurses made many contributions to improving the health care of communities, including participation in the hospice movement and the development of birthing centers, day care for elderly and disabled persons, drug-abuse treatment programs, and rehabilitation services in long-term care. Adequate funding for population health remained difficult to secure. Health care costs grew during the 1980s. Growing costs of acute hospital care, medical procedures, and institutional long-term care reduced funding for health promotion and disease prevention programs. The use of ambulatory services including health maintenance organizations was encouraged, and utilization of nurse practitioners (advanced practice nurses) increased. Despite unstable reimbursement, home health care began to increase its role in the care of the sick at home. By the 1980s, individuals and families assumed more responsibility for their own health, and health education—always a part of community health nursing—became more popular. Consumer and professional advocacy groups urged the passage of laws to prohibit unhealthy practices in public such as smoking and driving under the influence of alcohol. However, reduced federal and state funds led to decreases in the number of nurses in official public health agencies.

The Division of Nursing of the U.S. Public Health Service conducted and sponsored nursing research beginning in the late 1930s. This expanded in the late 1940s (Uhl, 1965). The National Center for Nursing Research (NCNR) was established in 1985 within the federal National Institutes of Health, reflecting the continued growth in nursing research. The NCNR focused attention on the value of nursing research and promoted the work of nurses. With the effort of many nurses the NCNR attained institute (rather than center) status in 1993 and became the National Institute of Nursing Research (NINR).

Healthy People 2010

History of the Development of *Healthy People 2010*

In 1979, the groundbreaking *Healthy People: The Surgeon Generals' Report on Health Promotion and Disease Prevention* asserted that "the health of the American people has never been better" (p. 3). But this was only the prologue to deep criticism of the status of American health care delivery. Between 1960 and 1978, health care spending increased 700% without striking improvements in mortality or morbidity. During the 1950s and 1960s, evidence accumulated about chronic disease risk factors, particularly cigarette smoking, alcohol and drugs, occupational risks, and injuries. These new research findings were not systematically applied to planning and improving the health of the population.

In 1974, the Government of Canada published *New Perspective on the Health of Canadians* (Lalonde, 1974), which considered death and disease to be the result of four contributing factors: inadequacies in the existing health care system, behavioral factors, environmental hazards, and human biological factors. Applying the Canadian approach, in 1976 U.S. experts analyzed the 10 leading causes of U.S. mortality and found that 50% of American deaths were caused by unhealthy behaviors and only 10% were the result of inadequacies in health care. Rather than just spending more to improve hospital care, clearly prevention was the key to saving lives, improving the quality of life, and saving health care dollars.

A multidisciplinary group of analysts conducted a comprehensive review of prevention activities. They verified that the health of Americans could be significantly improved through "actions individuals can take for themselves" and through actions public and private decision makers could take to "promote a safer and healthier environment" (p. 9). Like Canada's *New Perspectives, Healthy People* (1979) identified priorities and measurable goals. *Healthy People* grouped 15 key priorities into three categories: key preventive services that could be delivered to individuals by health providers, such as timely prenatal care; measures that could be used by governmental and other agencies, as well as industry, to protect people from harm, such as reduced exposure to toxic agents; and activities that individuals and communities could use to promote healthy lifestyles, such as improved nutrition.

In the late 1980s, success in addressing these priorities and goals was evaluated, new scientific findings were analyzed, and new goals and objectives were set for the period 1990-2000 through *Healthy People 2000: National Health Promotion and Disease Prevention Objectives* (U.S. Public Health Service, 1991b). This process was repeated 10 years later to develop goals and objectives for the period 2000-2010. Recognizing the continuing challenge to use emerging scientific research to encourage modification of health behaviors and practices, *Healthy People 2010* emphasizes reducing health disparities and increasing years of healthy life by focusing on the following:

- Active participation by individuals in decisions regarding their health and the health of their families.
- Encouragement of leadership roles in promoting healthier behaviors in clients, neighborhoods, or communities.
- The goal to improve the nation's health.
- Nurses who can improve health by beginning with the self and one client.
- Those factors that encourage health.
- The factors that determine health: the physical, social, and environmental factors related to individuals and communities, as well as the policies and interventions used to promote health, prevent disease, and ensure access to quality health care.

Like the nurse in the early twentieth century who spread the gospel of public health to reduce communicable diseases, today's community-oriented nurse uses *Healthy People* to reduce chronic and infectious diseases and injuries through health education, environmental modification, and policy development.

From Lalonde M: *New perspective on the health of Canadians,* Ottawa, Canada, 1974, Information Canada; U.S. Department of Health and Human Services: *Healthy People 2010: understanding and improving health,* ed 2, Washington, DC, 2000, U.S. Government Printing Office; U.S. Department of Health, Education, and Welfare: *Healthy people: the surgeon general's report on health promotion and disease prevention,* DHEW Publication No. 79-55071, Washington, DC, 1979, U.S. Government Printing Office; and U.S. Public Health Services: *Healthy people 2000: national health promotion and disease prevention objectives,* Washington, DC, 1991b, U.S. Government Printing Office.

By the late 1980s, public health had declined in its ability to implement its mission and influence the health of the public. The disarray resulting from reduced political support, financing, and effectiveness were clearly described by the Institute of Medicine (IOM) in *The Future of Public Health* (Institute of Medicine, 1988). Although many people agreed about what the mission of public health should be, there was much less agreement about how to turn the mission into action and effective programs. The IOM report emphasized the core functions of public health as assessment, policy development, and assurance (see Chapter 1). The *Healthy People* initiative has influenced goals and priority setting in public health and in public nursing. In 1979, *Healthy People* proposed a national strategy to improve significantly the health of Americans by preventing or delaying the onset of major chronic illnesses, injuries, and infectious diseases. Specific goals and objectives were established, and time frames for accomplishing them were set. Implementation of these strategies has considerably influenced the work of nurses, through their employment in health agencies or through participation in state or local *Healthy People* coalitions (*Healthy People 2010* box). Many *Healthy People 2010* objectives and intervention strategies are described in chapters throughout this text, and in *Healthy People 2010: Understanding and Improving Health* (U.S. Department of Health and Human Services, 2000). New *Healthy People* objectives for the next decade will be set for 2020.

During the 1990s and continuing at present, public concerns about health have focused on cost, quality, and access to services. Despite wide-spread interest in universal health insurance coverage, neither individuals nor employers are willing to pay for this level of service. The core debate of the economics of health care—who would pay for what— has emphasized the need for reform of medical care rather than comprehensive reform of health care. In 1993 a blue-ribbon group assembled by President Clinton, with First Lady Hillary Rodham Clinton serving as chair, proposed the American Health Security Act. This proposal led to broad

Table 2-3   Milestones in the History of Community Health and Public Health Nursing: 1946-2004

Year	Milestone
1946	Nurses classified as professionals by U.S. Civil Service Commission; Hill-Burton Act approved providing funds for hospital construction in underserved areas and requiring these hospitals to provide care to poor people; passage of National Mental Health Act
1950	25,091 nurses employed in public health
1951	National organizations recommended that college-based nursing education programs include public health content
1952	National Organization for Public Health Nursing merged into the new National League for Nursing; Metropolitan Life Insurance Nursing Program closed
1964	Passage of the Economic Opportunity Act; public health nurse defined by the American Nurses Association (ANA) as a graduate of a bachelor of science in nursing (BSN) program; Congress amended the Social Security Act to include Medicare and Medicaid
1965	ANA position paper recommended that nursing education take place in institutions of higher learning
1977	Passage of the Rural Health Clinic Services Act, which provided indirect reimbursement for nurse practitioners in rural health clinics
1978	Association of Graduate Faculty in Community Health Nursing/Public Health Nursing (later renamed *Association of Community Health Nursing Educators*)
1980	Medicaid amendment to the Social Security Act to provide direct reimbursement for nurse practitioners in rural health clinics; both ANA and the American Public Health Association (APHA) developed statements on the role and conceptual foundations of community and public health nursing, respectively
1983	Beginning of Medicare prospective payments
1985	National Center for Nursing Research (NCNR) established in the National Institutes of Health (NIH)
1988	Institute of Medicine published *The Future of Public Health*
1990	Association of Community Health Nursing Educators published *Essentials of Baccalaureate Nursing Education*
1991	More than 60 nursing organizations joined forces to support health care reform and published a document entitled *Nursing's Agenda for Health Care Reform*
1993	American Health Security Act of 1993 was published as a blueprint for national health care reform; the national effort, however, failed, leaving states and the private sector to design their own programs
1993	NCNR became the National Institute for Nursing Research, as part of the National Institutes of Health
1993	Public Health Nursing section of the American Public Health Association updated the definition and role of public health nursing
1996	Passage of the Health Insurance Portability and Accountability Act

discussion of the key issues and concerns in health care, especially the organization and delivery of medical care with an emphasis on managed care. When Congress failed to pass the American Health Security Act, considerable change followed in health care financing and the private sector assumed even greater control. As managed care grew, costs were contained, but constraints increased in terms of how to access care and how much and what kind of care would be paid for. Throughout these debates, public health was generally ignored. There was little attention given to ensuring that populations and the communities in which they lived were healthy. This omission reflected the large gap between the proposal and actual comprehensive health care reform.

In 1991 the American Nurses Association, the American Association of Colleges of Nursing, the National League for Nursing, and more than 60 other specialty nursing organizations joined to support health care reform. The coalitions of organizations emphasized the key health care issues of access, quality, and cost. Improved primary care and public health efforts would help build a healthy nation. Professional nursing continues to support revisions in health care delivery

and extension of public health services to prevent illness, promote health, and protect the public (Table 2-3).

During the late twentieth and early twenty-first century, challenges continued to trigger growth and change in nursing in the community. Nurse-managed centers now provide a diversity of nursing services, including health promotion and disease/injury prevention where existing organizations have been unable to meet community and neighborhood needs. These centers provide valuable services but typically face many challenges in securing adequate funding. As population needs continue to grow and change, schools of nursing, health departments, rural health clinics, migrant health and other community services are challenged to provide the range of services to meet specific needs. Transfer of official health services to private control has sometimes reduced professional flexibility and service delivery. A nursing shortage reduces staffing when community nurses look to employment in acute care facilities that often pay higher salaries. The Association of Community Health Nurse Educators recommends increased graduate programs to educate public health nurse leaders, educators, and researchers. Natural disasters (such as

HOW TO	**Conduct an Oral History Interview**

1. Identify an issue or event of interest.
2. Gather information from written materials.
3. Find a person to interview.
4. Get permission from the person to do the interview and make an appointment to do so.
5. Gather information about the person's background and the time period of interest.
6. Write an outline of your questions. Use open-ended questions, since they usually give you more information.
7. Meet with the person being interviewed; use a tape recorder and bring extra tapes.
8. Conduct the interview asking only one question at a time and allowing adequate time for the reply.
9. Clarify points when needed; ask for examples; remember, most people like to talk about themselves.
10. After the interview, write it up as soon as possible when your recall is best.
11. Compare your written report with the tape. There may be times when you can ask the person interviewed to read your report for accuracy.

floods, hurricanes, and tornados) and human-made disasters (including explosions, building collapses, airplane crashes, and toxic ingredients added to food) have required rapid, innovative, and time-consuming responses. Preparation for future disasters and possible bioterrorism requires well prepared nurses. Some states hear new calls to deploy school nurses in every school; a new recognition of the link between school success and health is making the school nurse essential. Many of these stories are detailed in the chapters that follow.

Public health nursing, historically and in the present, is characterized by its reaching out to care for the health of people in need (U.S. Public Health Service, 1993). At present, many nurses work in the community. Some bring a public health population-based approach and have as their goal preventing illness and protecting health. Other nurses have a community-oriented approach and deal primarily with the health care of individuals, families, and groups in a community. Still other nurses bring a community-based approach that focuses on "illness care" of individuals and families in the community. Each type of nurse is needed in today's communities. It is important that we learn from the past and not mis-use time and resources. The "How To" box describes how to conduct an oral history interview. This is one effective way to learn from the successes and failures of our predecessors.

Today, nurses look to their history for inspiration, explanation, and prediction. Information and advocacy are used to promote a comprehensive approach to address the multiple needs of the diverse populations served. Nurses seek to learn from the past and to avoid known pitfalls, even as they seek successful strategies to meet the complex needs of today's vulnerable populations. As plans for the future are made and as unmet public health challenges are acknowledged, the vision of what nurses in community health can accomplish serves as a sustaining force.

CLINICAL APPLICATION

Mary Lipsky has worked for a visiting nurse association in a large urban area for 2 years. She is responsible for a wide variety of services, including caring for older and chronically ill clients recently discharged from hospitals, new mothers and babies, mental health clients, and clients with long-term health problems, such as chronic wounds.

Daily when she leaves the field to go home, she finds that she continues to think about her clients. She keeps going over these and other questions in her mind: Why is it so difficult for mothers and new babies to qualify for and receive WIC (Women, Infant, and Children Nutrition) Services? Why must she limit the number of visits and length of service for clients with chronic wounds? Why are so few services available for clients with behavioral health problems? In particular, she thinks about the burdens and challenges that families and friends face in caring for the sick at home.

A. *Why might it be difficult to solve these problems at the individual level, on a case-by-case basis?*
B. *What information would you need to build an understanding of the policy background for each of these various populations?*

Answers are in the back of the book.

REMEMBER THIS!

- A historical approach can be used to increase the understanding of public and community health nursing in the past, as well as its contemporary dilemmas and future challenges.
- Public health and community health nursing are products of various social, economic, and political forces and incorporate public health science in addition to nursing science and practice.
- Federal responsibility for health care was limited until the 1930s, when the economic challenges of the Depression highlighted the need for federal assistance for health care.
- Florence Nightingale designed and implemented the first program of trained nursing, and her contemporary, William Rathbone, founded the first district nursing association in England.
- Urbanization, industrialization, and immigration in the United States increased the need for trained nurses, especially in public and community health nursing.
- Increasing acceptance of public roles for women permitted public and community health nursing employment for nurses, as well as public leadership roles for their wealthy supporters.
- Frances Root was the first trained nurse in the United States who was salaried as a visiting nurse. She was hired in 1887 by the Women's Board of the New York City Mission to provide care to sick persons at home.
- The first visiting nurse associations were founded in 1885 and 1886 in Buffalo, Philadelphia, and Boston.

- Lillian Wald established the Henry Street Settlement, which became the Visiting Nurse Service of New York City, in 1893. She played a key role in innovations that shaped public and community health nursing in its first decades, including school nursing, insurance payment for nursing, national organization for public health nurses, and the United States Children's Bureau.
- Founded in 1902, with the vision and support of Lillian Wald, school nursing tried to keep children in school so that they could learn.
- The Metropolitan Life Insurance Company established the first insurance-based program in 1909 to support community health nursing services.
- The National Organization for Public Health Nursing (founded in 1912) provided essential leadership and coordination of diverse public and community health nursing efforts, before the organization merged into the new National League for Nursing in 1952.
- Official health agencies slowly grew in numbers between 1900 and 1940, accompanied by a steady increase in public health nursing positions.
- The innovative Sheppard-Towner Act of 1921 expanded community health nursing roles for maternal and child health during the 1920s.
- Mary Breckinridge established the Frontier Nursing Service in 1925 to provide rural health care.
- Tension between the nursing roles of caring for the sick and of providing preventive care and the related tension between intervening for individuals and for groups have characterized the specialty since at least the 1910s.
- The challenges of World War II sometimes resulted in extension of community health nursing care and sometimes in retrenchment and decreased public health nursing services.
- By the mid-twentieth century, the reduced incidence of communicable diseases and the increased prevalence of chronic illness, accompanied by large increases in the population older than 65 years, led to re-examination of the goals and organization of community health nursing services.
- Between the 1930s and 1965, organized nursing and community health nursing agencies sought to establish health insurance reimbursement for nursing care at home.
- Implementation of Medicare and Medicaid programs in 1966 established new possibilities for supporting community-based nursing care but encouraged agencies to focus on postacute care services rather than prevention.
- Efforts to reform health care organization, pushed by increased health care costs during the past 40 years, have focused on reforming acute medical care rather than on designing a comprehensive preventive approach.
- The 1988 the *Future of Public Health* report documented the reduced political support, financing, and impact that increasingly limited public health services at national, state, and local levels.
- In the late 1990s federal policy changes dangerously reduced financial support for home health care services, threatening the long-term survival of visiting nurse agencies.
- The *Healthy People* program has brought renewed emphasis on prevention to public and community health nursing.
- In 2002 the Association of Community Health Educators revised its *Essentials of Master's Level Nursing Education for Advanced Community/Public Health Nursing Practice* (Association of Community Health Educators, 2002) and the Institute of Medicine published a guide to education in each of the public health disciplines entitled *Who will keep the public healthy?*
- In 2003 the Quad Council, an alliance of four national nursing organizations that addresses public health nursing issues, finalized its own set of public health nursing competencies.

WHAT WOULD YOU DO?

1. Interview three nurses who work in a community setting. Ask them to describe the changes they have seen in the way in which care is delivered in the community. Ask if they think the changes have been positive or negative, and ask them to discuss specifically how they view the changes in regard to improving the health of the community residents.
2. Interview older friends or relatives to see if they have had any experiences with nursing care in the community. Next, meet with three or four classmates and discuss the following: If the older people had received nursing care in the community, what type of care was it? Was the care useful? What suggestions do they have for how care could be more useful to them if provided in a community setting?
3. What part of community health practice interests you? If you were to work in a community setting, what would it be? What effect would your work likely have?
4. If you prefer not to work in a community setting now or in the future, what are the primary reasons for this decision? If you work in an institution, how will community health practice influence your patient care decisions?
5. This chapter has described the work and enormous contributions of several leaders in nursing. Which ones do you admire the most? Whose work would you like to continue in the present health care system? What do you see as strengths and limitations of previous community health nurses? Which one strikes you as most interesting? Why?

■ REFERENCES

Backer BA: Lillian Wald: connecting caring with action, *Nurs Health Care* 14:122–128, 1993.

Brainard A: *Evolution of public health nursing*, Philadelphia, 1922, Saunders.

Browne H: A tribute to Mary Breckinridge, *Nurs Outlook* 14(5):54–55, 1966.

Buhler-Wilkerson K: Public health nursing: in sickness or in health? *Am J Pub Health* 75:1155–1161, 1985.

Buhler-Wilkerson K: *False dawn: the rise and decline of public health nursing, 1900–1930*, New York, 1989, Garland Publishing.

Buhler-Wilkerson K: *No place like home: a history of nursing and home care in the United States*, Baltimore, 2001, Johns Hopkins.

Cohen IB: Florence Nightingale, *Sci Am* 3:128–137, 1984.

Deloughery GL: *History and trends of professional nursing*, ed 8, St. Louis, 1977, Mosby.

Dock LL: The history of public health nursing, *Public Health Nurs*, 1922. (Reprinted by the American Public Health Association).

Dolan J: *History of nursing*, ed 14, Philadelphia, 1978, Saunders.

Frachel RR: A new profession: the evolution of public health nursing, *Public Health Nurs* 5(2):86–90, 1988.

Goan MB: *Mary Breckinridge: the frontier nursing service and rural health in Appalachia*, Chapel Hill NC, 2008, The University of North Carolina.

Hawkins JW, Hayes ER, Corliss CP: School nursing in America—1902–1994: a return to public health nursing, *Public Health Nurs* 11(6):416–425, 1994.

Hine DC: *Black women in white: racial conflict and cooperation in the nursing profession, 1890–1950*, Bloomington, 1989, Indiana University Press.

Holloway JB: Frontier nursing service 1925–1975, *J Ky Med Assoc* 73(9):491–492, 1975.

Hostutler J et al: Nurses: then and now and models of practice, *Am J Nurs* 100(2):82–83, 2000.

Institute of Medicine: *The future of public health*, Washington, DC, 1988, National Academy of Science.

Kalisch PA, Kalisch BJ: *The advance of American nursing*, ed 3, Philadelphia, 1995, Lippincott.

Lalonde M: *New perspective on the health of Canadians*, 1974, Government of Canada.

Madsen W: Teaching history to nurses: will this make me a better nurse? *Nurse Educ Today* 28(5):524–529, 2008.

National Organization for Public Health Nursing: approval of Skidmore College of Nursing as preparing students for public health nursing, *Public Health Nurs* 36:371, 1944.

Nightingale F: Sick nursing and health nursing. In Billings JS, Hurd HM, editors: *Hospitals, dispensaries, and nursing*, Baltimore, 1894, Johns Hopkins. (Reprinted New York, 1984, Garland.)

Nightingale F: *Notes on nursing: what it is, and what it is not*, Philadelphia, 1946, Lippincott.

Nutting MA, Dock LL: *A history of nursing*, New York, 1935, GP Putnam's Sons.

Palmer IS: *Florence Nightingale and the first organized delivery of nursing services*, Washington, DC, 1983, American Association of Colleges of Nursing.

Pickett G, Hanlon JJ: *Public health: administration and practice*, St. Louis, 1990, Mosby.

Quad Council of Public Health Nursing Organizations: *Public health nursing competencies*, Washington, DC, 2003, American Nurses Association.

Roberts DE, Heinrich J: Public health nursing comes of age, *Am J Public Health* 75:1162–1172, 1985.

Roberts M: *American nursing: history and interpretation*, New York, 1955, Macmillan.

Rodabaugh JH, Rodabaugh MJ: *Nursing in Ohio: a history*, Columbus, Ohio, 1951, Ohio State Nurses Association.

Rosen G: *A history of public health*, New York, 1958, MD Publications.

Scutchfield FD, Keck CW: *Principles of public health practice*, Albany, NY, 1997, Delmar.

Shyrock H: *The history of nursing*, Philadelphia, 1959, Saunders.

Thoms AB: *Pathfinders: a history of the progress of colored graduate nurses*, New York, 1929, Kay Printing House.

Tirpak H: The Frontier Nursing Service: fifty years in the mountains, *Nurs Outlook* 33:308–310, 1975.

Uhl G: The Division of Nursing: USPHS, *Am J Nurs* 65(7):82–85, 1965.

U.S. Department of Health and Human Services: *Healthy People 2010: understanding and improving health*, Washington, DC, 2000, U.S. Government Printing Office.

U.S. Public Health Service: Division of Nursing: *A century of caring: a celebration of public health nursing in the United States, 1893–1993*, Washington, DC, 1993, U.S. Government Printing Office.

U.S. Public Health Service: *Healthy communities 2000: model standards*, Washington, DC, 1991a, U.S. Government Printing Office.

U.S. Public Health Service: *Healthy People 2000: national health promotion and disease prevention objectives*, Washington, DC, 1991b, U.S. Government Printing Office.

Wilner DM, Walkey RP, O'Neill EJ: *Introduction to public health*, ed 7, New York, 1978, Macmillan.

Zerwekh JV: Public health nursing legacy: historical practical wisdom, *Nurs Health Care* 13:84–91, 1992.

evolve   http://evolve.elsevier.com/stanhope/foundations

The U. S. Health and Public Health Care Systems

Bonnie Jerome-D'Emilia

ADDITIONAL RESOURCES

These related resources are found either in the appendix at the back of this book or on the book's website at http://evolve.elsevier.com/stanhope/foundations.

Appendix

- Appendix A.3: Declaration of Alma-Ata
- Appendix E.3: The Health Insurance Portability and Accountability Act (HIPAA): What Does It Mean for Public Health Nurses?

Evolve Website

- Community Assessment Applied

- Case Study, with Questions and Answers
- Quiz review questions
- WebLinks, including link to *Healthy People 2010* website

Real World Community Health Nursing: An Interactive CD-ROM, second edition

If you are using this CD-ROM in your course, you will find the following activities related to this chapter:
- *Dig for Data* in **Health Care Systems**
- *Agencies and Their Services* in **Health Care Systems**
- *The Health Care Services Challenge* in **Health Care Systems**

OBJECTIVES

After reading this chapter, the student should be able to:

1. Describe the events and trends that influence the status of the health care system.
2. Discuss key aspects of the private health care system.
3. Define public health care and explain the role nurses play in this care.
4. Describe the current public health care system in the United States and compare and contrast the responsibilities of the federal, state, and local public health systems.
5. Examine nursing roles in selected government agencies.

CHAPTER OUTLINE

FORCES STIMULATING CHANGE IN THE DEMAND FOR HEALTH CARE
Demographic Trends
Social and Economic Trends
Health Workforce Trends
Technological Trends
CURRENT HEALTH CARE SYSTEM IN THE UNITED STATES
Cost
Access
Quality

ORGANIZATION OF THE HEALTH CARE SYSTEM
Primary Health Care
Public Health System
The Federal System
The State System
The Local System
FORCES INFLUENCING THE HEALTH CARE SYSTEM OF THE FUTURE

KEY TERMS

advanced-practice nursing (APN): nurses who hold graduate preparation in a nursing specialty area.

community participation: involvement of members of the community in decision making and planning for meeting their needs.

Declaration of Alma-Ata: resolution supporting primary health care for all people by 2000.

disease prevention: activities that have as their goal the protection of people from becoming ill because of actual or potential health threats.

electronic medical record (EMR): a client safety-oriented system in which patient information is digital, privacy protected, and interchangeable.

health: a state of complete physical, mental, and social well-being; not merely the absence of disease or infirmity (World Health Organization, 1986a, p. 1).

health promotion: activities that have as their goal the development of human attitudes and behaviors that maintain or enhance well-being.

managed care: an integrated system for providing health care services in which consumers must abide by certain rules designed to achieve cost savings.

National Health Service Corps: a commissioned corps of health personnel who provides care in designated underserved areas.

primary care: the providing of integrated, accessible health care services by clinicians who are accountable for addressing a large majority of personal health care needs, developing a sustained partnership with patients, and practicing in the context of family and community.

primary health care (PHC): a combination of primary care and public health care made universally accessible to individuals and families in a community, with their full participation, and provided at a cost that the community and country can afford (World Health Organization, 1978).

public health: organized community efforts designed to prevent disease and promote health. It links disciplines, builds on the science of epidemiology, and focuses on the community.

root cause analysis: a technique for identifying prevention of error strategies and developing a culture of safety.

U.S. Department of Health and Human Services (USDHHS): the federal agency most heavily involved in health and welfare.

Despite the fact that health care costs in the United States are the highest in the world and comprise the greatest percentage of the gross domestic product, the indicators of what constitutes good health do not document that Americans are really getting their money's worth. In the first decade of the twenty-first century there have been massive and unexpected changes to health, economic, and social conditions as a result of terrorist attacks, hurricanes, fires, floods, infectious diseases, and an economic turndown. New systems have been developed to prevent and/or to deal with the onslaught of these horrendous events. Not all of the systems have worked, and many are regularly criticized for their inefficiency and costliness. Simultaneously, new, nearly miraculous advances have been made in treating health-related conditions. Organs and joints are being replaced and medicines are keeping people alive who only a few years ago would have suffered and died. These advances and "wonder drugs" save and prolong lives, and a number of deadly and debilitating diseases have been eliminated through effective immunizations and treatments. In addition, sanitation, water supplies, and nutrition have been improved, and animal cloning begun.

However, attention to all of these advances may overshadow the lack of attention to public health and prevention. We have still not embraced primary health care and an overall public health approach for our citizens. Several of the most destructive health conditions can be prevented either through changes in lifestyle or interventions such as

immunizations. The increasing rates of obesity, especially among children, substance use, lack of exercise, violence, and accidents are alarmingly expensive, particularly when they lead to disruptions in health.

This chapter describes a health care system in transition as it struggles to meet evolving global and domestic challenges. The overall health care and public health systems in the United States are described and differentiated, and the changing priorities are identified. Nurses play a pivotal role in meeting these needs, and the role of the nurse is described. Box 3-1 lists selected definitions that will help explain concepts introduced in this chapter.

FORCES STIMULATING CHANGE IN THE DEMAND FOR HEALTH CARE

In recent years, enormous changes have occurred in society, both in the United States and most other countries of the world. The extent of interaction among countries is stronger than ever, and the economies of countries depend on the stability of other countries. The United States has felt the effects of rising labor costs as many companies have shifted their production to other countries with lower labor costs. It is often less expensive to assemble clothes, automobile parts, and appliances and to have call distribution centers in a less-industrialized country and pay the shipping and other charges involved than to have the items fully assembled in the United States. In recent years the vacillating costs of fuel

Box 3-1   Definitions of Selected Terms

- **Disease prevention**: Activities whose goal is to protect people from becoming ill due to actual or potential health threats
- **Disparities**: Racial or ethnic differences in the quality of health care, not based on access or clinical needs, preferences, or appropriateness of an intervention
- **Electronic medical record**: A computer-based client medical record
- **Globalization:** A trend toward an increased flow of goods, services, money, and disease across national borders
- **Health**: A state of complete physical, mental, and social well-being; not merely the absence of disease or infirmity (World Health Organization, 1986a)
- **Health promotion**: Activities that have as their goal the development of human attitudes and behaviors that maintain or enhance well-being
- **Institute of Medicine**: A part of the National Academy of Sciences and an organization whose purpose is to provide national advice on issues relating to biomedical science, medicine, and health
- **Primary care**: The providing of integrated, accessible health care services by clinicians who are accountable for addressing a large majority of personal health care needs, developing a sustained partnership with clients, and practicing in the context of family and community
- **Primary health care**: A combination of primary care and public health care made universally accessible to individuals and families in a community, with their full participation, and provided at a cost that the community and country can afford (World Health Organization, 1978)
- **Public health**: Organized community and multidisciplinary efforts, based on epidemiology, aimed at preventing disease and promoting health (Institute of Medicine, 1988, p. 4)

has affected almost every area of the economy, leading to both higher costs of products and layoffs as some industries have struggled to stay solvent. This has affected the employment rate in the United States. The economic downturn of 2008 left many people unemployed, and many have lost their homes due to inability to pay their mortgages. When the unemployment rate is high, more people lack comprehensive insurance coverage, since in the United States this is typically provided by employers. In late November 2008, the U.S. unemployment rate was 6.7 percent. This represented an increase from 4.6 percent in 2007. Health care services and the ways in which they are financed are likely to change in the years to come as President Obama and his administration tackle this issue.

DEMOGRAPHIC TRENDS

The population of the world is growing as a result of increased fertility and decreased mortality rates. The largest growth is occurring in underdeveloped countries, and this is accompanied by decreased growth in the United States and other developed countries. The year 2000, however, marked the first time in more than 30 years that the total fertility rate in the United States was above the replacement

level. *Replacement* means that for every person who dies, another is born (Martin et al, 2002). Both the size and the characteristics of the population contribute to the changing demography.

Seventy-seven million babies were born between the years of 1946 and 1963, giving rise to the often discussed Baby Boomer generation (Center for Health Communication, 2004). The oldest of these boomers will be 65 years of age in 2011, and they are expected to live longer than people born in earlier times. The impact on the federal government's insurance program for people 65 years of age and older, Medicare, is expected to be enormous, and this population is expected to double between the years 2000 and 2030.

At the time of the 1990 census, African-Americans were the largest minority group in the United States (U.S. Bureau of the Census, 1996). However, in 2003, the Census Bureau announced that Hispanic persons now outnumbered African-Americans (Singer, 2004). It is predicted that whites will make up only 50.1% of the U.S. population by 2050 (U.S. Bureau of the Census, 2001). The nation's foreign-born population is growing, with 34.2 million or 12% of the population being foreign born in 2004; this is a 2.3% rise from 2003 figures (Bernstein, 2005). Within the foreign-born group, 53% were born in Latin America and 24% in Asia (Singer, 2004).

The composition of the U.S. household is also changing. Families make up about 69% of all households, down from 81% in 1970 (U.S. Bureau of the Census, 2001). A single parent, usually the mother, heads 3 of 10 families. Single-parent families now constitute 19% of all white families, 32% of Hispanic families, and 52% of African-American families (U.S. Bureau of the Census, 2001).

From 1990 to 2000, mortality for both genders in all age groups declined (U.S. Bureau of the Census, 2001). As a result of medical progress, the leading causes of death have changed from infectious diseases to chronic and degenerative diseases. New treatments for infectious diseases have resulted in steady declines of mortality among children. The mortality for older Americans has also declined, especially during the 1970s and 1980s. However, people 50 years of age and older have higher rates of chronic illness and they use a larger portion of health care services than other age-groups.

SOCIAL AND ECONOMIC TRENDS

In addition to the size and changing age distribution of the population, other factors also affect the health care system. Several social trends that influence health care include changing lifestyles, a growing appreciation of the quality of life, the changing composition of families and living patterns, changing household incomes, and a revised definition of quality health care.

Americans spend considerable money on health care, nutrition, and fitness (U.S. Department of Labor, 2004), because **health** is seen as an irreplaceable quality. To be healthy, people must take care of themselves. Many people combine traditional medical and health care practices with complementary and alternative therapies to achieve the highest level of health. Complementary therapies are those that are used in addition to traditional health care, and alternative therapies are those used instead of traditional care. People often spend a considerable amount of their own money for these types of therapies because few are covered by insurance. In recent years, some insurance plans have recognized the value of complementary therapies and have reimbursed for them. About 60 years ago, income was distributed in such a way that a relatively small portion of households earned high incomes; families in the middle-income range made up a somewhat larger proportion and households at the lower end of the income scale made up the largest proportion. By the 1970s, household income had risen, and income was more evenly distributed, largely as a result of dual-income families.

Since 1970, two trends in income distribution have been emerging. The first is that the average per-person income in America has been increasing. However, in recent years with layoffs, outsourcing, and other economic forces, many families are seeing decreases in wages. The second trend is that the gap between the richest 25% and the poorest 25% is widening because of the movement of middle-class families into higher income levels. Chapter 8 provides a detailed discussion of the economics of health care and how financial constraints influence decisions about public health services.

HEALTH WORKFORCE TRENDS

The health care workforce ebbs and flows. The early years of the twenty-first century saw the beginning of what is expected to be a long-term and sizable nursing shortage. Similarly, most other health professionals are documenting current and future shortages. Historically, nursing care has been provided in a variety of settings, primarily in the hospital. In 2008, 56% of all registered nurses (RNs) were employed in hospitals (American Nurses Association, 2008). A few years ago hospitals began reducing their bed capacity as care became more community based. Now they are expanding, including building for both acute and longer term chronic care. This growth is due to the factors previously discussed: the ability to treat and cure more diseases, the complexity of the care and the need for inpatient services, and the growth in the older age group. By 2016 there are expected to be 587,000 new nursing positions (Dehm and Shniper, 2007). In addition, 55% of surveyed nurses reported that they intended to retire between 2011 and 2020 (Orlovsky, 2006).

There tends to be periodic shortages, especially in the primary care workforce in the United States, as providers choose to be specialists in fields such as medicine and nursing. Primary care providers include generalists who are skilled in diagnostic, preventive, and emergency services. The health care personnel trained as primary care generalists include family physicians, general internists, general pediatricians, nurse practitioners (NPs), clinical nurse specialists (CNSs), physician assistants, and certified nurse-midwives (CNMs) (Steinwald, 2008).

NPs, CNSs, and CNMs, considered **advanced practice nursing (APN)** specialties, are vital members of the primary health care teams. NPs receive advanced graduate education, and pursue certification by examination in a specialty area such as pediatrics, adults, gerontology, obstetrics/gynecology, or family. Training emphasizes clinical medical skills (history, physical, and diagnosis) and pharmacology, in addition to the traditional psychosocial- and prevention-focused skills that are normally thought of as nursing. Studies have shown that much of the primary care can be provided by APNs with high quality and at an affordable cost (Hopkins et al, 2005). The cost-effectiveness of the advanced practice nurse reflects a variety of factors related to employment setting, liability insurance, and the cost of education. There are currently 7400 CNMs in clinical practice in the United States (American Nurses Association, 2008). In 2005, 11.2% of all vaginal births in the United States were attended by midwives (American College of Nurse-Midwives, 2008), CNM practitioners receive an average of 1.5 years of specialized education beyond nursing school, and all but 4 of the 43 accredited programs in the United States are at the master's level. They are required to pass a national certification examination before practice. CNMs provide well-woman gynecological and low-risk obstetrical care, including prenatal, labor and delivery, and postpartum care. They have prescriptive authority in more than 33 states. Medicaid reimbursement is mandatory in every state, and 33 states mandate private insurance reimbursement for midwifery services (American College of Nurse-Midwives, 2008).

CNSs are experts in a specialized area of clinical practice such as public health, mental health, gerontology, cardiac, and cancer care. Many provide primary care. They may also work in consultation, research, education, and administration. Some work independently or in private practice and can be reimbursed by Medicare and Medicaid (Zuzelo et al, 2004).

In terms of the nursing workforce, increasing the number of minority nurses remains a priority and a strategy for addressing the current nursing shortage. This will help close the health disparity gap for minority populations (National Advisory Council on Nurse Education and Practice, 2003). For example, persons from minority groups, especially when language is a barrier, often are more comfortable with and more likely to access care from a provider from their own minority group.

TECHNOLOGICAL TRENDS

The development and refinement of new technologies such as telehealth have opened up new clinical opportunities for nurses and their patients, especially in the areas of managing chronic conditions, assisting persons who live in rural areas, home health care, rehabilitation, and long-term care. On the positive side, technological advances promise improved health care services, reduced costs, and more convenience in terms of time and travel for consumers. Reduced costs result from a more efficient means of delivering care and from replacement of people with machines. Contradictory as it may seem, cost is also the most significant negative aspect of advanced health care technology. The more high-technology equipment and computer programs become available, the more they are used. High-technology equipment is expensive, quickly becomes outdated when newer developments occur, and often requires highly trained personnel. There are other drawbacks to new technology, particularly in the area of home health care. These include increased legal liability, the potential for decreased privacy, too much reliance on technological advances, and the inconsistent quality of resources available on the Internet and other places.

Advances in medical technology will continue. One example of an effective use of technology is the funding provided by the U.S. Department of Health and Human Services, Health Resources and Services Administration (HRSA) to fund health centers so they can adopt and implement Electronic Health Records (EHR) and other health information technology. HRSA's Office of Health Information Technology (HIT) was created in 2005 to promote the effective use of HIT as a mechanism for responding to the needs of the uninsured, underinsured, and special-needs populations (HRSA 2009). Specifically, in October 2008 when announcing the award of $18.9 million to expand health information technology in health centers, the HRSA administrator said, "Health information technology has the potential to transform care for underserved communities and its expansion is a priority for all Americans." (HRSA, 2008)

The **electronic medical record (EMR,)** a form of electronic health record, helps with ensuring patient safety and quality care. It is an expensive system to set up but has enormous potential for portability of patient records. In the United States, the Veterans Administration is a pioneer in having a complete EMR system. The EMR is an information system that is portable, digital, and privacy protected (Richwine, 2005). One innovative use of the EMR in public health is to imbed reminders or guidelines into the system. For example, the Centers for Disease Control and Prevention (CDC) published health guidelines that contain clinical recommendations for screening, prevention, diagnosis, and treatment. To find and keep current on these guidelines, clinicians must visit the CDC website. The availability of an EMR system allows the embedding of reminders so that the clinician can have access to practice guidelines at the very point of care for patients. Some additional benefits in public health, and these are some of the uses health centers make of such records, include

- 24-hour availability of records with downloaded laboratory results and up-to-date assessments,
- facilitation of interdisciplinary care,
- coordination of referrals,
- incorporation of protocol reminders for prevention, screening, and management of chronic disease,
- production of client reminders to improve compliance, and
- improved security when compared with paper records (Community Health Access Network, 2002).

Two federal programs, Medicaid and State Children's Health Insurance Program (SCHIP), have effectively used health information technology (HIT) in several key functions including outreach and enrollment, service delivery, and care management, as well as communications with families and the broader goals of program planning and improvement (Morrow, 2008). In early 2009, the surgeon general's office reopened a site that had been tried first in 2004, then closed: an electronic family tree for your health (MSNBC, 2009). This is described as an easy-to-use computer application for people to keep a personal record of their family health history (http://familyhistory.hhs.gov).

CURRENT HEALTH CARE SYSTEM IN THE UNITED STATES

Despite the many advances and the sophistication of the U.S. health care system, the system is also plagued with problems related to cost, access, and quality. These problems are different for each person and are affected by their health insurance. Most industrialized countries want the same things from their health care system. Several give their government a greater role in health care delivery and eliminate or reduce the use of market forces to control cost, access, and quality. Seemingly, there is no one perfect health care system in the world.

COST

In 2006, Americans spent $2.1 trillion, nearly 16% of the gross domestic product (GDP), on health care, or 16 cents from every dollar. This is $7,026 per person per year (Goodell and Ginsburg, 2008). As a percent of the GDP, the United States spends more than 6 percentage points higher on health care than the average percent spent by other developed countries. Yet unlike these other countries, which provide nearly universal coverage, 16% of Americans were uninsured in 2008 (Goodell and Ginsburg, 2008). This percent represents 45 million non-elderly uninsured people (Holahan and Garrett, 2009). Some people must choose between buying food and paying the utility bill and getting health care. Despite efforts to contain costs, this problem has not been solved. See Chapter 8 for details about the economics of health care.

Medical technology is the driving force in the growth of health care spending in the United States. Other contributing factors include the costs of drugs, hospital care, and physician and clinical services; efficiency as measured by excess capacity of services and facility; and the cost of the administration of health insurance (Goodell and Ginsberg, 2008). Note that none of these high-cost items are part of a public health approach to health care.

ACCESS

Another significant problem is poor access to health care (Case Study). The American health care system is described as a two-class system: private and public. People with insurance or those who can personally pay for health care are viewed as receiving superior care; those who receive

Box 3-2	Government-Financed Reimbursement Programs

Medicare
- Federal government pays
- People 65 years of age or older
- Some people under 65 years of age with disabilities
- People with end-stage renal disease requiring dialysis or a kidney transplant

Medicaid
- Federal and state share expenses
- State programs vary
- Low-income families with children who meet eligibility requirements
- Disabled who meet eligibility requirements
- Poor elderly

State Children's Health Insurance Program (SCHIP)
- Created by the Balanced Budget Act of 1997
- Builds on Medicaid to provide insurance coverage to low-income, uninsured children who are not eligible for Medicaid
- State administered
- Federal allocations are set and new costs to the program must be met by the states
- Coverage of children to age 19 if not already insured
- 43 states and the District of Columbia cover children in family of four with income below $42,406

CASE STUDY

Public health nurses who worked with local Head Start programs noted that many children had untreated dental caries. Despite qualifying for Medicaid, only two dentists in the area would accept appointments from Medicaid patients. Dentists asserted that Medicaid patients frequently did not show up for their appointments and that reimbursement was too low compared with other third-party payers. They also said the children's behavior made it difficult to work with them. So the waiting list for local dental care was approximately 6 years long. Although some nurses found ways to transport clients to dentists in a city 70 miles away, it was very time consuming and was feasible for only a small fraction of the clients. When decayed teeth abscessed, it was possible to get extractions from the local medical center. The health department dentist also saw children, but he, too, was booked for years.

Created by Deborah C. Conway, Assistant Professor,
University of Virginia School of Nursing.

lower-quality care are (1) those whose only source of care depends on public funds or (2) the working poor, who do not qualify for public funds either because they make too much money to qualify or because they are illegal immigrants. The number of uninsured Americans is rising, due largely to the loss of coverage by employment-based health plans. Either employers cannot afford to provide the coverage or workers are losing the jobs that include health care coverage (DeNavas-Walt, Proctor, and Mills, 2004). Employment-provided health care is tied to both the economy and to changes in health insurance premiums. As costs for premiums rise, employers need to shift more of the cost to their employees or cease providing this benefit. Health Insurance premiums increased 117% between 1997 and 2007, whereas worker's earnings grew only 27% (Goodell and Ginsburg, 2008). Consider that about 70% of the uninsured live in homes with at least one full-time worker, and only around 20% live in homes with no employed workers (Kaiser Commission on Medicaid and the Uninsured, 2003). Box 3-2 describes several government programs that help meet the health care needs of older adults, children, and the uninsured.

In 2006, 10.8% of white, non-Hispanic Americans were uninsured, compared with 20.5% of African-Americans and 34% of Hispanics (Center on Budget and Policy Priorities, 2007). The risk of being uninsured is particularly high for immigrants who are not citizens: 45% of noncitizens were uninsured in 2006 (Center on Budget and Policy Priorities, 2007). As discussed, there is a strong relationship between health insurance coverage and access to health care services. Insurance status determines the amount and kind of health care people are able to afford, as well as where they can receive care.

The uninsured receive less preventive care, are diagnosed at more advanced disease states, and once diagnosed tend to receive less therapeutic care in terms of surgery and treatment options. There is a safety net for the uninsured or underinsured. As will be discussed later in the chapter, there are more than 3800 federally funded community health centers throughout the country. Federally funded community health centers provide a broad range of health and social services, using nurse practitioners, physician assistants, physicians, social workers, and dentists. Community health centers primarily serve in medically underserved areas, which can be rural or urban. These centers serve people of all ages, races, and ethnicities and with or without health insurance.

BRIEFLY NOTED

HRSA supported health centers provide comprehensive primary health care services as well as education, translation and transportation to promote access to health care.

QUALITY

The quality of health care leaped to the forefront of concern following the 1999 release of the Institute of Medicine (IOM) report *To Err Is Human: Building a Safer Health System* (Institute of Medicine, 2000). As indicated in this groundbreaking report, as many as 98,000 deaths a year could be attributed to preventable medical errors. Some of the untoward events categorized in this report included adverse drug events and improper transfusions, surgical injuries and wrong-site surgery, suicides, restraint-related injuries or death, falls, burns, pressure ulcers, and mistaken client identities. It was further determined that high rates of errors with serious consequences are most likely to occur in intensive care units, operating rooms, and emergency departments. Beyond the cost in human lives, preventable medical errors result in the loss of several billions of dollars annually in hospitals nationwide. Categories of error include diagnostic, treatment, and prevention errors as well as failure of communication, equipment failure, and other system failures. Significant to nurses, the IOM estimated the number of lives lost to preventable errors in medication alone represented more than 7000 deaths annually, with a cost of about $2 billion nationwide. Although the IOM report made it clear that the majority of medical errors today were not produced by provider negligence, lack of education, or lack of training, questions were raised about the nurse's role and workload and its effect on client safety. In a follow-up report, *Keeping Patients Safe: Transforming the Work Environment of Nurses,* the IOM (2003) stated that nurses' long work hours pose a serious threat to patient safety, since fatigue slows reaction time, saps energy, and diminishes attention to detail. The group called for state regulators to pass laws barring nurses from working more than 12 hours a day and 60 hours a week—even if by choice (Kowalczyk, 2004). Although this information is largely related to acute care, many of the patients who survive medical errors are later cared for in the community.

BRIEFLY NOTED

Maintaining client privacy and confidentiality is more than good nursing practice; it is the law. Personal Digital Assistants (PDA) and use of the Internet and e-mail are becoming integral parts of nursing practice. Be sure to know your facility's policy and forms of privacy protection before you use a PDA or e-mail for client care.

Has this culture of safety resulted in a safer health care system? A safety report card presented in the journal *Health Affairs* in November 2004 gave the U.S. health system an overall grade of C+ on client safety, noting some improvement but showing considerable deficiencies in key categories (Wachter, 2004).

BRIEFLY NOTED

The process by which medical errors are identified and addressed in many facilities uses an approach called **root cause analysis**. As part of an overall process for identifying prevention strategies by looking at changes that need to be made, root cause analysis asks those most familiar with the problem to scrutinize a problem situation until there is no further room for questions. The goal of the root cause analysis is to generate specific prevention strategies, but it is also designed to engender a culture of safety in the organization that uses it. The technique is used in the Veterans Health Administration hospitals and clinics around the country, and has been recommended for use by The Joint Commission (TJC) (National Center of Continuing Education, 2000). Although this example is related to hospital-based practice, the concept applies in the community as well.

ORGANIZATION OF THE HEALTH CARE SYSTEM

An enormous number and range of facilities and providers make up the health care system. These include physicians' and dentists' offices, hospitals, nursing homes, mental health facilities, ambulatory care centers, freestanding clinics and clinics inside stores such as drug stores, as well as free clinics, public health, and home health agencies. Providers include nurses, advanced practice nurses, physicians and physician assistants, dentists and dental hygienists, pharmacists, and a wide array of essential allied health providers such as physical, occupational, and recreational therapists, nutritionists, social workers, and a range of technicians. In general, however, the American health care system is divided into the following two, somewhat distinct, components: a private or personal care component and a public health component, with some overlap, as discussed in the following sections. It is important to discuss primary health care and examine how it is part of both systems.

PRIMARY HEALTH CARE

Primary health care (PHC) includes a comprehensive range of services including public health and preventive, diagnostic, therapeutic, and rehabilitative services. A major part of the primary care system is the community health center, which should (1) be located in or serve a medically underserved area or population, (2) provide comprehensive primary care services and supportive services such as translation and transportation, and (3) be available to all residents of their service area and adjust fees based on the client's ability to pay (O'Malley et al, 2005).

From a conceptual point of view, PHC is essential care made universally accessible to individuals and families in a community. Health care is made available to them with their full participation and is provided at a cost that the community and country can afford. This care is not uniformly available and accessible to all people in many counties including the United States. Full **community participation** means that individuals within the community help in defining health problems and in developing approaches to address the problems. The setting for primary health care is within all communities of a country and involves all aspects of society (World Health Organization, 1978).

The primary health care movement officially began in 1977 when the 30th World Health Organization (WHO) Health Assembly adopted a resolution accepting the goal of attaining a level of health that permitted all citizens of the world to live socially and economically productive lives. At the international conference in 1978 in Alma-Ata, in the former Soviet Union (Russia), it was determined that this goal was to be met through PHC. This resolution, the **Declaration of Alma-Ata**, became known by the slogan "Health for All (HFA) by the Year 2000," which captured the official health target for all the member nations of the WHO. In 1998 the program was adapted to meet the needs of the new century and was deemed "Health for All in the 21st Century."

In 1981 the WHO established global indicators for monitoring and evaluating the achievement of HFA. In the *World Health Statistics Annual* (World Health Organization, 1986b), these indicators are grouped into the following four categories: health policies, social and economic development, provision of health care, and health status. The indicators suggest that health improvements are a result of efforts in many areas, including agriculture, industry, education, housing, communications, and health care. Because PHC is as much a political statement as a system of care, each United Nations member country interprets PHC according to its own culture, health needs, resources, and system of government. Clearly, the goal of PHC has not been met in most countries including the United States.

Promoting Health/Preventing Disease: Year 2010 Objectives for the Nation

As a WHO member nation, the United States has endorsed primary health care as a strategy for achieving the goal of "Health for All in the 21st Century." However, the PHC emphasis on broad strategies, community participation, self-reliance, and a multidisciplinary health care delivery team is not the primary strategy for improving the health of the American people. The national health plan for the United States focuses more on **disease prevention** and **health promotion** as the areas of most concern in the nation.

This focus is seen in the health objectives for the nation stated in *Healthy People 2010* (U.S. Department of Health and Human Services, 2000b). Each decade since the 1980s has been measured and tracked according to health objectives set at the beginning of the decade. The national health plan for the United States focuses on disease prevention and health promotion. The following are the two broad goals of *Healthy People 2010*:

1. Increasing the quality and years of healthy life
2. Eliminating health disparities (among racial and ethnic groups)

The *Healthy People 2010* goals also include leading health indicators that refer to 10 areas of health status. In general, the 10 leading health indicators are the following (U.S. Department of Health and Human Services, 2000b):

1. Physical activity
2. Injury and violence
3. Overweight and obesity
4. Environmental quality
5. Tobacco use
6. Immunization
7. Substance abuse
8. Responsible sexual behavior
9. Mental health
10. Access to health care

In the chapters throughout this book, the *Healthy People 2010* objectives are discussed in the context of the chapter (see the "*Healthy People 2010*" box).

● Healthy People 2010

Objectives Relative to Health
In January 2000, *Healthy People 2010* was released. The goals for this decade are even more ambitious than for previous decades. For example, instead of aiming to reduce health disparities, as was the goal for 2000, *Healthy People 2010* aims to eliminate health disparities. The objectives focus on the following two overarching goals (U.S. Department of Health and Human Services, 2000b):
• Help Americans of all ages increase life expectancy and improve their quality of life.
• Eliminate the health disparities that exist between different segments of the U.S. population.
The following are specific areas of concern for each of these goals:
• Health promotion: nutrition; physical activity and fitness; consumption of tobacco, alcohol, and other drugs; family planning; violent and abusive behavior; mental health; and educational and community-based programs
• Health protection: environmental health, occupational safety and health, accidental injuries, food and drug safety, and oral health
• Preventive services priorities: maternal and infant health; immunizations and infectious diseases, human immunodeficiency virus (HIV) infection; sexually transmitted diseases; heart disease and stroke; cancer, diabetes, and other chronic disabling disorders and clinical preventive services for these; and mental and behavioral disorders
• System improvement priorities: health education and preventive services and surveillance and data systems

From the U.S. Department of Health and Human Services: *Healthy People 2010: understanding and improving health,* ed 2, Washington, DC, 2000b, U.S. Government Printing Office.

Primary care, the first level of the private health care system, is delivered in a variety of community settings, such as physicians' offices, urgent care centers, in-store clinics, community health centers, and community nursing centers. Near the end of the past century, in an attempt to contain costs, managed care organizations grew. **Managed care** is defined as a system in which care is delivered by a specific network of providers who agree to comply with the care approaches established through a case management approach. The key factors are a specified network of providers and the use of a gatekeeper to control access to providers and services. This form of care has not become as prominent as the original concept outlined.

The government has tried to reap the benefits of cost savings by introducing the managed care model into Medicare and Medicaid with varying levels of success. Of the nation's 41.7 million Medicare enrollees in 2004, 4.7 million (11%) were enrolled in managed care plans. Participation in Medicare managed care increased steadily in the 1990s, reaching a peak of 6.3 million beneficiaries (16%) in 2000. Enrollment began to decline in 2000. Some of the reasons found for this decline included plan withdrawals from some areas because of inadequate levels of reimbursement, reduced benefits, and higher premiums. Medicaid, on the other hand, has made large-scale use of the managed care model within its various state programs. Medicaid managed care enrollment grew rapidly in the 1990s, with the percentage of beneficiaries enrolled in managed care plans increasing from 9% in 1990 to 59% of the Medicaid population in 2003. By 2005 all states enrolled a proportion of their Medicaid population in MCOs, and 14 states had more than 75% of their Medicaid recipients enrolled in MCOs. SCHIP programs tend to be managed similarly to state Medicaid program, thus resulting in the use of MCOs for these children as well.

PUBLIC HEALTH SYSTEM

The **public health** system is mandated through laws that are developed at the national, state, or local level. Examples of public health laws instituted to protect the health of the community include a law mandating immunizations for all children entering kindergarten and a law requiring constant monitoring of the local water supply. The public health system is organized into many levels in the federal, state, and local systems. At the local level, health departments provide care that is mandated by state and federal regulations.

THE FEDERAL SYSTEM

The **U.S. Department of Health and Human Services (USDHHS)** is the agency most heavily involved with the health and welfare concerns of U.S. citizens. The organizational chart of the HHS (Figure 3-1) shows the office of the secretary, 11 agencies, and a program support center. Ten regional offices are maintained to provide more direct assistance to the states. Their locations are shown in Table 3-1. The USDHHS is charged with regulating health care and overseeing the health status of Americans. See Box 3-3 for the HHS Strategic Plan Goals and Objectives-FY 2007-2012. Newer areas in the HHS are the Office of Public Health Preparedness, the Center for Faith-Based and Community Initiatives, and the Office of Global Affairs. The Office of Public Health Preparedness was added to assist the nation and states to prepare for bioterrorism after September 11, 2001. The Faith-Based Initiative Center was developed by President George W. Bush to allow faith communities to compete for federal money to support their community activities. The goal of the Office of Global Affairs is to promote global health by coordinating HHS strategies and programs with other governments and international organizations (U.S. Department of Health and Human Services, 2000). The USDHHS also provides a commissioned corps of uniformed personnel, the **National Health Service Corps,** who provide care to residents of medically underserved areas. The activities of several key agencies include the following:

1. The U.S. Public Health Service (PHS) is a major component of the Department of Health and Human Services. The PHS consists of eight agencies: Agency for Healthcare Research and Quality, Agency for Toxic Substances and Diseases Registry, Centers for Disease Control and Prevention, Food and Drug Administration, Health Resources and Services Administration, Indian Health Service, National Institutes of Health, and Substance Abuse and Mental Health Services Administration.

2. The Health Resources and Services Administration (HRSA) is the USDHHS agency with primary responsibility for improving access to health care of special populations, including people who are uninsured, isolated, or medically vulnerable (e.g., mothers and their children, people with HIV/AIDS, and rural residents) (HRSA, 2008). HRSA has four bureaus: Primary Health Care, Maternal and Child Health, Health Resources Development, and Health Professions. HRSA manages the Health Center Program, which funds over 3800 clinics. This program was created in the 1960s through legislation sponsored by Senator Edward Kennedy, and it was expanded by President George W. Bush. These clinics include community health centers, migrant health centers, centers for the homeless, and people who live in public housing. The mission of these centers is to provide preventive and primary care services to people regardless of their ability to pay (HRSA, 2009).

   To improve access to health care in health manpower shortage areas, the Bureau assists states and communities in the placement of physicians, dentists, and other health professionals through the National Health Service Corps (NHSC). The goal of the NHSC is to provide health care providers for placement in underserved areas. They operate an NHSC scholarship program and the NHSC loan repayment program. Nurses are represented throughout the ranks of HHS and particularly HRSA in many senior and policymaking positions, as well as staffing the centers that provide care to the underserved throughout the nation.

3. The Bureau of Health Professions, a component of HRSA, includes separate divisions for nursing, medicine, dentistry, public health, and allied health professions. The federal government looks to the Division of Nursing to provide the competence and expertise for administering nurse education legislation, interpreting trends and needs of the nursing component of the nation's health care delivery system, and maintaining a liaison with the nursing community and with international, state, regional, and local health interests. As the federal focus for nursing education and practice, the Division of Nursing identifies current and future nursing issues.

4. The National Institutes of Health (NIH) is the world's premier medical research organization, supporting research projects nationwide investigating diseases including cancer, Alzheimer's disease, diabetes, arthritis, heart ailments, and AIDS. Twenty-seven separate health institutes and centers are included in the NIH structure, including the National Institute for Nursing Research (NINR), which is the focal point of the nation's nursing research activities. The NINR promotes the growth and quality of research in nursing and client care, provides important leadership, expands the pool of experienced nurse researchers, and serves as a point of interaction with other bases of health care research.

5. The Agency for Healthcare Research and Quality (AHCRQ) supports research on health care systems, health care quality and cost issues, access to health care,

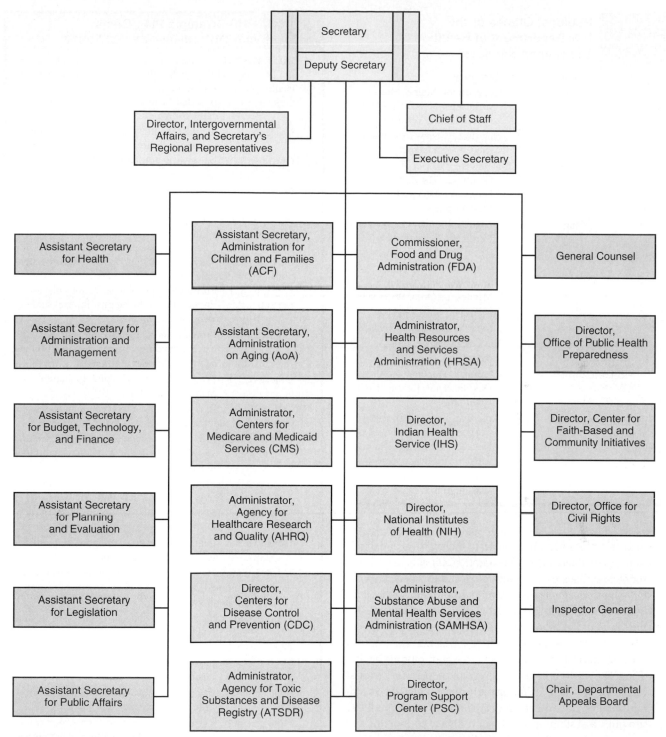

FIGURE 3-1 Organization of the U.S. Department of Health and Human Services. (From U.S. Department of Health and Human Services, available at www.hhs.gov/about/orgchart.html.)

and the effectiveness of medical treatments. It provides evidence-based information on health care outcomes and quality of care.

6. The Food and Drug Administration (FDA) ensures the safety of foods and cosmetics and the safety and efficacy of pharmaceuticals, biological products, and medical devices. In addition to the approval and monitoring of products, the FDA promotes food safety and tracks foodborne illnesses, and is also responsible for the safety of the nation's blood and plasma supply. Products that must have FDA approval before being sold in the United States include drugs, medical treatments, and food additives. For this reason, there are often restrictions on the import of drugs produced in foreign countries if they do not meet FDA standards. Some products that do not require approval, including cosmetics and dietary aids, are closely

Table 3-1	Regional Offices of the U.S. Department of Health and Human Services

Region	Location	Territory
1	Boston	Connecticut, Maine, Massachusetts, New Hampshire, Rhode Island, Vermont
2	New York	New Jersey, New York, Puerto Rico, Virgin Islands
3	Philadelphia	Delaware, District of Columbia, Maryland, Pennsylvania, Virginia, West Virginia
4	Atlanta	Alabama, Florida, Georgia, Kentucky, Mississippi, North Carolina, South Carolina, Tennessee
5	Chicago	Illinois, Indiana, Michigan, Minnesota, Ohio, Wisconsin
6	Dallas	Arkansas, Louisiana, New Mexico, Oklahoma, Texas
7	Kansas City	Iowa, Kansas, Missouri, Nebraska
8	Denver	Colorado, Montana, North Dakota, South Dakota, Utah, Wyoming
9	San Francisco	American Samoa, Arizona, California, Guam, Hawaii, Nevada, N. Mariana Islands, Trust Territories
10	Seattle	Alaska, Idaho, Oregon, Washington

monitored for safety. In addition to the approval and monitoring of products, the FDA promotes food safety and tracks foodborne illnesses. It regulates consumer labels, creating the guidelines that are used to monitor the information on (and the truthfulness of) the label. It is also responsible for the safety of the nation's blood and plasma supply.

7. The main job of the Centers for Disease Control and Prevention (CDC) is to protect lives and improve health. The CDC's two primary goals are to prepare for terrorist health threats and, at the same time, protect the health and quality of life across the United States. The CDC provides a system of health surveillance to monitor and prevent disease outbreaks (including bioterrorism), implement disease prevention strategies, and maintain national health statistics; it also provides for immunization services, workplace safety, and environmental disease prevention. The CDC also guards against international disease transmission, with personnel stationed in more than 25 foreign countries. In 2005 the CDC (Centers for Disease Control and Prevention, 2005) reorganized, creating four new coordinating centers and two national offices, to help it more efficiently and effectively deal with twenty-first century health threats. With the new coordinating centers, the CDC's scientists are better able to share their

Box 3-3	HHS Strategic Plan Goals and Objectives—FY 2007-2012

GOAL 1: Health Care: Improve the safety, quality, affordability, and accessibility of health care, including behavioral health care and long-term care.

Objective 1.1 Broaden health insurance and long-term care coverage.

Objective 1.2 Increase health care service availability and accessibility.

Objective 1.3 Improve health care quality, safety, cost, and value.

Objective 1.4 Recruit, develop, and retain a competent health care workforce.

GOAL 2: Public Health Promotion and Protection, Disease Prevention, and Emergency Preparedness: Prevent and control disease, injury, illness, and disability across the lifespan, and protect the public from infectious, occupational, environmental, and terrorist threats.

Objective 2.1 Prevent the spread of infectious diseases.

Objective 2.2 Protect the public against injuries and environmental threats.

Objective 2.3 Promote and encourage preventive health care, including mental health, lifelong healthy behaviors, and recovery.

Objective 2.4 Prepare for and respond to natural and manmade disasters.

GOAL 3: Human Services: Promote the economic and social well-being of individuals, families, and communities.

Objective 3.1 Promote the economic independence and social well-being of individuals and families across the lifespan.

Objective 3.2 Protect the safety and foster the well-being of children and youth.

Objective 3.3 Encourage the development of strong, healthy, and supportive communities.

Objective 3.4 Address the needs, strengths, and abilities of vulnerable populations.

GOAL 4: Scientific Research and Development: Advance scientific and biomedical research and development related to health and human services.

Objective 4.1 Strengthen the pool of qualified health and behavioral science researchers.

Objective 4.2 Increase basic scientific knowledge to improve human health and human development.

Objective 4.3 Conduct and oversee applied research to improve health and well-being.

Objective 4.4 Communicate and transfer research results into clinical, public health, and human service practice.

From the U.S. Department of Health and Human Services, 2008. Retrieved Oct 10, 2008, from http://www.hhs.gov/strategic_plan/.

expertise to solve public health problems, emergencies or not, streamline the flow of information for leadership decision making, and better leverage the expertise of partners.

Other HHS agencies outside of the PHS include the Centers for Medicare and Medicaid Services (CMS), which administers Medicare and Medicaid; the Administration for

Children and Families, which oversees 60 programs that promote the economic and social well-being of children, families, and communities, including the state-federal welfare program, Temporary Assistance for Needy Families, and Head Start; and the Administration on Aging, which supports a nationwide aging network, providing services to the elderly, in particular to enable them to remain independent, and providing policy leadership on issues concerning the aging. The U.S. Public Health Service Commissioned Corps is a uniformed service of more than 6000 health professionals who serve in many HHS and other federal agencies. The Surgeon General is head of the Commissioned Corps.

An important agency and a recent addition to the federal government, the Department of Homeland Security (DHS), was created in 2002. The mission of the DHS is to prevent and deter terrorist attacks and protect against and respond to threats and hazards to the nation. The goals for the department include awareness, prevention, protection, response, and recovery. The DHS works with first responders throughout the United States, and through the development of programs such as the Community Emergency Response Team (CERT) trains people to be better prepared to respond to emergency situations in their communities. Nurses working in state and local public health departments as well as those employed in hospitals and other health facilities may be called upon to respond to acts of terrorism or natural disaster in their careers, and the DHS, along with the FDA and CDC, is developing programs to ready nurses and other health care providers for an uncertain future.

Department of Agriculture

The Department of Agriculture is involved in health care primarily through administering the Food and Nutrition Service. Although plant, product, and animal inspections by the Department of Agriculture are also related to health, the Food and Nutrition Service oversees a variety of food assistance activities. This service collaborates with state and local government welfare agencies to provide food stamps to needy persons to increase their food-purchasing power. Other programs include school breakfast and lunch programs; the Supplemental Food Program for Women, Infants, and Children (WIC); and grants to states for nutrition education training.

Department of Justice

Health services to federal prisoners are administered by the Department of Justice. The Medical and Services Division of the Bureau of Prisons includes medical, psychiatric, dental, and health support services. It also administers environmental health and safety, farm operations, and food service, along with commissary, laundry, and other personal services for inmates.

Department of Commerce

The U.S. Census Bureau, a unit of the Department of Commerce, provides health information. This Bureau, established in 1902, conducts a census of the population every 10 years.

Box 3-4	**Typical Programs in a State Health Department**

- Disease information and prevention: researching diseases, monitoring their occurrences, and educating the public about preventing and controlling common and rare diseases
- Healthy living: including such programs as childhood lead poisoning prevention, child safety seat distribution, education and inspection program, dental health, immunizations, and Women's, Infant's and Children's program (WIC)
- Health records and statistics
- Preparing and responding to emergencies
- Hometown health: learn about what is available in the local community
- Protecting your environment, including food, water, and the overall environment
- Regulations and licensing, including the licensing of health care professionals
- Newsroom that provides media and public relations and other educational information

From the Virginia Department of Health. Retrieved Feb 1, 2009, from www.Vdh. See your own state department website for other examples.

The National Oceanic and Atmospheric Administration, also part of this Bureau, provides services that support the control of urban air quality.

Department of Defense

The Department of Defense provides health care for members of the military and their dependents. The assistant secretary of defense for health affairs administers the Civilian Health and Medical Program of the Uniformed Services (CHAMPUS). Also, each of the departments within the Department of Defense, including the Army, Navy, Air Force, and Marines, has a surgeon general and a chief nursing officer.

Department of Labor

Two agencies within this department have health functions: the Occupational Safety and Health Administration and the Mine Safety and Health Administration. Both develop safety and health standards and ensure compliance. Each coordinates its activities with state departments of labor and health.

THE STATE SYSTEM

The state public health system serves many purposes including those of preventing and responding to infectious disease outbreaks. State health departments have other important functions such as health care financing and administration for programs such as Medicaid, providing mental health and professional education, establishing health codes, licensing facilities and personnel, and regulating the insurance industry (Tulchinsky, 2000). State systems also have an important role in direct assistance to local health departments, including ongoing assessment of health needs. Box 3-4 provides a list of typical state health department programs and the Levels of Prevention box provides a list of interventions for levels of preventive care typically found in the public health system.

Levels of Prevention	Related to the Public Health Care System

PRIMARY PREVENTION

Counsel clients in health behaviors related to lifestyle.

SECONDARY PREVENTION

Implement a family-planning program to prevent unintended pregnancies for young couples who attend the primary clinic.

TERTIARY PREVENTION

Provide a self-management asthma program for children with chronic asthma to reduce their need for hospitalization.

Nurses serve in many capacities in state health departments; they are consultants, direct service providers, researchers, teachers, and supervisors. They also participate in program development, planning, and the evaluation of health programs.

Every state has a board of examiners of nurses. The board may be found either in the department of licensing boards of the health department or in an administrative agency of the governor's office. Created by legislation known as a *state nurse practice act,* the examiners' board is made up of nurses and consumers. A few states have other providers or administrators as members. The functions of this board are described in the practice act of each state and generally include licensing and examination of registered nurses and licensed practical nurses; approval of schools of nursing in the state; revocation, suspension, or denial of licenses; and writing of regulations about nursing practice and education.

THE LOCAL SYSTEM

The local health department has direct responsibility to the citizens in its community or jurisdiction. Services and programs offered by local health departments vary depending on the state and local health codes that must be followed, the needs of the community, and available funding and other resources. For example, one health department might be more involved with public health education programs and environmental issues, whereas another health department might emphasize direct client care. Local health departments vary in providing sick care or even primary care. A list of health department programs, taken from an urban-suburban county health department in a mid-Atlantic state, is shown in Box 3-5.

Public health nursing is defined as the practice of protecting and promoting the health of populations using knowledge from nursing, social, and public health sciences (American Public Health Association, 1996). More often than at other levels of government, public health nurses at the local level provide direct services. Some of these nurses deliver special or selected services, such as follow-up of contacts in cases of tuberculosis or venereal disease or providing child immunization clinics. Others provide more general care, delivering services to families in certain geographic areas. This method of delivery of nursing services involves broader needs and

Box 3-5	Examples of Programs That May Be Provided by Local Health Departments*

- Birth and death records
- Child health clinics
- Dental health clinics
- Environmental health
- Epidemiology and disease control
- Family planning
- Health education
- Home health agency
- Immunization clinics
- Information services
- Maternal health
- Nursing
- Nursing home licensure
- Nutrition
- Occupational therapy
- School health
- Services for children with special needs
- Speech and audiology

*Note that the range of services varies considerably depending on the size of the area served and the resources available to fund programs.

a wider variety of nursing interventions. The local level often provides an opportunity for nurses to take on significant leadership roles, with many nurses serving as directors or managers.

Since the tragedy of September 11, 2001, state and local health departments have increasingly focused on emergency preparedness and response. In case of an event, state and local health departments in the affected area will be expected to collect data and accurately report the situation, to respond appropriately to any type of emergency, and to ensure the safety of the residents of the immediate area, while protecting those just outside the danger zone. This level of knowledge—to enable public health agencies to anticipate, prepare for, recognize, and respond to terrorist threats or natural disasters such as hurricanes or floods—has required a level of interstate and federal-local planning and cooperation that is unprecedented for these agencies. Whether participating in disaster drills or preparing a local high school for use as a shelter, nurses will play a major role in meeting the challenge of an uncertain future.

FORCES INFLUENCING THE HEALTH CARE SYSTEM OF THE FUTURE

Although most people are personally satisfied with their own physicians or nurse practitioners, currently few people are satisfied with the health care system in general. Costs are high and keep rising and quality and access are uneven across the country and within communities depending on the ability to pay. What, then, are some of the factors that might influence health care? First, as a nation, citizens must decide what has to be provided for all people, who will be in charge of the system, and who will pay for what. In recent years, federal and state services have been reduced and more responsibility for health care delivery has been moved to the private sector. Health care has become big business. Health care company stocks are now traded by major stock exchanges, directors receive benefits when profits are high, and the locus of control has shifted from the provider to the payer. The following four major competing forces will influence the future design of the health care system: consumers, employers (purchasers), care delivery systems, and state and federal legislation.

First, consumers want lower costs and high-quality health care without limits and with an improved ability to choose the providers of their choice. They are becoming more knowledgeable about appealing health care decisions that are being made for them and are joining and appealing to consumer groups to help them fight their battles in and outside of the courtroom. Consumer groups will continue to play a major role in helping shape the future health care system. Consumers also seek health care with more information that they glean from reading, talking with others, and the Internet.

Second, employers (purchasers of health care) want to be able to obtain basic health care plans at reasonable costs for their employees. Many employers are seeing their profits diminish as they put more money into providing adequate health care coverage for employees. As mentioned earlier, many employers expect employees to pick up a greater share of this cost; some employers cover only the worker, leaving the family to find other and often expensive ways to cover health care costs.

Third, health care systems want a better balance between consumer and purchaser demands. Thus they continually watch their own budget and expenses. To maintain a profit while providing quality care, many health care delivery groups have downsized and created alliances, mergers, and other joint ventures. It is not uncommon for a hospital system to buy several hospitals in an area and begin to close those that are less profitable. This reduces the choices for consumers and also may mean that access is reduced when clients must travel much further to seek care.

Finally, legislation, especially concerning access and quality, continues to be enacted, thus creating one more force helping shape a health care system. The goal of this "evidence-based care" is to ensure quality.

Many say that solving the health care crisis requires the institution of a rational health care system that balances equity, cost, and quality. The fact that millions of people are uninsured, that wide disparities exist in access, and that a large proportion of deaths each year is attributable to preventable causes (errors as well as tobacco, alcohol abuse, preventable injuries, and obesity) indicates that the American system is currently not serving the best interests of the American population.

There are many expectations that a new federal administration in the United States will be able to find ways to deliver health care that takes into account the concerns described in this chapter about cost, access, and quality of care.

Evidence-Based Practice

A multicenter study of the use of Emergency Department visits for outreach for the State Children's Health Insurance Program (SCHIP) was conducted among uninsured children (under 18 years of age) who presented to four Emergency Departments (EDs) in 2001 and 2002. The intervention consisted of staff handing out SCHIP applications to children who were confirmed to be uninsured. The primary outcome was state-level confirmation of insured status at 90 days.

A group of 223 subjects (108 control, 115 intervention) were followed by both a phone interview and state records. Compared to control subjects, those receiving a SCHIP application were more likely to have state health insurance at 90 days, at a rate of 42% versus 28%. Although the intervention effect was prominent among 118 African-Americans (50% insured after intervention versus 31% of controls), lack of family enrollment in other public assistance programs was the primary predictor of intervention success. The conclusion from this study was that particularly among minority children not otherwise involved with the social welfare system, handing out insurance applications in the ED could be an effective SCHIP enrollment strategy. If this strategy was adopted nationwide, more than a quarter million additional children each year could receive insurance coverage.

Although SCHIP was authorized in 1997, and despite significant efforts within each state, over 7 million children remain uninsured, and many eligible families are still unaware of SCHIP enrollment opportunities. Although outreach and enrollment efforts have been put in place in the states with varying levels of success, there is limited evidence as to the effectiveness of specific recruitment and enrollment strategies. This study identified a simple method of outreach strategies, handing out SCHIP applications at locations frequented by uninsured children, while seeking to quantify its effectiveness.

Uninsured children make approximately 3 million ED visits annually. National estimates indicate that up to 30% of these, or nearly 1 million, will enroll in government-supported insurance programs without additional outreach. In this sample of inner-city sites, it was demonstrated that by simply handing out applications in the ED nearly four times as many children would be enrolled in Medicaid or SCHIP programs within 90 days of the ED visit. Since lack of participation in public assistance programs was the primary predictor of success among intervention subjects, this study concludes that subjects without ongoing connections with the health and welfare system would be most effectively targeted in this kind of an outreach program. Although this sample was a small one, this rather low cost intervention is capable of yielding a high return and should be considered at EDs across the United States.

NURSE USE: Because lack of participation in public assistance programs was the primary predictor of success among intervention subjects, this study concludes that subjects without ongoing connections with the health and welfare system would be most effectively targeted in this kind of an outreach program. Although this sample was a small one, this rather low-cost intervention is capable of yielding a high return and should be considered at EDs across the Untied States; nurses can implement this intervention.

From Gordon JA, Emond JA, Camargo CA: The state's children's health insurance program: a multicenter trial of outreach through the emergency department, *Am J Public Health* 95(2):250–253, 2005.

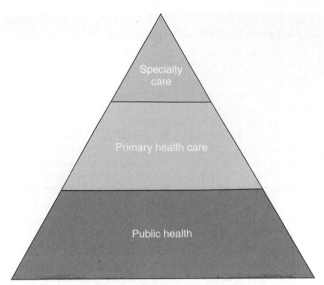

FIGURE 3-2 Health care pyramid.

In its 2005 Healthcare Agenda, the American Nurses Association (American Nurses Association, 2005b), promoted a blueprint for reform that includes the following:
- Health care is a basic human right, and so a restructured health care system with universal access to a standard package of essential health care services for all citizens and residents must be assured.
- The development and implementation of health policies that reflect the aims put forth by the Institute of Medicine (safe, effective, patient centered, timely, efficient, equitable) and are based on outcomes' research will ultimately save money.
- The overuse of expensive, technology-driven, acute, hospital-based services must give way to a balance between high-tech treatment and community-based and preventive services, with emphasis on the latter.
- A single-payer mechanism is the most desirable option for financing a reformed health care system.

These suggestions have merit but would require a cultural change in how we think about health care, the education and training of health care providers, and the financing of our health care system. A change of this magnitude, affecting so many aspects of citizens' lives, is not easily made, but there is hope that some changes will be made and that those made will place high value on the role of public health in the nation's health. However, we must remember that public health is heavily controlled by government influences. Since program funding comes from the federal, state, or local level and not from the private sector, programs are susceptive to political agendas and decisions. Programs are cut to balance a budget, and this is often without a thorough evaluation based on evidence of the usefulness (or lack thereof) of the program. What then, is needed to improve health care? It has always seemed that in the United States the health care pyramid was upside down. That is, the majority of funds were spent on high-cost reparative care. What would be more logical is to have a system that builds upon a base of public health followed by primary care and then specialty care. See Figure 3-2 for an idea of how we might have organized health care differently.

CLINICAL APPLICATION

During a well-child clinic visit, Jenna Wells, R.N., met Sandra Farr and her 24-month-old daughter, Jessica. The Farrs had recently moved to the community. Mrs. Farr stated that she knew that Jessica needed the last in a series of immunizations and because they did not have health insurance, she brought her daughter to the public health clinic. Upon initial assessment, Mrs. Farr told the nurse that her husband would soon be employed, but the family had no health care coverage for the next 30 days. The Farrs also needed to decide which health care package they wanted. Mr. Farr's company offers a preferred provider organization (PPO), an HMO, and a community nursing clinic plan to all employees. Neither Mr. nor Mrs. Farr has ever used an HMO or a community nursing clinic, and they are not sure what services are provided.

Mrs. Farr asks Nurse Wells what she should do.
Nurse Wells should do which of the following?
A. *Encourage Mrs. Farr to choose the HMO because it will pay more attention to the family's preventive needs, and direct Mrs. Farr to other sources of health care should the family need to see a provider while they are uninsured.*
B. *Encourage Mrs. Farr to choose the PPO because it will have a greater number of qualified providers from which to choose, and direct Mrs. Farr to other sources of health care should the family need to see a provider while they are uninsured.*
C. *Encourage Mrs. Farr to choose the local community nursing center because it is staffed with nurse practitioners who are well qualified to provide comprehensive health care with an emphasis on health education, and direct Mrs. Farr to other sources of health care should the family need to see a provider while they are uninsured.*
D. *Explain the differences between a PPO, HMO, and community nursing clinic and encourage Mrs. Farr to discuss the options with her husband, and direct Mrs. Farr to other sources of health care should the family need to see a provider while they are uninsured.*
Answer is in the back of the book.

REMEMBER THIS!

- Health care in the United States is made up of a personal care system and a public health system, with overlap between the two systems.
- Primary care is a personal health care system that provides for first contact and continuous, comprehensive, and coordinated care.
- Primary health care is essential care made universally accessible to individuals and families in a community. Health care is made available to them through their full participation and is provided at a cost that the community and country can afford.
- Primary care is part of primary health care.

- Public health refers to organized community efforts designed to prevent disease and promote health.
- Important trends that affect the health care system include the demographic, social, economic, political, and technological.
- More than 47 million people in the United States are uninsured, and many more simply lack access to adequate health care.
- Many federal agencies are involved in government health care functions. The agency most directly involved with the health and welfare of Americans is the U.S. Department of Health and Human Services (USDHHS).
- Most state and local jurisdictions have government activities that affect the health care field.
- Health care reform measures seek to make changes in the cost and quality of and access to the present system.
- To achieve the specific health goals of programs such as *Healthy People 2010*, primary care and public health must work within the community for community-based care.
- The most sustainable individual and system changes come when people who live in the community have actively participated.
- Nurses are more than able to fill the gap between personal care and public health because they have skills in assessment, health promotion, and disease and injury prevention; knowledge of community resources; and the ability to develop relationships with community members and leaders.

WHAT WOULD YOU DO?

1. Compare the local and state services where you live with those that have been presented in this chapter. How are they similar? How are they different? What changes would you recommend to your local health department to improve public health and primary health care?
2. Debate the following with a classmate: The major problem with the health care system is (choose one of the following topics):
   a. Escalating costs (including those from increased technology)
   b. Fragmentation of services
   c. Limited access to care
   d. Quality of care
3. Visit your local health department and determine how its services fit into a primary care, public health, community-based health care system. Illustrate what you mean by your answer with examples.
4. Determine if there is a federally funded health center in your community. If yes, learn what services are provided. Are there services that are needed in the community that are not being provided? If so, what are they?

■ REFERENCES

American College of Nurse-Midwives: *Midwifery 101: fast Facts about Midwives,* 2008, available at http://www.mymidwife.org/Midwifery_101.cfm#CGI.HTTP_REFERER.

American Nurses Association: *More about RNs and advanced practice RNs,* Silver Spring, Md, 2008, available at http://www.nursingworld.org/EspeciallyForYou/StudentNurses/RNsAPNs.aspx.

American Nurses Association: *Healthcare agenda 2005.* Retrieved Aug 2005 from http://www.nursingworld.org/readroom/anahca05.pdf.

American Public Health Association: *Public health nursing section: definition and role of public health nursing,* Washington, DC, 1996, American Public Health Association.

Bernstein R: Foreign-born population tops 34 million: census bureau estimates, *U.S. Census Bureau News,* February 2005. Retrieved Aug 2005 from http://www.census.gov/Press-Release/www/releases/archives/foreignborn_population/003969.html.

Center on Budget and Policy Priorities: *More Americans, now including more children, lack health insurance,* 2007, available at http://www.cbpp.org/8 28-07health.htm.

Centers for Disease Control and Prevention: Office of Communication: Division of Media Relations, 2005. Retrieved Aug 2005 from http://www.cdc.gov/od/oc/media/pressrel/r050421.htm.

Center for Health Communication, Harvard School of Public Health: *Reinventing aging: baby boomers and civic engagement,* Boston, Mass, 2004. Harvard School of Public Health. Retrieved Aug 2005 from http://www.hsph.harvard.edu/chc/reinventingaging/Report.pdf.

Community Health Access Network: *Integrated health center network information technology applications,* 2002. Retrieved Aug 2005 from http://bphc.hrsa.gov/chc/CHCInitiatives/emr.htm#Resource%20Documents.

Dehm A, Shniper L: Occupational employment projections to 2016, *Monthly Labor Review,* Nov 2007.

DeNavas-Walt C, Proctor BD, Mills RJ: *Income, poverty, and health insurance coverage in the United States: 2003,* U.S. Census Bureau, Current Population Reports, P60-226, Washington, DC, 2004. U.S. Government Printing Office.

Goodell S, Ginsburg PB: *High and rising health care costs: demystifying U.S. health care spending.* The Synthesis Project. Robert Wood Johnson Foundation, Policy Brief No 16, Oct 2008. Retrieved Jan 31, 2008, from www.policysynthesis.org.

Gordon JA, Emond JA, Camargo CA: The state's children's health insurance program: a multicenter trial of outreach through the emergency department, *Am J Public Health* 95(2):250–253, 2005.

Health Resources and Services Administration: *HRSA awards $18.9 million to expand use of health information technology* at health centers, 2008, *HRSA NEWS.* Retrieved Jan 21, 2009, from http://newsroom.hrsa.gov.

Health Resources and Services Administration: The health center program: what is a health center? Retrieved Jan 22, 2009, from http://bphc.hrsa.gov.

Holahan J, Garrett AB: *Rising unemployment, Medicaid and the uninsured,* Report 7850, January 2009. Kaiser Commission on Medicaid and the Uninsured. Retrieved Feb 1, 2009, from www.kff.org.

Hopkins SC et al: Context of care or provider training: the impact on preventive screening practices, *Prevent Med* 40(6):718-724, 2005.

Institute of Medicine: To err is human: building a safer health system, 2000. Retrieved Aug 2005 from http://www.iom.edu/Object.File/Master/4/117/0.pdf.

Institute of Medicine: *Keeping patients safe: transforming the work environment of nurses,* Washington, DC, 2003, National Academy Press.

Kaiser Commission on Medicaid and the Uninsured: *Distribution of nonelderly uninsured by employment status, state data 2002-2003,* 2003. Retrieved July 2005 from http://www.statehealth-facts.kff.org/cgi-bin/healthfacts.cgi?action=compare&category =Health+Coverage+%26+Uninsured&subcategory=Nonelderly +Uninsured+topic=Distribution+by+Employment+Status.

Kowalczyk L: Study links long hours, nurse errors, *Boston Globe,* July 7, 2004. Retrieved July 2005 from http://www.boston.com/business/articles/2004/07/07/study_links_long_hours_nurse_errors/.

Martin JA et al: Births: final data for 2001, *Natl Vital Stat Rep* 51(2):1–102, 2002.

MSNBC: *Grow an electronic family tree for your health.* Retrieved Jan 12, 2009, from http://www.msnbc.msn.com/id/2865176/print/1/displaymode/1098.

National Advisory Council on Nurse Education and Practice: *Third report to the secretary of health and human services and the congress,* Washington, DC, November 2003, available at ftp://ftp.hrsa.gov/bhpr/nursing/nacreport.pdf.

National Center of Continuing Education: *Patient fact sheet: 20 tips to help prevent medical errors,* AHRQ Publication No. 00-PO38, Rockville, Md, Feb 2000, Agency for Healthcare Research and Quality.

O'Malley AS et al: Health center trends, 1994-2001: what do they portend for the federal growth initiative? *Health Affairs* 24: 465-472, 2005.

Orlovsky C: Mass nurse retirement expected in 2011: survey, AMN, available at http://www.amnhealthcare.com/News.aspx?id=15444.

Richwine L: U.S. moves to spur digital healthcare network: *ABC News,* June 2005. Retrieved July, 2005 from http://abcnews.go.com/Health/wireStory?id=827024.

Singer A: The changing face of America, e-journal USA: society and values, 2004. Retrieved July 2008 from http://usinfo.state.gov/journals/itsv/1204/ijse/singer.htm.

Steinwald AB: *Primary care professionals: recent supply trends, projections, and valuation of services: testimony before the Committee on Health, Education, Labor, and Pensions,* U.S. Senate, Washington DC, 2008, U.S. Government Accountability Office.

Tulchinsky TH: *The new public health: an introduction to the 21st century,* San Diego, 2000, Academic Press.

U.S. Bureau of the Census: *Population projections of the United States by age, sex, race and Hispanic origin (1995-2050),* Washington, DC, 1996, Author.

U.S. Bureau of the Census: *Statistical abstract of the United States: 2001,* ed 21, Washington, DC, 2001. U.S. Government Printing Office.

U.S. Department of Health and Human Services: *Strategic plan goals and objectives, FY 2007-2012, 2008.* Retrieved Oct 10, 2008, from http://www.hhs.gov/strategic_plan/.

U.S. Department of Health and Human Services: *Healthy people 2010: understanding and improving health,* 2000, Washington, DC, U.S. Government Printing Office.

U.S. Department of Labor: *Bureau of Labor Statistics releases 2002-12 employment predictions, 2004,* Retrieved July 2005 from http://www.bls.gov.news.release/ecopro.nr0.htm.

Wachter RM: The end of the beginning: patient safety five years after 'To Err Is Human,' *Health Affairs,* 10.1377/hlthaff.w4.534, November 2004. Retrieved July 2005 from http://content.healthaffairs.org/cgi/content/abstract/hlthaff.w4.534.

World Health Organization: *Primary health care,* Geneva, 1978, WHO.

World Health Organization: *Basic documents,* ed 36, Geneva, 1986a, WHO.

World Health Organization: *World health statistics annual,* Geneva, 1986b, WHO.

Zuzelo P, Fallon R, Lang A et al Clinical nurse specialists: knowledge specific to Medicare structures and processes, *Clin Nurse Spec* 18:(4):207–217, 2004.

Influences on Health Care Delivery and Nursing

Chapter 4

Ethics in Community-Oriented Nursing Practice

Mary Cipriano Silva
James J. Fletcher
Jeanne Merkle Sorrell

ADDITIONAL RESOURCES

These related resources are found either in the appendix at the back of this book or on the book's website at http://evolve.elsevier.com/stanhope/foundations.

⊜ Evolve Website

• Community Assessment Applied

• Case Study, with Questions and Answers
• Quiz review questions
• WebLinks, including link to *Healthy People 2010* website

OBJECTIVES

After reading this chapter, the student should be able to:
1. Describe a brief history of the ethics of nursing in community health.
2. Discuss ethical decision-making processes.
3. Compare and contrast ethical theories and principles, virtue ethics, ethic of care, and feminist ethics.

4. Describe how ethics is part of the core functions of nursing in community health.
5. Analyze codes of ethics for nursing and for public health.
6. Apply the ethics of advocacy to nursing in community health.

CHAPTER OUTLINE

KEY TERMS

advocacy: the act of pleading for or supporting a course of action on behalf of a person, group, or community.

beneficence: a principle that is complementary to nonmaleficence and requires that we "do good." We are limited by time, place, and talents in the amount of good we can do. We have general obligations to perform those actions that maintain or enhance the dignity of other persons whenever those actions do not place an undue burden on health care providers. Health care professionals have special obligations of beneficence to clients.

bioethics: a branch of ethics that applies the knowledge and processes of ethics to the examination of ethical problems in health care.

code of ethics: moral standards that specify a profession's values, goals, and obligations.

communitarianism: maintains that abstract, universal principles are not an adequate basis for moral decision making. History, tradition, and concrete moral communities should be the basis of moral thinking and action.

consequentialism: an approach whereby the right action is the one that produces the greatest amount of good or the least amount of evil in a given situation.

deontology: an ethical theory that bases moral obligation on duty and claims that actions are obligatory irrespective of the good or bad consequences that they produce. Because humans are rational, they have absolute value. Therefore, persons should always be treated as ends in themselves and never only as means.

distributive justice: requires that there be a fair distribution of the benefits and burdens in society based on the needs and contributions of its members. This principle requires that consistent with the dignity and worth of its members and within the limits imposed by its resources, a society must determine a minimal level of goods and services to be available to its members.

ethical decision making: making decisions within an orderly framework that considers context, ethical approaches, client values, and professional obligations.

ethical dilemmas: puzzling moral problems in which a person, group, or community can envision morally justified reasons for both taking and not taking a certain course of action.

ethical issues: moral challenges facing the nursing profession.

ethics: a branch of philosophy that includes both a body of knowledge about the moral life and a process of reflection for determining what persons ought to do or be, regarding this life.

ethic of care: the belief in the morality of responsibility in relationships that emphasize connection and caring.

feminist ethics: knowledge and critique of classical ethical theories developed by men and women; entails knowledge about the social, cultural, political, economic, environmental, and professional contexts that insidiously and overtly oppress women as individuals, or within a family, group, community, or society.

feminists: women and men who hold a worldview advocating economic, social, and political status for women that is equivalent to that of men.

moral distress: uncomfortable state of self when one is unable to act ethically.

morality: shared and generational societal norms about what constitutes right or wrong conduct.

nonmaleficence: a principle, according to Hippocrates, that requires that we do no harm. It is impossible to avoid harm entirely, but this principle requires that health care professionals act according to the standards of due care and try to cause the least amount of harm possible.

principlism: an approach to problem solving in bioethics that uses the principles of respect for autonomy, beneficence, nonmaleficence, and justice as the basis for organization and analysis.

respect for autonomy: based on human dignity and respect for individuals and allows them to choose those actions and goals that fulfill their life plans unless those choices result in harm to another.

utilitarianism: an ethical theory based on the weighing of morally significant outcomes or consequences regarding the overall maximizing of good and minimizing of harm for the greatest number of people.

values: beliefs about the shared worth or importance of what is desired or esteemed within a society.

virtue ethics: asks "What kind of person should I be?" and purports that people should be allowed to flourish as human beings.

virtues: acquired traits of character that dispose humans to act in accord with their natural good.

The work of nurses in public health involves ethical activities. Nurses focus on protecting, promoting, preserving, and maintaining health while preventing disease. These goals reflect the ethical principles of promoting good and preventing harm. Nurses also struggle with the rights of individuals and families versus the rights of local groups within a community. These struggles reflect the tensions between respect for autonomy, rights-based ethical theory, and community-based ethical theory.

Nurses also deal with consequence-based ethical theory, obligation-based ethical theory, and the ethical components of advocacy, justice, health policy, caring, women's moral experiences, and the moral character of health care practitioners. They are guided by codes of ethics and ethical decision-making frameworks. **Ethics** is a body of knowledge and, as such, is more than "being a good person." Ethics is a part of clinical decision making and practice (Hamric, 2002). Stated differently, Chaloner says that "Ethics is a branch of philosophy concerned with determining right and wrong in relation to people's decisions and actions" (2007, p. 42). It is relevant to both the ordinary and profound aspects of life. Regardless, when persons are unable to act ethically, they experience **moral distress**. For example, in a survey Ulrich and colleagues (2007) found that when nurses and social workers felt powerless and overwhelmed with ethics issues, they experienced frustration and fatigue. These are two symptoms of moral distress. This chapter applies a core knowledge of ethics to nursing to help nurses develop effective coping strategies for ethical issues and moral distress.

HISTORY

Chapter 2 discussed the history of public health and of public and community health nursing. The focus here is a brief history of nursing and public health ethics and the relationship between them and nursing in community health.

Modern nursing has a rich heritage of ethics and **morality**, beginning with Florence Nightingale (1820–1910). The morals and **values** she gave to nursing have endured. She saw nursing as a call to service, and she thought that those who became nurses should be people of good moral character. She was passionate about the need to provide care to poor people and also about the importance of a sanitary environment as seen in her work with soldiers in the Crimean War (1854–1856). Because of her commitment to poor people in communities, her championing of primary prevention, and the work she did to show that healthy environments save soldiers' lives, she is seen as nursing's first moral leader and nurse in community health.

In the 1960s, two seminal events occurred. First, the American Nurses Association (ANA) recommended that all nursing education should occur in institutions of higher education. As this process slowly took place, ethics, as a course per se, was removed from many schools of nursing, although ethical values remained. Second, because of major advances in science and technology that affected health care, the field of bioethics began to emerge and was seen in nursing curricula. Today, most nursing programs integrate bioethical content into their courses or have separate courses on this topic.

Nurses' codes of ethics are important in the history of nursing practice in the community. The Nightingale Pledge is generally considered to be nursing's first **code of ethics** (American Nurses Association, 2001). After the Nightingale Pledge, a "suggested" code and a "tentative" code were published in the *American Journal of Nursing* but were not formally adopted. The *Code for Professional Nurses* was formally adopted by the ANA House of Delegates in 1950. It was amended and revised five more times until in 2001, after 5 years of work, the ANA House of Delegates adopted the *Code of Ethics for Nurses with Interpretive Statements*.

BRIEFLY NOTED

The Nightingale Pledge was written by Lystra Gretter in 1893.

The first known international code of ethics was developed by the International Council of Nurses (1953). Like the ANA code, it has undergone various revisions and adoptions. The most recent revision of the *ICN Code of Ethics for Nurses* was adopted in 2005 and copyrighted in 2006 (International Council of Nurses, 2006).

The **bioethics** movement of the late 1960s influenced both nursing ethics and public health ethics. Only recently has the relationship between public health and ethics been made explicit (Public Health Leadership Society, 2002). After input from many public health professionals and their associations, the Code of Ethics for Public health was approved in 2002 (Olick, 2005). This code was crafted in an interesting manner in that it began as a project of the graduating class of the Public Health Leadership Institute in 2002. The goal was to have a small initial group write the code and then take it to stakeholders to seek their input and further develop the code based on the feedback. That was done, and the code, which is titled "Principles of the ethical practice of public health" was endorsed in 2002 by the key public health associations beginning with the American Public Health Association (Thomas, 2002). For clarity in this chapter, this document is called the Code of Ethics for Public Health.

ETHICAL DECISION MAKING

Ethical decision making is that component of ethics that focuses on the process of how ethical decisions are made. The process is the thinking that occurs when health care professionals must make decisions about ethical issues and ethical dilemmas. **Ethical issues** are moral challenges facing our profession. In nursing one such challenge is how to prepare an adequate and competent workforce for the future. In contrast, **ethical dilemmas** are human dilemmas and puzzling moral problems in which a person, group, or community can envision morally justified reasons for both taking and not taking a certain course of action. One example of an ethical dilemma is how to allocate resources to two equally needy populations when the resources are sufficient to serve only one of the populations. Ethical theories, principles and decision-making frameworks help us think through these issues and dilemmas. Often this content is abstract, which makes decision making more difficult (Hentz, 2007).

Ethical decision-making frameworks use problem-solving processes. They provide guides for making sound ethical decisions that can be morally justified. Some of these frameworks are discussed in this chapter. It is important to remember that when all is said and done we each make our own decisions. Weston (2002) said, "Whether we admit it or not, we *do* make our own decisions. We cannot pretend that we

Table 4-1	Rationale for Steps of an Ethical Decision-Making Framework

Steps	Rationale
1. Identify the ethical issues and dilemmas.	Persons cannot make sound ethical decisions if they cannot identify ethical issues and dilemmas.
2. Place them within a meaningful context.	The historical, sociological, cultural, psychological, economic, political, communal, environmental, and demographic contexts affect the way ethical issues and dilemmas are formulated and justified.
3. Obtain all relevant facts.	Facts affect the way ethical issues and dilemmas are formulated and justified.
4. Reformulate ethical issues or dilemmas if needed.	The initial ethical issues and dilemmas may need to be modified or changed on the basis of context and facts.
5. Consider appropriate approaches to actions or options.	The nature of the ethical issues and dilemmas determines the specific ethical approaches used.
6. Make decisions and take action.	Professional persons cannot avoid choice and action in applied ethics.
7. Evaluate decisions and action.	Evaluation determines whether the ethical decision-making framework used resulted in morally justified actions related to the ethical issues and dilemmas.

Evidence-Based Practice

According to Hentz (2007), the clinical reality of nursing adds a level of complexity to ethical decision making. She states that the theories and principles inherent in ethics do not address the relational aspects, the contextual details, or the personal nature of the situation. It is the relational aspects of ethical situations as well as the human pain and suffering seen in the clinical setting that add to the moral anguish that some nurses experience. To this end, the author recommends that ethical decision making be taught more holistically, addressing both the subjective and objective aspects of the situation at hand. This shift, from ethical dilemmas to human dilemmas, offers a more person-centered approach that blends theory and reason with empathy and compassion.

NURSE USE: The cornerstone of nursing practice is the therapeutic relationship, or the view from the patient's bedside. Because ethics in the clinical setting is multifaceted, courses in nursing ethics must focus not only on the theoretical component of ethical decision making, but on the social and situational components as well.

From Hentz P: Ethical decision-making: blending the voice of reason and the voice of compassion, *Pennsylvania Nurse* 14–15, March 2007.

are simply obeying some rules (or authorities) that settle matters—ours only to obey. Choosing is inescapable" (p. 28).

Keeping this in mind, the following generic ethical decision-making framework is presented:
1. Identify the ethical issues and dilemmas.
2. Place them within a meaningful context.
3. Obtain all relevant facts.
4. Reformulate ethical issues and dilemmas, if needed.
5. Consider appropriate *approaches* to actions or options (utilitarianism, deontology, principlism, virtue ethics, ethic of care, feminist ethics).
6. Make the decision and take action.
7. Evaluate the decision and the action.

The steps of a generic ethics framework are often nonlinear, and with the exception of the ethical approach, they do not change substantially. Their rationales are presented in Table 4-1. Step 5 (the one exception) lists six approaches to the ethical decision-making process; these approaches are outlined throughout the chapter in the "How To" boxes.

Two factors affect this ethical decision-making framework: (1) the growing multiculturalism of the American society, and (2) moral distress. First, nurses often deal with ethical issues and dilemmas related to the diverse and at times conflicting values that result from ethnicity. From a moral perspective, what should the nurse do when facing conflicts in ethnicity?

Callahan (2000) offers useful insights into these conflicts. He describes the following four situations in which ethnic diversity can be judged in relationship to cultural standards:
1. Situations that place persons at direct risk of harm, whether psychological or physical
2. Situations in which ethnic cultural standards conflict with professional standards
3. Situations in which the greater community's values are jeopardized by specific ethnic values
4. Situations in which specific ethnic community customs are annoying but not problematic for the greater community

Callahan (2000) discusses how to judge diversity in the four situations. In situation 1, he says that "we in America imposed some standards on ourselves for important moral reasons; and there is no good reason to exempt [ethnic] subgroups from those standards" (p. 43). Regarding situations 2 and 3, he suggests a thoughtful tolerance, but also some degree of moral persuasion (not coercion) for ethnic groups to alter values so that they are more consistent with what is normative in the American culture. However, Callahan notes that "in the absence of grievous harm, there is no clear moral mandate to interfere with those values" (p. 43). Finally, regarding situation 4, he believes in moral tolerance

ETHICAL CASE

Jeff Williams, team leader in Home Health Care Services at the county health department, was preparing to visit Mr. Chisholm, a 59-year-old client recently diagnosed as having emphysema. Mr. Chisholm, who was unemployed because of a farming accident several years earlier, was well known to the health department. Hypertensive and overweight, he was also a heavy, long-term cigarette smoker despite his decreased lung function. Mr. Williams visited Mr. Chisholm to find out why the client had missed his latest chest clinic appointment. He also wanted to determine if the client was continuing his medications as ordered.

As Mr. Williams parked his car in front of his client's house, he could see Mr. Chisholm sitting on the front porch smoking a cigarette. A flash of anger made him wonder why he continued trying to encourage Mr. Chisholm to stop smoking and why he took the time from his busy home care schedule to follow up on Mr. Chisholm's missed clinic appointments. This client certainly did not seem to care enough about his own health to give up smoking.

During the home visit, Mr. Williams determined that Mr. Chisholm had discontinued the use of his prophylactic antibiotic and was not taking his expectorant and bronchodilator medication on a regular basis. Mr. Chisholm's blood pressure was 210/114 mm Hg, and he coughed almost continuously. Although he listened politely to Mr. Williams' concerns about his respiratory function and the continued use of his medications, Mr. Chisholm simply made no effort to take responsibility for his health care. Even so, another clinic appointment was made, and Mr. Williams encouraged the client to attend.

As he drove to his next home visit, Mr. Williams wondered to what extent he was obligated as a nurse to spend time on clients who took no personal responsibility for their health. He also wondered if there was a limit to the amount of nursing care a noncooperative client could expect from a service provided in the community.

1. What are Mr. Williams' professional responsibilities for Mr. Chisholm's rights to health care?
2. Is there a limit to the amount of care nurses should be expected to give to clients?
3. What authority defines the moral requirements and moral limits of nursing care to clients?

Modified from Veatch RM, Fry ST: *Case studies in nursing ethics*, Philadelphia, 1995, Lippincott Williams & Wilkins.

ETHICAL CASE 2

Ralph Bradley, a recently widowed man in his mid-60s, was discharged from the hospital after exploratory surgery that disclosed colon cancer with metastasis to the lymph nodes. His physician referred him to a home health agency for nursing care follow-up. In reading the referral, the nurse learned that Mr. Bradley had been living with a married daughter and her family since his wife's death. An unmarried daughter apparently lived nearby, visiting him regularly and helping with his daily care. The referral did not explain what, if anything, the client had been told by his physician concerning his condition.

During the first home visit, it became apparent that Mr. Bradley did not know that the tumor removed from his body had been diagnosed as cancerous or that it had metastasized to the lymph nodes. He did not realize the seriousness of his condition, but he did express concern about his health. He complained of vague pain in the abdomen, asked for information about the results of the tests performed before discharge from the hospital, and wanted to know how soon he would be able to return to his work as a cabinetmaker. When the nurse avoided a direct answer to these questions, Mr. Bradley asked directly, "Is everything all right?" The married daughter, who was present when her father was asking these questions, assured him that everything was all right and that he would soon be up and around.

Walking the nurse to her car when the visit was over, the married daughter confided that it was the family's wish that their father not be told how serious his condition was. She said that her mother's recent death had been very difficult for him to accept. They did not want him to be further burdened with the knowledge of his condition. The nurse listened, acknowledging the difficulties posed by the wife's recent death and the father's serious condition. She told the daughter, however, that it would be very difficult, if not impossible, for anyone from her agency to continue to provide nursing care to Mr. Bradley without his knowledge of his condition.

When she returned to her office, the nurse discussed Mr. Bradley's situation with her supervisor. The nurse did not want to continue visiting the client knowing he was being deceived by the physician and family. The supervisor suggested that she consult with the attending physician as soon as possible and explain that Mr. Bradley was asking questions about his condition. Luckily, the nurse was able to reach the physician before it was time to make the next home visit. She asked the physician what the client had been told about his condition. The physician said that at the family's request, Mr. Bradley had not been told that he had cancer. He said he agreed with the family that Mr. Bradley could probably not cope with the anxiety of knowing he had a terminal illness so soon after his wife's death. The physician also expressed concern about Mr. Bradley's daughters who, as he put it, "need a little time to accept the mother's death, as well as accept the impending death of the old man." The physician said that he would consider any act of disclosure on the nurse's part at this time to be inappropriate to her role as a visiting nurse and inconsistent with the well-being of the client and his family.

1. What is the professional duty of veracity?
2. What reasons might the nurse give for telling Mr. Bradley the truth?
3. What reasons might the nurse give for not telling Mr. Bradley the truth?
4. How does not telling the truth constrain nursing care in the community?

Modified from Veatch RM, Fry ST: *Case studies in nursing ethics,* Philadelphia, 1995, Lippincott Williams & Wilkins.

Apply the Utilitarian Ethics Decision Process

1. Determine moral rules that are important to society and that are derived from the principle of utility.*
2. Identify the communities or populations that are affected or most affected by the moral rules.
3. Analyze viable alternatives for each proposed action based on the moral rules.
4. Determine the consequences or outcomes of each viable alternative on the communities or populations most affected by the decision.
5. Select the actions on the basis of the rules that produce the greatest amount of good or the least amount of harm for the communities or populations that are affected by the action.
   NOTE: Remember that the utilitarian ethics decision process is one of the approaches in step 5 of the generic ethical decision-making framework.

*Moral rules of action that produce the greatest good for the greatest number of communities or populations affected by or most affected by the rules.

of nonthreatening ethnic traditions, because there is no moral mandate to do otherwise.

Second, since decision making is so central to the practice of nursing, and many decisions are not easy ones to make, spending more time on the experience of ethical or **moral distress** is useful. Moral or ethical distress occurs when a person is unable to act in a way that he or she thinks is right. You do not feel that you are able to act in a manner consistent with your own values, cultural expectations, and religious beliefs. When this conflict occurs, it can lead to a personal sense of failure in the kind of care you give and to subsequent performance issues and may lead to work and/ or career dissatisfaction. However, there are ways to handle moral distress:

1. Identifying the type(s) of situations that lead to distress
2. Communicating that concern to your manager and examining ways to work toward addressing the stressor
3. Seeking support from colleagues

It is often useful to talk with colleagues. You may learn that they have similar concerns or that they have found ways to interrupt the stressful situation(s) (Carlock and Spader, 2007). Understanding both multiculturalism and moral distress enhances ethical decision making.

ETHICS

DEFINITION, THEORIES, PRINCIPLES

Ethics is both a process for reflection and a body of knowledge that addresses questions such as the following: How should I behave? What actions should I perform? What kind of person should I be? What are my obligations to myself and to others? Chaloner says the word "should" involves ethical thinking since it indicates a perception of the right way to act (2007).

The remainder of this section of the chapter summarizes content about ethical theories and principles.

- Ethical judgments are concerned with values. The goal of an ethical judgment is to choose that action or state of affairs that is good or right in the circumstances.
- Ethical judgments generally do not have the certainty of scientific judgments. For example, nurses often diagnose a situation on the basis of the best available information and then choose the course of action that seems to provide the best ethical resolution to the issue.
- At times, the decision is based on outcomes or consequences. In this approach, called **consequentialism**, the right action is the one that produces the greatest amount of good or the least amount of harm in a given situation. **Utilitarianism** is a well-known consequentialist ethical theory that appeals exclusively to outcomes or consequences in determining which choice to make. In utilitarianism, "the moral value of an action is determined by its overall benefit" (Chaloner, 2007, p. 43). Stated differently, since the outcome is the key factor, then the end justifies the means (Hentz, 2007).
- In other situations, nurses touch upon options open to fundamental beliefs. In such circumstances, these nurses may conclude that the action is right or wrong in itself, regardless of the amount of good that might come from it. This is the ethical theory known as **deontology** or adhering to moral rules or duty rather than to the consequences of the actions. It is based on the premise that persons should always be treated as ends in themselves and never as mere means to the ends of others.
- Health professionals have specific obligations that exist because of the practices and goals of the profession. These health care obligations can be interpreted in terms of a set of principles in bioethics. The primary principles are **respect for autonomy**, **nonmaleficence**, **beneficence**, and **distributive justice**, as shown in Box 4-1. These principles have dominated the development of the field of bioethics since its inception in the 1960s (Evans, 2000). This approach has been called **principlism**, and one of its best descriptions and fullest articulations is given in the sixth edition of Beauchamp and Childress' *Principles of Biomedical Ethics* (2008). This approach to ethical decision making in health care arose in response to life-and-death decision making in acute care settings, where the question to be resolved tended to concern a single localized issue such as the withdrawing or withholding of treatment (Holstein, 2001). In these circumstances, preserving and respecting a patient's autonomy became the dominant issue.

BRIEFLY NOTED

Deontology comes from the Greek roots *deon* meaning duty and *logos* meaning study of.

Although principlism has been used effectively as a way to analyze situations in bioethics, it has come under attack (e.g., Boylan, 2000; Callahan, 2000; Clouser and Gert,

---

Box 4-1 Ethical Principles

Respect for autonomy. Based on human dignity and respect for individuals, autonomy requires that individuals be permitted to choose those actions and goals that fulfill their life plans unless those choices result in harm to another.

Nonmaleficence. According to Hippocrates, nonmaleficence requires that we do no harm. It is impossible to avoid harm entirely, but this principle requires that health care professionals act according to the standards of due care, always seeking to produce the least amount of harm possible.

Beneficence. This principle is complementary to nonmaleficence and requires that we do good. We are limited by time, place, and talents in the amount of good we can do. We have general obligations to perform those actions that maintain or enhance the dignity of other persons whenever those actions do not place an undue burden on health care providers.

Distributive justice. Distributive justice requires that there be a fair distribution of the benefits and burdens in society based on the needs and contributions of its members. This principle requires that consistent with the dignity and worth of its members and within the limits imposed by its resources, a society must determine a minimal level of goods and services to be available to its members.

1990), and there are grounds for the criticism. First, some people say the principles are too abstract to serve as guides for action. Second, the principles themselves can conflict in a given situation and there is no independent basis for resolving the conflict. Third, some persons claim that effective ethical problem solving must be rooted in concrete, individual experiences. Fourth, ethical judgments may depend more on the judgment of sensitive persons than on the application of abstract principles.

Autonomy is often emphasized in acute care settings, whereas beneficence and distributive justice are emphasized more in community and public health. For this reason, it is useful to consider other models for ethical decision making. Utilitarianism and deontology were developed from the Enlightenment's focus on universals, rationality, and isolated individuals. Each theory maintains that there is a universal first principle, the principle of utility for utilitarianism and the categorical imperative for deontology, that serves as a rational norm for our behavior and allows us to calculate the rightness or wrongness of each individual action. According to both utilitarianism and deontology, as in classic liberalism, the individual is the special center of moral concern (Steinbock, London, and Arras, 2008). Giving priority to individual rights and needs refers to the concept that a person's rights and dignity should never (or rarely) be sacrificed to the interests of society (Steinbock, London, and Arras, 2008). The focus on individual rights leads to complications in the interpretation of distributive or social justice.

Distributive or social justice refers to the allocation of benefits and burdens to members of society. Benefit refers to basic needs, including material and social goods, liberties, rights, and entitlements. Some benefits of society are wealth, education, and public services. Among the burdens to be

---

ETHICAL CASE 3

Because finding affordable housing was difficult, 26-year-old Terry White lived with her 6-month-old son, Tommy, and his father, Billy Smith, in one room of the landlord's own house. Ms. White was morbidly obese and was diagnosed with bipolar disease; Mr. Smith had served time for drug dealing and was out on parole and staying straight. Neither had finished high school. Mr. Smith's past drug use had rendered him unable to do much manual labor because of heart damage, but on occasion he would work in construction to support the family.

Public health nurse Jim Lewis had received a referral on Tommy when he was diagnosed with failure to thrive (FTT) 2 months earlier. Ms. White, who had had two children removed from her custody by child protective services (CPS) in the past, and Mr. Smith seemed to adore their baby, so much so that Ms. White would hold the baby all day long. In the past 2 months, the nurse had taught Ms. White about infant nutrition and gotten her enrolled in the Women's, Infants, and Children (WIC) nutrition program; as a result, Tommy had increased his rate of physical growth and was above the 5% level of his growth percentile. Yet he was not meeting his gross motor milestones per Denver Developmental Screening Test II (DDST II) testing. Mr. Lewis thought that Tommy was not allowed to play on the floor enough to progress in sitting, pushing his shoulders up, or crawling. Most of their small room was taken up with the bed and the boxes that stored their belongings. There wasn't really space for "tummy time" or play. When not in the room, the family would take the bus to a discount store and spend the day walking around to get a change of scene.

One week Ms. White told the nurse she was not taking her medications for bipolar disease anymore because they caused her to gain weight. The next week she confided that Mr. Smith had had a "dirty" urine specimen check and would have to return to prison in the near future. The following week Mr. Lewis found the family living in a run-down motel since they had been evicted by their landlord after a disagreement. Ms. White was agitated and she told the nurse that they had only $100, Mr. Smith was going to have to return to prison that week, and the motel bill was already $240. Ms. White knew she would be homeless soon without Mr. Smith's support but refused to talk with her social worker about her needs. She asked the nurse not to tell anyone about her situation because she was afraid CPS would take Tommy from her. It was clear to Mr. Lewis that she might not know where Tommy was after they left this motel.

1. What are Mr. Lewis' professional responsibilities to Ms. White, to Tommy, and to the social worker assigned to this family?
2. How should Mr. Lewis respond to Ms. White's request to not tell anyone about their situation?
3. What communication, if any, should the nurse initiate with the social worker? With others?

Created by Deborah C. Conway, Assistant Professor of Nursing, School of Nursing, University of Virginia.

---

shared are things such as taxes, military service, and the location of incinerators and power plants. Justice requires that the distribution of benefits and burdens in a society be fair or equal. It is widely agreed that the distribution should be based on what one needs and deserves, but there is considerable

HOW TO	**Apply the Deontological Ethics Decision Process**

1. Determine the moral rules (e.g., tell the truth) that serve as standards by which individuals can perform their moral obligations.
2. Examine personal motives for proposed actions to ensure that they are based on good intentions in accord with moral rules.
3. Determine whether the proposed actions can be generalized so that all persons in similar situations are treated similarly.
4. Select the action that treats persons as ends in themselves and never as mere means to the ends of others.
    NOTE: Remember that the deontological ethics decision process is one of the approaches in step 5 of the generic ethical decision-making framework.

HOW TO	**Apply the Principlism Ethics Decision Process**

1. Determine the ethical principles (respect for autonomy, non-maleficence, beneficence, justice) that are relevant to an ethical issue or dilemma.
2. Analyze the relevant principles within a meaningful context of accurate facts and other pertinent circumstances.
3. Act on the principle that provides, within the meaningful context, the strongest guide to action that can be morally justified by the tenets foundational to the principle.
    NOTE: Remember that the principlism ethics decision process is one of the approaches in step 5 of the general ethical decision-making framework.

disagreement as to what these terms mean. Three primary theories of distributive justice are defended today. They are the egalitarian, libertarian, and liberal democratic theories.

Egalitarianism is the view that everyone is entitled to equal rights and equal treatment in society. Ideally, each individual has an equal share of the goods of society, and it is the role of government to ensure that this happens. The government has the authority to redistribute wealth if necessary to ensure equal treatment. Thus, egalitarians are supportive of welfare rights—that is, the right to receive certain social goods necessary to satisfy basic needs. These include adequate food, housing, education, and police and fire protection (Boss, 1998). There are practical and theoretical weaknesses in egalitarianism. For example, it would be almost impossible to ensure the equal distribution of goods and services in any moderately complex society. Assuming that such a distribution could be accomplished, it would require a coercive authority to maintain it (Hellsten, 1998). Egalitarianism cannot provide an incentive for each of us to do our best, because there is no promise of our merit being rewarded. Also in a situation of egalitarianism, we would not have the huge number of underinsured and uninsured people we have at present.

According to the libertarian view of justice, the right to private property is the most important right. Libertarians recognize rights to liberty, for example, the right to be left alone to accomplish our goals. Hellsten (1998) notes, "The central feature of the libertarian view on distributive justice is that it is totally individualist. It rejects any idea that societies, states, or collectives of any form can be the bearers of rights or can owe duties" (p. 822). Libertarians see a limited role for government, namely the protection of property rights of individual citizens by providing police and fire protection. Although they also agree that there is a need for jointly shared, publicly owned facilities such as roads, they reject the idea of the rights to welfare and view taxes to support the needs of others as coercive taking of their property.

Rawls (2001), discussing the liberal democratic theory, attempts to develop a theory that values both liberty and equality. While commenting that inequities are inevitable in society, he tries to justify them by establishing a system in which everyone benefits, especially the least advantaged. This is an attempt to address the inequalities that result from birth, natural endowments, and historic circumstances. Imagining what he calls a "veil of ignorance" to keep us unaware of our actual advantages and disadvantages, Rawls would have us choose the basic principles of justice (p. 15). Once impartiality is guaranteed, Rawls maintains that all rational people will choose a system of justice containing the following two basic principles (Rawls, 2001, p. 42):
1. Each person has the same claim to a fully adequate scheme of equal basic liberties and this scheme is compatible with the same scheme of liberties for all; and
2. Social and economic inequalities are to satisfy two conditions: first, they are to be attached to offices and positions open to all under conditions of fair equality of opportunity; and second, they are to be to the greatest benefit of the least advantaged members of society (the difference principle).

As the veil of ignorance device and the justice principles indicate, Rawls and other justice theorists assume the Enlightenment concept of isolated selves (persons) in competition for scarce resources. In this view justice refers to ensuring fairness to individuals. The interests of the community may conflict with the interests of individuals; yet, from the Enlightenment ideal, the needs of society are neither directly addressed nor given any priority. This Enlightenment assumption has been challenged by a number of ethical theories loosely grouped together under the heading *communitarianism*. **Communitarianism** maintains that abstract, universal principles are not an adequate basis for moral decision making; instead, these theorists argue, history, tradition, and concrete moral communities should be the basis of moral thinking and action (Solomon, 1993). Among the theories with a communitarian focus are virtue ethics, feminism, and care.

VIRTUE ETHICS

Virtue ethics, one of the oldest ethical theories, dates back to the ancient Greek philosophers Plato and Aristotle. It is not concerned with actions, as utilitarianism and deontology are, but instead asks, What kind of person should I be? Virtue ethics seeks to enable persons to flourish as human beings. According to Aristotle, **virtues** are acquired, excellent traits of character that dispose humans to act in accord with their natural good. During the seventeenth and eighteenth centuries, the Greek concept of the good as a principle of explanation went out of favor. Because virtue ethics was closely tied to the concept of the good, interest in virtues as an element of normative ethics also declined. Examples of virtues include benevolence, compassion, discernment, trustworthiness, integrity, and conscientiousness (Beauchamp and Childress, 2008). The appeal to virtues results in a significantly different approach to moral decision making in health care (Fletcher, 1999). In contrast to moral justification via theories or principles, the emphasis is on practical reasoning applied to character development.

CARING AND THE ETHIC OF CARE

Caring in nursing, the **ethic of care**, and feminist ethics are all interrelated and converged between the mid-1980s and early 1990s. Nurses (Leininger, 1984; Watson, 1985) have written about caring as the essence of or the moral ideal of nursing. This view was a response to the technological advances in health care science and to the desire of nurses to differentiate nursing practice from medical practice. Caring and the ethic of care are core values of nursing in community health.

Carol Gilligan and Nel Noddings are considered to be the mothers of the *ethic of care* (Volbrecht, 2002). Their work can easily be used in nursing. Gilligan (1982) describes a personal journey in which, by listening and talking to people, she began to notice two distinct voices (those of women and men) and two distinct themes(those of affiliation and autonomy between women and men) She said (Gilligan, 1982, p. 2):

> *The different voice I describe is characterized not by gender but theme. Its association with women is an empirical observation, and it is primarily through women's voices that I trace its development. But this association is not absolute, and the contrasts between male and female voices are presented here to highlight a distinction between two modes of thought and to focus [on] a problem of interpretation rather than to represent a generalization about either sex.*

She went on to formulate basic premises about responsibility, care, and relationships (1982):

- "Sensitivity to the needs of others and the assumption of responsibility for taking care lead women to attend to voices other than their own" (p. 16).
- "Women not only define themselves in a context of human relationships but also judge themselves in terms of their ability to care" (p. 17).
- "The truths of relationship, however, return in the rediscovery of connection, in the realization that self and other are interdependent and that life, however valuable in itself, can only be sustained by care in relationships" (p. 127).

Noddings' (1984) personal journey started at a point different from that of Gilligan's. Noddings noted that ethics

---

HOW TO   **Apply the Virtue Ethics Decision Process**

1. Identify communities that are relevant to the ethical dilemmas or issues.
2. Identify moral considerations that arise from a communal perspective, and apply the consideration to specific communities.
3. Identify and apply virtues that facilitate a communal perspective.
4. Modify moral considerations as needed to apply to the specific ethical dilemmas or issues.
5. Seek ethical community support to enhance character development.
6. Evaluate and modify the individuals or community character traits that impede communal living.

NOTE: Remember that the virtue ethics decision process is one of the approaches in step 5 of the generic ethical decision-making framework.

Modified from Volbrecht RM: *Nursing ethics: communities in dialogue,* Upper Saddle River, NJ, 2002, Prentice Hall, p 138.

---

was described in the literature primarily using principles and logic and her goal was to express a feminine view that could be accepted or rejected by women *or* men. Noddings' (1984) basic premises are as follows:

1. "The essential elements of caring are located in the relation between the one caring and the cared-for" (p. 9).
2. "Caring requires me to respond . . . with an act of commitment: I commit myself either to overt action on behalf of the cared-for or I commit myself to thinking about what I might do" (p. 81).
3. "We are not 'justified'—we are *obligated*—to do what is required to maintain and enhance caring" (p. 95).
4. "Caring itself and the ethical ideal that strives to maintain and enhance it guide us in moral decisions and conduct" (p. 105).

Gilligan and Noddings have in common a feminine ethic because they believe in the morality of responsibility in relationships that emphasize connection and caring. To them, caring is not a mere nicety but a moral imperative. Nevertheless, a long-term healthy debate has surrounded their premises.

FEMINIST ETHICS

The beliefs of **feminist ethics** are relevant to nursing. Leipert (2001) says that a feminist perspective supports critical thinking and a focus on issues such as gender, power, and socioeconomic status. Clearly these issues affect health and the work of nurses. Defining the terms *feminists* and *feminist ethics* is helpful. **Feminists** are women *and* men who hold a worldview advocating economic, social, and political status for women that is equivalent to that of men. Consequently, feminists reject the devaluing of women and their experiences through systematic oppression based on gender. Volbrecht (2002) says, "A feminist is also someone who works to bring about the social changes necessary to promote more

HOW TO **Apply the Care Ethics Decision Process**

1. Recognize that caring is a moral imperative.
2. Identify personally lived caring experiences as a basis for relating to self and others.
3. Assume responsibility and obligation to promote and enhance caring in relationships.
   NOTE: Remember that the care ethics decision process is one of the approaches in step 5 of the generic ethical decision-making framework.

HOW TO **Apply the Feminist Ethics Decision Process**

1. Identify the social, cultural, political, economic, environmental, and professional contexts that contribute to the identified problem (e.g., underrepresentation of women in clinical trials).
2. Evaluate how the preceding contexts contribute to the oppression of women.
3. Consider how women's lives are defined by their status in subordinate social groups.
4. Analyze how social practices marginalize women.
5. Plan ways to restructure those social practices that oppress women.
6. Implement the plan.
7. Evaluate the plan, and restructure it as needed.
   NOTE: Remember that the feminist ethics decision process is one of the approaches in step 5 of the generic ethical decision-making framework.

Modified from Volbrecht RM: *Nursing ethics: communities in dialogue,* Upper Saddle River, NJ, 2002, Prentice Hall, p 219.

just relationships among women and men" (p. 160). Feminists believe in the ethic of care and think that the oppression of women is morally wrong.

ETHICS AND THE CORE FUNCTIONS OF PUBLIC HEALTH NURSING

In Chapter 1, the three core functions of public health nursing (i.e., assessment, policy development, and assurance) were discussed. The following discussion links these three core functions to ethics.

ASSESSMENT

"Assessment refers to systematically collecting data on the population, monitoring the population's health status, and making information available about the health of the community." (Williams and Stanhope, 2008, p. 7.)

The following three ethical tenets support these core functions:

1. *Competency related to knowledge development, analysis, and dissemination.* An ethical question related to competency is: Are the persons assigned to develop community knowledge adequately prepared to collect data on groups and populations? This question is important because the research, measurement, and analysis techniques used to gather information about groups and populations usually differ from the techniques used to assess individuals. Wrong research techniques can lead to wrong assessments, which in turn may hurt rather than help the intended group or population.

2. *Virtue ethics or moral character.* An ethical question related to moral character is: Do the persons selected to develop, assess, and disseminate community knowledge possess integrity? Beauchamp and Childress (2008) define integrity as the holistic integration of moral character. The importance of this virtue is clear: without integrity, the core function of assessment is endangered. Persons with compromised integrity are easy prey for potential or real scientific misconduct.

3. *"Do no harm."* An ethical question related to "do no harm" is: Is disseminating appropriate information about groups and populations morally necessary and sufficient? The answer to "morally necessary" is yes, but the answer to "morally sufficient" is no. The fallacy with dissemination is that there is no built-in accountability that what is disseminated will be read or understood. If it is not read or understood, harm could come to groups and populations regarding their health status.

POLICY DEVELOPMENT

"Policy development refers to the need to provide leadership in developing policies that support the health of the population, including the use of the scientific knowledge base in making decisions about policy" (Williams and Stanhope, 2008, p. 7). Underlying this core function are at least three ethical tenets. The first says that an important goal of both policy and ethics is to achieve the public good (Silva, 2002), which is a part of the concept of citizenship. To be an effective citizen, people must be both informed about policy and able and willing to do what is in the best interests of the community (Denhardt and Denhardt, 2000). The approach is basically one in which the voice of the community is the foundation upon which policy is developed, rather than the voice of community *and* public health administrators.

The second ethical tenet purports that service to others over self is a necessary condition of what is "good" or "right" policy (Silva, 2002). Denhardt and Denhardt (2000) offer three perspectives on this matter:

1. *Serve rather than steer.* An increasingly important role of the public servant (e.g., nurses and administrators) is to help citizens articulate and meet their shared interests rather than to attempt to control or steer society in new directions (p. 553).

2. *Serve citizens, not customers.* The public interest results from a dialogue about shared values rather than the aggregation of individual self-interests. Therefore public servants do not merely respond to the demands of "customers" but focus on building relationships of trust and collaboration with and among citizens (p. 555).

ETHICAL CASE   4

Autonomy and Distributive Justice

Amelia Lewis, a 31-year-old African-American woman with multiple diagnoses, has been followed in the local mental health system for over 10 years. Four years ago, while a patient at the local day hospital, she met and married another patient, James Wood. She became pregnant and now has Tyesha, who is 3 years old. Multiple agencies have followed Ms. Lewis and her little girl, who live in a sparsely furnished apartment in subsidized housing. Mr. Wood lives separately, and he and his family welcome contact with Tyesha, but the relationship between Ms. Lewis and Mr. Wood has deteriorated. A guardian handles all of Ms. Lewis's financial affairs.

Ms. Lewis has issues of trust, and she is often suspicious of the care providers who come to her home. She does rely on some of the professionals with whom she interacts on a weekly or biweekly basis. Her developmental level places her at a stage at which her own needs are her primary focus, and this is not expected to change; her interaction with Tyesha is perfunctory, involving little outward affection. She is unable to understand that Tyesha is not capable of self care, and that her 3-year-old child will not always obey when Ms. Lewis instructs her to do something. Tyesha's needs, level of functioning, and cognitive development are quickly surpassing her mother's ability to cope. Frustration and misunderstanding ensue when Ms. Lewis thinks that Tyesha doesn't listen to her, and encouragement and parent education have done little to improve the situation as Tyesha gets older and more assertive. This has made toilet training, provision of an appropriate diet, and other aspects of normal child care problematic.

Many services besides those for mental health are involved to help this family of two cope. There is concern about abuse or neglect due to Ms. Lewis's lack of understanding of how to be a parent. Supplemental Security Income provides monetary support because of her mental disability and they have Medicaid coverage for their health care needs, as well as food stamps and modest financial assistance through Temporary Assistance for Needy Families (TANF). Ms. Lewis cannot currently work and take care of her child due to her mental disability. Before Tyesha's birth, Ms. Lewis held a job and maintained self care, but the care of Tyesha has precluded her managing employment at this time. Child Protective Services are also monitoring Ms. Lewis's situation. Ms. Lewis attends a local program to complete her General Education Development (GED), which provides child care during the day. Though Ms. Lewis is not expected to complete her GED, this program provides structured time for Tyesha three times a week. The child is considered developmentally normal at this time, and she is being followed by an infant development program that monitors her progress on developmental issues. The Child Health Partnership, an agency that addresses the needs of challenged families, provides regular visits, family support, and parenting education, and the GED teachers make regular home visits to check on Ms. Lewis and Tyesha. Ms. Lewis thinks things are going just fine.

The Child Health Partnership nurse is concerned about this family, and thinks that some permanent resolution of the situation is inevitable. There is minimal coordination of services and there is no "lead agency" in the family's care.

1. Should the nurse involved in the Child Health Partnership program initiate any action to try to coordinate the work of the many agencies involved with this family?
2. Who has a professional responsibility to determine when the mother can no longer cope with the developing child?
3. Whose needs, Ms. Lewis's or Tyesha's, should take precedence?

Created by Mary E. Gibson, Assistant Professor, School of Nursing, University of Virginia.

---

3. *Value citizenship and public service above entrepreneurship.* The public interest is better advanced by public servants and citizens committed to making meaningful contributions to society rather than by entrepreneurial managers acting as if public money were their own (p. 556).

At the core of these three perspectives is service, and service always has been an enduring value of nursing.

The third ethical tenet purports that what is ethical is also good policy (Silva, 2002). What is ethical should be the sole foundational pillar upon which nursing is based. Moral leadership is critical to policy development because it is the highest human standard and therefore should result in ethical health care policies.

ASSURANCE

"*Assurance* refers to the role of public health in making sure that essential community-oriented health services are available, which may include providing essential personal health services for those who would otherwise not receive them. Assurance also refers to making sure that a competent public health and personal health care workforce is available" (Williams and Stanhope, 2008, p. 7). At least two ethical tenets underlie this core function:

1. All persons should receive essential personal health services or, put in terms of justice, "to each person a fair share" or, reworded, "to all groups or populations a fair share." This is an egalitarian perspective of justice. This perspective does not mean that all persons in a society should share all of society's benefits equally but that they should share at least those benefits that are essential. Many persons think that basic health care for all is essential for social justice.
2. Providers of public health services should be competent and available. Although the Code of Ethics for *Public Health* does not speak directly to workforce availability, it does speak directly to ensuring professional competency of public health employees. However, *Healthy People 2010* discusses both competencies and workforce as seen in the *Healthy People 2010* box.

NURSING CODE OF ETHICS

As noted in the "History" section of this chapter, the *Code of Ethics for Nurses With Interpretive Statements* was adopted by the ANA House of Delegates in 2001. There are three purposes of the 2001 code (American Nurses Association, 2001):

Healthy People 2010

Public Health Infrastructure and Workforce

The following are national goals (and their code numbers) for ensuring that all public agencies have the necessary infrastructure to provide essential and efficient public health services:

23-8 Increase the proportion of federal, tribal, state, and local agencies that incorporate specific competencies in the essential public health services into personnel systems.

23-9 Increase the proportion of schools for public health workers that integrate into their curricula specific content to develop competency in the essential public health services.

23-10 Increase the proportion of federal, tribal, state, and local public health agencies that provide continuing education to develop competency in essential public health services for their employees.

From the U.S. Department of Health and Human Services: *Healthy People 2010: understanding and improving health*, ed 2, Washington, DC, 2000, U.S. Government Printing Office.

1. To be a "succinct statement of the ethical obligations and duties of every individual who enters the nursing profession" (p. 5)
2. To be "the profession's nonnegotiable ethical standard" (p. 5)
3. To be "an expression of nursing's own understanding of its commitment to society" (p. 5)

These purposes are reflected in the nine provisional statements of the code, as identified in Box 4-2. The *Code of Ethics for Nurses* and its interpretive statements apply to nurses in community health, although the emphasis for each type of nursing sometimes varies. For example, provision 1 and its interpretive statement primarily address the individual but acknowledge that there are times when public health considerations override individual rights. Provisions 2 and 3 and their interpretive statements are pertinent to both nurses in community health and to public health nurses. Keep in mind, however, that in provision 3, *patient* means the recipient of nursing care, whether a group, family, or community.

Whereas provisions 1 through 3 focus on the recipients of nursing care, provisions 4 through 6 focus on the nurse. This focus addresses nurses' accountability, competency, and contributions to their employment conditions.

Provisions 7 through 9 focus on the bigger picture of both the nursing profession and national and global health concerns. In nursing, the emphasis is on professional standards, active involvement in nursing, and the integrity of the profession. All nurses have a responsibility to meet these obligations. Regarding national and global health concerns, the emphasis is on social justice and reform. According to the American Nurses Association (2001), "The nurse has a responsibility to be aware not only of specific health needs of individual patients but also of broader health concerns such as world hunger, environmental pollution, lack of access to

| Box 4-2 | **Code of Ethics for Nurses** |

1. The nurse, in all professional relationships, practices with compassion and respect for the inherent dignity, worth, and uniqueness of every individual, unrestricted by considerations of social or economic status, personal attributes, or the nature of the health problems.
2. The nurse's primary commitment is to the patient, whether an individual, family, group, or community.
3. The nurse promotes, advocates for, and strives to protect the health, safety, and rights of the patient.
4. The nurse is responsible and accountable for individual nursing practice and determines the appropriate delegation of tasks consistent with the nurse's obligation to provide optimal patient care.
5. The nurse owes the same duties to self as to others, including the responsibility to preserve integrity and safety, to maintain competence, and to continue personal and professional growth.
6. The nurse participates in establishing, maintaining, and improving health care environments and conditions of employment conducive to the provision of quality health care and consistent with the values of the profession through individual and collective action.
7. The nurse participates in the advancement of the profession through contributions to practice, education, administration, and knowledge development.
8. The nurse collaborates with other health professionals and the public in promoting community, national, and international efforts to meet health needs.
9. The profession of nursing, as represented by associations and their members, is responsible for articulating nursing values, for maintaining the integrity of the profession and its practice, and for shaping social policy.

From the American Nurses Association: *Code of ethics for nurses with interpretive statements*, Washington, DC, 2001, American Nurses Association. See also www.nursingworld.org.

health care, violation of human rights, and inequitable distribution of nursing and health care resources" (p. 23). The American Nurses Association Code (American Nurses Association, 2001) emphasizes political action as the mechanism to effect social justice and reform regarding homelessness, violence, and stigmatization. All of the preceding responsibilities typically fall more in the domain of public health nursing than nursing in community health, although nurses in community health should be aware of the social activism embedded in the 2001 Code.

PUBLIC HEALTH CODE OF ETHICS

The Code of Ethics for *Public Health* (Public Health Leadership Society, 2002) was noted in the "History" section of this chapter. This code consists of a preamble; 12 principles related to the ethical practice of public health (Box 4-3); 11 values and beliefs that focus on health, community, and action; and a commentary on each of the 12 principles. The preamble asserts the collective and societal nature of public health to keep people healthy. The 12 principles incorporate

Levels of Prevention — Related to Ethics

PRIMARY PREVENTION

Use the Code of Ethics for Nurses to guide your nursing practice.

SECONDARY PREVENTION

If you are unable to behave in accordance with the Code of Ethics for Nurses (e.g., you speak in a way that does not communicate respect for a patient), take steps to correct your behavior. You could explain to the patient your error and apologize.

TERTIARY PREVENTION

If you have treated a patient or staff member in a way that is inconsistent with ethics practices, seek guidance on other choices you could have made.

Box 4-3   Principles of the Ethical Practice of Public Health

1. Public health should address principally the fundamental causes of disease and requirements for health, aiming to prevent adverse health outcomes.
2. Public health should achieve community health in a way that respects the rights of individuals in the community.
3. Public health policies, programs, and priorities should be developed and evaluated through processes that ensure an opportunity for input from community members.
4. Public health should advocate and work for the empowerment of disenfranchised community members, aiming to ensure that the basic resources and conditions necessary for health are accessible to all.
5. Public health should seek the information needed to implement effective policies and programs that protect and promote health.
6. Public health institutions should provide communities with the information they have that is needed for decisions on policies or programs and should obtain the community's consent for their implementation.
7. Public health institutions should act in a timely manner on the information they have within the resources and the mandate given to them by the public.
8. Public health programs and policies should incorporate a variety of approaches that anticipate and respect diverse values, beliefs, and cultures in the community.
9. Public health programs and policies should be implemented in a manner that most enhances the physical and social environment.
10. Public health institutions should protect the confidentiality of information that can bring harm to an individual or community if made public. Exceptions must be justified on the basis of the high likelihood of significant harm to the individual or others.
11. Public health institutions should ensure the professional competencies of their employees.
12. Public health institutions and their employees should engage in collaborations and affiliations in ways that build the public's trust and the institution's effectiveness.

From the Public Health Leadership Society (PHLS): *Code of ethics for public health*, New Orleans, La, 2002, Louisiana Public Health Institute. The ethics project was funded in part by the Centers for Disease Control and Prevention.

---

the ethical tenets of preventing harm; doing no harm; promoting good; respecting both individual and community rights; respecting autonomy, diversity, and confidentiality when possible; ensuring professional competency; trustworthiness; and promoting advocacy for disenfranchised persons within a community. Examples of values and beliefs include a right to health care resources, the interdependency of humans living in the community, and the importance of knowledge as a basis for action.

When the *Code of Ethics for Nurses* and the Code of Ethics for *Public Health* are assessed, some commonalities emerge. Both provide general ethical principles and approaches that are enduring and dynamic. They force nurses to think about the underlying ethics of their profession. Although the two codes do not specify (nor should they specify) details for every ethical issue, other mechanisms such as standards of practice, ethical decision-making frameworks, and ethics committees help work out the details. Nevertheless, the preceding two codes address most approaches to ethical justification, including traditional and emerging ethical theories and principles, humanist and feminist ethics, virtue ethics, professional–individual and/or community relationships, and advocacy.

ADVOCACY AND ETHICS

DEFINITIONS, CODES, STANDARDS

Advocacy is a powerful ethical concept in nursing. But what does *advocacy* mean? Christoffel (2000) offers two definitions that are useful since they seem to differentiate between nursing in community health and in public health nursing. The following definition related to nursing in community health seems appropriate: "*Advocacy* is the application of information and resources (including finances, effort, and votes) to effect systemic changes that shape the way people in a community live" (p. 722). In contrast, "*Public health advocacy* is advocacy that is intended to reduce death or disability in groups of people. . . . Such advocacy involves the

use of information and resources to reduce the occurrence or severity of public health problems" (pp. 722–723). The former definition is intended to address the quality of life of individuals in a community, whereas the latter is intended to address the quality of life for aggregates or populations. As such, both definitions have an ethical basis grounded in quality of life. Several codes and standards of practice address advocacy. Three are noted here. Advocacy is addressed in the ANA and the Public Health Leadership Society's codes of ethics, as well as the ANA's *Public Health Nursing: Scope and Standards of Practice* (American Nurses Association, 2007).

According to the ANA's *Code of Ethics for Nurses with Interpretive Statements,* "The nurse promotes, advocates for, and strives to protect the health, safety, and rights of the patient" (American Nurses Association, 2001, p. 12). The focus of the interpretive statements regarding advocacy is the nurse's responsibility to take action when the patient's best interests are jeopardized by questionable practice on the part of any member of the health team, the health care system, or others.

According to the Public Health Leadership Society's Code of Ethics for Public Health, "Public health should advocate and work for the empowerment of disenfranchised community members, aiming to ensure that the basic resources and conditions necessary for health are accessible to all" (Public Health Leadership Society, 2002, p. 1). The Public Health Leadership Society's Code elaborates on the preceding principle by addressing the following two issues: that the voice of the community should be heard and that the marginalized or underserved in a community should receive "a decent minimum" (p. 4) of health resources.

According to the ANA's *Public Health Nursing: Scope and Standards of Practice* (American Nurses Association, 2007), public health nurses have a moral mandate to establish ethical standards when advocating for health care policy. The preceding standards extend the prior two concepts of advocacy by moving advocacy into the policy arena, particularly health and social policy as applied to populations.

COMPONENTS OF ADVOCACY

According to Christoffel (2000), public health advocacy is composed of the following two components: products and processes. The end products are decreased morbidity and mortality. The intermediate products occur at the individual/family level and at the extended family/community level. Examples of products at the individual/family level include healthy diet, stress reduction, and prenatal care. Examples of products at the extended family/community level include reduced dangers from the environment (e.g., pollution) and facilitation of community actions (e.g., school-based health services). To reduce public health problems effectively, multiple changes need to occur at both levels.

In addition, Christoffel (2000, p. 723) lists the following processes of public health advocacy:
1. Problem identification
2. Research and data gathering
3. Professional and clinical education, as well as education of those involved in the creation of public policy (including media coverage)
4. Development and promotion of regulations and legislation
5. Endorsement of regulations and legislation via elections and government actions
6. Enforcement of effective policies
7. Policy process and outcome evaluations

All seven processes are interwoven within a context that best reduces morbidity and mortality. Two ethical principles underlying these products and processes are promoting good and preventing harm.

Box 4-4	**Ethical Principles for Effective Advocacy**

1. Act in the client's (group's, community's) best interests.
2. Act in accordance with the client's (group's, community's) wishes and instructions.
3. Keep the client (group, community) properly informed.
4. Carry out instructions with diligence and competence.
5. Act impartially, and offer frank, independent advice.
6. Maintain client confidentiality.

Modified from Bateman N: *Advocacy skills for health and social care professionals*, p. 63, Philadelphia, 2000, Jessica Kingsley.

CONCEPTUAL FRAMEWORK FOR ADVOCACY

Christoffel's (2000) conceptual framework for advocacy has these three stages:
1. An *information stage* that focuses on gathering data about public health problems, including factors such as extent of the problem, patterns of frequency, and effectiveness of and barriers to public health programs.
2. A *strategy stage* that focuses on tactics such as disseminating the gathered information and policy statements to lay and professional audiences, identifying objectives, building and funding coalitions, and working with legislators.
3. An *action stage* that focuses on implementing the strategies through tactics such as lobbying, testifying, issuing press releases, passing laws, and voting.

Some of the principles that underlie this framework include scientific integrity in data gathering and dissemination, respect for persons (i.e., lay and professional audiences), honesty regarding fundraising, truthfulness in lobbying and testifying, and justice in passing laws.

PRACTICAL FRAMEWORK FOR ADVOCACY

Bateman (2000) takes a practical approach to advocacy. He places the advocate's core skills (i.e., interviewing, assertiveness and force, negotiation, self-management, legal knowledge and research, and litigation) within the context of six ethical principles for effective advocacy, as shown in Box 4-4. Although his focus is on the individual, it can also apply to groups and communities.

In the first ethical principle, Bateman (2000) is sensitive to the ethical conflict between clients' best interests and the best interests of groups, communities, or societies but does not elaborate on this conflict. The second ethical principle, which puts the client in charge, works in tandem with the first principle. It goes like this: "This is what I think we can do. What do you want me to do?" (Bateman, 2000, p. 51). Of course, the advocate can refuse the request if self or others may be harmed. By following the third ethical principle, the client is empowered to make knowledgeable decisions. The fourth ethical principle addresses standards of practice. The fifth ethical principle addresses fairness and respect for persons (nursing in community health is more collaborative in nature than independent). The last ethical principle, confidentiality, ensures that information will be shared only on a need-to-know basis.

CLINICAL APPLICATION

The retiring director of the Division of Primary Care in a state health department had recently hired Ann, a 34-year-old nurse with a master's degree in public health, to be director of the division. Ann's work involved the monitoring of millions of dollars of state and federal money and the supervising of the funded programs within her division.

Ann received many requests for funding from a particular state agency that served a poor, large district. The poor people of the district consisted primarily of young families with children and homebound older adults with chronic illnesses. Over the past 3 years, the federal government had allocated considerable money to the state agency to subsidize pediatric primary care programs, but no formal evaluation of these programs had occurred.

The director of the state agency was a physician who had been in this position for more than 20 years. He was good at obtaining funding for primary care needs in his district, but the statistics related to the pediatric primary care program seemed implausible—that is, few physical examinations were performed on the children, which had resulted in extra money in the budget. This unspent federal money was being used to supplement home health care services for the indigent homebound older adults in his district. The thinking of the physician was that he was doing good by providing some needed services to both indigent groups in his district. Ann felt moral discomfort because she did not have either the money or the personnel to provide both services.

What should she do?

A. *What facts are the most relevant in this scenario?*

B. *What are the ethical issues?*

C. *How can Ann resolve the issues?*

NOTE: The preceding case and answers are adapted and paraphrased from a real practice application shared by J. L. Chapin (Chapin, 1990).

Answers are in the back of the book.

REMEMBER THIS!

- Nursing has a rich heritage of ethics and morality, beginning with Florence Nightingale.
- During the late 1960s, the field of bioethics began to emerge and influence nursing.
- Ethical decision making is the component of ethics that focuses on the process of how ethical decisions are made.
- Many different ethical decision-making frameworks exist; however, the problem-solving process underlies each of them.
- Ethical decision making applies to all approaches to ethics: utilitarianism, deontology, principlism, virtue ethics, the ethic of care, and feminist ethics.
- Cultural diversity and moral distress make ethical decision making more challenging.

- Classical ethical theories are utilitarianism and deontology.
- Principlism consists of respect for autonomy, nonmaleficence, beneficence, and justice.
- Other approaches to ethics include virtue ethics, the ethic of care, and feminist ethics.
- The core functions of nursing in public health (i.e., assessment, policy development, assurance) are all grounded in ethics.
- *Healthy People 2010*, under public health infrastructure, addresses workforce competencies, training in essential public health services, and continuing education.
- The 2001 *Code of Ethics for Nurses* contains nine statements that address the moral standards that delineate nursing's values, goals, and obligations.
- The 2002 *Code of Ethics for Public Health* contains 12 statements that address the moral standards that delineate public health's values, goals, and obligations.
- Advocacy is the act of pleading for or supporting a course of action on behalf of a person, group, or community.
- The *Code of Ethics for Nurses,* the *Code of Ethics for Public Health,* and *Public Health Nursing: Scope and Standards of Practice* all address advocacy.
- Public health advocacy is composed of both products and processes.
- The products of advocacy are decreased morbidity and mortality.
- The processes of public health advocacy include, but are not limited to, identifying problems, collecting data, developing and endorsing regulations and legislation, enforcing policies, and assessing the policy process.

WHAT WOULD YOU DO?

1. You are interested in the extent to which clients' rights to privacy are respected and protected in a community health care agency and the extent to which the agency complies with the requirements of the Health Insurance Portability and Accountability Act (HIPAA). What questions would you ask? Examples: To what extent are the written and electronic communications of the agency protected from people who have no authority to access that information? If client records are used for research, are the correct permissions obtained?

2. How would you protect clients' rights to privacy about their personal health care information? Suggest two methods by which client privacy could be more adequately protected. What would be the relative costs and benefits of your proposed methods?

3. What if public opinion surveys about professional aid in dying suggested that 50% to 75% of adults favor allowing health care professionals to assist the suicide of those who are terminally ill? Nurses, however, are ethically and legally prohibited from assisting the suicide of anyone and participating in acts of euthanasia. What should the nurse do when a terminally ill and suffering client asks the nurse to help him die?

■ REFERENCES

American Nurses Association: *Public health nursing: the scope and standards of practice*, Washington, DC, 2007, American Nurses Publishing.

American Nurses Association: *Code of ethics for nurses with interpretive statements*, Washington, DC, 2001, American Nurses Publishing.

Bateman N: *Advocacy skills for health and social care professionals*, Philadelphia, 2000, Jessica Kingsley.

Beauchamp TL, Childress JF: *Principles of biomedical ethics*, ed 6, New York, 2008, Oxford University.

Boss J: *Ethics for life,* Mountain View, Calif, 1998, Mayfield.

Boylan M: Interview with Edmund D. Pellegrino. In Boylan M, editor: *Medical ethics: basic ethics in action*, Upper Saddle River, NJ, 2000, Prentice Hall.

Callahan D: Universalism and particularism fighting to a draw, *Hastings Center Rep* 30(1):37, 2000.

Carlock C, Spader C: Communication and understanding: best vs distress, *Nsg Spectrum.* Retrieved Oct 8, 2007, from www.nurse.com.

Chaloner C: An introduction to ethics in nursing, *Nurs Standard* 21(32):42–45, 2007.

Chapin JL: The inappropriate distribution of primary health care funds. In Silva M, editor: *Ethical decision making in nursing administration*, Norwalk, Conn, 1990, Appleton & Lange.

Christoffel KK: Public health advocacy: process and product, *Am J Public Health* 90(5):722–723, 2000.

Clouser KD, Gert B: A critique of principlism, *J Med Philos* 15:219, 1990.

Denhardt RB, Denhardt JV: The new public service: serving rather than steering, *Public Admin Rev* 60(6):549–552, 2000.

Evans JH: A sociological account of the growth of principlism, *Hastings Center Rep* 30(5):31, 2000.

Fletcher JJ: Virtues, moral decisions, and healthcare, *Nurs Connections* 12(4):26, 1999.

Gilligan C: *In a different voice: psychological theory and women's development*, Cambridge, 1982, Harvard University.

Hamric AB: Bridging the gap between ethics and clinical practice, *Nurs Outlook* 50(5):176–178, 2002.

Hellsten S: Theories of distributive justice. In Chadwick R, editor: *Encyclopedia of applied ethics*, vol 1, New York, 1998, Academic Press, pp 815–827.

Hentz P: Ethical decision-making: blending the voice of reason and the voice of compassion, *Pennsylvania Nurse,* March 2007, available at www.panurses.org.

Holstein MB: Bringing ethics home: a new look at ethics in the home and the community. In Holstein MB, Mitzen PB, editors: *Ethics in community-based elder care*, New York, 2001, Springer.

International Council of Nurses: *ICN code of ethics for nurses*, Geneva, 1953, ICN.

International Council of Nurses: *ICN code of ethics for nurses*, Geneva, 2006, ICN.

Leininger M, editor: *Care: the essence of nursing and health*, Thorofare, NJ, 1984, Slack.

Leipert BD: Feminism and public health nursing: partners for health, *Sch Inq Nurs Prac* 15(1):49, 2001.

Noddings N: *Caring: a feminine approach to ethics & moral education*, Berkeley, Calif, 1984, University of California.

Olick RS: From the column editor: ethics in public health, *J Public Health Manag Pract* 11:258–259, 2005.

Public Health Leadership Society: *Code of ethics for public health*, New Orleans, La, 2002, Louisiana Public Health Institute. Retrieved April 23, 2008, from http://phls.org/home/section/3-26.

Rawls J: *Justice as fairness: a restatement,* Kelly E, editor: Cambridge, Mass, 2001, Harvard University.

Silva MC: Ethical issues in health care, public policy, and politics. In Mason D, Leavitt J, Chaffee M, editors: *Policy and politics in nursing and health care*, ed 4, Philadelphia, 2002, Saunders.

Solomon RC: *Ethics: a short introduction*, Dubuque, Iowa, 1993, Brown & Benchmark.

Steinbock B, London AJ, Arras JD, editors: *Ethical issues in modern medicine*, ed 7, New York, 2008, McGraw-Hill.

Thomas JC et al: A code of ethics for public health, *Am J Public Health,* 92(7):1057–1059, 2002.

Ulrich C et al: Ethical climate, ethics stress, and the job satisfaction of nurse and social workers in the United States, *Soc Sci Med* 65(7):1708–1719, 2007.

U.S. Department of Health and Human Services: *Healthy People 2010: understanding and improving health*, ed 2, Washington, DC, 2000, U.S. Government Printing Office.

Veatch RM, Fry ST: *Case studies in nursing ethics*, Philadelphia, 1995, Lippincott Williams & Wilkins.

Volbrecht RM: *Nursing ethics: communities in dialogue*, Upper Saddle River, NJ, 2002, Prentice Hall.

Watson J: *Nursing: human science and human care*, Norwalk, Conn, 1985, Appleton-Century-Crofts.

Weston A: *A practical companion to ethics*, ed 2, New York, 2002, Oxford University.

Williams CA, Stanhope MK: Population-focused practice: the foundation of specialization in public health nursing. In Stanhope M, Lancaster J, editors: *Public health nursing: population-centered health care in the community*, ed 7, St. Louis, 2008, Elsevier.

Cultural Influences in Nursing in Community Health

Cynthia E. Degazon

ADDITIONAL RESOURCES

These related resources are found either in the appendix at the back of this book or on the book's website at http://evolve.elsevier.com/stanhope/foundations.

Appendix
- Appendix B.2: Multicultural Nursing Assessment: Cultural Assessment Guide

Evolve Website
- Community Assessment Applied
- Quiz review questions
- WebLinks, including link to *Healthy People 2010* website

OBJECTIVES

After reading this chapter, the student should be able to:
1. Discuss ways in which culture can affect nursing practice.
2. Describe methods for developing cultural competence.
3. Evaluate the effects of cultural organizational factors on health and illness.
4. Conduct a cultural assessment of a person from a cultural group other than yours.
5. Develop culturally competent nursing interventions to promote positive health outcomes for clients.

CHAPTER OUTLINE

IMMIGRANT HEALTH ISSUES

CULTURE, RACE, AND ETHNICITY
Culture
Race
Ethnicity
CULTURAL COMPETENCE
Developing Cultural Competence
Dimensions of Cultural Competence
INHIBITORS TO DEVELOPING CULTURAL COMPETENCE
CULTURAL NURSING ASSESSMENT
Using an Interpreter

CULTURAL GROUPS' DIFFERENCES
Communication
Space
Social Organization
Time Perception
Environmental Control
Biological Variations
CULTURE AND NUTRITION
CULTURE AND SOCIOECONOMIC FACTORS

KEY TERMS

biological variations: the physical, biological, and physiological differences that exist and distinguish one racial group from another.

cultural accommodation: negotiation with clients to include aspects of their folk practices with the traditional health care system to implement essential treatment plans.

cultural awareness: an appreciation of and sensitivity to a client's values, beliefs, practices, lifestyle, and problem-solving strategies.

cultural blindness: when differences between cultures are ignored and persons act as though these differences do not exist.

cultural brokering: advocating, mediating, negotiating, and intervening between the client's culture and the biomedical health care culture on behalf of clients.

cultural competence: an interplay of factors that motivates persons to develop knowledge, skill, and the ability to care for others.

cultural conflict: a perceived threat that may arise from a misunderstanding of expectations between clients and nurses when neither is aware of their cultural differences.

cultural desire: the nurse's intrinsic motivation to provide culturally competent care.

cultural encounter: interaction with a client related to all aspects of his or her life.

cultural imposition: the process of imposing one's values on others.

cultural knowledge: the information necessary to provide nurses with an understanding of the organizational elements of cultures and to provide effective nursing care.

cultural nursing assessment: a systematic way to identify the beliefs, values, meanings, and behaviors of people while considering their history, life experiences, and the social and physical environments in which they live.

cultural preservation: the use by clients of those aspects of their culture that promote healthy behaviors.

cultural repatterning: working with clients to make changes in health practices when the client's cultural behaviors are harmful or decrease their well-being.

cultural shock: the feeling of helplessness, discomfort, and disorientation experienced by an individual attempting to understand or effectively adapt to another cultural group that differs in practices, values, and beliefs. It results from the anxiety caused by losing familiar sights, sounds, and behaviors.

cultural skill: the effective integration of cultural knowledge and awareness to meet the needs of clients.

culture: the learned ways of behaving that are communicated by one group to another to provide tested solutions to vital problems.

environmental control: the ability of individuals to control nature and to influence factors in the environment that affect them.

ethnicity: shared feeling of peoplehood among a group of individuals.

ethnocentrism: belief that one's own group or culture is superior to others.

immigrants: people who come into a new country in order to settle there.

nonverbal communication: the use of body language or gestures to convey information that cannot or may not be indicated verbally.

prejudice: the emotional manifestation of deeply held beliefs about other groups; it involves negative attitudes.

race: a biological designation whereby group members share distinguishing features (e.g., skin color, bone structure, genetic traits such as blood groupings).

racism: a form of prejudice that refers to the belief that persons who are born into particular groups are inferior in intelligence, morals, beauty, and self-worth.

social organization: the way in which a cultural group structures itself around the family to carry out role functions.

space: the physical distance between individuals during an interaction.

stereotyping: the basis for ascribing certain beliefs and behaviors about a group to an individual without giving adequate attention to individual differences.

time: refers to past, present, and future times, as well as to the duration of and period between events. Some cultures assign greater or lesser value to events that occurred in the past, occur in the present, or will occur in the future.

verbal communication: the use of language in the form of words within a grammatical structure to express ideas and feelings and to describe objects.

Nurses have cared for culturally diverse groups since the beginning of the discipline. As early as 1893, nurses in New York City started public health nursing and provided home care to **immigrants,** particularly recent arrivals (Denker, 1994). When nurses were not from the same cultural background as the immigrants, they had to deal with the cultural differences between themselves and the persons in their care. Often the same situation still exists. That is, the nurse and client come from different cultural groups and may not recognize or understand their differences.

It is useful in talking about culture in this country to think back to the first wave of migration of people here, which took place from the 1680s to 1803. These first migrants were largely English-speaking white Protestants who thought of themselves as founders and settlers in a new country rather than as immigrants. The next wave was from the 1820s to the 1920s and was made up of immigrants who were different in color, language, place of origin, and religion. This group brought their own foreign cultures. At present, there is another increase in immigration. In 1995, there were 24 million foreign-born people in the United States, and of these, 30% were naturalized citizens, 47% were documented immigrants, and approximately 20% were undocumented immigrants. In 2005, the foreign-born population had increased to nearly 36 million with 35% naturalized citizens, 33% documented immigrants, and 31% undocumented immigrants (Center for

| Table 5-1 | **Immigrants by Country of Last Residence: 1961 to 2007 (numbers in thousands)** |

Region/Country of Last Residence	1961–1970	1971–1980	1981–1990	1991–2000	2001–2005	2006	2007
All countries	3321.7	4493.3	7388.1	9095.4	4914.1	1266.1	1052.405.8
Europe	1123.5	800.3	761.6	1359.7	768.1	422.3	120.8
Asia	427.6	1588.2	2738.2	2795.7	1635.1	422.3	383.5
Central America (excluding Mexico)	101.3	134.6	468.1	526.9	308.7	75.0	55.9
Mexico	453.9	640.3	1655.8	2249.4	873.9	173.8	148.6
Caribbean	470.2	741.1	872.0	978.8	456.7	146.8	119.1
South America	257.9	295.7	461.8	539.7	371.1	138.0	106.5
Africa	29.0	80.8	176.9	355.0	303.4	117.4	94.7
Canada	413.3	169.9	156.9	192.0	111.6	18.2	15.5
Oceania	25.1	41.2	45.2	55.8	31.4	7.4	6.1

From U.S. Department of Homeland Security, 2007 Yearbook of Immigration Statistics.Office of Immigration Statistics, Office of Management, Department of Homeland Security: *2003 Yearbook of immigration statistics,* Washington, DC, 2007, U.S. Government Printing Office.

American Progress, 2007). As of 2007, Hispanics made up the largest immigrant group in the United States. Specifically, 45.5 million, or 15.1%, of Americans were of Hispanic descent (U.S. Census Bureau, 2008). The current Hispanic wave differs from the two preceding ones. Latinos tend not to leave their culture behind. They also travel back to their homeland more often (Ledger, 2003). This wave is accompanied by a strong increase in Asians and a modest increase in Americans of African descent. These changes reflect a society that is becoming more diverse with regard to racial and ethnic groups. As a result, significant differences in beliefs about health and illness are becoming apparent among the various groups. Nurses who want to reflect their clients' beliefs of health and illness when intervening to promote and maintain wellness face many challenges.

This chapter discusses strategies to assist nurses in providing culturally competent care. The special concerns of immigrants are discussed and the following four groups are emphasized: African-Americans, Asians, Hispanics, and Native Americans.

IMMIGRANT HEALTH ISSUES

Recent changes in immigration laws have increased migration to the United States. The 1965 amendment of the Immigration and Nationality Act changed the quota system that discriminated against individuals from southern and eastern Europe. The Refugee Act of 1980 provided a uniform procedure for refugees (based on the United Nations definition) to be admitted to the United States (U.S. Census Bureau, 2001). This included refugees from Cuba, Vietnam, Laos, and Cambodia, as well as Russian Jewish refugees. The 1986 Immigration Reform and Control Act permitted illegal aliens already living in the United States to apply for legal status if they met certain requirements. People come to the United States for religious and political freedom and for economic opportunities. In 2007 the nation's immigrant population (legal and illegal) reached 37.9 million

(Camarota, 2007). Table 5-1 summarizes the immigration patterns of selected immigrants by country of origin for a 42-year period.

However, people in the United States are ambivalent in their attitudes and policies about immigrants. There is also some misunderstanding about what distinguishes an immigrant. The national debate about immigration policy has intensified since the events of September 11, 2001. More recently, many states have begun discussing whether nonlegal immigrants could work in the United States. The complex issues involved with immigrants and their health are beyond the scope of this discussion, but several are discussed and suggestions are made for nursing actions.

There are several categories of foreign-born persons. First are the *legal immigrants who are* also known as *lawful permanent residents.* These people are not citizens but they are by law allowed to both live and work in the United States, often because they have useful job skills or family ties. There has been a trend toward more immigrants being "low skill" workers, and they compete with native low skill workers for jobs. The argument has been made that low skill workers take jobs that other Americans and "lawful residents" do not want. Since 1997, immigrants must have lived in the United States for 10 years to be eligible for all entitlements, such as Aid to Families of Dependent Children, food stamps, Medicaid, and unemployment insurance (National Immigration Forum, 2005). The second category of foreign-born immigrants consists of refugees and people seeking asylum. Refugees are admitted outside the usual quota restrictions based on fear of persecution due to their race, religion, nationality, social group, or political views (Lipson and Dibble, 2005). These are people seeking protection because they fear harm if they return to their home country. A person who receives refugee status may receive Temporary Assistance for Needy Families, Supplemental Security Income, and Medicaid. The third category of foreign-born people are *nonimmigrants,* who are admitted to the United States for a limited duration of time and for a specific purpose. Examples include students, tourists, temporary workers, business executives, diplomats, artists, entertainers, and reporters. The fourth category consists of *unauthorized immigrants,* or undocumented or illegal aliens. They may have crossed a border into the United States illegally or their legal permission to stay may have expired. They are eligible only for emergency medical services, immunizations, treatment for the symptoms of communicable diseases, and access to school lunches. See *A Description of Immigrant Population Health* (Congress of the United States, 2004) for a description of immigrant populations and the benefits for which they are eligible. Huang, Yu, and Ledsky (2006), using the 1999 National Survey of America's Families, found that children from immigrant families used fewer health care resources and tended to be in worse physical health than nonimmigrant children.

There are several misperceptions about the economic value of allowing immigrants to enter or to stay in the United States. It is estimated that immigrants add about $10 billion to the economy annually, and that, in their lifetime in the United States, an immigrant family will pay $80,000 more in taxes than they consume in services (*Immigrants' Health Care Coverage and Access Fact Sheet,* 2001). This poses a dilemma for communities since these taxes are paid to the federal government while immigrants use services provided and paid for by states and localities. Despite the lack of federal matching funds for Medicaid for immigrants, some states, citing compelling public health reasons, use their own funds to cover groups such as children, pregnant women, the disabled, and older adults.

Carlock (2007) has compiled useful information on how to find and access information that is culturally suited to the nation's increasingly diverse population, including culturally and linguistically appropriate patient education. In addition to financial constraints on providing health care for immigrants, other factors need to be considered:

- Language barriers
- Differences in social, religious, and cultural backgrounds between the immigrant and the health care provider
- Providers' lack of knowledge about high-risk diseases in the specific immigrant groups for whom they care
- The fact that many immigrants rely on traditional healing or folk health care practices that may be unfamiliar to their U.S. health care providers

When working with immigrant populations, consider how your own background, beliefs, and knowledge may be significantly different from those of the people receiving care. *Language barriers* may interfere with efforts to provide assistance. Community members may be excellent resources as translators, not only of the actual words but also of the cultural beliefs, expectations, and use of nontraditional health practices.

The inability to speak English interferes with an immigrant's ability to access health care or even to seek health care (Steefel, 2007). Nurses need to know if there are *specific risk factors* for a given immigrant population. For example, Southeast Asians are often at risk for hepatitis B (with its attendant effects on the liver); tuberculosis; intestinal parasites; and visual, hearing, and dental problems. Most of these conditions are either preventable or treatable if managed correctly (Office of Minority Health, 2008).

Nurses need to understand the *nontraditional healing practices* that their clients use. Many of these treatments have proved effective and can be blended with traditional Western medicine. The key is to know what practices are being used so the blending can be knowledgeably done. Community members are excellent sources of this information, and nurses working with immigrant populations should use the community assessment, group work, and family techniques described in other chapters.

Often children and adolescents adjust to the new culture more easily than their elders. This can lead to *family conflict* and, at times, violence. Be alert for warning signs of family stress and tension. On the other hand, family members can help translate their culture, religion, beliefs, practices, support systems, and risk factors for the health care provider. They can also assist with decision making and provide support to enable the person or group seeking care to change behaviors to become more health conscious. Nurses need to understand the role of the family in immigrant populations and to treat individuals in the context of the families from which the immigrants come.

Similarly, the community plays a key role in the care of immigrants. Community members can help both clients and providers with communication, explanation, crisis intervention, emotional and other forms of support, and housing. Be sure to carefully assess the community and learn what strengths, resources, and talents are available. Horowitz (1998) has identified the following six steps that clinicians can take to more effectively work with immigrant populations:

1. Know yourself: providers, like clients, are influenced by culture, values, and language.
2. Get to know the families and their health-seeking behaviors. You might try using a simple genogram, which places family members on a diagram. Ask who the family members are, where they live, and who is missing or dead. You might also ask them to talk about holidays: who comes, who is missing, what do they do?
3. Get to know the communities common to your setting: read about them, take a course, get involved (e.g., volunteer to give talks), hold forums with free-flowing and two-way communication, and learn who the formal and informal resources are.
4. Get to know some of the traditional practices and remedies used by families and communities so you can work with, not against, them.
5. Learn how a community deals with common illnesses or events.
6. Try to see things from the viewpoint of the patient, family, or community.

Special note should be made about refugees. Unlike many of the immigrants, refugees may have left their homes as a result of a disaster and this might have led to physical or psychological consequences. Some may have been tortured; others may have lost family members in horrible ways. Still others may have lived in camps and lost all or most of their personal possessions. Some will have come from poor countries, and much of American culture will be alien to them. Sensitivity on the part of the nurse is essential as well as skill in finding resources to both help understand them and their needs and then meet those needs (Plumb, 2003).

BRIEFLY NOTED

Definitions for *immigrant* differ, and immigrants may be legal or illegal. They come from all parts of the world and bring with them unique cultural, health care, and religious backgrounds.

- Access to health care may be limited because of immigrants' lack of benefits, resources, language ability, and transportation.
- Nurses need to be astute in considering the cultural backgrounds of their immigrant clients and populations. Often, the family and community must be relied on to provide information, support, and other aid.
- Nurses need to know the major health problems and risk factors that are specific to immigrant populations.

CULTURE, RACE, AND ETHNICITY

The concepts of culture, race, and ethnicity influence our understanding of human behavior. These three terms are often used incorrectly. Nurses need to understand the meaning of each when providing culturally competent health care to clients of diverse cultures.

CULTURE

Culture is a set of beliefs, values, and assumptions about life that is widely held among a group of people and that is transmitted across generations (Leininger, 2002a). Burchum (2002) defines culture as a learned world view "shared by a population or group and transmitted socially that influences values, beliefs, customs, and behaviors, and is reflected in the language, dress, food, materials, and social institutions of a group" (p. 7).

Culture develops over time and is resistant to change. It takes many years for individuals to become familiar enough with a new value for it to become part of their culture. In response to the needs of its members and their environment, culture provides tested solutions to life's problems.

Individuals learn about their culture during the processes of learning language and becoming socialized, usually as children. Parents and family, the most important sources for the transfer of traditions, teach both explicit and implicit behaviors of the culture. The explicit behaviors, such as language, interpersonal distance, and kissing in public, can be observed and allow the individual to identify with other persons of the culture. In this way, people share traditions, customs, and lifestyles with others. The implicit behaviors are less visible and include the way individuals perceive health and illness, body language, difference in language

---

Box 5-1 Factors Influencing Individual Differences Within Cultural Groups

- Age
- Religion
- Dialect and language spoken
- Gender identity roles
- Socioeconomic background
- Geographic location in the country of origin
- Geographic location in the current country
- History of the subcultural group with which clients identify in their current country of residence
- History of the subcultural group with which clients identify in their country of origin
- Amount of interaction between older and younger generations
- Degree of assimilation in the current country of residence
- Immigration status*
- Conditions under which migration occurred*

Except where noted with an asterisk (*) from Orque M: Orque's ethnic/cultural system: a framework for ethnic nursing care. In Orque MS, Bloch B, Monrroy LSA, editors: *Ethnic nursing care: a multicultural approach*, St. Louis, 1983, Mosby.

---

expressions, and the use of titles. These behaviors are subtle and may be difficult for persons to state, yet they are very much a part of the culture. For example, deferring to older adults, standing when they enter the room, or offering them a seat suggests a cultural value related to older adults.

Another example of an implicit aspect of culture is the use of language to communicate. For instance, in one culture a sign might read "No smoking is permitted." In another culture the sign might read "Thank you for not smoking." The former statement represents a culture that values directness, whereas the latter values indirectness. Each culture has an organizational structure that distinguishes it from others and provides the structure for what members of the cultural group determine to be appropriate or inappropriate behavior. The organizational elements of cultures have been described by Andrews and Boyle (2007), Giger and Davidhizar (2004), Leininger (2002b), Purnell and Paulanka (2008), and Spector (2008). These elements include child-rearing practices, religious practices, family structure, space, and communication. In the case of language, there are characteristic expressions unique to each language. Nurses need to know these organizational elements to provide appropriate care to persons of diverse cultures. This does not mean, however, that you should overlook or fail to incorporate the individuality of any person within any culture when developing a plan of care. Just as all cultures are not alike, all individuals within a culture are not alike. Each person should be viewed as a unique human being with differences that are respected. Box 5-1 lists factors that may contribute to individual differences within cultures. For example, for some native Koreans going to a physician is a last resort. At The Johns Hopkins University School of Nursing researchers are promoting principles of "co-learning," in which both the investigators and clients are learning from one another in an effort to remove the stigma attached to having cancer and to encourage people to talk about the illness. Specifically, a man might decline to marry a woman if her parent was a cancer survivor, thinking that she may have inherited an inferior gene. Likewise, mental health carries a stigma (Steefel, 2007).

RACE

Race is primarily a social classification that relies on physical markers such as skin color to identify group membership (Bhopal and Donaldson, 1998). Individuals may be of the same race but of different cultures. For example, African-Americans, who may have been born in Africa, the Caribbean, North America, or elsewhere, are a heterogeneous group, but they are often viewed as culturally and racially homogeneous. This perception can cause providers to be unaware of cultural differences among individuals who come from different countries but who share similar racial characteristics. This often blurs an understanding of this culturally diverse group.

It is important to understand the growing numbers of interracial families. Physical changes in biracial and multiracial generations lead to changes in physical appearances of individuals and make race less important in ethnic identity. In the United States, children of biracial parents are assigned the race of the mother.

ETHNICITY

Ethnicity is the shared feeling of peoplehood among a group of individuals (Giger and Davidhizar, 2004). It reflects cultural membership and is based on individuals sharing similar cultural patterns (e.g., beliefs, values, customs, behaviors, traditions) that, over time, create a common history that is resistant to change. Ethnicity represents the identifying characteristics of culture (e.g., race, religion, national origin). It is influenced by education, income level, geographic location, and association with people from other ethnic groups. Therefore, a reciprocal relationship exists between the individual and society. Members of an ethnic group give up aspects of their identity and society when they adopt characteristics of the group's identity. However, when the ethnic identity is strong, the group maintains its values, beliefs, behaviors, practices, and ways of thinking.

CULTURAL COMPETENCE

Many people are taught by and have knowledge of a dominant culture. As long as the person operates within that culture, responses occur without thought to a variety of situations and do not require examination of the cultural context. However, in today's climate of multiculturalism, there is increasing emphasis from health care providers and organizations for nurses to provide quality and effective care. For example, a recent Mexican immigrant who speaks little English goes to a community health center because of a urinary infection. The nurse understands that she must use strategies that would allow her to effectively communicate with the client; the client has the right to receive effective care, to judge whether she had received the care she wanted, and to follow up with appropriate action if she did not receive the expected care. Culturally competent care is provided not only to individuals of racial or ethnic minority groups but also to individuals belonging to groups held together by factors such as age, religion, sexual orientation, and socioeconomic status. Nurses must be culturally competent to provide nursing care that meets the needs of these persons.

Cultural competence in nurses is a combination of culturally congruent behaviors, practice attitudes, and policies that allow nurses to work effectively in cross-cultural situations. The term *competence* refers to performance that is sufficient and adequate. Culturally competent nurses function effectively when caring for clients of other cultures. Nurses who strive to be culturally competent respect people from other cultures and value diversity; this helps them to provide more responsive care (Suh, 2004). Cultural competence includes acknowledging the fundamental differences in the ways clients and families respond to illness and treatment from what might be your response or a more typical Western health care response (Dreher and MacNaughton, 2002). This can include paying attention to dietary practices, pain, death and dying, modesty, eye contact, closeness, and touching others.

BRIEFLY NOTED

Standards for transcultural nursing have been developed to guide nurses in delivering culturally competent nursing care. The standards are available for all professional nurses to use as a basis for documenting, describing, teaching, and evaluating culturally competent care (Leininger, 2002b).

Culturally competent nursing care is guided by the following four principles (American Academy of Nursing Expert Panel Report, 1992):
1. Care is designed for the specific client.
2. Care is based on the uniqueness of the person's culture and includes cultural norms and values.
3. Care includes self-empowerment strategies to facilitate client decision making in health behavior.
4. Care is provided with sensitivity and is based on the cultural uniqueness of clients.

Nurses must be culturally competent for a number of key reasons:
- First, the nurse's culture often differs from that of the client, leading to different understandings of communication, behaviors, and plans for care.
- Second, care that is not culturally competent may increase the cost of health care and decrease the opportunity for positive client outcomes. Clients who do not feel understood may delay seeking care or may withhold key information. For example, for fear of disapproval, a person may not tell the nurse that he is using folk medicine as well as Western medicine. The two medicines may have cumulative effects that could be dangerous to the client.

Table 5-2	The Cultural Competence Framework: Stages of Competence Development		
	Culturally Incompetent	**Culturally Sensitive**	**Culturally Competent**
Cognitive dimension	Oblivious	Aware	Knowledgeable
Affective dimension	Apathetic	Sympathetic	Committed to change
Skills dimension	Unskilled	Lacking some skills	Highly skilled
Overall effect	Destructive	Neutral	Constructive

From Orlandi MA: Defining cultural competence: an organizing framework. In Orlandi MA, editor: *Cultural competence for evaluators,* Washington, DC, 1992, U.S. Department of Health and Human Services.

• Third, to meet some of the objectives for persons of different cultures as outlined in *Healthy People 2010* (see the *"Healthy People 2010"* box) (U.S. Department of Health and Human Services, 2000), lifestyle and personal choices must be considered. For example, in the U.S. health care system excessive drinking is seen as a sign of disease and alcoholism is considered a mental illness. However, in the Native American culture, this would signify a disharmony between the individual and the spirit world, and biomedical interventions alone may not be adequate to reduce alcoholism within this culture. Many Native Americans view alcohol consumption as an acceptable way to participate in family celebrations and tribal ceremonies (Orlandi, 1992), and refusal to drink with the family may be viewed as a sign of rejection. The second goal of *Healthy People 2010* deals with eliminating health disparities among people that occur due to gender, race or ethnicity, education or income, disability, geographic location, or sexual orientation. Diabetes is discussed in this context since its prevalence is associated with disparities of income and education and it is more prevalent among Hispanics living in the United States than among non-Hispanic whites. Diabetes is higher in American Indians and Alaska Natives than among whites, thereby demonstrating the need to look at culture when working with these populations.

DEVELOPING CULTURAL COMPETENCE

Developing cultural competence is an ongoing life process that involves every aspect of client care. It is challenging and at times painful as nurses struggle to adopt new ways of thinking and performing. Leininger (2002a) suggests that the following two principles are useful in developing cultural competence:
1. Maintain a broad, objective, and open attitude toward individuals and their cultures.
2. Avoid seeing all individuals as alike.

Nurses develop cultural competence in different ways, but the key elements are experience with clients of other cultures, an awareness of this experience, and the promotion of mutual respect for differences. Because degrees of cultural competence vary, not all nurses may reach the same level of development.

Orlandi (1992) suggests that there are three stages in the development of cultural competence: culturally incompetent, culturally sensitive, and culturally competent (Table 5-2).

Healthy People 2010

Objectives Related to Cultural Issues
Goal:
To eliminate health disparities among different segments of the population as defined by gender, race or ethnicity, education, income, disability, living in rural areas, and sexual orientation.

Objectives:
• Increase the proportion of persons with health insurance.
• Increase the proportion of insured persons with clinical preventive services coverage.
• Increase the proportion of persons who have a specific source of ongoing care.
• Increase the proportion of persons with a usual primary care provider.
• Reduce the proportion of families that experiences difficulties or delays in obtaining health care for one or more family members.
• Increase the proportion of all degrees awarded in the health professions to members of underrepresented racial and ethnic groups.

From U.S. Department of Health and Human Services: *Healthy People 2010: understanding and improving health,* ed 2, Washington, DC, 2000, U.S. Government Printing Office.

Each stage has three dimensions—cognitive (thinking), affective (feeling), and psychomotor (doing)—that together have an overall effect on nursing care.

Burchum (2002) used the method of concept analysis to identify the key attributes of cultural competence. The attributes form the meaning of the concept. The following six attributes were most frequently found in her review of the concept of cultural competence:
1. Cultural awareness
2. Cultural knowledge
3. Cultural understanding
4. Cultural sensitivity
5. Cultural interaction
6. Cultural skill

Table 5-3 presents the attributes and dimensions of cultural competence in a clear and easy-to-understand way.

Similarly, Campinha-Bacote (2002) describes five constructs that explain the process of developing cultural competence:
1. Cultural awareness
2. Cultural knowledge

Table 5-3	**Attributes and Dimensions of Culture**

Attributes	Dimensions
Cultural awareness	• Understand your own culture • Know your ethnocentric views, biases, and prejudices • Be aware of similarities and differences between and among cultures
Cultural knowledge	• Know about cultures other than your own • Be able to recognize differences in communication styles and etiquette between and among cultures • Acquire familiarity with conceptual and theoretical frameworks
Cultural understanding	• Understand that "Western medicine" does not have all the answers • Recognize how culture shapes our beliefs, values, and behavior • To avoid stereotyping, be aware that there are racial, ethnic, and cultural variations • Understand the concerns and issues that occur when your values, beliefs, and practices differ from those of the dominant culture • Know that marginalization influences patterns of seeking care
Cultural sensitivity	• Appreciate and respect your individual client's beliefs and values • Appreciate and value diversity • Appreciate and genuinely care about those of other cultures • Recognize how your own cultural background may influence professional practice
Cultural interaction	• Interact with those of other cultures • Engage in practice with those of other cultures
Cultural skill	• Perform cultural assessments that consider beliefs and values, family roles, health practices, and the meanings of health and illness • Perform physical assessments that incorporate knowledge of racial variations • Be sure to communicate, either personally or through appropriate use of interpreters and other resources, in a manner that is understood and that effectively responds to those who speak other languages • Make sure your nonverbal communication techniques take into consideration the client's use of eye contact, facial expressions, body language, touch, and space • Know how to provide care that incorporates the development of a respectful and therapeutic alliance with the client • Provide care that overcomes biases and is modified to respect and accommodate the values, beliefs, and practices of the client without compromising your own values • Provide care that is beneficial, safe, and satisfying to your client • Know how to provide care that elicits a feeling by the client of being welcome, understood, important, and comfortable • Provide care that addresses disadvantages arising from the client's position in relation to networks • Use self-empowerment strategies in your client care
Cultural proficiency	• Add new knowledge by conducting research, by developing new culturally sensitive therapeutic approaches, and by delivering this information to others • Evidence a commitment to change

Modified from Burchum JL: Cultural competence: an evolutionary perspective, *Nurs Forum* 37(4):5–15, 2002.

3. Cultural skill
4. Cultural encounter
5. Cultural desire

There is strong congruence between the works of Burchum and Campinha-Bacote.

Cultural Awareness

Cultural awareness is the self-examination and in-depth exploration of one's own beliefs and values as they influence behavior (Campinha-Bacote, 2002). Nurses who have developed cultural awareness are:

• Receptive to learning about the cultural dimensions of the client.
• Able to understand the basis for their own behavior and how it helps or hinders the delivery of competent care to persons from cultures other than their own (American Academy of Nursing Expert Panel Report, 1992).

• Able to recognize that health is expressed differently across cultures and that culture influences an individual's responses to health, illness, disease, and death.

For example, at a community outreach program, a nurse was teaching a racially mixed group the screening protocol for the detection of breast and cervical cancer. An African-American woman in the group refused to give the return demonstration for breast self-examination. When encouraged to do so, she said, "My breasts are much larger than those on the model. Besides, the models are not like me. They are all white." After hearing the client's comments, the nurse realized that she had made no reference in her talk to the influence of culture or race on screening for breast and cervical cancer.

The nurse talked with the client, asked for her recommendations, and encouraged her to return to the demonstration. The nurse coached the client through the self-examination

Box 5-2 Early Cultural Awareness

- Think about the first time you had contact with someone you realized was culturally different from you.
- Briefly describe the situation and/or the event. How old were you? What were your feelings? What were your thoughts?
- What did your parents and other significant adults say about those who were culturally different from your family? What adjectives were used? What attitudes were conveyed?
- As you got older, what messages did you get about minority groups from the larger community or culture?
- As an adult, how do you see others in the community talk about culturally different people? What adjectives are used? What attitudes are conveyed? How does this reinforce or contradict your earlier experience?
- What parts of this cultural baggage make it difficult to work with clients from different cultural groups?
- What parts of this cultural baggage facilitate your work with clients?

From Randall-David E: *Culturally competent HIV counseling and education*, McLean, Va, 1994, Maternal and Child Health Clearinghouse.

process while pointing out that regardless of breast size, shape, and color, the technique is the same for feeling the tissue and squeezing the nipple to make certain that there is no discharge. Because this nurse was culturally aware, she neither became angry with herself or the client nor imposed her own values on the client. Rather, the client talked about her beliefs, attitudes, and feelings about screening for cancer that may be influenced by her culture. Subsequently, the nurse purchased a model of an African-American woman's breast to be used in future health education programs with African-American women. If the nurse had not been culturally aware, she might have misunderstood the client's concerns and acted in a defensive manner. This may have led to lack of information being provided or a confrontation between the nurse and client.

Box 5-2 lists several factors that can guide nurses to understand their own culture and the implications of their cultural values.

Cultural Knowledge

Cultural knowledge is information about organizational elements of diverse cultures and ethnic groups. Emphasis is on learning about the clients' worldview from an emic (native) perspective. An understanding of the client's culture decreases misinterpretations and misapplication of scientific knowledge and facilitates the client's cooperation with the health care regimen (Campinha-Bacote, 2002; Leininger, 2002a). Leininger points out that nurses who lack cultural knowledge may develop feelings of inadequacy and helplessness because they are often unable to effectively help their clients. Studies have shown that when students are not exposed to a variety of cultures, they may have gaps in their cultural knowledge and ability to care for diverse clients (Jones, Cason, and Bond, 2004). Although it is unrealistic to expect that nurses will have knowledge of all cultures, they

should be aware of and know how to obtain knowledge of cultural influences that affect groups with whom they most frequently interact.

Cultural Skill

Cultural skill refers to the effective integration of cultural awareness and cultural knowledge to obtain relevant cultural data and meet the needs of culturally diverse clients. Culturally skillful nurses use appropriate touch during conversation, modify the physical distance between themselves and others, and use strategies to avoid cultural misunderstandings while meeting mutually agreed-upon goals.

Cultural Encounter

A cultural encounter is the fourth construct essential to becoming culturally competent. **Cultural encounter** is the process that permits nurses to seek opportunities to engage in cross-cultural interactions (Munoz and Luckmann, 2005). The most important ones are those in which nurses engage in effective communication, use appropriate language and literacy level, and learn directly from clients about their life experiences and the significance of these experiences for health (Leininger, 2002a).

BRIEFLY NOTED

Nurses can help clients who come from different cultures as they attempt to recover from similar illnesses. Through educational groups, the clients from different cultures can learn from one another new survival strategies and a variety of ways to relate to families, community, and workplace.

In some communities, nurses may have few opportunities to develop cultural competence by working directly with persons of other cultures. When nurses come into contact with persons who are culturally different from themselves, they should adapt general cultural concepts to the situation until they are able to learn directly from the clients about their culture (Figure 5-1). Nurses can develop cultural competence by reading about, taking courses on, and discussing different cultures within multicultural settings.

A successful encounter may be judged on the basis of the following four aspects (Brislin, 1993):
1. The nurse feels successful about the relationship with the client.
2. The client feels that interactions are warm, cordial, respectful, and cooperative.
3. Tasks are done efficiently.
4. The nurse and client experience little or no stress.

Cultural Desire

Cultural desire is the fifth construct in the development of cultural competence. It refers to the nurse's intrinsic motivation to provide culturally competent care (Campinha-Bacote, 2002). Nurses who desire to become culturally competent do so because they want to rather than because they are directed

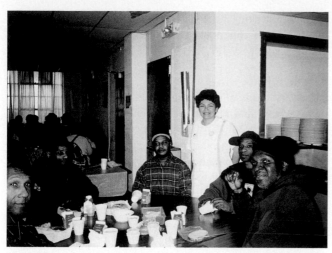

FIGURE 5-1 An Hispanic nursing student interacting with African-American men at a nutrition center. To interact in a culturally competent manner, the student needs to have an awareness of and knowledge about the differences between her culture and the men's culture and the skill to portray this in her behavior toward them.

to do so. They are energetic, enthusiastic, and goal directed in providing culturally competent care. Unlike the other constructs, cultural desire cannot be directly taught in the classroom or other educational settings. However, nurses are more likely to demonstrate cultural desire when their work environment reflects a philosophy that values cultural competence at all levels of the organization and for all its clients. Campinha-Bacote (1998) cautions nurses not to be afraid of making mistakes, and she provides a list of nine do's and six don'ts that could be helpful as they undertake the journey toward cultural competency. For example, Campinha-Bacote (1998) encourages nurses to develop a culture habit or desire to want to build relationships with people of other cultures. She also suggests that we not assume that people who look and act like us are culturally the same.

DIMENSIONS OF CULTURAL COMPETENCE

Nurses integrate their professional knowledge with the client's knowledge and practices to negotiate and promote culturally relevant care. Leininger (2002a) suggests the following three modes of action, based on negotiation between the client and nurse, that guide the nurse to deliver culturally competent care: cultural preservation, cultural accommodation, and cultural repatterning. When these decisions and actions are used with cultural brokering, the nurse is able to fulfill the various roles vital to providing holistic care for culturally diverse clients.

Cultural Preservation
Cultural preservation means that the nurse supports and facilitates the use of scientifically supported cultural practices, such as acupuncture and acupressure, together with interventions from the biomedical health care system. Acupuncture is an ancient Chinese practice of inserting needles at specific points in the skin to cure disease or relieve pain.

These practices are being accepted by increasing numbers of Western practitioners as a legitimate method of health care.

For example, Ms. Lin, a 73-year-old Chinese woman, is discharged to home care after surgery for cancer of the large intestine. The nurse found her at home alone with her 76-year-old husband. After the physical assessment, the nurse discussed making a referral for Ms. Lin to have a home health aide to assist her with physical care and light housekeeping chores. The family was gracious but seemed hesitant to accept the referral. The nurse knew that Chinese people often value the extended family network and family decision making. She asked the couple if they would like to discuss the situation with their daughters. Both the client and her husband seemed pleased with the idea, and the nurse promised to return the next day. When the nurse returned for her visit, one of Ms. Lin's daughters was present and told the nurse that the family could manage without additional help. The three daughters had made a schedule to take turns caring for their parents. The nurse accepted and supported the family's decision and told them that if they decided at a later time to have the home health aide, they should call the agency, and she gave them the telephone number. She then scheduled the next follow-up visit with them.

Cultural Accommodation
Cultural accommodation means that the nurse supports and facilitates the use of cultural practices, such as home burial of the placenta (Helsel and Mochel, 2002), when such cultural practices are not harmful to clients. For example, the delivery nurse was helpful when Ms. Sanchez asked her not to discard a piece of the amniotic sac that was present on her grandbaby's face immediately after birth. Ms. Sanchez asked the nurse to give it to her instead. The grandmother believed that being born with a piece of the amniotic sac on the face was a visible sign that something special was going to happen in the person's life. The grandmother explained that after she dried the piece of the amniotic sac, she would keep it in a safe place. She would also spend extra time protecting the baby to prevent her from being harmed. Although the delivery room nurse did not know about this practice, she gave the grandmother the piece of the sac as she requested. As another example, using cultural accommodation, nurses can assist older Chinese clients to more effectively manage their hypertension by modifying their use of high sodium soy sauce by substituting low sodium soy sauce in their cooking. Similarly, African-Americans can be guided to use more broiled and boiled foods and eat fewer fried foods.

Cultural Repatterning
Cultural repatterning means that the nurse works with clients to help them reorder, change, or modify their cultural practices when these practices are harmful to them. For example, a culturally competent nurse knows of the high incidence of obesity among Mexican-American women 20 years of age and older. A school nurse was invited to develop a health education program for Mexican teenagers in the local high school. While respecting their cultural traditions, the

Evidence-Based Practice

From 1995 to 1999, a research team in Philadelphia sought to determine the epidemiology of type 1 diabetes in children aged 0–14 years. To conduct the study, the team examined records obtained from hospitals regarding newly diagnosed patients and those diagnosed from January 1995 to December 1999. Additional records from school nurses working for the School District of Philadelphia were reviewed in the study.

Two hundred and thirty-four subjects were included in the study, with an average age of 14.8 years. In white and Hispanic children, incidence rates for type 1 diabetes remained relatively stable, continuing a 15-year trend; however, the incidence of the disease in the Hispanic population remains the highest in any racial group in the United States for children aged 0–14 years. In black children, the team found an alarming increase in those diagnosed with type 1 diabetes. The findings stated that the incidence of the disease has increased dramatically to 64% in black children aged 5–9 years, which is the highest increase ever reported in children in this age group, and to 37% in black children aged 10–14 years.

The researchers called the risk of type 1 diabetes for black children "a tremendous public health problem" because of the racial disparities existent in the treatment of children with type 1 diabetes (Lipman et al., 2006, p. 2394). Previous studies have found poor metabolic control in children with the disease and a significantly higher mortality rate for black diabetics, both of which add to the complexity of the problem.

NURSE USE: As the incidence of type 1 diabetes increases in the black population, the development of culturally relevant interventions are crucial in order to minimize racial disparities in treatment and outcomes. Additionally, greater efforts are needed in the epidemiology of diabetes to clarify the causes of epidemics and to uncover trends occurring in populations worldwide. Finally, the researchers state that type 1 diabetes should be declared a reportable disease so that genetic and environmental risk factors can be defined and thoroughly explored.

Data from Lipman TH et al: Incidence of type 1 diabetes in Philadelphia is higher in black than white children from 1995 to 1999: epidemic or misclassification? *Diabetes Care* 11(29):2391–2395, 2006.

nurse discussed weight management strategies with the teenagers. The nurse understood the teenagers' cultural issues pertaining to food and knew how to negotiate with them. She discouraged the use of fried foods (such as tortillas), sour cream, and regular cheese and encouraged and demonstrated the use of baked tortillas and salsa as dip and topping.

In another example, a nurse who has been giving prenatal instructions to pregnant Haitian women discovered that many of them were visiting an herbalist to obtain teas that would contribute to their having a "strong baby." The nurse asked for the names of the herbs in the teas that they were drinking and scheduled a conference with the pharmacist to discuss the specific ingredients in the herbs and ways that they might help the client meet her cultural needs. The nurse found that one of the herbs contributed to high blood pressure, a problem that many of the women were experiencing. She explained to the women why they should not drink the tea with the specific herb. The nurse sought

cooperation from the herbalist because she understood the importance of supernatural causes of illness in the Haitian culture (Miller, 2000).

Cultural Brokering

Culturally competent nurses use cultural brokering to make certain that clients receive culturally competent care (Leininger, 2002a). **Cultural brokering** is advocating, mediating, negotiating, and intervening between the client's culture and the biomedical health care culture on behalf of clients. It is important to understand both cultures and to resolve or decrease problems that result from individuals in either culture not understanding the other person's values. To illustrate, migrant workers tend to have high occupational mobility; many are poor and have limited formal education. They may seek health care only when they are ill and cannot work. Whenever a nurse interacts with them, it is important to teach them about prevention, health maintenance, environmental sanitation, and nutrition, because it may be the only opportunity that the nurse will ever have to treat a particular migrant worker. Nurses should also advocate for the rights of the migrant worker to receive quality health care. For example, the nurse may contact the migrant health services for follow-up or referral care for the migrant worker.

INHIBITORS TO DEVELOPING CULTURAL COMPETENCE

Nurses may fail to provide culturally competent nursing care if they do not understand transcultural nursing, their supervisors are pressuring them to increase productivity by increasing their case loads, or they are pressured by colleagues who are not knowledgeable about other cultures and who are offended when others use these concepts. These and similar issues can inhibit delivery of culturally competent care and may result in nurse behaviors such as stereotyping, prejudice and racism, ethnocentrism, cultural imposition, cultural conflict, and cultural shock.

- **Stereotyping** means attributing certain beliefs and behaviors about a group to an individual without giving adequate attention to individual differences. An example of a stereotype is "All Asian people are hard-working."
- **Prejudice** refers to having a deeply held reaction, often negative, about another group or person. For example, a person may be viewed negatively because of skin color, race, religion, or social standing with no regard for the worth of the person as an individual.
- **Racism** is a form of prejudice and refers to the belief that persons who are born into a particular group are inferior, for example, in intelligence, morals, beauty, or self-worth (Brislin, 1993). See Box 5-3 for examples of prejudice and racist behaviors.
- **Ethnocentrism,** a type of cultural prejudice at the population level, is the belief that one's own group determines the standards for behavior by which all other groups are to be judged. Ethnocentric nurses are unfamiliar and uncomfortable with anything that is different from their culture. Some

Box 5-3	**Types of Prejudice and Racist Behaviors**

Overt Intentional Prejudice/Racism

Two homeless women, one African-American and the other Irish, are clients at the neighborhood health care center. Both women are having financial difficulty. The African-American client's husband was laid off 4 years ago after his company merged with another company. The Irish client is undergoing radiation treatment for metastatic cancer and has lost her job as a result of her prolonged illness. Both women are without health insurance. A nurse referred the Irish client to social services but did not refer the African-American woman. The nurse believed that minority clients have direct experience with some local and national government programs. Therefore these clients know about available resources and can negotiate the social system for themselves and their family. In contrast, the nurse believed that the Irish woman had a catastrophic illness, she had no experience negotiating government programs, and therefore the nurse needs to advocate for her. The nurse, not knowing the health-seeking behaviors of either client, stereotyped both women and intentionally used her informational power to help one client while denying assistance to the other client.

Overt Unintentional Prejudice/Racism

A nurse was assigned to make an initial visit to two clients recently discharged from the hospital with a diagnosis of hypertension. The nurse performed physical assessments on both clients. He developed an extensive culturally relevant teaching plan with the Filipino client that included information on sodium restriction and the effect on kidney functioning, ways to integrate cultural foods into the diet, and support in lifestyle changes. With the Puerto Rican client, the nurse performed a routine physical assessment and did not discuss the client's culturally special dietary requirements. The nurse believed that the Puerto Rican client was not capable of understanding such complex information and was going to continue to seek help from her *curandera* (a folk practitioner) to manage the hypertension.

At the end of his visit, the nurse said to this client, "Take care of yourself. See you next time." This nurse did not realize that he had stereotyped the client and that his actions were hurtful. He believed that he was providing quality care on the basis of the client's needs.

Covert Intentional Prejudice/Racism

A Native American nurse works in a home health agency that serves an ethnically diverse community. The nurse has observed that the clients are always among the poorest and live in the unsafe areas of the community, and she is very concerned about her client care assignment. Her nonminority colleagues are not assigned to those sections of the community. In a recent staff meeting, she raised the concerns with her nursing supervisors. On hearing her observations, the supervisors looked at her in a skeptical manner and asked what she was talking about. This is covert racism because the nursing supervisors were aware of the informal policy dictating that they assign minority nurses to clients in a particular area of the community. They had discussed the practice among themselves but would never admit to it. The supervisors believed that the best way to ensure that minority clients would be the recipients of culturally competent care was to assign a minority nurse to care for them.

Covert Unintentional Prejudice/Racism

A lesbian middle-class couple legally adopted a physically challenged child. Their insurance refuses to pay for the child's medical care. The nurse, who has been working for the agency for many years, is aware but failed to tell the parents that the baby can qualify for Medicaid through the handicapped insurance program, even though both parents work and their income is above the Medicaid guidelines limit. This nurse was unaware that her dislike for the parent's sexual lifestyle influenced her thinking (she had in the past provided heterosexual couples with information on how to apply for Medicaid).

American nurses may think that the way we do it is the best (or only) way to provide this care (Sutherland, 2002).

- **Cultural blindness** is the tendency to ignore all differences among cultures, to act as though these differences do not exist, and as a result to treat all people the same (when in truth each person is an individual with unique needs).
- **Cultural imposition** is the process of imposing one's values on others. Nurses impose their values on clients when they forcefully promote Western medical traditions while ignoring the clients' value of non-Western treatments such as acupuncture, herbal therapy, or spiritual remedies.
- **Cultural conflict** is a perceived threat that may arise from a misunderstanding of expectations between clients and nurses when either group is not aware of cultural differences (Andrews and Boyle, 2007).
- **Cultural shock** is the feeling of helplessness, discomfort, and disorientation experienced by an individual attempting to understand or effectively adapt to another cultural group that differs in practices, values, and beliefs. It results from the anxiety caused by losing familiar sights, sounds, and behaviors.

BRIEFLY NOTED

Being aware of the clients' cultural beliefs and knowing about other cultures may help nurses to be less judgmental, more accepting of cultural differences, and less likely to engage in the behaviors just listed that inhibit cultural competence.

CULTURAL NURSING ASSESSMENT

A **cultural nursing assessment** is a systematic way to identify the beliefs, values, meanings, and behaviors of people while considering their history, life experiences, and the social and physical environments in which they live.

Skills such as listening, explaining, acknowledging, recommending, understanding, and negotiating help the nurse to be nonjudgmental. It is vital that nurses listen to clients' perceptions of their problems and, in turn, that nurses explain to clients the nurses' perceptions of the problems. Nurses and clients should acknowledge and discuss similarities and differences between the two perceptions to develop suggestions and recommendations for managing problems. Nurses also negotiate with clients on nursing care actions to meet the needs of the clients.

Many tools are available to assist nurses in conducting cultural assessments (Andrews and Boyle, 2007; Leininger, 2002b; Tripp-Reimer et al., 1997). The focus of such tools varies, and selection is determined by the dimensions of culture to be assessed.

During initial contacts with clients, nurses should perform a cultural assessment that may be brief or may be just the beginning of an in-depth assessment (Tripp-Reimer et al., 1997). In a brief cultural assessment, nurses ask clients about the following issues:

- Ethnic background
- Religious preference
- Family patterns
- Food patterns
- Health practices

Such basic data help nurses understand the client from the client's point of view and recognize what is unique about the person, thus avoiding stereotyping. Data from a brief assessment help determine the need for an in-depth cultural assessment. An in-depth cultural assessment should be conducted over a period of time and should not be restricted to the first encounter with the client. This gives both clients and nurses time to get to know each other and gives clients a chance to see nurses in helping relationships. Tripp-Reimer et al (1997) suggest that an in-depth cultural assessment should be conducted in two phases: a data-collecting phase and an organizing phase. The data collection phase consists of the following three steps:

1. The nurse collects self-identifying data similar to what was collected in the brief assessment.
2. The nurse raises a variety of questions that seek information on clients' perception of what brings them to the health care system, the illness, and previous and anticipated treatments.
3. After the nursing diagnosis is made, the nurse identifies cultural factors that may influence the effectiveness of nursing care actions.

In the organization phase, data related to the client's and family's views on optimal treatment choices are routinely examined and areas of difference between the client's cultural needs and the goals of Western medicine are identified. (See Appendix B.2 for the Cultural Assessment Guide.)

The key to a successful cultural assessment lies in nurses being aware of their own culture. Randall-David (1989) developed a variety of principles that may be helpful as nurses conduct cultural assessments. Nurses should do the following:

1. *Be aware of the environment.* Look around and listen to what is being said and understand nonverbal communications before taking action.
2. *Know about community social organizations* such as schools, churches, hospitals, tribal councils, restaurants, taverns, and bars.

3. *Know the specific areas on which the nurse wants to focus* before beginning the cultural assessment.
4. *Select a strategy to help gather cultural data.* Strategies may include in-depth interviews, informal conversations, observations of everyday activities or specific events in the life of the client, survey research, and a case method approach to study certain aspects of a client.
5. *Identify a confidante* who will help "bridge the gap" between cultures.
6. *Know the appropriate questions* to ask without offending the client.
7. *Interview other nurses or health care professionals* who have worked with the client to get their input.
8. *Talk with formal and informal cultural leaders* to gain a comprehensive understanding about significant aspects of community life.
9. *Be aware that all information has both subjective and objective data,* and verify and cross-check the information that is collected before acting on it.
10. *Avoid pitfalls* in making premature generalizations.
11. *Be sincere, open, and honest* with yourself and with the clients.

USING AN INTERPRETER

Communication with the client or family is required for a cultural assessment. When nurses do not speak or understand the client's language, they should obtain an interpreter. The amount of accommodation that an agency must provide is guided by the proportion of people using the service overall as compared with those who need special assistance. Depending on the volume of clients who cannot speak English, agencies may be required to have all of their written materials translated and regularly use interpreters or have only portions of the materials translated. Using translators and interpreters is not without risk. They may not understand all the terms, especially the medical ones that are used, so they may omit, substitute, condense, or change the client's response in order to make sense of what they do not understand. They may also answer for the patient instead of working toward greater understanding of all participants (Flaskerud, 2007). Interpreters may emphasize their personal preferences by influencing both nurses' and clients' decisions to select and participate in treatment modalities. Nurses may minimize this by learning basic words and sentences of the most commonly spoken languages in the community and by having key written materials translated into the language of sizable client populations. Strategies that nurses may use to select and effectively use an interpreter are listed in the "How To" box.

BRIEFLY NOTED

Health care agencies are responsible for effectively communicating with their clients. When an interpreter is not available to translate, the client may view this behavior as unacceptable and bring legal action against the agency.

HOW TO   Select and Use an Interpreter

1. When feasible, select an interpreter who has knowledge of health-related terminology.
2. Use family members with caution because of the client's need for privacy when discussing intimate matters, because family members may lack the ability to communicate effectively in both languages, and because family members may exhibit a bias that influences the client's decisions.
3. The sex of the interpreter may be of concern; in some cultures, women may prefer a female interpreter and men may prefer a male interpreter.
4. The age of the interpreter may also be of concern. For example, older clients may want a more mature interpreter. Children tend to have limited understanding and language skills, and when used as interpreters, they may have difficulty interpreting the information.
5. Differences in socioeconomic status, religious affiliation, and educational level between the client and the interpreter may lead to problems in translation of information.
6. Identify the client's origin of birth and language or dialect spoken before selecting the interpreter. For example, Chinese clients speak different dialects depending on the region in which they were born.
7. Avoid using an interpreter from the same community as the client to avoid a breach of confidentiality.
8. Avoid using professional jargon, colloquialisms, abstractions, idiomatic expressions, slang, similes, and metaphors (Randall-David, 1994). Speak slowly, and use words that are common in the client's culture.
9. Clarify roles with the interpreter.
10. Introduce the interpreter to the client, and explain to the client what the interpreter will be doing.
11. Observe the client for nonverbal messages, such as facial expressions, gestures, and other forms of body language (Giger and Davidhizar, 2004). If the client's responses do not fit with the question, the nurse should check to be sure that the interpreter understood the question.
12. Increase accuracy in transmission of information by asking the interpreter to translate the client's own words, and ask the client to repeat the information that was communicated.
13. At the end of the interview, review the material with the client to ensure that nothing has been missed or misunderstood.

Data from Giger JN, Davidhizar R: *Transcultural nursing: assessment and intervention*, ed 4, St. Louis, 2004, Mosby; Randall-David E: *Culturally competent HIV counseling and education*, McLean, Va, 1994, Maternal and Child Health Clearinghouse.

CULTURAL GROUPS' DIFFERENCES

Although all cultures are not the same, all cultures have the same basic organizing factors (Giger and Davidhizar, 2004). These factors should be explored in a cultural assessment because of the potential for differences among groups. Some of these differences among cultural groups are presented in Table 5-4. See the Levels of Prevention box for preventions related to cultural differences.

Levels of Prevention   Related to Cultural Differences (Hypertension, Stroke, and Heart Disease)

PRIMARY PREVENTION

Provide health teaching about balanced diet and exercise.

SECONDARY PREVENTION

Teach clients and/or family to monitor blood pressure. Teach about diet, keeping in mind the client's cultural preferences. Talk about health beliefs and cultural implications, such as the use of alternative therapies; make sure alternative therapies are compatible with any medications that may be prescribed.

TERTIARY PREVENTION

If blood pressure cannot be controlled by diet, refer the client to a physician for medication; advise the client to engage in a cardiac program that will oversee diet and exercise.

COMMUNICATION

Understanding variations in patterns of **verbal communication** and **nonverbal communication** is the basis for achieving therapeutic goals. Variations among cultures are reflected in verbal styles (e.g., pronunciation, word meaning, voice quality, humor) and in nonverbal styles (e.g., eye contact, gestures, touch, interjecting during conversation, body posture, facial expression, silence). For example, when gathering data from an Hispanic woman, the nurse should be aware that the style may be low-key and that the woman may avoid eye contact and be hesitant to respond to questions. This behavior should not be interpreted as either a lack of interest or an inability to relate to others (Randall-David, 1989).

Another example occurred when a nurse gave instructions to Asian clients about taking antituberculin drugs. The clients smilingly responded with "yes, yes." The nurse interpreted this response to mean that the clients understood the instructions and that they accepted the treatment protocol. A week later, when the clients returned for a follow-up visit, the nurse discovered that the medications had not been taken. The nurse knew that acceptance by and avoidance of confrontation or disagreement with those in authority are important behaviors in the Asian culture; interventions were therefore adjusted accordingly. The nurse repeated the medication instructions and gave the clients an opportunity to raise questions and concerns and to repeat the instructions that were given. The nurse also discussed the cultural meaning and treatment of tuberculosis.

BRIEFLY NOTED

Respect all information that a client shares with you, even when the information is in conflict with your own value system.

Table 5-4   Cultural Variations among Selected Groups

	African-Americans	Asians	Hispanics	Native Americans
Verbal communication	Asking personal questions of someone you have met is seen as improper and intrusive	High level of respect is shown for others, especially those in positions of authority	Expression of negative feelings is considered impolite	Low tone of voice is used and the listener is expected to be attentive
Nonverbal communication	Direct eye contact in conversation is often considered rude	Direct eye contact among superiors may be considered disrespectful	Avoidance of eye contact is usually a sign of attentiveness and respect	Direct eye contact is often considered disrespectful
Touch	Touching someone else's hair is often considered offensive	It is not customary to shake hands with persons of the opposite sex	Touching is often observed between two persons in conversation	A light touch of the person's hand instead of a firm handshake is often used as a greeting
Family organization	Usually have close extended family networks; women play key roles in health care decisions	Usually have close extended family ties; emphasis may be on family needs rather than individual needs	Usually have close extended family ties; all members of the family may be involved in health care decisions	Usually have a close extended family; emphasis tends to be on the needs of the family rather than on individual needs
Time	Often present oriented	Often present oriented	Often present oriented	Often past oriented
Perception of health	Harmony of mind, health, body, and spirit with nature	When the "yin" and "yang" energy forces are balanced	Balance and harmony among mind, body, spirit, and nature	Harmony of mind, body, spirit, and emotions with nature
Alternative healers	"Granny," "root doctor," voodoo priest, spiritualist	Acupuncturist, acupressurist, herbalist	*Curandero, espiritualista, yerbero*	Medicine man, shaman
Self-care practices	Poultices, herbs, oils, roots	"Hot" and "cold" foods, herbs, teas, soups, cupping, burning, rubbing, pinching	"Hot" and "cold" foods, herbs	Herbs, cornmeal, medicine bundle
Biological variations	Sickle cell anemia, mongolian spots, keloid formation, inverted "T" waves, lactose intolerance, skin color	Thalassemia, drug interactions, mongolian spots, lactose intolerance, skin color	Mongolian spots, lactose intolerance, skin color	Cleft uvula, lactose intolerance, skin color

SPACE

Personal **space** is the physical area that persons need between themselves and others to feel comfortable. When this space is violated, the client may become uncomfortable. Nurses should take cues from clients to place themselves in the appropriate spatial zone and avoid misinterpretation of clients' behavior as they handle their spatial needs. Most cultural groups have spatial preferences. Some groups typically stand close to one another. However, one group may be comfortable with only a 9-inch distance between faces, whereas another group might find that small distance threatening and overly aggressive.

SOCIAL ORGANIZATION

Social organization refers to the way in which a cultural group structures itself around the family to carry out role functions. In some cultures, family may include people who are not actually related to one another. Find out who is considered to be in the family, who the key decision makers are, and if the needs of the family supersede those of the individuals in the family. Nurses should advocate for the individual,

so that when families make decisions, the individual's needs are also considered.

TIME PERCEPTION

Regarding **time,** cultures are considered to be either future, past, or present oriented. The American middle-class culture tends to be future oriented, and individuals are willing to delay immediate gratification until future goals are accomplished. In contrast, African-American and Hispanic families may place greater value on quality of life and view present time as being more important than future time. The future is unknown, but the present is known. When nurses discuss health promotion and disease prevention strategies with persons from a present orientation, they should focus on the immediate benefits these clients would gain rather than emphasizing future outcomes.

In cultures that focus on a past orientation (e.g., the Vietnamese culture), individuals may focus on wishes and memories of their ancestors and look to them to provide direction for current situations (Giger and Davidhizar, 2004).

In a past-oriented culture, time is viewed as being more flexible than in a present-oriented culture. Nurses socialized in the Western culture may view time as money and equate punctuality with goodness and being responsible. Working with clients who have a different perception of time than the nurse can be problematic. Nurses should clarify the clients' perception to avoid misunderstanding. It is not realistic to expect clients to change their behavior and adopt the nurse's schedule.

ENVIRONMENTAL CONTROL

Environmental control refers to the relationships between humans and nature. Cultural groups might perceive humans as having mastery over nature, being dominated by nature, or having a harmonious relationship with nature. Those who view nature as dominant (e.g., African-Americans and Hispanics) believe that they have little or no control over what happens to them. They may not adhere to a cancer treatment protocol because of the belief that nothing will change the outcome because it is their destiny. These individuals are less likely to engage in illness prevention activities than those who have other worldviews.

Persons who view a human harmony with nature (e.g., Asians and Native Americans) may perceive that illness is disharmony with other forces and that medicine can relieve the symptoms but cannot cure the disease. They would seek treatment for the malignancy from the mind, body, and spirit connection, because they believe that healing comes from within. These groups are likely to look to naturalistic solutions, such as herbs, acupuncture, and hot and cold treatments, to resolve or cure a cancerous condition.

BRIEFLY NOTED

Some clients may view their illness as punishment for misdeeds and may have difficulty accepting care from nurses who do not share their belief.

BIOLOGICAL VARIATIONS

Biological variations are the physical, biological, and physiological differences that exist and distinguish one racial group from another. They occur in areas of growth and development, skin color, enzymatic differences, and susceptibility to disease (Andrews and Boyle, 2007; Giger and Davidhizar, 2004). Other common and obvious variations include eye shape, hair texture, adipose tissue deposits, shape of earlobes, thickness of lips, and body configuration. For example, Western-born neonates are slightly heavier at birth than those born in non-Western cultures. Another variation is mongolian spots, which are present on the skin of African-American, Asian, Hispanic, and Native American babies. These are bluish discolorations that may be mistaken for bruises. When nurses are exposed to situations involving biological variations of which they are unfamiliar, they may create embarrassing situations. Consider the following scenario: The school nurse observes a bluish discoloration on the thigh of a Filipino child that she mistook for a bruise. The nurse reported her observation to the child protective agency in her state. When the child's mother arrived to pick her child up at the end of the school day, she was accused of child abuse. The mother had to disprove the allegation before her child could be released into her care.

Variations in growth and development may be influenced by environmental conditions such as nutrition, climate, and disease. Research findings suggest that sensitivity to codeine varies with ethnic background, and that Asian men experience significantly weaker effects from the drug than do European men (Wu, 1997). Asian men are missing an enzyme called *CYP2D6* that allows the body to metabolize codeine into morphine, which is responsible for the pain relief provided by codeine. When an individual is missing the enzyme, no amount of codeine will lessen the pain, and other pain-reducing medicines should be explored. A more common enzyme deficiency is glucose-6-phosphate dehydrogenase (G6PD) deficiency, which is responsible for lactose intolerance in many ethnic groups (Giger and Davidhizar, 2004).

CULTURE AND NUTRITION

Nutritional practices are an integral part of the assessment process for all families, especially since they play a prominent role in the health problems of some groups (Kaplan et al, 2004). Efforts to understand dietary patterns of clients should go beyond relying on membership in a defined group. Knowing clients' nutrition practices makes it possible to develop treatment regimens that would not conflict with their cultural food practices (Figure 5-2). Box 5-4 identifies several questions that nurses should ask when conducting

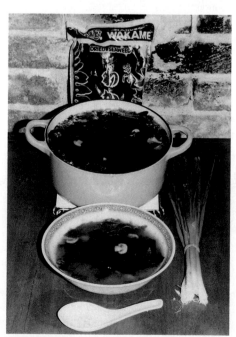

FIGURE 5-2 Mi-yuk kook (seaweed soup) is a Korean dish eaten by postpartum women to stop bleeding and to cleanse body fluids. It is also eaten on every birthday.

a nutritional assessment. Table 5-5 identifies the nutritional disadvantages to health of selected food preferences associated with four cultural groups.

BRIEFLY NOTED

Many people who subscribe to the Buddhist religion are vegetarian. Their faith teaches self-control as a means to search for happiness. The Buddhist code of morality is in their Five Moral Precepts, and eating meat would conflict with both the first and the fifth (i.e., meat is seen as an intoxicant). These precepts are as follows:

1. Do not harm or kill living things
2. Do not steal
3. Do not engage in sexual misconduct
4. Do not lie
5. Do not consume intoxicants such as alcohol, tobacco, or mind-altering drugs (ElGindy, 2005)

CULTURE AND SOCIOECONOMIC FACTORS

Socioeconomic factors contribute greatly to understanding perceptions of health and illness among minority groups. These groups may not have opportunities for education,

---

Box 5-4   Assessment of Dietary Practices and Food Consumption Patterns

- What is the social significance of food in the family?
- What foods are most frequently bought for family consumption?
- What foods, if any, are taboo (prohibited) for the family?
- Does religion play a significant role in food selection?
- Who prepares the food? How is it prepared?
- How much food is eaten? When is it eaten and with whom?
- Where does the client live and what types of restaurants does he or she frequent?
- Has the family adopted foods of other cultural groups?
- What are the family's favorite recipes?

---

occupation, income earning, and property ownership similar to those of the dominant group. Socioeconomic status is a critical factor in determining access to health care and the development of some chronic health problems (Kington and Smith, 1997). According to the U.S. Census Bureau (2001), in 1999 more white families than minorities were below the poverty level. However, the proportion of poor families in a minority group is greater. For example, white families represent 7.3% of those in poverty, whereas African-Americans represent 21.9% and Hispanics represent 20.9%. Consequently, minority families are disproportionately represented on the lower tiers of the socioeconomic ladder. Poor economic achievement is also a common characteristic found among populations at risk, such as those in poverty, the homeless, migrant workers, and refugees. Data suggest that when nurses and clients come from the same social class, it is more likely that they operate from the same health belief model and consequently there is less opportunity for misinterpretation and problems in communication.

There is also a danger in believing that certain cultural behaviors, such as folk practices, are restricted to lower socioeconomic classes. For example, health professionals, such as nurses and physicians, may also use folk systems in conjunction with the biomedical system to promote their health and prevent disease. Therefore nurses must conduct a cultural assessment for all individuals when they first come in contact with them. Nurses should have guidance in integrating cultural concepts with other aspects of client care to meet their clients' total health care needs. Nurses should be able to distinguish between issues of culture and socioeconomic class and not misinterpret behavior as having a cultural origin, when in fact it should be attributed to socioeconomic class.

CLINICAL APPLICATION

Shu Ping was concerned about her father's deteriorating health and contacted her church friend, Ms. Johnson, a registered nurse, for advice. A public health nurse had been visiting the father since his recent discharge from the hospital, but the father had asked this nurse not to discuss

---

Table 5-5   Food Preferences and Associated Risk Factors in Selected Cultural Groups

Cultural Group	Food Preferences	Nutritional Excess	Risk Factors
African-American	Fried foods, greens, bread, lard, pork, rice, foods with high sodium and starch content	Cholesterol, fat, sodium, carbohydrates, calories	Coronary artery disease, obesity
Asians	Soy sauce, rice, pickled dishes, raw fish, teas, balance between yin (cold) and yang (hot) concepts	Cholesterol, fat, sodium, carbohydrates, calories	Heart disease, liver disease, cancer of the stomach, ulcers
Hispanics	Fried foods, beans and rice, chili, carbonated beverages, high-fat and high-sodium foods	Cholesterol, fat, sodium, carbohydrates, calories	Heart disease, obesity
Native Americans	Blue cornmeal, fruits, game and fish	Carbohydrates, calories	Diabetes, malnutrition, tuberculosis, infant and maternal mortality

Data from Andrews MM, Boyle JS: *Transcultural concepts in nursing care,* ed 5, Philadelphia, 2007, Lippincott Williams & Wilkins; Giger JN, Davidhizar R: *Transcultural nursing: assessment and intervention,* ed 4, St. Louis, 2004, Mosby.

his diagnosis with his family. After several weeks with the family, Ms. Johnson was able to establish a close enough relationship with the father so that she could engage him in a private discussion about his health. He confided in Ms. Johnson that he was diagnosed with cancer of the small intestine, and he feared he was dying. He did not want the family to know the "bad news." He refused treatment because his view was that people never got better after they were diagnosed with cancer; they always died.

Which of the following actions best characterizes the public health nurse's willingness to provide culturally competent care to the family?

A. *Discussing the medical treatment and surgical intervention for cancer of the small intestine*
B. *Discussing with Shu Ping's father the prognosis for a person diagnosed with cancer of the small intestine in the United States*
C. *Requesting a conference involving the primary physician, the father, and the family to discuss the diagnosis and treatment options*
D. *Contacting the public health agency and discussing the problem with them*

Answer is in the back of the book.

REMEMBER THIS!

- The population of the United States is increasingly diverse. Changes in immigration laws and policies have increased migration, contributed to changes in community demographics, and heightened the need to recognize the impact of culture on health care and the need for nurses to learn about the culture of the individuals to whom they give care.
- Culture is a learned set of behaviors that is widely shared among a group of people; the culture of people helps guide individuals in problem solving and decision making.
- Culturally competent nursing care is designed for a specific client, reflects the individual's beliefs and values, and is provided with sensitivity. Such nursing care helps improve health outcomes and reduce health care costs.
- A culturally competent nurse uses cultural knowledge as well as specific skills, such as intracultural communication and cultural assessment, in selecting interventions to care for clients.
- The four modes of action that nurses may use to negotiate with clients and give culturally competent care are cultural preservation, cultural accommodation, cultural repatterning, and cultural brokering.
- Barriers to providing culturally competent care are stereotyping, prejudice and racism, ethnocentrism, cultural imposition, cultural conflict, and cultural shock.
- Nurses should perform a cultural assessment on every client with whom they interact. Cultural assessments help nurses understand clients' perspectives of health and illness and thereby guide them in discussing culturally appropriate interventions. The needs of clients vary with their age, education, religion, and socioeconomic status.

- When nurses do not speak or understand the client's language, they should use an interpreter. In selecting an interpreter, nurses should consider the clients' cultural needs and respect their right to privacy.
- Dietary practices are an integral part of the assessment data. Efforts to understand dietary practices should go beyond relying on membership in a defined group and should include individual nutritional practices and religious requirements.
- Members of minority groups are overrepresented on the lower tiers of the socioeconomic ladder. Poor economic achievement is also a common characteristic among populations at risk, such as those in poverty, the homeless, migrant workers, and refugees. Nurses should be able to distinguish between cultural issues and socioeconomic class issues and not interpret behavior as having a cultural origin when in fact it is based on socioeconomic class.

WHAT WOULD YOU DO?

1. Select a culture that you would like to learn more about. Go to an appropriate website and gather information about the cultural group. Identify the group's health-seeking behaviors. Validate this information with a member of the group. List differences between the two sources of data. How do you explain these findings? Explain how you can use this information in your clinical practice.
2. Recall a first meeting with a client whose culture differed from yours. Did you form an immediate impression about the reason for the individual's contact with the health care system? Discuss your assumptions about this client. What led you to make them? How did your assumptions influence your interaction with the client or family member? Give specific examples.
3. Interview an older person. What would you do to prepare for this interview? Discuss the individual's perspective of health and illness. Explore the use of Western and alternative health practices, and determine the individual's decision-making process in seeking out these health services. Prepare a list of alternative health care specialists who practice in your community.
4. With your community health agency explore the availability of culturally relevant policies and approaches for providing health care to the major cultural groups in the population it serves. On the basis of your findings, what gaps in services were evident? What input would you give the agency to augment services?
5. Which major ethnic and religious groups are represented in the community in which you live? What resources are available to meet their needs? What mechanisms are in place to facilitate access to these services by these groups?
6. On the basis of *Healthy People 2010* objectives, identify an at-risk aggregate in your community. Develop a health education program that utilizes cultural interventions to promote positive health behaviors for the group.

■ *REFERENCES*

American Academy of Nursing Expert Panel Report: Culturally competent health care, *Nurs Outlook* 40(6):277, 1992.

Andrews MM, Boyle JS: *Transcultural concepts in nursing care,* ed 5, Philadelphia, 2007, Lippincott Williams & Wilkins.

Bhopal R, Donaldson L: White, European, Western, Caucasian, or what? Inappropriate labeling in research on race, ethnicity, and health, *Am J Public Health* 88(9):1303, 1998.

Brislin R: *Understanding culture's influence on behavior,* Fort Worth, Tex, 1993, Harcourt Brace.

Burchum JL: Cultural competence: an evolutionary perspective, *Nurs Forum* 37(4):5–15, 2002.

Camarota SA: Immigrants in the United States, 2007: a profile of America's foreign born population, Centers for Immigration Studies. Released Nov 2007. Retrieved May 15, 2009, from http://www.cis.org/.

Campinha-Bacote J: *The process of cultural competence in the delivery of healthcare services: a culturally competent model of care,* ed 3, Cincinnati, Ohio, 1998, Transcultural CARE Associates.

Campinha-Bacote J: The process of cultural competence in the delivery of healthcare services: a model of care, *J Transcult Nurs* 13:181, 2002.

Carlock DM: Finding information on immigrant and refugee health, *J of Transcult Nurs* 18:373, 2007. http://tcn.sagepub.com/cgi/content/abstract/18/4/373.

Center for American Progress: *Immigrants in the US health care system,* Washington, DC, 2007.

Congress of the United States: *A description of the immigrant population,* Washington, DC, 2004, U.S. Government Printing Office.

Denker EP, editor: *Healing at home: Visiting Nurse Service of New York, 1893-1993,* Dalton, Mass, 1994, Studley.

Dreher M, MacNaughton N: Cultural competence in nursing: foundation or fallacy, *Nurs Outlook* 50(5):181–186, 2002.

ElGindy G: Understanding Buddhist patients' dietary needs, *Minority Nurse* 49-52, Spring 2005.

Flaskerud JH: Cultural competence column: What else is necessary? *Issues in Ment Health Nurs* 28(2):219–222, 2007.

Giger JN, Davidhizar R: *Transcultural nursing: assessment and intervention,* ed 4, St. Louis, 2004, Mosby.

Helsel DG, Mochel M: Afterbirth in the afterlife: cultural meaning of placental disposal in a Hmong American community, *J Transcult Nurs* 13:282, 2002.

Horowitz C: The role of the family and the community in the clinical setting. In Loue S, editor: *Handbook of immigrant health,* New York, 1998, Plenum, pp 163–182.

Huang ZJ, Yu SM, Ledsky R: Health status and health service access and use among children in US immigrant families, *Am J Public Health* 96(4):634-640, 2006.

Immigrants' Health Care Coverage and Access Fact Sheet, Washington, DC, 2001, Kaiser Commission on Medicaid and the Uninsured.

Jones ME, Cason CL, Bond ML: Cultural attitudes, knowledge, and skills of a health workforce, *J Transcult Nurs* 158:283–290, 2004.

Kaplan MS, Huguent N, Newman J et al: The association between length of residence and obesity among Hispanic immigrants, *Am J Preventive Med* 27:323–326, 2004.

Kington RS, Smith JP: Socioeconomic status and racial ethnic differences in functional status associated with chronic diseases, *Am J Public Health* 8(5):805, 1997.

Ledger MA: *The transformers,* Philadelphia, 2003, Pew Charitable Trusts 6(3):3–9.

Leininger M: Essential transcultural nursing care concepts, principles, examples, and policy statements. In Leininger MM, McFarland M, editors: *Transcultural nursing: concepts, theories, research, and practices,* ed 3, New York, 2002a, McGraw-Hill, pp 45–69.

Leininger M: The theory of culture care and the ethnonursing research method. In Leininger MM, McFarland M, editors: *Transcultural nursing: concepts, theories, research, and practices,* ed 3, New York, 2002b, McGraw-Hill, pp 71–98.

Lipman TH et al: Incidence of type 1 diabetes in Philadelphia is higher in black than white children from 1995 to 1999: Epidemic or misclassification? *Diabetes Care* 11(29):2391–2395, 2006.

Lipson JG, Dibble SL: *Providing culturally appropriate health care in cultural and clinical care,* San Francisco, 2005, University of San Francisco Nursing Press, pp XII-XVII.

Miller NK: Haitian ethnomedical systems and biomedical practitioners: directions for clinicians, *J Transcult Nurs* 11:204, 2000.

Munoz CC, Luckmann J: *Transcultural communication in nursing,* ed 2, Clifton Park, NY, 2005, Thompson Delmar.

National Immigration Forum: *Immigration basics 2005,* Washington, DC, 2005, National Immigration Forum. Retrieved May 15, 2009, from http://www.immigrationforum.org/documents/Publications/ImmigrationBasics2005.pdf.

Office of Minority Health: *Asian American/Pacific Islander profile.* Retrieved April 11, 2008 at http://www.omhrc.gov/templates/browse.aspx?lvl=2&lvlID=53.

Orlandi MA, editor: *Cultural competence for evaluators,* Washington, DC, 1992, U.S. Department of Health and Human Services.

Orque M: Orque's ethnic/cultural system: a framework for ethnic nursing care. In Orque MS, Bloch B, Monrroy LSA, editors: *Ethnic nursing care: a multi-cultural approach,* St. Louis, 1983, Mosby.

Plumb AL: Refuges for refugees and their caregivers, *Am J Nurs* 103(12):98–99, 2003.

Purnell LD, Paulanka BJ: *Transcultural health care,* ed 3, Philadelphia, 2008, FA Davis.

Randall-David E: *Strategies for working with culturally diverse communities and clients,* Bethesda, MD, 1989, Washington, DC, U.S. Department of Health and Human Services.

Spector RE: *Cultural diversity in health and illness,* ed 7, Upper Saddle River, NJ, 2008, Prentice Hall.

Steefel L: Caring the Korean way, *Nursing Spectrum,* 32–33, 2007, Washington, DC.

Suh EE: The model of cultural competence through an evolutionary concept analysis, *J Transcult Nurs* 152:93–102, 2004.

Sutherland LL: Ethnocentrism in a pluralistic society: a concept analysis, *J Transcultural Nursing* 13(4):274–281, 2002.

Tripp-Reimer T, Brink PJ, Saunders JM: Cultural assessment: content and process. In Spradley BW, Allender JA, editors: *Readings in community health,* ed 5, Philadelphia, 1997, Lippincott Williams & Wilkins.

U.S. Census Bureau: *Statistical abstract of the United States,* ed 121, Washington, DC, 2001, U.S. Government Printing Office.

U.S. Census Bureau: *Data interval from April 1, 1990 to September 20, 1990.* Released Feb 8, 2002. Retrieved March 2, 2004, from http://www.census.gov/population/documentation/twps0051/tab05.pdf.

U.S. Census Bureau: *Annual estimates of the Hispanic population by sex and age for the United States April 1, 2000 to July 1, 2007,* U.S. Census Bureau, Population Division, 2008. Retrieved May 15, 2009, from http://www.census.gov/

U.S. Department of Health and Human Services: *Healthy People 2010: understanding and improving health,* ed 2, Washington, DC, 2000, U.S. Government Printing Office.

Wu C: Drug sensitivity varies with ethnicity, *Science News* 152:165, 1997.

Chapter 6

Environmental Health

Barbara Sattler
Brenda Afzal
Lillian H. Mood

ADDITIONAL RESOURCES

These related resources are found either in the appendix at the back of this book or on the book's website at http://evolve.elsevier.com/stanhope/foundations.

Appendix

• Appendix G.3: Comprehensive Occupational and Environmental Health History

Evolve Website

• Community Assessment Applied
• Quiz review questions
• WebLinks, including link to *Healthy People 2010* website

Real World Community Health Nursing: An Interactive CD-ROM, second edition

If you are using this CD-Rom in your course, you will find the following activities related to this chapter:

• *Lead Levels: How Do States Rank?* in **Environmental Health**
• *Get the Lead Out: Identify the Hazards* in **Environmental Health**
• *Water, Water Everywhere* in **Environmental Health**
• *How Polluted Is Your Community?* in **Environmental Health**
• *Assess Environmental Hazards in the Home* in **A Day in the Life of a Community Health Nurse**

OBJECTIVES

After reading this chapter, the student should be able to:

1. Explain how the environment influences human health and disease.
2. Know which disciplines work most closely with nurses in environmental health.
3. Describe legislative and regulatory policies that have influenced the effect of the environment on health and disease patterns.
4. Describe the skills needed by nurses practicing in environmental health and apply the nursing process to the practice of environmental health.

CHAPTER OUTLINE

HEALTHY PEOPLE 2010 OBJECTIVES FOR ENVIRONMENTAL HEALTH
HISTORICAL CONTEXT
ENVIRONMENTAL HEALTH SCIENCES

The authors wish to thank Robyn Gilden and Laura Anderko for their assistance with this chapter.

Toxicology
Epidemiology
Multidisciplinary Approaches Including Nursing Competencies
ENVIRONMENTAL HEALTH COMPETENCIES FOR NURSES
Basic Knowledge
Assessment and Referral

ENVIRONMENTAL HEALTH ASSESSMENT
Environmental Exposure History
Environmental Health Assessment
The Right to Know
Risk Assessment
Assessing Risks in Vulnerable Populations: Children's Environmental Health
REDUCING ENVIRONMENTAL HEALTH RISKS
Risk Communication

Ethics
Government Environmental Protection
ADVOCACY
Environmental Justice
Unique Environmental Health Threats in the Health Care Industry: New Opportunities for Advocacy
REFERRAL RESOURCES
ROLES FOR NURSES IN ENVIRONMENTAL HEALTH

KEY TERMS

agent: causative factor invading a susceptible host through an environment favorable to produce disease, such as a biological or chemical agent.

compliance: processes for ensuring that permitting requirements are met.

consumer confidence report (CCR): a report that began in 1996 when Congress amended the Safe Drinking Water Act to add a provision that required all community water systems to deliver a brief annual water quality report to their customers. The CCR includes information on the water source, the levels of any detected contaminants, and compliance with drinking water rules, plus some educational material. The rationale for these reports is that consumers have a right to know what is in their drinking water. The reports help consumers make informed choices that affect their health.

enforcement: occurs when formal actions are taken to control environmental damage. Examples include fines or penalties, suspension of specific operations, or closure of the facility.

environment: all of those factors internal and external to the client that constitute the context in which the client lives and that influence and are influenced by the host and agent–host interactions; the sum of all external conditions affecting the life, development, and survival of an organism.

environmental epidemiology: the study of the effect on human health of physical, chemical, and biological factors in the external environment.

environmental justice: equal protection from environmental hazards for individuals, groups, or communities regardless of race, ethnicity, or economic status. This applies to the development, implementation, and enforcement of environmental laws, regulations, and policies and implies that no population of people should be forced to shoulder a disproportionate share of negative environmental effects of pollution or environmental hazard because of a lack of political or economic strength levels.

environmental standards: norms that impose limits on the amount of pollutants or emissions produced. The Environmental Protection Agency establishes minimum standards, but states are allowed to be stricter.

epidemiologic triangle: infectious agent, host, and environment,

epidemiology: the science that explains the strength of association between exposures and health effects in human populations.

host: a living human or animal organism in which an infectious agent can exist under natural conditions.

indoor air quality: a measure of the breathable air inside a habitable structure or conveyance. A measure of the chemical, physical, or biological contaminants in indoor air.

methyl mercury: an organic form of mercury. Methyl mercury may be formed when inorganic mercury enters lakes and combines with bacteria. It can then build up in the tissues of fish. Larger and older fish tend to have the highest levels of methyl mercury. Methyl mercury is highly toxic to humans and causes a number of adverse effects. It is a potent neurotoxicant.

monitoring: periodic or continuous surveillance or testing to determine the level of compliance with statutory requirements and/or pollutant levels in various media or in humans, plants, and animals.

nonpoint source: diffuse pollution source (i.e., without a single point of origin or not introduced into a receiving stream from a specific outlet). The pollutants may be carried off the land by storm water. Examples of nonpoint sources are traffic, fertilizer or pesticide run-off, and animal wastes.

permitting: the first step in the process of controlling pollution. A process by which the government places limits on the amount of pollution emitted into the air or water.

persistent bioaccumulative toxins (PBTs): highly toxic, long-lasting substances that can build up in the food chain to levels that are harmful to human health and cause environmental harm. These contaminants can be transported long distances and move readily from land to air and water.

persistent organic pollutants (POPs): toxic substances composed of organic (carbon-based) chemical compounds and mixtures. They include industrial chemicals such as polychlorinated biphenyl (PCB) and pesticides such as dichlorodiphenyltrichloroethane (DDT). They are primarily products and by-products from industrial processes, chemical manufacturing, and resulting wastes. These pollutants are persistent in the environment and have the ability to travel through the air and water to regions far from their original source. POPs are highly toxic; at very low concentrations they can injure wildlife and human health.

point-source: stationary location or fixed facility from which pollutants are discharged; any single identifiable source of pollution (e.g., a pipe, ditch, ship, ore pit, factory smokestack).

right to know: the right of citizens to have direct access to information about issues of environmental concern such as information on the quality of drinking water, the use of food additives, and chemical use in the workplace and community.

risk assessment: qualitative and quantitative evaluation of the risk posed to human health and/or the environment by the actual or potential presence and/or use of specific pollutants.

risk communication: the exchange of information about health or environmental risks among, for example, risk assessors and managers, the general public, news media, and interest groups.

toxicology: the basic science that studies the health effects associated with chemical exposures.

The environment is everything around us, and the quality of our lives depends heavily on the quality of our environment. A healthy environment is essential for optimal health and health care (Olshansky, 2008). The environments in which most of us spend time are our homes, schools, workplaces, and communities. We often take the environment for granted and may fail to see the hazards in front of us. For example, how many of us know for certain that our drinking water is safe, or that the air we breathe is free from pollutants that aggravate our individual respiratory functions? If children are in the home, are all the toxic cleaning materials and insecticides out of reach? Lead-based paint is in more than 52 million homes in the United States, and we know that exposure to lead can cause premature births, learning disabilities in children, hypertension in adults, and other health problems. Of the top 20 environmental pollutants reported to the Environmental Protection Agency (EPA), nearly 75% were known or suspected neurotoxins, that is, toxins that destroy nerves or nervous tissue. In 2004, U.S. facilities led by the chemical and paper industries released more than 70 million pounds of recognized carcinogens to the air and water (Cassady and Fidis, 2007). Thirty million Americans drink water that exceeds one or more of the EPA's safe drinking water standards, and 50% of Americans live in areas that exceed current national ambient air quality standards. Given such reported exposures, what is the role of nurses in community health?

What exposures can you identify in your own home? Do you use pesticides? Does your home have lead-based paint? Is the paint chipping or peeling? Have you checked your home for radon, the second largest cause of lung cancer in the United States? How about our workplaces? Do we continue to use medical equipment that contains mercury, such as mercury thermometers and sphygmomanometers, which later contribute to the environmental mercury load that has contaminated fish in lakes and streams in 40 states?

Chemical, biological, and radiological exposures that affect our health come from the air we breathe, the water we drink, the food we eat, and the products we use. Nurses need to know how to assess for environmental health risks and develop educational and other preventive interventions to help individuals, families, and communities understand and, where possible, decrease the risks. The National Academy of Science's Institute of Medicine (IOM) recommends that all nurses have a basic understanding of environmental health principles and that these principles be integrated into all aspects of practice, education, advocacy, policies, and research. This chapter explores the basic competencies recommended by the IOM (Box 6-1).

HEALTHY PEOPLE 2010 OBJECTIVES FOR ENVIRONMENTAL HEALTH

Environmental health is one of the priority areas of the *Healthy People 2010* objectives (see *Healthy People 2010* box). The federal government has long recognized the importance of the relationship between environmental risks and diseases.

Box 6-1 | **General Environmental Health Competencies for Nurses**

Basic Knowledge and Concepts

All nurses should understand the scientific principles and underpinnings of the relationship between individuals or populations and the environment (including the work environment). This understanding includes the basic mechanisms and pathways of exposure to environmental health hazards, basic prevention and control strategies, the interdisciplinary nature of effective interventions, and the role of research.

Assessment and Referral

All nurses should be able to successfully complete an environmental health history, recognize potential environmental hazards and sentinel illnesses, and make appropriate referrals for conditions with probable environmental causes. An essential component is the ability to locate referral sources, access them, and provide information to clients and communities.

Advocacy, Ethics, and Risk Communication

All nurses should be able to demonstrate knowledge of the role of advocacy (case and class), ethics, and risk communication in client care and community intervention with respect to potential adverse effects of the environment on health.

Legislation and Regulation

All nurses should understand the policy framework and major pieces of legislation and regulations related to environmental health.

From Pope AM, Snyder MA, Mood LH, editors: *Nursing, health, and environment*, Washington, DC, 1995, Institute of Medicine, National Academy Press.

HISTORICAL CONTEXT

Nurses, like physicians, have been taught little about the environment and environmental threats to health. This recognition led the IOM to evaluate the current state of environmental health knowledge and skills applied in nursing. The IOM report *Nursing, Health, and Environment* (Pope, Snyder, and Mood, 1995) noted that the environment, as a determinant of health, is deeply rooted in nursing's heritage. As mentioned in Chapter 2, Florence Nightingale, well known for her work in Crimea, is called by some "the mother of biostatistics" for her skilled use of data, both her own observations and the aggregate compilation of information, to compel action on conditions affecting health. She made it clear in her work and her writings that the quality of the environment influenced health and recovery from illness. She talked about the importance to the patient's health of fresh air, pure water, adequate food, good drainage, cleanliness, and light, especially good sunlight (Olshansky, 2008). Early in the twentieth century, Lillian Wald, who coined the term *public health*

Healthy People 2010

Selected Objectives Related to Environmental Health

8-1 Reduce the proportion of persons exposed to air that does not meet the U.S. EPA health- based standards for harmful air pollutants

8-2 Increase the use of alternative modes of transportation to reduce motor vehicle emissions and improve the nation's air quality

8-3 Improve the nation's air quality by increasing the use of cleaner alternative fuels

8-4 Reduce air toxic emissions to decrease the risk of adverse health effects caused by airborne toxicants

8-5 Increase the proportion of persons served by community water systems that receive a supply of drinking water that meets the regulations of the Safe Drinking Water Act

8-6 Reduce the waterborne disease outbreaks arising from water intended for drinking among persons served by community water systems

8-7 Reduce the per capita domestic water withdrawals

8-8 Increase the proportion of assessed rivers, lakes, and estuaries that is safe for fishing and recreational purposes

8-9 Reduce the number of beach closings that result from the presence of harmful bacteria

8-10 Reduce the potential human exposure to persistent chemicals by decreasing fish- contaminant levels

8-11 Eliminate elevated blood levels of lead in children

8-12 Minimize the risks to human health and the environment posed by hazardous sites

8-13 Reduce pesticide exposures that result in visits to a health care facility

8-14 Reduce the amount of toxic pollutants released, disposed of, treated, or used for energy recovery

8-15 Increase recycling of municipal solid waste

8-16 Reduce indoor allergen levels

From U.S. Department of Health and Human Services: *Healthy People 2010: understanding and improving health*, ed 2, Washington, DC, 2000, U.S. Government Printing Office.

nurses, and her colleague, Mary Brewster, worked tirelessly to improve the environment of the Henry Street neighborhood and used their network of influential contacts to make changes in the physical environment and social conditions that affected health (Wright, 2003). The need to pay close attention to the environment and its effect on health is as crucial today as it was in earlier times. In fact, it is important to note how radically different our environment is compared with how it was a century ago. In addition to environmental contamination, many of the human-made chemicals can now also be found in our bodies (including breast milk) in measurable amounts. To understand the relationship between the environment and health, some knowledge about toxicology and other environmental sciences is necessary.

BRIEFLY NOTED

"In watching diseases, both in private homes and in public hospitals, the thing which strikes the experienced observer most forcibly is this, that the symptoms or the sufferings generally considered to be inevitable and incident to the disease are very often not symptoms of the disease at all, but of something quite different—of the want of fresh air, or of light, or of warmth, or of quiet, or of cleanliness, or of punctuality and care in the administration of diet, of each or of all of these" (Nightingale, 1859, p. 8).

ENVIRONMENTAL HEALTH SCIENCES

TOXICOLOGY

Toxicology is the basic science that studies the health effects associated with chemical exposures. Its corollary in health care is pharmacology, which studies the human health effects, both desirable and undesirable, associated with drugs. In toxicology, only the negative effects of chemical exposures are studied. However, the key principles of pharmacology and toxicology are the same. Just as the dose of a drug influences its effectiveness and its toxicity, the quantity of an air or water pollutant to which we may be exposed will determine the risk of experiencing a negative health effect.

Both drugs and pollutants can enter the body by a variety of routes. Most drugs are given orally and are absorbed via the gastrointestinal tract. Water- and food-associated pollutants, including pesticides and heavy metals, enter the body via the digestive tract. Some drugs are administered as inhalants, and some pollutants in the air (including indoor

BRIEFLY NOTED

"Environmental health is in the midst of a paradigm shift. Today, features of the built environment, such as architecture and urban planning, are considered as important to human health as features of the natural environment, such as air quality and water pollution" (Lopez and Welker-Hood, 2007, p. 56).

air) enter the body via the lungs. Some drugs are applied topically. In work settings, employees can receive dermal exposures from toxic chemicals when they immerse their unprotected hands in chemical solutions. Pollution can enter the body via the lungs (inhalation), gastrointestinal tract (ingestion), and skin and mucous membranes (dermal absorption). Some chemicals can cross the placental barrier and affect the fetus.

When we administer medications to patients, we consider age, weight, other drugs taken, and the underlying health status of the person. We should also make it clear to patients that taking the prescription or over-the-counter drug more often than recommended can have a toxic effect on them. Likewise, we must also consider how environmental exposures affect community members. For example, children are more vulnerable to almost all pollutants. More vulnerable to foodborne and waterborne pathogens are immunocompromised people such as (1) those infected with the human immunodeficiency virus (HIV), (2) those who have acquired immunodeficiency syndrome (AIDS), (3) those who are taking chemotherapeutic drugs, or (4) those who are organ recipients. When assessing a community's environmental health status, be sure to review the general health status of the community to identify members who may have higher risk factors as well as to assess the environmental exposures.

Knowing about chemicals and using that information in practice can seem like a huge task. Fortunately, chemicals can be grouped into families so that it is possible to understand the actions and risks associated within these groups. The following are examples:

1. Metals and metallic compounds such as arsenic, cadmium, chromium, lead, mercury
2. Hydrocarbons such as benzene, toluene, ketones, formaldehyde, trichloroethylene
3. Irritant gases such as ammonia, hydrochloric acid, sulfur dioxide, chlorine
4. Chemical asphyxiants including carbon monoxide, hydrogen sulfide, cyanides
5. Pesticides such as organophosphates, carbamates, chlorinated hydrocarbons, bipyridyls

Technology helps us understand environmental threats. The National Library of Medicine (NLM) databases are user friendly and accessible on the Internet. The NLM website provides access to medical databases such as PubMed and GratefulMed. The databases can be searched for possible environmental linkages to illnesses using illness and symptom search terms. A convenient way to access the NLM toxicology databases is through the WebLinks on this book's website at http://evolve.elsevier.com/stanhope/foundations or at www.nlm.nih.gov. Using chemical name search terms and display options of health effects, some potential environmental threats to health can be understood or ruled out.

EPIDEMIOLOGY

Whereas toxicology is the science that studies the poisonous effects of chemicals, **epidemiology** is the science that helps us understand the strength of the association between exposures and health effects in human populations. Chapter 9 discusses epidemiology in detail. However, a few points are relevant here since epidemiology is an applied science used in environmental health. Epidemiologic studies associated some learning disabilities and exposure to lead-based paint dust, and epidemiology is important for examining occupation-related illnesses.

Environmental epidemiology, a useful tool for nurses, is the study of the effect on human health of physical, chemical, and biological factors in the external environment. By examining specific populations or communities exposed to different ambient environments, environmental epidemiology seeks to clarify the relationships between physical, chemical, and biological factors and human health. Environmental epidemiology explains the risk of lead poisoning, exacerbation of asthma from air pollution, and an outbreak of cryptosporidiosis from water contamination with *Cryptosporidium* (Goldman, 2000). Environmental surveillances, such as childhood lead registries, use epidemiologic methods to track and analyze incidence, prevalence, and health outcomes.

As discussed in Chapter 9, three major concepts—agent, host, and environment—form the classic **epidemiologic triangle**. This simple model belies the often-complex relationships among **agent**, which may include chemical mixtures (i.e., more than one agent); **host**, which may refer to a community spanning different ages, genders, ethnicities, cultures, and disease states; and **environment**, which may include dynamic factors such as air, water, soil, and food, as well as temperature, humidity, and wind. Limitations of environmental epidemiologic data include a reliance on occupational health studies to characterize certain toxic exposures. Studies are usually performed on healthy adults whose biological systems are quite different from those of neonates, pregnant women, children, the immunosuppressed, and older adults.

MULTIDISCIPLINARY APPROACHES INCLUDING NURSING COMPETENCIES

In addition to toxicology and epidemiology, a number of earth sciences help explain how pollutants travel in air, water, and soil. Geologists, meteorologists, and chemists all contribute information to help understand how and when humans may be exposed to hazardous chemicals, radiation (such as radon), and biological contaminants. The public health field also depends on food safety specialists, sanitarians, radiation specialists, and industrial hygienists.

The nature of environmental health requires a multidisciplinary approach to assess and decrease environmental health risks. For instance, to assess and address a case of lead-based paint poisoning, the team might include a housing inspector with expertise in lead-based paint or a sanitarian to assess the lead-associated health risks in the home; clinical specialists to manage the clients' health needs; laboratory workers to assess lead levels in the clients' blood as well as in the paint, house dust, and drinking water; and lead-based paint remediation specialists to reduce the lead-based paint risk in the home. This approach could potentially involve the local health department, the state department of environmental protection, the housing department, a tertiary care setting, and public or private sector laboratories. It is important that nurses understand the roles of each respective agency and organization, know the public health laws (particularly as they pertain to lead-based paint poisoning), and work with the community to coordinate services to address the community's needs. The nurse might also set up a blood-lead screening program through the local health department, educate local health providers to encourage them to systematically test children for lead poisoning, or work with local landlords to improve the condition of their housing stock.

BRIEFLY NOTED

Factors contributing to the reduction of lead levels in the United States include elimination of lead in paint, reduction of lead in gasoline, reduction in the number of manufactured food and drink cans and household plumbing components containing lead solder, lead screening laws, and lead paint-abatement programs in communities.

ENVIRONMENTAL HEALTH COMPETENCIES FOR NURSES

Because nurses play a role in environmental health, what do they need to know to be effective partners in this work? The 1995 IOM study *Nursing, Health, and Environment* (Pope, Snyder, and Mood, 1995) identifies four general environmental health competencies for nurses, which are presented in Box 6-1 and discussed in the following sections.

BASIC KNOWLEDGE

Even though selected environmental sciences are summarized above, it is important to remember that the science base is large and constantly changing. Although interdisciplinary practice makes it unnecessary for the nurse to be an in-depth expert in environmental science, knowledge of four principles and how they explain environmental threats to health is useful.

Environmental Principle 1: Everything Is Connected to Everything Else

This principle is introduced in elementary school science when students are taught about the water cycle of evaporation and condensation. The consequences of the connectedness of all things in the environment can be seen in Figure 6-1. Lead in paint is a good example, banned in 1978 but still present in older homes in poorer neighborhoods and in restored homes in more affluent communities. As indicated in a recent report by the U.S. Department of Housing and Human Development, 24 million American homes have hazards that could put children at risk for lead poisoning (Laraque and Trasande, 2005). The lead-containing paint chips are scraped, become airborne in the breathing space for a brief time, and then end up in nearby soil. Children play in the soil, where their hand-to-mouth activity results in exposure

to lead, which has developmental and behavioral effects on them, both known and being discovered through research.

In a 2005 study, lead-based paint hazards were estimated to be present in 38 million housing units, a decrease from 64 million in 1990 (Laraque and Trasande, 2005). This decrease could be attributed to advocacy efforts that brought forth legislation to reduce exposure and force compliance with lead removal from the environment. Additional efforts to combat lead contamination include education for prevention, screening (both the victim and the source), and treatment (in the individual and the environment). The principle of connectedness is the essence of tracking exposures and risks (Box 6-2).

Environmental Principle 2: Everything Has to Go Somewhere

Again, this principle can be traced to science taught in elementary education: matter cannot be created or destroyed. Once waste products are generated, they must be disposed of in one of the following three ways:

1. *Incineration.* Burning can change the chemical composition through heat, but the products of burning such as ash and air emissions must be controlled and disposed of in one of the following two options.
2. *Water discharge.* To interrupt the exposure pathway, the products to be disposed of in water must be treated to ensure that the dose in the water is not great enough to do harm.
3. *Landfilling or burial in the soil.* Protections must be put in place, such as liners and leachate pumps and monitors, to avoid seepage of harmful doses into the groundwater or air.

Each of the options for waste disposal is intended to provide a way either to alter the waste product to a less toxic form through chemical intervention (biodegradation) or to store the product in a biounavailable form or place. Because either of the options for disposal can be a problem, prevention is desirable.

Remember that human effects are intensified in the most sensitive, vulnerable environments, such as estuaries, the nurseries for much of sea and coastal plant and animal life. Some of the most valued food sources are also the most sensitive to pollution. Shellfish are efficient filters of contaminants in the water in which they live. For example, oysters filter and retain almost all contaminants from the water in which they grow. It is impossible to rid them of contaminants after harvesting. The only protection for humans is to grow oysters in environments free from harmful contamination. Safe seafood depends on clean water. This example leads to the third principle.

Environmental Principle 3: The Solution to Pollution Is Dilution

Reflecting on the element of dose in human exposure reveals the truth in this principle. The use of this principle can be seen in historic environmental and sanitation measures. Garbage was moved from streets to the nearest body of water. Early

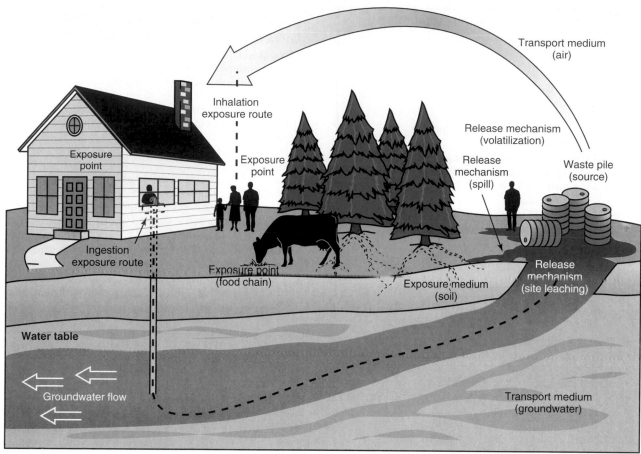

FIGURE 6-1 Exposure pathways. (From the Agency for Toxic Substances and Disease Registry: Identifying and evaluating exposure pathways. In *Public health assessment guidance manual*, Atlanta, Ga, 1992, ATSDR.)

Box 6-2   **Environmental Harm**

For persons to be harmed by something in the environment, several factors must be in place and connected (see Figure 6-1):
- A source of harm that has chemical and/or physical properties
- An environmental medium for transport—air, water (surface and/or groundwater), or soil
- A receptor population within the exposure pathway for harm to human health
- A route of exposure. Humans can be exposed to environmental contaminants through only three routes: inhalation, ingestion, and skin absorption
- An adequate amount (dose) of the chemical to result in human harm

---

industries went from dumping wastes outside their buildings to piping them to the nearest stream or river. Human wastes followed the same paths and pipelines. The problem with this principle is that it was tied to a world view that saw the environment as an unlimited resource, a limitless repository for whatever was useless. The dilution capacity of large rivers and certainly the ocean seemed boundless. The belief in the capacity of air to dilute resulted in "solutions" such as taller smoke stacks to release pollutants higher into the atmosphere. The reality, which becomes more evident every day, is that this planet's capacity to assimilate by-products of human civilization is not limitless. It is, in fact, fragile and delicately balanced, and the knowledge and practice about how to live peacefully within that balance without doing harm is far from adequate. The fourth principle reflects this insight.

Environmental Principle 4: Today's Solution May Be Tomorrow's Problem

As in almost every aspect of life, environmental scientists and regulators deal with incomplete information and insufficient science. The brief history of organized environmental protection is filled with examples. Garbage that went from the streets into unlined landfills is now a source of groundwater contamination. Gasoline tanks that were buried underground to avoid an ugly landscape were found to leak over time. New solutions of lined landfills and double-walled storage tanks, with sensors for leaks and monitoring wells, have emerged, as has the increasing work of cleaning up the earlier "mistakes."

What can now be called *mistakes* were not necessarily the result of malicious carelessness or insensitivity. Decisions were based on the best information available at the time. The "best information" may be incomplete and imperfect. That is why research is so necessary. An encouraging trend in

Box 6-3	Information and Guidance Sources for Referrals

Federal Agencies
- Agency for Toxic Substances and Disease Registry
- Centers for Disease Control and Prevention
- Consumer Product Safety Commission
- Environmental Protection Agency
- Office of Children's Environmental Health
- Food and Drug Administration
- National Institute for Occupational Safety and Health
- National Institute of Environmental Health Sciences
- National Institutes of Health
- National Cancer Institute
- National Institute of Nursing Research
- Occupational Safety and Health Administration

State Agencies
- State Health Departments
- State Environmental Protection Agencies

Associations and Organizations
- American Association of Poison Control Centers
- American College of Occupational and Environmental Medicine
- American Cancer Society
- American Lung Association
- Association of Occupational and Environmental Clinics
- Center for Health and Environmental Justice
- Children's Environmental Health Network
- Children's Health and the Environment Coalition
- National Environmental Education and Training Foundation
- Pesticide Education Center
- Society for Occupational and Environmental Health
- Teratogen Exposure Registry and Surveillance

industry's new product development is engineering analysis of the full life-cycle of the product, from raw material to waste disposal. Up-front consideration of the costs and effects throughout the cycle can lead to choices that prevent future problems.

One of the greatest challenges and a major source of concern in today's environmental picture are solutions themselves. The growing number and complexity of chemicals that are part of everyday life exemplify this. Citizens have enthusiastically embraced "better living through chemistry," with more than 65,000 new chemical compounds introduced into the environment between 1950 and 1984 (Pope, Snyder, and Mood, 1995). An estimated 1000 or more have been added each year since. The uses range from industry to household to medical, and there is no doubt that chemicals have been a part of the solution to numerous problems.

The problem with the enormous growth in chemicals is that the effects of new chemicals on the environment are unknown. People in neighborhoods near industrial parks are concerned that even when only allowable levels of each chemical are released, no one is able to say what the health effects of exposure to the combination of small amounts of chemicals may be over time.

HOW TO   Apply the Nursing Process to Environmental Health

If you suspect that a client's health problem is being influenced by environmental factors, follow the nursing process and note the environmental aspects of the problem in every step of the process as follows:
1. *Assessment.* Include inventories and history questions that cover environmental issues as a part of the general assessment.
2. *Diagnosis.* Relate the disease and the environmental factors in the diagnosis.
3. *Goal setting.* Include outcome measures that mitigate and eliminate the environmental factors.
4. *Planning.* Look at community policy and laws as methods to facilitate the care needs for the client; include environmental health personnel in the planning.
5. *Intervention.* Coordinate medical, nursing, and public health actions to meet the client's needs.
6. *Evaluation.* Examine criteria that include the immediate and long-term responses of the client, as well as the recidivism of the problem for the client.

ASSESSMENT AND REFERRAL

The second general environmental health competency cited in the IOM study is assessment and referral. Both of these activities are familiar parts of nursing practice, but they have specific meaning in environmental health. *Assessment* activities of nurses can range from individual health assessments to being full participants in community assessment or partners in a specific environmental site assessment. *Referral* resources may vary in communities. One starting point may be the environmental epidemiology or toxicology unit of the state health department or environmental agency. Box 6-3 lists several good referral sources.

ENVIRONMENTAL HEALTH ASSESSMENT

When assessing environmental exposures, the environment can be divided into functional locations such as home, school, workplace, and community. In each of these locations, there may be unique environmental exposures as well as overlapping exposures. For instance, ethylene oxide, the toxic gas that is used to sterilize equipment in hospitals, is typically found only in a workplace. However, pesticides might be found in all four areas. When assessing environments, determine whether an exposure is in the air, water, soil, or food (or a combination) and whether it is a chemical, biological, or radiological exposure. The key questions in any assessment should cover past as well as present conditions in work, home, and community environments (Pope, Snyder, and Mood, 1995):
1. What are your longest held jobs, current and past?
2. Have you been exposed to any radiation or chemical liquids, dusts, mists, or fumes?
3. Is there any relationship between current symptoms and activities at work or at home?

The "How To" box demonstrates how to apply the nursing process to environmental health.

Box 6-4	The "I PREPARE" Mnemonic

An exposure history should identify current and past exposures, have a preliminary goal of reducing or eliminating current exposures, and have a long-term goal of reducing adverse health effects. The "I PREPARE" mnemonic consigns the important questions to categories that can be easily remembered.

I   Investigate Potential Exposures

Investigate potential exposures by asking,
- Have you ever felt sick after coming in contact with a chemical, pesticide, or other substance?
- Do you have any symptoms that improve when you are away from your home or work?

P   Present Work

At your present work,
- Are you exposed to solvents, dusts, fumes, radiation, loud noise, pesticides, or other chemicals?
- Do you know where to find material data safety sheets on the chemicals with which you work?
- Do you wear personal protective equipment?
- Are work clothes worn home?
- Do co-workers have similar health problems?

R   Residence

At your place of residence,
- When was your residence built?
- What type of heating do you have?
- Have you recently remodeled your home?
- What chemicals are stored on your property?
- Where does your drinking water come from?

E   Environmental Concerns

In your living environment,
- Are there environmental concerns in your neighborhood (i.e., air, water, soil)?
- What types of industries or farms are near your home?
- Do you live near a hazardous waste site or landfill?

P   Past Work

About your past work,
- What are your past work experiences?
- What is the longest job you held?
- Have you ever been in the military, worked on a farm, or done volunteer or seasonal work?

A   Activities

About your activities,
- What activities and hobbies do you and your family engage in?
- Do you burn, solder, or melt any products?
- Do you garden, fish, or hunt?
- Do you eat what you catch or grow?
- Do you use pesticides?
- Do you engage in any alternative healing or cultural practices?

R   Referrals and Resources

Use these key referrals and resources.
- Environmental Protection Agency (www.epa.gov)
- National Library of Medicine, Toxnet programs (www.nlm.nih.gov)
- Agency for Toxic Substances and Disease Registry (www.atsdr.cdc.gov)
- Association of Occupational and Environmental Clinics (www.aoec.org)
- Material safety data sheets (www.hazard.com/msds)
- Occupational Safety and Health Administration (www.osha.gov)
- EnviRN website (www.envirn.umaryland.edu)
- Local health department, environmental agency, poison control center

E   Educate

Use this checklist of educational materials:
- Are materials available to educate the client?
- Are alternatives available to minimize the risk of exposure?
- Have prevention strategies been discussed?
- What is the plan for follow-up?

Prepared by Grace Paranzino, R.N., M.P.H., for the Agency for Toxic Substances and Disease Registry. For more information, contact ATSDR at 1-888-42-ATSDR, or visit ATSDR's website at www.atsdr.cdc.gov.

ENVIRONMENTAL EXPOSURE HISTORY

A mnemonic was developed to help health professionals remember the questions to ask when taking an environmental history. Exposures may occur in any setting in which people spend time; be sure to assess them all. The "I PREPARE" mnemonic can be used when assessing an individual, family, or community (Box 6-4). Figure 6-1 shows various pathways for toxic chemicals in our environment.

ENVIRONMENTAL HEALTH ASSESSMENT

A windshield survey is a helpful first step to understanding the potential environmental health risks in a community. If the community is urban, the age and condition of the housing and potential trash problems (and the associated pest problems) can be easily determined by driving around the neighborhood. Note also the proximity to factories, dumpsites, major transportation routes, and other sources of pollution.

In rural communities, pay attention to the use of aerial and other types of pesticide and herbicide spraying.

In addition to the tools used for a general community assessment, some specific tools are available to detect the environmental health risks within a community. The Right to Know section (p. 95) describes the types of information that are available to the public about air and water emissions, drinking water quality, and other environmental sources. In addition, Appendix G.3 is a community health assessment tool that provides an example of an environmental health assessment form with Internet resources for each of the potential exposures being assessed.

Air

The Clean Air Act regulates air pollution from both point sources (smokestacks) and nonpoint sources (automobiles, trucks, buses). The EPA uses a set of pollutants ("criteria

is responsible for testing the water according to EPA standards. The results of the testing must be reported to those who purchase the water, in the form of a **consumer confidence report (CCR)**. Nurses should review consumer confidence reports, sometimes referred to as *right-to-know reports,* to determine what pollutants have been found in the drinking water. If the drinking water poses an immediate health threat, the water provider must send emergency warnings to the community via the local newspapers, radio, and television. The Freedom of Information Act is a federal law that allows citizens to request public documents.

Employees have the right to know, through the federal Hazard Communication Standard, about hazardous chemicals with which they work. This standard requires employers (including hospitals) to maintain a list of all hazardous chemicals used on site. Each of these chemicals should have an associated chemical information sheet, known as a *material safety data sheet* (MSDS), written by the chemical manufacturer. These safety sheets, available to any employee or his or her representative, should provide information about the chemical makeup, the health risks, and any special guidance on safe use and handling (e.g., requirements for protective gloves or respiratory protection). This standard is enforced by the Occupational Safety and Health Administration (OSHA) (see www.osha.gov).

RISK ASSESSMENT

Currently, the EPA uses a process called risk assessment when they develop health-based standards. The term **risk assessment** refers to a process to determine the probability of a health threat associated with an exposure. The following describes the four phases of a risk assessment related to chemical exposures.

First, access toxicologic and/or epidemiologic data to learn if a chemical is known to be associated with negative health effects (in animals or humans). Remember, the available toxicologic data will probably be based on animal studies (from which the potential effects on humans are estimated), whereas the results of the epidemiologic studies will be for human health effects.

Second, determine if the chemical has been released into the environment via the air, water, soil, or food. Environmental professionals such as sanitarians, food inspectors, air and water pollution scientists, and environmental engineers can test for the presence of the suspected chemical in the various media (air, water, soil, food). In performing a risk assessment, determine if multiple sources of the questionable chemical are present. For example, is lead found in the drinking water, in the ambient air, *and* in the paint in houses in a given community? If so, the lead will have a cumulative effect and be more of a danger.

In the third phase, estimate how much of the chemical might enter the human body, and by which route. This estimate can be based on a one-time exposure, a short-term exposure, or a projected lifetime exposure. Federal standards created for air, water, and other pollutants are based on an estimation of a lifetime exposure. However, in workplace settings, the chemical exposure standards are based on an average exposure during a typical work shift or they are set for a maximum exposure at any given time.

Pollution sources are characterized as point sources. A **point-source** pollutant is released into the environment from a single site, such as a smoke stack, a hazardous waste site, or an effluent pipe into a waterway. A **nonpoint source** of pollution is more diffuse—for example, traffic, fertilizer, or pesticide run-off into waterways (whether from large-scale farming operations or from individual lawns and gardens). Another nonpoint source is animal waste, from wildlife or confined animal operations for food production (e.g., swine, poultry), that can get into nearby water bodies, resulting in coliform contamination and nutrient overload. The result can be illness from ingestion of contaminated water and the creation of conditions amenable to growth of toxic algae such as *Pfiesteriae piscicida* (Burkholder et al, 2005).

The final stage of the risk assessment process takes into account all three of the previous steps and asks the following questions:

- Is the chemical toxic?
- What is the source and amount of the exposure?
- What is the route and duration of the exposure for humans?

The final synthesis attempts to predict the potential for harm on the basis of the estimated exposure. Like all science, risk assessment is subject to interpretation. In translating the risk assessment results for the purposes of policy development and recommendations for risk reduction activities, there are often several interpretations for each risk assessment step and the result is different recommendations. Furthermore, areas of scientific uncertainty contribute to variations in assessment of risk. Also, environmental laws are often contentious not only because of public or ecological health concerns but also economic interests are at stake.

ASSESSING RISKS IN VULNERABLE POPULATIONS: CHILDREN'S ENVIRONMENTAL HEALTH

Children today are especially at risk for environmental hazards because of factors such as poverty, lack of access to health care, and the dangerous environmental situations in the communities in which they live. Environmental toxins, such as lead, pesticides, mercury, air pollution, solvents, asbestos, and radon, get into homes, schools, childcare centers, and playgrounds. Children exposed to environmental hazards are at risk for developing learning disabilities, behavioral disorders, chronic diseases such as asthma and cancer, and illness resulting from central nervous system damage (Massey-Stokes, 2002).

In childhood cancer, the good news is that successes in treatment are mounting; however, the bad news is that cancer is still the leading cause of death from disease in children younger than 15 years (Massey-Stokes and Lanning, 2002). Leukemia and tumors of the central nervous system combined account for approximately 50%. The list of possible causes of children's cancer includes genetic abnormalities, ultraviolet and ionizing radiation, electromagnetic fields, viral infections, certain medications, food additives, tobacco, alcohol, and industrial and agricultural chemicals (Ross and Olshan, 2004). Clearly, the environment is playing an important role.

Children are not just little adults with regard to their responses to environmental exposures. Infants and young children breathe more rapidly than adults and thus have a proportionally greater exposure to air pollutants. While infants' lungs are developing, they are particularly susceptible to environmental toxicants. Because children are short, their breathing zones are lower than those of adults, so they have closer contact to the chemical and biological agents that accumulate on floors and carpeting.

Children's bodies also operate differently. Some protective mechanisms that are well developed in adults, such as the blood brain barrier, are immature in young children, making them more vulnerable to the effects of toxic chemicals. And, finally, the kidneys of young children are less effective at filtering out undesirable, toxic chemicals, which then continue to circulate and accumulate.

BRIEFLY NOTED

Children's ability to readily absorb calcium and other nutrients is important for their growing bodies. But this mechanism also enhances the uptake of unwanted chemicals such as lead and other heavy metals.

Infants and young children drink more fluids per kilogram of body weight than do adults, thus increasing their dose of contaminants found in their drinking water, milk (hormones, antibiotics), and juices (particularly pesticides). (To drink an amount equivalent to an infant's intake, an adult would have to drink about 50 glasses of water a day.) Children also eat more per kilogram of body weight than do adults in order to maintain homeostasis (Illig and Haldeos, 2004). Children consume more fruits and fruit juices than do adults, once again increasing their exposure to pesticide residues.

Toxic chemicals can have different effects depending on the timing of exposure (Table 6-1). During fetal development, there are periods of great sensitivity to the effects of toxic chemicals. During such times, even small exposures can prevent or change a process that may permanently affect normal development. The brain undergoes rapid structural and functional changes during late pregnancy and in the neonatal period. Therefore it is extremely important to safeguard women's environments when they are pregnant.

BRIEFLY NOTED

Developmental toxicants such as lead, mercury, and pesticides (all found in hospitals and their waste streams) may directly interfere with processes required for normal brain development.

Table 6-1 Environmental Agents Implicated in Adverse Reproductive Outcomes

Exposure	Known/Suspected Effect
Anesthetic compounds	Infertility, spontaneous abortion, fetal malformations, low birthweight
Antineoplastics	Infertility, spontaneous abortion
Dibromochloropropane	Sperm abnormalities, infertility
Ionizing radiation	Infertility, microcephaly, chromosomal abnormalities, childhood malignancies
Lead	Infertility, spontaneous abortion, developmental disabilities
Manganese	Infertility
Organic mercury	Developmental disabilities, neurological abnormalities
Organic solvents	Congenital malformations, childhood malignancies
Chlorinated biphenyls, polybrominated biphenyls	Fetal mortality, low birthweight, congenital abnormalities, developmental disabilities

From Aldrich T, Griffith J: *Environmental epidemiology and risk assessment,* New York, 1993, Van Nostrand Reinhold.

It is alarming that 23 states have issued mercury contamination advisories for fish in *every* lake and river within their borders (Environmental Protection Agency, 2006). According to the EPA, more than 1 million women of childbearing age in the United States eat sufficient amounts of mercury-contaminated fish to risk damaging the brain development of their children. A nutritionally balanced diet is important, and fish is a good source of protein; however, the effects of mercury are important. Remember that waterfowl and other wildlife also eat contaminated fish and may be additional sources of mercury to people. Mercury accumulates in muscle tissue and is linked to neurological and renal disorders, as well as the fetal and neonatal risks just described.

BRIEFLY NOTED

A fish alert warns pregnant women (or women who wish to become pregnant) to limit their fish consumption to one portion a week for certain fish, including tuna. Both the EPA and the Food and Drug Administration (FDA) have issued alerts because dangerously high amounts of mercury are in these fish that create risks for the unborn child's developing nervous system. (See www.epa.gov/ost/fish or www.cfsan.fda.gov.)

Of the tens of thousands of synthetic chemicals that are in air, water, food, workplaces, and products, 75% have undergone little or no toxicity testing. Based on recent laboratory models, many additional chemicals are said to cause neurotoxic effects in adults (Grandjean and Landrigan, 2006). Companies are not required to divulge all the results of their private testing. A full battery of neurotoxicity tests is not

---

Box 6-7 **Food Quality Protection Act of 1996**

New provisions under the Food Quality Protection Act are related to protection of infants and children from pesticide exposure from multiple sources:

- *Health-based standard:* A new standard of a reasonable certainty of "no harm" that prohibits taking into account economic considerations when children are at risk
- *Additional margin of safety:* Requires that the Environmental Protection Agency (EPA) use an additional tenfold margin of safety when there are adequate data to assess prenatal and postnatal developmental risks
- *Account for children's diet:* Requires the use of age-appropriate estimates of dietary consumption in establishing allowable levels of pesticides on food to account for children's unique dietary patterns
- *Account for all exposures:* In establishing acceptable levels of a pesticide on food, the EPA must account for exposures that may occur through other routes, such as drinking water and residential application of the pesticide
- *Cumulative impact:* The EPA must consider the cumulative impacts of all pesticides that may share a common mechanism of action
- *Tolerance reassessments:* All existing pesticide food standards must be reassessed over a 10-year period to ensure that they meet the new standards to protect children
- *Endocrine disruption testing:* The EPA must screen and test all pesticides and pesticide ingredients for estrogen effects and other endocrine disruptor activity
- *Registration renewal:* Establishes a 15-year renewal process for all pesticides to ensure that they have up-to-date scientific evaluations over time

From the Environmental Protection Agency, Office of Pesticide Programs, available at http://www.epa.gov/oppfead1/fqpa.

Box 6-8 **Industrial Hygiene Controls**

- Substitute less hazardous or nonhazardous substances for hazardous ones (e.g., use water-based instead of solvent-based products)
- Isolate the hazardous chemicals from human exposure (closed systems)
- Apply engineering controls (e.g., ventilation systems, including exhausts)
- Reduce the exposures through administrative controls (rotating employees)
- Utilize personal protective equipment (gloves, respirators, protective clothing)
- Educate employees about controls

From Levy B, Wegman D: *Occupational health: recognizing and preventing work-related disease and injury,* ed 4, Philadelphia, 2000, Lippincott Williams & Wilkins.

---

required, even for pesticides that may be sprayed in nurseries and labor and delivery areas of hospitals, not to mention in our homes. Complicating matters even further, risks from multiple chemical exposures are rarely considered when regulations are drafted. Such an omission ignores the reality that children (as well as adults) are exposed to many toxic chemicals, often concurrently. The only exception to this is in the case of regulations regarding pesticides that are used on food supplies. This exception was created by the 1996 Food Quality Protection Act, in which Congress acknowledged that children eat foods that may be contaminated by more than one pesticide residue (Box 6-7). Remember, with thousands of chemical compounds now creating a chemical "soup" in air and water (in our bodies, in our breast milk), it is increasingly difficult to prove a relationship between exposure to a single chemical and disease outcome in humans.

REDUCING ENVIRONMENTAL HEALTH RISKS

Preventing problems is less costly, whether the cost is measured in resources consumed or health effects. Education is a primary preventive strategy. When examining the sources of environmental health risks in communities and planning

intervention strategies, it is important to apply the basic principles of disease prevention. For a home with lead-based paint, apply the primary prevention strategy of removing that specific source of lead. Good surveillance, a secondary prevention strategy, will not prevent lead exposure, but it may help with early identification of rising blood lead levels. For a symptomatic child brought to a health care provider, a system should be in place for specialists familiar with lead poisoning to provide immediate care; swift medical interventions to reduce blood levels of lead can reduce the risk of further harm. This might be a tertiary prevention response.

For workplace exposures, industrial hygienists have developed a list of precautions for avoiding or minimizing employee exposures to potentially hazardous chemicals. Industrial hygienists are public health professionals who specialize in workplace exposures to hazards—physical, chemical, and biological—that create conditions of health risk (Box 6-8). Once we have established that a human health threat exists, we must develop a plan of action to eliminate or manage (reduce) the risk. Risk management, which should be informed by the risk assessment process, involves the selection and implementation of a strategy to reduce risks, and this can take many forms. For example, the "Three R's for Reducing Environmental Pollution" are as follows:

1. *Reduce:* Reducing consumption reduces waste and unnecessary packaging and nonessentials.
2. *Reuse:* Choosing reusable rather than disposable products creates less waste (e.g., using glass dishes rather than paper ones).
3. *Recycle:* Recycling paper, glass, cans, and plastic decreases pollution.

Another form of risk reduction is to reduce the risk from exposure to ultraviolet rays. People need to avoid being outside during peak sun hours and need to wear protective clothing and/or sun block. To reduce exposure to dangerous heavy metals, special processes can be used at the water filtration plant that supplies the public water. In the home, running the cold water tap for 1 or 2 minutes each morning before collecting water for coffee or drinking will reduce the presence of lead that may have leached from old pipes

Levels of Prevention **Related to the Environment**

PRIMARY PREVENTION

To prevent lead poisoning, instruct families not to use lead-based paint. If such paint has been used, instruct them in removing it and repainting with a non-lead-based paint.

SECONDARY PREVENTION

Identify any household members whose blood lead level is rising.

TERTIARY PREVENTION

Initiate treatment for lead poisoning that will reduce blood lead levels.

Box 6-9 Outrage Factors: Characteristics of Risk that Contribute to the Public's Feeling of Outrage

Twelve Principal Outrage Components

SAFER (LESS OUTRAGE)	LESS SAFE (MORE OUTRAGE)
Voluntary	Involuntary (coerced)
Natural	Industrial (artificial)
Familiar	Exotic
Not memorable	Memorable
Not dreaded	Dreaded
Chronic	Catastrophic
Knowable (detectable)	Unknowable (undetectable)
Controlled by the individual	Controlled by others
Fair	Unfair
Morally irrelevant	Morally relevant
Trustworthy sources	Untrustworthy sources
Responsive process	Unresponsive process

Eight Secondary Outrage Components

SAFER (LESS OUTRAGE)	LESS SAFE (MORE OUTRAGE)
Affects average populations	Affects vulnerable populations
Immediate effects	Delayed effects
No risk to future generations	Substantial risk to future generations
Victims statistical	Victims identifiable
Preventable	Not preventable (only reducible)
Substantial benefits	Few benefits (foolish risk)
Little media attention	Substantial media attention
Little opportunity for collective action	Much opportunity for collective action

---

(or the solder used on them) overnight. In communities that report in the local media pollution levels, it is important to encourage residents to exercise or not walk excessively outside when the air pollution index is high. Individuals, communities, and nations can reduce risks. In recent years, there have been global agreements to reduce persistent pollutants and decrease global warming.

Climate changes around the world are leading to global warming. The greenhouse effect is influencing the prevalence of global warming. The greenhouse effect refers to the rise in temperature that occurs when the Earth experiences certain gases in the atmosphere, such as water vapor, carbon dioxide, nitrous oxide, and methane, that trap incoming solar radiation from the sun (Afzal, 2007). A certain amount of the greenhouse effect is essential for human life; however, an excess is dangerous. The goal is to reduce the amount of heat in the environment since high temperatures in the presence of sunlight and certain air pollutants can lead to the formation of ground level ozone. Increased exposure to ozone is associated with increased risk of premature mortality. This risk supports the growing trend toward actions such as walking not driving; recycling; and purchasing energy-efficient cars, appliances, and light bulbs.

Nursing interventions to reduce environmental health risks can also take many forms. Education is a key mode of nursing action. By working with a variety of community members, nurses can explain the relationship between harmful environmental exposures and human health and guide the community toward risk reduction based on both changes in individual behavior and community-wide approaches.

RISK COMMUNICATION

Risk is a familiar term in nursing practice. We counsel people about risks of pregnancy, communicable disease (especially sexually transmitted disease), unintentional injury, and personal health-related choices (e.g., smoking, alcohol consumption, diet). Risk assessment in environmental health has focused on characterizing the hazard (i.e., the source), its physical and chemical properties, its toxicity, and the presence of (or potential for) other elements in the exposure pathway—mode of transmission, route of exposure, receptor population, and dose. Risk has traditionally been formulated

as the process of estimating the likelihood of an unwanted, adverse effect and the probable magnitude and intensity of that effect (Fairbrother and Turnley, 2005). For example, an environmental risk assessment of a contaminated site includes a calculation of the dose that might be received through all routes of exposure, the toxicity of the chemical, the size and vulnerability (age, health) of the population potentially exposed (resident, future resident, transient), and the likelihood of exposure.

Sandman, Chess, and Hane (1991) noted that, in their experience, the reaction to things that scare people and the things that kill people are often not related to the actual hazard. They have gone further to probe what is behind those differences and have identified 20 "outrage" factors to explain people's responses to risk (Box 6-9). They maintain that the outrage is just as predictable and open to intervention as the science of addressing the hazard.

Communication of risk is both an area of practice and a skill. It involves understanding the outrage factors relevant to the risk being addressed so that both can be incorporated in the message, with the result that either action is taken to ensure safety or unnecessary fear is reduced. An example of raising outrage to produce action can be seen in the shift from emphasis on smokers (voluntary) to victims of passive smoking (involuntary) to stimulate public policy that limits or bans smoking in public places. When the emphasis on risk went from a voluntary choice of smokers to an involuntary exposure of nonsmokers, the outrage level of the nonsmoking public became high enough to result in legislation guaranteeing smoke-free public spaces (e.g., public buildings, airplanes, restaurants). On the other hand, outrage diminishes when people obtain information about a situation from a trusted source, and doctors and nurses are often cited in surveys as trusted sources of information on environmental risks (University of Newcastle upon Tyne, 2001–2002).

Risk communication includes general principles of good communication. It is a combination of the following:

- *The right information:* accurate, relevant, and in a language that audiences can understand. A good risk assessment is essential information for shaping the message.
- *To the right people:* those affected and those who may not be affected but are worried. Information about the community is essential: the geographic boundaries, who lives there (demographics), how they get information (flyers, newspapers, radio, television, the Internet, word of mouth), where they get together (school, church, community center), and who within the community can help plan the communication.
- *At the right time:* for timely action or to allay fear.

ETHICS

As discussed in Chapter 4, understanding ethics is essential for nurses making their own choices, in describing issues and options within groups, and in advocating for ethical choices. When the sticking points are around competing commodities (e.g., jobs vs. environmental protection; production vs. conservation), the skillful nurse can change the discussion from "either/or" to "both" by opening new possibilities for ethical and mutually satisfactory outcomes. The following ethical issues may arise in environmental health decisions:

- Who has access to information and when?
- How complete and accurate is the available information?
- Who is included in decision making and when?
- What and whose values and priorities are given weight in decisions?
- How are short-term and long-term consequences considered?

GOVERNMENT ENVIRONMENTAL PROTECTION

The federal government is involved with many major pieces of environmental legislation (Box 6-10). The government manages environmental exposures through the development and enforcement of standards and regulations that limit a polluter's ability to put hazardous chemicals into our food, water, air, or soil. The government may also be involved in educating the public about risks and risk reduction. Several federal agencies are involved in environmental health

regulation, including the EPA, the Food and Drug Administration, and the Department of Agriculture. In every state, an equivalent state agency exists as well. At the city or county level, environmental health issues are most often managed by the local health department. However, environmental protection issues are typically directed by the state using both federal and state laws. The organization and approach to environmental protection vary somewhat among states, but the common essential strategies of prevention and control via the permitting process, establishment of environmental standards, and monitoring, as well as compliance and enforcement, are found in every state.

Potentially harmful pollution that cannot be prevented must be controlled. The first step in the process of controlling pollution is **permitting**, a process by which the government places limits on the amount of pollution emitted into the air or water. Industries and businesses whose processes will result in releases (discharges, emissions) that have the potential for harm are required to obtain environmental permits to construct and operate. A range of permits may be required (e.g., storm water control, construction, operations for air and wastewater discharges, waste management). It is in the permitting process that maximum opportunities to incorporate prevention strategies can be exercised. For example, waste minimization can be included as a permit condition, with the agreement of the industry, even if it is not required by a law or regulation. Once a condition exists in the permit, it has the force of law.

The permitting process includes submission of an application, which requires details on the proposed operation. Plans are studied, engineering processes are modeled and validated, and other technical requirements are reviewed by appropriate regulatory experts. Usually some form of public participation is required or included voluntarily. The public involvement can include public notice, public comment, and public meetings and hearings initiated by the regulatory agency. Public involvement can also take the form of voluntary agreements and dispute resolution between the industry and the community, which may or may not involve a government entity. Limits on what an industry or business can release or emit lawfully are based on environmental standards.

Environmental standards may be expressed as a permitted level of emissions, a maximum contaminant level (MCL) allowed, an action level for environmental cleanup, or a risk-based calculation. A standard often reflects the level of pollution that will limit a number of excess deaths at a given level of exposure over a specified period of time. For example, the MCL for a contaminant in drinking water may be the level of exposure that would produce one excess (over the expected rate) cancer death if a person drank 1 liter of the water a day for 70 years. Cancer deaths have been the most frequently used outcome measure in environmental standards, but the risk calculations are now expanding to include birth defects, reproductive disorders, immune function disorders, and morbidity (kidney, liver, respiratory, neurotoxicity) (Pope, Snyder, and Mood, 1995).

Box 6-10 Environmental Laws

National Environmental Policy Act—12 USC § 4321-4375 (1969)

The National Environmental Policy Act (NEPA) established the Environmental Protective Agency (EPA) and a national policy for the environment and provides for the establishment of a Council on Environmental Policy. All policies, regulations, and public laws shall be interpreted and administered in accordance with the policies set forth in this act.

Federal Insecticide, Fungicide, and Rodenticide Act—7 USC § 135 et seq. (1972)

The Federal Insecticide, Fungicide, and Rodenticide Act (FIFRA) provides federal control of pesticide distribution, sale, and use. The EPA was given the authority to study the consequences of pesticide usage and requires users such as farmers and utility companies to register when using pesticides. Later amendments to the law required of applicators (1) certification examinations, (2) registration of all pesticides used in the United States, and (3) proper labeling of pesticides that, if in accordance with specifications, will cause no harm to the environment. (Summary from FIFRA 1972.)

Clean Water Act—USC § 1251 et seq. (1977)

The Clean Water Act (CWA) sets basic structure for regulating pollutants to U.S. waters. The law gave the EPA authority to set effluent standards on an industry basis and continued the requirements to set water quality standards for all contaminants in surface water. The 1977 amendments focused on toxic pollutants. Reauthorized in 1987, the CWA again focused on toxic pollutants, authorized citizen suit provisions, and funded sewage treatment plants.

Clean Air Act—42 USC § 7401 et seq. (1970)

The Clean Air Act regulates air emissions from area, stationary, and mobile sources. The EPA was authorized to establish National Ambient Air Quality Standards (NAAQS) to protect public health and the environment. The goal was to set and achieve the NAAQS by 1975. The law was amended in 1977 when many areas of the country failed to meet the standards. The 1990 amendments to the Clean Air Act intended to meet unaddressed or insufficiently addressed problems, such as acid rain, ground-level ozone, stratospheric ozone depletion, and air toxics. Also included in the 1990 reauthorization was a mandate for chemical risk management plans. This mandate requires industry to identify worst-case scenarios regarding the hazardous chemicals that they transport, use, or dispose of. (Summary from Clean Air Act 1970.)

Occupational Safety and Health Act—29 USC § 651 et seq. (1970)

The Occupational Safety and Health Act (OSHA) was established to ensure worker and workplace safety. The goal was to make sure employers provide an employment place free of hazards to health and safety, such as chemicals, excessive noise, mechanical dangers, heat or cold extremes, and unsanitary conditions. To establish standards for the workplace, OSHA also created the National Institute for Occupational Safety and Health (NIOSH) as the research institution for OSHA.

Safe Drinking Water Act—42 USC § 300f et seq. (1974)

The Safe Drinking Water Act (SDWA) was passed to protect the quality of U.S. drinking water. SDWA authorized the EPA to establish safe standards of purity and required all owners or operators of public water systems to comply with primary (health-related) standards.

Resource Conservation and Recovery Act—42 USC § 321 et seq. (1976)

The Resource Conservation and Recovery Act (RCRA) gave the EPA the authority to control the generation, transportation, treatment, storage, and disposal of hazardous waste. The RCRA also set forth a framework to manage nonhazardous waste. The 1984 Federal Hazardous and Solid Waste amendments to this Act required phasing out land disposal of hazardous waste. The 1986 amendments enabled the EPA to address problems of underground tanks storing petroleum and other hazardous substances.

Toxic Substances Control Act—15 USC § 2601 et seq. (1976)

The Toxic Substances Control Act (TSCA) gives the EPA the ability to track the 75,000 industrial chemicals currently produced or imported into the United States. The EPA can require reporting or testing of chemicals that may pose environmental health risks and can ban the manufacture and import of those chemicals that pose an unreasonable risk. The TCSA supplements the Clean Air Act and the Toxic Release Inventory.

Comprehensive Environmental Response, Compensation, and Liability Act—42 USC § 9601 et seq. (1980)

The Comprehensive Environmental Response, Compensation, and Liability Act (CERCLA), known as the Superfund, created a tax on the chemical and petroleum industries and provided broad federal authority to respond directly to releases or threatened releases of hazardous substances that may endanger public health or the environment.

Superfund Amendments and Reauthorization Act (SARA)—42 USC § 9601 et seq. (1986)

The Superfund Amendments and Reauthorization Act (SARA) amended CERCLA. Changes increased the size of the trust fund, encouraged greater citizen participation in decision making about site cleanup, and increased state involvement in every phase of the Superfund program. Other changes focused on human health programs related to hazardous waste sites. The amendments focused on permanent remedies as well as innovative treatment technologies in the cleanup of hazardous waste sites. (Under Superfund legislation, the federal Agency for Toxic Substances and Disease Registry was established.)

Emergency Planning and Community Right-to-Know Act—42 USC § 11011 et seq. (1986)

The Emergency Planning and Community Right-to-Know Act (EPCRA), also known as Title III of SARA, was enacted to help local communities protect public health safety and the environment from chemical hazards. Each state was required to appoint a state Emergency Response Commission, and these were required to divide their states into emergency planning districts and establish a local emergency planning committee for each district.

National Environmental Education Act—Public Law 101-619, Nov. 16, 1990

The National Environmental Education Act created the National Environmental Education and Training Foundation, which resulted in a new and better-coordinated environmental education emphasis at the EPA.

Box 6-10 Environmental Laws—cont'd

Pollution Prevention Act—42 USC § 13101 and 13012 et seq. (1990)

The Pollution Prevention Act (PPA) focused industry, government, and public attention on reducing pollution through cost-effective changes in production, operation, and raw materials use. Other practices that increase efficient use of energy, water, and water resources include recycling, source reduction, and sustainable agriculture.

Food Quality Protection Act—Public Law 104-170, Aug. 3, 1996

The Food Quality Protection Act (FQPA) amended FIFRA and the Federal Food, Drug, and Cosmetic Act. The FQPA changed the way the EPA regulates pesticides. The requirements include a new safety standard—reasonable certainty of no harm—to be applied to all pesticides used on foods.

Chemical Safety Information, Site Security and Fuels Regulatory Act—Public Law 106-40, Jan. 6, 1999

The Chemical Safety Information, Site Security and Fuels Regulatory Act (an amendment to Section 112 of the Clean Air Act) removed from coverage by the Risk Management Plan (RMP) any flammable fuel when used as fuel or held for sale as fuel by a retail facility (flammable fuels held for sale at a wholesale facility are still covered). The law also limits access to off-site consequence analyses, which are reported in RMPs by covered facilities.

Once environmental standards are set, both for permitting and in individual facility permits, the next step in control is **monitoring**. Monitoring procedures, which must use methods approved by the EPA or scientific consensus, must follow accepted protocols (e.g., maintaining a documented chain of custody of samples to ensure accuracy and protection from contamination at the laboratory after sampling).

Environmental monitoring takes two main forms. One is actual inspections of permitted facilities to observe whether the plans submitted in the permit application are being implemented as approved. In addition to unannounced inspections, continuous monitoring of data and operating procedures required in permits is studied for any variations from what is allowed. Finally, periodic measurements of the facility outputs in air and water emissions are calculated or taken directly to ensure compliance with laws and regulations. An alternative or adjunct monitoring method is self-reported data from the regulated facility. Factors such as costs, reliability, and public trust and acceptance must be considered in deciding how much of the monitoring requirement can be met through self-reporting.

Beyond the monitoring of individual permitted facilities, official regulatory agencies design sampling networks for measuring the quality of water and air throughout the geographic area for which they have responsibility. Routine samples of air and water are taken at designated monitoring sites and analyzed.

Compliance and enforcement are the next building blocks in controlling environmental damage. **Compliance** refers to the processes for ensuring that permitting requirements are met. When permit or other legally defined violations are found, the first effort is to obtain quick, voluntary compliance from the violator. Incentives in the form of reducing or eliminating fines and penalties may be negotiated in return for rapid and effective action to correct the problem. Formal enforcement actions are taken when voluntary compliance is not achieved. **Enforcement** tools may include fines or penalties, suspension of specific operations, or closure of the

facility. If the violation is deemed to be willful and with full knowledge that it was unlawful, criminal law may provide for incarceration of the owners or operators, in addition to the other consequences.

Enforcement processes may also include provision for public involvement, although this is less common. The public often does not feel included at the level they desire in enforcement or changes to procedure. The public may be excluded if the problem is quickly resolved or the time for public comment would delay the solution. Also, industry may guard information for fear of private party lawsuits. Another view, however, is that public involvement is essential to ensure aggressive enforcement.

Cleanup or remediation of environmental damage is the final step. The authority to direct and ensure adequate restoration of environmental quality may be entirely in the hands of state or federal government agencies, or it may be contracted out to private companies, with official oversight. Public information and involvement processes, such as citizen advisory panels or community forums, are integral to remediation where implications for future land use and remedies acceptable to the affected community are part of the decision process.

ADVOCACY

The more than 2.7 million nurses in the United States today can and should be a strong voice for change. As informed citizens, nurses can take a variety of actions to protect the environmental health of families, clients, and communities. Nurses are seen as trusted sources of information and they need to serve as reliable sources of environmental health information. They can act in the best interest of public health, and use their abilities as educators, advocates, and communicators to affect public policy, laws, and regulations that protect public health. Nurses can serve as a resource for state and federal legislators and their staff. Often, legislators are asked to vote on environmental legislation without a sound understanding of how the legislation may affect public health. Although not every nurse can be an expert in all aspects of environmental health, every nurse has a basic education in human health and can identify people who may be most vulnerable to environmental insult. Nurses' thoughts about the potential effects of new laws on the health of individuals and communities are valuable to legislators. As communicators and educators, nurses can do the following:

- Write letters to local newspapers responding to environmental health issues affecting the community.
- Serve as a credible source of information at community gatherings, formal governmental hearings, and professional nursing forums.
- Volunteer to serve on state, local, or federal commissions. Know the zoning and permit laws that regulate the effects of industry and land use on the community.
- Read, listen, and ask questions. As informed citizens nurses can lead in fostering community action to address threats to environmental health.

ENVIRONMENTAL JUSTICE

Some diseases differentially affect different populations. Certain environmental health risks disproportionately affect poor people and people of color in the United States. A poor person of color is more likely to (1) live near a hazardous waste site or an incinerator, (2) have children who are lead poisoned, and (3) have children with asthma, which has a strong association with environmental exposures. Campaigns in communities of color and poor communities to improve the unequal burden of environmental risks strive to achieve **environmental justice** or environmental equity (Mood, 2002).

In 1993 the Environmental Justice Act was passed, and in 1994 Executive Order 12898, Federal Actions to Address Environmental Justice in Minority Populations, was signed. These created policies to more comprehensively reduce the incidence of environmental inequity by mandating that every federal agency act in a manner to address and prevent illnesses and injuries.

UNIQUE ENVIRONMENTAL HEALTH THREATS IN THE HEALTH CARE INDUSTRY: NEW OPPORTUNITIES FOR ADVOCACY

We seldom think of health care settings as sources of environmental pollution. However, the use of mercury-containing thermometers, sphygmomanometers, and esophageal dilators poses risks if they are broken and the mercury escapes (Shaner and Botter, 2003). (Even though this mercury-containing equipment is reliable, mercury-free alternatives are available.) Further, if the facility incinerates waste, the mercury will be released into the air. This airborne mercury will come down in raindrops, and when it lands in bodies of water (lakes, rivers, oceans), it is converted by microorganisms in the water to **methyl mercury**, which is highly toxic to humans. The methyl mercury is then bioaccumulated in fish; as larger fish eat smaller fish, the body burden of methyl mercury increases significantly.

Evidence-Based Practice

Grineski (2007) used an environmental justice frame to explore the sociodemographic, indoor hazard, and air quality factors that affect hospitalizations for asthma in Phoenix, Arizona. The researcher obtained data from the Arizona Department of Health about uncontrolled hospitalizations for asthma in which the patient was not receiving medication or treatment for the disease before being admitted to the hospital.

The study had four key findings that emerged from the data. First, air pollution is an important predictor of hospitalizations for asthma when sociodemographic factors are controlled. Second, indoor (and in some cases, outdoor) hazards are another significant predictor, with some struggling with indoor hazards such as mold as well as outdoor hazards such as ozone. Third, neighborhood social class diminished as a predictor when coupled with environmental conditions; however, Grineski notes that this is not surprising considering the linkages between the location of available housing for those of low social class and the location of areas that are highly polluted. Fourth, race is significant when considering uncontrolled asthma because of the high rates of asthma and hospitalizations for asthma in the African-American community, which is consistent with the literature in this area.

NURSE USE: This study examined the relationship between the environment and health care as it explored the causes for hospitalizations for asthma. The researcher concludes that more work must be done to determine the connection between poor quality housing and polluted environments, which she sees as an environmental justice issue. These predictors affect uncontrolled asthma in individuals in a particular population who happen to be of a particular social class. Further research linking issues of environmental justice and health care will add to a small but growing body of knowledge; this, in turn, can greatly affect future policies, research, and practice.

From Grineski SE: Incorporating health outcomes into environmental justice research: the case of children's asthma and air pollution in Phoenix, Arizona, *Environ Hazards* 7:360–371, 2007.

Many synthetic chemicals that contaminate the environment are referred to as **persistent bioaccumulative toxins (PBTs)** or **persistent organic pollutants (POPs)**. These are chemicals that do not break down, either in the air, water, or soil, or in the plant, animal, or human bodies to which they may be passed. Ultimately, because humans are at the top of the food chain, these chemicals may come to reside in our bodies. For instance, lead, which should not be found in the human body, can be found in the long bones of almost any human in the world because of its frequent use and presence in the environment.

Dioxin is another pollutant that contaminates our communities. It is created, in part, by the health care industry. Dioxin is an unintentional by-product of combusting chlorine compounds, and it is stored in fat cells as it works its way up the food chain. This phenomenon has resulted in dioxin deposition in breast tissue and then its expression in milk (both cow's milk and human milk). Almost all women on earth now have dioxin in their breast tissue. Dioxin, which is an endocrine-disrupting chemical, a carcinogen, and is associated with several neurodevelopmental problems including learning disabilities, is often expressed in human milk. The solution to this concern is pollution prevention to remove the dioxin from our environment, not to stop breastfeeding, which is still the best nutritional choice for the baby.

An international campaign called *Health Care Without Harm* is working on the reduction and elimination of mercury and polyvinyl chloride (PVC) plastic in the health care industry, as well as the elimination of incineration of medical waste. These plastics comprise about 25% of all health care products and packaging (Shaner and Botter, 2003). When PVC plastic is incinerated, an unintentional by-product of its combustion is dioxin, which is then released into the environment. The American Nurses Association (ANA) was a founder of the Health Care Without Harm campaign, and nurses have taken many leadership roles in the activities in the United States and around the world. The Health Care Without Harm website (www.noharm.org) and the ANA's website (www.nursingworld.org, navigate to Occupational and Environment, then RNnoHarm) provide outstanding information and resources about the prevention of pollution in the health care sector.

REFERRAL RESOURCES

No single source of information about environmental health is available, nor is there a single resource to which individuals or a community can be referred if they suspect an environmental problem. Information is widely accessible on the World Wide Web, but finding an actual person to assist you or the communities you serve may not be as easy. One starting point may be the environmental epidemiology unit or toxicology unit of your state health department or environmental agency. Another local or state resource may be environmental health experts in nursing or medical schools or schools of public health. The Association of Occupational and Environmental Clinics (www.AOEC.org) is a national network of specialty clinics and individual practitioners available for consultation and sometimes for provision of educational programs for health professionals.

Local resources include local health and environmental protection agencies, poison control centers, agricultural extension offices, and occupational and environmental departments in schools of medicine, nursing, and public health. Some local and state agencies have developed topical directories to assist in accessing the appropriate staff for specific questions. Many resources have websites that allow ready access through the Internet and can be located by using any of the popular search methods (see Boxes 6-3 and 6-6 and the WebLinks at http://evolve.elsevier.com/stanhope/foundations).

ROLES FOR NURSES IN ENVIRONMENTAL HEALTH

Nurses can be involved in a number of roles in environmental health, in full-time work, as an adjunct to existing roles, and as informed citizens:

Evidence-Based Practice

While it is commonly understood that the quality of the air we breathe and the water we drink can impact our health, it is often more difficult to recognize that our choices of health care products, along with the way we dispose of them, and the chemicals we spray on our foods or use to clean and disinfect may actually compromise the environment and consequently our health.

Nurses can transform the health care sector into a model sector whose goals include promoting environmental health for patients, employees, and communities. This can be accomplished as nurses help institutions adhere to environmentally preferable purchasing policies, follow environmentally conscious waste management strategies, decrease the use of chemical pollutants, promote the use of healthy foods, and provide leadership in environmental stewardship. By taking positive steps, however modest, nurses can begin to have a serious impact on the quality of our environmental health.

NURSE USE: Nurses can be the catalyst to transform their workplace into an environmentally healthy and safe place by promoting environmentally preferable purchasing policies and suggesting environmentally friendly products. Even in a bustling hospital, taking strides to reduce the amount of waste, properly disposing of potentially toxic materials such as batteries, and initiating recycling programs can work to improve environmental and workplace health. Nurses can take leadership in decreasing the use of chemical pollutants by helping purchasing and environmental services staff understand the connection between safe products and good health and working together with them to seek safe alternatives. What we put into our bodies is also key; supporting sustainable food programs, where the food is free of harmful chemicals, antibiotics, and hormones, is another area in which nurses can work with dietary departments to effect change. Nurses are the most appropriate personnel to demonstrate leadership in environmental stewardship as they are at the hub of all hospital activity. Nurses need to learn more about the health of the environment in which they work and direct change to improve this environment for their patients and themselves.

From Sattler B, Hall K: Healthy choices: transforming our hospitals into environmentally healthy and safe places, *OJIN: The Online Journal of Issues in Nursing* (12) 2, 2007. Retrieved November 26, 2007 from http://www.nursingworld.org/MainMenuCategories/ANAMarketplace/ANAPeriodicals/OJIN/TableofContents/Volume122007/May31/HealthyChoices.aspx.

- *Community involvement and public participation.* Organizing, facilitating, and moderating. Making public notices effective, public forums accessible and welcoming input. Making information exchange understandable and problem solving acceptable to culturally diverse communities are valuable contributions made by nurses. Skills in community organizing and mobilizing can be essential to the ability of a community to have a meaningful voice in decisions that affect it.
- *Individual and population risk assessment.* Using nursing assessment skills to detect potential and actual exposure pathways and outcomes for clients cared for in the acute, chronic, and healthy communities of practice.

- *Risk communication.* Interpreting, and applying principles to practice. Nurses may serve as skilled risk communicators within agencies, working for industries, or working as independent practitioners. Amendments to the Clean Air Act require major industrial sources of air emissions to have risk management plans and to inform their neighbors of specifics of the risks and plans (Clean Air Act, 1996).
- *Epidemiologic investigations.* Having the skills to respond in scientifically sound and humanly sensitive ways to community concerns about cancer, birth defects, and stillbirths that citizens fear may have environmental causes.
- *Policy development.* Proposing, informing, and monitoring action from agencies, communities, and organization perspectives.

The assimilation of the concepts of environmental health into a nurse's daily practice gives new life to the traditional public health values of prevention, building community, and social justice. There is great congruence with many personal, religious, and spiritual values of stewardship of creation, preserving the gifts of nature, and decision making that provides for quality of life for present and future generations. It is a context for practice in which nurses are welcomed and valued for their contribution.

As nurses learn more about the environment, opportunities for integration into their practice, educational programs, research, advocacy, and policy work will become evident. Opportunities abound for those pioneering spirits within the nursing profession who are dedicated to creating healthier environments for their clients and communities.

CLINICAL APPLICATION

Two case scenarios related to exposure pathways are presented here. The first involves lead poisoning and the second involves gasoline contamination of groundwater.

At the county health department, a 3-year-old boy presents with gastric upset and behavior changes that have persisted for several weeks. Billy's parents report that they have been renovating their home to remove lead paint. They had been discouraged from routinely testing their child because their insurance does not cover testing and they could not find information on where to have the test done. Their concern has heightened with Billy's persistent symptoms.

You test the level of lead in Billy's blood and find it to be 45 μg/dl. You research lead poisoning and discover that children are at great risk because of their inclination to absorb lead into their central nervous systems. You also find that chronic lead poisoning may have long-term effects, such as developmental delays and impaired learning ability. You refer Billy to his primary care physician. On further investigation, you find that Billy's home was built before 1950 and is still under renovation. The sanitarian tests the interior paint and finds a high lead content. Ample amounts of sawdust from sanding are noted in various rooms of the home.

You determine that a completed exposure pathway exists.

A. *What would you include in an assessment of this situation?*
B. *What prevention strategies would you use to resolve this issue?*
  1. *At the individual level?*
  2. *At the population level?*

A citizen calls the local health department to report that his drinking water, from a private well, "smells like gasoline." A water sample is collected, and analysis reveals the presence of petroleum products. A nearby rural store with a service station has removed its old underground gasoline storage tanks and replaced them, as required by law. Contaminated soil from the old leaking tank has been removed, and a well to monitor groundwater contamination is scheduled for installation. However, sandy soil has allowed rapid movement of the contamination through the groundwater, and the plume has reached the neighbor's drinking-water well at levels that exceed the drinking-water standard.

What are some possible responses?
Answers are in the back of the book.

REMEMBER THIS!

- Nurses have responsibilities to be informed consumers and to be advocates for citizens in their community regarding environmental health issues.
- Models describing the determinants of health acknowledge the role of the environment in health and disease.
- For many chemical compounds, whether new or familiar, scientific evidence of possible health effects is lacking.
- Prevention activities include education, waste minimizing, and land use planning. Control activities include environmental permitting, environmental standards, monitoring, compliance and enforcement, and cleanup and remediation.
- Each nursing assessment should include questions and observations about intended and unintended environmental exposures.
- Environmental databases facilitate the easy and immediate access to environmental data useful in assessment, diagnosis, intervention, and evaluation.
- Both case advocacy and class advocacy are important skills for nurses in environmental health practice.
- Risk communication is an important skill and must acknowledge the outrage factor experienced by communities with environmental hazards.
- Federal, state, and local laws and regulations exist to protect citizens from environmental hazards.

- Environmental health practice engages multiple disciplines, and nurses are important members of the environmental health team.
- Environmental health practice includes principles of health promotion, disease prevention, and health protection.
- The objectives of both *Healthy People 2000* and *Healthy People 2010* address targets for the reduction of risk factors and diseases related to environmental causes.

WHAT WOULD YOU DO?

1. If you think that the drinking water in your community is contaminated from polluted sources, how would you go about verifying your concern? Who would you contact? What would your sources of information be? If you find that you are correct, what steps would you take to remedy this environmental health problem?
2. Determine if your jurisdiction has a law or regulation for the disclosure of radon levels on personal property as part of a real estate sale. If your community does not, investigate with the government officials of the community the reasons for the lack of a disclosure requirement.
3. Do you think that waste materials from another country should be accepted into a landfill in the United States even if the other country is willing to pay an acceptable fee for this service? Justify your answer. If you found that this practice was taking place in your community, would you do anything? If so, what?

■ *REFERENCES*

Afzal, BM: Global warming: a public health concern, *OJIN: The Online Journal of Issues in Nursing*, 12(2). Retrieved November 26, 2007, from www.nursingworld.org/MainMenuCategories/ANAMarketplace/ANAPeriodicals?OJIN/TableofContents?Volume122007/May31/GlobalWarming.aspx

Agency for Toxic Substances and Disease Registry: Identifying and evaluating exposure pathways. In *Public health assessment guidance manual*, Atlanta, Ga, 1992, ATSDR.

Aldrich T, Griffith J: *Environmental epidemiology and risk assessment*, New York, 1993, Van Nostrand Reinhold.

Burkholder JM et al: Demonstration of toxicity to fish and to mammalian cells by Pfiesteria species comparison of assay methods and strains, *Proc Natl Acad Sci USA* 102:3471-3476, 2005.

Cassady A, Fidis A: *Toxic pollution and health: An analysis of toxic chemicals released in communities across the United States*, Washington, DC, 2007, U.S. Public Interest Research Group Education Fund.

Clean Air Act: Risk Management Programs, Section 112(7), Fed Regist, Part III EPA, 40 CFR, Part 68, June 20, 1996.

Dove A: Drugs down the drain, *Nat Med* 11:376-377, 2005.

Environmental Protection Agency: *Fact sheet national listing of fish advisories*, 2006, available at http://www.epa.gov/waterscience/fish/.

Fairbrother A, Turnley JG: Predicting risks of uncharacteristic wildfires: Application of the risk assessment process, *Forest Ecol and Mgmt* 211:28-35, 2005.

Goldman LR: Chemicals and children's environment: what we don't know about risks, *Environ Health Perspect* 106:875-879, 1998.

Goldman LR: Environmental health and its relationship to occupational health. In Levy BS, Wegman DH, editors: *Occupational health: recognizing and preventing work-related disease and injury*, Philadelphia, 2000, Lippincott Williams & Wilkins.

Grandjean P, Landrigan PJ: Developmental neurotoxicity of industrial chemicals, *The Lancet* DOI:10.1016/50140–6736(06)69665-7, 2006.

Grineski SE: Incorporating health outcomes into environmental justice research: The case of children's asthma and air pollution in Phoenix, Arizona, *Environ Hazards* 7:360-371, 2007.

Ilig P, Haldeos DP: Children's health and the environment, *Dev* 47:104-108, 2004.

Kinnula VL: Focus on antioxidant enzymes and antioxidant strategies in smoking related airway diseases, *Thorax* 60:693-700, 2005.

Laraque D, Trasande L: Lead poisoning: Successes and 21st century challenges, *Pediatr Rev* 26:435-443, 2005.

Levy B, Wegman D: *Occupational health: recognizing and preventing work-related disease and injury*, ed 4, Philadelphia, 2000, Lippincott Williams & Wilkins.

Lopez R, Welker-Hood K: Urban sprawl and the built environment, *Am Nurse Today* 2(1):56, 2007.

Massey-Stokes M: Foreword, Fam Community Health 24(4): viii, 2002.

Massey-Stokes M, Lanning B: Childhood cancer and environmental toxins: the debate continues, *Fam Community Health* 24(4):27-39, 2002.

Mood LH: Environmental health policy: environmental justice. In Mason DJ, Leavitt JK, editors: *Policy and politics in nursing and health care*, ed 4, Philadelphia, 2002, Saunders.

Nightingale F: *Notes on nursing: what it is and what it is not*, London, 1859, Harrison.

O'Connor AB, Roy C: Electric power plant emissions and public health, *AJN* 108(2):62-70, 2008.

Olshansky E: Why nurses need to be concerned about the environment, *J of Professional Nurs* 24(1):1-2, 2008.

Pope AM, Snyder MA, Mood LH, editors: *Nursing, health, and the environment*, Washington, DC, 1995, Institute of Medicine, National Academy Press.

Rosenthal LD: Carbon monoxide poisoning, *AJN* 106(3):40-46, March 2006.

Ross JS, Olshan AF: Pediatric cancer in the United States: the Children's Oncology Group Epidemiology Research Program, *Cancer Epidemiol, Biomarkers Prevention* 13:1552-1554, 2004.

Sandman PM, Chess C, Hane BJ: *Improving dialogue with communities*, New Brunswick, NJ, 1991, Rutgers University.

Sattler B, Hall K: Healthy choices: Transforming our hospitals into environmentally healthy and safe places. *OJIN: The Online Journal of Issues in Nursing*, (12) 2, 2007. Retrieved November 26, 2007, from http://www.nursingworld.org/MainMenuCategories/ANAMarketplace/ANAPeriodicals/OJIN/TableofContents/Volume122007/May31/HealthyChoices.aspx.

Sattler B, Lipscomb L, editors: *Environmental health and nursing practice*, New York, 2002, Springer.

Schettler T et al: *"In harm's way: toxic threats to development,"* a report by Greater Boston Physicians for Social Responsibility, prepared for a joint project with Clean Water, Cambridge, Mass, 2000, Physicians for Social Responsibility, available at http://www.igc.org/psr/pubs.htm.

Shaner H, Botter ML: Pollution: health care's unintended legacy, *Am J Nurs* 103(3):79-84, 2003.

University of Newcastle upon Tyne, School of Population and Health Sciences: Barriers to effective risk communication: study of the role of a local public health department in a controversial environmental investigation—2001-2002. Retrieved 11/10/06, from http:www.ncl.uk/pahs/research/project/811. (not found 8/08).

U.S. Department of Health and Human Services: *Healthy People 2010: understanding and improving health*, ed 2, Washington, DC, 2000, U.S. Government Printing Office.

Wright DJ: Collaborative learning experiences for nursing students in environmental health, *Nurs Educ Perspect* 24(4):189-191, 2003.

Government, the Law, and Policy Activism

Marcia Stanhope

ADDITIONAL RESOURCES

These related resources are found either in the appendix at the back of this book or on the book's website at http://evolve.elsevier.com/stanhope/foundations.

Appendix

- Appendix A.2: Schedule of Clinical Preventive Services
- Appendix A.3: Declaration of Alma Ata

Evolve Website

- Community Assessment Applied
- Case Study, with Questions and Answers
- Quiz review questions
- WebLinks, including link to *Healthy People 2010* website

OBJECTIVES

After reading this chapter, the student should be able to:

1. Discuss the structure of the U.S. government and health care roles.
2. List the functions of key governmental and quasigovernmental agencies that affect public health systems and nursing, both around the world and in the United States.
3. Identify the primary bodies of law that affect nursing and health care.
4. Define key terms related to policy and politics.
5. Describe the relationships between nursing practice, health policy, and politics.
6. Develop and implement a plan to communicate with policymakers on a chosen public health issue.

CHAPTER OUTLINE

KEY TERMS

advanced practice nurses: nurses with advanced education beyond the baccalaureate degree who are prepared to manage and deliver health care services to individuals, families, groups, communities, and populations; includes clinical nurse specialists, nurse practitioners, nurse midwives, nurse anesthetists, and others.

Agency for Healthcare Research and Quality (AHRQ): a division of the U.S. Department of Health and Human Services, formerly known as the Agency for Health Care Policy and Research (AHCPR), whose mission is to support research designed to improve the outcomes and quality of health care, reduce its costs, address patient safety and medical errors, and broaden access to services.

American Nurses Association (ANA): the national professional association of registered nurses in the United States, founded in 1896.

block grants: a predetermined amount of money based on previous spending and availability of funds that is given to a state by the federal government for designated purposes such as state health care programs.

board of nursing: a group created in each state by legislation known as a state nurse practice act. The board is made up of nurses and consumers who operationalize, implement, and enforce the statutory law by writing explicit statements (called rules) regarding nursing and nursing practice.

categorical programs/funding: federal, state, or local funds used to conduct a specific program such as tuberculosis screening, HIV/AIDS home care, or prenatal care. The money cannot be used for any other program or purpose.

constitutional law: branch of law dealing with the organization and function of a government.

devolution: the process of shifting, planning, delivering, and financing responsibility for programs from the federal to the state level.

health policy: public policy that affects health and health services. Delineates options from which individuals and organizations make their health-related choices. Made within a political context.

judicial law: law based on court or jury decisions.

legislation: bills introduced by Congress for the purpose of establishing laws that direct policy.

legislative staff: an individual or groups of individuals who perform duties such as research and writing, which helps the legislator move policy ideas through the legislative processes and into law.

licensure: legal sanction to practice a profession after attaining the minimum degree of competence to ensure protection of public health and safety.

National Institute of Nursing Research (NINR): one of the National Institutes of Health charged with promoting the growth and quality of research in nursing.

nurse practice act: state law that governs the practice of nursing.

Occupational Safety and Health Administration (OSHA): federal agency charged with improving worker health and safety by establishing standards and regulations and by educating workers.

Office of Homeland Security: an office of the executive branch designed to protect citizens from terrorist threats or attacks, including bioterrorism.

police power: states' power to act to protect the health, safety, and welfare of their citizens.

policy: settled course of action to be followed by a government or institution to obtain a desired end.

politics: the art of influencing others to accept a specific course of action.

regulations: specific statements of law that relate to and clarify individual pieces of legislation.

U.S. Department of Health and Human Services (USDHHS): a regulatory agency of the executive branch of government charged with overseeing the health and welfare needs of U.S. citizens.

World Health Organization (WHO): an arm of the United Nations that provides worldwide services to promote health.

Nurses are an important part of the health care system and are greatly affected by governmental and legal systems. Nurses who select the community as their area of practice must be especially aware of the impact of government, law, and health policy on nursing, health, and the communities in which they practice. Knowing how government, law, and political action have changed over time is necessary to understand how the health care system has been shaped by these factors. Also, understanding how these factors have influenced the current and future roles for nurses and the public health system is critical for establishing a better health policy for the nation.

Nurses have historically viewed themselves as advocates for the health of the population. It is this heritage that has moved the discipline into the policy and political arenas. To secure a more positive health care system, nurse professionals must develop a working knowledge of government, key governmental and quasigovernmental organizations and agencies, health care law, the policy process, and the political forces that are shaping the future of health care. This knowledge and the motivation to be an agent of change in the discipline and in the community are necessary ingredients for success as a nurse working in the community.

DEFINITIONS

To understand the relationship between health policy, politics, and laws, it is first necessary to understand the definitions of the terms.

1. **Policy** is a settled course of action to be followed by a government or institution to obtain a desired end.
2. **Health policy** is a set course of action to obtain a desired health outcome, for an individual, family, group, community, or society.

Policies are made not only by governments but also by institutions such as a health department or other health care agency, a family, or a professional organization.

Politics plays a role in the development of such policies. It is found in families, professional and employing agencies, and governments. Politics is the art of influencing others to accept a specific course of action. Therefore political activities are used to arrive at a course of action (the policy). Law is a system of privileges and processes by which people solve problems based on a set of established rules.

Laws govern the relationships of individuals and organizations to other individuals and to government. Through political action a policy becomes a law. After a law is established, regulations further define the course of action (policy) to be taken by organizations or individuals in reaching an outcome. Government is the ultimate authority in society and is designated to enforce the policy whether it is related to health, education, economics, social welfare, or any other society issue. The following discussion explains the role of government in health policy.

GOVERNMENTAL ROLE IN U.S. HEALTH CARE

In the United States, the federal and most state and local governments are composed of three branches, each of which has separate and important functions. The executive branch is composed of the president (or governor or mayor) along with the staff and cabinet appointed by this executive, various administrative and regulatory departments, and agencies such as the **U.S. Department of Health and Human Services (USDHHS)**. The legislative branch (i.e., Congress at the federal level) is made up of two bodies: the Senate and the House of Representatives, whose members are elected by the citizens of particular geographic areas. The judicial branch is composed of a system of federal, state, and local courts guided by the opinions of the Supreme Court.

- The executive branch suggests, administers, and regulates policy.
- The legislative branch identifies problems and proposes, debates, passes, and modifies laws to address those problems.
- The judicial branch interprets laws and their meaning and interprets states' rights to provide health services to citizens of the states.

BRIEFLY NOTED

One of the first constitutional challenges to a federal law passed by Congress was in the area of health and welfare in 1937, after the 74th Congress had established unemployment compensation and old-age benefits for U.S. citizens (U.S. Law, 1937b). Although Congress had created other health programs previously, its legal basis for doing so had never been challenged. In *Stewart Machine Co. v. Davis* (U.S. Law, 1937a), the Supreme Court (judicial branch) reviewed this legislation and determined, through interpretation of the Constitution, that such federal governmental action was within the powers of Congress to promote the general welfare.

Most legal bases for the actions of Congress in health care are found in Article I, Section 8 of the U.S. Constitution, including the following:

1. Provide for the general welfare.
2. Regulate commerce among the states.
3. Raise funds to support the military.
4. Provide spending power.

Through a continuing number and variety of cases and controversies, these Section 8 provisions have been interpreted by the courts to appropriately include a wide variety of federal powers and activities. State power concerning health care is called **police power**. This power allows states to act to protect the health, safety, and welfare of their citizens. Such police power must be used fairly, and the state must show that it has a compelling interest in taking actions, especially actions that might infringe on individual rights. Examples of a state using its police powers include requiring immunization of children before being admitted to school and requiring case finding, reporting, treating, and follow-up care of persons with tuberculosis. These activities protect the health, safety, and welfare of state citizens.

TRENDS AND SHIFTS IN GOVERNMENTAL ROLES

The government's role in health care at both the state and federal level began gradually. Wars, economic instability, and political differences between parties all shaped the government's role. The first major federal governmental action relating to health was the creation in 1798 of the Public Health Service (PHS). In 1934 Senator Wagner of New York initiated the first national health insurance bill. The Social Security Act of 1935 was passed to provide assistance to older adults and the unemployed; it also offered survivors' insurance for widows and children. In addition, it provided for child welfare, health department grants, and maternal and child health projects. In 1948 Congress created the National Institutes of Health (NIH). In 1965 it passed the most important health legislation to date—creating Medicare and Medicaid to provide health care service payments for older adults, the disabled, and the categorically poor.

The USDHHS was created in 1953. The Health Care Financing Administration (HCFA) was created in 1977 as the key agency within the USDHHS to provide direction for Medicare and Medicaid.

In 2002 HCFA was renamed the Centers for Medicare and Medicaid Services (CMS).

During the 1980s, a major effort of the administration was to shift federal government activities, including federal programs for health care, to the states. The process of shifting the responsibility for planning, delivering, and financing programs from the federal level to the states level is called **devolution**. From 1980 until the present, Congress has increasingly funded health programs by giving **block grants** to the states. Devolution processes including block granting should alert professional nurses that state and local policy is growing in importance in the health care arena.

The role of government in health care is shaped both by the needs and demands of its citizens and by the citizens' beliefs and values about personal responsibility and self-sufficiency. These beliefs and values often clash with society's sense of responsibility and need for equality for all citizens. A recent federal example of this ideological debate occurred in the 1990s over health care reform. The Democrats proposed the Health Security Act of 1993, which failed to gain Congress's approval. In an effort to make some incremental health care changes, both the Democrats and the Republicans in Congress passed two new laws.

The Health Insurance Portability and Accountability Act (HIPAA) allows working persons to keep their employee group health insurance for up to 16 months after they leave a job (U.S. Law, 1996).

The State Child Health Improvement Act (SCHIP) of 1997 provides insurance for children and families who cannot otherwise afford health insurance (U.S. Law, 1997).

This discussion has focused primarily on trends in and shifts between different levels of government. An additional aspect of governmental action is the relationship between government and individuals. Freedom of individuals must be balanced with governmental powers. After the terrorist attacks on the United States in September (World Trade Center attack) and October (anthrax outbreak) of 2001, much government activity is being conducted in the name of protecting the safety of U.S. citizens. Yet it remains unclear just how much governmental intervention is necessary and effective and how much will be tolerated by citizens.

BRIEFLY NOTED

Government has a great deal of influence on the way health care services are delivered and on who receives care.

It is interesting to note that before September 11, 2001, recognizing that the public health system infrastructure needed help, the Congress and President, in 2000, passed a law—"The Public Health Threats and Emergencies Act"

(PL 106-505). This was the "first federal law to comprehensively address the public health system's preparedness for bioterrorism and other infectious disease outbreaks" (Frist, 2002). This legislation is said to have signaled the beginning of renewed interest in public health as the protector for entire communities. In June 2002 the Public Health Security and Bioterrorism Preparedness and Response Act was signed into law (PL 107-188) with 3 billion dollars appropriated by Congress in December 2002 to implement the following antibioterrorism activities:

• Improving public health capacity
• Upgrading of the ability of health professionals to recognize and treat diseases caused by bioterrorism
• Speeding the development of new vaccines and other countermeasures
• Improving water and food supply protection
• Tracking and regulating the use of dangerous pathogens within the United States (Frist, 2002)

GOVERNMENT HEALTH CARE FUNCTIONS

Federal, state, and local governments carry out five health care functions, which fall into the general categories of direct services, financing, information, policy setting, and public protection.

Direct Services

Federal, state, and local governments provide direct health services to certain individuals and groups. For example, the federal government provides health care to members and dependents of the military, certain veterans, and federal prisoners. State and local governments employ nurses to deliver a variety of services to individuals and families, frequently on the basis of factors such as financial need or the need for

Evidence-Based Practice

The purpose of this study was to examine the changes in access to care, use of services, and quality of care among children enrolled in Child Health Plus (CHPlus), a state health insurance program for low-income children that became a model for the State Child Health Insurance Program (SCHIP). A before-and-after design was used to evaluate the health care experience of children the year before enrollment and the year after enrollment in the state health insurance program. The study consisted of 2126 children from New York State, ranging from birth to 12.99 years of age. Results indicated that the state health insurance program for low-income children was associated with improved access, use, and quality of care. The development and implementation of SCHIP were an outcome of the soaring costs of health care and the fact that there are 11 million uninsured children in the United States. It was the largest public investment in child health in 30 years.

NURSE USE: This study supports the value of health policy and the need to evaluate the effectiveness of policy in accomplishing the purposes of the policy.

From Szilagyi PG et al: Evaluation of a state health insurance program for low-income children: implications for state child health insurance programs, *Pediatrics* 105(2):363–371, 2000; U.S. Census Bureau Current Population Survey, 2004.

a particular service, such screening for hypertension or tuberculosis, immunizations for children and older adults, and primary care for inmates in local jails or state prisons. The Evidence-Based Practice box presents a study that examined the use of a state health insurance program.

Financing

Governments pay for some health care services. The government also pays for training some health personnel and for biomedical and health care research (U.S. Department of Health and Human Services, Centers for Medicare and Medicaid Services, 2005). Support in these areas has greatly affected both consumers and health care providers. State and federal governments finance the direct care of clients through the Medicare, Medicaid, Social Security, and SCHIP programs. Many nurses have been educated with government funds through grants and loans. Schools of nursing, in the past, have been built and equipped using federal funds. Governments have also financially supported other health care providers, such as physicians, most significantly through the program of Graduate Medical Education funds. The federal government invests in research and new program demonstration projects, with the NIH receiving a large portion of the monies. The **National Institute of Nursing Research (NINR)** is a part of the NIH and, as such, provides a substantial sum of money to the discipline of nursing for the purpose of developing the knowledge base of nursing and promoting nursing services in health care.

Information

All branches and levels of government collect, analyze, and disseminate data about health care and the health status of the citizens. An example is the annual report *Health: United States, 2007,* compiled each year by the USDHHS (U.S. Department of Health and Human Services, 2008). Collecting vital statistics, including mortality and morbidity data, gathering of census data, and conducting health care status surveys are all government activities. Table 7-1 lists examples of available federal and international data sources on the health status of populations in the United States and around the world. These sources are available on the Internet and in the governmental documents' section of most large libraries. This information is especially important because it can help nurses understand the major health problems in the United States and those in their own states and local communities.

Policy Setting

Policy setting is a primary government function. Governments at all levels and within all branches make policy decisions about health care. These health policy decisions have broad implications for financial expenses, resource use, delivery system change, and innovation in the health care field. One law that has played a very important role in the development of public health policy, public health nursing, and social welfare policy in the United States is the Sheppard-Towner Act of 1921 (U.S. Department of Health and Human Services, 1992; U.S. Department of Health and Human Services Human Resources and Services Administration, 2002) (Box 7-1).

Table 7-1	International and National Sources of Data on the Health Status of the U.S. Population
Organization	**Data Sources**
International	
United Nations	http://www.un.org/ *Demographic Yearbook*
World Health Organization	http://www.who.int/en/ *World Health Statistics Annual*
Federal	
Department of Health and Human Services	http://www.DHHS.gov National Vital Statistics System National Survey of Family Growth National Health Interview Survey National Health Examination Survey National Health and Nutrition Examination Survey National Master Facility Inventory National Hospital Discharge Survey National Nursing Home Survey National Ambulatory Medical Care Survey National Morbidity Reporting System U.S. Immunization Survey Surveys of Mental Health Facilities Estimates of National Health Expenditures AIDS Surveillance Nurse Supply Estimates
Department of Commerce	http://www.commerce.gov U.S. Census of Population Current Population Survey Population Estimates and Projections
Department of Labor	http://www.dol.gov Consumer Price Index Employment and Earnings

Public Protection

The U.S. Constitution gives the federal government the authority to provide for the protection of the public's health. This function is carried out in numerous ways, such as by regulating air and water quality and by protecting the borders from an influx of diseases by controlling food, drugs, and animal transportation. The Supreme Court interprets and makes decisions related to public health, for example, affirming a woman's rights to reproductive privacy (*Roe v. Wade*), requiring vaccinations, and setting conditions for states to receive public funds for highway construction and repair by requiring a minimum drinking age.

HEALTHY PEOPLE 2010: AN EXAMPLE OF NATIONAL HEALTH POLICY GUIDANCE

In 1979 the surgeon general issued a report that began a 20-year focus on promoting health and preventing disease for all Americans (Department of Health, Education and

---

Box 7-1   The Sheppard-Towner Act

The Sheppard-Towner Act did the following:
- Made nurses available to provide health services for women and children, including well-child and child-development services
- Provided adequate hospital services and facilities for women and children
- Provided grants-in-aid for establishing maternal and child welfare programs
- Set precedents and patterns for the growth of modern-day public health policy
- Defined the role of the federal government in creating standards to be followed by states in conducting categorical programs, such as today's Women, Infants, and Children (WIC) and Early Periodic Screening and Developmental Testing (EPSDT) programs
- Defined how the consumer could influence, formulate, and shape public policy
- Defined the government's role in research
- Developed a system for collecting national health statistics
- Explained how health and social services could be integrated
- Established the importance of prenatal care, anticipatory guidance, client education, and nurse–client conferences, all of which are viewed today as essential nursing responsibilities

---

Healthy People 2010

Goals
- Increase quality and years of healthy life
- Eliminate health disparities

Focus Areas
- Access to quality health services
- Arthritis, osteoporosis, and chronic back conditions
- Cancer
- Chronic kidney disease
- Diabetes
- Disability and secondary conditions
- Educational and community-based programs
- Environmental health
- Family planning
- Food safety
- Health communication
- Heart disease and stroke
- Human immunodeficiency virus
- Immunization and infectious diseases
- Injury and violence prevention
- Maternal, infant, and child health
- Medical product safety
- Mental health and mental disorders
- Nutrition and overweight
- Occupational safety and health
- Oral health
- Physical activity and fitness
- Public health infrastructure
- Respiratory diseases
- Sexually transmitted diseases
- Substance abuse
- Tobacco use
- Vision and hearing

From the U.S. Department of Health and Human Services: *Healthy People 2010: understanding and improving health,* ed 2, Washington, DC, 2000, U.S. Government Printing Office.

Welfare, 1979). In 1989 *Healthy People 2000* became a national effort with many stakeholders representing the perspectives of government, state, and local agencies; advocacy groups; academia; and health organizations (U.S. Department of Health and Human Services, 1991).

Throughout the 1990s states used *Healthy People 2000* objectives to identify emerging public health issues. The success of this national program was accomplished and measured through state and local efforts. The *Healthy People 2010* box shows the document's two overarching goals, with a vision of healthy people living in healthy communities.

ORGANIZATIONS AND AGENCIES THAT INFLUENCE HEALTH

INTERNATIONAL ORGANIZATIONS

In June 1945, following World War II, many national governments joined together to create the United Nations (UN). By charter, the aims and goals of the UN deal with human rights, world peace, international security, and the

BRIEFLY NOTED

With the approval and support of the UN Commission on the Status of Women, four world conferences on women have been held. At these conferences, the health of women and children and their rights to personal, educational, and economic security as well as initiatives to achieve these goals at the country level are debated and explored, and policies are formulated (United Nations, 1975, 1980, 1985, 1995).

promotion of economic and social advancement of all the world's peoples. The UN, headquartered in New York City, is made up of six principal divisions, several subgroups, and many specialized agencies and autonomous organizations.

One of the special autonomous organizations growing out of the UN is the **World Health Organization (WHO)**. Established in 1946, WHO works with the UN to achieve its goal to attain the highest possible level of health for all persons. "Health for All" is the creed of the WHO. Headquartered in Geneva, Switzerland, the WHO has six regional offices. The office for the Americas, in Washington, DC, is known as the Pan American Health Organization (PAHO). The WHO provides the following services worldwide (United Nations, 2002):
- Promotes health
- Cooperates with member countries in promoting their health efforts
- Coordinates the collaborating efforts among countries
- Disseminates biomedical research

Its services, which benefit all countries, include the following:
- Providing day-to-day information service on the occurrence of internationally important diseases
- Publishing the international list of causes of disease, injury, and death
- Monitoring adverse reactions to drugs
- Establishing world standards for antibiotics and vaccines

Assistance available to individual countries includes the following:
- Supporting national programs to fight disease
- Training health workers
- Strengthening the delivery of health services

The World Health Assembly (WHA) is the WHO's policymaking body, and it meets annually. The WHA's health policy work provides policy options for many countries of the world in their development of in-country initiatives and priorities; however, although important everywhere, WHA policy statements are guides and not law. The WHA's latest policy statement on nursing and midwifery was released in 2001 as Resolution WHA.49.1, and the worldwide shortage of professional nurses was on the WHO agenda for further action in 2003 (World Health Assembly, 2001).

The presence of nursing in international health is increasing to include the following:
- Direct health services in every country in the world
- Consultants
- Educators
- Program planners
- Evaluators

Nurses focus their work on a variety of public health issues:
- Health care workforce and education
- Environment
- Sanitation
- Infectious diseases
- Wellness promotion
- Maternal and child health
- Primary care

FEDERAL HEALTH AGENCIES

Laws passed by Congress may be assigned to any administrative agency within the executive branch of government for implementing, supervising, regulating, and enforcing. Congress decides which agency will monitor specific laws. For example, most health care legislation is delegated to the USDHHS. However, legislation concerning the environment would most likely be implemented and monitored by the Environmental Protection Agency (EPA), and legislation concerning occupational health by the **Occupational Safety and Health Administration (OSHA)** in the U.S. Department of Labor.

U.S. Department of Health and Human Services

The USDHHS is the agency most heavily involved with the health and welfare of U.S. citizens. It touches more lives than any other federal agency. The organizational chart of the USDHHS (see Figure 3-1 in Chapter 3) shows and

provides more discussion for the key agencies within the organization. The following agencies have been selected for their relevance to this chapter.

HEALTH RESOURCES AND SERVICES ADMINISTRATION. The Health Resources and Services Administration (HRSA) has been a long-standing contributor to the improved health status of Americans through the programs of services and health professions education that it funds. The HRSA contains the Bureau of Health Professions (BHPr), which includes the Division of Nursing as well as the Divisions of Medicine, Dentistry, and Allied Health Professions.

The Division of Nursing has the following specific goals (U.S. Department of Health and Human Services, 2007):
- Increase access to quality care through improved composition, distribution, and retention of the nursing workforce.
- Identify and use data, program performance measures, and outcomes to make informed decisions on nursing workforce issues.
- Increase the supply, distribution, and retention of the nursing workforce through additional financing.
- Improve the quality of nursing education and practice.
- Increase cultural competence in the nursing workforce.
- Increase diversity in the nursing workforce.

CENTERS FOR DISEASE CONTROL AND PREVENTION. The Centers for Disease Control and Prevention (CDC) serves as the national focus for developing and applying disease prevention and control, environmental health, and health promotion and education activities designed to improve the health of the people of the United States. The mission of the CDC is to promote health and quality of life by preventing and controlling disease, injury, and disability. The CDC seeks to accomplish its mission by working with partners throughout the nation and the world in the following ways:
- To monitor health
- To detect and investigate health problems
- To conduct research that will enhance prevention
- To develop and advocate sound public health policies
- To implement prevention strategies
- To promote healthy behaviors
- To foster safe and healthful environments
- To provide leadership and training

The mumps outbreak of Spring 2006 is an example of how CDC fulfills its mission. The outbreak of mumps began in Iowa among college students. The CDC regularly collects data about mumps through the National Notifiable Disease Surveillance System on a weekly basis (MMWR Dispatch, 2006). Because of the recognized increase in cases of mumps, states were asked to report aggregate numbers of cases twice a week along with mumps-related hospitalizations and complications. The CDC implemented an investigation to track the mumps cases and worked with state and local health departments to
- conduct mumps surveillance,
- assist with prevention and control activities,
- evaluate vaccine effectiveness,
- determine the duration of immunity, and
- evaluate risk factors for mumps.

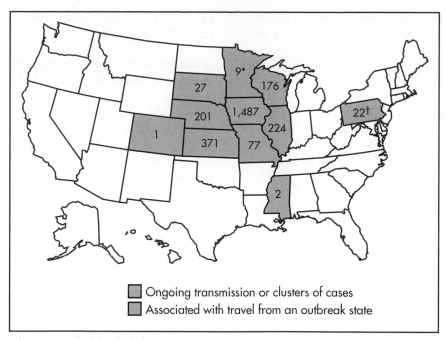

Ongoing transmission or clusters of cases

Associated with travel from an outbreak state

*Three cases related to the outbreak.
†Twelve cases related to the outbreak.
NOTE: The total number of cases represented on the map is 2,597.

FIGURE 7-I The number of reported mumps cases linked to multistate outbreak, by state—United States, January 1 to May 2, 2006. (From Centers for Disease Control and Prevention: Epidemiology of mumps and multistate mumps outbreak, United States, Atlanta, 2006, U.S. Department of Health and Human Services.)

Before January 1, 2006, there had been about 300 cases of mumps per year between 2001 and 2003. In 5 months there were 2067 cases involving 10 states. Figure 7-1 presents a CDC map indicating cases per state (MMWR Dispatch, 2006).

NATIONAL INSTITUTES OF HEALTH. Founded in 1887, the NIH today is one of the world's foremost biomedical research centers and the federal focus point for biomedical research in the United States. The NIH is composed of 27 separate institutes and centers. The goal of NIH research is to acquire new knowledge to help prevent, detect, diagnose, and treat disease and disability, from the rarest genetic disorder to the common cold, to lead to better health for everyone. The NINR, the focal point of the nation's nursing research activities, does the following:

• Promotes the growth and quality of research in nursing and client care
• Provides important research leadership
• Expands the pool of funded nurse researchers
• Serves as a point of interaction with other health care researchers and projects

AGENCY FOR HEALTHCARE RESEARCH AND QUALITY. The mission of the **Agency for Healthcare Research and Quality (AHRQ)** is to do the following:

• Support research designed to improve the outcomes and quality of health care
• Reduce health costs
• Address patient safety and medical errors
• Broaden access to effective services

By examining what works and what does not work in health care, the AHRQ fulfills its missions of translating research findings into better patient care and providing consumers, policymakers, and other health care leaders with information needed to make critical health care decisions.

CENTERS FOR MEDICARE AND MEDICAID SERVICES. One of the most powerful agencies within the USDHHS is the Centers for Medicare and Medicaid Services (CMS), which administers Medicare and Medicaid accounts and guides payment policy and delivery rules for services for the poor, elderly, disabled, and unemployed. In addition to providing health insurance, the CMS also performs a number of quality-focused health care or health-related activities, including the following:

• Regulates laboratory testing
• Develops coverage policies
• Improves quality of care
• Maintains oversight and provides information about surveying and certifying nursing homes and continuing care providers (including home health agencies, intermediate care facilities for the mentally retarded, and hospitals)

Specifically, the CMS administers the following programs:

• Old Age Survivors and Disability Insurance (OASDI)
• Aid to Families with Dependent Children (AFDC)
• Supplemental Security Income (SSI)

OASDI provides monthly benefits to retired and disabled workers, their spouses and children, and survivors of insured workers. AFDC, which is a federal and state program, helps needy families with children. It subsidizes children deprived of the financial support of one of their parents as a result of death, disability, absence from the home or, in some states, unemployment. SSI is a federal program for the aged, blind, and disabled that may be supplemented by state support.

FEDERAL NON-HEALTH AGENCIES

Although the USDHHS has the primary responsibility for federal health functions, several other departments of the executive branch carry out important health functions for the nation. Among these are the Departments of Commerce, Defense, Labor, Agriculture, and Justice.

- *Department of Commerce.* Within the Department of Commerce (DOC) is the Census Bureau, which carries out an information function in health care. Also a part of the DOC is the National Oceanic and Atmospheric Administration, which provides special services to control urban air quality, a major factor in community health today.
- *Department of Defense.* The Department of Defense delivers health care to members of the military and their dependents. In each command, nurses of high military rank, including brigadier general, are part of the administration of health services.
- *Department of Labor.* The Department of Labor has two agencies with health functions: OSHA and the Mine Safety and Health Administration. Both are charged with writing safety and health standards and ensuring compliance in the workplace.
- *Department of Agriculture.* The Department of Agriculture is involved in health care primarily by administering the Food and Nutrition Service. This service collaborates with state and local government welfare agencies to provide food stamps to needy persons to increase their food purchasing power. Other programs include school breakfast and lunch programs, the Women, Infants, and Children (WIC) nutrition program, and grants to states for nutrition education and training.
- *Department of Justice.* Health services to federal prisoners are administered within the Department of Justice. The Medical and Services Division of the Bureau of Prisons includes medical, psychiatric, dental, and health support services.

STATE AND LOCAL HEALTH DEPARTMENTS

Depending on funding, public commitment and interest, and access to other resources, programs offered by state and local health departments vary greatly. At the local and state levels, coordinating health efforts between health departments and other county or city departments is necessary. Gaps in community coordination are showing up in glaring ways as states and communities scramble to address bioterrorism preparedness since September 11, 2001.

Most state and local (county and city) areas perform government activities that affect the health care field. More often than at other levels of government, nurses at the local level provide direct services. Some nurses deliver special or selected services, such as follow-up of contacts in cases of tuberculosis or venereal disease or providing child immunization clinics. Other nurses have a more general

practice, delivering services to families in certain geographic areas (Nicola, 2002).

CASE STUDY

Tammy Jones is the school nurse at Caseyville Middle School. The state requires all entering sixth-grade students to have a current immunization certificate on file before the student's enrollment. It is now 6 months into the school year, and Ms. Jones is reviewing the students' records. Ms. Jones finds that several students do not have current immunization certificates on file. Although the state law requires immunization certificates, it does not specify the course of action in cases of noncompliance.

Ms. Jones goes to her supervisor to discuss possible resolutions to the situation. Should they suspend the noncompliant students since the law states the certificate for immunization is required for enrollment? This solution could mean many missed days of valuable lessons for the students. What implications for the students and the community could arise if the students continue to go without immunizations?

Ms. Jones and her supervisor decide to contact each student and meet with their family individually. The meetings reveal that many of the parents have tried to get their child immunized but have not been able to do so because of the costs of the shots or the inability to make an appointment at the busy doctor's office. Ms. Jones works with these families to make appointments at the local health department to fulfill the immunization requirement.

IMPACT OF GOVERNMENT HEALTH FUNCTIONS AND STRUCTURES ON NURSING

The variety and range of functions of governmental agencies have had a major impact on the practice of nursing. Funding, in particular, has shaped roles and tasks of population-centered nurses. The designation of money for specific needs, or **categorical programs/funding**, has led to special and more narrowly focused nursing roles. Examples are in emergency preparedness, school nursing, and family planning. Funds assigned to antibioterrorism cannot be used to support unrelated communicable disease programs or family planning.

As a result of the events of September 11, 2001, the public and the profession of nursing are concerned about the ability of the present public health system and its workforce to deal with bioterrorism, especially outbreaks of deadly and serious communicable diseases. For example, smallpox vaccinations stopped in 1972, but immunity lasts for only 10 years; as a result, although there have been no reported cases of smallpox since the early 1970s, almost no one in the United States retains their immunity. Thus the population is vulnerable to an outbreak of smallpox. Few public health professionals are knowledgeable about the symptoms, treatment, or mode of transmission of this disease. Most health professionals, including registered nurses (RNs), currently working in the

United States have never seen a case of anthrax, smallpox, or plague, the three major biological weapons of concern in the world today. The USDHHS and the new federal **Office of Homeland Security** have provided funds to address this serious threat to the people of the United States. One of the first things being done is the rebuilding of the crumbling public health infrastructures of each state to provide surveillance, intervention, and communication in the face of future bioterrorism events (Frist, 2002).

THE LAW AND HEALTH CARE

The United States is a nation of laws, which are subject to the U.S. Constitution. The law is a system of privileges and processes by which people solve problems on the basis of a set of established rules. It is intended to minimize the use of force. Laws govern the relationships of individuals and organizations to other individuals and to government. After a law is established, regulations further define the course of actions to be taken by the government, organizations, or individuals in reaching an agreed-on outcome. Government and its laws are the ultimate authority in society and are designed to enforce official policy whether it is related to health, education, economics, social welfare, or any other societal issue. The number and types of laws influencing health care are ever increasing. Definitions of law (Catholic University of America, 2002) include the following:

- A rule established by authority, society, or custom
- The body of rules governing the affairs of people, communities, states, corporations, and nations
- A set of rules or customs governing a discrete field or activity (e.g., criminal law, contract law)

These definitions reflect the close relationship of law to the community and to society's customs and beliefs. The law has had a major impact on nursing practice. Although nursing emerged from individual voluntary activities, society passed laws to give formality to public health and, through legal mandates (i.e., laws), positions and functions for nurses in community settings were created. These functions in many instances carry the force of law. For example, if the nurse discovers a person with smallpox, the law directs the nurse and others in the public health community to take specific actions. In the mumps outbreak, a nurse and other health professionals are required to report cases of mumps. This requirement for reporting helps locate and treat cases as they occur, thus preventing further spreading of disease. Three types of laws in the United States have particular importance to the nurse. They are constitutional law, legislation and regulation, and judicial or common law.

BRIEFLY NOTED

Persons with communicable diseases such as tuberculosis may be confined to a prison hospital if they are considered a threat to their community by failing to follow their treatment regimen.

CONSTITUTIONAL LAW

Constitutional law derives from federal and state constitutions. It provides overall guidance for selected practice situations. For example, on what basis can the state require quarantine or isolation of individuals with tuberculosis? The U.S. Constitution specifies the explicit and limited functions of the federal government. All other powers and functions are left to the individual states. The major constitutional power of the states relating to population-centered nursing practice is the state's right to intervene in a reasonable manner to protect the health, safety, and welfare of its citizens. The state has police power to act through its public health system, but it has limits. First, it must be a "reasonable" exercise of power. Second, if the power interferes or infringes on individual rights, the state must demonstrate that there is a "compelling state interest" in exercising its power. Isolating an individual or separating someone from a community because that person has a communicable disease has been deemed an appropriate exercise of state powers. The state can isolate an individual, even though it infringes on individual rights (such as freedom and autonomy), under the following conditions (Khan, Morse, and Lillibridge, 2000):

1. There is a compelling state interest in preventing an epidemic.
2. The isolation is necessary to protect the health, safety, and welfare of individuals in the community or the public as a whole.
3. The isolation is done in a reasonable manner.

BRIEFLY NOTED

The community's rights are more important than the individual's rights when there is a threat to the health of the public.

LEGISLATION AND REGULATION

Legislation is law that comes from the legislative branches of the federal, state, or local government. Much legislation has an effect on nursing. **Regulations** are specific statements of law related to defining or implanting individual pieces of legislation. For example, state legislatures enact laws (statutes) establishing boards of nursing and defining terms such as registered nurse and nursing practice. Every state has a **board of nursing**. The board may be found either in the department of licensing boards of the health department or in an administrative agency of the governor's office. Created by legislation known as a state nurse practice act, the board of nursing is made up of nurses and consumers. The functions of this board are described in the **nurse practice act** of each state and generally include licensing and examination of registered nurses and licensed practical nurses; approval of schools of nursing in the state; revocation, suspension, or denying of licenses; and writing of regulations about nursing practice and education. The state boards of nursing operationalize, implement, and enforce the statutory law by writing explicit statements (called rules) on what it means to be a registered nurse, and on the nurse's rights and responsibilities in delegating work to others and in meeting continuing requirements for education.

All nurses employed in community settings are subject to legislation and regulations. For example, home health care nurses employed by private agencies must deliver care according to federal Medicare or state Medicaid legislation and regulations, so the agency can be reimbursed for those services. Private and public health care services rendered by nurses are subject to many governmental regulations for quality of care, standards of documentation, and confidentiality of client records and communications.

JUDICIAL AND COMMON LAW

Both judicial law and common law have great impact on nursing. **Judicial law** is based on court or jury decisions. The opinions of the courts are referred to as case law. The court uses other types of laws to make its decisions, including previous court decisions or cases. Precedent, one principle of common law, means that judges are bound by previous decisions unless they are convinced that the older law is no longer relevant or valid. This process is called distinguishing, and it usually involves a demonstration of how the current situation in dispute differs from the previously decided situation. Other principles of common law, such as justice, fairness, respect for individual's autonomy, and self-determination, are part of a court's rationale and the basis upon which to make a decision.

LAWS SPECIFIC TO NURSING PRACTICE

Despite the broad nature and varied roles of nurses in practice, two legal arenas are most applicable to nurse practice situations. The first is the statutory authority for the profession and its scope of practice, and the second is professional negligence or malpractice.

SCOPE OF PRACTICE

The issue of scope of practice involves defining nursing, setting its credentials, and then distinguishing between the practices of nurses, physicians, and other health care providers. The issue is especially important to nurses in community settings, who have traditionally practiced with much autonomy.

Health care practitioners are subject to the laws of the state in which they practice, and they can practice only with a license. The states' nurse practice acts differ somewhat, but they are the most important statutory law affecting nurses. The nurse practice act of each state accomplishes at least four functions: defining the practice of professional nursing, identifying the scope of nursing practice, setting educational qualifications and other requirements for **licensure**, and determining the legal titles nurses may use to identify themselves. The usual and customary practice of nursing can

be determined through a variety of sources, including the following:

1. Content of nursing educational programs, both general and special
2. Experience of other practicing nurses (peers)
3. Statements and standards of nursing professional organizations
4. Policies and procedures of agencies employing nurses
5. Needs and interests of the community
6. Updated literature, including research, books, texts, and journals

All of these sources can describe, determine, and refine the scope of practice of a professional nurse. Every nurse should know and follow closely any proposed changes in the practice acts of nursing, medicine, pharmacy, and other related professions. The nurse should always examine all legislation, rules, and regulations related to nursing practice. For example, a review of the Pharmacy Act will let the nurse know whether to question the right to dispense medications in a family planning clinic in a local health department. Defining the scope of practice makes it necessary to clarify independent, interdependent, and dependent nursing functions.

Just as practice acts vary by state, so do the evolving issues and tensions of scopes of practice among the health professions. In the past few years, several state legislatures (working closely with the National Council of State Boards of Nursing) have embarked on a legislative effort to develop the Interstate Nurse Licensure Compact (American Nurses Association, 2000). The compact allows mutual recognition of generalist nursing licensure across state lines in the compact states. By 2006, 19 states had adopted the compact (American Nurses Association, 2007).

PROFESSIONAL NEGLIGENCE

Professional negligence, or malpractice, is defined as an act (or a failure to act) that leads to injury of a client. To recover money damages in a malpractice action, the client must prove all of the following:

1. The nurse owed a duty to the client or was responsible for the client's care.
2. The duty to act the way a reasonable, prudent nurse would act in the same circumstances was not fulfilled.
3. The failure to act reasonably under the circumstances led to the alleged injuries.
4. The injuries provided the basis for a monetary claim from the nurse as compensation for the injury.

Reported cases involving negligence and population-centered nurses are very few in number. However, the following is an example:

In *Williams v. Metro Home Health Care Agency et al* (U.S. Law, 2002), the patient brought a malpractice action against Edward Schiro, RN, and his employer, a home health agency, alleging that the nurse's failure to visit and treat the patient (a paraplegic) in a manner that followed the orders of the physician caused the progression of a decubitus ulcer on his hip to the extent that surgical intervention was required. The orders of the physician called for three visits per week, and the patient testified that the RN visited only once per week and had falsified the record as to the other visits.

The court determined that it was the nurse's duty to exercise the degree of skill employed by other nurses in the community, along with his best judgment on patient care to promote skin integrity. The failure of the nurse both to care for the patient's decubiti and to instruct the patient and his family concerning proper methods for self-care and assessment for decubitus ulcers contributed to the patient's deteriorating skin integrity and condition.

BRIEFLY NOTED

In the eyes of the law, the "prudent nurse" used as the example, or standard, by which to judge the competency of a nurse's practice can be practicing anywhere in the United States and not just in the community in which the nurse works.

An integral part of all negligence actions is the question of who should be sued. When a nurse is employed and functioning within the scope of employment, the employer is responsible for the nurse's negligent actions. This is referred to as the doctrine of *respondeat superior.* By directing a nurse to carry out a particular function, the employer becomes responsible for negligence, along with the individual nurse. Because employers are usually better able to pay for the injuries suffered by clients, they are sued more often than the nurses themselves, although an increasing number of judgments include the professional nurse by name as a codefendant.

Thus it is imperative that all nurses engaged in clinical practice carry their own professional liability insurance. Nurses may have personal immunity for particular practice areas, such as giving immunizations. In some states, the legislature has granted personal immunity to nurses employed by public agencies to cover all aspects of their practice under the legal theory of *sovereign immunity* (Shinn, Gaffney, and Curtin, 2003).

Nursing students need to be aware that the same laws and rules that govern the professional nurse govern them. Students are expected to meet the same standard of care as that met by any licensed nurse practicing under the same or similar circumstances. Students are expected to be able to perform all tasks and make clinical decisions on the basis of the knowledge they have gained or been offered, according to their progress in their educational programs and along with adequate educational supervision.

LEGAL ISSUES AFFECTING HEALTH CARE PRACTICES

Specific legal issues of nursing vary depending on the setting in which care is delivered, the clinical arena, and the nurse's functional role. The law, including legislation and judicial opinions, significantly affects each of the following areas of nursing practice. Nurses responsible for setting and implementing program priorities need to identify and monitor laws related to each special area of practice.

SCHOOL AND FAMILY HEALTH

School and family health nursing may be delivered by nurses employed by health departments or boards of education. School health legislation establishes a minimum of services that must be provided to children in public and private schools:
- Children must have had immunizations against certain communicable diseases before entering school.
- Children must have had a physical examination before entering school.
- Some types of health screening are conducted in schools (e.g., vision and hearing testing).
- Most states require nurses to notify police or a social service agency of any situation in which they suspect a child is being abused or neglected.

Child abuse and neglect constitute one instance in which society permits a professional to breach confidentiality to protect someone who may be in a helpless and vulnerable position. There is civil immunity for such reports, and the nurse may be called as a witness in any court hearing. The majority of legal cases involving community health nurses concern child abuse.

The following are other examples of federal legislation affecting nursing practice in schools and families:
- Head Start
- Early diagnostic screening programs
- Nutritional programs
- Services for the handicapped
- Special education

OCCUPATIONAL HEALTH

Occupational health is another special area of practice that is affected greatly by state and federal laws. OSHA imposes many requirements on industries. The following requirements shape the functions of nurses and the types of services given to workers:
- A required reporting system for workers exposed to toxic agents in the workplace
- A required recordkeeping system for health records in the workplace
- State monitoring and inspecting of industries, as well as the health services rendered to them by nurses
- A "worker's right to know" law requiring employers to provide employees with information concerning the nature of toxic substances in the workplace (most states)
- Compensation statutes that provide a legal opportunity for claims of workers injured on the job

Access to records, confidentiality, and the use of standing orders are legal issues of great significance to nurses employed in industries.

HOME CARE AND HOSPICE

State laws that require licensing and certification have a significant effect on home care and hospice services rendered by nurses. Compliance with these laws is directly linked to the method of payment for the services. For example, a provider must be licensed and certified to obtain payment for services through Medicare. Federal regulations implementing Medicare have an effect on much of nursing practice, including how nurses record details of their visits.

Legislation affecting home care and hospice services is related to issues such as the following:
- The right to death with dignity
- Rights of residents of long-term facilities and home-health clients
- Definitions of death
- Required use of living wills, specifically advance directives
- Requirement that nurses report elder abuse to the proper authorities

CORRECTIONAL HEALTH

Nursing practice in correctional health systems is controlled by federal and state laws and regulations and by recent Supreme Court decisions. The laws and decisions relate to the type and amount of services that must be provided for incarcerated individuals. For example, physical examinations are required of all prisoners after they are sentenced. Regulations specify basic levels of care that must be provided for prisoners, and care during illness is particularly addressed. Court decisions requiring adequate health services are based on constitutional law.

Each nurse working within a service based on legislation should be oriented to the legislation. It is advisable that the legislation and its regulations be included in the nursing agency's manual of policies and procedures so that the nurse may refer to it.

THE NURSE'S ROLE IN THE POLICY PROCESS

The number and types of laws influencing health care are increasing. Because of this, nurses need to be involved in the policy process and understand the importance of involvement to nursing to the clients they serve.

For nurses to effectively care for their client populations and their communities in the complex U.S. health care system, professional advocacy for logical health policy that considers equality is essential. Professional nurses working in the community know all too well about the health care problems they and their clients encounter daily, and it is through policy and political activism that both big-picture and long-term solutions can be developed.

Although the term policy may sound rather lofty, health policy is quite simply the process of turning health problems into workable action solutions. Health policy is developed on the three-legged stool of access, cost, and quality.

The policy process, which is very familiar to professional nurses, includes the following:
- Statement of a health care problem
- Statement of policy options to address the health problem
- Adoption of a particular policy option
- Implementation of the policy product
- Evaluation of the policy's intended and unintended consequences in solving the original health problem

Thus the policy process is very similar to the nursing process, but the focus is on the level of the larger society and the adoption strategies require political action. For most professional nurses, action in the policy arena comes most easily and naturally through participation in nursing organizations such as the **American Nurses Association (ANA)** at the state level and in certain specialty organizations.

BRIEFLY NOTED

The nurse's basic understanding of the political process should include knowing who the lawmakers are, how bills become laws (see Figure 7-2), the process of writing regulations (see Figure 7-3), and methods of influencing the process and shaping of health policy. With this knowledge, nurses can influence nursing practice.

LEGISLATIVE ACTION

The people within geographic jurisdictions elect their legislative representatives and senators. An important part of the legislative process is the work of the **legislative staff.** These individuals do the legwork, research, paperwork, and other activities that move policy ideas into bills and then into law. In addition to the individual legislator's office, the congressional committee staffs are also important. They are usually experts in the content of the work of a committee, such as a health and welfare committee. Frequently, developing a working relationship with key legislative staffers can be as important to achieving a policy objective as the relationship with the policymaker (i.e., the legislator).

BRIEFLY NOTED

As a former Speaker of the House of Representatives noted, "all politics is local." Therefore should nurses focus their political activities only in the local community?

The legislative process begins with ideas (policy options) that are developed into bills. After a bill is drafted, it is introduced to the legislature, given a number, read, and assigned to a committee. Hearings, testimony, lobbying, education, research, and informal discussions follow. If the bill is passed from the legislative committee, the entire House hears the bill, amends it as necessary, and votes on it. A majority vote moves the bill to the other House, where it is read and amended, and then a vote is taken. Figure 7-2 shows the necessary formal process of the legislative pathway.

Nurses can be involved in the legislative process at any point. Many professional nursing associations have legislative committees made up of volunteers, governmental relations staff professionals, and sometimes political action committees (PACs), all engaged in efforts to monitor, analyze, and shape health policy.

The Federal Level

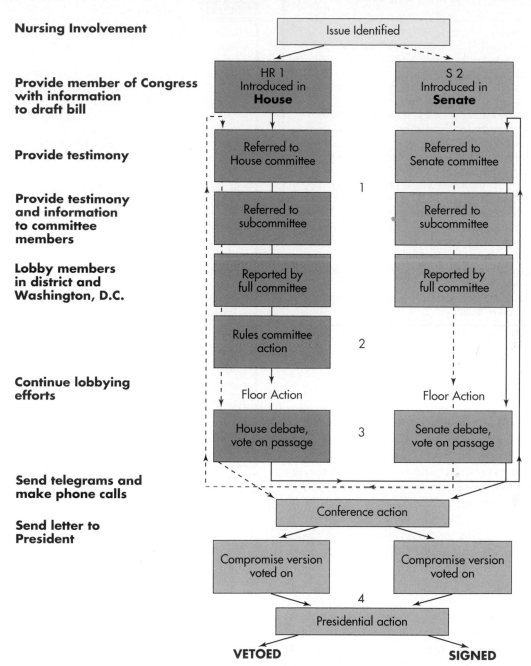

Nursing Involvement

Provide member of Congress with information to draft bill

Provide testimony

Provide testimony and information to committee members

Lobby members in district and Washington, D.C.

Continue lobbying efforts

Send telegrams and make phone calls

Send letter to President

[1] A bill goes to full committee first, then to special subcommittees for hearings, debate, revisions, and approval. The same process occurs when it goes to full committee. It either dies in committee or proceeds to the next step.
[2] Only the House has a Rules Committee to set the "rule" for floor action and conditions for debate and amendments. In the Senate, the leadership schedules action.
[3] The bill is debated, amended, and passed or defeated. If passed, it goes to the other chamber and follows the same path. If each chamber passes a similar bill, both versions go to conference.
[4] The President may sign the bill into law, allow it to become law without his signature, or veto it and return it to Congress. To override the veto, both houses must approve the bill by a two-thirds majority vote.

FIGURE 7-2 How a bill becomes a law. (From Mason DJ, Keavitt JK, Chaffee MW: *Policy and politics in nursing and health care,* ed 4, Philadelphia, 2002, Saunders.)

Box 7-2   **Tips for Visits with Legislators**
• Call ahead and ask how much time the staff or legislator is able to give you.
• When you arrive, ask if the appointment time is the same or if a scheduled vote on the house or senate floor is going to need the legislator's attention.
• Engage in small talk at the beginning of the conversation only if the staff or legislator has time.
• Structure time so that the issue can be presented briefly.
• Allow an opportunity for the staff or Congress member to seek clarity or ask questions.
• Do not assume that the legislator or the legislator's staff is well informed on the issue.
• Numbers count. If the views you express are shared by a local nurses' organization or by nurses employed at a health care facility, let the legislator know.
• Invite Congress members and their staffs to conferences or meetings of nurses' organizations or to tour nursing education facilities to meet others interested in the same policy issues.
• If appropriate, invite the media and let the legislator know.
• Send future invitations.
• Provide a one-page summary that gives key points at the conclusion of every meeting.

Modified from Milstead J: *Healthy policy and politics: a nurse's guide,* Gaithersburg, Md, 2004, Aspen.

Common methods of influencing health policy outcomes include face-to-face encounters, personal letters, mailgrams, electronic mail, telephone calls, testimony, petitions, reports, position papers, fact sheets, letters to the editor, news releases, speeches, coalition building, demonstrations, and law suits. Depending on the issue, any of these can be effective. Guidelines on communication are provided in the How To box. Tips on communication and visiting legislators and their staffs, as well as general tips on political action, are presented in Boxes 7-2, 7-3, and 7-4. Political activities in which nurses can and should be involved include a wide variety of activities such as being informed voters (A MUST!), participating in a political party, registering others to vote, getting out the vote, fundraising for candidates, building networks or communication links for issues (e.g., a phone tree), and participating in organizations to ensure their effective involvement in health policy and politics.

BRIEFLY NOTED

Which special interest group/groups has/have the most political influence in Washington, DC, today? Why did you choose your answer?

The ANA was a strong supporter of the Patient Safety Act of 1997 (American Nurses Association, 1997). This law requires health care agencies to make public some information on nurse staff levels, staff mix, and outcomes, and it

Box 7-3   **Tips for Written Communication with Legislators**
• Communicate in writing to express opinions.
• Acknowledge the Congress member's work as positive or negative, but be courteous.
• Follow-up on meetings or phone calls with a letter or e-mail.
• Share knowledge about a particular problem.
• Recommend policy solutions.
• The letter should be typed, a maximum of two pages, and focused on one or two issues at most.
• The purpose of the letter should be stated at the beginning.
• Present clear and compelling rationales for your concern or position on an issue.
• If the purpose of the letter is to express disappointment regarding a stance on an issue or a vote that has been cast, the letter should be as positive as possible.
• Write letters thanking a Congress member for taking a particular position on an issue.
• A letter to the editor of the local newspaper or a nursing newsletter praising a legislator's position (with a copy forwarded to the legislator) is welcome publicity, especially during an election year.
• Review the major points covered in person and answer any questions that were raised during conversation.
• Have business cards for yourself and include them with letters.
• Address written correspondence as follows (the same general format applies to state and local officials):

U.S. Senator	U.S. Representative
Honorable Jane Doe	Honorable Jane Doe
United States Senate	House of Representatives
Washington, DC 20510	Washington, DC 20515
Dear Senator Doe:	Dear Representative Doe:

Modified from Milstead J: *Healthy policy and politics: a nurse's guide,* Gaithersburg, Md, 2004, Aspen.

HOW TO   **Be an Effective Communicator**
• Use simple communications that will be readily understood.
• Choose language that clearly conveys information to individuals of diverse cultures, different ages, and different educational backgrounds.
• Oral or written communication needs to be targeted to the issue and free of terminology unique to medicine and nursing (i.e., jargon).
• State your expertise on the issue first.
• Describe briefly your education and experience.
• Identify the relevance of the issue beyond nursing.
• Provide information regarding the impact of the issue on the legislator's constituents.
• Present accurate, credible data.
• Do not oversell or give inaccurate information about the problem.
• Present information in an organized, thorough, concise form that is based on factual data (when it is available).
• Give examples.

Modified from Milstead J: *Healthy policy and politics: a nurse's guide,* Gaithersburg, Md, 1999, Aspen.

Box 7-4	Tips for Action

- Become involved in the state nurses' association.
- Build communication and leadership skills.
- Increase your knowledge about a range of professional issues.
- Expand and strengthen your professional network.
- Serve on committees and in elected positions.
- Build relationships within the profession and with representatives of public and private sector organizations with an interest in health care.
- Participate in political activities.
- Be aware of what is taking place in health care beyond the environment and the practice in which you work.
- Be well informed across a range of health-related issues.
- Identify yourself as a nurse with associated education and expertise.
- Let people know that nurses are capable of functioning in many different roles and making substantial contributions.
- Be confident.
- Do not burn bridges behind you. On another occasion, they may provide the only route to your destination.
- Be friendly.
- Lend a hand to other nurses. It benefits all of us.
- If you are new to the policy arena, seek support from many people of diverse backgrounds. Accomplished people, whether nurses or not, often value mentoring others.

Modified from Milstead J: *Healthy policy and politics: a nurse's guide,* Gaithersburg, Md, 2004, Aspen.

requires the USDHHS to review and approve all health care acquisitions and mergers. All of these requirements are to determine any long-term effect on the health and safety of clients, communities, and staff.

On the state legislative level, all 50 states have passed title protection for registered nurses; this was achieved by individual nurses, state nurses associations, and various nursing specialty groups participating in the legislative process with the 50 state legislators. Title protection means that only certain nurses who meet state criteria can call themselves **advanced practice nurses**.

REGULATORY ACTION

The regulatory process, although it may not be as visible a process as legislation, can also be used to shape laws and dramatically affect health policy. This process should be on the radar screen of professional nurses who wish to successfully participate in policy activity.

At each level of government, the executive branch can and, in most cases, must prepare regulations for implementing policy and new programs. These regulations are detailed, and they establish, fix, and control standards and criteria for carrying out certain laws. Figure 7-3 shows the steps in the typical process of writing regulations. When the legislature passes a law and delegates its oversight to an agency, it gives that agency the power to make regulations. Because regulations flow from legislation, they have the force of law.

THE PROCESS OF REGULATION

After a law is passed, the appropriate executive department begins the process of regulation by studying the topic or issue. Advisory groups or special taskforces are sometimes formed to provide the content for the regulations. Nurses can influence these regulations by writing letters to the regulatory agency in charge or by speaking at open public hearings. After rewriting, the proposed regulations are put into final draft form and printed in the legally required publication (e.g., at the federal level, the *Federal Register*). Similar registers exist in most states, where regulations from state executive departments, including state health departments, are published. Public comment is called for in written form within a given period.

Revisions made to proposed regulations are based on public comment and public hearing. Depending on the amount and content of the public reaction, final regulations are prepared or the area and issues are studied further. Final published regulations carry the force of law. When regulations become effective, health care practice is changed to conform to the new regulations. Monitoring administrative regulations is essential for the professional nurse, who can influence regulations by attending the hearings, providing comments, testifying, and engaging in lobbying aimed at individuals involved in the writing. Concrete written suggestions for revision submitted to these individuals are frequently persuasive and must be acknowledged by government in publishing the final rules.

Final regulations, published in a *Code of Regulations* (both federal and state), usually lead to changes in practice. For example, Medicare regulations setting standards for nursing homes and home health are incorporated into these agencies' manuals.

NURSING ADVOCACY

Advocacy begins with the art of influencing others (politics) to adopt a specific course of action (policy) to solve a societal problem. This is accomplished by building relationships with the appropriate policymakers—the individuals or groups that determine a specific course of action to be followed by a government or institution to achieve a desired end (policy outcome). Relationships for effective advocacy can be built in a number of ways.

BRIEFLY NOTED

In January 2006, Medicare Part D—the prescription drug benefit policy—became effective. Public health professionals will need to assist approximately 8 million vulnerable persons to understand the value of enrolling in Part D, to educate them on how to use the benefits, and to ensure that the populations who are "dually" enrolled in both Medicare and Medicaid are registered. Coordinating efforts among civic, religious, and health care agencies to provide health education is a necessity (Rosenbaum and Teitelbaum, 2005).

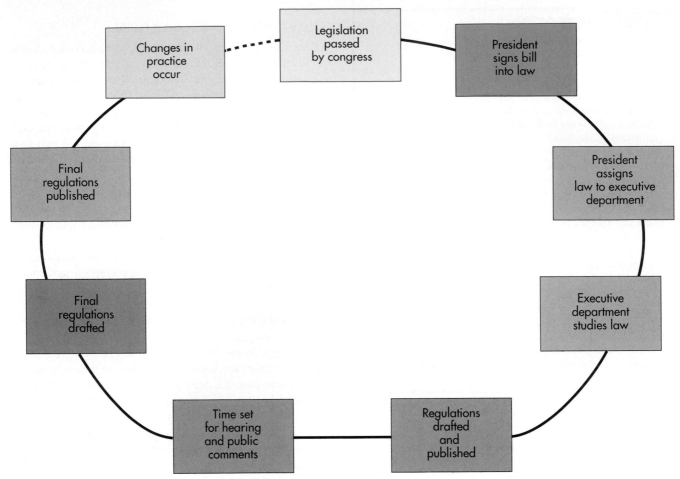

FIGURE 7-3 The process of writing regulations.

A letter or visit to the district, state, or national office of a legislator to discuss a particular policy or health care issue can be interesting, educational, and effective. Contributions of money, labor, expertise, or influence may also be welcomed by the policymakers involved in setting a course of action to obtain a desired health outcome, for an individual, a family, a group, a community, or society (health policy). Additionally, it is possible to develop a grassroots network of community and professional friends with a mutual interest in health policy advocacy. The network may be able to promote health policy initiatives for the community.

Many special-interest groups in health care have the potential, desire, and resources to influence the health policy process. A tremendous advantage that nursing has in advocating for issues and in influencing policymakers is the force of its numbers, as nursing is the largest of the health professions. However, nursing must organize its numbers in such a way that each nurse joins with others to speak with one voice. The greatest effect will be had when all nurses make similar demands for policy outcomes.

During 2002, nursing spoke clearly, distinctly, and together on a serious problem for the health arena and for the profession: the nursing shortage. Health care facilities and employers were having ever-increasing difficulty finding experienced nurses to employ. In addition, the need for RNs was predicted to balloon in the next 20 years because of the aging of the U.S. population, technological advances, and economic factors. Demand for RNs is expected to increase by 29% by the year 2029 (U.S. Department of Health and Human Services, 2007). This increased demand for professional nurses, coupled with the expected retirement of a rapidly aging nursing workforce, placed a tremendous stress on the health care system. A workforce supply study estimated that by 2020 the number of nurses per capita (client) will fall 20% short of demand. The workforce shortage results from a complex set of factors such as fewer young people entering the profession, declining nursing school enrollment, the aging of the current nurse workforce, and uncomfortable working conditions in which nurses feel pressured to "do more with less" (Bloom, 2002).

Advocacy by expert and committed health professionals works; it can bring about positive change for the profession, the community, and the clients that nurses serve. Keeping up to date on issues within government, professional organizations, law, and public policy is vitally important. Informed activism directed toward a professional role, image, and value for professional nurses and toward a health care system in the United States that provides universal access to health care that is of high quality and is affordable should be a lifelong commitment for all professional nurses.

CLINICAL APPLICATION

Larry was in his final rotation in the Bachelor of Science in Nursing program at State University. He was anxious to complete his final nursing course, because upon graduation he would begin a position as a staff nurse specializing in school health at the local health department. His wife was expecting their first child, and she had been receiving prenatal care at the health department.

Larry was aware that a few years ago, the federal government had, by law, provided block grants to states for primary care, maternal–child health programs, and other health care needs of states. He had read the *Federal Register* and knew that the regulations for these grants had been written through USDHHS departments. He was aware that these regulations did not require states to fund specific programs.

Larry read in the local newspaper that the health department was closing its prenatal clinic at the end of the month. When his state had received its block grant, they decided to spend the money for programs other than prenatal care. Larry found that a 3-year study in his own state showed improved pregnancy outcomes as a result of prenatal care. The results were further improved when the care was delivered by population-centered nurses.

Larry was concerned that as a student, he would have little influence. However, he decided to call his classmates together to plan a course of action.

What would such an action plan include?
Answers are in the back of the book.

REMEMBER THIS!

- The legal basis for most congressional action in health care can be found in Article I, Section 8, of the U.S. Constitution.
- The four major health care functions of the federal government are direct service, financing, information, and policy setting.
- The goal of the World Health Organization is the attainment by all people of the highest possible level of health.
- Many federal agencies are involved in government health care functions. The agency most directly involved with the health and welfare of Americans is the U.S. Department of Health and Human Services (USDHHS).
- Most state and local governments have activities that affect nursing practice.
- The variety and range of functions of governmental agencies have had a major impact on nursing. Funding, in particular, has shaped the role and tasks of nurses.
- The private sector (of which nurses are a part) can influence legislation in many ways, especially through the process of writing regulations.
- The number and types of laws influencing health care are increasing. Because of this, involvement in the political process is important to nurses.

- Professional negligence and the scope of practice are two legal aspects particularly relevant to nursing practice.
- Nurses must consider the legal implications of their own practice in each clinical encounter.
- The federal and most state governments are composed of three branches: the executive, the legislative, and the judicial.
- Each branch of government plays a significant role in health policy.
- The U.S. Public Health Service was created in 1798.
- The first national health insurance legislation was challenged in the Supreme Court in 1937.
- *Health: United States* (U.S. Department of Health and Human Services, 2008) is an important source of data about the nation's health care problems.
- In 1921 the Sheppard-Towner Act was passed, and it had an important influence on child health programs and community-oriented nursing practice.
- The Division of Nursing, the National Institute of Nursing Research, and the Agency for Healthcare Policy and Research are governmental agencies important to nursing.
- Nurses, through state and local health departments, function as consultants, direct care providers, researchers, teachers, supervisors, and program managers.
- The state governments are responsible for regulating nursing practice within the state.
- Federal and state social welfare programs have been developed to provide monetary benefits to the poor, older adults, the disabled, and the unemployed.
- Social welfare programs affect nursing practice. These programs improve the quality of life for special populations, thus making the nurse's job easier in assisting the client with health needs.
- The nurse's scope of practice is defined by legislation and by standards of practice within a specialty.

WHAT WOULD YOU DO?

1. Find and review your state nurse practice act and define your scope of practice. Give examples of your practice boundaries.
2. Contact your local public health agency to discuss the state's official powers in regulating epidemics, such as a West Nile virus outbreak and anthrax exposures related to bioterrorism.
   - Explore the state's right to protect the health, safety, and welfare of its citizens.
   - Ask about the conflict between the state's rights and individual rights and how such issues are resolved.
   - Ask about the standards of care that apply to this issue and how it is decided which services offered to clients should be mandatory and which should be voluntary.
   - Explore how the role of public health differs in these epidemics compared with the past epidemics of smallpox and tuberculosis. Be specific.

■ REFERENCES

American Nurses Association: Press release, *ANA applauds introduction of Patient Safety Act of 1997,* March 1997, available at http://www.nursingworld.org.

American Nurses Association: *Talking points on nurse licensure compacts.* Retrieved May 22, 2009, from www.neslon.org.

Bloom B: Crossing the quality chasm: a new health system for the 21st century, *JAMA* 287:646-647, 2002.

Catholic University of America: *Definitions of law, 2002.* Retrieved March 2002 from http://www.faculty.cua.edu.

Centers for Disease Control and Prevention: *Epidemiology of mumps and multistate mumps outbreak,* United States, Atlanta, 2006, U.S. Department of Health and Human Services.

Department of Health, Education and Welfare: Improving health. In *Healthy People: the surgeon general's report on health promotion and disease prevention,* DHEW Publication No. 79-55-71, Washington, DC, 1979, U.S. Government Printing Office. Retrieved July 2002 from http://www.census.gov/statab/www.

Frist B: Public health and national security: the critical role of increased federal support, *Health Aff* 21:117-130, 2002.

Khan A, Morse S, Lillibridge S: Public-health preparedness for biological terrorism in the USA, *Lancet* 356:1179-1182, 2000.

Mason DJ, Keavitt JK, Chaffee MW: *Policy and politics in nursing and health care,* ed 4, Philadelphia, 2002, Saunders.

Milstead J: *Healthy policy and politics: a nurse's guide,* Gaithersburg, Md, 2004, Aspen.

MMWR Dispatch: Update: multistate outbreak of mumps: United States, January 10, May 2, 2006. Retrieved May 28, 2006, from http://www.cdc.gov/mmwr/preview/mmwrhtml/mm55d518a1.htm.

Nicola B: The Model State Emergency Health Powers Act: turning point. In *Nursing concepts and challenges,* Philadelphia, 2002, Saunders, pp 529-549.

Rosenbaum S, Teitelbaum J: Law and the public's health, *Public Health Rep* 120:467-469, 2005.

Shinn L, Gaffney T, Curtin L: *An overview of risk management: an American Nurses Association educational program.* Retrieved February 2003 from http://nursingworld.org/mods/working/rskmgt1/cerm1ful.htm.

Szilagyi PG et al: Evaluation of a state health insurance program for low-income children: implications for state child health insurance programs, *Pediatrics* 105:363-371, 2000.

United Nations: *Report of the World Conference of the International Women's Year,* Mexico City, June 19 to July 2, Chapter I, Section A.2, Publication No. E.76.IV.1, New York, 1975, UN.

United Nations: *Report of the World Conference of the United Nations Decade for Women: Equality, Development and Peace,* Copenhagen, July 24-30, Chapter I, Section A, Publication No. E.80.IV.3, New York, 1980, UN.

United Nations: *Report of the World Conference to Review and Appraise Achievements of the United Nations Decade for Women: Equality, Development and Peace,* Nairobi, July 15-26, New York, 1985, UN.

United Nations: *Report of the Fourth World Conference on Women, Beijing,* Sept 4-15, Chapter I, Resolution 1, Annex I, Publication No. E.96.IV.13, New York, 1995, UN.

United Nations: *Basic facts about the UN,* New York, 2002, UN.

U.S. Department of Health and Human Services: *Healthy People 2000: national health promotion and disease prevention objectives,* Washington, DC, 1991, U.S. Government Printing Office, available at http://www.health.gov/healthypeople.

U.S. Department of Health and Human Services: *Neonatal intensive care: a history of excellence,* NIH Publication No. 92-2786, Oct 1992, available at http://www.nichd.nih.gov/publications/pubs/neonatal/nic.htm.

U.S. Department of Health and Human Services: *The division of nursing resource and information guide,* Rockville, Md, 2007, Division of Nursing.

U.S. Department of Health and Human Services: Leading indicators. In *Healthy People 2010: understanding and improving health,* ed 2, Washington, DC, 2000, U.S. Government Printing Office.

U.S. Department of Health and Human Services: *Health: United States,* 2007, Hyattsville, Md, 2008, National Center for Health Statistics with Chartbook on Trends on Health of Americans.

U.S. Department of Health and Human Services: *The registered nurse population: findings from the 2004 National Sample Survey,* 2007, Hyattsville, Md, National Center for Health Workforce Analysis.

U.S. Department of Health and Human Services, Centers for Medicare and Medicaid Services: *National health care expenditures projections:* 2005-2015, 2005. Retrieved May 30, 2006 from http://www.cms.hhs.gov/NationalHealthExpendData/downloads/proj2005.pdf.

U.S. Department of Health and Human Services, Health Resources and Services Administration (HRSA): *Community-based abstinence education program, Maternal and Child Health Bureau (MCHB) overview, Special Projects of Regional and National Significance (SPRANS),* Dec 2002, available at http://www.hrsa.gov.

U.S. Law: *42 SC 301, Stewart Machine Co. v. Davis,* 1937a.

U.S. Law: *49 Stat 622,* Title II, 1937b.

U.S. Law *(Public Law 107-105):* Health Insurance Portability and Accountability Act (HIPAA), 1996.

U.S. Law *(Title XXI of the Social Security Act, BBA '97):* State Child Health Improvement Act (SCHIP), 1997.

U.S. Law *(wl 1044712 La. App. 4 Cir.):* Williams v. Metro Home Health Care Agency et al, 2002.

World Health Assembly: *Strengthening nursing and midwifery: progress and future,* Resolution 49.1, 2001, WHA, available at http://www.who.org.

Chapter 8

evolve http://evolve.elsevier.com/stanhope/foundations

Economic Influences

Marcia Stanhope

ADDITIONAL RESOURCES

These related resources are found either in the appendix at the back of this book or on the book's website at http:// evolve.elsevier.com/stanhope/foundations.

Appendix

- Appendix E.3: The Health Insurance Portability and Accountability Act (HIPAA): What Does It Mean for Public Health Nurses?

Evolve Website

- Community Assessment Applied

- Case Study, with Questions and Answers
- Quiz review questions
- WebLinks, including link to *Healthy People 2010* website

Real World Community Health Nursing: An Interactive CD-ROM, second edition

If you are using this CD-ROM in your course, you will find the following activities related to this chapter:

- *The Money Challenge* in **Economics of Health Care Delivery**
- *Rate Your State* in **Economics of Health Care Delivery**

OBJECTIVES

After reading this chapter, the student should be able to:

1. Relate public health and economic principles to nursing and health care.
2. Identify major factors influencing national health care spending.
3. Describe the role of government and other third-party payers in health care financing.
4. Identify mechanisms for public health financing of services.
5. Discuss the implications of health care rationing from an economic perspective.
6. Evaluate levels of prevention as they relate to public health economics.

CHAPTER OUTLINE

HEALTH CARE PAYMENT SYSTEMS
Paying Health Care Organizations
Paying Health Care Practitioners

ECONOMICS AND THE FUTURE OF NURSING PRACTICE

KEY TERMS

capitation: a payment system whereby one fee is charged the client to pay for all services received or needed.

covered lives: persons enrolled in a health care plan who are eligible for services under that plan.

diagnosis-related groups (DRGs): a patient classification scheme that defines 468 illness categories and the corresponding health care services that are reimbursable under Medicare.

economics: social science concerned with the problems of using or administering scarce resources in the most efficient way to attain maximum fulfillment of society's unlimited wants.

effectiveness: a measure of an organization's performance as compared with its philosophy, goals, and objectives.

efficiency: the process of meeting goals in a way that minimizes costs and maximizes benefits.

enabling: the act of shielding or preventing the addict from experiencing the consequences of the addiction. Also applies to shielding individuals from the consequences of their actions more generally.

fee-for-service: list of health care services with monetary or unit values attached that specifies the amounts third parties must pay for specific services.

gross domestic product (GDP): a statistical measure used to compare health care spending among countries.

health care rationing: a method to reduce health care costs by controlling the use of health care services and technologies.

health economics: branch of economics concerned with the problems of producing and distributing the health care resources of the nation in a way that provides maximum benefit to the most people.

human capital: a measure of macroeconomic theory that involves improving human qualities, such as health, and is a focus for developing and spending money on goods and services because health is valued, it increases productivity, enhances the income-earning ability of people, and improves the economy.

inflation: a sustained upward trend in the prices of goods and services.

intensity: the use of technologies, supplies, and health care services by or for the client.

managed care: a method of organizing a number of different health care services together along a continuum of care, for example, from physician's office, to hospital, to home health, to nursing home. The client pays for services through an insurance plan.

means testing: a method used to assess whether a client's income level qualifies him or her for Medicare and/or Medicaid.

Medicaid: a jointly sponsored state and federal program that pays for medical services for the aged, poor, blind, disabled, and families with dependent children.

medical technology: the set of techniques, drugs, equipment, and procedures used by health care professions in the delivery of medical care to individuals.

Medicare: a federally funded health insurance program for the elderly and disabled and persons with end-stage renal disease.

prospective payment system (PPS): the diagnosis-related group payment mechanism for reimbursing hospitals for inpatient health care services through Medicare.

public health economics: focuses on the producing, distributing, and consuming of goods and services as related to public health.

retrospective reimbursement: method of payment to an agency based on units of service delivered.

return on investment: improved health outcomes as a result of the resources provided for a program or intervention. Resources include money, providers, time, equipment.

safety net providers: those community providers that offer services to the uninsured and underinsured.

third-party payers: reimbursement made to health care providers by an agency other than the client for the care of the client (e.g., insurance companies, governments, employers).

There is strong evidence to suggest that poverty can be directly related to poorer health outcomes. Poorer health outcomes lead to reduced educational outcomes for children, poor nutrition, low productivity in the adult workforce, and unstable economic growth in a population, community, or nation. However, improving health status and economic health is dependent on the "degree of equality" in policies that improve living standards for all members of a population, including the poor. To move toward improving a population's health there must be an "investment in public health" by all levels of government (Gupta, Verhoeven, and Tiongson, 2002; Subramanian, Belli, and Kawachi, 2002).

Estimates indicate that public spending on health care makes a difference but needs the support of increased private health care spending to improve the overall health status of populations (Gupta et al, 2002). Several facts are known from the literature (Epstein, 2001; Gwatkin, 2000;

Institute of Medicine, 2003; Makinem et al, 2000; Mantone, 2006; Wagstaff, 2000):

Approximately 47 million of 298 million people in the United States are without health insurance (U.S. Census Bureau, 2008). This number is expected to increase with the downward spiraling of the economic condition of the United States that occurred in summer and fall of 2008.

- About 40.4% of working adults were uninsured for at least part of a year in 2006.
- The poor are not as healthy as persons with middle to higher incomes.
- Persons with money and/or health insurance are more likely to seek health care.
- The poor are more likely to receive health care through publicly funded agencies.
- Preventable hospitalizations can be reduced in vulnerable populations when public health and ambulatory clinics are available.
- An emphasis on individual health care will not guarantee improvements in a population or in a community's health.

Approximately 95% of all health care dollars are spent for individual care while only 5% is spent on population-level health care. The 5% includes monies spent by the government on public health as well as the preventive health care dollars spent by private sources. The conclusion from these figures is that there is not a large investment in the public's health or population health in the United States.

The United States spends more on health care than any other nation. The cost of health care has been rising more than the rate of **inflation** since the mid-1960s. Yet the U.S. population does not enjoy better health as compared to nations that spend far less than the United States. The current health care system is at a point at which it is not affordable (Turnock, 2004). Knowledge about health economics is particularly important to community-oriented nurses because they are the ones who are often in a position to allocate resources to solve a problem or to design, plan, coordinate, and evaluate community-based health services and programs.

PUBLIC HEALTH AND ECONOMICS

Economics is the science concerned with the use of resources, including the producing, distributing, and consuming of goods and services. **Health economics** is concerned with how scarce resources affect the health care industry (Jacobs, 2002). **Public health economics** then focuses on the producing, distributing, and consuming of goods and services as related to public health (Moulton et al, 2004). Economics provides the means to evaluate society's attainment of its wants and needs in relation to limited resources. In addition to the day-to-day decision making about the use of resources, there is a focus on evaluating economics in health care. Until recently there has been limited focus on evaluating public health economics (Trust for America's Health, 2008). This report indicates that costs can be saved by adopting community-based programs that can improve

health through changes in lifestyle. While this information is needed to show the value of public health, it will continue to present challenges to public policy makers (legislators). Public health financing often causes conflict because the views and priorities of individuals and groups in society may differ with those of the public health care industry. If money is spent on public health care, then money for other public needs, such as education, transportation, recreation, and defense, may be limited. When trying to argue that more money should be spent for population-level health care or prevention, data must be available from this report and more like it to show the investment is a good one.

For many years it was thought that the public health system involved only government public health agencies, such as health departments; however, today it is known that the public health system is much broader and includes schools, industry, media, environmental protection agencies, voluntary organizations, civic groups, local police and fire departments, religious organizations, industry and business, and private sector health care systems, including the insurance industry. All can play a key role in improving population health (Institute of Medicine, 2003; Moulton et al, 2004).

BRIEFLY NOTED

In 2005, $33.8 billion was allocated for Homeland Security and bioterrorism initiatives for states to prepare for emergencies (GPO Access, 2006).

The goal of public health finance is "to support population focused preventive health services" (Moulton et al., 2004). Four principles are suggested that explain how public health financing may occur.

- The source and use of monies are controlled solely by the government.
- The government controls the money, but the private sector controls how the money is used.
- The private sector controls the money, but the government controls how the money is used.
- The private sector controls the money and controls how it is used (Gillespie et al, 2004; Moulton et al, 2004).

When the government provides the funding and controls the use, the monies come from taxes, user fees (e.g., license fees and purchase of alcohol and/or cigarettes), and charges to consumers of the services. Services offered at the federal government level include the following:

- Policymaking
- Public health protection
- Collecting and sharing information about U.S. health care and delivery systems
- Building capacity for population health
- Direct care services (Boufford and Lee, 2001)

Select examples of services offered at the state and local levels include the following:

- Maternal and child health
- Family planning

- Counseling
- Preventing communicable and infectious diseases
- Direct care services

When the government provides the money but the private sector decides how it is used, the money comes from business and individual tax savings related to private spending for illness prevention care. When a business provides disease prevention and health promotion services to their employees, and sometimes families, such as immunizations, health screening, and counseling, the business taxes owed to the government are reduced. This is considered a means by which the government provides money through tax savings to businesses to use for population health care.

When the private sector provides the money but the government decides how it is used, either voluntarily or involuntarily, the money is used for preventive care services for specific populations.

- A voluntary example is the private contributions made to reaching *Healthy People 2010* goals.
- An involuntary example is the fact that the Occupational Safety and Health Administration requires industry to adhere to certain safety standards for the use of machinery, air quality, ventilation, and eyewear protection to reduce disease and injury. This, for example, has the effect of reducing occupation-related injuries in the population as a whole.

When the private sector is responsible for both the money and its use of resources, the benefits incurred are many. For example, an industry may offer influenza vaccine clinics for workers and families that may lead to "herd immunity" in the community (see Chapter 9 on epidemiology). A business or community may institute a "no smoking" policy that reduces the risk of smoking-related illnesses to workers, family, and the consumers of the businesses' services. A voluntary philanthropic organization may give a local school money to provide preventive care and health education for the children of the school (Gillespie et al., 2004; Institute of Medicine, 2003; Moultin et al., 2004; Stanhope, 2006).

These are but a few examples of how public health services and the ensuring of a healthy population are not only government related. The partnerships between government and the private sector are necessary to improve the overall health status of populations.

BRIEFLY NOTED

The value of money varies over time. Today's dollar is worth more than tomorrow's dollar. The causes include inflation and interest rates.

FACTORS AFFECTING RESOURCE ALLOCATION IN HEALTH CARE

The distribution of health care is affected largely by the way in which health care is financed in the United States. Third-party coverage, whether public or private, greatly affects the distribution of health care. Also, socioeconomic status affects health care consumption, as it determines the ability to purchase insurance or to pay directly out-of-pocket expenses. The effects of barriers to health care access and the effects of **health care rationing** on the distribution of health care follow.

THE UNINSURED

In 1996 68% of the total U.S. population had private health insurance. An additional 15% received insurance through public programs, and 17%, or 37 million people, were uninsured. In 2008 the number of uninsured persons had increased to 47 million. The typical uninsured person is a member of the workforce or a dependent of this worker. Uninsured workers are likely to be in low-paying jobs, part-time or temporary jobs, or jobs at small businesses (Kaiser Family Foundation, 2005a). These uninsured workers cannot afford to purchase health insurance, or their employers may not offer health insurance as a benefit. Others who are typically uninsured are young adults (especially young men), minorities, persons less than 65 years of age in good or fair health, and the poor or near poor. These individuals

- may be unable to afford insurance,
- may lack access to job-based coverage, or
- because of their age or good health status, may not perceive the need for insurance.

Because of the eligibility requirements for Medicaid, the near poor are actually more likely to be uninsured than the poor.

Because of frustrations with the problems of lack of health insurance

- twenty-five states are considering making it mandatory for employers to provide coverage;
- seven states are looking at approaches to universal coverage; and
- six states are considering the development of universal health care plan commissions.

Examples of approaches in place in 2006 were the Massachusetts Expansion plan, the Maryland Employer mandate law, the West Virginia commission for developing a universal health care plan by 2010, and the New York law that limits medical debt (Mantone, 2006).

THE POOR

Socioeconomic status is inversely related to mortality and morbidity for almost every disease. Poor Americans with an income below poverty level have a mortality rate nearly three times that of middle-income Americans, even after accounting for age, sex, race, education, and risky health behaviors (such as smoking, drinking, overeating, and lack of exercise) (National Center for Health Statistics [NCHS], 2005). Historically, the link between poor health and socioeconomic status resulted from poor housing, malnutrition, inadequate sanitation, and hazardous occupations. Today, explanations include the cumulative effects of a number of characteristics that explain the concept of poverty. These characteristics include low educational levels, unemployment or low occupational status (blue collar or unskilled laborer), and low wages.

ACCESS TO CARE

Access to care is a public health issue (*Healthy People 2010*, *Healthy People 2000*). **Medicaid** is intended to improve access to health care for the poor. Although persons with Medicaid have improved access (approximately twofold) when compared to the uninsured, Medicaid recipients are only about half as likely to obtain needed health services (such as medical-surgical care, dental care, prescription drugs, and eyeglasses) as the privately insured. Specifically, the poorest Americans have Medicaid insurance, yet they also have the worst health.

The primary reasons for delay, difficulty, or failure to access care include the inability to afford health care and a variety of insurance-related reasons, such as
- the insurer not approving, covering, or paying for care;
- the client having preexisting conditions; and
- physicians refusing to accept the insurance plan.

Other barriers include lack of transportation, physical barriers, communication problems, childcare needs, lack of time or information, or refusal of services by providers. Additionally, lack of after-hours care, long office waits, and long travel distance are cited as access barriers. Community characteristics also contribute to the ability of individuals to access care. For example, the prevalence of managed care and the number of **safety net providers**, as well as the wealth and size of the community, affect accessibility.

Because reimbursement for services provided to Medicaid recipients is low, physicians are discouraged from serving this population. Thus people on Medicaid frequently have no primary care provider and may rely on the emergency department for primary care services. Although physicians can choose clients based on their ability to pay, emergency departments are required by law to evaluate all clients regardless of their ability to pay. Emergency department co-payments are modest and are frequently waived if the client is unable to pay. Thus low out-of-pocket costs provide incentives for Medicaid clients and the uninsured to use emergency departments for primary care services.

RATIONING HEALTH CARE

Escalating health care spending has spurred renewed interest in health care rationing. With unsuccessful attempts at controlling and reducing costs, new plans are being considered to control the use of services and technologies.

Rationing health care in any form implies reduced access to care and potential decreases in the acceptable quality of services offered. For example, a health provider's refusal to accept Medicare or Medicaid clients is a form of rationing. Like access to care, rationing health care is a public health issue. Where care is not provided, the public health system and nurses must ensure that essential clinical services are available. Managed care was thought to offer the possibility of more appropriate health care access and better-organized care to meet the basic health care needs

Healthy People 2010

Objectives Related to Public Health Infrastructure

Goal 23: Ensure that federal, tribal, state, and local health agencies have the infrastructure to provide essential public health services effectively.

23-16 Increase the proportion of all the above agencies that gather accurate data on public health expenditures.

23-17 Increase the proportion of all the above agencies that conduct or collaborate on population-based prevention research.

From the U.S. Department of Health and Human Services: *Healthy People 2010: understanding and improving health,* ed 2, Washington, DC, 2000, U.S. Government Printing Office.

Levels of Prevention   Economic Prevention Strategies

PRIMARY PREVENTION

Work with legislators and insurance companies to provide coverage for health promotion to reduce the risk of diseases.

SECONDARY PREVENTION

Encourage clients who are pregnant to participate in prenatal care and WIC to increase the number of healthy babies and reduce the costs related to preterm baby care.

TERTIARY PREVENTION

Participate in home visits to mothers who are at risk for neglecting babies to reduce the costs related to abuse.

From Folland S, Goodman AC, Stano M: *The economics of health and health care,* New York, 1993, Macmillan; U.S. Department of Health and Human Services: *Health: United States, 1998,* DHHS Publication No. (PHS) 98-1232, Washington, DC, 1998, U.S. Government Printing Office.

of the total population. A shift in the general approach to health care from a reactionary, acute-care orientation toward a proactive, primary prevention orientation is necessary to achieve not only a more cost-effective but also a more equitable health care system in the United States.

HEALTHY PEOPLE 2010

Healthy People 2010 goals are examples of strategies to provide better access for all people. The "Levels of Prevention" box shows the levels of economic prevention strategies.

PRIMARY PREVENTION

Society's investment in the health care system has been based on the premise that more health services will result in better health, but factors not related to health care also have an effect. Of the four major factors that affect health—personal behavior (or lifestyle), environmental factors (including physical, social, and economic environments), human biology, and the health care system—medical services are said to have the least effect. Behavior and lifestyle have been shown to have the greatest effect, with the environment and biology accounting for 70% of all illnesses (U.S. Department of Health and Human Services, 2000).

Despite the significant impact of behavior and environment on health, estimates indicate that most of the health care dollars are spent on secondary and tertiary care. Such a reactionary, secondary-care system results in high-cost, high-technology, and disease-specific care and is consistent with the U.S. system's traditional emphasis on "sickness care." A more proactive investment in disease prevention and health promotion targeted at improving health behaviors, lifestyle, and the environment has the potential to improve the health status of populations, thereby improving the quality of life while reducing health care costs. It has been argued that a higher value should be placed on primary prevention (Trust for America's Health, 2008). The goal of this approach is to preserve and maximize **human capital** by providing health promotion and social practices that result in less disease. An emphasis on primary prevention may reduce dollars spent and increase the quality of life.

The **return on investment** in primary prevention through gains in human capital has, unfortunately, not been acknowledged. Consequently, large investments in primary prevention and public health care have not been made. Reasons given for this lack of emphasis on prevention in clinical practice and lack of financial investment in prevention include the following (Chattopadhyay and Carande-Kulis, 2004):

- Provider uncertainty about which clients should receive services and at what intervals
- Lack of information about preventive services
- Negative attitudes about the importance of preventive care
- Lack of time for delivery of preventive services
- Delayed or absent feedback regarding the success of preventive measures
- Less reimbursement for these services than for curative services
- Lack of organization to deliver preventive services
- Lack of use of services by the poor and the elderly

A focus on prevention could mean reducing the need for and use of medical, dental, hospital, and health provider services. Under fee-for-service payment arrangements, this would mean that the health care system, the largest employer in the United States, would be reduced in size and would become less profitable. However, with the increasing costs of health care and consumer demand and the changes in financing mechanisms, there is a new trend toward financing more preventive care services.

Today, **third-party payers** are beginning to cover preventive services, recognizing that the growth of the health care system can no longer be supported. Under capitated health plans, health care providers stand to make money by keeping clients healthy and reducing health care use. Through combining client interests with financial interests of the health care industry, primary prevention and public health can be raised to the status and priority of acute care and chronic care. Support for an increasing national investment in primary prevention is sound and long-standing.

Since the public health movement of the mid-nineteenth century, public health officials, epidemiologists, and nurses have been working to advance the agenda of primary prevention to the forefront of the health care industry. Today, these efforts continue across a number of disciplines and in both the public and the private sectors.

THE CONTEXT OF THE U.S. HEALTH SYSTEM

The U.S. health care system is a diverse collection of industries that is involved directly or indirectly in providing health care services. The major players in the industry are the health professionals who provide health care services, pharmacy and equipment suppliers, insurers (public and/or government as well as private), managed care plans (health maintenance organizations, preferred provider organizations), and other groups, such as educational institutions, consulting and research firms, professional associations, and trade unions. Today, the health care industry is large, and its characteristics and operations differ between rural and urban geographic areas.

In the twenty-first century, health policy and national politics reflect the importance of health care delivery in the general economy. Conflicts arise between competing special-interest groups that have different goals and objectives when it comes to the producing and consuming of health services. To some degree this is caused by federal and state policy changes about how health services are financed (public and private).

Figure 8-1 illustrates the four basic components that make up the framework of health services delivery: service needs and intensity, facilities, technology, and labor. **Intensity** is

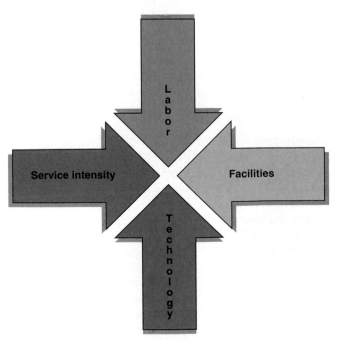

FIGURE 8-1 Components of health services development.

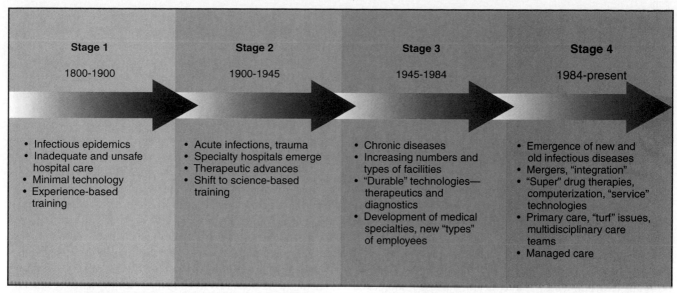

FIGURE 8-2 Developmental framework for health service needs and intensity, facilities, technology, and labor.

the extent of use of technologies, supplies, and health care services by or for the client. Intensity includes and is a partial measure of the use of technology (Kropf, 2005). **Medical technology** refers to the set of techniques, drugs, equipment, and procedures used by health care professionals in delivering medical care to individuals. It also includes information technology and the system within which such care is delivered (Kropf, 2005).

Health care systems have developed in four phases from the 1800s to today. These developmental stages correspond to different economic conditions. Developmentally, the four components of the health services delivery framework have changed over time, reflecting changes in morbidity and mortality, national health policy, and economics (Figure 8-2).

FIRST PHASE

The first developmental stage (1800 to 1900) was characterized by epidemics of infectious diseases, such as cholera, typhoid, smallpox, influenza, malaria, and yellow fever. Health concerns of the time related to social and public health issues, including contaminated food and water supplies, inadequate sewage disposal, and poor housing conditions (Lee and Estes, 2003). Family and friends provided most health care in the home. Hospitals were few in number and suffered from overcrowding, disease, and unsanitary conditions. Sick persons who were cared for in hospitals often died as a result of these conditions. Most people avoided being cared for in a hospital unless there was no alternative. In this first developmental phase, health care was paid for by individuals who could afford it, through bartering with physicians, or through charity from individuals or organizations. The first county health departments were established in 1908.

Technology to aid in disease control was very basic and practical but in keeping with the knowledge of the time. The physician's "black bag" contained the few medicines and tools available for treatment. The economics of health

care was influenced by the types of health care providers and the number of practitioners, with the labor force composed mostly of physicians and nurses who attained their skills through apprenticeships or on-the-job training. Nurses in the United States were predominantly female, and education was linked to religious orders that expected service, dedication, and charity (Kovner, 2005). The focus of nursing was primarily to support physicians and assist clients with activities of daily living.

SECOND PHASE

The second developmental stage (1900 to 1945) of U.S. health care delivery was focused on the control of acute infectious diseases. Environmental conditions influencing health began to improve, with major advances in water purity, sanitary sewage disposal, milk and water quality, and urban housing quality. The health problems of this era were no longer mass epidemics but individual acute infections or traumatic episodes (Lee and Estes, 2003).

Hospitals and health departments experienced rapid growth during the late 1800s and early 1900s as technological advances in science were made (Kovner, 2005). In addition to private and charitable financing of health care, city, county, and state governments were beginning to contribute by providing services for poor persons, state mental institutions, and other specialty hospitals, such as tuberculosis hospitals. Public health departments were emphasizing case finding and quarantine. Although health care was paid for primarily by individuals, the Social Security Act of 1935 signaled the federal government's increasing interest in addressing social welfare problems.

Clinical medicine entered its golden age during this period. Major technological advances in surgery and childbirth and the identification of disease processes, such as the cause of pernicious anemia, increased the ability to diagnose and treat diseases. The first serological tests used as a tool for diagnosis and control of infectious diseases were developed in 1910 to detect syphilis and gonorrhea (Lee and Estes, 2003). The first virus isolation techniques were also developed to filter yellow fever virus, for example. The discovery and development of pharmacological agents, such as insulin in 1922 for the control of diabetes, sulfa drugs in 1932 for the treatment of infectious diseases, and antibiotics such as penicillin in the 1940s, eradicated certain infectious diseases, increased treatment options, and decreased morbidity and mortality (Lee and Estes, 2003).

Advances in technology and knowledge shifted physician education away from apprenticeships to scientifically based college education, which occurred as a result of the Flexner Report in 1910. Nurses were trained primarily in hospital schools of nursing, with an emphasis on following and executing physicians' orders. Nurses in training were unmarried and under the age of 30. They provided the bulk of care in hospitals (Kovner, 2005). Public health nurses, who tracked infectious diseases and implemented quarantine procedures, worked more collegially with physicians (Kovner, 2005). In this period the university-based nursing programs were established to accommodate the expanding practice base of nursing. Client education became a nursing function early in the development of the health care delivery system.

THIRD PHASE

The third developmental stage (1945 to 1984) included a shift away from acute infectious health problems of previous stages toward chronic health problems such as heart disease, cancer, and stroke. These illnesses resulted from increasing wealth and lifestyle changes in the United States. To meet society's needs, the number and types of facilities expanded to include, for example, hospital clinics and long-term care facilities. The Joint Commission on Accreditation of Hospitals, established in 1951 and later renamed The Joint Commission on Accreditation of Healthcare Organizations (and now called The Joint Commission [TJC]), focused on the safety and protection of the public and the delivery of quality care.

Changes in the overall health of the American society also shifted the focus of technology, research, and development. Major technological advances included developments in the realms of chemotherapeutic agents; immunizations; anesthesia; electrolyte and cardiopulmonary physiology; diagnostic laboratories with complex modalities such as computerized tomography; organ and tissue transplants; radiation therapy; laser surgery; and specialty units for critical care, coronary care, and intensive care. The first "test tube baby" was born via *in vitro* fertilization, and other fertility advances soon emerged. Negative staining techniques for screening viruses via the electron microscope became available in the 1960s (Lee and Estes, 2003).

Health care providers constituted more than 5% of the total U.S. workforce during this period. The three largest health care employers were hospitals, convalescent institutions, and physicians' offices. Between 1970 and 1984 alone, the number of persons employed in the health care industry grew by

90%. The number of personnel employed in the community also increased. The expanding of care delivery into other sites, such as community-based clinics, increased not only the number but also the types of health care employees.

Technological advances brought about increased special training for physicians and nurses, and care was organized around these specialties. The ongoing shortage of nurses throughout the century was being seen in the 1970s and early 1980s. Nursing education expanded from hospital-based diploma and university-based baccalaureate education to include associate degree programs at the entry level. As the diploma schools of nursing began closing in the early-to-mid-1980s, the number of baccalaureate and associate degree programs began to increase. Graduate nursing education expanded to include the nurse practitioner (NP) and clinical nurse specialist (CNS) to meet increasing demands for the education of nurses in a specialty such as public health. The first doctoral programs in nursing were instituted to build the scientific base for nursing, and to increase the number of nurse faculty members.

The role of the commercial health insurance industry increased, and a strong link between employment and the providing of health care benefits emerged. Furthermore, the federal government's role expanded through landmark policymaking that would affect health care delivery well into the twenty-first century. Specifically, the passage of Titles XVIII and XIX of the Social Security Act in 1965 created the Medicare and Medicaid programs, respectively. The health care system appeared to have access to unlimited resources for growing and expanding.

Throughout the twentieth century, many public health advances were achieved. The life expectancy of U.S. citizens increased and has been related to public health activities. The most important achievements were in vaccinations, improved motor vehicle safety, safer workplaces, safer and healthier foods, healthier mothers and babies, family planning, fluoride in drinking water, and recognition of tobacco as a health hazard (Centers for Disease Control and Prevention, 2001).

FOURTH PHASE

The fourth developmental stage (1984 to the present) has been a period of limited resources, with an emphasis on containing costs, restricting growth in the health care industry, and reorganizing care delivery. For example, amendments were made to the Social Security Act in 1983 that created diagnostic-related groups and a prospective system of paying for health care provided to Medicare recipients. The 1997 Balanced Budget Act legislated additional federal changes in Medicare and Medicaid. Private-sector employer concerns about the rising costs of health care for employees and fear of profit losses spurred a major change in the delivery and financing of health care. Managed care systems were developed.

This period has included drastic change in the settings and organization of health care delivery. Transforming health care organizations became commonplace, and buzz words of the period were reorganization, reengineering, restructuring, and downsizing. Organization mergers occurred at an increased rate to consolidate care, to save money, and to coordinate care across the continuum (i.e., from "cradle to grave"). Merger discussions focused on horizontal integration, which indicated the union of similar agencies (e.g., a merger of hospitals), and vertical integration between different types of organizations (e.g., an acute care hospital, long-term care institution, and a home health facility).

Initially these pressures brought about hospital closings and a shifting of care to other settings, such as ambulatory and community-based clinics and specialty diagnostic centers that offer technologies such as magnetic resonance imaging (MRI) and sonography. Rehabilitative, restorative, and palliative care, once delivered in the hospitals, was shifted to other settings, such as subacute care hospitals, specialty rehabilitation hospitals, long-term care institutions, and even individual homes. Although the basis of care delivery was no longer the traditional acute care hospital, the nature of the care delivered in hospitals changed remarkably, as evidenced by the following:

- Patients admitted to hospitals were more acutely ill
- The length of stay for patients admitted to hospitals became shorter
- Care delivery became more intense as a result of the first two items

The widespread use of computers and the Internet has enabled society to become increasingly sophisticated about health. The public's increasing knowledge about health care and their awareness of health care advances have influenced the demand for health care, such as diagnostic and therapeutic services for treatment. Furthermore, pharmaceutical companies and other technological suppliers actively market their products through television, printed advertisements, the Internet, and other sources, so clients rapidly become aware of the new technologies.

Health professionals are dependent on technology to care for clients. Distance, as a barrier to the diagnosis and treatment of disease, had been overcome through the use of telehealth. The insurance industry has become the principal buyer of technology for the client. They often make decisions about when and if a certain technology will be used for a client problem. Nurses have become dependent on technologies to monitor client progress, make decisions about care, and deliver care in innovative ways.

The shift away from traditional hospital-based care to the community, together with the need to consider new models of care, brought about an increased emphasis on providing primary care, on developing care delivery teams, and on collaborating in practice and education. The substitution of one type of health personnel for another was occurring to control care delivery costs. As examples, the nurse practitioners (NPs) were replacing physicians as primary care providers, and unlicensed personnel were replacing staff nurses in hospitals and long-term care facilities. These replacements caused much debate, with territorial, or "turf," battles, for example, between physicians and nurses.

The increase in specialization by health professionals has led to changes in certification, qualifications, education, and standards of care in health professions. These factors, in turn, have caused an increase in the number and kinds of providers to meet the demands of the health care system. The Bureau of Labor Statistics predicts that health care employment will be among the top eight professional and related industries, with significant employment growth through 2014 (Bureau of Labor Statistics, 2006).

In the last part of the twentieth century, molecular tools were developed that provide a means of detecting and characterizing infectious disease pathogens and a new capacity to track the transmission of new threats, such as bioterrorism, and determine new ways to treat them.

TRENDS IN HEALTH CARE SPENDING

Much has been written in the popular and scientific literature about the costs of U.S. health care and how society makes decisions about using available and scarce resources. Given that economics in general and health care economics in particular are concerned with resource use and decision making, any discussion of the economics of health care must consider past and current health care spending. The trends shown here reflect public and private decisions about health care and health care delivery in the past. Past spending reflects past decision making; likewise, past decisions reflect the values and beliefs held by society and policymakers that underlie policymaking at any given point in time.

BRIEFLY NOTED

Only 5% of all health care dollars are spent for the public's health. Is this a concern to you? Justify your answer.

According to the Centers for Medicare and Medicaid Services (CMS), national health expenditures will reach $2.8 trillion in 2011 (Heffler et al, 2002). By 2007 the spending had reached $2.3 trillion (National Coalition for Health Care, 2008). Health spending will outpace increases in the gross domestic product by 2.5% per year, accounting for 17% of the **gross domestic product (GDP)** by 2011. This means that $17 of every $100 spent will be for health care. CMS relates the spending growth to new Medicare, Medicaid, and State Child Health Insurance Plans (SCHIP) (Balanced Budget Act, 1997). The effect of this economic growth represents a large increase in contrast to the approximately 13% GDP spent on health care between 1992 and 2001. The GDP was at 16% in 2007 (National Center for Health Statistics, 2008).

Table 8-1 shows the growth in U.S. health care expenditures between 1960 and 2015 (National Center for Health Statistics, 2005): spending for health care increased from approximately $27 billion in 1960 to over $1.8 billion in 2004. These numbers reflect per-person spending amounts of $143 in 1960 and $9173 in 2004. By 2008 the amount per person had exceeded $12,000. In 2003 approximately $1 to $20 was spent per person for public health activities depending on the geographic location of the person (National Center for Health Statistics, 2008).

Table 8-1	Health Care Expenditures: 1960-2015*		
Calendar Year	Total Health Expenditures (in Billions)	Total Health Expenditures per Capita (per Person) (in Billions) ($)	Percent (%) of Gross Domestic Product
1960	$26.7	$143	5.1
1970	$73.1	$348	7.0
1980	$245.8	$1,067	8.8
1990	$696.0	$2,738	12.0
2000	$1,309.9	$4,560	13.3
2004	$1,877.6	$6,280	16.0
2010*	$2,887.3	$9,173	18.0
2015*	$4,043.6	$12,357	20.0

From Centers for Medicare and Medicaid Services, Office of the Actuary, June 13, 2006: *National health care expenditures projections: 2005–2015,* available at http://www.cms.hhs.gov/NationalHealthExpendData/downloads/proj2005.pdf.
*Projected.

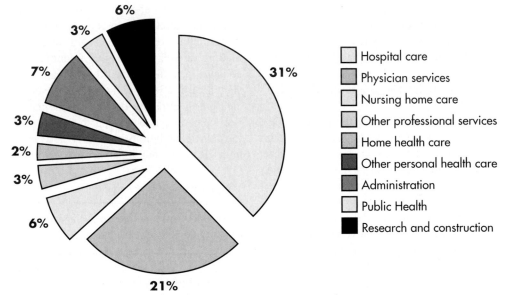

FIGURE 8-3 Distribution of U.S. health care expenditures, 2005. (From National Center for Health Statistics: *Health: United States, 2007, with chartbook on trends in the health of Americans,* Hyattsville, Md, 2008, U.S. Government Printing Office.)

Figure 8-3 shows a breakdown of the distribution in health care expenses for 2005 (National Center for Health Statistics, 2008). The largest portion of health care expenses was for hospital care and physician services, respectively. Although percentages for both of these categories have fluctuated over time, it is interesting to note that they have both changed since 1980, with hospital care declining and physician care increasing (National Center for Health Statistics, 2008). Only a small fraction of total health care dollars was spent on home health, public health, and research and construction in 2005.

FACTORS INFLUENCING HEALTH CARE COSTS

Health economists, providers, payers, and politicians have explored a variety of explanations for the rapid rate of increase in health expenses as compared to population growth. That individuals have, over time, consumed more health care is not an adequate explanation. The following factors are frequently cited as having caused the increases in total and per capita health care spending over 40 years (Levit, Lazenby, and Braden, 2002): inflation, changes in population demography, and technology and intensity of services.

DEMOGRAPHICS AFFECTING HEALTH CARE

A major demographic change under way in the United States is the aging of the population. Population changes are also affected by illnesses such as acquired immunodeficiency syndrome and by chemical dependency epidemics. These changes have implications for providers' health services, and they affect the overall costs of health care. Because the majority of older adults and other special populations receive services through publicly funded programs, the growing health needs among these populations have a great impact on costs, payments, and providers associated with Medicaid and Medicare programs. As the population ages and the baby boom generation ages and retires, federal expenses for Social Security will increase (Congressional Budget Office, 2001).

Although many older adults are independent and active, they are likely to experience multiple chronic conditions that may become disabling. They are admitted to hospitals three times more often than the general population, and their average length of stay is more than 3 days longer than the overall average. They visit physicians more often and make up a larger percentage of nursing home residents than the general population (Maddox, 2001).

Life expectancy and health status have been increasing in the United States. However, older adults continue to consume a large portion of financial resources. Health care providers are concerned about the growth in the older adult population because public funding sources, such as **Medicare**, have not been increasing their reimbursement rates sufficiently to cover inflation, and thus providers collect a smaller amount for visits by older adult clients each year.

The aging of the population also spurs concerns about funding their health care because of changes in the proportion of employed individuals to retired individuals. Persons in the workforce pay the majority of income taxes and all Social Security payroll taxes. The funding base for Medicare decreases as the population ages, as retirement rates increase, and as the numbers in the workforce decrease. As a result, some policy makers believe that Medicare and system reforms are needed to ensure adequate financing and delivery of health care services to an aging population (Maddox, 2001).

Health policy reform options being considered include increased age limits to become eligible for Medicare, **means testing** (i.e., determining a lack of financial resources) for Medicare eligibility, increased coverage for long-term care insurance, increased incentives for prevention, and less expensive and more efficient delivery arrangements and care settings (e.g., managed care arrangements). Meanwhile, the debate continues over how to best handle the future funding of the growing Medicare program.

BRIEFLY NOTED

One example of a policy change to reduce the Medicare program burden is the new prescription plan (Medicare D) that was passed by Congress in 2005 and became effective in January 2006. This plan, although complicated, requires most Medicare recipients to provide a copayment for prescription medications. Although controversial, the plan is thought to provide a positive impact for the elderly who could not afford to pay for their prescriptions, while reducing the cost burden for those who had to pay full price for prescriptions.

TECHNOLOGY AND INTENSITY

The introduction of new technology enhances the delivery of care, but it also has the potential to increase the costs of care. As new and more complex technology is introduced

Evidence-Based Practice

Los Angeles County instituted a study to assess the burden of disease and disability using a new tool called disability-adjusted life-years, or DALYs. This tool is a composite measure of premature mortality and disability that equals years of healthy life lost. The investigators looked at 105 health conditions and stratified the groups by gender and race and ethnicity of the individuals with these conditions. They also examined county mortality statistics. The results of the study provided a different ranking of disease and injury burden than simply looking at the leading causes of death alone, which is the usual approach.

The investigators found the leading causes of DALYs for men to be ischemic heart disease, violence, alcohol dependence, substance overdose, and depression. For females the five leading DALYs were ischemic heart disease, alcohol dependence, diabetes, depression, and osteoarthritis.

NURSE USE: This study can help nurses and health agency administrators examine the health of the population they are serving and use evidence-based approaches to develop programs and interventions for their populations. Improvement in functioning for persons with chronic disease leads to improved health outcomes, reduced costs of care, and economic growth.

Kominski GF et al: Assessing the burden of disease and injury in Los Angeles County using disability-adjusted life years, *Public Health Rep* 117:185-191, 2002.

into the system, the cost is typically high. However, clients often demand access to the technology, and providers want to use it. In an effort to keep health care costs down, however, payers have attempted to restrict the use of certain technologies. For example, the drug Viagra, developed for the treatment of impotence by Pfizer Pharmaceuticals, is an example of a controversial technological advance that, as soon as it was available to the public, was in high demand and prescribed by providers. Initially, use was restricted by payers because of cost. It is now covered by health insurance plans.

The adopting of new technology demands investment in personnel, equipment, and facilities. Furthermore, new technology adds to administrative costs, especially if the federal government provides financial coverage for the service or is involved in regulating the technology. Table 8-2 outlines federal policy that has impacted technology and the cost of health care over time.

CHRONIC ILLNESS

Chronic illness is a new factor affecting health care spending, with more than 50% of Americans reporting having a chronic disease. Chronic disease accounted for 75% of total health care spending in 2003 (Chattopadhyay and Carande-Kullis, 2004). Using Medical Expenditure Panel Survey (MEPS) data, chronic medical conditions are identified by those costing the most, the number of bed days, work-loss days, and activity impairments. The most costly (ischemic heart disease) was ranked tenth in terms of impairment of activities of daily living/instrumental activities of daily living (ADLs/IADLs).

| Table 8-2 | Federal Regulations Contributing to Technology and Cost Controls |

Year	Federal Regulation
1906	Prescription drug regulation: Food, Drug, and Cosmetic Act, now the U.S. Food and Drug Administration (FDA)
1935	Social Security Act (PL 74-271): Provides grants-in-aid to states for maternal and childcare, aid to crippled children, and aid to the blind and aged
1938	Food, Drug, and Cosmetic Act PL 75-540: Establishes federal FDA protections for drug safety and protections for misbranded goods, drugs, and cosmetics
1946	Hill-Burton Act (PL 79-725): Enacts Hospital Survey and Construction Act providing national direct support for community hospitals; establishes rudimentary standards for construction and planning; establishes community service obligation
1954	Hill-Burton Act amended (PL 83-482): Expands the scope of the program for nursing homes, rehabilitation facilities, chronic disease hospitals, and diagnostic or treatment centers
1963	Community Mental Health and Mental Retardation Center Construction Act (PL 88-164)
1965	Medicare Title 18; Medicaid Title 19 (PL 89-97): Amendments to Social Security Act provide Medicare and Medicaid to support health care services for certain groups
1966	Comprehensive Health Planning Act (PL 89-749): For health services, personnel, and facilities in federal, state, and local partnerships
1971	President Nixon introduces the concept of HMOs as the cornerstone of his administration's national health insurance proposal
1972	Social Security Act amendments (PL 92-603): Extend coverage to include new treatment technologies for end-stage renal disease; provide for professional standards review organizations to review the appropriateness of hospital care for Medicare and Medicaid recipients
1973	HMO Act (PL 93-222): Provides assistance and expansion for HMOs
1975	National Health Planning and Resources Development Act (PL 93-641): Designates local health system areas and establishes a national certificate-of-need (CON) program to limit major health care expansion at local and state levels
1978	Medicare End-Stage Renal Disease Amendment: Provides payment for home dialysis and kidney transplantation; Health Services Research, Health Statistics, and Health Care Technology Act establishes a national council on health care technology to develop standards for use
1981	Omnibus Budget Reconciliation Act of 1981 (PL 97-351): Consolidates 26 health programs into four block grants (preventatives, health services, primary care, and maternal and child health)
1982	Tax Equity and Fiscal Responsibilities Act (PL 97-248): Seeks to control costs by limiting hospital costs per discharge adjusted to hospital case mix
1983	Amended Social Security Act (PL 98-21): Establishes a new Medicare hospital prospective payment system based on diagnosis-related groups (DRGs)
1986	1974 Health Planning and Resource Development Act (PL 93-641): Moves CON program to states
1989	Omnibus Reconciliation Act of 1989 (PL 101-239): Creates a physician resource-based fee schedule to be implemented by 1992, with emphasis on high-tech specialties of surgery; creates the Agency for Health Care Policy and Research to research the effectiveness of medical and nursing services, interventions, and technologies
1990	Ryan White Care Act (PL 101-381): Authorizes formula-based and competitive supplemental grants to cities and states for HIV-related outpatient medical services
1990	Safe Medical Devices Act (PL 101-629): Gives the FDA authority to regulate medical devices and diagnostic products
1993	Omnibus Budget Reconciliation Act (OBRA 93) (PL 103-66): Cuts Medicare funding and ends ROE payments to skilled nursing facilities; provides support for immunizations for Medicaid children
1996	Health Insurance Portability and Accountability Act: Protects health insurance coverage for laid-off or displaced workers
1997	Balanced Budget Act of 1997: Creates a new program for states to offer health insurance to children in low-income and uninsured families
1998	PL 105-33: Authorizes third-party reimbursement for Medicare Part B services for NPs and CNSs
2003	Medicaid Nursing Incentive Act (HR 2295): Expands direct reimbursement to all nurse practitioners and clinical nurse specialists and recognizes specialized services offered by advanced practice registered nurses such as primary care case management, pain management, and mental health services
2006	Medicare Part D: Provides a plan for prescription payments

FINANCING OF HEALTH CARE

Against the backdrop of today's chronic conditions, it must be appreciated that financing for health care has evolved through the twentieth century from a system supported primarily by consumers to a system financed by third-party payers (public and private). From 1980 to 2005, the percent of third-party public insurance payments increased dramatically. Combined state and federal government payments are currently higher than those of private payers. In 2005 public sources paid the most (National Center for Health Statistics, 2008).

Table 8-3 **Comparison of Medicare and Medicaid Program Features**

Feature	Medicare	Medicaid
Where to obtain information	Local Social Security Administration office	State welfare office
Recipients	Client is 65 years of age or older, is disabled, or has permanent kidney failure	Specified low-income and needy, children, aged, blind, and/or disabled; those eligible to receive federally assisted income
Type of program	Insurance	Insurance
Government affiliation	Federal	All states
Availability	All states	All states
Financing of hospital insurance	Medicare Trust Fund, mandatory payroll deduction, recipient deductibles, trust fund interest	Federal and state governments
Financing of medical insurance	Recipient premium payments; general revenue, U.S. Treasury	Federal and state governments
Types of coverage	Inpatient and outpatient hospital services, skilled nursing facilities (SNFs), limited home health services	Inpatient and outpatient hospital services; prenatal care; vaccines for children; physician, dental, nurse practitioner, and nurse-midwife services; SNF services for persons 21 years of age or older; family services; rural health clinic

From U.S. Department of Health and Human Services, Centers for Medicare and Medicaid Services: *National trends 1966–2005*. Retrieved June 13, 2006, from www.cms.hhs.gov/MedicareEnRpts.

PUBLIC SUPPORT

The U.S. federal government became involved in health care financing for population groups early in its history. In 1798 the federal government created the Marine Hospital Service to provide medical care for sick and disabled sailors, and to protect the nation's borders against the importing of disease through seaports. The Marine Hospital Service is considered the first national health insurance plan in the United States. The National Health Board was established in 1879 and was later renamed the United States Public Health Service (PHS). Within the PHS, the federal government developed a public health liaison with state and local health departments for the purpose of controlling communicable diseases and improving sanitation. Additional health programs were also developed to meet obligations to federal workers and their families within the PHS, the Department of Defense, and the Veterans Administration.

Medicare and Medicaid, two federal programs administered by the Centers for Medicare and Medicaid Services (CMS), account for the majority of public health care spending. Table 8-3 compares these programs. The CMS is the federal regulatory agency within the U.S. Department of Health and Human Services that is responsible for overseeing and monitoring Medicare and Medicaid spending. This agency routinely collects and reports actual health care use and spending and projects future spending trends. Through these programs, the federal government purchases health care services for population groups through independent health care systems, such as managed care organizations, private practice physicians, and hospitals.

Medicare

The Medicare program, established in Title XVIII of the Social Security Act of 1965, provides hospital insurance and medical insurance to persons aged 65 years and older,

to permanently disabled persons, and to persons with end-stage renal disease—altogether approximately 43 million people in 2006 (National Center for Health Statistics, 2008). Medicare has two parts: Part A (hospital insurance) covers hospital care, home care, and skilled nursing care (limited); Part B (noninstitutional care insurance) covers medical care, diagnostic services, and physiotherapy.

Medicare Part A is primarily financed by a federal payroll tax that is paid by employers and employees. The proceeds from this tax go to the Hospital Insurance Trust Fund, which is managed by CMS. Part A coverage is available to all persons who are eligible to receive Medicare. Older adults comprise the majority of individuals eligible. There is concern about the future of the Medicare Trust Fund, as projected expenses may be more than the resources of the trust fund. Payments to hospitals for covered services have been and continue to be higher than fund growth. Thus the Medicare reimbursement policy has been changing in an attempt to control increasing hospital costs. Part A requires a deductible from recipients for the first 60 days of services with a reduced deductible for 61 to 90 days of service, based on a rate equal to a 1-day stay in the hospital. The deductible has increased as daily hospital costs have increased (Centers for Medicare and Medicaid Services, 2006). For skilled nursing facility care, persons pay nothing for the first 20 days and a cost per day for days 21 through 100.

The medical insurance package, Part B, is a supplemental (voluntary) program that is available to all Medicare-eligible persons for a monthly premium. The majority of Medicare covered persons elect this coverage. Part B provides coverage for services (other than hospital, physician care, outpatient hospital care, outpatient physical therapy, and home health care) that are not covered by Part A, such as laboratory services, ambulance transportation, prostheses, equipment, and some supplies. After a deductible, up to 80% of reasonable

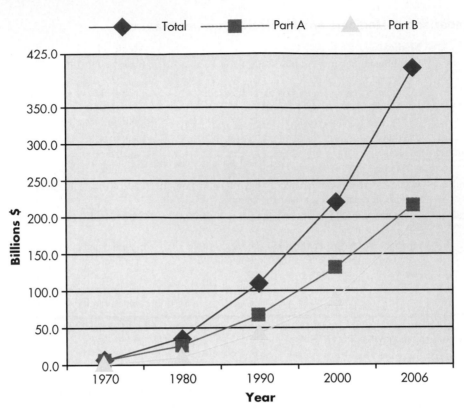

FIGURE 8-4 Medicare expenditures for selected years from 1970 to 2006. (From National Center for Health Statistics: *Health: United States, 2007 with chartbook on trends in the health of Americans,* Hyattsville, Md, 2008, U.S. Government Printing Office.)

charges are paid for these services. Part B resembles the major medical insurance coverage of private insurance carriers. Figure 8-4 shows the total expenses of the Medicare program from 1970 to 2006.

Since the passing of the Medicare amendments to the Social Security Act in 1965, the cost of Medicare has increased dramatically. Hospital care continues to be the major factor contributing to Medicare costs. However, because of shorter hospital stays, home health and nursing home costs have increased dramatically. As a result of rising health costs, Congress passed a law in 1983 that radically changed Medicare's method of payment for hospital services. In 1983 federal legislation (PL98-21) mandated an end to cost-plus reimbursement by Medicare and instituted a 3-year transition to a **prospective payment system (PPS)** for inpatient hospital services. The purpose of the new hospital payment scheme was to shift the cost incentives away from providing of more care and toward more efficient services. The basis for prospective reimbursement is the 468 **diagnosis-related groups (DRGs)**. Also, the Balanced Budget Act of 1997 determined that payments to Medicare skilled nursing facilities (SNFs) would be made on the basis of the PPS, effective July 1, 1998. The PPS payment rates cover SNF services, including routine, ancillary, and capital-related costs (Health Care Financing Administration, 1998). In 2001 CMS developed a PPS DRGs for home health with Health Insurance Prospective Payment System (HIPPS) codes.

In 2002 Medicare beneficiaries on average paid 19% of all medical costs out of pocket, approximately $2223 (Kaiser Family Foundation, 2005b). The average out-of-pocket spending is skewed to those beneficiaries who are older or have declining health (Kaiser Family Foundation, 2005b). This is because of the limits in Medicare coverage, including certain preventive care, and the limited number of physicians and agencies that accept Medicare and Medicaid payment. Older adults who do not have supplemental insurance must cover the difference between the Medicare payment and the additional costs for services.

Medicaid

The Medicaid program, Title XIX of the Social Security Act of 1965, provides financial assistance to states and counties to pay for medical services for poor older adults, the blind, the disabled, and families with dependent children. The Medicaid program is jointly sponsored and financed with matching funds from the federal and state governments. In 2003 more than 50 million people were enrolled in Medicaid (Kaiser Family Foundation, 2005c). Medicaid expenditures from 1980 to 2004 are shown in Figure 8-5. Since the beginning of Medicaid, full payment has been provided for five types of services (National Center for Health Statistics, 2008):

1. Inpatient and outpatient hospital care
2. Laboratory and radiology services
3. Physician services
4. Skilled nursing care at home or in a nursing home for people more than 21 years of age
5. Early periodic screening, diagnosis, and treatment (EPSDT) for people less than 21 years of age

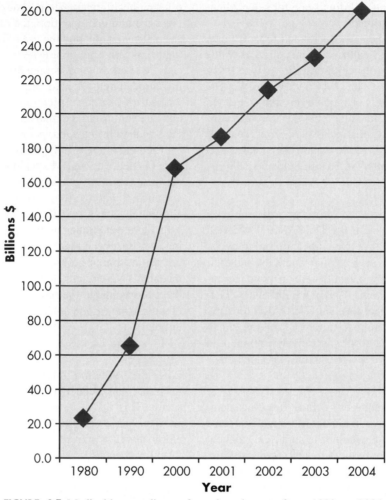

FIGURE 8-5 Medicaid expenditures for selected years from 1980 to 2004. (From National Center for Health Statistics: *Health: United States, 2007, with chartbook on trends in the health of Americans,* Hyattsville, Md, 2008, U.S. Government Printing Office.)

The 1972 Social Security amendments added family planning to the list of full-pay services. States can choose to add prescriptions, dental services, eyeglasses, intermediate care facilities, and coverage for the medically indigent as program options. By law, the medically indigent are required to pay a monthly premium.

Any state participating in the Medicaid program is required to provide the six basic services to persons who are below state poverty income levels. Optional programs are provided at the discretion of each state. In 1989 changes in Medicaid required states to provide care for children less than 6 years of age and to pregnant women under 133% of the poverty level. For example, if the poverty level were $12,000, a pregnant woman could have a household income as high as $16,000 and still be eligible to receive care under Medicaid. These changes also provided for pediatric and family nurse practitioner reimbursement. In the 1990s states were allowed to petition the federal government for a waiver. If the waiver was approved, the states could use their Medicaid monies for programs other than the six basic services. The first waiver

to be approved was given to Oregon for their health care reform plan. Other states have received waivers to develop Medicaid-managed care programs for special populations.

The major expense categories for the Medicaid program have historically been skilled and intermediate nursing home care and inpatient hospital care (National Center for Health Statistics, 2005).

PUBLIC HEALTH

Most public government agencies operate on an annual budget, and they plan for costs by estimating salaries, expenses, and costs of services for a year. Public health agencies, such as health departments and WIC programs (for women, infants, and children), receive primary funding from taxes, with additional money for select goods and services through private third-party payers. Selected public health programs receive reimbursement for services as follows: through grants given by the federal government to states for prenatal and child health; through Medicare and Medicaid for home health, nursing homes, WIC programs, and EPSDT; and through collecting of fees on a sliding scale for select client services, such as immunizations.

In 2006 only 5% of all health care-related federal funds were expended for federal health programs such as WIC, versus 95% for other types of health and illness care (such as hospital and physician services). In addition to this 5% allotment, public health funds also come through states and territorial health agencies. State and local governments contributed 17.2% to public and general assistance, maternal and child health, public health activities, and other related services in 2003 (National Center for Health Statistics, 2008).

OTHER PUBLIC SUPPORT

The federal government finances health services for military persons and dependents through the TRICARE. TRICARE is the Department of Defense's health care program for members of the uniformed services, their families, and their survivors. TRICARE also offers health care programs for retired service members, including TRICARE Pharmacy, TRICARE Dental (United Concordia), and TRICARE for Life, as well as the Veteran's Administration (VA) and the Indian Health Service (IHS). These programs are very important in providing needed health care services to these populations.

PRIVATE SUPPORT

Private health care payer sources include insurance, employers, managed care, and individuals. Although insurance and consumers have been prominent health care payment sources for some time, the role of employers, managed care, and consumers became increasingly prominent and powerful during the first decade of the twenty-first century, particularly as concerns grew about the use and changing nature of health insurance.

Evolution of Health Insurance

Insurance for health care was first offered for the private sector in 1847 by a commercial insurance company. The purpose of the insurance was to provide security and protection when health care services were needed by individuals. The idea behind insurance was that it provided security, guaranteeing (within certain limits) monies to pay for health care services to offset potential financial losses from unexpected illness or injury related to accidents, catastrophic communicable diseases (such as smallpox and scarlet fever), and recurring (but unexpected) chronic illnesses.

The Depression of the 1930s, rising medical costs, and the need to spread financial risk across communities spurred the development of the third-party payment system. The system began as a major industry in the 1930s with the Blue Cross system, which initially provided prepayment for hospital care. In 1939 Blue Shield created plans to provide physician payment. The Blue Cross plans began as tax-free, nonprofit organizations established under special **enabling** legislation in various states.

In the 1940s and 1950s, hospital and medical-surgical coverage increased. Employee group coverage appeared, and profit-making commercial insurance underwriters began offering health insurance packages with competitive premiums. Premium competition, the offering of health insurance as a fringe benefit, and the use of health insurance as a negotiable collective bargaining item led to an increase in covered benefits, first-dollar coverage for medical care expenses, and increased employer-paid premiums. In turn, these factors pushed up insurance premium costs and health care costs and enabled insurance plans to cover high-cost segments of the population (the aged, poor, or disabled).

The health needs of high-risk populations led to the passage of Medicare and Medicaid legislation. These and other national health programs targeted health care coverage for specific population groups. Because these programs directed additional money into the health care system to subsidize care, there were financial incentives to encourage the providing of services (i.e., the more services that were ordered, the greater the amount of money that would be received). Other incentives were related to the use of services by clients (i.e., the more available the payment was for services that might otherwise have gone unused, the more services that were requested).

Employers

Since the beginning of Blue Cross and Blue Shield, health insurance has been tied to employment and the business sector. This tie was strengthened during World War II to compensate, attract, and retain employees. Since that time, employers have played the major role in determining health insurance benefits.

BRIEFLY NOTED

If a client has health insurance, the payment to the provider is less than the payment made by the client who does not have health insurance.

Before the growth of insurance (i.e., before 1930 and the beginning of Blue Cross), the health care consumer had more influence over health care costs because payment was out-of-pocket. Consumers made decisions about how they would spend their money, making certain tradeoffs—for example, about the type of health care they were willing to buy and how much they would pay. Entering the system was restricted in large part to those who could afford to pay for care, or to those few who could find care financed through charitable and philanthropic organizations. With the beginning of the insurance (or third-party payer) system, health care costs were set by payers, and they determined the type of care or service that would be offered and its price. This began to change somewhat in the 1980s with the increased use of managed care.

As the cost of health insurance has increased, some employers, in an effort to bypass the costs established by insurers, have found it less costly to self-insure. The employer does this by contracting directly with providers to obtain health care services for employees rather than going through health insurance companies. Some large businesses directly employ on-site providers for care delivery or offer on-site wellness programs. These programs within the private sector offer opportunities for nurses to provide wellness programs and health assessments to screen and monitor employees and their families. This move to self-insure has resulted in savings to companies and has reduced overall sick care costs (Hunt and Knickman, 2005).

Individuals

In 2005 individuals paid only approximately 15% of total health expenditures out of pocket (National Center for Health Statistics, 2008). However, these figures do not reflect the amount of money the consumer pays in taxes to finance government-supported programs such as Medicare and Medicaid, insurance premiums, and money paid for supplemental insurance to cover the gaps in a primary health insurance policy or Medicare.

The average monthly cost for private health insurance has increased greatly through the years. Premiums reflect a shift of the health care cost burden from employers to employees as the percent of employer contributions to health care declines. The decrease in employer contribution to health insurance premiums parallels the move away from traditional insurance plans and toward managed care plans by both small and large employers, or to dropping health insurance as a benefit.

Managed Care Arrangements

Managed care is the term used for a variety of health care arrangements that integrate the financing and the delivery of health care. Managed care offers an array of services to purchasers, such as employers or Medicare, for a set fee. This fee, in turn, is used to pay providers through preset arrangements for services delivered to individuals who are covered (U.S. Department of Health and Human Services, 1998). The concept of managed care is based on the notion that the use of costly care could be reduced if consumers had access to care and services that would prevent illness through consumer education and health maintenance. Therefore managed care uses disease prevention, health promotion, wellness, and consumer education (Hunt and Knickman, 2005).

Two common types of managed care are health maintenance organizations (HMOs) and preferred provider organizations (PPOs). Box 8-1 provides an overview of HMOs and PPOs. Although they seem relatively new to many clients of care, HMOs have actually been around since the 1940s. The Health Maintenance Organization Act was enacted in 1972, and since that time the number of individuals receiving care through HMOs and other types of managed care organizations has increased considerably: between 1976 and 2004, the number of individuals enrolled in an HMO increased from 6 million to almost 69 million; the percent of the population enrolled in an HMO increased from approximately 3% to 23% (National Center for Health Statistics, 2005).

Box 8-1 Types of Managed Care

1. Health Maintenance Organization (HMO)
An HMO is a provider arrangement whereby comprehensive care is provided to plan members for a fixed, "per member per month" fee. Common features include the following:
   a. Capitation
   b. Use of designated providers
   c. Point-of-service care, or receiving care from nondesignated plan providers
   d. One of the following models:
      (1) Staff model, whereby physicians are HMO employees
      (2) Group model, whereby a physician group practice contracts with the HMO to provide care
      (3) Individual practice association (IPA), whereby the HMO contracts with physicians in solo, small group practices, or physician networks to provide care
      (4) Mixed model, whereby the HMO uses a combination group/IPA arrangement
2. Preferred Provider Organization (PPO)
A PPO is a provider arrangement whereby predetermined rates are established for services to be delivered to members. Common features include the following:
   a. Hospital and physician providers
   b. Discounted rate setting
   c. Financial incentives to encourage plan members to select PPO providers
   d. Expedited claims' payment to providers

From Folland S, Goodman AC, Stano M: *The economics of health and health care*, New York, 1993, Macmillan; U.S. Department of Health and Human Services: *Health: United States, 1998, DHHS Publication No. (PHS) 98-1232,* Washington, DC, 1998, U.S. Government Printing Office.

Medical Savings Accounts

Another insurance reform discussion at the political level concerns medical savings accounts (MSAs). MSAs are touted as a way of turning health care decision-making control over to the individuals receiving care. MSAs are tax-exempt accounts available to individuals who work for small companies, established usually through a bank or insurance company, that enable the individuals to save money for future medical needs and expenses (Internal Revenue Service, 2005). Money is contributed to an MSA by the employer, and the initial money put into an MSA does not come out of taxable income. Also, interest earned in MSAs is tax free, and unused MSA money can be held in the account from year to year until the money is used. MSAs, in theory, would allow individuals to make tradeoffs between cost and quality and would require that individuals become knowledgeable about health care, become involved in health care decision making, and take responsibility for the decisions made. Providers, in turn, must be willing to provide and disclose information to individuals and give up control of health care decision making. The HIPAA and MSAs are examples of health insurance reform efforts, and these efforts will very likely remain in the forefront of political discussions for some time to come.

HEALTH CARE PAYMENT SYSTEMS

Several methods have been used by public and private sources to pay health care providers for health care services. These include **retrospective reimbursement** and prospective reimbursement for paying health care organizations, and fee for service and capitation for paying health care practitioners (Hunt and Knickman, 2005).

PAYING HEALTH CARE ORGANIZATIONS

Retrospective reimbursement is the traditional reimbursement method, whereby fees for the delivery of health care services in an organization are set after services are delivered (Hunt and Knickman, 2005).

Prospective reimbursement, or payment, is a more recent method of paying an organization, whereby the third-party payer establishes the amount of money that will be paid for the delivery of a particular service before offering the services to the client (Hunt and Knickman, 2005). Since the establishment of prospective payment in Medicare in 1983, private insurance has followed by requiring preapprovals before clients can receive certain services, such as hospital admission or mammograms more than once a year (Hunt and Knickman, 2005).

Similarly, ambulatory care services received by Medicare recipients are classified into ambulatory payment classes (APCs), which reflect the type of ambulatory clinical services received and resources required (Centers for Medicaid and Medicare Services, 2005a). Prospective payment to skilled nursing facilities is also adjusted for case mix and geographic variations (Centers for Medicaid and Medicare Services, 2005b).

A growth in contracting, or competitive bidding, for health care services, intended to create incentives for providers to compete on price, has occurred as managed care has increased in health care markets. For example, contracting has been used by states to provide Medicaid services to eligible persons. Hospitals and other health care providers who do not have a contract with the state to provide services are not eligible to receive Medicaid payments for client care. Managed care organizations also use this approach to negotiate with health care organizations, such as hospitals, for coverage of services to be provided to covered enrollees, often called **covered lives**.

PAYING HEALTH CARE PRACTITIONERS

The traditional method of paying health care practitioners is known as **fee-for-service** payment (Hunt and Knickman, 2005) and is like the retrospective method just described. The practitioner determines the costs of providing a service, delivers the service to a client, and submits a bill for the delivered service to a third-party payer, and the payer pays the bill. Historically, Medicare, Medicaid, and private insurance companies have used this method of reimbursing physicians.

Capitation is similar to prospective reimbursement for health care organizations. Specifically, third-party payers determine the amount that practitioners will be paid for a unit of care, such as a client visit, before the delivery of the service, thereby placing a limit on the amount of reimbursement received per patient (Hunt and Knickman, 2005). In contrast to a fee-for-service arrangement, in which the practitioner determines both the services that will be provided to clients and the charges for those services, practitioners being paid through capitation are given the rate they will be paid for a client's care, regardless of specific services provided. Therefore, for example, physicians and nurse practitioners are aware, in advance, of the payment they will receive to perform a routine, uncomplicated physical examination or a more complex, detailed physical examination, diagnosis, and treatment (Hunt and Knickman, 2005).

In capitated arrangements, physicians and other practitioners are paid a set amount to provide care to a given client or group of clients for a set period of time and amount of money. This arrangement, typically used by managed care organizations, is one whereby the practitioner contracts with the managed care organization to provide health care services to plan members for a preset and negotiated fee. The agreed-on fee is negotiated between the practitioner and the managed care organization before the delivery of services and is set at a discounted rate, and the practitioner and managed care organization come to a legal agreement, or contract, for the delivery and payment of services. The managed care organization pays the predetermined fee to the practitioner, often before the delivery of services, to provide care to plan members for a set period of time (Hunt and Knickman, 2005).

Reimbursement for Nursing Services

Historically, practitioners eligible to receive reimbursement for health care services included physicians only. However, nurses who function in certain capacities, such as NPs, CNSs, and midwives, also provide primary care to clients and receive reimbursement for their services. Being recognized as primary care providers and eligible to receive reimbursement has not been an easy achievement.

Hospital nursing care costs have traditionally been included as part of the overall patient room charge and reimbursed as such. Other agencies, such as home health care agencies, include nursing care costs with administrative costs, supplies, and equipment costs. Nursing organizations, such as the American Nurses Association, have long advocated that nursing care should become a separate budget item in all organizations so that cost studies can show the **efficiency** and **effectiveness** of the nursing profession.

Spurred by efforts to control the costs of medical care, effective January 1, 1998, NPs and CNSs were granted third-party reimbursement for Medicare Part B services only, under Public Law 105-33 (American Nurses Association [ANA], 1999b). This new law sets reimbursement for NPs and CNSs at 85% of physician rates for the same service, an extension of previous legislation that allowed the same reimbursement rate to NPs and CNSs practicing in rural areas (Buppert, 1999). This law was passed after years of work in this area, including research documenting NP and CNS contributions to health care delivery and client outcomes, and after active lobbying efforts by professional nursing organizations.

Today, more than 200 nurse-managed clinics provide health care services to individuals in the United States who might not otherwise have access to health care, such as older adults, the homeless, and schoolchildren. All of these events have moved the discipline toward more autonomy in nursing practice and are serving as a means for evaluating and documenting nurses' contributions to health care delivery (Sebastian and Stanhope, 2005).

ECONOMICS AND THE FUTURE OF NURSING PRACTICE

The balance of interest within society and health care will continue to shift toward a focus on quality, safety, and eliminating health disparities through public and private sector partnerships. Health care system concerns of the twenty-first century are expected to focus on examining the quality of health care relative to the costs of care delivered. These changes will result from continued efforts of both the public and private sectors to reform the U.S. health care system. The current era of health care delivery will be noted as a time of vast changes in all sectors of health care delivery.

Nurses must plan for future changes in health care financing by becoming aware of the costs of nursing services, identifying aspects of care in which cost savings can be safely achieved, and developing knowledge on how nursing practice affects and is affected by the principles of economics. Nursing must continue to focus on improving the overall health of the nation, defining its contribution to the health of the nation, deriving the value of nursing care, and ensuring its economic viability within the health care marketplace. Nurses must effect changes in the health care system by providing leadership in developing new models of care delivery that provide effective, high-quality care and by assuming a greater role in evaluating client care and nurse performance. It is through their leadership that nurses will contribute to improved decision making about allocating scarce health care resources and will promote primary prevention as an answer to improve many of the current population-level health outcomes.

CLINICAL APPLICATION

Connie, a nursing student, has identified a caseload of five families in a chronic disease program offered by the local public health department. She is interested in assessing the costs of care to her clients and to the agency.

Connie approaches the public health nurse administrator and asks the following questions:

A. *How is the agency reimbursed for chronic disease management?*

B. *Does the client have a responsibility for paying for services?*

C. *Are nursing care costs known?*

D. *Are services rationed to clients?*

E. *What affect will the chronic disease management program have on the community population?*

Answers are in the back of the book.

REMEMBER THIS!

- From 1800 to the 1980s, the U.S. health care delivery system experienced three developmental stages, with different emphases on health care economics. In 1985 the health care delivery system entered a fourth developmental stage.
- Four basic components provide the framework for the development of the delivery of health care services: service needs and intensity, facilities, technology, and labor (workforce).
- Three major factors have been associated with the growth of the health care delivery system: price inflation, changes in population demographics, and technology and service intensity.
- Chronic disease is becoming a major health factor affecting health care spending.
- Health care financing has evolved through the twentieth century from a system financed primarily by the consumer to a system financed primarily by third-party payers. In the twenty-first century, the consumer is being asked to pay more.
- To solve the problems of rising health care costs, a number of plans for future payment of health care are being considered; all include some form of rationing.
- Excessive and inefficient use of goods and services in health care delivery has been viewed as the major cause of rising health care costs.
- Economics is concerned with the use of resources, including money, to fulfill society's needs and wants.
- Health economics is concerned with the problems of producing services and programs and distributing them to clients.
- The goal of public health economics is maximum benefits from services of public health providers, leading to health and wellness of the population.
- The goal of public health is providing the most good for the most people.
- Nurses need to understand basic economic principles to avoid contributing to rising health care costs.
- The GNP reflects the market value of goods and services produced by the United States.
- The GDP reflects the market value of the output of labor and property located in the United States.
- Social issues, economic issues, and communicable disease epidemics mark the problems of the twenty-first century.
- Medicare and Medicaid are two government-funded programs that help meet the needs of high-risk populations in the United States.
- A majority of the U.S. population has health insurance. The remaining uninsured segment represents millions of people, mostly the working poor, older adults, and children.
- Poverty has a detrimental effect on health.
- Health care rationing has always been a part of the U.S. health care system.

- Nurses are cost-effective providers and must be an integral part of health care delivery.
- *Healthy People 2010* is a document that has established U.S. health objectives.
- Human life is valued in health economics, as is money. An emphasis on changing lifestyles and preventive care will reduce the unnecessary years of life lost to early and preventable death.

WHAT WOULD YOU DO?

1. Define the following terms in your own words: economics, health economics, public health economics, public health finance, gross national product, gross domestic product, consumer price index, and human capital. How do these terms relate to your work as a nurse?
2. Compare the advantages and disadvantages of applying economics to public health care issues. Be specific.
3. Compare and contrast efficiency and effectiveness of a public health program. What factors make these difficult to control?
4. Apply the concepts of supply and demand to an example from population health. Be exact in your answer.
5. Review Chapter 4 (ethics). Debate in the class the ethical implications of the goal of rationing. Focus your debate on the implications for nursing practice. What are some of the complexities of this question?
6. Invite a public health nurse administrator to meet with your class or clinical conference group. Ask how inflation, changes in population, and technology have changed the public health care delivery system and nursing practice. How could we check for ourselves to find the answers?

■ *REFERENCES*

American Nurses Association: *Medicare reimbursement for NPs and CNSs,* 1999b, available at www.nursingworld.org/gova/medreimb.htm.

Balanced Budget Act: *State Children's Health Insurance Program,* Title XXI, Social Security Act, 1997, Section 210(a).

Boufford JL, Lee P: *Healthy Policies for the 21st century: challenges and recommendations for the U.S. Department of Health and Human Services,* New York, 2001, Milbank Memorial Fund.

Buppert C: HEDIS for the primary care provider: getting an "A" on the managed care report card, *Nurse Pract* 24(1):84–94, 1999.

Bureau of Labor Statistics: U.S. Department of Labor: *Occupational outlook handbook, 2004-2005 edition,* Washington, DC, 2006, Superintendent of Documents, U.S. Government Printing Office.

Centers for Disease Control and Prevention: Ten great public health achievements—United States 1900-1999. In Lee P, Estes C, editors: *The nation's health,* Boston, 2001, Jones and Bartlett.

Centers for Disease Control and Prevention (CDC): *Past avian influenza outbreaks,* 2006. Retrieved June 15, 2006, from http://www.cdc.gov/flu/avian/outbreaks/past.htm, page last updated February 17, 2006.

Centers for Medicaid and Medicare Services (CMS): *Medicare hospital outpatient payment system,* 2005a. Retrieved June 14, 2006, from http://www.cms.hhs.gov/apps/media/press/release.asp?Counter=376.

Centers for Medicaid and Medicare Services (CMS): *Overview: case mix prospective payment for SNFs balanced budget,* 2005b. Retrieved June 14, 2006, from http://www.cms.hhs.gov/SNFPPS/01_overview.asp.

Centers for Medicare and Medicaid Services, Office of the Actuary: *National health care expenditures projections: 2005-2015,* June 13, 2006. Retrieved from http://www.cms.hhs.gov/NationalHealthExpendData/downloads/proj2005.pdf.

Chattopadhyay SK, Carande-Kulis VG: Economics of prevention: the public health research agenda, *J Public Health Manag Pract* 10:467–471, 2004.

Congressional Budget Office: *The budget and economic outlook,* Washington, DC, Aug 2001, U.S. Government Printing Office.

Epstein AJ: The role of public clinics in preventable hospitalizations among vulnerable populations, *Health Serv Res* 36: 405–420, 2001.

Gillespie KN et al: Competencies for public health finance: an initial assessment and recommendations, *J Public Health Manag Pract* 10:458–466, 2004.

GPO Access: *Budget of the United States government: fiscal year 2005, homeland security,* 2006. Retrieved June 14, 2006, from http://www.gpoaccess.gov/usbudget/fy05/browse.html.

Gupta S, Verhoeven M, Tiongson R: Public spending on the poor, *Health Econ* 12:685–696, 2002.

Gwatkin DR: Health inequalities and the health of the poor: what do we know? What can we do? *Bull WHO* 78:19–29, 2000.

Health Care Financing Administration: *Case mix prospective payment for SNF's Balanced Budget Act of 1997.* Retrieved June 24, 1998, from www.hcfa.gov/medicare/overview.html.

Heffler S et al: Health spending projections for 2001-2011: the latest outlook, *Health Aff* 21(2):201–218, 2002.

Hunt KA, Knickman JR: Financing for health care. In *Health care delivery in the United States,* New York, 2005, Springer.

Institute of Medicine: *The future of the public's health in the 21st century,* Washington, DC, 2003, The National Academic Press.

Internal Revenue Service (IRS): *Publication 969: health savings accounts and other tax-favored health plans,* 2005. Retrieved June 13, 2006, from http://www.irs.gov/publications/p969/ar02.html.

Jacobs P: *The economics of health and medical care,* ed 5, Gaithersberg, Md, 2002, Aspen.

Kaiser Family Foundation: *The Kaiser Family Foundation and Health Research and Education Trust. Employee health benefits: 2005 summary of findings,* 2005a. Retrieved June 13, 2006, from http://www.kff.org/insurance/7315/sections/upload/7316.pdf.

Kaiser Family Foundation: *Medicare chartbook,* ed 3, 2005b, Henry J. Kaiser Family Foundation. Retrieved June 13, 2006, from http://www.kff.org/medicare/upload/Medicare-Chart-Book-3rd-Edition-Summer-2005-Report.pdf.

Kaiser Family Foundation: *Medicaid facts: Medicaid enrollment and spending trends,* 2005c. Retrieved June 13, 2006, from http://www.kff.org/medicaid/upload/Medicaid-Enrollment-and-Spending-Trends-Fact-Sheet.pdf.

Kovner C: The health care workforce in the United States. In Kovner A, editor: *Health care delivery in the United States,* New York, 2005, Springer.

Kropf R: Technology assessment in health care. In *Health care delivery in the United States,* New York, 2005, Springer.

Lee P, Estes C: *The nation's health,* Boston, 2003, Jones and Bartlett.

Levit KR, Lazenby HC, Braden BR: National health spending trends, *Health Aff* 21, 2002.

Maddox PJ: Impact of financing arrangements and economics on nursing. In Doechterman G, editor: *Current issues in nursing,* ed 6, St Louis, 2001, Mosby.

Makinem M et al: Inequalities in health care use and expenditures: empirical data from eight developing countries in transition, *Bull WHO* 78:55–65, 2000.

Mantone J: Stating the case for coverage, *Mod Health Care* 16:6–7, 2006.

Moulton AD et al: Public health finance: a conceptual framework, *J Public Health Manag Pract* 10:377–382, 2004.

National Center for Health Statistics: *Health: United States, 2005, with chartbook on trends in the health of Americans,* Hyattsville, Md, 2005, U.S. Government Printing Office.

National Center for Health Statistics: *Health: United States, 2007, with chartbook on trends in the health of Americans*, Hyattsville, Md, 2008, U.S. Government Printing Office.

National Coalition on Health Care: Health Insurance Costs, Washington, DC, 2008. Retrieved from info@nchc.org, October 6, 2008.

Sebastian J, Stanhope M: *Survey of academic primary care nurse managed centers, a joint project of the Michigan Consortium Group and the University of Kentucky College of Nursing,* 2005.

Stanhope M: *Good Samaritan Nursing Center Annual Report*, Jan 2006.

Subramanian SV, Belli P, Kawachi I: The macroeconomic determinants of health, *Annu Rev Public Health* 23:287–302, 2002.

Trust for America's Health: *Prevention for a healthier America,* Washington, DC, July 2008. Retrieved October 6, 2008, from www.healthyamericas.org.

Turnock BJ: *Public health: What it is and how it works,* Boston, 2004, Jones and Bartlett.

U.S. Census Bureau: *Number of US Uninsured Rises.* Retrieved October 6, 2008, from http://www.census.gov.

U.S. Department of Health and Human Services: *Healthy People 2000: national health promotion and disease prevention objectives,* Washington, DC, 1990, USDHHS, Public Health Service.

U.S. Department of Health and Human Services: *Health: United States, 1998, DHHS Publication No. (PHS) 98–1232,* Washington, DC, 1998, U.S. Government Printing Office.

U.S. Department of Health and Human Services: *Healthy People 2010: understanding and improving health*, Washington, DC, 2000, Public Health Service.

Wagstaff A: Socioeconomic inequalities in child mortality: comparisons across nine developing countries, *Bull WHO* 78:19–29, 2000.

PART III

Conceptual Frameworks Applied to Nursing Practice in the Community

evolve   http://evolve.elsevier.com/stanhope/foundations

Epidemiologic Applications

Robert E. McKeown
DeAnne K. Hilfinger Messias

ADDITIONAL RESOURCES

These related resources are found either in the appendix at the back of this book or on the book's website at http://evolve.elsevier.com/stanhope/foundations.

Evolve Website

- Community Assessment Applied
- Case Study, with Questions and Answers
- Quiz review questions
- WebLinks, including link to *Healthy People 2010* website

Real World Community Health Nursing: An Interactive CD-ROM, second edition

If you are using this CD-ROM in your course, you will find the following activities related to this chapter:
- *Epidemiology: Calculate and Compare Rates* in **Epidemiology**
- *Epidemiology Crossword Puzzles* in **Epidemiology**
- *HIV/AIDS Epidemiology: Evaluate the Trends* in **Epidemiology**
- *Epidemiology: Report It* in **Epidemiology**
- *Investigation of an Outbreak* in **Epidemiology**

OBJECTIVES

After reading this chapter, the student should be able to:
1. Define epidemiology and describe how it has developed over time.
2. Describe the essential elements of epidemiology and an epidemiologic approach.
3. Discuss the steps in the epidemiologic process.
4. Explain the basic epidemiologic concepts of population at risk, natural history of disease, levels of prevention,

host–agent–environment relationships, and the web-of-causation model.
5. Differentiate between descriptive and analytic epidemiology.
6. Explain how nurses use epidemiology in community health practice.

CHAPTER OUTLINE

DEFINITIONS
HISTORY
HOW NURSES USE EPIDEMIOLOGY
BASIC CONCEPTS IN EPIDEMIOLOGY
Measures of Morbidity and Mortality
Epidemiologic Triangle: Agent, Host, and Environment
Levels of Preventive Interventions
AN INTERVENTION SPECTRUM

SCREENING
Reliability and Validity
BASIC METHODS IN EPIDEMIOLOGY
Sources of Data
Rate Adjustment
Comparison Groups
DESCRIPTIVE EPIDEMIOLOGY
Person
Place

Time
ANALYTIC EPIDEMIOLOGY
Cohort Studies
Prospective Cohort Studies
Case-Control Studies
Cross-Sectional Studies
Ecological Studies
EXPERIMENTAL STUDIES

Clinical Trials
Community Trials
CAUSAL INFERENCE
Statistical Associations
Bias
Assessing Evidence of Causal Associations
APPLICATIONS OF EPIDEMIOLOGY IN NURSING

KEY TERMS

agent: causative factor invading a susceptible host through an environment favorable to produce disease, such as a biological or chemical agent.

analytic epidemiology: a form of epidemiology that investigates causes and associations between factors or events and health.

attack rate: a type of incidence rate defined as the proportion of persons who are exposed to an agent and who develop the disease, usually for a limited time in a specific population.

bias: in determining causality, a systematic error because of the way the study is designed, how it was carried out, or some unplanned events that occurred and affected the study.

case-control study: an epidemiologic study design in which subjects with a specified disease or condition (cases) and a comparable group without the condition (controls) are enrolled and assessed for the presence or history of an exposure or characteristic.

case fatality rate: the proportion of persons diagnosed with a specific disorder who die within a specified time.

causal inference: using epidemiologic, clinical, statistical, and other scientific evidence to judge if a causal association exists between two or more factors or events. Guidelines for evaluation of evidence are often used in making causal inference. Different levels of evidence may be required for different settings, for example, clinical decisions versus policy determinations.

cohort study: an epidemiologic study design in which subjects without an outcome of interest are classified according to past or present (or future) exposures or characteristics and followed over time to observe and compare the rates of some health outcome in the various exposure groups.

confounding: a bias that results from the relationship between both the outcome and study factor (exposure or characteristic) and some third factor not accounted for in analysis.

cross-sectional study: an epidemiologic study in which health outcomes and exposures or characteristics of interest are simultaneously ascertained and examined for an association in a population or sample, providing a picture of existing levels of all factors.

descriptive epidemiology: a form of epidemiology that describes a disease according to dimensions of person, place, and time.

determinants: factors that influence the risk for or distribution of health outcomes.

distribution: a pattern of a health outcome in a population; the frequencies of the outcome according to various personal characteristics, geographic regions, and time.

ecological model: a multidimensional model of determinants of health and disease that spans many levels from individual genetic and physiologic characteristics to broader contextual influences (e.g., neighborhood characteristics and social context). This model encompasses a broader spectrum of systems and etiologic factors than the web of causality model and includes a lifespan perspective.

environment: for public health refers to all factors that constitute the context in which persons or animals live and that influence and are influenced by the host and agent–host interactions.

epidemic: a rate of disease clearly in excess of the usual or expected frequency in that population.

epidemiology: the study of the distribution and factors that determine health-related states or events in a population and the use of this information to control health problems.

host: a human or animal that provides adequate living conditions for any given infectious agent.

incidence proportion: the proportion of the population at risk who experience the event over some period of time.

incidence rate: the frequency or rate of new cases of an outcome in a population; it provides an estimate of the risk of disease in that population over the period of observation.

levels of prevention: a three-level model of interventions based on the stages of disease, designed to halt or reverse the process of pathological change as early as possible, thereby preventing damage.

natural history of disease: the course or progression of a disease process from onset to resolution.

negative predictive value: the proportion of persons with a negative test who are disease free.

point epidemic: a concentration in space and time of a disease event, such that a graph of the frequency of cases over time shows a sharp point, usually suggestive of a common exposure.

positive predictive value: the proportion of persons with a positive screening or diagnostic test who do have the disease (the proportion of "true positives" among all who test positive).

prevalence proportion: a measure of existing disease in a population at a given time.

primary prevention: a type of intervention that seeks to promote health and prevent disease from the beginning.

proportion: a type of ratio in which the denominator includes the numerator.

proportionate mortality ratio: the proportion of all deaths due to a specific cause.

rate: a measure of the frequency of a health event in a defined population during a specified period.

reliability: the precision, stability, agreement, or replicability of a measuring instrument when repeatedly used; an indication of consistency from time to time or from person to person.

risk: the probability of some event or outcome occurring within a specified period.

screening: the application of a test to people who are as yet asymptomatic for the purpose of classifying them with respect to their likelihood of developing a particular disease.

secondary prevention: an intervention that seeks to detect disease early in its progression (early pathogenesis) before clinical signs and symptoms become apparent in order to make an early diagnosis and begin treatment.

secular trends: long-term patterns of morbidity or mortality (i.e., over years or decades).

sensitivity: the extent to which a test identifies those individuals who have the condition being examined.

specificity: the extent to which a test identifies those individuals who do not have the disease or condition being examined.

surveillance: systematic and ongoing observation and collection of data concerning disease occurrence in order to describe phenomena and detect changes in frequency or distribution.

tertiary prevention: intervention that begins once the disease is obvious; the aim is to interrupt the course of the disease, reduce the amount of disability that might occur, and begin rehabilitation.

validity: the accuracy of a test or measurement; how closely it measures what it claims to measure. In a screening test, validity is assessed in terms of the probability of correctly classifying an individual with regard to the disease or outcome of interest, usually in terms of sensitivity and specificity.

web of causality: complex interrelations of factors interacting with each other to influence the risk for or distribution of health outcomes.

Epidemiology is the study of the distribution and factors that determine health-related states or events in a population and the use of this information to control health problems. The term originally referred to the spread of infectious epidemics such as cholera or tuberculosis (TB). Now the term is much more inclusive, involving infectious diseases and chronic diseases, such as cancer and cardiovascular disease, as well as mental health and other health-related events, such as intentional injuries (accidents), violence, occupational and environmental exposures and their effects, and positive health states. The public health science of epidemiology has made major contributions to (1) the understanding of factors that contribute to health and disease, (2) the development of health promotion and disease-prevention measures, (3) the detection and characterization of emerging infectious agents, (4) the evaluation of health services and policies, and (5) the practice of nursing in community health.

DEFINITIONS

Epidemiology investigates the **distribution** or the patterns of health events in populations and the determinants or the factors that influence those patterns. When using **descriptive epidemiology**, health outcomes are considered in terms of what, who, where, and when. That is: What is the disease? Who is affected? Where are they? When do events occur? Descriptive epidemiology discusses a disease in terms of person, place, and time. On the other hand, **analytic epidemiology** looks at the "why" or the etiology (origins or

causes) of the disease and deals with determinants of health and disease. The **determinants** of health events are the factors, exposures, characteristics, and behaviors that determine (or influence) the patterns: How does it occur? Why are some people affected more than others? Determinants may be individual, relational or social, communal, or environmental.

Epidemiology, like both the research process and nursing process, consists of a set of steps. The first step is to define the outcome. The health outcome can be a disease, or it can refer to both intentional and unintentional injuries or even wellness. Using epidemiologic methods, a nurse describes the distribution or the who, where, and when of a disease, event, or injury and searches for factors that explain the pattern or risk of occurrence. The nurse asks what influences the occurrence of this disease or injury or why and how events occurred as they did.

Like nursing, epidemiology builds on and draws from other disciplines and methods, including clinical medicine and laboratory sciences, social sciences, quantitative methods (especially biostatistics), and public health policy and goals. Epidemiology focuses on populations, whereas clinical medicine focuses on the diagnosis and treatment of disease in *individuals*. Epidemiology studies *populations* to determine the causes of health and disease in communities and to investigate and evaluate interventions that will prevent disease and maintain health. Epidemiologic methods are used extensively to determine to what extent the goals of *Healthy People 2010* (U.S. Department of Health and

Categories with Objectives Related to Epidemiology
1. Access to quality health services
2. Arthritis, osteoporosis, and chronic back conditions
3. Cancer
4. Chronic kidney disease
5. Diabetes
6. Disability and secondary conditions
7. Educational and community-based programs
8. Environmental health
9. Family planning
10. Food safety
11. Health communication
12. Heart disease and stroke
13. Human immunodeficiency virus infection
14. Immunization and infectious diseases
15. Prevention of injury and violence
16. Maternal, infant, and child health
17. Medical product safety
18. Mental health and mental disorders
19. Nutrition and overweight
20. Occupational safety and health
21. Oral health
22. Physical activity and fitness
23. Public health infrastructure
24. Respiratory disease
25. Sexually transmitted diseases
26. Substance abuse
27. Tobacco use
28. Vision and hearing

From U.S. Department of Health and Human Services: *Healthy People 2010: understanding and improving health,* ed 2, Washington, DC, 2000, U.S. Government Printing Office.

Human Services, 2000) have been met and to monitor the progress of those objectives not fully met at present.

As noted, epidemiology differs from clinical medicine, which focuses on the diagnosis and treatment of disease in individuals. Epidemiology is the study of populations to (1) monitor the health of the population, (2) identify the determinants of health and disease in communities, and (3) investigate and evaluate interventions to prevent disease and maintain health. Effective nursing in community health bridges these disciplines in its focus on individual clients and services provided for them, as well as on the broader context in which they live and the complex interplay of social and environmental factors that affect their well-being. This task involves using epidemiologic methods and findings in community health programs and using preventive measures. Epidemiology is true detective work. For example, consider a man who visits a country other than where he lived. Within 3 days, he was experiencing nausea and diarrhea. The epidemiologic process could help determine what action should be taken. Specifically, what did he eat or drink? Did others eat or drink the same things? Are other people with him experiencing the same symptoms? After a thorough review of the "what, who, where, and when" he realizes that the only thing he did differently from others with him was use

water from the bathroom faucet to brush his teeth. Others in his group had used bottled water. Although he knew that people often react negatively to water that is different from their own, he was so accustomed to drinking tap water to brush his teeth that he did so in this new location without thinking about the effects it might have for him.

HISTORY

In the fourth century BCE, Hippocrates was one of the first people to use the ideas that are now part of epidemiology (Timmreck, 2002). He examined health and disease in a community by looking at geography, climate, the seasons of the year, the food and water consumed, and the habits and behaviors of the people. His approach, like descriptive epidemiology, looked at how health is influenced by personal characteristics, place, and time. Notable events in the history of epidemiology are shown in Table 9-1.

During the nineteenth century, Louis Pasteur developed both the germ theory and pasteurization. In the latter, he made an enormous contribution to the safety of milk. Pasteur also recognized the role of personal characteristics, such as immunity and host resistance, in explaining why some people were susceptible to disease and others were not (Vandenbroucke, 1990). Other examples of major discoveries during this century were made by Joseph Lister, the British surgeon who developed antiseptic surgery, and Robert Koch, a German scientist who developed pure culture and identified the organisms that cause TB, anthrax, and cholera.

In the eighteenth and nineteenth centuries, comparison groups began to be used to measure change or the effects of some action or treatment on an experimental group. Also at this time, quantitative methods (numeric measurements or counts) were beginning to be used. One of the most famous studies using a comparison group is the mid-nineteenth century investigation of cholera by John Snow, whom some call the "father of epidemiology" (Timmreck, 2002). Snow observed that cholera rates were higher among households supplied by water companies whose water came from downstream than among households whose water came from farther upstream, where it was subject to less contamination. Because in some areas, households near each other had different sources of water, differences observed in rates of cholera could not be attributed to location or economic status. Snow showed that households receiving water from the Lambeth Company, whose intake had been moved away from sewage contamination, had cholera rates considerably lower than those supplied by Southwark and Vauxhall, a company whose water intake was still in a contaminated section of the river. Snow conducted a "natural experiment" as seen in Table 9-2 and documented that foul water was the vehicle for transmission of the agent that caused cholera (Rothman, 2002).

In response to an outbeak in the Golden Square area of London, in 1854 Snow drew a map of cholera deaths and found that they were clustered around a a single public water pump, supporting his theory that the spread of cholera was related to the water supply. Clearly Snow's work can

Table 9-1 **Significant Milestones in the History of Epidemiology**

Date	Investigator	Contribution
1662	John Graunt	Used Bills of Mortality (forerunner of modern vital records) to study patterns of death in various populations in England. Published early form of life table analysis.
1760	Daniel Bernoulli	Used life table technique to demonstrate that smallpox inoculation conferred lifelong immunity.
1798	Edward Jenner	Demonstrated the effectiveness of smallpox vaccination.
1836		Marine Hospital Service was opened; forerunner of the U.S. Public Health Service (1912). Establishment of Registrar-General's Office in England as a registry for births, deaths, marriages.
1840s	William Farr	Developed the forerunner of a modern vital records system in the Registrar-General's Office. Study of mortality in Liverpool led to significant public health reform. Pioneered mortality surveillance and anticipated many of the basic concepts in epidemiology. His data provided much of the basis for Snow's work on cholera.
1850	Lemuel Shattuck	Reported on sanitation and public health in Massachusetts. The London Epidemiological Society was founded. Known for influential reports on smallpox vaccination and studies of cholera.
1850s	John Snow	Conducted epidemiologic research on transmission of cholera. Used mapping and natural experiment, comparing rates in groups exposed to different water supplies.
1870-1880s	Robert Koch	Discovered causal agents for anthrax, tuberculosis, and cholera; development of causal criteria.
1887	Joseph Kinyuon	Founded the "Laboratory of Hygiene," forerunner of the National Institutes of Health (1930). The United States Public Health Service (USPHS) assumed the work previously done by the Marine Hospital Service.
1921	Wade Hampton Frost	Founded the first U.S. academic program in epidemiology at Johns Hopkins. The National Institutes of Health (NIH) was created.
1942		The Office of Malarial Control in War Areas was established; it became the Communicable Disease Center (CDC) in 1946; then the Centers for Disease Control (1973); now the Centers for Disease Control and Prevention.
1948		Framingham Heart Study began.
1950s	A. Bradford Hill and Richard Doll Jerome Cornfield	Pioneering studies on smoking and lung cancer were conducted. A method of estimating comparative rates from clinical data (use of odds ratio from a case-control study as an estimate of relative risk).
1964		The Surgeon General's report on smoking and health was released.
1975		CDC biomedical scientists/epidemiologists identified *Legionella* bacteria as the cause of an outbreak of a "flu-like" syndrome, later named *legionnaires' disease*, after the American Legion commanders who fell ill at a meeting in Philadelphia from this then-unknown disease.
1980		American Psychiatric Association *Diagnostic and Statistical Manual of Mental Disorders, 3rd ed (DSM-III)* was published, which for the first time provided consistent, reliable, and generally accepted criteria for the diagnosis of psychiatric disorders that could be used in epidemiologic research as well as clinical practice. Led to the development of assessment instruments that could be used in epidemiologic studies. Followed by *DSM-III-R* (revised, 1987), *DSM IV* (1994), and *DSM-IV-TR* (text revision, 2000).
1981		The CDC's *Morbidity and Mortality Weekly Report* (MMWR) ran an article on *Pneumocystis* pneumonia that announced the new disease of acquired immunodeficiency syndrome (AIDS).
1983		The Public Health Service (PHS) published its first guidelines on AIDS prevention, recommending that people refrain from donating blood and modify their sexual practices.
1988		The Institute of Medicine published *The Future of Public Health*. This report says that the core public health functions are assessment, policy development, and assurance. Epidemiology and statistics are established as the basis for the assessment function.
1990		Ryan White Comprehensive AIDS Resources Emergency Act.
1991		Publication of *Healthy People 2000: National Health Promotion and Disease Prevention Objectives* by the U.S. Department of Health and Human Services, Public Health Service.
1995		Hantavirus respiratory disease, an acute disease usually fatal and caused by human exposure to mouse droppings, was declared a notifiable disease by the CDC.
1996		Health Insurance Portability and Accountability Act PL 104-191.

Continued

Table 9-1   Significant Milestones in the History of Epidemiology—cont'd

Date	Investigator	Contribution
2000		Establishment of a task force to prepare the Guide to Community Prevention Services to spell out ways to implement the objectives of *Healthy People 2010*.
		Publication of *Healthy People 2010: Understanding and Improving Health* by the U.S. Department of Health and Human Services.
		American College of Epidemiology. Publication of Ethics Guidelines for Epidemiology (*Ann Epidemiol* 10[8]:485–497, 2000).
2001		Emergency Supplemental Appropriations Act of Recovery from and Response to Terrorist Attacks on the United States.
2003		Completion of the Human Genome Project, which provided breakthroughs in information that will aid in predicting the potential for disease, prevention, and treatment.
2004		Publication by the Agency for Healthcare Research and Quality: "Child Health Care Quality Toolbox: Why Child Health Measures?"
2006		Publication of the "Essential Nursing Competencies and Curricula Guidelines for Genetics and Genomics" by the American Nurses Association, Silver Spring, Md.
2007		Publication by the Centers for Disease Control and Prevention of "Epidemiology and Prevention Vaccine-Preventable Diseases" or "The Pink Book."
		Publication by the Agency for Healthcare Research and Quality: "2007 National Healthcare Quality & Disparities Report" and "Guide to Clinical Preventive Services, 2007."

Data from Benedict I et al: Developing the guide to community preventive services: overview and rationale, *Am J Prev Med* 18(1S):18–26, 2000; Institute of Medicine: *The future of public health,* Washington, DC, 1988, National Academy Press; Lilienfeld DE, Stolley PD: *Foundations of epidemiology,* ed 3, New York, 1994, Oxford University Press; Mullan F: *Plagues and politics: the story of the United States Public Health Service,* New York, 1989, Basic Books; Schneider MJ: *Introduction to public health,* Gaithersburg, Md, 2000, Aspen; Susser M: Epidemiology in the United States after World War II: the evolution of technique, *Epidemiol Rev* 7:147, 1985; Timmreck TC: *An introduction to epidemiology,* Boston, 1994, Jones & Bartlett; U.S. Department of Health and Human Services: *Public Health Service fact sheet,* Washington, DC, 1984, U.S. Department of Health and Human Services, Public Health Service.

Table 9-2   Household Cholera Death Rates by Source of Water Supply in John Snow's 1853 Investigation

Company	Number of Houses	Deaths from Cholera	Deaths per 10,000 Households
Southwark and Vauxhall	40,046	1263	315
Lambeth	26,107	98	37
Rest of London	256,423	1422	59

From Snow J: On the mode of communication of cholera. In *Snow on cholera,* New York, 1855, The Commonwealth Fund.

be compared with that of a detective and also is much like putting a puzzle together. That is, he had many pieces of the puzzle concerning the disease, and his task was to assemble the pieces to find an explanation for the outbreak of cholera.

In nursing, Florence Nightingale contributed to the development of epidemiology in her work with British soldiers during the Crimean War (1854 to 1856). At this time, sick soldiers were cared for in cramped quarters that had poor sanitation, were overrun with lice and rats, and had insufficient food and medical supplies. She looked at the relationship between the conditions of the environment and the recovery of the soldiers. Using simple epidemiologic measures of rates of illness per 1000 soldiers, she was able to show

that improving environmental conditions and adding nursing care decreased the mortality rates of the soldiers (Cohen, 1984; Palmer, 1983). These same principles can be applied today in the many countries that experience war leading to poor food, water, and sanitary conditions. That is, if the environment could be improved and better care provided, the rate of illnesses and death would be reduced.

During the twentieth century, several changes in society influenced the further development of epidemiology. Some of these were the Great Depression of the 1920s in the United States; World War II; a rising standard of living for many but abject poverty for others; improved nutrition; better sanitation; the development of antibiotics, vaccines, and cancer chemotherapies; decreased birth rates in some countries; and decreases in infant and child mortality in many nations. People began to live longer, and the rates of several chronic diseases such as coronary heart disease (CHD), stroke, cancer, and senile dementia increased (Susser, 1985). Figure 9-1 shows the 10 leading causes of death in the United States in 1900, 1950, 2001 and 2005, with the percentage of all deaths attributed to each.

During the twentieth century a shift occurred from looking for single agents, such as the infectious agent that causes cholera, to determining the multifactorial etiology or the many factors or combinations of factors that contribute to disease. An example of multifactorial etiology is to look at the complex number and type of factors that cause cardiovascular disease. People began to realize that not all the diseases of older people were the result of the degenerative processes of aging. Rather, it became clear that many behavioral and environmental factors supported or encouraged the development of diseases. This information led to the belief that some diseases could be prevented and other diseases could at least be delayed (Susser, 1985).

In addition, the development of genetic and molecular techniques increased the ability of the epidemiologist to classify persons in terms of exposures or inherent susceptibility to disease. Examples included the identification of genetic traits that indicated an increased risk for breast cancer and markers that identified exposures to environmental toxins such as lead or pesticides. These developments are of particular interest to nurses who work with people in their living and work environments and understand the interaction of the environment(s) on health and well-being. Furthermore, nurses in the community can assess a broad range of health outcomes as well as factors that contribute to wellness and illness.

Unfortunately, in recent years new infectious diseases (e.g., Lyme disease, legionnaires' disease, hantavirus, Ebola virus, severe acute respiratory syndrome [SARS], human immunodeficiency virus/acquired immunodeficiency syndrome [HIV/AIDS], methicillin-resistant *Staphylococcus aureus* [MRSA], as well as new forms of old diseases [e.g., drug-resistant strains of TB, new forms of *Escherichia coli*]) have emphasized the dangers that can occur with these

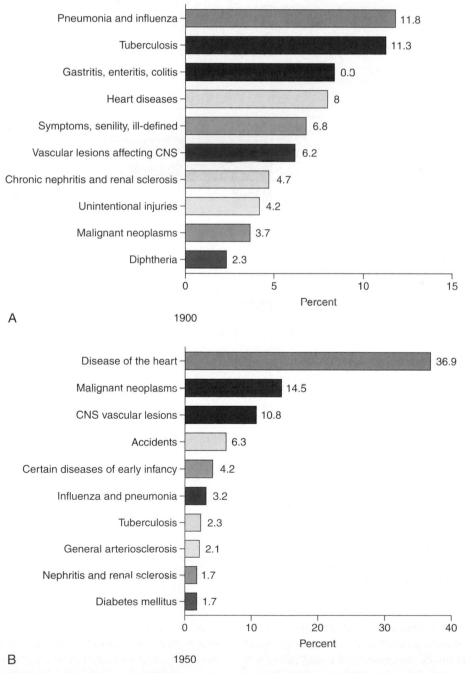

FIGURE 9-1 Ten leading causes of death as a percentage of all deaths, United States. **A**, 1900; **B**, 1950;

Continued

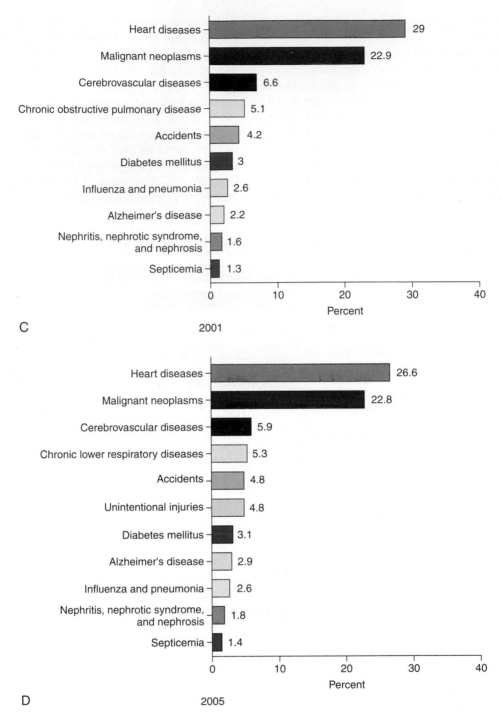

FIGURE 9-I, cont'd **C,** 2001; **D,** 2005. (Data from Anderson RN: Deaths: leading causes for 2000, *Natl Vital Stat Rep* 50(16), 2002; Brownson RC, Remington PL, Davis JR: *Chronic disease epidemiology and control,* ed 2, Washington, DC, 1998, American Public Health Association; U.S. Department of Health, Education, and Welfare: *Vital statistics of the United States: 1950,* vol 1, Washington, DC, 1954, USDHEW, Public Health Service. Centers for Disease Control and Prevention: Deaths: leading causes for 2001, *Natl Vital Stat Rep* 52(9):7–14, 2003; Centers for Disease Control and Prevention: National Center for Health Statistics, 2005. Retrieved September 1, 2008, from http://www/cdc/gov. nchs.FASTATS/lcod.htm.

diseases. Also, potential threats from terrorist use of infectious agents (e.g., anthrax, smallpox) have once again placed the epidemiology of infectious disease in the spotlight. There is an urgency to use the tools provided by epidemiology to improve the control and management of health care. As mentioned, epidemiologic methods also have been applied to a broader spectrum of health-related outcomes including accidents, injuries and violence, occupational and environmental exposures, psychiatric and sociological phenomena, health-related behaviors, and health services research.

Following the terrorist attacks of September 11, 2001, and the apparently unrelated anthrax letters that appeared, public health took on a broader mission, with increased public awareness of its importance. Centers of public health preparedness are funded by the federal government, with both researchers and practitioners focusing on preparation, prevention, and response to attacks. There is renewed awareness of the importance of a sound public health infrastructure, especially with regard to surveillance and outbreak investigations, which can carry on critical day-to-day public health functions while also monitoring, alerting, and responding to events. Epidemiologists were among the first to respond to both the terrorist attacks of 9/11 and the anthrax letters, and they remain at the center of public health planning and the design of response plans using epidemiologic methods.

HOW NURSES USE EPIDEMIOLOGY

Nurses are a key part of the interdisciplinary team in community settings, looking at health and at disease causation and at how to both prevent and treat illness. In the community, nurses often use epidemiology, since the factors that affect the individual, family, and population group cannot be as easily controlled as in acute care settings. That is, it is difficult, for example, to control the environment including water and food supplies, air quality conditions including pollutants, disposal of garbage and trash, quality of paint used to ensure it contains no lead, or what comes in the mail. Therefore community residents are often exposed to many factors affecting their health.

Nurses are involved in the surveillance and monitoring of disease trends. In settings such as homes, schools, work places, clinics, and other and health care organizations, nurses can identify patterns of disease in a group. For example, if several children in a school become sick with abdominal problems within a short period (e.g., a 24-hour period), the nurse would try to determine what these children had in common. For instance, did they eat the same food, drink from the same source of water, or swim in the same pool? Likewise, if workers in a plant displayed a similar pattern of symptoms, the nurse would look for factors in the workplace to locate the cause. The reason for looking at the workplace first is that it is the setting the individuals have in common.

Care of clients, families, and population groups in the community uses the following steps of the nursing process: (1) assessment, (2) planning, (3) implementation, and (4) evaluation. When using the nursing process, epidemiology provides baseline information for assessing needs, identifying problems, designing appropriate strategies to evaluate the problems, setting priorities to develop a plan of care, and evaluating how effective the care was. The information learned from the Human Genome Project completed in 2003 will continue to be the basis of new discoveries about the consequences of genetic variations and the outcomes of the interaction between genes and the environment. Nurses, in their focus on health, can use the information that is now available and will increasingly become available as a result of further research. The "Essential nursing competencies and curricula guidelines for genetics and genomics" will help nurses care for individuals, families, communities, and populations by including genetic and genomic information in their practice. For example, this information could assist a nurse in recognizing a newborn who is at risk for morbidity or mortality due to errors in genetic metabolism (American Nurses Association, 2006). The sections that follow discuss the "tools of epidemiology" that are needed by nurses who work in community settings.

CASE STUDY

Mary Miles is the nurse epidemiologist for the Warren County Health Department. A local church contacted Ms. Miles when several church members became sick after the annual church picnic. Of the 200 people who attended the picnic, 100 were ill with diarrhea, nausea, or vomiting. Ten people required emergency medical treatment or hospitalization. Incubation periods ranged from 1½ hours to 30 hours, with a mean of 6 hours and a median of 3½ hours. Duration of illness ranged from 1 to 80 hours, with a mean of 30 hours and a median of 15 hours.

The annual church picnic is a potluck lunch buffet. The menu included macaroni casserole (brought by the Joneses), turkey with gravy and stuffing (brought by the Smiths), potato salad (brought by the Changs), green bean casserole (brought by the Champs), chili (brought by the Turners), homemade bread (brought by Granny Ivy), chocolate cake (brought by the Bushes), and cookies (brought by the Beckmans). Ms. Miles interviewed the church members who were ill and found that three food items were significantly associated with illness: turkey, gravy, and stuffing.

Ms. Miles interviewed the Smiths, who brought the turkey, gravy, and stuffing to the picnic. Review of food-handling procedures indicated that the turkey had cooled for 4 hours at room temperature after cooking—a time and temperature sufficient for bacterial growth and toxin production. Furthermore, the same utensils were used for both the turkey and other foods before and after cooking.

Ms. Miles talked with the Smiths about proper food-handling practices, emphasizing hand washing, proper cooling and preserving methods, and better equipment and utensil sanitation. Ms. Miles also offered a similar class to the church congregation.

BASIC CONCEPTS IN EPIDEMIOLOGY

MEASURES OF MORBIDITY AND MORTALITY

Rates, Proportions, and Risk

Epidemiology looks at the distribution of health states and events. Because people differ in their probability or risk of disease, the primary concern is how they differ. Mapping cases of a disease in an area, as John Snow mapped cases of cholera in one area of London and as many epidemiologists now map various health-related events, can be instructive even though it is limited in what it can reveal. A larger number of cases may simply be the result of a larger population with more potential cases or the result of a longer period of observation. Any description of disease patterns should take into account the size of the population at risk for the disease. That is, we should look not only at the numerator (the number of cases) but also at the denominator (the number of people in the population at risk) and at the amount of time each was observed. For example, 50 cases of influenza might be seen as a serious epidemic in a population of 250 but would be a low rate in a population of 250,000. Using rates and proportions instead of simple counts of cases takes the size of the population at risk into account.

Epidemiologic studies rely on rates and proportions. A **proportion** is a type of ratio in which the denominator includes the numerator. For example, in the year 2000 there were 2,404,624 deaths recorded in the United States, of which 709,894 were reported to have been caused by diseases of the heart. Therefore, the proportion of deaths caused by heart disease in the year 2000 was 709,894/2,404,624 = 0.295, or 29.5%. Because the numerator must be included in the denominator, proportions can range from 0 to 1. Proportions are often multiplied by 100 and expressed as a percent, literally meaning *per 100*. In public health statistics, however, if the proportion is very small, we use a larger multiplier to avoid small fractions, so the proportion may be expressed as a number per 1000 or per 100,000.

A **rate** is a measure of the frequency of a health event in different populations at certain periods of time (Dawson and Trapp, 2004). A rate is a ratio but it is not a proportion because the denominator is a function of both the population size and the dimension of time, whereas the numerator is the number of events. Furthermore, depending on the units of time and the frequency of events, a rate may exceed 1. As its name suggests, a rate is a measure of how quickly something is happening: how rapidly a disease is developing in a population or how rapidly people are dying. Rates deal with change: moving from one state of being to another, from well to ill, from alive to dead, or from ill to cure. Because they deal with events (moving from one state of being to another), time is involved. We must follow a population over time to observe the changes in state, and we typically exclude from the population being followed those persons who have already experienced the event.

Risk refers to the probability that an event will occur within a specified period. A population at risk is the population of persons for whom there is some finite probability (even if small) of that event occurring. For example, although the risk of breast cancer in men is small, a few men do develop breast cancer and therefore are part of the population at risk. There are some outcomes for which certain people would never be at risk (e.g., men cannot be at risk of ovarian cancer nor can women be at risk of testicular cancer). A high-risk population, on the other hand, would include those persons who, because of exposure, lifestyle, family history, or other factors, are at greater risk for disease than the population at large. It seems that all persons are susceptible to HIV infection, although the degree of susceptibility

may vary. Therefore everyone is in the population at risk for HIV and AIDS. Persons who have multiple sexual partners without adequate protection or who use intravenous drugs are in the high-risk population for HIV infection. However, others who do not fit these categories may unknowingly be at high risk. An example is women who consider themselves to be in monogamous relationships but are unaware that their partners have sexual relations with other women or men. As proportions, risk estimates have no dimensions, but they are a function of the length of time of observation. Given a continuous rate, increasing time will mean that a larger proportion of the population will eventually become ill.

Epidemiologists and other health professionals are interested in measures of morbidity, especially incidence proportions, incidence rates, and prevalence proportions. These measures provide information about the risk of disease, the rate of disease development, and the levels of existing disease in a population, respectively.

BRIEFLY NOTED

Genetic testing is becoming more common, but most tests for disease indicate only susceptibility to disease, not certainty. Similarly, screening tests are never perfect so there is always some probability of misclassifying a person.

Measures of Incidence

Measures of incidence reflect the number of new cases or events in a population at risk during a specified time. An **incidence rate** quantifies the rate of development of new cases in a population at risk (Greenberg et al., 2005), whereas an incidence proportion indicates the proportion of the population at risk that experiences the event over some period of time (Rothman, 2002). The population at risk is considered to be persons without the event or outcome of interest but who are at risk of experiencing it. Note that existing (or prevalent) cases are excluded from the population at risk for this calculation because they already have the condition and are no longer at risk of developing it. The **incidence proportion** is also referred to as the *cumulative incidence rate* because it reflects the cumulative effect of the incidence rate over the time period. The risk of disease is a function of both the rate of new disease development and the length of time the population is at risk. The interpretation can be for an individual (i.e., the probability that the person will become ill) or for a population (i.e., the proportion of a population expected to become ill over that period). In epidemiology, we often calculate proportions on the basis of population frequencies. These frequencies are then translated into personal risk statements for people representative of the population on which the estimates are based.

For example, suppose a health department and community hospital jointly begin an intensive, broad-based screening program in an area that had overcrowded housing, limited access to services, and underuse of preventive health practices. Their program includes physical examinations; tuberculin skin tests with follow-up chest radiography where indicated; cardiovascular, glaucoma, and diabetes screening; and mammography for women and prostate screening for men older than 45 years of age. Of the 8000 women screened, 35 were previously diagnosed with breast cancer; by screening and follow-up, 20 with no history of breast cancer were found to have cancer of the breast. We could follow the 7945 women in whom no breast cancer was detected and note the number of new cases of breast cancer detected over the following 5 years. Assuming no losses to follow-up (moved away or died from other causes), if 44 women were diagnosed over the 5-year period, the 5-year incidence proportion of breast cancer in this population would be as follows:

$$\frac{44}{7945} = 0.005538, \text{ or } 553.8 \text{ per } 100,000$$

Note the multiplication by 100,000, so that the number of cases is expressed as per 100,000 women. A cumulative incidence rate estimates the risk of developing the disease in that population during that time. Also, as a proportion, each event in the numerator must be represented in the denominator, and only those persons at risk for the event counted in the numerator may be included in the denominator.

We estimate incidence rates by counting events relative to the total amount of time that persons in a population are observed, referred to as *person-time*. For many calculations it is generally assumed that rates are constant over the period of observation. A true incidence rate is an instantaneous rate of disease development, often approximated by incidence density. In calculating the person-time of observation for a denominator, we count the amount of time each person contributes from the time the observation of that person begins until the person (1) experiences the event, (2) is lost to follow-up or dies from some other cause or otherwise is no longer at risk, or (3) reaches the end of observation. Incidence density is an estimate of the instantaneous rate (or hazard) of the event. It is an indication of how rapidly disease is developing in a population.

To continue the previous example, suppose the 7945 women we follow for 5 years accumulate a total of 39,615 person-years of observation. Remember, the assumption was that there was no loss to follow-up or deaths from other causes. Note that the total person-time is not equivalent to 5×7945 (which is 39,725), because we stop counting time for the 44 women who developed breast cancer at the time of diagnosis. (You can imagine that determining the exact time of disease onset is often a problem in epidemiologic studies. Using the time of diagnosis can be biased because diagnosis occurs at different stages of disease in populations.) So the incidence rate for the diagnosis of breast cancer in this population, after 5 years of observation, would be estimated as 44 newly diagnosed cases per 39,615 person-years of observation, or 0.0011107, which we could express as 11.1 cases per 10,000 person-years.

We often want to know about the risk—that is, the probability of disease occurring over some defined period of time, such as a year or several years. Earlier we estimated the risk

directly as the number of new cases over a 5-year period in a population at risk. That was straightforward because we had no losses and observation began at the same time for all the women. A more common situation is that people come under observation at different times and losses occur as a result of attrition or competing risks (i.e., other events or deaths). We can handle those easily by counting the amount of time that is observed and calculating the incidence density as an estimate of the incidence rate. The question is how the incidence density rate is related to an estimate of risk. We can say that the risk for individuals, accumulated over a population, gives rise to the rate observed in that population. In epidemiology, however, it is the observed rate in a population that allows us to estimate the risk of an event in that population, both in terms of the expected proportion of the population that would become ill and in terms of the risk to a representative member of the population. When certain assumptions are met, primarily a constant rate, the average incidence density over a period of time is related to the cumulative risk for that period by the following equation:

$$\text{Risk} = 1 - e^{[-I \times T]}$$

where I is the mean per-person-time incidence rate, T is the period of observation in the same units of time, and e is the base of the natural logarithm. Again, to return to the example, suppose we observed the 44 new cases in 39,615 person-years of follow-up, but there were losses to follow-up and women entered and left the population at different times. Assuming that the rate of new breast cancer is fairly constant over that 5-year period, the cumulative risk over 5 years is estimated as follows:

$$\text{Risk} = 1 - e^{[-0.0011107 \times 5]} = 0.005538$$

which is the same as the risk we calculated for the simpler situation.

Note that the rate used is *not* the incidence proportion but the mean incidence densities for intervals of time comprising the total period, and the formula assumes that the rates do not vary over the period. Also, risk is a probability whose value depends on both the incidence rate and the period of observation, but not on the units of measurement for time, and whose range is restricted to between 0 and 1. The value of incidence density, on the other hand, does depend on the units of time and, because it is not a probability, it is not restricted to the 0 to 1 range. Furthermore, when the incidence rate is low or the period of observation is short—so that, relative to the size of the population, few people are removed from the population at risk by disease—the product of the per-person rate and the period of observation approximates the risk for the period (Greenberg et al, 2005; Rothman, 2002).

A ratio can be used as an approximation of a risk. For example, the infant mortality "rate" is the number of infant deaths (i.e., infants are defined as being younger than 1 year of age) in a given year divided by the number of live births in that same year. It approximates the risk of death in the first year of life for live-born infants in a specific year. Some of the infants who die that year were born in the previous year, and some of the infants born that year may die in the following year before their first birthday. However, because about two-thirds of infant deaths occur within the first 28 days of life, the number of infants in the numerator (deaths in a given year) but not in the denominator (live births in that same year) will be small. It can be assumed that current year deaths from the previous year's cohort approximately equal the deaths from the current year's cohort occurring in the following year. Although technically a ratio, this is an approximation to the true proportion and, therefore, an estimate of the risk.

An **epidemic** occurs when the rate of disease, injury, or other condition exceeds the usual (endemic) level of that condition. No specific threshold of incidence indicates that an epidemic exists. Because smallpox has been eradicated, any occurrence of smallpox might be considered an epidemic by this definition. In contrast, given the high rates of ischemic heart disease in the United States, an increase of many cases would be needed before an epidemic was noted, although some might argue that the current high rates compared with earlier periods already indicate an epidemic.

Prevalence Proportion

The **prevalence proportion** is a measure of existing disease in a population at a particular time (i.e., the number of existing cases divided by the current population). It is also possible to calculate the prevalence of a specific risk factor or exposure. In the breast cancer example given earlier, the screening program discovered 35 of the 8000 women screened had previously been diagnosed with breast cancer and 20 women with no history of breast cancer were diagnosed as a result of the screening. The prevalence proportion of current and past breast cancer events in this population of women would be as follows:

$$\frac{55}{8000} = 0.006875, \text{ or } 687.5 \text{ per } 100,000$$

A prevalence proportion is not an estimate of the risk of developing disease, because it is a function of both the rate at which new cases of the disease develop and how long those cases remain in the population. In this example, the prevalence of breast cancer in this population of women is a function of how many new cases develop and how long women live after the diagnosis of breast cancer. A fairly constant prevalence might be seen, for example, if improved survival after diagnosis were offset by an increasing incidence rate. The duration of a disease is affected by case fatality and cure. (For simplicity, in this example, women with a history of the disease are counted in the prevalence proportion even though they may have been cured.) A disease with a short duration (e.g., an intestinal virus) may not have a high prevalence proportion even if the rate of new cases is high, because cases do not accumulate (see the discussion of point epidemic). A disease with a long course will have a higher prevalence proportion than a rapidly fatal disease that has the same rate of new cases.

In their 2007 study, Valdez et al. sought to test the association between stratified levels of familial risk of diabetes and the prevalence of the disease in the United States population. The research team used results from the National Health and Nutrition Examination Survey taken between 1999 and 2004. The sample included 16,388 adults; a subsample of 6004 participants was selected based on the availability of their fasting glucose. Familial risk of diabetes was categorized as average, moderate, or high based on the prevalence and the odds of having the disease.

The study found that 69.8% of adults were of average risk for diabetes overall, 22.7% were of moderate risk, and 7.5% were of high familial risk. The crude prevalence for each category was 5.9, 14.8, and 30%, respectively. Once sex, race and ethnicity, age, body mass index (BMI), hypertension, income, and education were accounted for, the graded association between familial risk and prevalence of diabetes remained constant. Percentages for the moderate and high-risk groups were 2.3 and 5.5% higher than those in the average risk group.

The researchers concluded that based on the data, a family history of diabetes has a significant, independent, and graded association with the prevalence of diabetes in the American population. This association therefore highlights the importance of family history, shared genes, and environment in the development of diabetes.

NURSE USE: This study found that family history is a powerful independent risk factor for diabetes and recommends that this knowledge be used in public health programs that address the disease. Incorporating family history into screening programs is another recommendation, and evaluating both types of programs to determine their usefulness and cost effectiveness is key. Further studies on family history are recommended in order to create a universal, quantifiable definition to use in future research. This research could also help identify segments of the population that are at greater risk for the disease.

From Valdez R et al: Family history and prevalence of diabetes in the U.S. population: The 6-year results from the National Health and Nutrition Examination Survey (1999-2004), *Diabetes Care* 30:2517-2522, 2007.

Incidence and Prevalence Compared

The prevalence proportion measures existing cases of disease. The prevalence odds ($P[1-P]$) are roughly proportional to the incidence rate multiplied by the average duration of disease (Rothman, 2002). The prevalence proportion is, therefore, affected by factors that influence risk (incidence) and by factors that influence survival or recovery (duration). For that reason, prevalence measures are less useful when looking for factors related to disease etiology. Because prevalence proportions reflect duration in addition to the risk of getting the disease, it is difficult to sort out what factors are related to risk and what factors are related to survival or recovery. In mathematical notation,

$$P/(1-P) \cong I \times D,$$
$$\text{or, when } P \text{ is small } (<0.1), \text{ the } P \cong I \times D,$$

where P = prevalence, I = incidence rate, and D = average duration.

Determine If a Health Problem Exists in the Community

Planning for resources and personnel often requires quantifying the level of a problem in a community. For example, to know how different districts compare in the rates of very-low-birthweight infants, you would calculate the prevalence of very-low-birthweight births in each district:

1. Determine the number of live births in each district from birth certificate data obtained from the vital records division of the health department.
2. Use the birthweight information from the birth certificate data to determine the number of infants born weighing less than 1500 grams in each district.
3. Calculate the prevalence of very-low-birthweight births by district as the number of infants weighing less than 1500 grams at birth divided by the total number of live births.
4. If the number of very-low-birthweight births in each district is small, use several recent years of data to obtain a more stable estimate.

For example, the 5-year survival rate for breast cancer is about 85%, but the 5-year survival rate for lung cancer in women is only about 15%. Even if the incidence rates of breast and lung cancer were the same in women (and they are not), the prevalence proportions would differ because, on average, women live longer with breast cancer (i.e., it has a longer duration). Incidence rates and incidence proportions, on the other hand, are the measure of choice to study etiology because incidence is affected only by factors related to the risk of developing disease and not to survival or cure. Prevalence is useful in planning health care services because it is an indication of the level of disease existing in the population and therefore of the size of the population in need of services. In the previous example about screening, the health department would want to know both the existing level of TB in the area (the prevalence), to plan services and direct prevention and control measures, and the rate at which new cases are developing (the incidence), to study risk factors and evaluate the effectiveness of prevention and control programs (see How To Box).

Attack Rate

One final measure of morbidity, often used in infectious disease investigations, is the **attack rate**, or the proportion of persons who are exposed to an agent and develop the disease. Attack rates are often specific to an exposure; food-specific attack rates, for example, are the proportion of persons becoming ill after eating a specific food item.

Mortality Rates

Several key mortality rates are shown in Table 9-3. Many commonly used mortality rates are not true rates but are proportions. Although measures of mortality reflect serious health problems and changing patterns of disease, they have limited usefulness. They provide information only about fatal diseases and do not provide direct information about either the level of existing disease in the population or the risk of getting a particular disease. Also, a person may have

one disease (e.g., prostate cancer) yet die from a different cause (e.g., stroke).

Because the population changes during the course of a year, the usual practice is to estimate the population at midyear as the denominator for annual rates. The crude annual mortality rate is an estimate of the risk of death for a person in a given population for that year. These rates are multiplied by a scaling factor, usually 100,000, to avoid small fractions. The result is then expressed as the number of deaths per 100,000 persons. Although a crude mortality rate is calculated easily and represents the actual death rate for the total population, it has certain limitations. It does not reveal specific causes of death, which change in relative importance over time. Also, the mortality rate is affected by the population's age distribution, since older people are at much greater risk of death than younger people.

Mortality rates are also calculated for specific groups (e.g., age-specific, gender-specific, or race-specific rates). In these instances, the number of deaths occurring in the specified group is divided by the population at risk, now restricted to the number of persons in that group. This rate is then viewed as the risk of death for persons in the specified group during the period of observation.

The cause-specific mortality rate is an estimate of the risk of death from some specific disease in a population. It is the number of deaths from a specific cause divided by the total population at risk, usually multiplied by 100,000. Two related measures should be distinguished from the cause-specific mortality rate. The **case fatality rate** (CFR) is the proportion of persons diagnosed with a particular disorder (i.e., cases) who die within a specified period. It is considered an estimate of the risk of death within that period for a person newly diagnosed with the disease (e.g., the proportion of persons with a disease who die during the natural history of the disease). Since the CFR is the proportion of diagnosed persons who die within the period, 1 minus the CFR yields the survival rate. For example, if the CFR for 15 women diagnosed with an illness is 40% ($n = 6$), the survival rate is 60%, or $n = 9$ (Greenberg et al, 2005). Persons diagnosed with a particular disease often want to know the probability of surviving. These rates provide that information.

The second measure to be distinguished from the cause-specific mortality rate is the **proportionate mortality ratio** (PMR), the proportion of all deaths resulting from a specific cause. Some sources, especially those used in occupational health, say it is the proportion of all deaths resulting from a specific cause divided by the same proportion in a standard population. The denominator is not the population at risk of death but the total number of deaths in the population; therefore the PMR is not a rate nor does it estimate the risk of death. The magnitude of the PMR is a function of both the number of deaths from the cause of interest and the number of deaths from other causes. If deaths from certain causes decline over time, deaths from other causes that remain fairly constant may have increasing PMRs. For example, motor vehicle accidents accounted for 3.9 deaths per 100,000 persons ages 5 to 14 years in the United States in 2002. This was

Table 9-3 **Common Mortality Rates**

Rate/Ratio	Definition and Example
Crude mortality rate	Usually an annual rate that represents the proportion of a population that dies from any cause during the period, using the midyear population as the denominator. **Example:** In 2000 there were 2,403,351 deaths in a total population of 275,264,999, or 873.1 per 100,000
Age-specific rate	Number of deaths among persons of a given age group per midyear population of that age group. **Example:** 2000 age-specific mortality rate for persons ages 20 to 24 years: per 100,000 persons aged 20 to 24 years. $$\frac{17,744}{18,484,615} = 96 \text{ per } 100,000 \text{ persons ages 20 to 24 years}$$
Cause-specific rate	Number of deaths from a specific cause per midyear population. **Example:** 2000 cause-specific rate for accidents: $$\frac{97,900 \text{ accidental deaths}}{275,264,999 \text{ midyear population}} = 35.6 \text{ per } 100,000$$
Case fatality rate	Number of deaths from a specific disease in a given period/Number of persons diagnosed with that disease. **Example:** If 87 of every 100 persons diagnosed with lung cancer die within 5 years, the 5-year case fatality rate is 87%; the 5-year survival rate is 13%
Proportionate mortality ratio	Number of deaths from a specific disease per total number of deaths in the same period. **Example:** In 2000, there were 710,760 deaths from diseases of the heart and 2,403,351 deaths from all causes: $$\frac{710,760}{2,403,351} = 0.296 \text{ or } 29.6\% \text{ of all deaths were due to heart disease}$$
Infant mortality ratio	Number of deaths of infants under 1 year of age in a year per number of live births in the same year. **Example:** In 2000, there were 28,035 infant deaths and 4,058,814 live births: $$\frac{28,035}{4,058,814} = 0.0069 \text{ or } 6.9 \text{ per } 1000 \text{ live births}$$
Neonatal mortality rate	Number of deaths of infants under 28 days of age in a year per number of live births in the same year. **Example:** In 2000, there were 18,776 neonatal deaths and 4,058,814 live births: $$\frac{18,776}{4,058,814} = 4.63 \text{ per } 1000 \text{ live births}$$
Postneonatal mortality rate	Number of deaths of infants from 28 days to 1 year of age in a year per number of live births in the same year. **Example:** In 2000, there were 9259 postneonatal deaths and 4,058,814 live births: $$\frac{9295}{4,058,814} = 2.28 \text{ per } 1000 \text{ live births}$$

From Anderson RN: Deaths: leading causes for 2000, *Natl Vital Stat Rep* 50(16), 2002; Martin JA et al.: Births: final data for 2000, *Natl Vital Stat Rep* 50(5), 2002; National Center for Health Statistics: *Health, United States,* 1998, Hyattsville, Md, 1998, Public Health Service.

22.4% of all deaths in this age group (the PMR). By comparison, motor vehicle accidents caused 25.7 deaths per 100,000 persons 75 to 84 years of age in 2002, which was less than 0.5% of all deaths in the older age group (Kochanek et al, 2004). This demonstrates that although the risk of death from a motor vehicle accident was more than four times as great in the older group (based on the rates), such accidents accounted for a far greater proportion of all deaths in the younger group (based on the PMR). This is because of the much greater risk of death from other causes in the older group.

Infant mortality is used around the world as an indicator of overall health and availability of health care services. The most common measure, the infant mortality rate, is the number of deaths to infants in the first year of life divided by the total number of live births. Because the risk of death declines considerably during the first year of life, neonatal (i.e., newborn) and postneonatal mortality rates are also of interest.

BRIEFLY NOTED

Epidemiologic concepts and data are used in ongoing assessments of both community and individual health problems. An initial component of a community health assessment is the collection of incidence, morbidity, and mortality rates for specific diseases. Health service data, such as immunization rates, causes of hospitalization, and emergency department visits, are also obtained.

EPIDEMIOLOGIC TRIANGLE: AGENT, HOST, AND ENVIRONMENT

Epidemiologists understand that disease results from complex relationships among causal agents, susceptible persons, and environmental factors. These three elements—agent, host, and environment—are called the *epidemiologic triangle* (Figure 9-2A). Changes in one of the elements of the

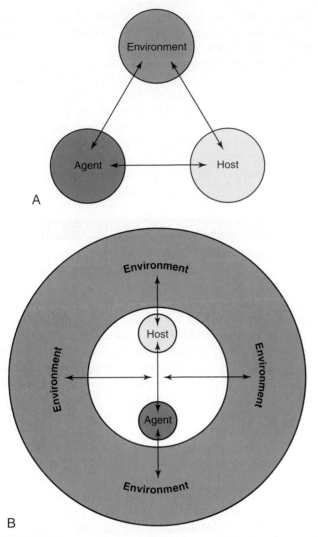

A

B

FIGURE 9-2 Two models (**A** and **B**) of the agent–host–environment interaction (the epidemiologic triangle).

Box 9-1	Examples of Agent, Host, and Environmental Factors in the Epidemiologic Triangle

Agent
- Infectious agents (bacteria, viruses, fungi, parasites)
- Chemical agents (heavy metals, toxic chemicals, pesticides)
- Physical agents (radiation, heat, cold, machinery)

Host
- Genetic susceptibility
- Immutable characteristics (age, sex)
- Acquired characteristics (immunological status)
- Lifestyle factors (diet, exercise)

Environment
- Climate (temperature, rainfall)
- Plant and animal life (agents or reservoirs or habitats for agents)
- Human population distribution (crowding, social support)
- Socioeconomic factors (education, resources, access to care)
- Working conditions (levels of stress, noise, satisfaction)

---

triangle can influence the occurrence of disease by increasing or decreasing a person's risk for disease. Figure 9-2B shows that agent and host, as well as their interaction, are influenced by the environment in which they exist. They also may influence the environment. Specifically, these elements or variables are defined as follows:

- **Agent:** an animate or inanimate factor that must be present or lacking for a disease or condition to develop
- **Host:** a living species (human or animal) capable of being infected or affected by an agent
- **Environment**: all that is internal or external to a given host or agent and that is influenced and influences the host and/or agent

Some examples of these three components are listed in Box 9-1.

Causal relationships (one thing or event causes another) are often more complex than the epidemiologic triangle conveys. The term **web of causality** recognizes the complex interrelationships of many factors interacting, sometimes in subtle ways, to increase (or decrease) the risk of disease. Also, associations are sometimes mutual, with lines of causality going in both directions. Recently some researchers advocated for a new paradigm that goes beyond the two-dimensional causal web and considers multiple levels of factors that affect health and disease (Krieger, 1994; Macintyre and Ellaway, 2000). This is consistent with the **ecological model** for population health supported by the Institute of Medicine's report (IOM, 2002), which expands epidemiologic studies both upward to broader contexts such as neighborhood characteristics and social context and downward to the genetic and molecular level. The ecological model treats the multiple determinants of health as interrelated and acting synergistically (or antagonistically), rather than as discrete factors. This model encompasses determinants at many levels: biologic, mental, behavioral, social, and environmental factors, including policy, culture, and economic environments, and includes a lifespan perspective. The IOM's vision of "healthy people in healthy communities" requires a model that recognizes that healthy communities are more than a collection of healthy individuals and that the characteristics of communities affect the health of people who live in them.

LEVELS OF PREVENTIVE INTERVENTIONS

The goal of epidemiology is to identify and understand the causal factors and mechanisms of disease, disability, and injuries so that effective interventions can be implemented to prevent the occurrence of these adverse processes before they begin or before they progress. The **natural history of disease** is the course of the disease process from onset to resolution (Greenberg et al, 2005). The three **levels of prevention,** primary, secondary and tertiary, provide a framework often used in public health practice. As practicing epidemiologists, nurses in community health are involved in all three levels of prevention, and at all levels, nurses engage in the core public health functions of *assessment, policy development,* and *assurance* (Institute of Medicine, 1988). These functions are discussed in Chapter 1.

Primary prevention refers to interventions that promote health and prevent the occurrence of disease, injury, or disability. Primary prevention is aimed at individuals and groups who are susceptible to disease but have no discernible pathology (i.e., they are in a state of prepathogenesis). This first level of prevention includes broad efforts such as the following:

- *Health promotion,* includes nutrition education and counseling, sex education, family planning, and the promotion of physical activity. An example is the nurse who provides health education and training for day care workers about issues of health and hygiene, such as proper hand hygiene, diapering, and food preparation and storage. Another example is the nurse who teaches an asthmatic client to recognize and avoid exposure to asthma triggers and assists the family in implementing specific protection strategies such as replacing carpets, keeping air systems clean and free of mold, and avoiding pets.

- *Environmental protection* ranges from basic sanitation and food safety, to home and workplace safety plans, to air quality control. An example is the nurse who develops and advocates for policies and legislation that lead to prevention of environmental hazards. Another example is the nurse who consults with industries, local governments, and groups of concerned citizens and provides public education about preventable environmental health problems.

- *Specific protection against disease or injury* includes immunizations, proper use of seatbelts and infants' car seats, preconception folic acid supplementation to prevent neural tube defects, fluoridation of water supplies to prevent dental caries, and actions taken to reduce human exposure to agents that may cause cancer.

Nurses are actively involved in the primary prevention in homes, community settings, and at the primary level of health care (e.g., in public health clinics, physicians' offices, community health centers, and rural health clinics).

Secondary prevention refers to interventions designed to increase the probability that a person with a disease will have that condition diagnosed early enough that treatment is likely to result in cure. Health screenings are at the core of secondary prevention. Early and periodic screenings are critical for diseases for which there are few specific primary prevention strategies, such as breast cancer. Screening programs are discussed in the "Screening" section that follows.

Interventions at the secondary level of prevention often take place in community settings. For example, in developing countries, if there is some available water that is safe to drink, oral rehydration therapy (ORT) is a low-cost and effective way to treat infant diarrheal disease. A nurse can teach mothers to recognize the early signs of infant dehydration and give the child a homemade ORT solution of water, sugar, and salt. Again using secondary prevention, the nurse might ask a family about their history of cancer, heart disease, diabetes, and mental illness as part of a client's health history and then follow up with education about appropriate screening procedures. Other secondary prevention interventions include mammography to detect breast cancer, Papanicolaou (Pap) smears to detect cervical

cancer, colonoscopy for early detection of colon cancer, and prenatal screening of pregnant women to screen for gestational diabetes.

Tertiary prevention includes interventions aimed at limiting disability and interventions that enhance rehabilitation from disease, injury, or disability. Interventions for tertiary prevention occur most often at secondary and tertiary levels of care (e.g., specialized clinics, hospitals, rehabilitation centers) but may also occur in community and primary care settings. Examples of tertiary prevention are medical treatment, physical and occupational therapy, and rehabilitation.

AN INTERVENTION SPECTRUM

The standard classification in prevention: primary, secondary and tertiary has been refined for application to diverse settings and health issues. Specifically, in mental health, three generations of prevention have been identified, ranging from pre-intervention prevention to acute care (Figure 9-3). The Institute of Medicine publication on prevention research in mental disorders classified an intervention as *universal* when it was directed to the general population and provided general benefit with little risk and at low cost; *selective* when it was directed toward persons or groups who were at increased risk for developing a problem, with risk and harms justified on the basis of the potential reduction in adverse outcomes; and *indicated* when more costly or higher-risk interventions target high-risk persons who already have a problem. This report reserved the term *prevention* for those interventions that occur before the onset of a disorder. The two components of *treatment interventions* include case identification and standard treatment for known disorders. Lastly, the components of maintenance in an ongoing disorder are *compliance with long-term treatment* and *provision of aftercare services, including rehabilitation*. Although this classification system was designed for use in mental health, it can be applied to other public health issues and used by nurses.

SCREENING

Screening, a key component of many secondary prevention interventions, involves the testing of groups of individuals who are at risk for a specific condition but do not have symptoms. The goal is to determine the likelihood that these individuals will develop the disease. From a clinical perspective, the aim of screening is early detection and treatment when these result in a more favorable prognosis. From a public health perspective, the objective is to sort out efficiently and effectively those who probably have the disease from those who probably do not, again to detect early cases for treatment or begin public health prevention and control programs. A screening test is not a diagnostic test. Effective screening programs must include referrals for diagnostic evaluation for those who screen positive, to determine if they actually have the disease and need treatment.

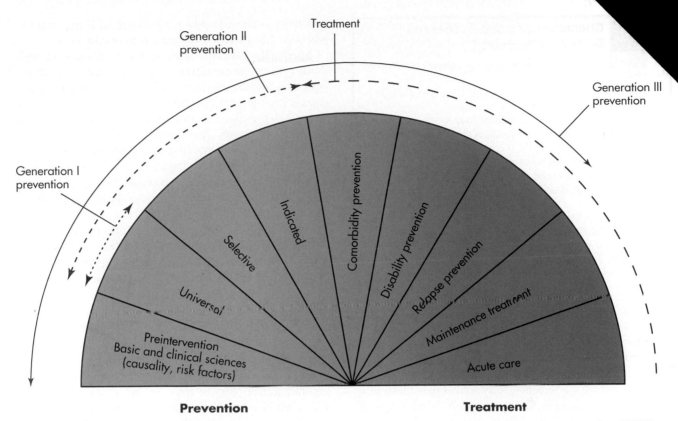

FIGURE 9-3 Health intervention spectrum. (From National Institute of Mental Health: *Priorities for prevention research at NIMH: a report by the National Advisory Health Council Workgroup on Mental Disorders Prevention Research,* Publication No. 98-4321, Washington, DC, 1998, NIH.)

Nurses must stay current about screening guidelines since these are regularly reviewed and revised on the basis of epidemiologic research results. For example, the latest U.S. Preventive Services Task Force (2008) strongly recommends routine screening for lipid disorders in men ages 35 years and older and women ages 45 years and older. Screening for younger adults (men ages 20 to 35 years and women ages 20 to 45 years) is recommended when any of the following risk factors are present: diabetes, family history of cardiovascular disease before age 50 years in male relatives or age 60 years in female relatives, family history suggestive of familial hyperlipidemia, or multiple risk factors for CHD (e.g., tobacco use, hypertension). The Task Force also noted that all clients, regardless of lipid levels, should be offered counseling about the benefits of a diet low in saturated fat and high in fruits and vegetables, regular physical activity, avoidance of tobacco, and maintenance of a healthy weight. The rationale for the current guidelines is explained as follows.

The clearest benefit of lipid screening is identifying individuals whose near-term risk of CHD is sufficiently high to justify drug therapy or other intensive lifestyle interventions to lower cholesterol. Screening men older than 35 years and women older than 45 years will identify nearly all individuals whose risk of CHD is as high as that of the subjects in the existing primary prevention trials. Younger people typically have a substantially lower risk unless they have other important risk factors for CHD or a family history of hyperlipidemia. The primary goal of screening younger people is to promote lifestyle changes, which may provide long-term benefits later in life. The average effect of diet interventions is small, and screening is not needed to advise young adults about the benefits of a healthy diet and regular exercise, since this advice is considered useful for all age groups.

As community health advocates, nurses are responsible for planning and implementing screening and prevention programs targeted to higher risk populations, such as prostate-screening programs among African-American men. Occupational nurses and nurses in community health may work together to target populations on the basis of occupational risk. Men with questionable prostate-specific antigen (PSA) levels need to be referred, especially if they have increased risk factors for prostate cancer, such as African-American race or a family history of prostate cancer. Successful screening programs have several characteristics that depend on the tests and on the population screened (Box 9-2). Desirable traits include the availability of reliable and valid screening tests (Gordis, 2004).

RELIABILITY AND VALIDITY

Reliability

It is important to pay attention to the precision, or **reliability,** of the measure (its consistency or repeatability) and the accuracy of the measure, its validity (whether it is really measuring what we think it is, and how exactly). Suppose you

tics of a Successful
'rogram

probability of correct classification

ults are consistent from place to
person to person

administration:

a. Fast in both the administration of the test and the obtaining of results
b. Inexpensive in both personnel required and the materials and procedures used
4. *Innocuous*: Few if any side effects, and the test is minimally invasive
5. *High yield*: Able to detect enough new cases to warrant the effort and expense (*yield* defined as the amount of previously unrecognized disease that is diagnosed and treated as a result of screening)

want to screen for blood pressure in a community. You will take blood pressure readings on a large number of people, perhaps following up with repeated measures for individuals with higher pressures. If the readings of the sphygmomanometer used for the screening vary so that two consecutive readings are not the same for the same person, the sphygmomanometer lacks reliability. The instrument would be unreliable even if the overall mean of repeated measurements was close to the true overall mean for the persons measured. The problem would be that the readings would not be reliable for any individual, which is what a screening program requires.

On the other hand, suppose the readings are reliably reproducible, but, unknown to you, they tend to be about 10 mm Hg too high. This instrument is producing precise readings, but the uncorrected (or uncalibrated) instrument lacks accuracy. In short, a measure can be consistent without producing valid results.

The following three major sources of error can affect the reliability of tests:
1. Variation inherent in the trait being measured (e.g., blood pressure changes with time of day, activity, level of stress, and other factors)
2. Observer variation, which can be divided into intraobserver reliability (consistency by the same observer) and interobserver reliability (level of consistency from one observer to another)
3. Consistency in the instrument, which includes the level of internal consistency of the instrument (e.g., whether all items in a questionnaire measure the same thing) and the stability (or test–retest reliability) of the instrument over time

Validity: Sensitivity and Specificity

Validity in a screening test is typically measured by sensitivity and specificity. **Sensitivity** quantifies how accurately the test identifies those *with* the condition or trait. Sensitivity represents the proportion of persons *with* the disease whom the test correctly identifies as positive (true positives). High

sensitivity is needed when early treatment is important and when identification of every case is important.

Specificity indicates how accurately the test identifies those *without* the condition or trait (i.e., the proportion of persons whom the test correctly identifies as negative for the disease [true negatives]). High specificity is needed when rescreening is impractical and when it is important to reduce false-positive results. The sensitivity and specificity of a test are determined by comparing the results from the test with results from a definitive diagnostic procedure (sometimes called the *gold standard*). For example, the Pap smear is used frequently to screen for cervical dysplasia and carcinoma. The definitive diagnosis of cervical cancer requires a biopsy with histological confirmation of malignant cells.

The ideal for a screening test is 100% sensitivity and 100% specificity. That is, the test is positive for 100% of those who actually have the disease and it is negative for all those who do not have the disease. In practice, sensitivity and specificity are often inversely related. That is, if the test results are such that it is possible to choose some point beyond which a person is considered positive (a "cutpoint"), as in a blood pressure reading to screen for hypertension or a serum glucose reading to screen for diabetes, then moving that critical point to improve the sensitivity of the test will result in a decrease in specificity or an improvement in specificity can be made only at the expense of sensitivity.

A third measure associated with sensitivity and specificity is the predictive value of the test. The **positive predictive value** (also called *predictive value positive*) is the proportion of persons with a positive test who actually have the disease, interpreted as the probability that an individual with a positive test has the disease. The **negative predictive value** (or *predictive value negative*) is the proportion of persons with a negative test who are actually disease free. Although sensitivity and specificity are relatively independent of the prevalence of disease, predictive values are affected by the level of disease in the screened population and by the sensitivity and specificity of the test. When the prevalence is very low, the positive predictive value is likely to be low, even with tests that are sensitive and specific. In addition, lower specificity produces lower positive predictive values because of the increase in the proportion of false-positive results.

Two or more tests can be combined, in series or in parallel, to enhance sensitivity or specificity. In series testing, the final result is considered positive only if all tests in the series were positive, and it is considered negative if any test was negative. For example, if a blood sample were screened for HIV, a positive enzyme-linked immunosorbent assay (ELISA) might be followed up with a Western blot and the sample would be considered positive only if both tests were positive. Series testing enhances specificity, producing fewer false positives, but sensitivity will be lower. In series testing, sequence is important; a very sensitive test is often used first to pick up all cases including false positives, and then a second, very specific test is used to eliminate the false positives. In parallel testing, the final result is considered positive if *any* test was positive and is considered negative only if *all* tests were negative. To return to the example of a blood sample being tested for HIV, a blood bank might consider a sample positive if a positive result was found on either the ELISA or the Western blot. Parallel testing enhances sensitivity, leaving fewer false negatives, but specificity will be lower.

BASIC METHODS IN EPIDEMIOLOGY

SOURCES OF DATA

It is important to know early in any epidemiologic study how the data will be obtained (Koepsell and Weiss, 2003; Gordis, 2004). The following three major categories of data sources are commonly used in epidemiologic investigations:

1. Routinely collected data: census data, vital records (birth and death certificates), and **surveillance** data (systematic collection of data concerning disease occurrence) as carried out by the Centers for Disease Control and Prevention (CDC)
2. Data collected for other purposes but useful for epidemiologic research: medical, health department, and insurance records
3. Original data collected for specific epidemiologic studies

Routinely Collected Data

The United States census is conducted every 10 years and provides population data, including demographic distribution (age, race, sex), geographic distribution, and additional information about economic status, housing, and education. These data provide denominators for various rates.

Vital records are the primary source of birth and mortality statistics. Registration of births and deaths is mandated in most countries and provides one of the most complete sources of health-related data. However, the quality of specific information varies. For example, on birth certificates, sex and date of birth are fairly reliable, whereas gestational age, level of prenatal care, and smoking habits of the mother during pregnancy are less reliable. On death certificates, the quality of the cause-of-death information varies over time and from place to place, depending on diagnostic capabilities and custom. Vital records are readily available in most areas; they are inexpensive and convenient and allow study of long-term trends. Mortality data, however, are informative only for fatal diseases.

Data Collected for Other Purposes

Hospital, physician, health department, and insurance records provide information on morbidity, as do surveillance systems, such as cancer registries and health department reporting systems, which solicit reports of all cases of a particular disease within a geographic region. Other information, such as occupational exposures, may be available from employer records.

Epidemiologic Data

The National Center for Health Statistics sponsors periodic health surveys and examinations in carefully drawn samples of the U.S. population. Examples are the National Health and Nutrition Examination Survey (NHANES), the National Health Interview Survey (NHIS), and the National Hospital Discharge Survey (NHDS). The CDC also conducts or contracts for conduct of surveys such as the Youth Risk Behavior Surveillance Survey (YRBSS), Pregnancy Risk Assessment Monitoring System (PRAMS), and the Behavioral Risk Factor Surveillance System (BRFSS). These surveys provide information on the health status and behaviors of the population. For many studies, however, the only way to obtain the needed information is to collect the required data in a study specifically designed to investigate a particular question. The design of such studies is discussed on pp. 171

RATE ADJUSTMENT

Rates, which are essential in epidemiologic studies, can be misleading when compared across different populations. For example, the risk of death increases considerably after 40 years of age, so a higher crude death rate is expected in a population of older people compared with a population of younger people (Gordis, 2004; Rothman, 2002; Koepsell and Weiss, 2003). Comparing the overall mortality rate in an area with a large population of older adults with the rate in a younger population would be misleading. Methods that adjust for differences in populations can be used to compare death rates. Age adjustment is based on the assumption that a population's overall mortality rate is a function of the age distribution of the population and the age-specific mortality rates.

Age adjustment can be performed by direct or indirect methods. Both methods require a *standard population,* which can be an external population, such as the U.S. population for a given year (not usually year 2000); a combined population of the groups under study; or some other standard chosen for relevance or convenience.

HOW TO	**Assess Health Problems in a Community**

1. Examine local epidemiologic data (e.g., incidence, morbidity, and mortality rates) to identify major health problems.
2. Examine local health services data to identify major causes of hospitalizations and emergency department visits. Consult with key community leaders (e.g., political, religious, business, educational, health, and cultural) about their perceptions of identified community health problems.
3. Mobilize community groups to elicit discussions and identify perceived health priorities within the community (e.g., focus groups, neighborhood or community-wide forums).
4. Analyze community environmental health hazards and pollutants (e.g., water, sewage, air, toxic waste).
5. Examine indicators of community knowledge and practices of preventive health behaviors (e.g., use of infant car seats, safe playgrounds, lighted streets, seatbelt use, designated driver programs).
6. Identify cultural priorities and beliefs about health among different social, cultural, racial, or national origin groups.
7. Assess community members' interpretation of and degree of trust in federal, state, and local assistance programs.
8. Engage community members in conducting surveys to assess specific health problems.

A direct adjusted rate applies the age-specific death rates from the study population to the age distribution of the standard population. The result is the (hypothetical) death rate of the study population if it had the same age distribution as the standard population.

The indirect method, as the name suggests, is more complicated. The age-specific death rates of the standard population applied to the study population's age distribution result in an index rate that is used with the crude rates of both the study and standard populations to produce the final indirect adjusted rate, which is also hypothetical. The indirect method may be required when the age-specific death rates for the study population are unknown or unstable (e.g., based on relatively small numbers).

Often, instead of an indirect adjusted rate, a standardized mortality ratio (SMR) is calculated. This is the number of observed deaths in the study population divided by the number of deaths expected on the basis of the age-specific rates in the standard population and the age distribution of the study population (Gordis, 2004; Greenberg et al, 2005).

COMPARISON GROUPS

Comparison groups are often used in epidemiology. To decide if the rate of disease is the result of a suspected risk factor, the exposed group should be compared with a group of comparable unexposed persons. For example: you might investigate the effect of smoking during pregnancy on the rate of low-birth-weight infants by calculating the rate of low-birth-weight infants born to women who smoked during their pregnancy. However, the hypothesis that smoking during pregnancy is a risk factor for low birth weight is supported only when the low-birth-weight rate among smoking women is compared with the (lower) rate of low-birth-weight infants born to nonsmoking women.

Ideally you want to compare one group of people who all have a certain characteristic, exposure, or behavior with a group of people *exactly* like them except they all *lack* that characteristic, exposure, or behavior. In the absence of that ideal, you can either randomize people to exposure or treatment groups in experimental studies or select comparison groups that are comparable in observational studies. It is especially important in observational studies to control for confounding variables or factors.

DESCRIPTIVE EPIDEMIOLOGY

Descriptive epidemiology describes the distribution of disease, death, and other health outcomes in the population according to person, place, and time. This type of epidemiology provides a picture of how things are or have been—the who, where, and when of disease patterns. Analytic epidemiology, on the other hand, searches for the determinants of the patterns observed—the how and why. That is, epidemiologic concepts and methods are used to identify what factors, characteristics, exposures, or behaviors might account for differences in the observed patterns of disease occurrence. Descriptive and analytic studies are observational. In these studies the investigator observes events as they are or have been and does not intervene to change anything or to introduce a new factor. Experimental or intervention studies, however, include interventions to test preventive or treatment measures, techniques, materials, policies, or drugs.

BRIEFLY NOTED

Lung cancer has now surpassed breast cancer as the leading cause of cancer mortality among women. The rapidly increasing rate of lung cancer deaths in women mirrors the patterns of increased rates of smoking among women and increased cigarette advertising directed toward women.

PERSON

Personal characteristics of interest in epidemiology include race, sex, age, education, occupation, income (and related socioeconomic status), and marital status. Age is the most important predictor of overall mortality. The mortality curve by age drops sharply during and after the first year of life to a low point in childhood, then it begins to increase through adolescence and young adulthood, and after that it increases sharply through middle and older ages (Gordis, 2004).

Mortality and morbidity differ by sex. Female infants have a lower mortality rate than do comparable male infants, and the survival advantage continues throughout life (Case and Paxson, 2004). However, patterns for specific diseases vary. For example, women have lower rates of CHD until menopause, after which the gap narrows. For rheumatoid arthritis, the prevalence among women is greater than among men (Case and Paxson, 2004).

Although the concept of race as a variable for public health research has been questioned (Bussey-Jones et al, 2005), there are clear differences in morbidity and mortality rates by race in the United States (National Center for Health Statistics, 2004; Greenberg et al, 2005). According to the *2007*

| HOW TO | Assess Health Problems in an Individual |

1. Obtain a history of physical and mental health problems.
2. Ask the individual to identify major health problems. Always start interventions with what the individual views as important.
3. Obtain a family history of diseases. Identify a possible genetic link based on early age of onset of a disease or multiple family members with a disease.
4. Perform clinical examination, including laboratory work.
5. Evaluate health risk based on lifestyle. Include smoking status, dietary patterns of fiber and fat, exercise patterns, stress factors, and risk-taking behaviors.
6. Identify immediate and long-range safety concerns.
7. Assess individual's cultural beliefs about health.
8. Assess social support.
9. Examine the knowledge and practice of preventive health care.
10. Provide appropriate age-based screening (e.g., cancer screening, hypertension screening).

National Healthcare Disparities Report, although racial and ethnic minority groups are among the fastest-growing populations in the United States, they have poorer health and remain chronically underserved by the health care system (Agency for Healthcare Research and Quality, 2007). Data in the report highlighted some of the significant health disparities within the leading categories of death in the United States. For example, in 2002, the overall U.S. infant mortality rate (IMR) was 7.0 deaths per 1000 live births, but the IMR among African-Americans was 14.4 per 1000 live births. The incidence and prevalence of diabetes among ethnic and racial minorities are another example of health disparities. African-Americans experience diabetes at a rate that is 70% higher than white Americans, whereas Native Americans and Native Alaskans experience a diabetes death rate that is 3.5 times that of the rest of the U.S. population. The burden of HIV/AIDS is also greater among minority communities, which in official estimates account for 25% of the total U.S. population but 50% of all cases of AIDS. A National Center for Health Statistics (NCHS) study of progress toward meeting the *Healthy People 2000* goal of eliminating racial and ethnic disparities found that although rates for most health status indicators did improve for all racial and ethnic groups, the improvements have not been uniform across groups and "substantial differences among racial/ethnic groups persist" (Keppel, Pearcy, and Wagener, 2002). Among Native Americans and Native Alaskans, several health indicators actually worsened from 1990 to 1998. The infant morality rate declined in all groups, but it remains 2.3 times higher for infants born to non-Hispanic African-American mothers than for those born to non-Hispanic white mothers. Similarly, the overall age-adjusted mortality rate was 30% higher in the African-American population than in the white population in 2000, and it was higher for 10 of the 15 leading causes of death (Kochanek et al., 2004). Reports from the NCHS provide further insight into health disparities across socioeconomic and racial and ethnic groups (Fuller et al, 2005; Krieger, 2000).

PLACE

In looking at the distribution of a disease, it is useful to examine geographic patterns. Does the rate of disease differ from place to place (e.g., with local environment)? If geography had no effect on disease occurrence, random geographic patterns might be seen, but that is often not the case. For example, at high altitudes, oxygen tension is lower, which might result in smaller babies. Other diseases reflect distinctive geographic patterns. For example, Lyme disease is transmitted from animal reservoirs to humans by a tick vector. Disease is more likely to be found in areas in which there are animals carrying the disease, a large tick population for transmission to humans, and contact between the human population and the tick vectors (Chin, 2000). Geographic variations can be caused by the following:

- Differences in the chemical, physical, or biological environment
- Differences in population densities, or in customary patterns of behavior and lifestyle, or in other personal characteristics

Geographic variations might occur because of high concentrations of a religious, cultural, or ethnic group that practices certain health-related behaviors. The high rates of stroke found in the southeastern United States are likely to be the result of a number of social and personal factors that have little to do with geographic features per se. Other neighborhood-level variables include the unemployment and crime rate, social cohesion, and access to important services (see the "How To" boxes on pp. 167 and 168) (Bradman et al, 2005; Fuller et al, 2005; McLafferty and Grady, 2005).

TIME
Secular Changes
Time is the third component of descriptive epidemiology. Is there an increase or decrease in the frequency of the disease over time, or are other temporal patterns evident? Long-term patterns of morbidity or mortality rates (i.e., over years or decades) are called **secular trends**. Secular trends may reflect changes in social behavior or practices. For example, increased lung cancer mortality rates in recent years reflect a delayed effect of the increased smoking in prior years. Also, the decline in cervical cancer deaths is primarily the result of widespread screening with the Pap test (Centers for Disease Control and Prevention, 2008).

Some secular trends may result from an increased diagnostic capability or changes in survival (or case fatality) rather than in incidence. For example, case fatality from breast cancer has decreased in recent years, although the incidence of breast cancer has increased. Some, though not all, of the increased incidence is the result of improved diagnostic capability. These two trends result in a breast cancer mortality curve that is flatter than the incidence curve (Bray, McCarron, and Parkin, 2004). Relying on mortality data alone does not accurately reflect the true situation. Secular trends are affected also by changes in case definition or revisions in the coding of a disease according to the International Classification of Diseases (ICD).

Point epidemic is a time-and-space-related pattern that is important in infectious disease investigations and as an indicator for toxic exposures. A point epidemic is most clearly seen when the frequency of cases is graphed against time. The sharp peak characteristic of such graphs indicates a concentration of cases over a short interval of time. The peak often indicates the population's response to a common source of infection or contamination to which they were all simultaneously exposed. Knowledge of the incubation or latency period (the time between exposure and development of signs and symptoms) for the specific disease entity can help determine the probable time of exposure. A common example of a point epidemic is an outbreak of gastrointestinal illness from a foodborne pathogen. Nurses who are alert to a sudden increase in the number of cases of a disease can chart the outbreak, determine the probable time of exposure, and, by careful investigation, isolate the probable source of the agent.

In addition to secular trends and point epidemics, there are also cyclical time patterns of disease. Seasonal fluctuation is a common type of cyclical variation in some infectious illnesses. Seasonal changes may be influenced by changes in the agent itself, changes in population densities or behaviors of animal reservoirs or vectors, or changes in human behaviors resulting in changing exposures (being outdoors in warmer weather and indoors in colder months). Also, calendar events may create artificial seasons, such as holidays and tax-filing deadlines, that are associated with patterns of stress-related illness. Patterns of accidents and injuries may also be seasonal, reflecting differing employment and recreational patterns. Some disease cycles, such as influenza, have patterns of smaller epidemics every few years, depending on strain, with major pandemics occurring at longer intervals (Chin, 2000). Attention to cyclical patterns is especially important for people who work in public health, to enable them to prepare adequately to meet possible increased demands for service.

A third type of temporal pattern is nonsimultaneous, event-related clusters. These are patterns in which time is not measured from fixed dates on the calendar but from the point of some exposure, event, or experience presumably held in common by affected persons, though not occurring at the same time. An example of this pattern would be vaccine reactions during an immunization program. Clearly, if vaccinations are being given on a regular basis, nonspecific symptoms, such as fever, headaches, or rashes, might be seen fairly consistently over time, making identification of a cluster related to the vaccinations difficult. If, however, the occurrence of symptoms is plotted against the amount of time since vaccination, the number of vaccine reactions is likely to peak at some period after the immunization.

ANALYTIC EPIDEMIOLOGY

Descriptive epidemiology deals with the *distribution* of health outcomes. The goal of *analytic* epidemiology is to discover the *determinants* of outcomes, the how and the why. Analytic epidemiology deals with the factors that influence the observed patterns of health and disease and increase or decrease the risk of adverse outcomes. This section discusses analytic study designs and the related measures of association derived from them. Table 9-4 summarizes the advantages and disadvantages of each design.

COHORT STUDIES

The **cohort study** is the standard for observational epidemiologic studies. It comes closest to the idea of a natural experiment (Rothman, 2002). The term *cohort* is used in epidemiology to describe a group of persons who are born at about the same time. In analytic studies, cohort refers to a group of persons generally sharing some characteristic of interest. They are enrolled in a study and followed over time to observe some health outcome. Because of this ability to observe the development of new cases of disease, cohort study designs allow for calculation of incidence rates and therefore estimates of risk of disease. Cohort studies may be prospective or retrospective (Rothman, 2002; Gordis, 2004).

PROSPECTIVE COHORT STUDIES

In a prospective cohort study (also called a *longitudinal* or *follow-up study*), subjects determined to be free of the outcome under investigation are classified on the basis of the exposure of interest at the beginning of the follow-up period. The subjects are then followed for some period of time to determine the occurrence of disease in each group. The question is "Do persons with the factor (or exposure) of interest develop (or avoid) the outcome more frequently than those without the factor (or exposure)?"

For example, a cohort of subjects could be recruited who would be classified as physically active ("exposed") or sedentary ("not exposed"). One might further quantify the amount of the "exposure" if there were sufficient information. These subjects would then be followed over time to determine the development of CHD. This study design avoids the problem of selective survival seen in other designs. The cohort study also has the advantage of allowing estimation of the risk of acquiring disease for those who are exposed compared to those who are unexposed (or less exposed). This ratio of cumulative incidence rates is called the *relative risk.*

Suppose 1000 physically active and 1000 sedentary middle-aged men and women were enrolled in a prospective cohort study. All were free of CHD at enrollment. Over a 5-year follow-up period, regular examinations detect CHD in 120 of the sedentary men and women and in 48 of the active men and women. Assuming no other deaths or losses to follow-up, the data could be presented as shown in Figure 9-4.

The incidence of CHD in the active group is $[a/(a + b)] = 48/1000$, and the incidence of CHD in the sedentary group is $[c/(c + d)] = 120/1000$. The relative risk is

$$(48/1000) \div (120/1000) = 0.4$$

Because physical activity is protective for CHD, the relative risk is less than 1. The interpretation for this hypothetical example is that over a 5-year period, the risk of CHD in persons who are physically active compared to the risk among sedentary persons was 0.4. If the risk were greater for those exposed, the relative risk would be greater than 1. For example, if the relative risk of CHD for smokers compared to nonsmokers were 3.5, it would be interpreted to mean that the risk of CHD among smokers is 3.5 times the risk among nonsmokers. The null value indicating no association is 1, since the incidence rates and thus the risk would be equal in the two groups if there were no association.

In the cohort study design, subjects are enrolled before disease onset. This pattern of subject recruitment allows the researcher to study more than one outcome, calculate incidence rates and estimate risk, and establish the temporal sequence of exposure and outcome with greater clarity and certainty. As a result, the researcher may avoid many of the problems of other study designs with selective survival or exposure misclassification. On the other hand, large samples are often necessary to ensure that enough cases are observed to provide statistical power to detect meaningful differences between groups. This is complicated by the long period required for some diseases

| Table 9-4 | **Comparison of Major Epidemiologic Study Designs** | |

Study Design	Advantages	Disadvantages
Ecological	Quick, easy, inexpensive first study Uses readily available existing data May prompt further investigation or suggest other or new hypotheses May provide information about contextual factors not accounted for by individual characteristics	Ecological fallacy: the associations observed may not hold true for individuals Problems in interpreting temporal sequence (cause and effect) More difficult to control for confounding and "mixed" models (ecological and individual data); more complex statistically
Cross-sectional (correlational)	Gives general description of the scope of problem; provides prevalence estimates Often based on population (or community) sample, not just who sought care Useful in health service evaluation and planning Data obtained at once; less expense and quicker than cohort because of no follow-up Baseline for prospective study or to identify cases and controls for case-control study	No calculation of risk; prevalence, not incidence Temporal sequence unclear Not good for rare disease or rare exposure unless there is a large sample size or stratified sampling Selective survival can be a major source of selection bias; surviving subjects may differ from those who are not included (e.g., death, institutionalization) Selective recall or lack of past exposure information can create bias
Case-control (retrospective, case comparison)	Less expensive than cohort; smaller sample required Quicker than cohort; no follow-up Can investigate more than one exposure Best design for rare diseases If well designed, it can be an important tool for etiologic investigation Best suited to a disease with a relatively clear onset (timing of onset can be established so that incident cases can be included)	Greater susceptibility than cohort studies to various types of bias (selective survival, recall bias, selection bias in choice of both cases and controls) Information on other risk factors may not be available, resulting in confounding Antecedent-consequence (temporal sequence) not as certain as in cohort Not well suited to rare exposures Gives only an indirect estimate of risk Generally limited to a single outcome because of sampling effect on disease status
Prospective cohort (concurrent cohort, longitudinal, follow-up)	Best estimate of disease incidence Best estimate of risk Fewer problems with selective survival and selective recall Temporal sequence more clearly established Broader range of options for exposure assessment	Expensive in terms of time and money More difficult organizationally Not good for rare diseases Attrition of participants can bias the estimate Latency period may be very long; may miss cases May be difficult to examine several exposures
Retrospective cohort (nonconcurrent cohort)	Combines advantages of both prospective cohort and case-control Shorter time (even if follow-up into the future) than prospective cohort Less expensive than prospective cohort because it relies on existing data Temporal sequence may be clearer than case-control	Shares some disadvantages with both prospective cohort and case-control Subject to attrition (loss to follow-up) Relies on existing records that may result in misclassification of both exposure and outcome May have to rely on a surrogate measure of exposure (e.g., job title) and vital records information on cause of death

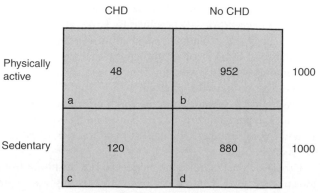

FIGURE 9-4 Cohort study.

to develop (the latency period). Also, the number of subjects required to observe sufficient cases makes longitudinal studies unsuitable for very rare diseases unless they are part of a larger study of a number of outcomes.

Retrospective Cohort Studies

Retrospective cohort studies combine some of the advantages and disadvantages of case-control studies and prospective cohort studies. These studies rely on existing records, such as employment, insurance, or hospital records, to define a cohort that is classified as having been exposed or unexposed at some time in the past. The cohort is followed over time using the records to determine if the outcome occurred.

Retrospective cohort (also called *historical cohort*) studies may be conducted entirely using past records or may include current assessment or additional follow-up time after study initiation. The obvious advantage of this approach is the savings in time, because it is not necessary to wait for new cases of disease to develop. The disadvantages are largely related to the reliance on existing historical records. Retrospective cohort studies frequently are used in occupational epidemiology where industrial records are available to investigate work-related exposures and health outcomes.

CASE-CONTROL STUDIES

In the **case-control study**, subjects are enrolled *because* they are known to have the outcome of interest (these are the cases) or they are known *not* to have the outcome of interest (these are the controls). Case-control status is verified using a clear case definition and some previously determined method or protocol (e.g., by an examination, laboratory test, or medical chart review). Information is then collected on the exposures or characteristics of interest, frequently from existing sources, subject interview, or questionnaire (Rothman, 2002). The question in a case-control study is "Do persons with the outcome of interest (cases) have the exposure characteristic (or a history of the exposure) more frequently than those without the outcome (controls)?"

Because of the method of subject selection in case-control studies, neither incidence nor prevalence can be calculated directly. In a case-control study, an odds ratio tells us how much more (or less) likely the exposure is to be found among cases than among controls. The odds of exposure among cases (*a* and *c* in the table that follows) are compared with the odds of exposure among controls (*b* and *d*). The ratio of these two odds provides us with an estimate of the relative risk.

Suppose a research group wanted to study risk factors for suicide attempts among adolescents. To do so they would enroll 100 adolescents who had attempted suicide, and select 200 adolescents from the same community with no history of a suicide attempt. The research group's goal is to determine if the adolescents had a history of substance abuse (SA). Through a questionnaire and use of medical records they learned that 68 of the 100 adolescents who had attempted suicide had a history of substance abuse. They also found that 36 of the 200 adolescents with no suicide attempt had a history of substance abuse. The information could be presented as follows:

	Suicide attempt	*No attempt*
History of Substance Abuse	68 (a)	36 (b)
No History of Substance Abuse	32 (c)	164 (d)

The odds of a history of substance abuse among suicide attempters are *a/c* or 68/32, whereas the odds of substance abuse among controls are *b/d* or 36/164. The odds ratio (equivalent to *ad/bc*) is the following:

$$\frac{68 \times 164}{36 \times 32} = 9.68$$

This would be interpreted to mean that adolescents who attempted suicide are almost 10 times more likely to have a history of substance abuse than are adolescents who have not attempted suicide. Note that an odds ratio of 1 is indicative of no association (i.e., the odds of exposure are similar for cases and controls). An odds ratio less than 1 suggests a protective association, that is, cases are less likely to have been exposed than controls.

Because the number of cases is known or actively sought out, case-control studies do not require large samples or the long follow-up time that is often required for prospective cohort studies. For these reasons, many important cancer studies have used the case-control design.

Case-control studies can have a number of biases. (*Bias*, a systematic deviation from the truth, is discussed on p. 174) Because these studies begin with existing diseases, differential survival can produce biased results. The use of recently diagnosed (or "incident") cases may reduce this bias. Because exposure information is obtained from subject recall or past records, there may be errors in exposure assessment or misclassification.

CROSS-SECTIONAL STUDIES

The **cross-sectional study** provides a snapshot, or cross section, of a population or group (Gordis, 2004). Information is collected on current health status, personal characteristics, and potential risk factors or exposures all at once. In the cross-sectional study there is a simultaneous collection of information necessary for the classification of exposure. Historical information can also be collected (e.g., past diet, history of radiation exposures).

One way cross-sectional studies evaluate the association of a factor with a health problem is to compare the prevalence of the disease in those with the factor (or exposure) with the prevalence of the disease in the unexposed. The ratio of the two prevalence rates is an indication of the association between the factor and the outcome. If the prevalence of CHD in smokers were twice as high as the prevalence among nonsmokers, the prevalence ratio would be 2. If a factor is unrelated to the prevalence of a disease, the prevalence ratio will be close to 1. A value less than 1 may suggest a protective association. For example, the prevalence of CHD is lower among physically active people than among sedentary persons. Thus the prevalence ratio for the association between physical activity and CHD should be less than 1. Use caution in interpreting prevalence ratios because the prevalence measure is affected by cure, survival, and migration and does not estimate the risk of *getting* the disease.

Cross-sectional studies are subject to bias resulting from selective survival. That is, persons with existing cases who have survived to be in the study may be different from those diagnosed at about the same time who have died and are not available for inclusion. Suppose physical activity not only reduced the risk of heart disease but also markedly improved survival among those with heart disease. Sedentary persons with heart disease would then have higher fatality rates than physically active persons who developed heart disease. Higher rates of physical activity might be observed in a group of heart disease survivors than in a general population without heart disease. This might occur because of the survival advantage and also because of the participation of the survivors in cardiac rehabilitation programs. It might, however, erroneously appear that physical activity was a risk factor for heart disease.

ECOLOGICAL STUDIES

An ecological study bridges descriptive and analytic epidemiology. The descriptive component looks at variations in disease rates by person, place, or time. The analytic component tries to determine if there is a relation of disease rates to variations in rates for possible risk (or protective) factors or characteristics. The identifying characteristic of ecological studies is that only aggregate data, such as population rates, are used rather than data on individuals' exposures, characteristics, and outcomes. Examples include the following:

1. Examination of information on per capita cigarette consumption in relation to lung cancer mortality rates in several countries, or several groups of people, or in the same population at different times
2. Comparisons of rates of breastfeeding and of breast cancer
3. Average dietary fat content and rates of CHD
4. Unemployment rates and level of psychiatric disorder

Ecological studies often use existing readily available rates and are therefore quick and inexpensive to conduct. They are subject, however, to ecological fallacy (i.e., associations observed at the group level may not hold true for the individuals that comprise the groups, or associations that actually exist may be masked in the grouped data). This can occur when other factors operate in these populations for which the ecological correlations do not account. For that reason, ecological studies may suggest possible answers, but they require confirmation in studies that use individual data (Gordis, 2004; Koepsell and Weiss, 2003).

EXPERIMENTAL STUDIES

The study designs discussed so far are called *observational studies* because the investigator observes the association between exposures and outcomes as they exist but does not intervene to alter the presence or level of any exposure or behavior. In contrast, in experimental or intervention studies, the investigator initiates a treatment or intervention to influence the risk or course of disease. These studies test whether interventions can prevent disease or improve health. Both observational and experimental studies generally use comparison (or control) groups. In experimental studies, persons can be randomly assigned to a particular group; an

intervention (a treatment or exposure) is applied, and the effects of the intervention are measured. There are two types of intervention studies: clinical trials and community trials.

BRIEFLY NOTED

Epidemiology uses a process similar to the nursing process.

CLINICAL TRIALS

The goal of a clinical trial is generally to evaluate the effectiveness of an intervention such as a medical treatment for disease, a new drug or existing drug used in a new or a different way, a surgical technique, or other treatment. In clinical trials, subjects should be randomly assigned to groups. In randomization, treatments are assigned to patients (subjects) so that all possible treatment assignments have a predetermined probability but neither subject nor investigator determines the actual assignment of any participant. Randomization avoids the bias that may result if subjects choose to be in one group or the other or if the investigator or clinician chooses subjects for each group.

Masking or "blinding" treatment assignments is a second aspect of treatment allocation. Generally it is best to use a double-blinded study in which neither subject nor investigator knows who is getting which treatment. Clinical trials usually are the best way to show causality because of the objective way in which subjects are assigned and the greater control over other factors that could influence outcome. Like cohort studies, they are prospective and provide the clearest evidence of correct temporal sequence.

They do tend to be conducted in a contrived (versus natural) situation, under controlled conditions, and with patient populations. That means that treatment may not be as effective when applied under more realistic clinical or community conditions in a more diverse patient population. There are also more ethical considerations involved in experimental studies than in observational studies. For example, is it fair to withhold a treatment if the treatment truly appears to have the potential to alleviate a disease in order to evaluate systematically this treatment using both an experimental and a control group? Finally, clinical trials are expensive in terms of time, personnel, facilities, and, in some cases, supplies.

COMMUNITY TRIALS

Community trials are similar to clinical trials in that an investigator determines what the exposure or intervention will be. However, community trials often deal with health promotion and disease prevention rather than treatment of existing disease. The intervention is usually undertaken on a large scale, and the unit of treatment is a community, region, or group rather than individuals. Although a pharmaceutical product such as fluoridation of water or mass immunizations may be involved in a community trial, these trials often involve educational, programmatic, or policy interventions. Examples of community interventions would be measuring the rates of diabetes or cardiovascular disease in a community in which the availability of exercise programs and facilities was increased or in which a much larger supply of healthful fresh foods were made available.

Although community trials provide the best means of testing whether changes in knowledge or behavior, policy, programs, or other mass interventions are effective, they do present some problems. For many interventions, it may take years for the effectiveness to be evident, for example, the effect of changing the availability of exercise and healthful food on the rates of either diabetes or heart disease. While the study is being carried out over time, other factors can influence the outcome either positively (making the intervention look more effective than it really is) or negatively (making the intervention look less effective than it really is). Comparable community populations without similar interventions for comparative analysis are often difficult to find. Even when comparable comparison communities are available—especially when the intervention is improved knowledge or changed behavior—it is difficult and unethical to prevent the control communities from making use of generally available information, effectively making them less different from the intervention communities. Finally, because community trials are often undertaken on a large scale and over long periods, they can be expensive, require a large staff, have complicated logistics, and need extensive communication about the study.

CAUSAL INFERENCE

STATISTICAL ASSOCIATIONS

Sample size, strength of association, and variance of measures can all affect statistical significance. For example, to determine if eating habits affect the onset of hypertension a statistical association between the factor (diet) and the health outcome (hypertension) would need to be established. If the probability of disease seems unaffected by the presence or level of the factor, no association is apparent. If, on the other hand, the probability of disease does vary according to whether the factor is present, there is a statistical association. The earlier discussion of null values is pertinent at this point. When an observed measure of association (e.g., a risk ratio) does not differ from the null value, there is no evidence of an association between the factor and the outcome being studied. To say a result is statistically significant means that the observed result is unlikely to be due to chance. Sample size affects statistical significance.

BIAS

A statistically significant result may also be observed because of **bias**, a systematic error as a result of the study design, the way it is conducted, or a **confounding** factor. For example, if there were a gumball machine with colors randomly mixed and three red ones in a row came out, that would be due to chance. If, however, the person loading the gum ball machine had poured in a bag of red ones first, then green ones, then yellow ones, it would not be surprising to get three red ones in a row because of the way the machine was loaded. In epidemiologic

studies, results are sometimes biased because of the way the study was "loaded" (i.e., the way the study was designed or the way subjects were selected, information was collected, and subjects were classified). Although the types of bias are numerous, there are three general categories of bias (Rothman, 2002). Bias can be attributed to the following:

1. *Selection or the way subjects enter a study.* Selection bias has to do with selection procedures, the population from which subjects are drawn, and may involve self-selection factors. *Example:* are teenagers who agree to complete a questionnaire on alcohol, tobacco, and other drug use representative of the total teenage population?

2. *Misclassification of subjects once they are in the study.* This is information, or classification (or misclassification), bias. It is related to how information is collected, including the information that subjects supply or how subjects are classified.

3. *Confounding or bias resulting from the relationship between the outcome and study factor and some third factor not accounted for. Example:* there is a well-known association between maternal smoking during pregnancy and low-birth-weight babies. There is also an association between alcohol consumption and smoking that is not due to chance nor is it causal (i.e., drinking alcohol does not cause a person to smoke, nor does smoking cause a person to drink alcohol). If we were to investigate the association between alcohol consumption and low birth weight, smoking would be a confounder because it is related to both alcohol consumption and low birth weight. Failure to account for smoking in the analysis would bias the observed association between alcohol use and low birth weight. In practice, we can often identify potentially confounding variables and adjust for them in analysis.

ASSESSING EVIDENCE OF CAUSAL ASSOCIATIONS

The existence of a statistical association does not necessarily mean that a causal relationship exists or that causality is present. As just discussed, the observed association may be a random event (due to chance) or may be the result of bias from confounding or from some aspect of the study design or execution. Statistical associations, although necessary to an argument for **causal inference**, are not adequate proof. Some epidemiologists refer to guidelines, a term originally established to evaluate the link between an infectious agent and a disease but revised and elaborated to apply also to other outcomes. Although various lists of guidelines have been proposed, the seven guidelines listed in Box 9-3 are often used (Gordis, 2004; Koepsell and Weiss, 2003).

APPLICATIONS OF EPIDEMIOLOGY IN NURSING

Both knowledge and practical application of epidemiology are essential competencies for nurses (Gebbie and Hwang, 2000). Nurses use epidemiology in their practices and function in epidemiologic roles in a variety of ways. In many

Box 9-3   Guidelines for Causal Inference

1. *Strength of association:* A strong association between a potential risk factor and an outcome supports a causal hypothesis (i.e., a relative risk of 7 provides stronger evidence of a causal association than a relative risk of 1.5).
2. *Consistency of findings:* Repeated findings of an association with different study designs and in different populations strengthen a causal inference.
3. *Biological plausibility:* Demonstration of a physiological mechanism by which the risk factor acts to cause disease enhances the causal hypothesis. Conversely, an association that does not initially seem biologically defensible may later be discovered to be so.
4. *Demonstration of correct temporal sequence:* For a risk factor to cause an outcome, it must precede the onset of the outcome.
5. *Dose-response relationship:* The risk of developing an outcome should increase with increasing exposure (either in duration or quantity) to the risk factor of interest. For example, studies have shown that the more a woman smokes during pregnancy, the greater the risk of delivering a low-birthweight infant.
6. *Specificity of the association:* The presence of a one-to-one relationship between an agent and a disease (i.e., the idea that a disease is caused by only one agent and that agent results in only one disease lends support to a causal hypothesis, but its absence does not rule out causality). This criterion grows out of the infectious disease model in which it is more often though not always satisfied and is less applicable in chronic diseases.
7. *Experimental evidence:* Experimental designs provide the strongest epidemiologic evidence for causal associations, but they are not feasible or ethical to conduct for many risk factor–disease associations.

Levels of Prevention   Related to Cardiovascular Disease

PRIMARY PREVENTION

Discuss a low-fat diet and the need for regular physical exercise with clients.

SECONDARY PREVENTION

Implement blood pressure and cholesterol screening; give a treadmill stress test.

TERTIARY PREVENTION

Provide cardiac rehabilitation, medication, and surgery.

settings, nurses regularly collect, report, analyze, interpret, and communicate epidemiologic data. Nurses involved in the care of persons with communicable diseases use epidemiology daily as they identify, report, treat, and provide follow-up on cases and contacts of TB, gonorrhea, and gastroenteritis. School nurses also function as epidemiologists, collecting data on the incidence and prevalence of accidents, injuries, and illnesses in the school population. They are also key players in the detection and control of local epidemics, such as outbreaks of lice. As described earlier in this chapter, nurses across practice settings are actively involved in activities related to primary, secondary, and tertiary prevention (see the "Levels of Preventive Interventions" section and Levels of Prevention Box).

Some nursing jobs are specifically based in epidemiologic practice. These include nurse epidemiologists and environmental risk communicators employed by local health departments as well as hospital infection control nurses. Nurses are key members of local fetal and infant mortality review boards, which examine cases of newborn deaths for identifiable risk factors and quality of care measures. Members of these review boards may include public health and maternal child nurses, as well as representatives from hospital labor and delivery and neonatal intensive care units. Nurses play a key role in disaster preparedness in their communities and this work includes knowledge of epidemiology.

Nursing documentation on patient charts and records is an important source of data for epidemiologic reviews. Patient demographics and health histories are often collected or verified by nurses. As nurses collect and document patient information, they might not be thinking about the epidemiologic connection. However, the reliability and validity of such data can be key factors in the quality of future epidemiologic studies.

CLINICAL APPLICATION

You are a nurse at a local health department where Rob Jones, a 46-year-old African-American, comes for a routine blood pressure check. He mentions that his father recently died from prostate cancer and that he is worried about himself. Further assessment reveals that his father was diagnosed with prostate cancer when he was 52 and that Mr. Jones's uncle, who is 56 years old, was recently diagnosed with prostate cancer. You know from Mr. Jones' health history that he smokes a pack of cigarettes a day and eats fried food frequently.
Which action would be your best choice?
A. *Give Mr. Jones a digital rectal examination and prostate-specific antigen (PSA) test immediately to screen for prostate cancer.*
B. *Do not discuss or provide prostate cancer screening with him, because he is younger than 50 years.*
C. *Advise Mr. Jones to be tested immediately for the prostate cancer gene, because of his family history.*
D. *Inform him of the risks and benefits of prostate cancer testing and of his increased personal risk of prostate cancer because of his family history, smoking, and dietary habits. Involve him in the decision-making process about prostate cancer screening.*
Answer is in the back of the book.

REMEMBER THIS!

- Epidemiology is the study of the distribution and determinants of health-related events in human populations and the application of this knowledge to improving the health of communities.

- Epidemiology is a multidisciplinary science that recognizes the complex interrelationships of factors that influence disease and health at both the individual and the community level; it provides the basic tools for the study of health and disease in communities.
- Epidemiologic methods are used to describe health and disease and to investigate the factors that promote health or influence the risk or distribution of disease. This knowledge can be useful in planning and evaluating programs, policies, and services and in clinical decision making.
- Basic epidemiologic concepts include the interrelationships between agent, host, and environment (the epidemiologic triangle); the interactions of factors, exposures, and characteristics in a causal web affecting the risk of disease; and the levels of prevention corresponding to stages in the natural history of disease.
- Primary prevention involves interventions to reduce the incidence of disease by promoting health and preventing disease processes from developing.
- Secondary prevention includes programs (e.g., screening) designed to detect disease in the early stages, before signs and symptoms are clinically evident, to intervene with early diagnosis and treatment.
- Tertiary prevention provides treatments and other interventions directed toward persons with clinically apparent disease, with the aim of lessening the course of the disease, reducing disability, or rehabilitating the client.
- Epidemiologic methods are also used in the planning and design of screening (secondary prevention) and community health intervention (primary prevention) strategies and in the evaluation of their effectiveness.
- Basic epidemiologic methods include the use of existing data sources to study health outcomes and related factors and the use of comparison groups to assess the association between exposures or characteristics and health outcomes.
- Epidemiologists use rates and proportions to quantify levels of morbidity and mortality.
- Prevalence proportions provide a picture of the level of existing cases in a population at a given time.
- Incidence rates and proportions measure the rate of new case development in a population and provide an estimate of the risk of disease.
- Descriptive epidemiologic studies provide information on the distribution of disease and health states according to personal characteristics, geographic region, and time. This knowledge enables practitioners to target programs and allocate resources more effectively and provides a basis for further study.
- Analytic epidemiologic studies investigate associations between exposures or characteristics and health or disease outcomes, with the goal of understanding the etiology of disease. Analytic studies provide the foundation for understanding disease causality and for developing effective intervention strategies aimed at primary, secondary, and tertiary prevention.

WHAT WOULD YOU DO?

1. Read your local newspaper for a week and see if you can find any reports that use epidemiologic methods. If yes, what was the health risk? What was the intervention? What might have prevented the disease or accident? Discuss this with two classmates to see if they agree or disagree with you.
2. Identify a current health issue in your local community (e.g., childhood lead poisoning, diabetes, HIV/AIDS, *Escherichia coli,* childhood obesity).
   a. Describe primary, secondary, and tertiary prevention interventions related to this health issue.
   b. How could nurses improve the effectiveness of their prevention activities related to this health issue?
3. Look at a recent issue of the *Morbidity and Mortality Weekly Report* (www.cdc.gov/mmwr) and find one health issue that is or could possibly affect your community. Work with a group of your classmates and identify the most useful nursing and public health interventions.
4. Think about the last time you used public transportation (bus, train, airplane). What were likely sources of disease transmission? How could you protect yourself from getting a disease if, while you were present, another passenger was sneezing and spraying droplets through the air?

■ *REFERENCES*

Agency for Healthcare Research and Quality, *Key themes and highlights from the National Healthcare Disparities Report,* Rockville, Md, 2007, available at http://www.ahrq.gov.qual/qrdr.07.htm. Accessed September 1, 2008.

American Nurses Association: *Essential nursing competencies and curricula guidelines for genetics and genomics,* Silver Spring, Md, *ANA,* 2006.

Anderson RN: Deaths: leading causes for 2000, *Natl Vital Stat Rep* 50(16):1–85, 2002.

Bradman A et al: Association of housing disrepair indicators with cockroach and rodent infestations in a cohort of pregnant Latina women and their children, *Environ Health Perspect* 113:1795–1801, 2005.

Bray F, McCarron P, Parkin DM: The changing global patterns of female breast cancer incidence and mortality, *Breast Cancer Res* 6:229–239, 2004.

Brownson RC, Remington PL, Davis JR: *Chronic disease epidemiology and control,* ed 2, Washington, DC, 1998, American Public Health Association.

Bussey-Jones J et al: The meaning of race: Use of race in the clinical setting, *J of Lab and Clin Med* 146(4):205–209, 2005.

Case A, Paxson C: *Sex differences in morbidity and mortality, NBER Working Paper 10653, 2004,* available at http://www.nber.org/papers/w10653. Accessed September 1, 2008

Centers for Disease Control and Prevention: *National Center for Health Statistics, 2005,* available at http://www/cdc/gov.nchs.FASTATS/lcod.htm. Accessed September 1, 2008.

Centers for Disease Control and Prevention: *Cervical cancer statistics, 2008,* available at http://www.cdc.gov/cancer/cervical/statistics. Accessed September 1, 2008.

Centers for Disease Control and Prevention: Deaths: Leading causes for 2001, *Natl Vital Stat Rep* 52(9):7–14, 2003.

Chin J, editor: *Control of communicable diseases manual,* ed 17, Washington, DC, 2000, American Public Health Association.

Cohen IB: Florence Nightingale, *Sci Am* 250(3):128–137, 1984.

Dawson B, Trapp RG: *Basic and clinical biostatistics*, ed 4, Columbus, Ohio, 2004, McGraw-Hill.

Fuller CM et al: Effects of race, neighborhood, and social network on age at initiation of injection drug use, *Am J Public Health* 95:689–695, 2005.

Gebbie KM, Hwang I: Preparing currently employed public health nurses for changes in the health system, *Am J Public Health* 20:716–721, 2000.

Gordis L: *Epidemiology*, ed 3, Philadelphia, 2004, Elsevier/Saunders.

Greenberg RS, Daniels SR, Flanders WD et al: *Medical epidemiology*, ed 4, Columbus, Ohio, 2005, McGraw-Hill.

Institute of Medicine: *The future of public health*, Washington, DC, 1988, National Academy Press.

Keppel KG, Pearcy JN, Wagener DK: *Trends in racial and ethnic-specific rates for the health status indicators: United States, 1990-98, Healthy People 2000 Stat Notes* Jan(23):1–16, Hyattsville, Md, 2002, National Center for Health Statistics.

Kochanek KD et al: *Deaths: final data for 2002,* Natl Vital Stat Rep 53, 2004.

Koepsell TD, Weiss NS: *Epidemiologic methods: Studying the occurrence of illness,* New York, 2003, Oxford University Press.

Krieger N: Discrimination and health. In Berkman LF, Kawachie I, editors: *Social epidemiology*, Oxford, 2000, Oxford University Press, pp 36–75.

Krieger N: Epidemiology and the web of causation: has anyone seen the spider? *Soc Sci Med* 39:887, 1994.

Macintyre S, Ellaway A: Ecological approaches: rediscovering the role of the physical and social environment. In Berkman LF, Kawachi I, editors: *Social epidemiology*, New York, 2000, Oxford University Press, pp 332–348.

McLafferty S, Grady S: Immigration and geographic access to prenatal clinics in Brooklyn, NY: A geographic information systems analysis, *Am J Public Health* 95:638–640, 2005.

National Center for Health Statistics: *Health: United States, 2004, with chartbook on trends in the health of Americans*, Hyattsville, Md, 2004, Public Health Service.

Palmer IS: *Florence Nightingale and the first organized delivery of nursing services*, Washington, DC, 1983, American Association of Colleges of Nursing.

Rothman KJ: *Epidemiology: an introduction*, New York, 2002, Oxford University Press.

Snow J: On the mode of communication of cholera. In *Snow on cholera*, New York, 1855, The Commonwealth Fund.

Susser M: Epidemiology in the United States after World War II: the evolution of technique, *Epidemiol Rev* 7:147, 1985.

Timmreck TC: *An introduction to epidemiology*, ed 3, Boston, 2002, Jones & Bartlett.

U.S. Department of Health, Education, and Welfare: *Vital statistics of the United States: 1950, vol 1*, Washington, DC, 1954, USDHEW, Public Health Service.

U.S. Department of Health and Human Services: *Healthy People 2010: understanding and improving health*, ed 2, Washington, DC, 2000, U.S. Government Printing Office.

U.S. Department of Health and Human Services: *Public Health Service: Healthy People 2000: national health promotion and disease prevention objectives*, Washington, DC, 1991, U.S. Government Printing Office.

U.S. Preventive Services Task Force: *Screening for lipid disorders in adults: Summary of recommendations, 2008,* available at http://www.ahrq.gov/clinic/uspstf/uspschol.htm. Accessed September 1, 2008.

Valdez R et al: Family history and prevalence of diabetes in the U.S. population: The 6-year results from the National Health and Nutrition Examination Survey (1999–2004), *Diabetes Care* 30:2517–2522, 2007.

Vandenbroucke JP: Epidemiology in transition: a historical hypothesis, *Epidemiol* 1(2):164, 1990.

Evidence-Based Practice

Sharon E. Lock

ADDITIONAL RESOURCES

These related resources are found either in the appendix at the back of this book or on the book's website at http://evolve.elsevier.com/stanhope/foundations.

Appendix

- Appendix H.1: Examples of Public Health Nursing Roles and Implementing Public Health Functions
- Appendix H.2: American Nurses Association Standards of Care of Public Health Nursing Practice

- Appendix H.3: Quad Council Public Health Nursing Core Competencies and Skill Levels

Evolve Website

- Community Assessment Applied
- Case Study, with questions and answers
- Quiz review questions
- WebLinks, including link to *Healthy People 2010* website

OBJECTIVES

After reading this chapter, the student should be able to:
1. Define evidence-based practice.
2. Understand the history of evidence-based practice in health care.
3. Assess the relationship between evidence-based practice and the practice of nursing in the community.
4. Provide examples of evidence-based practice in the community.
5. Identify barriers to evidence-based practice.
6. Identify resources for evidence-based practice.

CHAPTER OUTLINE

KEY TERMS

evidence-based medicine: being "aware of the evidence on which one's practice is based, the soundness of the evidence, and the strength of inference the evidence permits" (Guyatt and Rennie, 2002, p. xiv).

evidence-based nursing: "an integration of the best evidence available, nursing expertise, and the values and preferences of the individuals, families, and communities who are served" (Honor Society of Nursing, Sigma Theta Tau, *Position Statement*, 2005).

evidence-based practice: includes the best available evidence from a variety of sources, including research studies, evidence from nursing experience and expertise, and evidence from community leaders.

evidence-based public health: "a public health endeavor in which there is an informed, explicit, and judicious use of evidence that has been derived from any of a variety of science and social science research and evaluation methods" (Rychetnik et al., 2003, p. 538).

grading the strength of evidence: determining the quality, quantity, and consistency of research studies in order to make recommendations for practice.

meta-analysis: a specific method of statistical synthesis used in some systematic reviews, in which the "results from several studies are quantitatively combined and summarized" (Rychetnik et al., 2003, p. 542).

randomized controlled trial (RCT): generally ranks as the highest level of evidence followed by other RCTs, nonrandomized clinical trials, prospective cohort studies, case-control studies, case reports, and expert opinion (Akobeng, 2005).

research utilization: "the process of transforming research knowledge into practice" (Stetler, 2001, p. 272) and "the use of research to guide clinical practice" (Estabrooks, Winther, and Derksen, 2004, p. 293).

systematic review: a summary of the research evidence that relates to a specific question and to the effects of an intervention.

Nurses use various sources of knowledge to make clinical decisions. Intuition, trial and error, tradition, authority, and clinical experience are often used as sources of knowledge in clinical settings. However, not all sources of knowledge are reliable and all do not consistently produce the desired outcomes (Ledbetter and Stevens, 2000). A procedure done by trial and error might be performed successfully sometimes and other times it might not. Intuition and authority may lead to faulty clinical decision making. Although experience can be a good teacher, it can contain bias (Ledbetter and Stevens, 2000). For example, just because a nurse has experience in successfully performing an intervention a certain way does not mean it is the best way or that it will be successful every time.

Research evidence provides a scientific basis for practice; thus using research to support practice will result in better client outcomes and more efficient practice. Research evidence is not always available to use for decision making. When that is the case, other sources of evidence are used to make clinical decisions.

DEFINITION OF EVIDENCE-BASED PRACTICE

Evidence-based medicine is the "integration of best research evidence with clinical expertise and client values" (Sackett et al., 2000, p. 1). Rychetnik et al. (2003) defined **evidence-based public health** as "a public health endeavor in which there is an informed, explicit, and judicious use of evidence that has been derived from any of a variety of science and social science research and evaluation methods" (Rychetnik et al., 2003, p. 538). In a position statement on evidence-based practice, the Honor Society of Nursing, Sigma Theta Tau International, defined **evidence-based nursing** as "an integration of the best evidence available, nursing expertise, and the values and preferences of the individuals, families, and communities who are served" (Honor Society of Nursing, Sigma Theta Tau International, *Position Statement*, 2005).

Applied to nursing, **evidence-based practice** includes the best available evidence from a variety of sources, including research studies, evidence from nursing experience and expertise, and evidence from community leaders. Culturally and financially appropriate interventions need to be identified when working with communities. The use of evidence to determine the appropriate use of interventions that are culturally sensitive and cost-effective is a must.

Evidence-based practice includes clients and communities in decisions, presenting evidence to them in an understandable fashion, informing them of the pros and cons of an intervention, and basing practice decisions on the values of the clients (Jennings and Loan, 2001).

HISTORY OF EVIDENCE-BASED PRACTICE

During the mid to late 1970s there was growing consensus among nursing leaders that scientific knowledge should be used as a basis for nursing practice. During that time, the Division of Nursing in the U.S. Public Health Service began funding research utilization projects. **Research utilization** has been defined as "the process of transforming research knowledge into practice" (Stetler, 2001, p. 272) and "the use of research to guide clinical practice" (Estabrooks, Winther, and Derksen, 2004, p. 293).

As nursing began to focus on research utilization projects, medicine also began to call for physicians to increase their use of scientific evidence to make clinical decisions. In the late 1970s, David Sackett, a medical doctor and clinical epidemiologist at McMaster University, published a series of articles in the *Canadian Medical Association Journal* describing how to read research articles in clinical journals (Guyatt and Rennie, 2002). Later Sackett proposed the phrase "bringing critical appraisal to the bedside" to describe the application of evidence from medical literature to client care. This concept was used to train resident physicians at McMaster University and evolved into a "philosophy of medical practice based on knowledge and understanding of the medical literature supporting each clinical decision" (Guyatt and Rennie, 2002, p. xiv).

Guyatt and Rennie (2002) described the goal of evidence-based medicine as being "aware of the evidence on which one's practice is based, the soundness of the evidence, and the strength of inference the evidence permits" (p. xiv).

In 1992 the Evidence-Based Medicine Working Group published an article in the *Journal of the American Medical Association* expanding the concept of evidence-based medicine and calling it a "paradigm shift." According to the Working Group (Evidence-Based Medicine Working Group, 1992), the old paradigm viewed unsystematic clinical observations as a valid way for "building and maintaining" knowledge for clinical decision making (p. 2421). In addition, principles of pathophysiology were seen as a "sufficient guide for clinical practice" (p. 2421). Training, common sense, and clinical experience were considered sufficient for evaluating clinical data and developing guidelines for clinical practice. The Working Group cited developments in research over the past 30 years as providing the foundation for the paradigm shift and a "new philosophy of medical practice" (p. 2421).

The new paradigm, evidence-based medicine, acknowledges clinical experience as a crucial, but not sufficient, part of clinical decision making. Systematic and unbiased recording of clinical observations in the form of research will increase confidence in the knowledge gained from clinical experience. Principles of pathophysiology are seen as necessary but not sufficient knowledge for making clinical decisions. The Working Group also stressed that physicians need to be able to critically appraise the research literature in order to appropriately apply research findings in practice. Knowledge gained from authoritative figures was also not sufficient for practice in the new paradigm (Evidence-Based Medicine Working Group, 1992).

In the years since, the term *evidence-based practice* has been proposed as a term that integrates all health professions. The underlying principle is that high-quality care is based on evidence rather than on tradition or intuition (Beyers, 1999). The current nursing literature on evidence-based practice is primarily associated with applications in the acute and primary care settings and little is reported about its use in community settings. However, the basic principles of evidence-based practice can be applied at the individual level or at the community level (Youngblut and Brooten, 2001).

BRIEFLY NOTED

Systematic reviews of research evidence can potentially overcome barriers to putting evidence into practice. Systematic reviews, also known as evidence summaries and integrative reviews, have been called the heart of evidence-based practice (Stevens, 2001).

TYPES OF EVIDENCE

No matter which definition is supported, what counts as evidence has been the issue most hotly debated. Estabrooks et al. (2004) recognized two broad categories of evidence—research evidence (research synthesis and individual studies)

and nonresearch evidence (clinical experience, colleagues, and clinical judgment). Although it could be argued that other types of nonresearch evidence, such as intuition, should be included, the notion of Estabrooks that nurses should learn to integrate research evidence with nonresearch evidence is a valid point.

Two approaches are described that allow the nurse to read research evidence in a condensed format. A **systematic review** is "a method of identifying, appraising, and synthesizing research evidence. The aim is to evaluate and interpret all available research that is relevant to a particular research question" (Rychetnik et al, 2003, p. 542). A systematic review is usually done by more than one person and describes the methods used to search for and evaluate the evidence. Systematic reviews can be accessed from most databases, such as Medline and CINAHL. The Cochrane Library is an electronic database that contains regularly updated evidence-based health care databases maintained by the Cochrane Collaboration, a not-for-profit organization (http://www.cochrane.org). The Cochrane Library publishes systematic reviews on a wide variety of topics. Systematic reviews, as opposed to traditional literature review publications, require more rigor and contain less opinion of the author.

Meta-analysis is "a specific method of statistical synthesis used in some systematic reviews, where the results from several studies are quantitatively combined and summarized" (Rychetnik et al, 2003, p. 542). A well-designed systematic review or meta-analysis can provide stronger evidence than a single **randomized controlled trial (RCT),** which is the gold standard in research.

What counts as evidence has also been debated in the public health literature (Victora and Habicht, 2004). RCTs are appropriate for evaluating many interventions in medicine, but are often inappropriate for evaluating public health interventions. For example, an RCT can be ethically designed to test a new medication for diabetes, but not for a smoking cessation intervention. In a smoking cessation intervention, subjects could not be randomly assigned to smoking or nonsmoking groups. In this situation, a case-control study would be most appropriate (see Chapter 9).

HOW TO	Perform a Systematic Review

- Develop a conceptual approach to organize, group, and select the evidence.
- Systematically search for and retrieve evidence.
- Assess the quality of and summarize the strength of the evidence.
- Assess cost and cost-effectiveness data (when available) for recommended interventions.
- Identify issues of applicability and barriers to implementation (when available) for recommended interventions.
- Summarize information regarding other benefits or harms potentially resulting from the intervention.
- Identify and summarize the evidence.

From the Task Force on Community Prevention Services, National Center for Chronic Disease Prevention and Health Promotion. Retrieved March 6, 2006, from http://www.cdc.gov.

<table>
<tr><td>HOW TO</td><td>Develop an Evidence-Based Practice Guide to a Community Preventive Service</td></tr>
</table>

- Form a development team, preferably interdisciplinary, to choose a topic based on a community issue that needs to be addressed.
- Develop a structured approach to organize, group, select, and evaluate the interventions from the literature that work to address the issue.
- Select the interventions that the group wishes to evaluate for use.
- Assess the quality of the evidence found in the literature.
- Summarize the findings.
- Make recommendations.
- Write a protocol or step-by-step guide to resolving the community issue.

Adapted from Briss P et al: Developing an evidence-based guide to community preventive services and methods, *Am J Prevent Med* 18(15):35–43, 2000.

EVALUATING EVIDENCE

Several variables are considered important in determining the quality of evidence used to make clinical decisions (Polit and Beck, 2003):

- *Sample selection:* Sample selection should be as unbiased as possible. For example, a sample is randomly selected when each subject has an equal chance of being selected from the population of interest. Random selection offers the least bias of any type of sample selection. Other types of sample selection, such as convenience sampling, contain researcher or evaluator bias.
- *Randomization*: For a study that is testing an intervention, participants should be randomly assigned to the intervention or control group. This type of assignment is less biased than if participants are allowed to choose the group they want to join.
- *Blinding*: The researcher or evaluator should not know which participants are in the experimental (treatment) group or which are in the control group. The researcher or evaluator is "blinded" as to who is and who is not receiving the treatment.
- *Sample size*: The sample size should be large enough to show an effect of the intervention. In general, the larger the sample size, the better.
- *Description of intervention:* The intervention should be described in detail and explicitly enough that another person could duplicate the study if desired.
- *Outcomes*: The outcomes should be measured accurately.
- *Length of follow-up*: Depending on the intervention, the participants should be followed for a long enough period of time to determine if the intervention continued to work or if the results were just by chance.
- *Attrition*: Few subjects should have dropped out of the study.
- *Confounding variables:* Variables that could affect the outcome should be accounted for either by statistical methods or by study measurements.
- *Statistical analysis*: Statistical analysis should be appropriate to determine the desired outcome.

BRIEFLY NOTED

It can take 16 to 20 years for research to change practice.

Shaughnessy, Slawson, and Bennett (1994) proposed criteria for evaluating the usefulness of evidence, calling the process *patient-oriented evidence that matters* (POEM). In general, the reader should ask the following questions: "What are the results? Are the results valid? How can the results be applied to client care?" (p. 489).

GRADING THE STRENGTH OF EVIDENCE

When evidence is graded, the evidence is assigned a "grade" based on the quality of the evidence, the number of well-designed studies, and the presence of similar findings in all of the studies. **Grading the strength of evidence** has been debated so strongly that in 2002 the Agency for Healthcare Research and Quality (AHRQ) commissioned a study to describe existing systems used to evaluate the quality of studies and the strength of evidence. The report reviewed 40 systems and identified 3 domains for evaluating systems that grade the strength of evidence: quality, quantity, and consistency. The quality of a study refers to the extent to which bias is minimized. Quantity refers to the number of studies, the magnitude of the effect, and the sample size. Consistency refers to studies that have similar findings, using similar and different study designs (West et al, 2002). A link to an example of how the U.S. Preventive Services Task Force graded the strength of evidence for the *Guidelines for Clinical Preventive Services* can be found in the WebLinks section on the book's website.

IMPLEMENTATION

The first step toward implementing evidence-based practice in nursing is recognizing the current status of your own practice and believing that care based on the best evidence will lead to improved client outcomes (Melnyk et al, 2000). Implementation will be successful only when nurses practice in an environment that supports evidence-based care. Nurses consider evidence-based practice as a process to improve practice and outcomes and use evidence to influence policies that will improve the health of communities.

Melnyk and Fineout-Overholt (2005) have outlined steps for evidence-based practice.

The first step involves asking a clinical question. The format of the question should include the problem, the population, the intervention or exposure, the comparison (if relevant), and outcomes. In the second step, the most relevant and best evidence is collected. In the third step, evidence is critically appraised. In the fourth step, a clinical decision or change is made by integrating all the evidence with clinical expertise, client preferences, and values. Finally, the clinical decision or change is evaluated.

In a busy community practice setting, it is often difficult for nurses to access evidence-based resources. Using evidence-based clinical practice guidelines is one way for nurses to provide evidence-based nursing care in an efficient manner. Clinical practice guidelines are usually developed by a group of experts in the field who have reviewed the evidence and have made recommendations based on the best available evidence. The recommendations are usually graded according to the quality and quantity of the evidence.

BRIEFLY NOTED

Many clinical practice guidelines of interest to nurses working in the community can be easily downloaded to a handheld device for easy access in the community without having to have a computer available (see How To Box, p. 181).

BARRIERS TO IMPLEMENTATION

Barriers of evidence-based practice "occur when time, access to journal articles, search skills, critical appraisal skills, and an understanding of the language used in research are lacking" (Ciliska et al, 2001, p. 525). Common barriers

Evidence-Based Practice

This study used a population-based descriptive survey design to describe access to health care services and perceived health care needs of people who live in coal-producing counties in southwest Virginia. A researcher-developed survey was mailed to a random sample of people who lived in the area. One person in the household was asked to complete the survey about household demographics, health insurance coverage, and needs such as prescription and health care services, family health problems, and health behaviors. In all, 922 surveys were completed. The respondents had an average age of 54 years and an annual income range of $25,000 to $29,000. Most of the respondents were employed and had health insurance, usually Medicare or Medicaid; however, 80% of other people in the households did not have health insurance.

The top 10 health problems in order of prevalence were hypertension, arthritis, obesity, back problems, tooth cavities, depression, loss of many teeth, diabetes, heart disease, and asthma. Most did not see a health care provider or dentist regularly. About half of the respondents had problems paying for health needs not covered by insurance such as prescription medications and dental, vision, and preventive care. Family members often shared medications. There was also concern about the costs, lack of specialty providers, and long waits for appointments. About one-third of the respondents thought they had fair or poor health and 50% smoked cigarettes.

NURSE USE: Nurses can screen for depression and work with pharmacists in the community to develop educational programs to explain the dangers of medication sharing. They can also work with community leaders to overcome problems with transportation.

From Huttlinger K, Schaller-Ayers J, Lawson T: Health care in Appalachia: a population-based approach, *Public Health Nurs* 21(2):103–110, 2004.

to implementing evidence-based practice in nursing include misunderstood communication among nursing leaders about the process involved, the inferior quality of available research or other types of evidence, an inability to assess and use the evidence, an unwillingness of organizations to fund research and make decisions based on research or other evidence, and a concern that evidence-based practice will lead to a cookbook approach to nursing while ignoring individual client needs and the nurse's ability to make clinical decisions (McCloughen, 2001; Melnyk et al, 2000).

Although a community agency may subscribe in theory to the use of evidence-based practice, actual implementation may be affected by the realities of the practice setting. Community-focused nursing agencies may lack the resources needed for its implementation in the clinical setting, such as time, funding, computer resources, and knowledge. Nurses may be reluctant to accept the findings and feel threatened when long-established practices are questioned. "The challenge for the clinician is how to access the evidence and integrate it into practice, thus moving beyond practice based solely on experience, tradition or ritual" (Barnsteiner and Prevost, 2002, p. 18).

BRIEFLY NOTED

An organization must value evidence-based practice for it to be fully implemented. What factors do you think support the development of an environment in which nurses can implement evidence-based practice in the community?

Cost can also be a barrier if the clinical decision or change will require more funds than the agency has available. Compliance can be a barrier if the client will not follow the recommended intervention (McKenna, Ashton, and Keeney, 2004).

Levels of Prevention | Using Evidence-Based Practice

According to evidence collected and averaged by the Task Force on Community Preventive Services, the following are interventions supported by the literature at each level of prevention:

PRIMARY PREVENTION

Extended and extensive mass media campaigns reduce youth initiation of tobacco use.

SECONDARY PREVENTION

Client reminders and recalls via mail, telephone, e-mail, or a combination of these strategies are effective in increasing compliance with screening activities such as those for colorectal and breast cancer.

TERTIARY PREVENTION

Diabetes self-management education in community gathering places improves glycemic control.

From the Task Force on Community Prevention Services, National Center for Chronic Disease Prevention and Health Promotion. Retrieved March 6, 2006 from http://www.cdc.gov.

CURRENT PERSPECTIVES

Cost versus quality. Much of the pressure to use evidence-based practice comes from third-party payers and is a response to the need to contain costs and reduce legal liability. Nurses must question whether the current agenda to contain health care costs creates pressure to focus on those research results that favor cost saving at the expense of quality outcomes for clients. Outcomes include client and community satisfaction and the safety of care. Costs can be weighed against outcomes when evidence-based practice is used to show the best practices available to reduce possible harm to clients (Youngblut and Brooten, 2001).

Individual differences. Evidence-based practice cannot be applied as a universal remedy without attention to client differences. When evidence-based practice is applied at the community level, the best evidence may point to a solution that is not sensitive to cultural issues and distinctions and thus may not be acceptable to the community. Ethical practice in communities requires attention to community differences.

Appropriate evidence-based practice methods for community-oriented nursing practice. Gaining a number of perspectives in a situated community is important for nurses using evidence-based practice. Nursing has a legitimate role to play in interdisciplinary community health practice and can contribute to its evidence base. Nurses are obliged to ensure that the evidence applied to practice is acceptable to the community. Establishing an evidence-based practice culture depends on the use of both qualitative and quantitative research approaches, or the best evidence available at the time. For example, a quantitative research study of a community health center could provide information about patterns of client use, the cost of various services, and the use of different health care providers. However, when quantitative research is combined with qualitative research, the nurse can gain an understanding of why clients use or do not use the services and can help the health center be both clinically effective and cost-effective. Evidence from multiple research methods has the potential to enrich the application of evidence and improve nursing practice (Wittemore, 2005).

FUTURE PERSPECTIVES

Nurses need to acknowledge and understand evidence-based practice. They can participate by using it or they can add to the research base for the public's health through active programs of research, or reviewing the best available evidence. Nurses should demonstrate leadership in supporting evidence-based practice. Using evidence in practice will demonstrate its value, but implementation can be difficult because of the sheer volume of evidence and increasing population needs (Melnyk et al, 2000). Nurses active in the evidence-based practice movement should devote attention to understanding how best to incorporate the guidelines into practice (Kitson, 2001).

The rising cost of health care will demand a more critical look at benefits and costs of evidence-based practice. Finding resources to implement evidence-based practice will continue to be a challenge requiring creative strategies (Cook and Grant, 2002). An emphasis on quality care, equal distribution of health care resources, and cost control will continue. Implementing evidence-based practice can assist nurses in addressing these issues in the clinical setting.

Nurses must use caution in adopting evidence-based practice in a prescriptive manner in different community environments.

One source of evidence data is the Internet (Box 10-1); however, there may be a lack of quality indicators to evaluate the myriad of websites claiming to contain evidence-based information.

It is essential to evaluate the quantity of the information on the website, whether it comes from a reputable agency or scholar, and whether the source of the website has a financial interest in the acceptance of the evidence presented.

HEALTHY PEOPLE 2010 OBJECTIVES

Healthy People 2010 objectives offer a systematic approach to health improvement. These objectives provide general direction and focus for measuring progress in improving health status within a specific amount of time. The National Center for Health Statistics, Centers for Disease Control and Prevention, developed a data system to track all 467 objectives. The data are available for the public on the National Center for Health Statistics website. An organization known as Partners in Information Access for the Public Health Workforce was formed to make information and evidence-based strategies related to the *Healthy People 2010* objectives easier to find.

● *Healthy People 2010*

The Information Access Project

The Information Access Project (http://phpartners.org/hp/) is a resource for population-centered nurses. It helps them identify research findings that have direct links to population-focused and community-based care. The project has identified evidence-based strategies that assist in evaluating progress toward the achievement of *Healthy People 2010* goals and objectives. The Information Access Project can be described as follows:

- It draws its citations from peer-reviewed literature available through PubMed.
- It is designed to yield more information about interventions and models than the extent or nature of the problems addressed by a *Healthy People* objective.
- All preformulated searches are reviewed by the staff of the Public Health Foundation (a nonprofit organization) or by external subject matter experts to ensure that searches adequately capture the largest amount of published research related to achieving the objective.
- The project provides links to relevant guidelines related to the focus area.

| Box 10-1 | Resources for Implementing Evidence-Based Practice |

The following resources can assist nurses in developing an evidence-based nursing practice:

1. **The Evidence-Based Practice for Public Health Project** at the University of Massachusetts Medical School Library has developed a website for evidence-based practice in public health (http://library.umassmed.edu/ebpph/). Many bibliographic databases, such as Medline, do not list all the journals of interest to public health workers. The project provides access to numerous databases of interest concerning public health. From the project's website, nurses can access free public health online journals and databases.

2. The **Agency for Healthcare Quality and Research** (AHRQ) developed clinical guidelines based on the best available evidence for several clinical topics, such as pain management. The guidelines are accessible via the agency's website (http://www.ahrq.gov) and serve as a resource to nurses involved in individual client care.

3. The **National Guideline Clearinghouse** (http://www.guideline.gov/), an initiative of the Agency for Healthcare Research and Quality (AHRQ), is an online resource for evidence-based clinical practice guidelines. AHRQ also supports Evidence-Based Practice Centers, which write evidence reports on various topics.

4. **PubMed** (http://www.pubmed.gov/) is a bibliographic database developed and maintained by the National Library of Medicine. Bibliographic information from Medline is covered in PubMed and includes references for nursing, medicine, dentistry, the health care system, and preclinical sciences. Full texts of referenced articles are often included. Searches can be limited to type of evidence (e.g., diagnosis, therapy) and systematic reviews.

5. The **Cochrane Database of Systematic Reviews** is a collection of more than 1000 systematic reviews of effects in health care internationally. These reviews are accessible at a cost via the website (http://www.cochrane.org). Nurses may also have free access from a medical library.

6. The **University of Iowa Health Center, Department of Nursing,** gained national recognition for its use of evidence-based practice to improve care. The success is attributed to an organization culture that supports evidence-based practice (Titler et al., 2001). These resources can be accessed at http://www.uihealthcare.com/depts/nursing/rqom/evidencebasedpractice/index.html.

7. The *Evidence-Based Nursing Journal* (http://ebn.bmjjournals.com/) is published quarterly. The purpose of the journal is to select articles reporting studies and reviews from health-related literature that warrant immediate attention by nurses attempting to keep pace with advances in their profession. Using predefined criteria, the best quantitative and qualitative original articles are abstracted in a structured format, commented on by clinical experts, and shared in a timely fashion. The research questions, methods, results, and evidence-based conclusions are reported. The website for the journal is http://www.evidencebasednursing.com.

8. The Honor Society of Nursing, Sigma Theta Tau International, sponsors the online peer-reviewed journal *Worldviews on Evidence-Based Nursing,* which publishes systematic reviews and research articles on best evidence that supports nursing practice globally. The journal is available by subscription (http://www.nursingsociety.org/).

9. The **Task Force on Community Preventive Services** is an independent, nonfederal task force appointed by the director of the Centers for Disease Control and Prevention. Information about the Task Force may be found at the website http://www.thecommunityguide.org. The Task Force is charged with determining the topics to be addressed by the CDC's Community Guide and the most appropriate means to assess evidence regarding population-based interventions. The Task Force reviews and assesses the quality of available evidence on the effects of essential community preventive services. The multidisciplinary Task Force determines the scope of the Community Guide that will be used by health departments and agencies to determine best practices for preventive health in populations.

10. The **U.S. Preventive Services Task Force** (USPSTF) is an independent panel of private-sector experts in prevention and primary care. The USPSTF conducts rigorous, impartial assessments of the scientific evidence for the effectiveness of a broad range of clinical preventive services, including screening, counseling, and preventive medications. Its recommendations are considered the "gold standard" for clinical preventive services. The mission of the USPSTF is to evaluate the benefits of individual services based on age, gender, and risk factors for disease; make recommendations about which preventive services should be incorporated routinely into primary medical care and for which populations; and identify a research agenda for clinical preventive care. Recommendations of the USPSTF are published as the Guide to Clinical Preventive Services. The guide is available online at http://www.ahrq.gov/clinic/uspstfix.htm.

11. The **Centers for Disease Control and Prevention** (www.CDC.gov) publishes guidelines on immunizations and sexually transmitted diseases. Guidelines are developed by experts in the field appointed by the U.S. Department of Health and Human Services and the CDC.

From Titler MG et al: The Iowa model of evidence-based practice to promote quality care, *Crit Care Nurs Clin North Am* 13:497–509, 2001.

NURSING INTERVENTIONS RELATED TO CORE PUBLIC HEALTH FUNCTIONS

The core functions of public health are to assess the health of a community or population, develop comprehensive public health policy, and ensure that services are provided to the community (Table 10-1) (Institute of Medicine, 1988). These core functions have been expanded to include 10 public health services (Public Health Functions Steering Committee, 1994). Services related to assessment include monitoring health and diagnosis and investigation. Services related to policy development include informing and educating the public and mobilizing the community. Services related to assurance include linking or providing care to the community, ensuring a competent workforce, and evaluation.

Beginning in 1994, the Minnesota Department of Health nursing staff embarked on a project to develop a model of

Table 10-1	Core Public Health Functions and Related Evidence-Based Nursing Interventions
Core Functions	**Related Nursing Interventions**
Assessment	Diagnose and investigate health problems and hazards in the community
	Mobilize community partnerships to identify and solve health problems
	Link people to needed health services
	Use evidence-based practice for new insights and innovative solutions to health problems
Policy development	Inform, educate, and empower communities about health issues
	Develop policies and plans using evidence-based practice that supports individual and community health efforts
Assurance	Monitor health status to identify community health problems
	Enforce laws and regulations that protect health and ensure safety
	Ensure the provision of health care that is otherwise unavailable
	Ensure a competent public health and personal health care workforce
	Use evidence-based practice to evaluate effectiveness, accessibility, and quality of personal and population-based services

From U.S. Department of Health and Human Services: *Healthy People 2010: national health promotion and disease prevention objectives,* Washington, DC, 2000, U.S. Government Printing Office.

public health nursing interventions. They received support from educators in Minnesota and public health nurses and educators from Minnesota and four other states: Iowa, North Dakota, South Dakota, and Wisconsin. The resulting model was based on the following evidence:

- Input from more than 200 public health nurses who defined 17 interventions common to public health nursing practice
- A rigorous and systematic search of the literature to support the interventions
- A review of the most frequently used public health nursing textbooks for content regarding the 17 interventions identified
- An expert panel of 42 nurses, clinicians, and educators from the five states to review the 201 articles identified in the literature search to determine whether the content of the articles could be applied in practice
- The presenting of a continuing education curriculum to determine the ability to use the model
- A national expert panel to prepare the final draft of the model

The final model defines the scope of public health nursing practice by type of intervention and the client level of practice. The model describes the practice of the nurse at the community and systems level, as well as practice with individuals and families. The final 17 interventions were as follows:

1. Surveillance
2. Disease and health event investigation
3. Outreach
4. Screening
5. Case finding
6. Referral and follow-up
7. Case management
8. Delegated functions
9. Health teaching
10. Counseling
11. Consultation
12. Collaboration
13. Coalition building
14. Community organizing
15. Advocacy
16. Social marketing
17. Policy development and enforcement

Each intervention is listed, and the following actions are taken:
- The intervention is defined.
- Assumptions about the intervention are given.
- Practice examples are given for type of client.
- How the intervention relates to other interventions is explained.
- Basic steps are given for implementing the intervention.
- Best practices are explained.
- The evidence used to develop the intervention is given.

The model of interventions in Appendix H.4 is shown as a wheel of interventions and how each intervention interacts with client levels is identified (Minnesota Department of Health, 2003).

CASE STUDY

Jamie Lee is the occupational health nurse at the T-shirt factory in town. Recently, the health clinic at the T-shirt factory had budget cuts, resulting in the reduction of services and personnel. The once full-time clinic is now open only 3 days a week, and Ms. Lee no longer has support staff to help her with her paperwork responsibilities.

From her interactions with the workers, Ms. Lee has observed several risky health behaviors (e.g., unhealthy diets, smoking) among them. Although she is very busy in the clinic, Ms. Lee would like to develop a health promotion program to address these risky health behaviors, but she is not sure where to start.

CLINICAL APPLICATION

A nurse who is the director of a part-time, nurse-managed clinic is in the process of analyzing how best to expand services to operate as a full-time clinic in the most cost-effective and clinically effective manner. The director gathers evidence from the literature on nurse-managed clinics in other rural settings to evaluate the cost and clinical effectiveness of various models. The nurse also considers evidence from the following sources in the decision-making process: client satisfaction research data, knowledge of clinic staff, expert opinion of community advisory board members, evidence from community partners, and data on service needs in the state. Having examined the evidence, the nurse decides that incremental (step-by-step) growth toward full-time status is warranted. Evidence of needs in the community and analysis of statistical data indicate that the addition of services for children is a priority and a pediatric nurse practitioner is hired as a first step while planning for full-time status continues.

Evaluation of the evidence gathered demonstrates which of the following?

    A. *Effectiveness of the intervention in communities*
    B. *Application of the data to populations and communities*
    C. *Existence of positive or negative health outcomes*
    D. *Economic consequences of the intervention*
    E. *Barriers to implementation of the interventions in communities*

Explain how this example applies principles of evidence-based practice.
Answers are in the back of the book.

REMEMBER THIS!

- Evidence-based practice was developed in other countries before its use in the United States.
- Application of evidence-based practice in relation to clinical decision making in population-centered nursing concentrates on interventions and strategies geared to communities and populations rather than to individuals.
- The goals, as evidenced through *Healthy People 2010*, are to increase the quality and years of healthy life and to eliminate health disparities in populations (U.S. Department of Health and Human Services, 2000).
- Cost and quality of care are issues in evidence-based practice.
- Evidence-based practice includes interventions based on theory, expert opinions, provider knowledge, and research.

WHAT WOULD YOU DO?

1. Give an example of how undergraduates can be involved in evidence-based practice.
2. Explain how the nurse's knowledge of the community relates to evidence-based practice. Give examples.
3. What are the barriers to implementing evidence-based practice? How can these barriers be resolved?
4. Is the cost or quality of care more important in evidence-based practice? Debate this issue with classmates.
5. When working with a community to improve its health, is it more important to consider the perspectives of the community or those of the provider when defining health problems? Elaborate.

6. Invite the director of nursing from the local health department to speak to your class. Ask if evidence is used to develop nursing policies and practice guidelines. If not, why not?
7. Explain how you can apply evidence to your practice.

■ REFERENCES

Akobeng AK: Principles of evidence based medicine, *Arch Dis Child* 90:837-840, 2005.

Barnsteiner JP, Prevost S: How to implement evidence-based practice: some tried and true pointers, *Reflect Nurs Leadership* 28:18-21, 2002.

Beyers M: About evidence-based nursing practice, *Nurs Manag* 30:56, 1999.

Briss P et al: Developing an evidence-based guide to community preventive services and methods, *Am J Prevent Med* 18:35-43, 2000.

Ciliska D et al: Resources to enhance evidence-based nursing practice, *Am Assoc Crit Care Nurs Clin Issues* 12:520-528, 2001.

Cook L, Grant M: Support for evidence-based practice, *Oncol Nurs* 18:71-78, 2002.

Estabrooks CA, Winther C, Derksen L: Mapping the field: a biliometric analysis of the research utilization literature in nursing, *Nurs Res* 53:293-303, 2004.

Evidence-Based Medicine Working Group: Evidence-based medicine: a new approach to teaching the practice of medicine, *JAMA* 268:2420-2425, 1992.

Guyatt G, Rennie D, editors: *Users' guides to the medical literature: a manual for evidence-based clinical practice*, Chicago, Ill, 2002, American Medical Association.

Honor Society of Nursing, Sigma Theta Tau International: *Position statement on evidence-based nursing,* Indianapolis, Ind, 2005. Retrieved January 26, 2006, from http://www.nursingsociety.org.

Huttlinger K, Schaller-Ayers J, Lawson T: Health care in Appalachia: a population-based approach, *Public Health Nurs* 21:103-110, 2004.

Institute of Medicine: *The future of public health*, Washington, DC, 1988, National Academy Press.

Jennings BM, Loan LA: Misconceptions among nurses about evidence-based practice, *J Nurs School* 33:121-127, 2001.

Kitson AL: Approaches used to implement research findings into nursing practice: report of a study tour to Australia and New Zealand, *Int J Nurs Pract* 7:392-405, 2001.

Ledbetter CA, Stevens KR: Basics of evidence-based practice part 2: unscrambling the terms and processes, *Semin Periop Nurs* 9:98-104, 2000.

McCloughen A: Identifying barriers to the application of evidence-based practice in mental health nursing, *Contemp Nurs* 11:226-230, 2001.

McKenna HP, Ashton S, Keeney S: Barriers to evidence-based practice in primary care, *J Adv Nurs* 45:178-189, 2004.

Melnyk BM, Fineout-Overholt E: *Evidence-based practice in nursing and healthcare: a guide to best practice*, Philadelphia, 2005, Lippincott Williams & Wilkins.

Melnyk B et al: Evidence-based practice: the past, the present, and recommendations for the millennium, *Pediat Nurs* 26:77-81, 2000.

Minnesota Department of Health: Public health interventions: applications for public health nursing practice, St. Paul, Minn, 2003, the department.

Polit DF, Beck CT: *Nursing research principles and methods*, ed 7, New York, 2003, Lippincott Williams & Wilkins.

Public Health Functions Steering Committee: *Public health in America,* 1994. Retrieved January 28, 2006, from http://www.health.gov/phfunctions/public.htm.

Rychetnik L et al: A glossary for evidence-based public health, *J Epidemiol Comm Health* 58:538-545, 2003.

Sackett DL et al: *Evidence-based medicine: how to practice and teach EBM*, London, 2000, Churchill Livingstone.

Shaughnessy AF, Slawson DC, Bennett JA: Becoming an information master: a guidebook to the medical information jungles, *J Fam Pract* 39:489-499, 1994.

Stetler CB: Updating the Stetler model of research utilization to facilitate evidence-based practice, *Nurs Outlook* 49:272-279, 2001.

Stevens KR: Systematic reviews: the heart of evidence-based practice, *AACN Clin Issues* 12:529-538, 2001.

Task Force on Community Preventive Services: *Guide to community preventive services,* July 27, 2005. Retrieved January 26, 2006, from http://www.thecommunityguide.org/diabetes/default.htm.

Task Force on Community Preventive Services, National Center for Chronic Disease Prevention and Health Promotion: *The community guide: what works to promote health.* Retrieved March 6, 2006, from www.cdc.gov.

Titler MG et al: The Iowa model of evidence-based practice to promote quality care, *Crit Care Nurs Clin North Am* 13:497-509, 2001.

U.S. Department of Health and Human Services: *Healthy People 2010: national health promotion and disease prevention objectives*, Washington, DC, 2000, U.S. Government Printing Office.

Victora CG, Habicht JP: Evidence-based public health: moving beyond randomized trials, *Am J Public Health* 94:400-405, 2004.

West S et al: *Systems to rate the strength of scientific evidence,* Evidence Report/Technology Assessment No. 47, AHRQ Publication No. 02-E016, Rockville, Md, 2002, Agency for Healthcare Research and Quality.

Wittemore R: Combining evidence in nursing research: methods and implications, *Nurs Res* 54:56-62, 2005.

Youngblut JM, Brooten D: Evidence-based nursing practice: why is it important? *Am Assoc Crit Care Nurs Clin Issues* 12:468-476, 2001.

Using Health Education and Group Process in the Community

Lisa L. Onega
Edie Devers Barbero

ADDITIONAL RESOURCES

These related resources are found either in the appendix at the back of this book or on the book's website at http://evolve.elsevier.com/stanhope/foundations.

e Evolve Website

- Community Assessment Applied
- Case Study, with Questions and Answers
- Quiz review questions
- WebLinks, including link to *Healthy People 2010* website

Real World Community Health Nursing: An Interactive CD-ROM, second edition

If you are using this CD-ROM in your course, you will find the following activities related to this chapter:
- *Educational Assessment* in **Health Education**
- *Health Education Movie Theater* in **Health Education**
- *Health Risk Appraisal: How Healthy are You?* in **Health Education**

OBJECTIVES

After reading this chapter, the student should be able to:
1. Discuss the ways in which people learn.
2. Describe effective principles and methods of instruction.
3. Identify factors that affect group functioning including purpose, development, cohesion, norms, structure, interaction, and management of conflict.
4. Examine ways in which nurses can use groups to promote the health education of individuals.
5. Describe ways in which nurses can work with groups to meet health goals.

CHAPTER OUTLINE

EDUCATIONAL ISSUES
Population Considerations
Barriers to Learning
Technological Issues
THE EDUCATIONAL PROCESS
Identify Educational Needs
Establish Educational Goals and Objectives

Select Appropriate Educational Methods
Implement the Educational Plan
Evaluate the Educational Process
THE EDUCATIONAL PRODUCT

KEY TERMS

affective domain: a domain of learning that includes changes in attitudes and the development of values.

andragogy: the art and science of teaching adults and individuals with some knowledge about a health-related topic.

cognitive domain: a domain of learning that includes memory, recognition, understanding, and application and is divided into a hierarchical classification of behaviors.

cohesion: the attraction between individual members and between each member and the group.

communication structure: a descriptive framework that identifies message pathways and member participation in sending and receiving messages utilized for a group or groups.

conflict: the opposite of harmony; a state of interference that people want to guard against; antagonistic points of view.

education: the establishment and arrangement of events to facilitate learning.

established groups: an existing group of persons linked by membership and group purpose.

group: a collection of interacting individuals who have a common purpose or purposes.

group culture: a composite of the group norms that come to dictate perceptions and behaviors.

group purpose: the reason two or more people come together; it may be subtle or obvious and is easily stated by members.

group structure: the particular arrangement of group parts that constitute the whole.

leadership: influencing others to achieve a goal.

learning: the process of gaining knowledge and skills that lead to behavioral changes.

long-term evaluation: geared toward following and assessing the behavior of an individual, family, community, or population over time.

maintenance functions: behaviors that provide physical and psychological support and therefore hold the group together.

maintenance norms: norms that create group pressures to ensure affirming actions for members and are helpful in maintaining comfort.

member interaction: the ways that group members behave and relate toward each other.

norms: standards that guide, regulate, and control.

pedagogy: the art and science of teaching children and individuals with little knowledge about a health-related topic.

psychomotor domain: a domain of learning that includes the performance of skills that require some degree of neuromuscular coordination.

reality norms: group members' perceptions of reality, upon which daily behavior is based; influence decision-making and action-taking processes.

role structure: the arrangement of group member positions according to the expected functions of members.

short-term evaluation: focuses on identifying behavioral effects of health education programs and determining whether changes are caused by the educational program.

task function: behaviors that focus or direct movement toward the main work of the group.

task norm: a group's commitment to return to the central goals of the group when it has strayed from its purpose.

Nurses working in the community regularly use health education to help clients promote, maintain, and restore health. As discussed in Chapter 1, community health clients include individuals, families, communities, and populations. Nurses often educate clients across three levels of prevention: primary, secondary, and tertiary. See the Levels of Prevention box. Nurses provide information to enable clients to attain optimal health, prevent health problems, identify and treat health problems early, and minimize disability. Education allows individuals to make informed health-related decisions, assume personal responsibility for their health, and cope effectively with alterations in their health and lifestyles.

The following list identifies the sequence of actions that a nurse follows when developing an educational program. The typical steps include the following:

1. Identify a population-specific learning need for the community health client.
2. Select one or more learning theories to use in the educational program. Examples include behavioral, cognitive, critical, developmental, humanistic, or social learning theories.
3. Consider educational principles that will increase learning, and choose those that are most appropriate. They could include those that are related to domains of

Levels of Prevention	Related to Community Health Education

PRIMARY PREVENTION

Education at health fairs regarding immunizations for children, older adults, and people with chronic illnesses.

SECONDARY PREVENTION

Education at health fairs regarding early diagnosis and treatment of diabetes and hypercholesterolemia, along with providing health screenings, with the goal of shortening disease duration and severity.

TERTIARY PREVENTION

Education in rehabilitation centers or adult day care centers to help individuals who have had a stroke maximize their functioning.

learning, associated with the events of learning, or guide the educator.
4. Examine educational issues such as population-specific concerns, barriers to learning, and technological strategies to facilitate learning.
5. Design and implement an educational program using a variety of strategies.
6. Evaluate the effects of the educational program on learning and behavior.

HEALTHY PEOPLE 2010 EDUCATIONAL OBJECTIVES

As discussed throughout the text, The *Healthy People 2010* document identifies national health needs and outlines goals and objectives designed to improve health. Community-based educational programs can often be used to meet and maintain many of these objectives. Settings such as schools, worksites, community centers, and health care agencies can be used as learning sites. The *Healthy People 2010* box outlines the objectives that specifically address health education (U.S. Department of Health and Human Services, 2000).

These objectives emphasize the importance of educating various populations (based on age and ethnicity) about health promotion activities such as avoiding cigarette smoking and illegal drug use, drinking alcohol in moderation, eating a well-balanced diet, exercising routinely, avoiding injuries, and making responsible sexual choices (U.S. Department of Health and Human Services, 2000). The objectives can be addressed through primary and secondary prevention. Health fairs are useful avenues for prevention, since they are generally held in locations that attract many people; they may have health demonstrations to identify possible problems, provide easy-to-understand educational materials, and encourage positive actions related to diet, exercise, and stress management. See the "How To" box for information on how to set up a health fair.

Typically, a nurse identifies a health need or problem in a particular population. Then health education programs are

Healthy People 2010

Educational and Community-Based Programs

Goal: To increase the quality, availability, and effectiveness of educational and community-based programs designed to prevent disease and improve the health and quality of life

School Setting
7-1 Increase completion of high school
7-2 Increase the proportion of middle, junior high, and senior high schools that provide comprehensive school health education to prevent health problems in the following areas: (1) unintentional injury, violence, and suicide; (2) tobacco use; (3) alcohol and other drug use; (4) unintended pregnancy and sexually transmitted infections; (5) unhealthy dietary patterns; and (6) inadequate physical activity
7-3 Increase the proportion of college and university students who receive information from their institution on each of the six priority health-risk behavior areas listed above
7-4 Increase the proportion of elementary, middle, junior high, and senior high schools that have a nurse-to-student ratio of at least 1:750

Worksite Setting
7-5 Increase the proportion of worksites that offer a comprehensive employee health promotion program to their employees
7-6 Increase the proportion of employees who participate in employer-sponsored health promotion activities

Health Care Setting
7-7 Increase the proportion of health care organizations that provide client and family education
7-8 Increase the proportion of clients who report that they are satisfied with the client education that they receive from their health organization
7-9 Increase the proportion of hospitals and managed care organizations that sponsor community disease prevention and health promotion activities that address the priority health needs identified by their community

Community Setting and Select Populations
7-10 Increase the proportion of tribal and local health service areas that establish community health promotion programs
7-11 Increase the proportion of local health departments that establish culturally appropriate and linguistically competent community health promotion and disease prevention programs
7-12 Increase the proportion of older adults who have participated during the preceding year in at least one organized health promotion activity

Modified from the U.S. Department of Health and Human Services: *Healthy People 2010: understanding and improving health,* ed 2, Washington, DC, U.S. Government Printing Office, November 2000.

designed to meet that health need or problem. Generally these programs involve educating individual members of the population about health promotion, illness prevention, and treatment. For example, in a community in which there is documented air pollution and in which increased morbidity, mortality, and health care costs associated with childhood

HOW TO	Set Up a Health Fair

- Establish goals, outcomes, and screening activities in conjunction with desires of the population or community.
- Recruit a variety of health care professionals and sponsors to participate in the fair.
- Reserve the location and set the date and time of the fair approximately 1 year in advance.
- At least 6 months in advance, obtain a financial commitment from sponsors and develop a budget.
- About 4 months in advance, send letters to health care professionals and agencies verifying their participation and informing them of the location, date, and time of the fair.
- Approximately 2 months in advance, obtain tables, chairs, trash cans, decorations, and equipment needed for exhibits. Prepare program handouts and advertisements. Begin advertising for the fair. Verify that parking and security personnel are available.
- Approximately 1 week in advance, confirm that health care professionals and agency participants are planning to participate.
- The day before the health fair, set up tables, chairs, decorations, and equipment.
- On the day of the fair, greet health care professionals, agency representatives, sponsors, and members of the population being served. Solve problems as needed during the course of the day.
- Between 1 week and 1 month after the fair, send thank-you letters to health care professionals, agencies, and sponsors. Pay all bills associated with the fair.
- Work with the population of interest to evaluate the effectiveness of the health fair.

Modified from Kelemen A: Wellness promotion: how to plan a college health fair, *Am J Health Studies* 17(1):31-36, 2001; Lyman S, Benedik JR: Health fairs: timetable, pitfalls, & burnout, *College Student J* 33(4):534, 1999.

and adolescent asthma exist, a community-based asthma education and training program could be established. Also if there is a documented number of obese children in the public schools, nurses could campaign for reduced calorie foods, more physical education, and better student and parent education about diet and exercise, and their effects on health.

EDUCATION AND LEARNING

Acquiring information about health provides people with tools to make better health decisions and to understand why they might want to change their behavior. There is a difference between education and learning (Knowles, Holton, and Swanson, 2005) and between knowing and doing. **Education** is the establishment and arrangement of events to facilitate learning, including providing knowledge and teaching skills. **Learning** is defined in many ways. Most definitions of the learning process include measurable change in behavior that continues over time. Thus learning is the process of gaining knowledge and expertise. Once an individual has learned or gained specified knowledge and expertise, the process is complete and behavioral change results (Palazzo, 2001).

HOW PEOPLE LEARN

There has been a shift in ideas about how people learn. Learning previously used what might be called either a sponge or a vessel approach. In the former the instructor spread out the information and the learner soaked it up. In the vessel approach, information is poured out and the learner has to collect it. The more viable thinking about ways to learn is that it is an active process between instructor and learner. Learners accept information based on a range of factors including what they know, what they believe, the culture in which they were raised and live, as well as how they process the information they receive. No doubt all of us have been in a small group in which we all heard the same facts, but we each took away a somewhat different interpretation of those facts. What we hear is filtered through our assumptions, values, level of attention, and knowledge (Wilson and Peterson, 2006). Also, social groups play a key role in the development of understanding. This is partially because learning is a social process that takes place in the communities in which we live and the groups with which we associate. We respond in different ways to information based on the esteem in which we hold the speaker. Furthermore, a variety of educational principles can assist in selecting health information for individuals, families, communities, and populations. Three of the most useful categories of educational principles include those associated with the nature of learning, the events of instruction, and guidelines for the effective educator.

THE NATURE OF LEARNING

One way to think about the nature of learning is to examine the cognitive (thinking), affective (feeling), and psychomotor (acting) domains of learning. Each domain has specific behavioral components that form a hierarchy of steps, or levels. Each level builds on the previous one. Understanding these three learning domains is crucial in providing effective health education (Bloom et al, 1956).

Cognitive Domain

The **cognitive domain,** which includes memory, recognition, understanding, reasoning, application, and problem solving, is divided into a hierarchical classification of behaviors. Learners master each level of cognition in order of difficulty (Bloom et al, 1956; Dembo, 1994). Start by assessing the cognitive abilities of the learner so that the instructor's expectations and plans are directed toward the correct level. Teaching above or below the client's level of understanding may lead to frustration and discouragement. The cognitive domain has the following elements (Bloom et al, 1956):

- Knowledge: requires recall of information
- Comprehension: combines recall with understanding
- Application: new information is taken in and used in a different way
- Analysis: breaks communication down into parts to understand both the parts and their relationships
- Synthesis: builds on the prior four levels by assembling them into a unified whole
- Evaluation: judges the value of what has been learned

Affective Domain

The **affective domain** includes changes in attitudes and the development of values. For affective learning, nurses consider and try to influence what clients feel, think, and value. Because the attitudes and values of the nurse may differ from those of the clients, be sure to listen carefully to detect clues to feelings that learners have that may influence learning. It is difficult to change deeply rooted attitudes, beliefs, interests, and values. People need support and encouragement from those around them to make such changes and to reinforce new behaviors. Like cognitive learning, affective learning consists of a series of steps. Steps in the affective domain as modified from Krathwohl, Bloom, and Masia (1964) have the learner doing the following in this sequence:

1. Knowledge: receives the information
2. Comprehension: responds to what is being taught
3. Application: values the information
4. Analysis: makes sense of the information
5. Synthesis: organizes the information
6. Evaluation: adopts behaviors that are consistent with the new values

Psychomotor Domain

The **psychomotor domain** includes the performance of skills that require some degree of neuromuscular coordination and that emphasize motor skills (Bloom et al, 1956). Clients are taught a variety of psychomotor skills including bathing infants, changing dressings, giving injections, measuring blood sugars, taking blood pressures, and walking with crutches.

In learning a skill, the first step is to show learners the skill either in person, using pictures, a video, a CD, or the Internet. Next, allow learners to practice and immediately correct any errors in performing the skill. The following three conditions must be met before psychomotor learning occurs (Bloom et al, 1956; Dembo, 1994):

1. The learner must have the necessary ability. For example, someone with Alzheimer disease may be able to follow only one-step instructions. Adapt the educational plan to fit this person's abilities.
2. The learner must have a sensory image of how to carry out the skill. For example, when educating a group of pregnant women about ways to manage labor, ask the women to visualize themselves in calm control of their delivery.
3. The learner must have opportunities to practice the new skills being learned. Provide practice sessions during the program because many people may not have the facilities, motivation, support from others, or time to practice at home what they have learned. Nor will they have their skill evaluated by a person who understands what the performance goal is.

In assessing a person's ability to learn a skill, evaluate intellectual, emotional, and physical ability. Some clients do not have the intellectual ability to learn the steps that make up a complex procedure. Others may have cultural beliefs that conflict with healthy behaviors. A tremulous person with poor eyesight may not be able to learn insulin self-injection. Be careful to teach at the level of the learner's ability and use words at the level of their understanding of the language. This is true for native English speakers whose literacy level is low, as well as for people for whom English is a second language and who may have limited understanding of the spoken or written word. Also, be sure that the learner has the equipment to use the learning resource. For example, if you are asking the person to view a CD, make sure the person has a CD player with visual capability.

Read the three examples below and identify how the cognitive, affective, and psychomotor domains are being used:

Clinical example 1: A nurse works with a group of women who do not perform monthly breast self-examinations (BSEs). She instructs them in how to do so. The nurse seeks to change their thought patterns by providing information about BSEs in a variety of ways. First, the nurse tells the women about the procedure, explains the reasons for doing BSEs, and shows them a video. Next, she watches each woman practice breast examinations on a breast model. Finally, the nurse gives each woman a handout with the procedure written and diagrammed on it and instructs the women to hang the handout next to the bathroom mirror to remind them to do monthly BSEs. By using a variety of environmental cues and sensory input, the women's thought patterns can be changed, thereby influencing their behavior related to BSEs.

Clinical example 2: The nurse wants a newly diagnosed group of diabetic clients to be able to manage their diabetes. The nurse asks them what they know about diabetes. They demonstrate that they can check their own blood sugar and prepare their own insulin injections. However, on further questioning, the nurse learns that they do not know about the long-term complications of diabetes. The nurse then educates them about these complications. Next, the clients ask questions about ways they can prevent long-term complications. As a result of this discussion and exchange of information, the clients begin to go to an ophthalmologist every year and to check their feet daily for alterations in skin color or integrity.

Clinical example 3: To help a family with a toddler prevent accidents in the home, nurses educate parents about safety practices. They also discuss how to teach the toddler simply and clearly about safety according to the child's developmental stage and readiness to understand concepts and to change behavior. The nurses recognize that the parents' and the toddler's levels of readiness to learn are quite different. Because the toddler cannot reach the stove top, teaching about the dangers of a hot stove at this stage of physical development is unnecessary. However, the toddler is at risk for accidental poisoning. Although the parents may teach the toddler not to open bottles and jars without their help, all poisons must be removed from the toddler's possible reach as a necessary precaution. The risk of poison ingestion is incomprehensible to the toddler because of the child's language and cognitive development. Thus, the parents and

Box 11-1	Six Principles That Guide the Educator

1. *Message.* Sending a clear message to the learner
2. *Format.* Selecting the most appropriate learning format
3. *Environment.* Creating the best possible learning environment
4. *Experience.* Organizing positive and meaningful learning experiences
5. *Participation.* Engaging the learner in participatory learning
6. *Evaluation.* Evaluating and giving objective feedback to the learner

Modified from Knowles M: *The adult learner: a neglected species,* ed 4, Houston, 1990, Gulf.

Box 11-2	Guidelines for Clear Educational Programs

- *Begin strongly.* People remember the first point.
- *Use a clear, direct, succinct style.* This helps the learner remain focused.
- *Use the active voice.* For example, the educator may say "We will discuss relaxation techniques" instead of "Relaxation techniques will be discussed."
- *Accentuate the positive.* For example, the educator may say "The majority of individuals are able to lose weight with a well-balanced diet and exercise" instead of "A few people have not been able to lose weight with a well-balanced diet and exercise."
- *Use vivid communication, not statistics or jargon.* Stories or examples are often more meaningful than dry statistics or general, nonspecific terms.
- *Refer to trustworthy sources.* For example, "the surgeon general" is a more credible source than "some people."
- *Base strategies on knowledge of the audience.* Be aware of the perspectives and preferences of the audience.
- *Use aids to highlight key points.* Provide a handout with learning objectives and an outline of the major points.
- *Make points explicitly.* Be direct and give clear instructions.
- *End strongly.* The last point made is likely to be remembered.

Modified from Babcock DE, Miller MA: *Client education: theory and practice,* St. Louis, 1994, Mosby; Palazzo M: Teaching in crisis: patient and family education in critical care, *Crit Care Nurs Clin North Am* 13(1):83–92, 2001.

the toddler receive different information depending on their stage of development.

COMMUNITY HEALTH EDUCATION

Understanding the basic sequence of instruction is essential in effective education. The following nine steps for instructing others are useful guides in planning effective health education (Driscoll, 1994; Knowles, Holton, and Swanson, 2005):

1. *Gain attention.* Before learning can take place, you need to gain the learner's attention. One way to do this is by convincing the learner that the information about to be presented is important and beneficial.
2. *Inform the learner of the objectives of instruction.* Before teaching begins, outline the major goals and objectives of instruction so that learners develop expectations about what they are supposed to learn.
3. *Stimulate recall of prior learning.* Have the learners recall previous knowledge related to the topic of interest. This assists them in linking new knowledge with prior knowledge.
4. *Present the material.* The essential elements of a topic should be presented in a clear, organized, and simple manner. The material should be presented in a way that is congruent with the learner's strengths, needs, and limitations.
5. *Provide learning guidance.* For long-lasting behavioral changes to occur, the learner must store information in long-term memory. Help the learner find ways to transform the information so it will be stored in memory.
6. *Elicit performance.* Encourage learners to demonstrate what they have learned. Expect that during the educational process, learners will need to correct errors and improve skills.
7. *Provide feedback.* Provide feedback to assist learners in improving their knowledge and skills. Feedback enables learners to modify their thinking patterns and behaviors.
8. *Assess performance.* Evaluate learning. Knowledge and skills should be formally assessed with the expectation that new information has been understood.
9. *Enhance retention and transfer of knowledge.* Once a baseline level of knowledge and skills has been attained, assist learners in applying this information to new situations.

By using these instructional principles, nurses can help clients obtain the most from the learning experiences. The omission of steps can lead to superficial and fragmented learning.

THE EFFECTIVE EDUCATOR

Nurse educators must be effective teachers. Six basic principles guide the effective educator (Box 11-1).

Send a Clear Message

Regardless of the importance of the content or the interest level of learners, material must be presented in a clear and logical manner for learners to both receive and retain the information. At various stages in the educational process, reassess the learners' readiness and be aware of possible barriers to effective communication. Both emotional stress and physical illness may limit the amount of information that learners can absorb. Also, learners' receptivity may vary from session to session depending on various internal and external factors. Educational strategies and activities can be developed and adjusted to fit the dynamic needs of learners (Palazzo, 2001). Provide information that is understandable (Box 11-2). Medical jargon and technical terms can interfere with the clarity of the intended message. For example, when teaching about interactions among diet, exercise, and blood pressure, the term *high blood pressure* may be more familiar than *hypertension.*

WORKING TO EFFECTIVELY EDUCATE GROUPS

Groups can be used to initiate and implement changes for individuals, families, organizations, and the community. People naturally form groups in their homes, and groups in the community influence the community's health. Groups form for various reasons: (1) to achieve a stated purpose or goal, or (2) naturally as a result of shared values, interests, and activities, or (3) because personal characteristics attract individuals to each other.

Some groups are ongoing, i.e., the family, while others such as a project in a community are short term. Some have clear goals and a specified timeline. Groups may be physically together or may meet in a virtual way such as in an Internet chat room via a podcast or video conferencing.

Community groups represent the collective interests, needs, and values of individuals; they provide a link between the individual and the larger social system. Throughout life, membership in groups influences thoughts, choices, behaviors, and values as people socialize and interact. Groups can bring about changes to improve the health and well-being of individuals and communities. Some individual changes for health are difficult or impossible to achieve without group support and encouragement. In daily practice, nurses plan and use health-focused action with clients, other nurses, and other health care workers. Understanding the community and assessing its health begin by identifying groups and their goals, member characteristics, and their place in the community structure. Through community groups, nurses help people identify priority health needs and capabilities and make valuable community changes.

GROUP CONCEPTS

To work effectively with groups and use them to improve the health of community members, it is helpful to understand core group concepts. These include defining the group and understanding group purpose, membership, cohesion, and task and maintenance functions.

DEFINITIONS

A **group** is a collection of interacting individuals who have common purposes. Each member influences and is in turn influenced by every other member to some extent. Key elements are **member interaction** and **group purpose**. Groups form for a variety of reasons. Families, a familiar community group, share kinship bonds, living space, and economic resources. They have many purposes such as providing psychological support and socialization for their members.

Groups may engage in problem solving, decision making, planning, or implementation of a goal (London, 2007), and often form in response to community needs, problems, or opportunities. For example, residents in a community may come together to oppose zoning changes, the building of a road, or the closing of a valued community resource. Other groups in the community form spontaneously because of mutual attraction between individuals and for socialization and recreation. Health-promoting groups may form when people meet in community and health care settings and discover common challenges to their physical and emotional well-being. Health-promoting groups such as Alcoholics Anonymous, Parents without Partners, and the La Leche League improve members' health and deal with specific threats to health. Members support one another in the attainment of goals.

GROUP PURPOSE

Once a health change goal is specified and group work is chosen as the medium, a clear statement and presentation of the proposed group's purpose must be developed. A clear purpose helps establish criteria for member selection. A clear statement of purpose was valuable in forming a new group in one city's housing development. The local social services department had received numerous reports of child abuse and neglect. Routine home visits for well-child care documented high stress levels between parents and their offspring. Some parents asked the nurse to teach and guide them in child discipline. The nurse proposed that a parent group address this community need and chose this purpose for the group: dealing with kids to achieve child and parent satisfaction. The purpose indicated both the process (to help parents deal with children) and the desired outcome (satisfaction for parents and children). As potential members were approached, the stated purpose for the group helped individuals decide if they wanted to join.

BRIEFLY NOTED

When the purpose for a group is clearly stated and agreed on, the group becomes increasingly attractive to members.

When a group makes a public appeal for members and accepts everyone who wants to join, the membership is self-selected on the basis of the group's stated purpose. In this type of recruitment, publicity must reach those who need to make specific health changes. Prospective members may want to discuss the purpose with leaders or clarify questions about the purpose at the first group meeting. A commitment to group health is partly based on individual goals and how well the group goal satisfies personal objectives.

GROUP DEVELOPMENT

There are a variety of ways to discuss group development. Berman-Rossi (1992) says that how the group develops is related to two internal processes: that of member-to-authority and member-to-member relationships. These relationships can change over time. A feared group member can become a confidant and an overbearing leader may later seem helpful and supportive. He notes five commonly accepted stages of group development:

1. *Pre-Affiliation*—the group has not formed; potential participants do not know if they can trust one another; relationships are individual not collective. The primary task of the leader at this point is to clarify the purpose and arrive at agreement with members about this.

2. *Power and Control*—it must become clear at this point where the authority for leading the group lies and what the power and control issues among members are, including status, ranking, and the development of norms.
3. *Intimacy*—members begin to need one another and rely on one another for support; helping relationships are part of this stage and the leader has a less hierarchical role and is more of a partner in helping members attain their goals.
4. *Differentiation*—where the roles of the members differ from one another and each one uniquely contributes to the goal of the group.
5. *Separation*—where the work is largely complete and the group relies less on one another.

Each stage must be mastered before the group can move to the next level. Feinberg (1980) applies Tuckman's (1965) developmental sequence in groups to a self-help group. This application can be used by nurses in the community. For example, in the first, or "forming" stage, members identify, try-out, and change behavior based on group goals and accepted group behaviors (Feinberg, 1980). It is in the second, or "storming" stage, that the members express their hostility to one another and tend to move toward polar opposite views. Harmony can be present once again in the third, or "norming" stage. At this time members accept one another, become cohesive, and develop norms and roles. Finally, in the fourth, or "performing" stage, members use the interpersonal structure developed in stage three to accomplish the group's work goals. In a later work, Tuckman and Jensen (1977) added a fifth stage, "adjourning," that coincides with the last stage of separation.

COHESION

Cohesion is the attraction between individual members and between each member and the group (Figure 11-1). Individuals in a highly cohesive group identify themselves as a unit,

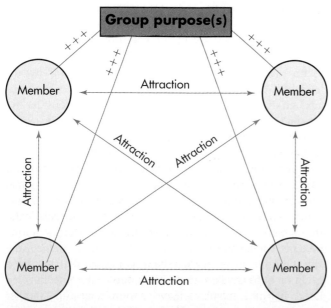

FIGURE 11-1 Cohesion is the measure of attraction between members, and of member attraction to group purpose(s).

work toward common goals, endure frustration for the sake of the group, and defend the group against outside criticism. Attraction increases when members feel accepted and liked by others, see similar qualities in one another, and share similar attitudes and values. Group effectiveness also improves as members work together toward group goals while still satisfying the needs of individual members (Brandler, 1999).

BRIEFLY NOTED

Because the mood and behavior of the leader affect the way in which the group functions, leaders need to assess and modify, where indicated, their mood, attitude, and behaviors.

Members' traits that increase group cohesion and productivity include the following:
- Compatible personal and group goals
- Attraction to group goals
- Attraction to selected members
- Appropriate mix of leading and following skills
- Good problem-solving skills

A **task function** is anything a member does that deliberately contributes to the group's purpose. Members with task-directed abilities are attractive to the group. These traits include strong problem-solving skills, access to material resources, and skills in directing. Of equal importance are abilities to affirm and support individuals in the group. These functions are called **maintenance functions** because they help other members remain in the group and feel accepted. Another maintenance function is that of helping people resolve conflicts and ensuring social and environmental comfort. Both task and maintenance functions are necessary for group progress. Naturally, members who provide such group requirements are attractive, and an abundance of such traits within the membership tends to increase group cohesion.

The following group members' traits may decrease cohesion and productivity:
- Conflicts between personal and group goals
- Lack of interest in group goals and activities
- Poor problem-solving and communication abilities
- Lack of both leadership and supporter skills
- Disagreement about types of leadership
- Aversion to other members
- Behaviors and attributes that are poorly understood by others

Similarity among members tends to increase group attraction while differences tend to decrease attractiveness. Members' perceptions of differences can create competition and jealousy. At the same time personal differences can increase group cohesion if they support complementary functioning or provide contrasting viewpoints necessary for decision making. Cohesive factors are complex, and many factors influence member attraction to each other and to the group's goal. High group cohesion positively affects productivity and member satisfaction. The following example illustrates factors that influence group cohesion:

Case Example: *A nurse initiated a group for clients who had been treated for burns. Ten residents, all from one city, had been discharged after a month in the local burn unit. The stated purpose for the group was to teach coping skills to assist members in the difficult transition from hospital to home. Each person had (1) been treated for extensive burns in an intensive care treatment center; (2) relied heavily on health care workers for physical, social, and emotional rehabilitation; and (3) faced the challenge of resuming work and family roles. Although they shared some similar experiences and hopes for the future, their amounts of trauma and stress varied. They also differed widely in psychological readiness for a return to ordinary daily routines. One woman in the group was able to return quickly to her job as a cashier in a large supermarket. The strength of her determination to overcome public reaction to her scars, coupled with an ability to "use the right words" and an empathy for others, distinguished her from others in the group. These differences proved attractive to other members, inspiring them to work toward a return to their own roles in life. These members saw her differences as attainable.*

This group's cohesion was provided by the members' attraction to the common purpose of returning to successful life patterns and managing relationships with others. Each member also believed that interaction with others with similar burn experiences could help them reach that goal. This example shows that certain member experiences such as crises or traumas may help individuals identify with each other and may increase member attraction.

Being different from the general population and similar to the other group members is, for some, a compelling force for membership in the group. Others are repelled by the group because they do not want to be identified by an aversive characteristic such as disfigurement. Empathy for another's pain, learned only through mutual experience, may provide each individual with a required perspective for problem solving or affirming another's view. This nurse helped members use common experiences and learn from their differences. The group was effective.

Members' attraction to the group also depends on the nature of the group. Factors include the group's programs, size, type of organization, and position in the community. Attraction to the group is increased when individuals perceive goals clearly and see group activities as effective.

The concept of cohesion helps to explain group productivity. Some cohesion is essential for people to remain with a group and accomplish its goals. Attractiveness positively influences members' motivation and commitment to work on the group task. Group cohesion may be increased as members better understand the experiences of others and identify common ideas and reactions to various issues. Nurses facilitate this process by pointing out similarities, contrasting supportive differences, or helping members redefine differences in ways that make those dissimilarities compatible.

NORMS

Norms are standards that guide, control, and regulate individuals and communities. Group norms set the standards for group members' behaviors, attitudes, and perceptions. They suggest what a group believes is important, what it finds acceptable or objectionable, or what it perceives as having no consequence. This commonly held view of what ought to be provides motivation for the members to use the group for their mutual benefit (Northen and Kurland, 2001). All groups have norms and mechanisms to accomplish conformity. Group norms serve three functions:

1. They ensure movement toward the group's purpose or tasks.
2. They maintain the group through various supports to members.
3. They influence members' perceptions and interpretations of reality.

Even though certain norms keep the group focused on its task, a certain amount of diversion is permitted as long as members respect central goals and are committed to return to them. This commitment to return to the central goals is the **task norm**; its strength determines the group's ability to adhere to its work.

Maintenance norms create group pressures to affirm members and maintain their comfort. Individuals in groups are most productive and at ease when psychological and social well-being is nurtured. Maintenance behaviors include identifying the social and psychological tensions of members and taking steps to support members at high-stress times. Members may pay attention to temperature, space, and seating when attending to health-supportive maintenance norms. Attention to comfort and the role of arrangements may include meeting in places that are easily accessible and comfortable to the participants, providing refreshments, and scheduling meetings at convenient times.

A third and equally important function of group norms relates to members' perceptions of reality (Figure 11-2). Daily behavior is largely based on the way each aspect of life is understood. Through socialization, individuals learn how to gather information, assign meaning, and react to situations in a way that satisfies needs. Decision-making and action-taking processes are influenced by the meanings ascribed by a group's **reality norms**. Individuals look to others to reinforce or to challenge and correct their ideas of what is real. Groups serve to examine the life situations confronting individuals. As individuals gather information, attempt to understand that information, make decisions, and consider the facts and their implications, they can take responsible action, not only in relation to themselves and their group but also for the community. Group (task, maintenance, and reality) norms combine to form a **group culture**. Although working with a group does not mean dictating its norms, the nurse can support helpful rules, attitudes, and behaviors. Norms form when rules, attitudes, and behaviors become part of the life of the group, independent of the nurse. Reality norms influence each member to see relevant situations in the same way the other members see them. For example, suppose a group of individuals with diabetes defines an uncontrolled diet as harmful; members may try to influence one another to maintain diet control. The nurse's role in this group is to provide accurate information about diet and the disease

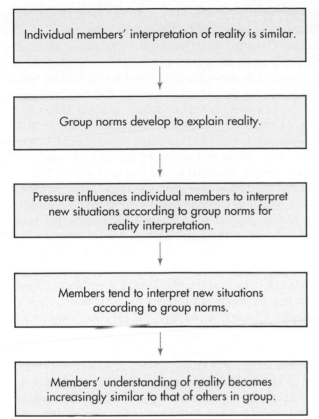

FIGURE 11-2 Influence of group reality norms on individual members.

process while continually displaying a belief that health through diet control is attainable and desirable.

When group members have similar backgrounds, their scope of knowledge may be limited. For example, women in a spouse abuse group may believe that men are exploitive and harmful based on their common childhood and marriage experiences. Such a stereotypical view of men could be reinforced by similar perceptions in other members; this might lead to continuing anger, fear of interactions with men, and a hostile or helpless approach to family affairs. Nurses or group members who have known men in loving, helpful, and collaborative ways can describe their different and positive perceptions of men, thereby adding information and challenging beliefs. The health and condition of members improve as their perceptions of reality are based on a more complete range of data. Nurses bring an important perspective to groups in which similar backgrounds limit the understanding and interpretation of personal concerns.

LEADERSHIP

Leadership is a complex concept. It consists of behaviors that guide or direct members and determine and influence group action. Positive leadership defines or negotiates the group's purpose, selects and helps implement tasks that accomplish the purpose, maintains an environment that

affirms and supports members, and balances efforts between task and maintenance. An effective leader pays attention to member communications and interactions as they unfold in the here and now. Attention to both spoken words and body language provides continuous feedback to leaders and members. This attention alerts members to changing group needs and encourages them to take responsibility and pride in their own involvement. Leader directiveness in group processes improves group satisfaction and group performance (Peterson, 1997).

Leading may be concentrated in one or a few persons, or it may be shared by many. Generally, shared leadership increases productivity, cohesion, and satisfying interactions among members.

BRIEFLY NOTED

Leading community groups is best done when leaders have a degree of emotional intelligence, are aware of their own emotional skills, and modify strategies to meet the evolving needs of the group.

After initiating or establishing a group, nurses may facilitate leadership within and among members, frequently relinquishing central control and encouraging members to determine the ultimate leadership pattern for their group. In some settings and circumstances, a single authority seems necessary (e.g., when members have limited skills or limited time, or when groups say they are uncomfortable with shared responsibility for leading). A leadership style that shares leading functions with other group members is effective when there are many alternatives and issues of values and ethics are involved in the group's action. Leadership can be described as patriarchal, paternal, or democratic. Each style has a particular effect on members' interaction, satisfaction, and productivity. Groups may reflect one or a combination of styles.

A patriarchal or paternal style is seen when one person has the final authority for group direction and movement. Patriarchal leadership may control members through rewards and threats, often keeping them in the dark about the goals and rationale behind prescribed actions. Paternal leadership wins the respect and dependence of its followers by parent-like devotion to members' needs. The leader controls group movement and progress through interpersonal power. Patriarchal and paternal styles of leadership are authoritarian. These styles are effective for groups such as a disaster team in which immediate task accomplishment or high productivity is the goal. Group morale and cohesiveness are typically low under sustained authoritarian styles of leadership, and members may not learn how to function independently. Also, issues of authority and control may disrupt productivity if the group members challenge the power of the leader.

Democratic leadership is cooperative in nature and promotes and supports members' involvement in all aspects of decision making and planning. Members influence each other

---

Box 11-5	Examples of Group Role Behavior

- *Follower:* Seeks and accepts the authority or direction of others
- *Gatekeeper:* Controls outsiders' access to the group
- *Leader:* Guides and directs group activity
- *Maintenance specialist:* Provides physical and psychological support for group members (i.e., holds the group together)
- *Peacemaker:* Tries to reconcile conflict between members or acts in response to influences that disrupt the group process and threaten its existence
- *Task specialist:* Focuses or directs movement toward the main work of the group

---

as they explore goals, plan steps toward the goals, implement those steps, and evaluate progress.

GROUP STRUCTURE

Structure describes the arrangement of group parts as they combine to make up the group as a whole. A **communication structure** identifies message pathways and member participation in sending and receiving messages. It is important that the structure include people who actively receive and send messages and who serve as channels for messages. These "central" individuals influence the group because of their access to and control over communication flow. Communication and role structures are interrelated.

Role structure refers to the expected behaviors of members in relation to each other as the group interacts. The role assumed by each member serves a purpose in the life of the group. Leader, follower, task specialist, maintenance specialist, evaluator, peacemaker, and gatekeeper are examples of roles (Box 11-5). Members' roles in the group may be described by their predominant actions. Identification of communication patterns helps to determine roles because people occupying particular roles characteristically use certain kinds of communication.

A person occupying a gatekeeper's role controls outsiders' access to the group. Gatekeepers either facilitate or block communication between outsiders and group members. Identification of those in gatekeeper roles is crucial when established groups are used for community health. The gatekeeper usually confronts the nurse after beginning contacts are attempted. An invitation to communicate further with group members is extended only after the nurse and gatekeeper determine mutual benefits and possible risks from continued contact between the nurse and the group.

Group structure emerges from various member influences including the members' understanding and support of the group purpose. Nurses assess the group structure as it relates to goal accomplishment. Many groups also consider their own structure, assess its usefulness in relation to member comfort and productivity, and then plan for a different division of tasks that is agreeable to the whole.

CASE STUDY

Tammy Edwards' social history included being molested by her father when she was 12, her mother dying when she was 13, and then living with several foster families. Subsequently she dropped out of school (where she had been studying in the special education track), married, and was beaten by her first husband to the point that she was hospitalized. At 26, Ms. Edwards is remarried and expecting her third child. When the nurse, Mary Morgan, visited, she saw that the mother was caring, yet overwhelmed by the young children's behavior, and that the family was eating nonnutritious, convenience foods, despite not having much income. Ms. Edwards told Ms. Morgan that she wanted to be a good mother but thought that she was not. The nurse assessed that Ms. Edwards needed some education and support, since she did not have any family or friends to help her and few resources.

Ms. Morgan brought Ms. Edwards a children's cookbook that she had used to cook with her children when they were Ms. Edwards' children's ages. The nurse talked about how much fun it was to cook with children and to see them grow healthily from good nutrition. The cookbook gave Ms. Edwards an age-appropriate activity to do with her children, as well as information on nutritious food for the family. Suggesting a children's cookbook for Ms. Edwards could have been seen as an insult had the nurse not combined learning to cook with a way to encourage productive activities with the children. When Ms. Morgan returned the next week, Ms. Edwards proudly reported on the several recipes she had cooked successfully with her children.

Created by Deborah C. Conway, Assistant Professor,
University of Virginia School of Nursing

PROMOTING HEALTH THROUGH GROUP EDUCATION

Health behavior is influenced by the groups to which people belong. Individuals live within a social structure of significant others such as family members, friends, co-workers, and acquaintances. The patterns and directions of everyday activities are learned in a family, and these are later reinforced or challenged by new groups. These groups constitute the context in which values, beliefs, and attitudes are formed; individuals usually consider the responses of others in all types of decisions regarding personal welfare.

Groups that will support a person's health changes are unavailable to some people because of their social or emotional isolation. Isolated individuals may have low self-esteem, be mentally ill, or occupy positions of low status in their family or community. They may be disadvantaged, gifted, or deviant, or they may simply live in a rural area or be engaged in solitary work. These individuals often benefit from newly organized groups established for specific purposes.

Although social support is basic to health, the absence of negative social interactions is equally important to well-being. Groups sometimes oppose health, i.e., friends who

Evidence-Based Practice

This study explored the opinions, behaviors, and expectations of nurse-facilitators and participants following a small-group health education program aimed at managing patient hypertension. As noted by the authors, effective blood pressure control is essential in the reduction of hypertension-related morbidity and mortality, and small group educational interventions were cited as having positive relationship outcomes for nurses and patients. In this study, patients failed to adopt health-enhancing behaviors. Additionally, the study revealed gaps in program expectations between nurses and their patients as well as lack of peer support felt by program participants. Although nurses and patients concurred on knowledge acquisition in managing hypertension, patients failed to mention intermediate health outcomes, such as behavior change, as their objective postprogram, whereas nurses saw this as a primary goal of the program. Thus, the authors suggest that the goals and purposes of such interventions be clarified in order to develop realistic expectations that are achievable (Leung et al, 2005). Lastly, both nurses and patients were dissatisfied with the lack of information about hypertensive medications provided by the program.

NURSE USE: Clear expectations and goals are essential to the success of small-group education. To prevent a mismatch in expectations and to organize those with similar backgrounds, a prior assessment of potential participants is encouraged by the authors.

From Leung CM et al: Small-group hypertension health education programme: a process and outcome evaluation, *J Adv Nurs* 52(6):631–639, 2005.

use addictive drugs. It may be impossible for an individual to quit drug use while associating with such friends. To effect a lasting change in behavior, an addicted person needs support and new friends who do not abuse drugs. Through participation with others, meaning is confirmed, confounded, contradicted, or compromised. This is how social reality is created. Within groups, people believe or are encouraged to believe in their created, shared realities (Goldberg and Middleman, 1997).

CHOOSING GROUPS FOR HEALTH CHANGE

Nurses may use groups to help individuals within a community after studying the overall needs of the community and its people. Such a study is based on client contacts, expressed concerns from various community spokespersons, health statistics for the area, available health resources, and the community's general well-being. These data point to the community's strengths and critical needs. Just as other nursing interventions are based on the assessment of needs and knowledge of effective treatment, group formation is determined by the assessment of priority community needs for individual health change.

At times nurses work with existing groups, and at other times they form new groups. Initiation of change and recruitment of a nurse may come not just from the nurse but from individuals, the affected groups, or a related organization. A decision about whether to work in established groups or to begin new ones is based on the clients' needs, the purpose of existing groups, and the membership ties in existing groups.

ESTABLISHED GROUPS

Some of the advantages to using **established groups** for individual health change are:
- Membership ties already exist.
- The existing structure can be used.
- It is not necessary to find new members because compatible individuals already form a working group.
- Established groups often have operating methods that have been successful; an approach for a new goal is built on this history.
- Members are aware of one another's strengths, limitations, and preferred styles of interaction.
- Members' comfort levels, stemming from their experience together, help them focus on the new goal.

Established groups have a strong potential for influencing members. Ties between members often are enhanced by successful group work. Their bonds are usually multidimensional because of the length of time they have spent together. Such rich ties support group change efforts for individuals' health.

Before deciding to work with particular established groups, the nurse must judge if introducing a new focus is compatible with existing group purposes. In some cases individual health goals will enhance existing group purposes, and the nurse is an important resource for bringing information for health, behavior, and group process.

How can the nurse enter existing groups and direct their attention to individual health needs? One nurse employed by an industrial firm noted the harmful effect of managerial stress on several individuals. They had elevated blood pressure, stomach pain, and emotional tension. The nurse learned that the employees with stress were all members of a jogging team that met weekly for conversation in addition to regular workouts. High-level health had been a value shared by all team members, but although jogging was seen as an enjoyable and health-promoting activity, they had never talked about a shared purpose for improved health. In this circumstance the nurse saw a need for stress reduction, thought that the individuals at risk could achieve stress reduction if supported through a group process from valued friends, and proposed that a new purpose be added to the jogging team's activities. All in the group readily accepted this.

SELECTED MEMBERSHIP GROUPS

If it is not desirable or possible to use existing groups, then select members for a new group. Some groups form because of a similar health concern. For instance, individuals with diabetes can meet to discuss diet management and physical care and to share problem-solving remedies, community residents can meet for social support and rehabilitation after treatment for mental illness, or isolated older adults can meet to socialize and eat nutritious meals.

Be sure to consider members' attributes when assembling a new group. Members are attracted to others from similar backgrounds, with similar experiences, and with common interests and abilities. Individual behavior is influenced not only by the membership, purpose, attraction, norms, leadership, and structure of the group, but also by those processes remembered from other valued group memberships. It is important to select members so that common ties or interests balance out dissimilar traits.

When the nurse is able to arrange it, the membership for selected groups should contain one or more individuals with expressive and problem-solving skills and others who are comfortable in supportive roles. People have varying degrees of competence in task and maintenance functions. Support and training for group effectiveness within the unit build cohesion.

The size of the group influences effectiveness; generally, 8 to 12 is a good number for group work focused on individual health change. Groups of up to 25 members can be effective when their focus is on community needs. Large groups often divide and assign tasks to smaller subgroups, with the original large groups meeting less frequently for reporting and evaluation.

Setting member criteria can facilitate recruitment and selection of the most appropriate members for any group. The criteria usually suggest a mixture of member traits, allowing for balance for the processes of decision making and growth.

BRIEFLY NOTED

A group is often more valuable to members when the group's purpose is clearly stated and mutually adopted by members.

BEGINNING INTERACTIONS

As soon as the group forms, begin to work on the purpose of the group. First, clarify both individual and group goals. Members vary in their degree of openness about themselves and their backgrounds. They may begin by seeking and giving information about themselves and move toward problem solving. The role of the nurse is to:
- Support ideas and feelings
- Invite participation
- Give information
- Seek and provide clarification
- Suggest structure

Subsequent steps are then planned according to the skill of the nurse and the composition of the group. Early in the process the nurse can help members interact with a degree of satisfaction. This requires close attention to maintenance tasks of attending, eliciting information, clarifying, and recognizing contributions of members. Attending includes simple responses to people such as listening carefully and observing their dress, mood, and nonverbal actions. A first step might be asking what brought each of them to the group.

Be sure to encourage member-to-member exchanges and recognize and support members when they assume leadership functions. Even in beginning sessions, roles and a structure for the new group begin to take shape. Members try out familiar roles and test their individual abilities. Those approaches to member support, leadership, and decision

---

Box 11-6	**Core Competencies for Communication Skills**

Communication Skills
- Communicates effectively in writing, words, and other ways
- Seeks input from individuals and organizations
- Advocates for public health programs and resources
- Leads and participates in groups to address specific issues
- Uses the media, advanced technologies, and community networks to communicate information
- Effectively presents accurate demographic, statistical, programmatic, and scientific information for professional and lay audiences

Attitudes
- Listens to others in an unbiased manner
- Respects the points of view of others
- Promotes the expression of diversion opinions and perspectives

From the Council on Linkages between Academia and Public Health Practice: *Core competences for public health professionals,* Washington, DC, Public Health Foundation. Retrieved June 12, 2008, from www.trainingfinder.org/competencies/list_nolevels.htm.

---

making that are comfortable and productive become normative ways for the group to work. The nurse helps by creatively evaluating the appropriateness of style and productivity of roles. The work of the group is begun even as the goals for health change are examined carefully and are realistically accepted. During this early period, members' attractions to one another and to the group begin to develop. The core competency skills for communication recommended by the Public Health Foundation are useful to nurses engaged in group work in the community. Box 11-6 lists these competencies. Subsequent steps are then planned not only according to the nurse's skill and preference but also according to the group composition and the skills brought by members.

CONFLICT

Conflict occurs normally in all human relations. However, people generally see conflict as the opposite of harmony and try to guard against it. This is an unfortunate view because the tensions of difference and potential conflict actually help groups work toward their purposes. Understanding common causes of conflict, conflict management approaches, and conflict resolution models is especially important during times of challenges to health and health care systems and increasingly violent expressions of community conflict.

Conflict occurs when group members feel obstructed or irritated by one or more other group members (Northen and Kurland, 2001). Conflict signals that antagonistic points of view must be considered and that it is necessary to reexamine beliefs and assumptions underlying relationships. Some people are concerned about security, control of self and others, respect between parties, and access to limited resources. In groups, members may express frustrations about trust, closeness and separation, and dependence and independence.

These themes of interpersonal conflict operate to some extent in all interactions and are not unique to groups. Within a group, because members are working toward a common purpose, such issues are important and responding to them appropriately encourages personal growth and the examination of frustrations in the group.

People tend to repeat the same patterns of behavior in conflicts. Sometimes the pattern works; other times it does not. The best approach is to match the response style to the situation (Sportsman and Hamilton, 2007). This requires personal awareness as well as awareness of those involved in the conflict. Specifically, when you respond to conflict by avoidance, forcing with power, capitulation, or excluding a member, the behaviors fail to satisfy the concerns of those involved. Assertiveness (attempting to satisfy one's own concerns) and cooperativeness (attempting to satisfy the concerns of others) are two potentially positive dimensions of response to conflict. Behaviors that reflect either assertiveness or cooperativeness and also potentially may satisfy the frustrated parties include confrontation, competition, compromise, reconciliation, and collaboration. Resolving conflict within groups depends on open communication among all parties, diffusion of negative feelings and perceptions, concentration on the issues, and use of fair procedures and a structured approach to the process.

Conflict can be overwhelming, especially when members view the expression of controversy as unacceptable or unremitting. Conflict suppressed over time tends to build up and finally explode out of proportion to the current frustration. A group that repeatedly avoids expressing conflict becomes fragile, unable to adapt, and helpless in facing challenges. Conflict may be destructive if contentious parties fail to respect the rights and beliefs of others or ignore commonly accepted standards of civility.

Approaches for conflict-acknowledging and problem-solving situations that respect others and represent self-concerns are first learned in families and other small groups. These lessons teach people to see conflict as a natural occurrence that supports growth and change. Other people learn to avoid conflict or to disregard others in the promotion of self. Teams that embrace a united desire for harmony to the extent of avoiding conflict in interactions may hinder collaboration and personal growth (Gerow, 2001). A useful way to deal with a conflict is through collaboration and cooperation in mutually beneficial problem-solving (Sportsman and Hamilton, 2007). Using collaboration as a tool for conflict resolution requires time and energy. Also, it may be useful to have a neutral party help those involved in the conflict move toward understanding one another's point of view and work toward a solution that will at least be tolerable for the involved parties. People often forget that when working with others, it is almost impossible to always get your own way.

STRATEGIES FOR CHANGE

Nurses can help groups meet established health goals through their knowledge of health and health risks for individuals, groups, and communities. Skill in problem solving for change is essential for accomplishing health goals. Change, whether welcome or not, is disruptive to the client. Even though moving from a familiar way of being and interacting with others is uncomfortable (and resisted), all human systems do change over time because of development within the system and adaptation to outside stimuli. A change for one person in a group affects each other member. Change creates an opportunity for learning that is more than mastery of new information and identification of appropriate adjustment resources.

Healthful change requires knowledge, practice of new skills, examination of attitudes and values about the change, and adjustment of roles in your personal group or network. Helping people accomplish needed changes is ideally done in a small-group context.

Basic teaching helps members understand the known associations among environment, body response, wellness, and pathological states that are pertinent to desired changes. Together, group members focus on the reality of the problems and ways to understand them. A group reaches its full potential for effecting individual change when members work actively and directly through discussion and other approaches to problem solving. Teaching is an appropriate method to use in expectant-parent groups. Participants need to understand facts about pregnancy, labor and delivery, self-care, infant care, parenting, and adjustment to change. They also need to practice the new skills that will be required and examine their attitudes and emotional responses to the anticipated family changes. Specific learning activities include diaper changes, swaddling, feeding, and bathing the baby. Often members can provide tips to others in the group based on what works for them. Some will have babysitting experience or care of siblings that they can share with group members.

Group support may help people make needed changes for health that they are unable to accomplish on their own or with the help of just one individual. Skillful use of group methods can help a person analyze the problem, sustain motivation for change, support the client during vulnerable periods, and provide quick interpersonal feedback for success and failure. The discomfort associated with change can be reduced through the relationships with others in beneficial groups. Most of the *Healthy People 2010* priorities may be addressed in health promotion and disease prevention groups in which individuals learn healthier behaviors and gain support from others in changing from risky to healthy lifestyle choices. For example, groups may support physical activity and fitness, sound nutrition, and safe sexual practices. Through group support, individuals may conquer smoking, drug abuse, or abusive relationship problems. They may identify and reduce exposure to environmental hazards and promote safer physical settings for all.

EVALUATION OF GROUP PROGRESS

Evaluation of individual and group progress toward health goals is important. Action steps toward the goal are identified early in the planning stage. These small steps may be responses to learning objectives (listed action steps designed to support facilitative forces and deal with resistive forces), or they may reflect the group's problem-solving plan. The action steps and the indicators of achievement are discussed and written in a group record. Recognition of accomplishments in the group and of the group is built into the group's evaluation system. Recognition may include concrete rewards such as special foods and drinks, or it may be the personal expression of joy and member-to-member approval. Celebration for group accomplishments marks progress, rewards members, and motivates each person to continue.

COMMUNITY EDUCATION AND ITS CONTRIBUTION TO COMMUNITY LIFE

Each community consists of related and integrated parts. These components fit within the community according to residents' beliefs and definitions of who belongs there, who is included within an organization or group, and how they relate to each other. Community organizations include service sectors, neighborhood sectors, and professional, social, employment, worship, and cultural associations. Community components reflect the major social institutions of society: economy, government, family, education, religion, and medicine (Renzetti and Curran, 2000).

An understanding of group concepts provides a starting point for identifying community groups and describing how they function as components of the community. Because individuals develop, refine, and change their ideas within the context of the groups to which they belong, groups are vital to community well-being. Groups help identify community health concerns and are important in the management of interactions within the community and between the community and the larger society.

Community groups may be informal or formal. Formal groups have a defined membership and a specific purpose. They may or may not have an official place in the community's organization. In informal groups, the ties between members are multiple, and the purposes are unwritten yet understood by members. Informal groups can be identified through interviews with key spokespersons. Information about when and why they gather is learned through interviews or by observing gatherings to which the nurse is invited. Informal groups are often featured in the news when they are distinguished for community action or service. Formal groups can usually be identified in a variety of community media with meetings announced and business reported publicly. Typically, residents willingly describe the informal and formal groups in their communities after they learn the nurse's purpose for entering and studying their community. Nurses have traditionally facilitated linkages or initiated new ones between community groups (Schulte, 2000). See the "How To" box for information on how to initiate and conduct group work in the community setting.

Community residents' interactions across groups influence the overall harmony and free exchange in the community. When citizens experience threats to community well-being, they seek others with similar concerns to collectively explore the problem and consider relevant action. Citizens use focal concern groups to address perceived threats to community well-being.

HOW TO	Initiate and Conduct Group Work in the Community Setting

Example: Group work to address disease prevention through a community agency

Purposes for Group Members
1. To increase awareness of common risks to health
2. To improve health through problem solving
3. To foster health promotion behaviors

Planning and Implementation Steps
1. Seek consultation from community agency staff about priority health concerns and interests of the population that the agency serves.
2. Determine times when members can meet, when meetings can be held, and standards and procedures related to working within the agency.
3. Select a health-focused topic of interest. Develop a teaching plan; submit the plan to a designated agency contact for information and approval.
4. Market group teaching through a variety of strategies. Make the purpose, benefits to members, and length, place, and time of the meeting clear in the recruitment. Group members may volunteer, be referred, or be selected through leaders' interviews. The number should be limited to 10 to 15 members per group.
5. Meet with the group at designated times. Stick to the teaching plan; submit needed revisions to the agency contact.
6. Record and evaluate the process and outcome of group teaching. Keep a meeting journal.
7. Keep the agency staff up to date on progress throughout the group meeting block of time.
8. Meet with agency staff for a summary report of the group project; make recommendations for continued teaching or other health-focused follow-up for members.
9. Write a summary report.

Focal concern groups provide a context through which persons influence and are influenced by the community.

Nurses have a historical role and acceptance in communities. Nurses are in a privileged position to work with and assist community groups as they respond to actual and potential threats to their health (Powell, 1999). For example, when populations are exposed to environmental toxins, nurses provide information and links to information and they encourage community groups to organize and address such threats.

The nurse identifies goals for the community and for various groups through media reports, from community informants, and from local archives. These goals report resources and visions for change as perceived by the people living and working in the local community. Data may be organized according to the opinions and behaviors of the identified groups. Such information about community groups and assessment data are used with community representatives to plan desired interventions. Community working alliances or coalitions unite diverse groups that share a common interest in perceived threats to community health. Nurses and other professionals are active in groups formed to address community issues. Groups are both units of community analysis and vehicles for change.

Extensive research has been done on the hazardous effects of tobacco use. More recently, attention has focused on the harmful effects of secondhand smoke (SHS). A growing body of research supports best practices for eliminating SHS. This article describes the evaluation and outcomes of a community-based coalition in the Midwest that used such practices to educate the public and change attitudes about SHS, thereby promoting social policy change for tobacco-free environments. The evaluation model used in the study incorporated evidence-based indicators as measures for coalition goal achievement and found the best practices program to be effective for eliminating exposure to SHS.

NURSE USE: This study brought together a number of different elements to create a conceptual framework that could evaluate the community coalition's efforts to combat SHS. The usage of local data coupled with this framework created a roadmap for researchers to follow as they continue to evaluate the program and examine issues such as SHS-related health effects and the economic outcomes associated with SHS. This unique approach could be a useful model for other researchers seeking to evaluate similar programs.

From Cramer M, Roberts S, Xu L: Evaluating community-based programs for eliminating secondhand smoke using evidence-based research for best practices, *Family Commun Health* (30):129–143, 2007.

Small groups can influence and change the larger social community of which they are a part. The social system depends on groups for governing, making policy, determining community needs, taking steps to alleviate those needs, and evaluating program outcomes. The small group is a mechanism for interrelatedness between community subsystems, certain subsystems and their counterparts in the larger social structure, and factions within subsystems. Change in the composition and function of strategic small groups may produce change for the wider social system that depends on small groups for direction and guidance (Benne, 1976). See the "Evidence-Based Practice" box for suggestions about how to use a coalition.

WORKING WITH GROUPS TO MEET COMMUNITY HEALTH GOALS

Nurses use their understanding of group principles to work with community groups to make needed health changes. The groupings appropriate for this work include both established, community-sanctioned groups and groups for which nurses select members representing diverse community sectors.

Existing community groups formed for community-wide purposes such as elected executive groups, health-planning groups, better business clubs, women's action groups, school boards, and neighborhood councils are excellent resources for community health assessment, because part of their ongoing purpose is to determine and respond to community needs. In addition, they are already established as part of the community structure. When a group representing one community sector is selected for community health intervention,

the total community structure is studied. Groups reflect existing community values, strengths, and normative forces.

How might nurses help established groups to work toward community goals? The same interventions recommended for groups formed for individual health change can be used for groups focused on community health. Such interventions include the following:

- Building cohesion through clarifying goals and individual attraction to groups
- Building member commitment and participation
- Keeping the group focused on the goal
- Maintaining members through recognition and encouragement
- Maintaining member self-esteem during conflict and confrontation
- Analyzing forces affecting movement toward the goal
- Evaluating progress

When nurses enter established groups, they need to assess the leadership, communications, and normative structures. This facilitates group planning, problem solving, intervention, and evaluation. The steps for community health changes parallel those of decision making and problem solving in other methodologies.

Case Example: *A nurse was asked to meet with a neighborhood council to help members study and "do something about" the number of homeless living on the streets. Residents knew this nurse from a local clinic and from his consulting work at a shelter for the homeless in an adjacent community. When the council invited him, they stated that "our intent is to be part of the solution rather than part of the problem." The nurse accepted the invitation to visit. He learned that the neighborhood council had addressed concerns of the neighborhood for 20 years—protecting zoning guidelines, setting up a recreational program for teens, organizing an after-school program for latchkey children, and generally representing the homeowners of the area. The neighborhood was composed of low-income families who took great pride in their homes. After meeting with the council and listening to their description of the situation, the nurse agreed to help, and he joined the council.*

As the first step in addressing the problem, the council conducted a comprehensive problem analysis of the homeless situation. All known causes and outcomes of homeless persons on the street were identified, and the relationships between each factor and the problem were documented from literature and from the local history. The nurse brought expertise in health planning and knowledge of the homeless and their health risks. He suggested negotiation between the council and the local coalition for the homeless, recognizing that planning would be most relevant if homeless individuals participated. The council was cohesive and committed to the purpose, had developed working operations, and did not need help with group process. They made adjustments in their usual group operation to use the knowledge and health-planning skills of the nurse. Interventions for the homeless included establishing temporary shelters at homes on a rotating basis, providing daily meals through the city council or churches, and joining the area coalition for the homeless.

This example shows how an established, competent group addressed a new goal successfully by building on existing strengths in partnership with the nurse. Community groupings, because of their interactive roles, are logical and natural ways for people who work together for community health change. As the decision-making and problem-solving capabilities of community groups are strengthened, the groups become more able representatives for the whole community. Nurses improve the community's health by working with groups toward that goal. Since many of the skills used in working with groups in the community require educational strategies, issues related to teaching and learning are discussed in the next sections.

EDUCATIONAL ISSUES

In planning educational programs for individuals and groups, consider three important issues: (1) different populations of learners require different teaching strategies; (2) educators need to be prepared to overcome barriers to learning; and (3) educators need to consider how to use technological advances in their educational programs appropriately.

POPULATION CONSIDERATIONS

Nurses working in community health need to use educational skills effectively. The increase in populations of varying cultural and ethnic backgrounds and the aging of baby boomers require that community health education be pertinent to different age-groups, different cultural groups, and groups with varying levels of literacy, especially health literacy.

Children, adults, and older adults have different learning needs and respond to different educational strategies. In each age group, nurses need to realize that learners vary in the following three ways (Knowles, Holton, and Swanson, 2005):
1. By cognitive ability, each person has different innate intellectual abilities
2. By personality, people need different amounts of encouragement and support
3. By prior knowledge, participants have previously learned different amounts of information on a health topic

The learning strategies for children and individuals with little knowledge about a health-related topic are characterized as **pedagogy.** The learning strategies for adults, older adults, and individuals with some health-related knowledge about a topic are called **andragogy** (Table 11-2). Each model has useful elements (Knowles, Holton, and Swanson, 2005). For example, when learners are dependent and entering a totally new content area, they may require more pedagogical experiences. In addition to considering the age of the population to be educated, nurses think about the learning needs of the population and use the pedagogical and andragogical principles that will best meet these needs.

When educating children, provide educational programs suited to their developmental abilities. The following age-specific strategies may help the nurse tailor educational programs for children (Whitener, Cox, and Maglich, 1998). Use concrete examples and word choices for young children. For example, the nurse might tell a group of 3-year-old children that brushing

Table 11-2	**Pedagogy versus Andragogy**
Pedagogy	**Andragogy**
Learners need to know that they must learn what the instructor teaches.	Learners need to know why they need to learn something before undertaking it.
Learners depend on teachers to teach them.	Learners seek self-direction.
Learners' experience is of little value as a resource for learning.	Learners have a variety of life experiences that need to be incorporated into learning experiences.
Learners need to be ready to learn when the teacher tells them they are ready.	Learners become ready to learn the things that they need to know to cope effectively with real-life situations.
Learners have a subject-centered orientation to learning.	Learners have a life-centered or problem-centered orientation to learning.
Learners are motivated to learn by external motivators such as grades.	Learners are motivated to learn by intrinsic motivators such as a sense of satisfaction.

Modified from Knowles MS, Holton III EF, Swanson RA: *The adult learner: the definitive classic in adult education and human resource development,* ed 6, San Diego, Calif, 2005, Elsevier; Palazzo M: Teaching in crisis: patient and family education in critical care, *Crit Care Nurs Clin North Am* 13(1):83-92, 2001.

their teeth twice a day is good to do. When discussing health promotion activities such as brushing teeth with 10-year-old children, the nurse might explain to them the benefits of brushing their teeth and the risks of not brushing and discuss issues such as the care of teeth if they wear braces. A group of students used skits to demonstrate to children in a migrant farm workers camp the importance of good health behaviors such as brushing teeth, eating proper foods, and getting adequate sleep.

The use of objects with children increases their attention. This is especially true when they can interact with the objects. For example, when teaching a group of children with asthma how to use inhalers, it is better to hand out inhalers to each participant and have them practice proper technique with the inhalers than it is to give them a handout with instructions or to demonstrate how to use an inhaler while they observe.

Incorporating repetitive health behaviors into games helps children retain knowledge and acquire skills. For example, singing songs while acting out healthy activities such as washing hands before eating helps children develop the habit of washing their hands and makes this health promotion behavior fun.

Populations Based on Culture
As discussed in Chapter 5, the cultural makeup of the United States is changing. Culture influences family structure and interactions and views about health and illness. These demographic changes present new challenges. Nurses must understand the health belief systems of the ethnic populations they serve. They also need to be familiar with populations that are prone to develop certain health problems. Multilinguistic

presentations of health education seminars and written materials need to be available to provide culturally competent health education (Go, 1998; Palazzo, 2001).

For example, in a rural area, a large number of Mexican migrant crop workers may attend health education programs. Knowing that this Spanish-speaking group is more likely to have tuberculosis (TB) than are other segments of the community, nurses may visit the migrant worker camp to present information on TB, such as prevention, symptoms, early diagnosis, and treatment. An interpreter may accompany the nurses and provide oral content in Spanish. Written handouts should be in Spanish and designed to be read and understood on a second-grade or third-grade reading level. Posters and pictures may also convey the message. Try to avoid using complex health terms and verify with the listeners that they do understand what you are saying.

BARRIERS TO LEARNING

Barriers to learning fall into two broad categories one having to do with the educator and the other having to do with the learner.

Educator-Related Barriers

Some common educator-related barriers to learning, together with strategies to minimize each barrier, follow. Educators may be affected as follows (Knowles, Holton, and Swanson, 2005):

- *Fear public speaking.* Strategies to minimize fear include being well prepared, using icebreakers, acknowledging the fear, and practicing in front of a mirror or video camera or with a friend.
- *Think that they are not credible with respect to a certain topic.* Strategies to increase confidence include preparing for the talk and learning about the topic, not apologizing for not being an expert. Convey the attitude of an expert and share personal and professional backgrounds.
- *Have a limited number of professional experiences related to a health topic.* Strategies to deal with this obstacle are to share personal experiences; share the experiences of others; and use analogies, illustrations, or examples from movies or famous people.
- *Have to deal with difficult people who need to learn health-related information.* One strategy that may help with handling difficult learners is to confront the problem learner directly. Other strategies include using humor, using small groups to foster participation of timid people, asking disruptive people to give others a chance to speak or, if this fails, asking them to leave, and circumventing dominating behavior, thereby enabling everyone to participate.
- *Not knowing how to get participation.* Strategies to foster participation include asking open-ended questions, inviting participation, and planning small-group activities whereby a person responds based on the group not his or her own information.
- *Be concerned about timing a presentation so that it is not too long and not too short.* Strategies to be sure that the length of the presentation is appropriate include planning well and practicing the presentation.

- *Feel uncertain about how to adjust instruction.* Strategies that can help the educator adjust instruction include knowing the participants' needs, requesting feedback, and redesigning during breaks.
- *Be uncomfortable when learners ask questions.* Strategies to help include anticipating questions, concisely paraphrasing questions to be sure that the question is correctly understood, and recognizing that it is appropriate to admit that you do not know the answer to a question.
- *Want to obtain feedback from learners.* Strategies to obtain feedback are to solicit informal feedback and to do program evaluations.
- *Be concerned about whether media, materials, and facilities will function properly.* Strategies include having equipment ready and knowing how it works, having backup plans, obtaining assistance, being prepared, visiting the facility in advance to practice using the equipment, and arriving early.
- *Have difficulty with openings and closings.* Strategies to foster successful openings and closings include developing a repertoire of openings and closings, memorizing the opening and closing, relaxing learners, concisely summarizing information, and thanking participants.
- *Be overly dependent on notes.* Useful strategies are using note cards or visual aids as prompts, and practicing.

Learner-Related Barriers

Two of the most important learner-related barriers are low literacy and lack of motivation to learn information and make needed behavioral changes.

LOW LITERACY INCLUDING HEALTH LITERACY LEVELS. Nurses often deal with individuals and populations who are illiterate or have low literacy levels. People who are functionally illiterate are often embarrassed to admit this to health care providers and educators. They may not ask questions to clarify information and may have problems understanding health education materials. The 2003 National Assessment of Adult Literacy (NAAL) was released in late 2005 and provided the first look at the literacy of America's adults in the twenty-first century. The 1992 National Adult Literacy Survey, the largest literacy assessment study that has been done in the United States, showed that 50% of Americans fell into the two lowest levels of literacy; the other 50% of Americans fell into the top three levels of literacy (levels 3, 4, and 5). Level 3 proficiency is the minimal standard needed to function in the workplace. This comprehensive survey, which goes beyond self-report of one's literacy, is now called the National Assessment of Adult Literacy. In 2003 the assessment instrument, designed to measure the literacy of American adults, was given to more than 19,000 adults ages 16 years of age and older. This instrument requires those taking it to perform tasks to demonstrate their health literacy. The definition used describes health literacy as the ability that a person has to access and understand health information that is necessary for health-related decision making (U.S. Department of Health and Human Services, 2000). This tool measured literacy in terms of *Below Basic, Basic, Intermediate,* and *Proficient.*

They found that the majority of adults (53%) had *Intermediate* health literacy; 12% were *Proficient,* 22% were *Basic,* and 14% had *Below Basic* levels of literacy. To summarize some of their findings: women had higher average health literacy than men; white and Asian/Pacific Islander adults had higher scores than black, Hispanic, American Indian/Alaska Native, and multiracial adults; and adults 65 years of age or older had lower average health literacy (Kutner et al, 2006).

Flaskerud (2007) found that even high school graduates had average reading levels of grade 6 or below. This issue of reading levels becomes more complex when cultural differences are present (see Chapter 5). In the United States a person's ability to understand and act on health care information and instructions is a stronger predictor of health status than age, income, employment, education, race or ethnicity. Most health information is printed at a tenth-grade reading level, yet the average U.S. adult reads at the eighth-grade level and 40% of adults over age 65 years read below the fifth-grade level (Health Literacy Innovations, 2007).

Although using pictures, computer and video presentations, and models to educate clients with low literacy is helpful, a focus on individual learning capacity is essential to understand the knowledge and beliefs of clients with low literacy and tailor educational programs to their needs. A series of educational sessions may be needed. At the first session, identify learning ability and provide a small amount of basic information. During later sessions, new information that builds on existing knowledge and skills is provided and evaluated. Additional information is not provided until the nurse is sure that knowledge and skills are understood and are being incorporated into learners' lives (Davis et al, 2002). In 2007, The Joint Commission, the accreditation agency for hospitals, and their affiliated agencies released a white paper called *'What Did the Doctor Say?' Improving Health Literacy to Protect Patient Safety.* This paper, which was consistent with the work of the 2003 National Assessment of Adult Literacy (2005) mentioned above, also recommended the following actions, which apply to the community as well as to in-patient encounters:

1. Make effective communication an organizational priority.
   - Train all staff to recognize and respond appropriately to patients with literacy and language needs.
   - Use well-trained medical interpreters for patients with low proficiency in English.
2. Address patient's communication needs across the continuum of care.
   - Use plain language and "teach back" techniques (have the person repeat what was taught to verify understanding).
   - Limit information to three important points.
   - Encourage people to ask questions.
   - Regularly place outreach calls to patients to ensure understanding of, and adherence to, the self-management regimen.
3. Pursue policy changes that promote improved practitioner-patient communications.
   - Refer persons with low literacy to adult learning centers.

- Expand the development of patient educational materials and programs (The Joint Commission, 2007).

LACK OF MOTIVATION. Some clients are not motivated to make behavioral changes; therefore, nurses need to understand the importance of motivating clients whom they seek to educate. Motivation is influenced by the following three factors (Dembo, 1994):

1. The value component (Why am I learning this?)
2. The expectancy component (Can I do this?)
3. The affective component (How do I feel about this?)

Learned helplessness occurs when individuals realize that, over time, they cannot control the outcome of events affecting their lives; there is no relation between effort and attainment of goals. Self-efficacy is individuals' evaluation of their performance capabilities related to a particular type of task. Motivation occurs when goal-directed behavior is initiated and sustained. Learners' beliefs about themselves in relation to task difficulty and outcome are important and influence self-efficacy. Strategies to increase motivation and self-efficacy include the following (Driscoll, 1994):

- Enhance relevance. The educator should explain how instruction relates to learners' goals and should build on learners' previous experiences.
- Build confidence. The educator should create positive expectations for success, provide opportunities for learners to successfully attain goals, and enable learners to exert control over their learning.
- Generate satisfaction. The educator should provide learners with opportunities to use newly acquired skills and should provide them with positive feedback.

TECHNOLOGICAL ISSUES

Many kinds of technologies such as computer games and programs, videos, CDs, and Internet resources can increase learning. These technologies may enable the learner to control the pace of instruction, offer flexibility in the time and location of learning, are engaging, provide immediate feedback, and may be more consistent with how the learner prefers to receive other kinds of information. See the "How To" box for information on how to produce videotapes for health education. Also, a computer-based educational program can be tailored to meet the needs of specific populations.

Increasingly, people rely on the Internet for health information. Although this is often a good source of information, people need to assess reliability. The following are some general questions to ask when evaluating health information on the web:

- What organization sponsors the website? Does the organization have a vested interest? For example, is the content of the website supported by political or marketing groups or is the site hosted by a health provider association?
- Is there a list of people who review information for the site? What are their credentials to do so?
- Are there links to other related sources?
- When was the site updated?

The Agency for Health Care Research and Quality has suggested the following criteria for assessing the quality of

HOW TO
Produce Videotapes for Health Education

Health education videos are a useful strategy for providing education in a low-cost, efficient manner. The following is a list of the steps needed to produce videotapes for health education:

1. Determine the need for a health education video on a specific topic.
2. Know the target audience, and involve them in the planning and production process.
3. Develop goals of the educational videotape, and know how these goals are going to be measured.
4. Identify stakeholders and key personnel who will be involved in the project.
5. Develop a budget, and find funding.
6. Develop a timeline for production.
7. Develop the script and information that will be included.
8. Make sure that the content is appropriate for the target audience. Consider the educational levels, cultural background, and age of the target audience.
9. Actively involve the production team.
10. Plan for the filming of the video.
11. Film the video.
12. When editing, add narration, music, and graphics.

Modified from Meade CD: Producing videotapes for cancer education: methods and examples, *Patient Educ* 23(5):837–846, 1996.

Internet health information (Assessing the Quality of Internet Health Information, 1999):

- *Authorship.* Are the authors and contributors, as well as their credentials and affiliations, listed?
- *Caveats.* Does the site clarify whether its function is to provide information or to market products?
- *Content.* Is the information accurate and complete, and is an appropriate disclaimer provided?
- *Credibility.* Does the site include the source, currency, relevance, and editorial review process for the information?
- *Currency.* Are dates that the content was posted and updated listed?
- *Design.* Is the site accessible, capable of internal searches, easy to navigate, and logically organized?
- *Disclosure.* Is the user informed about the purpose of the site and about any profiling or collection of information associated with using the site?
- *Interactivity.* Does the site include feedback mechanisms and opportunities for users to exchange information?
- *Links.* Have the links been evaluated according to back linkages, content, and selection?
  Clearly both lists have elements in common.

BRIEFLY NOTED

Since millions of Americans seek health information on the Internet, either instead of seeing their health care provider or in addition to doing so, be sure to encourage patients to tell you and other health care providers what they have read. Also instruct them in how to effectively evaluate what they read on the Internet.

THE EDUCATIONAL PROCESS

The five steps of the educational process (identify educational needs, establish educational goals and objectives, select appropriate educational methods, implement the educational plan, and evaluate the educational process), are discussed next.

IDENTIFY EDUCATIONAL NEEDS

Nurses perform systematic needs assessments to identify the health education needs of their clients (Bartholomew et al., 2000). This assessment is much like the nursing process in that you begin by (1) identifying what the client wants to know; (2) collecting data about learning needs, readiness and willingness to learn, and barriers to learning; (3) evaluating what you have learned to identify any cognitive, affective, or psychomotor learning needs; (4) think about ways to enhance the client's ability and motivation to learn; and (5) in collaboration with the client prioritize the learning needs. Factors that may influence clients' learning needs and their ability to learn are demographic, physical, geographic, economic, psychological, social, and spiritual (Babcock and Miller, 1994; Bartholomew et al, 2000).

Be sure to consider the learner's knowledge, skills, and motivation to learn. Sometimes it takes a frightening event such as a heart attack to motivate people to eat healthy foods and exercise regularly. Also identify resources for and barriers to learning. Resources include printed materials, equipment, agencies, and other individuals. Barriers include lack of time, money, space, energy, confidence, and organizational support (Rankin and Stallings, 1996). Some communication barriers can be avoided by paying close attention to how print materials are structured. Health Literacy Innovations (2007) provides 10 tips for print materials:

- Use an active voice and a conversational tone.
- Make the piece personal.
- Eliminate jargon, technical terms, or slang words.
- Avoid multisyllable words and use simple terms.
- Use a size of type that is readable to the average person such as 12 point for most and 14 point for older people.
- Use upper and lower case letters; all capital letters is hard to read.
- Use examples to show the desired behavior.
- Have plenty of white space.
- Choose ink that markedly contrasts with the color of the background.

ESTABLISH EDUCATIONAL GOALS AND OBJECTIVES

Once learner needs are determined, goals and objectives to guide the educational program must be identified. Goals are broad, long-term expected outcomes such as "Mr. Williams will be able to independently take care of his ostomy bag within 3 months." Goals should directly address the client's learning needs.

Table 11-3   The Four Elements of an Objective*

Element	Example
Who is expected to exhibit the behavior?	(a) Ms. Smith (b) Each member of the Jones family (c) 80% of the target population
What behavior is expected?	(a) will do breast self-examinations (b) will give an insulin injection to Billy (c) will take their children to receive immunizations
Conditions and qualifiers of the behavior	(a) correctly on the same day each month (b) with accuracy regarding the dosage and procedure (c) within 1 month of the immunization due date
Standards of the behavior or performance	(a) 100% of the time for 1 year (b) 100% of the time for 10 consecutive trials (c) for 100% of the standard childhood disease immunizations

Modified from Babcock DE, Miller MA: *Client education: theory and practice,* St. Louis, 1994, Mosby; Bartholomew LK et al: Watch, discover, think, and act: a model for patient education program development, *Patient Educ Couns* 39:253–268, 2000.
*Instructions: String all "a" phrases together to make one sentence for the first example. String all "b" phrases together for the second example, and all "c" phrases for the third.

BRIEFLY NOTED

Consider the target audience carefully when developing a community health education project. Determine educational needs, educational and literacy levels, cultural backgrounds, health beliefs, and what existing groups might be useful.

Objectives are specific, short-term criteria that must be met in order to achieve the long-term goal, such as "Within 2 weeks, Mr. Williams will properly reattach his own ostomy bag, after the nurse has cleaned the site, five consecutive times." Objectives are written statements of an intended outcome or expected change in behavior and should define the minimum degree of knowledge or ability needed by a client. Objectives must be stated clearly and defined in measurable terms (Bartholomew et al, 2000; Wolf, 2001). The four elements of an objective are listed in Table 11-3.

SELECT APPROPRIATE EDUCATIONAL METHODS

Choose educational methods that will lead to the efficient and successful accomplishment of program goals and objectives. The methods should be appropriately matched to the client's strengths and needs. Use complex designs with care. Try to choose a simple, clear, and succinct manner of presentation. A few examples of strategies that may be used to enhance learning are listed in Box 11-7.

Box 11-7   Strategies to Enhance Learning

- Audiovisual materials
- Brainstorming
- Case studies
- Computer-assisted learning
- Demonstrations
- Field trips
- Games
- Group participation
- Guest speakers
- Peer counseling and tutoring
- Peer presentations
- Printed materials
- Role plays
- Simulation

Modified from Dobbins KR: Applying learning theories to develop teaching strategies for the critical care nurse: don't limit yourself to the formal classroom lecture, *Crit Care Nurs Clin North Am* 13(1):1–11, 2001; Johnson PH, Kittleson MJ: A content analysis of health education teaching strategy/idea articles: 1970–1998, *J Health Educ* 31(5):282–298, 2000; Knowles M: *The adult learner: a neglected species,* ed 4, Houston, 1990, Gulf.

Box 11-8   How to Effectively TEACH Clients

Use the TEACH mnemonic, as follows:

Tune in. Listen before you start teaching. Client's needs should direct the content.
Edit information. Teach necessary information first. Be specific.
Act on each teaching moment. Teach whenever possible. Develop a good relationship.
Clarify often. Make sure your assumptions are correct. Seek feedback.
Honor the client as a partner. Build on the client's experience. Share responsibility with the client.

Modified from Hansen M, Fisher J: Patient-centered teaching from theory to practice, *Am J Nurs* 98(1):56–60, 1998.

Educators need to implement various strategies for different learning orientations: for example, activity-oriented learners enjoy participation; goal-oriented learners want to achieve a specific outcome; and learning-oriented learners enjoy learning new things. The following are some important skills for educators to develop (Knowles, Holton, and Swanson, 2005):
- Match media and other tools to the needs of the learner
- Be able to give examinations, deliver presentations, lead group discussions, organize role plays, provide feedback to learners, share case studies, and use media and materials
- Know the benefits of group teaching such as cohesiveness among members, increased number of clients seen, clients' learning from each other, and cost-effectiveness
- Use educational methods such as structuring content, organizing the instructional sequence, planning for the rate of delivery, identifying amounts of repetition, practicing, evaluating the results, and providing reinforcement and rewards (Box 11-8)

BRIEFLY NOTED

When developing a health education presentation, use assorted methods, involve the audience, and make sure the presentation fits the level of comprehension of the audience.

Also be sure to consider age, developmental disabilities, educational level, knowledge of the subject, size of the group, and the ability to access the information. For example, clients with a visual impairment may need more verbal description. Clients with hearing impairments may need increased visual material, and speakers or translators who can use sign language may be necessary. Also, if clients have limited spans of attention and concentration you may need to use creative methods and tools to keep the learner focused. Examples include frequent breaks; plain, nondistractive surroundings; small-group interactions that keep the learner involved and interested; and the use of hands-on equipment such as mannequins, models, and other materials that the learner can physically manipulate. The amount of learner involvement is often related to the comprehension and retention of the learner. Interactive strategies include discussion, games, and role playing. Noninteractive strategies include demonstrations, films, and lectures (Knowles, 1990).

People living in rural areas may find it hard to access health information. For this reason, technology-based delivery methods such as use of a videophone and other forms of telecommunication may help you individualize information for distant learners (Buckwalter et al, 2002).

IMPLEMENT THE EDUCATIONAL PLAN

After educational methods have been selected, the following suggestions can guide the implementation (Knowles, 1990):

- Maintain control over starting, sustaining, and stopping each method and strategy in the most effective and appropriate time and manner.
- Coordinate and control environmental factors, the flow of the presentation, and other contributory facets of the program.
- Keep the materials logically related to the core theme and overall program goals.
- Be flexible and modify methods and strategies to meet unexpected challenges such as time limitations, expense, administrative and political factors, and unanticipated learner needs.

EVALUATE THE EDUCATIONAL PROCESS

Evaluation is as important in the educational process as it is in the nursing process. Evaluation provides a systematic and logical method for making decisions to improve the educational program (Babcock and Miller, 1994). Educational evaluation involves three areas:

1. Educator evaluation
2. Process evaluation
3. Product evaluation

Educator and process evaluation are described next. Product evaluation is described later in the "Educational Product" section.

Educator Evaluation

Feedback helps the educator modify the teaching process and, if needed, find ways to better meet the learner's needs. Learner evaluation occurs continuously throughout the educational program and may come in writing such as in an evaluation sheet. Or feedback may be conveyed verbally or nonverbally, such as in return demonstrations or by facial expressions (Palazzo, 2001).

When evaluation reveals that the learning objectives are not being met, try to determine why the instruction is not effective. It is best to assume that inadequate learner responses reflect an inadequate program, not an inadequate learner. The educator is responsible for presenting the material creatively and meaningfully in new ways to increase learner retention and the ability to apply the new knowledge (Knowles, 1990). Ultimately, the educator is responsible for the success or failure of the educational process and the development of learner knowledge, skills, and abilities.

Process Evaluation

Process evaluation examines the dynamic components of the educational program. It follows and assesses the movements and management of the transfer of information and attempts to keep the objectives on track. Process evaluation is necessary throughout the educational program to determine whether goals and objectives are being met and the time required for their accomplishment. Ongoing evaluation also allows the teacher to correct misinformation, misinterpretation, or confusion (Palazzo, 2001).

Goals and objectives should be periodically reconsidered. Ask if the desired change in health behavior is really necessary. This question inevitably leads back to the original learning objectives and enables the nurse to rethink the practicality and merit of each of the objectives. Finally, factors that influence learner readiness and motivation should be reassessed if teaching seems to be ineffective. Process evaluation uses information gathered from the educator as well as from learner evaluations and assesses the dynamics of their interactions (Knowles, 1990).

THE EDUCATIONAL PRODUCT

The educational product is the outcome of the educational process. The product is measured both qualitatively and quantitatively (Krathwohl, Bloom, and Masia, 1964). For example, a qualitative assessment should answer the following question: "How well does the learner appear to understand the content?" A quantitative assessment should answer the following question: "How much of the content does the learner retain?" Thus the quality of the product is measured by improvement and increase, or the lack thereof, in the learner's knowledge, skills, and abilities related to the content of the educational program. Selected outcomes for the population of interest need to be identified when the educational program is conceived. Measurement of changes in these outcomes determines the effectiveness of the program (Babcock and Miller, 1994). The educational product is assessed as a measurable change in the health or behavior of the client.

A variety of approaches, methods, and tools can be used to evaluate health and behavioral changes. These include questionnaires, rating scales, surveys, checklists, skills demonstrations, testing, subjective client feedback, and direct observation of improvements in client mastery of materials (Babcock and Miller, 1994). Qualitative or quantitative strategies may be used, depending on the nature of the expected educational outcome. Evaluation of outcomes measured includes changes in knowledge, skills, abilities, attitudes, behavior, health status, and quality of life (Krathwohl, Bloom, and Masia, 1964). Approaches to evaluating health education effects will vary, depending on the situation. For example, when considering a client's ability to perform a psychomotor skill, such as changing a dressing, watching the person perform the skill is the most effective way to evaluate skill attainment.

When evaluation of the educational product shows positive changes in health status and health-related behaviors, you can expect good results in similar health educational programs. If evaluation of the educational product shows that either no changes or negative changes in health status and health-related behaviors resulted, examine and modify the process.

It is important to evaluate short-term health and behavioral effects of health education programs and to determine if they are really caused by the educational program. Short-term objectives are often easy to evaluate (Babcock and Miller, 1994). For example, a **short-term evaluation** of whether a client can perform a return demonstration of breast self-examination requires minimal energy, expense, or time; skill mastery can be determined within a matter of minutes. If the short-term objective is not met, the nurse determines why and identifies possible solutions so that successful learning can occur. If the short-term objective is met, then focus on long-term evaluation to assess the lasting effects of the education program—in this case, that of ongoing monthly breast self-examinations performed by the learner independently at home.

The ultimate goal of health education is to help people make lasting behavioral changes to improve their overall health status. Long-term follow-up is a challenging task. When clients make positive behavioral changes and their health status improves, they may no longer require the health care services of the nurse. Other reasons long-term evaluation can be challenging are listed in Box 11-9.

Long-term evaluation is geared toward following and assessing the status of an individual, family, community, or population over time. The tools of evaluation are designed to assess whether specific goals and objectives were met. Also, the extent and direction of changes in health status and health behaviors that the client has experienced are monitored (Babcock and Miller, 1994; Kleinpell and Mick, 2001).

Often, for nurse educators in community health, the goal of long-term evaluation is an analysis of the effectiveness of the education program for the entire community, not

---

Box 11-9   Long-Term Evaluation Is Challenging

Cooperation
Clients may show a lack of interest in their own health care.
   Clients may think that it is too time consuming or expensive to follow up.
   Clients may not keep scheduled appointments or return phone calls.

Time
Follow-up requires that the educator keep track of clients and locate those who have moved.
   Follow-up requires making phone calls, evaluating clients, and reviewing and analyzing the results of the evaluation.

Energy
The nurse must obtain the cooperation of clients.
   The nurse must balance long-term evaluation responsibilities with other demands.

Expense
Mail, phone calls, staff time, and travel are expenses related to long-term evaluation.

Modified from Kleinpell RM, Mick DJ: Evaluating outcomes. In Fulmer TT, Foreman MD, Walker M, editors: *Critical care nursing of the elderly,* ed 2, New York, 2001, Springer; Redman BK: Patient education at 25 years: where we have been and where we are going, *J Adv Nurs* 18(5):725, 1993.

---

the health status of a specific individual. Nurses track the achievement of community objectives over time but not that of individual community members. Thus, in a changing population, long-term evaluation of the results of an education program is still possible. The percentage of objectives and goals met by sampling the target population provides valid statistics for program assessment even though the population of individuals may have experienced a complete turnover (Kleinpell and Mick, 2001).

For example, a nurse sees that according to annual health department data, 60% of all pregnant women in the nurse's catchment area received some prenatal care. The nurse wanted to increase this percentage to 90%, so she tried an educational intervention in which radio and television stations made public service announcements about the importance and availability of prenatal services. After 1 year, the nurse discovered that 80% of all pregnant women received prenatal care. The nurse continued using public service announcements the next year, since the results were so good. However, the long-term goal of the education program to influence the behavior of 90% of the pregnant women in the community had not yet been met. Therefore the nurse asked volunteers to put informational posters in shopping malls, grocery stores, public transportation stops, laundries, and public transportation vehicles. In the second year after implementing the revised educational program the nurse used statistics from the health department and found that 95% of all pregnant women in the target area had received prenatal care. The nurse can next evaluate and modify a community educational program over time to increase the rate, range, and consistency of progress made toward meeting the long-term goals of the project.

CLINICAL APPLICATION

Kristi is working toward her Bachelor of Science in Nursing (BSN) degree in a community health practicum at a local health department. The health department has received several calls from people wanting information about anthrax, smallpox, and other potential weapons of biological warfare. For Kristi's community health intervention project, she decides to do a community education piece on this topic.

What is her best course of action?

A. *Develop a poster presentation to have on display at the health department.*

B. *Put together an educative pamphlet to mail to anyone calling with questions.*

C. *Work with the health department staff to develop a community forum-style presentation and information brochures on biological warfare weapons.*

D. *Develop an inservice program for health department staff on potential weapons of biological warfare so that they can provide accurate information to callers.*

Answer is in the back of the book.

REMEMBER THIS!

- Health education is a vital component of nursing, because the promotion, maintenance, and restoration of health rely on clients' understanding of health care topics.
- The nurse educator in the community identifies a learning need, selects aspects from the theories of learning, considers educational principles, examines educational issues, designs and implements an educational program, and evaluates the effects of the educational program on learning and behavior.
- The nurse often uses the *Healthy People 2010* educational objectives as a guide to identifying learning needs.
- Education and learning are different. Education is the establishment and arrangement of events to facilitate learning. Learning is the process of gaining knowledge and expertise and results in behavioral changes.
- The three domains of learning are cognitive, affective, and psychomotor. Depending on the needs of the learner, one or more of these domains may be important for the nurse educator to consider as learning programs are developed.
- Nine principles associated with instruction are gaining attention, informing the learner of the objectives of instruction, stimulating recall of prior learning, presenting the stimulus, providing learning guidance, eliciting performance, providing feedback, assessing performance, and enhancing the retention and transfer of knowledge.
- Principles that guide the effective educator include message, format, environment, experience, participation, and evaluation.
- Working with groups is an important skill for nurses.

- Groups are an effective and powerful way to initiate and promote health.
- A group is a collection of interacting individuals with a common purpose. Each one influences and is influenced by others in the group.
- Leadership is an important group concept; effective leaders are essential to highly functioning groups.
- Educational issues include population considerations, barriers to learning, and technological issues.
- The five phases of the educational process are identifying educational needs, establishing educational goals and objectives, selecting appropriate educational methods, implementing the educational plan, and evaluating the educational process and product.
- Evaluation of the product includes the measurement of short-term and long-term goals and objectives related to improving health and promoting behavioral changes.

WHAT WOULD YOU DO?

1. You need to develop an educational program to help a group of Hispanic Americans recently diagnosed with diabetes mellitus. What would be the six most important principles of health education for your work? How would you change your plan if you were working with a community in which adolescent cigarette smoking is on the rise or with families caring for an individual with Alzheimer disease? What different choices would you use for each population?

2. Recall an educational interaction that you had with each type of client (individual, family, community, and population) that did not seem to go well. For each type of client, and on the basis of educational principles, identify what might have been the problem. Develop a plan for ways in which the interaction could have been improved, again on the basis of educational principles.

3. Recall a learning experience in which either the message, format, environment, experience, participation, or evaluation was unsatisfactory. Then develop a plan for how the problem could have been overcome and turned from a negative or neutral learning situation into a positive one.

4. Select one of the *Healthy People 2010* educational objectives and design a population-specific education program to meet that objective. Include the educational principles, educational issues, educational process including teaching strategies, and evaluation procedures that you would use.

5. Consider the groups in which you are a member. What qualities make them successful? What are barriers to success? What role do you play in general?

■ REFERENCES

Assessing the Quality of Internet Health Information. Summary. Agency for Health Care Policy and Research, Rockville, Md, and Mitretek Systems, McLean, Va. Retrieved June 1999 from http://www.ahrq.gov/data/infoqual.htm.

Babcock DE, Miller MA: *Client education: theory and practice,* St. Louis, 1994, Mosby.

Bandura A: *Social foundations of thought and action: a social cognitive theory*, Englewood Cliffs, NJ, 1986, Prentice Hall.

Bartholomew LK et al: Watch, discover, think, and act: a model for patient education program development, *Patient Educ Couns* 39:253–268, 2000.

Benne KD: The current state of planned changing in persons, groups, communities, and societies. In Benne KD, Chin R, Carey KE, editors: *The planning of change*, New York, 1976, Holt, Rinehart & Winston.

Berman-Rossi T: Empowering groups through understanding stages of group development, *Social Work With Groups* 15(2-3): 239–255, 1992.

Bloom BS et al: *Taxonomy of educational objectives: the classification of educational goals—handbook 1: cognitive domain*, White Plains, NY, 1956, Longman.

Brandler S: *Group work: skills and strategies for effective intervention*, ed 2, New York, 1999, Haworth Press.

Buckwalter KC et al: Telehealth for elders and their caregivers in rural communities, *Fam Comm Health* 25(3):31–40, 2002.

Council on Linkages between Academia and Public Health Practice: Core competencies for public health professionals. Washington DC, Public Health Foundation. Retrieved June 12, 2008, from www.trainingfinder.org/competencies/list_nolevels.htm.

Cramer M, Roberts S, Xu L: Evaluating community-based programs for eliminating secondhand smoke using evidence-based research for best practices, *Fam Com Health* (30):129–143, 2007.

Davis TC et al: Health literacy and cancer communication, *Cancer* 52(3):134–153, 2002.

Dembo MH: *Applying educational psychology*, ed 5, White Plains, NY, 1994, Longman.

Dobbins KR: Applying learning theories to develop teaching strategies for the critical care nurse: don't limit yourself to the formal classroom lecture, *Crit Care Nurs Clin North Am* 13(1):1–11, 2001.

Driscoll MP: *Psychology of learning for instruction*, Boston, 1994, Allyn & Bacon.

Edelman CL, Mandle CL, editors: *Health promotion throughout the lifespan*, ed 6, St. Louis, 2006, Mosby.

Feinberg N: A study of group stages in a self-help setting, *Social Work with Groups* 3(1):41–50, 1980.

Flaskerud JH: Cultural competence column: what else is necessary? *Issues in Ment Health Nurs* 28(2):219–222, 2007.

Gerow SJ: Teachers in school-based teams: contesting isolation in schools. In Sockett HT et al, editors: *Transforming teacher education: Lessons in professional development,* Westport, Conn, 2001, Bervin & Garvey.

Go GV: Changing populations and health. In Edelman CL, Mandle CL, editors: *Health promotion throughout the lifespan*, ed 4, St Louis, 1998, Mosby.

Goldberg G, Middleman RR: Constructivism, power, and social work with groups. In Parry JK, editor: *From prevention to wellness through group work*, New York, 1997, Haworth Press.

Hansen M, Fisher J: Patient-centered teaching from theory to practice, *Am J Nurs* 98(1):56–60, 1998.

Health Literacy Innovations: *10 tips for print materials*. Press release, May 8, 2007. Retrieved Feb 22, 2008, from http://www.HealthLiteracyInnovations.com.

Johnson PH, Kittleson MJ: A content analysis of health education teaching strategy/idea articles: 1970-1998, *J Health Educ* 31(5):282–298, 2000.

Kelemen A: Wellness promotion: how to plan a college health fair, *Am J Health Studies* 17(1):31–36, 2001.

Kleinpell RM, Mick DJ: Evaluating outcomes. In Fulmer TT, Foreman MD, Walker M, editors: *Critical care nursing of the elderly*, ed 2, New York, 2001, Springer.

Knowles M: *The adult learner: a neglected species*, ed 4, Houston, 1990, Gulf.

Knowles MS, Holton III EF, Swanson RA: *The adult learner: the definitive classic in adult education and human resource development*, ed 5, San Diego, Calif, 2005, Elsevier.

Krathwohl DR, Bloom BS, Masia BB: *Taxonomy of educational objectives: the classification of educational goals—handbook 2: affective domain*, New York, 1964, David McKay.

Kutner M et al: The health literacy of today's adults: results from the 2003 national assessment of adult literacy, September 2006, U.S. Department of Education. Retrieved Feb 17, 2009, from http://www.nces.ed.gov/naal/related_pubs.asp.

Leung CM et al: Small-group hypertension health education programme: A process and outcome evaluation, *J of Adv Nurs* 52(6):631–639, 2005.

London M: Performance appraisal for groups: Models and methods for assessing group processes and outcomes for development and evaluation, *Consult Psychol J* 59(3):175–188, 2007.

Lyman S, Benedik JR: Health fairs: timetable, pitfalls, & burnout, *College Student J* 33(4):534, 1999.

Meade CD: Producing videotapes for cancer education: methods and examples, *Patient Educ* 23(5):837–846, 1996.

Musinski B: The educator as facilitator: a new kind of leadership, *Nurs Forum* 34(1):23–29, 1999.

Northen H, Kurland R: *Social work with groups*, ed 3, New York, 2001, Columbia University Press.

Palazzo M: Teaching in crisis: patient and family education in critical care, *Crit Care Nurs Clin North Am* 13(1):83–92, 2001.

Peterson RS: A directive leadership style in decision making can be both virtue and vice: evidence from elite and experimental groups, *J Personality Soc Psych* 72:1107, 1997.

Powell DL: Environmental justice. In Howard University Division of Nursing: *Environmental health and nursing: the Mississippi Delta project, a modular curriculum*, Atlanta, Ga, 1999, Agency for Toxic Substances and Disease Registry.

Rankin SH, Stallings KD: *Patient education: issues, principles, and practices*, ed 3, New York, 1996, Lippincott Williams & Wilkins.

Redman BK: Patient education at 25 years: where we have been and where we are going, *J Adv Nurs* 18(5):725, 1993.

Renzetti CM, Curran DJ: *Living sociology*, ed 2, Boston, 2000, Allyn & Bacon.

Schulte JA: Finding ways to create connections among communities: partial results of an ethnography of urban public health nurses, *Public Health Nurs* 17:3, 2000.

Sportsman S, Hamilton P: Conflict management styles in the health professions, *J Prof Nurs* 23(3):157–166, 2007.

The Joint Commission: What did the doctor say? *Improving health literacy to protect patient safety,* Oakbrook Terrace Ill, 2007. Retrieved Feb 22, 2008, from http://www.jointcommission.org/PublicPolicy/health_literacy.htm.

Tuckman BW: Developmental sequence in small groups, *Psychol Bull* 63(6):384–399, 1965.

Tuckman BW, Jensen M: Stages of small-group development revisited, *Group Org Studies* 2(4):419–427, 1977.

U.S. Department of Health and Human Services: *Healthy People 2010: understanding and improving health,* ed 2, Washington, DC: U.S. Government Printing Office, November 2000. Retrieved Jan 30, 2001, from http://www.health.gov/healthypeople/document/tableofcontents.htm and http://www.healthypeople.gov/document/html/volume1/11HealthCom.htm#_Toc490471359).

Whitener LM, Cox KR, Maglich SA: Use of theory to guide nurses in the design of health messages for children, *Adv Nurs Sci* 20(3):21–35, 1998.

Wilson SM, Peterson PL: *Theories of learning and teaching: what do they mean for educators?* Washington, DC, 2006, National Education Association.

Wolf MS: Patient education. In Fulmer TT, Foreman MD, Walker M, editors: *Critical care nursing of the elderly*, ed 2, New York, 2001, Springer.

PART IV

Issues and Approaches in Health Care Populations

Community Assessment and Evaluation

George F. Shuster

ADDITIONAL RESOURCES

These related resources are found either in the appendix at the back of this book or on the book's website at http://evolve.elsevier.com/stanhope/foundations.

Evolve Website

- Community Assessment Applied
- Case Study, with questions and answers
- Quiz review questions
- WebLinks, including link to *Healthy People 2010* website

Real World Community Health Nursing: An Interactive CD-Rom, second edition

If you are using this CD-ROM in your course, you will find the following activities related to this chapter:
- *Keys to the Community* in **Community as Client**
- *Community Assessment* in **Community as Client**
- *Assess a Real Community* in **Community as Client**

OBJECTIVES

After reading this chapter, the student should be able to:
1. Decide whether nursing practice is community oriented.
2. Understand selected concepts basic to community-oriented nursing practice: community, community client, community health, and partnership for health.
3. Compare the nursing process to community-oriented nursing practice.
4. Decide which methods of assessment, intervention, and evaluation are most appropriate in selected situations.
5. Develop a community-oriented nursing care plan.

CHAPTER OUTLINE

WHAT IS A COMMUNITY?
COMMUNITY AS CLIENT
The Community as Client and Partner in Nursing Practice
GOALS AND MEANS OF COMMUNITY-ORIENTED PRACTICE
Community Health
Healthy People 2010
Community Partnerships

COMMUNITY-FOCUSED NURSING PROCESS: AN OVERVIEW OF THE PROCESS FROM ASSESSMENT TO EVALUATION
Assessing Community Health
Identifying Community Problems
Planning for Community Health
Implementation in the Community
Evaluating the Intervention for Community Health
PERSONAL SAFETY IN COMMUNITY PRACTICE

KEY TERMS

aggregate: population or defined group.

change agent: nursing role that facilitates change in client or agency behavior to more readily achieve goals. This role stresses gathering and analyzing facts and implementing programs.

change partner: a nursing role that facilitates change in client or agency behavior to more readily achieve goals. This role includes the activities of serving as an enabler-catalyst, teaching problem-solving skills, and acting as an activist advocate.

community: people and the relationships that emerge among them as they develop and use in common some agencies and institutions and a physical environment.

community assessment: process of critically thinking about the community and getting to know and understand the community as a client. Assessments help identify community needs, clarify problems, and identify strengths and resources.

community health: meeting collective needs by identifying problems and managing interactions within the community and larger society. The goal of community-oriented practice.

community health problems: actual or potential difficulties within a target population with identifiable causes and consequences in the environment.

community health strengths: resources available to meet a community health need.

community-oriented practice: a clinical approach in which the nurse and community join in partnership and work together for healthful change.

community partnership: collaborative decision-making process participated in by community members and professionals.

confidentiality: information kept private, such as between the health care provider and client.

database: collection of gathered and generated data.

data collection: the process of acquiring existing information or developing new information.

data gathering: the process of obtaining existing, readily available data.

data generation: the development of data, frequently qualitative rather than numerical, by the data collector.

evaluation: provision of information through formal means, such as criteria, measurement, and statistics, for making rational judgments necessary about outcomes of care.

goals: the end or terminal point toward which intervention efforts are directed.

implementation: carrying out a plan that is based on careful assessment of need.

informant interviews: directed conversation with selected members of a community about community members or groups and events; a direct method of assessment.

interdependent: the involvement among different groups or organizations within the community that are mutually reliant upon each other.

intervention activities: means or strategies by which objectives are achieved and change is effected.

objectives: a precise behavioral statement of the achievement that will accomplish partial or total realization of a goal; includes the date by which the achievement is expected to be completed.

participant observation: conscious and systematic sharing in the life activities and occasionally in the interests and activities of a group of persons; observational methods of assessment; a direct method of data collection.

partnership: a relationship between individuals, groups, or organizations in which the parties are working together to achieve a joint goal. Often used synonymously with coalitions and alliances, although partnerships usually have focused goals, such as jointly providing a specific program.

problem analysis: process of identifying problem correlates and interrelationships and substantiating them with relevant data.

problem prioritizing: evaluating problems and establishing priorities according to predetermined criteria.

secondary analysis: analysis using previously gathered data.

setting for practice: the community.

surveys: method of assessment in which data from a sample of persons are reported to the data collector.

target of practice: population group for whom healthful change is sought.

value: ideas of life, customs, and ways of behaving that members of a society regard as desirable.

windshield survey: a community assessment, the motorized equivalent of a physical assessment for an individual; windshield refers to looking through the car windshield as the nurse in community health drives through the community collecting data.

In the past, nurses have viewed the community as a client and as a partner in improving the health status of its citizens. Since the days of Florence Nightingale and Lillian Wald, nurses have looked at what is going on in the communities and environments in which they found their clients. Florence Nightingale defined her community as war-torn Crimea and discovered that the lack of fresh air, sanitation, and hygiene was contributing to the illnesses of the soldiers. Lillian Wald found that the neighborhoods around the Henry Street Settlement were impoverished with poor housing conditions and sanitation, improper nutrition, and crowding contributing to the problems of new mothers and children. Both women became political activists, worked with the leaders in their communities, and even solicited help from their respective governments to help change the conditions for the individuals and families in their communities.

Although, in the past, nurses have sometimes viewed the community as a client, many community-oriented nurses have come to consider the community their most important client and, more recently, their partner (Anderson and McFarlane, 2004; Saunders, Greaney, and Lees, 2003; Westbrook and Schultz, 2000). This chapter clarifies community concepts and provides a guideline for nursing practice with the community client. The core functions of public health nursing include assessment, policy development, and assurance. A public and private group partnership called the *Council on Linkages Between Academia and Public Health Practice* (2001) has defined competencies for the core functions of public health practice (see Chapter 1 for more details). In the area of assessment, 11 competencies for the nurse and other health providers working in the community are listed (Box 12-1).

The nursing process from assessment through evaluation is used to promote community health. This process begins with **community assessment**, one of the core functions, which involves getting to know the community. It is a logical, systematic approach to identifying community needs, clarifying problems, and identifying community strengths and resources. This chapter provides the nurse with the knowledge necessary to develop the community assessment core competencies. Nurses in community health are interested in these concepts because they want to know how the community's health affects their individual, family, and group clients.

Box 12-1 Core Competencies for Public Health Professionals

Public health professionals should be able to do the following:
- Define a problem
- Determine appropriate uses and limitations of both quantitative and qualitative data
- Select and define variables relevant to the defined public health problems
- Identify relevant and appropriate data and information sources
- Evaluate the integrity and comparability of data and identify gaps in data sources
- Apply ethical principles to the collection, maintenance, use, and dissemination of data and information
- Partner with communities to attach meaning to collected quantitative and qualitative data
- Make relevant inferences from quantitative and qualitative data
- Obtain and interpret information regarding risks and benefits to the community
- Apply data collection processes, information technology applications, and computer systems storage and retrieval strategies
- Recognize how the data illuminate ethical, political, scientific, economic, and overall public health issues

From Council on Linkages between Academia and Public Health Practice: *Core competencies for public health professionals,* Washington, DC, 2001, USDHHS and Public Health Foundation, available at www.phf.org/Link.htm.

WHAT IS A COMMUNITY?

The concept of *community* varies widely. The expert committee report on community health nursing by the World Health Organization (WHO) (World Health Organization, 1974) includes this definition: "A community is a social group determined by geographic boundaries and/or common values and interests. Its members know and interact with one another. It functions within a particular social structure and exhibits and creates norms, values and social institutions" (p. 7).

The most frequently used single definition of community is "community of place" or geographic boundaries. With agency interactions (e.g., among schools, social services, and governmental agencies) extending the ability to solve problems, nurses working in communities quickly learn that society consists of many different kinds of communities. Neighborhood and face-to-face communities are two examples. Some other types of communities are listed in Box 12-2.

Other communities, such as communities of special interest or resource communities, are spread out across widely scattered geographic areas. They are brought together by long-term or short-term common concerns and interests. An example of another type of community is a community of problem ecology, which is created when environmental problems affect a widespread area. For instance, a problem such as water pollution can bring people together from areas that would not normally share a common interest. Nurses also may work in partnership with political communities, such as school districts, townships, or counties. Because the nature of each type of community varies, nurses planning interventions with communities must take into account the characteristics of that specific community. Each community is unique, and its defining characteristics will affect the nature of the partnership.

In most definitions, the concept of community includes three dimensions—*people, place,* and *function*—as follows:
1. The *people* are the community residents.
2. *Place* refers both to geographic and time dimensions.
3. *Function* refers to the aims and activities of the community.

Box 12-2 Types of Communities

- Face-to-face community
- Neighborhood community
- Community of identifiable need
- Community of problem ecology
- Community of concern
- Community of special interest
- Community of viability
- Community of action capability
- Community of political jurisdiction
- Resource community
- Community of solution

From Blum HL: *Planning for health,* New York, 1974, Human Sciences Press.

Table 12-1   Concepts of Community Specified

Dimensions	Measures	Examples of Data Sources
Place	Geopolitical boundaries	Maps
	Local or folk name for area	Local newspaper
	Size in square miles, acres, blocks, or census tracts	Census data
	Transportation avenues, such as rivers, highways, railroads, and sidewalks	Chamber of Commerce
		City, county, or township government
	History	Library archives and local histories
	Physical environment such as land use patterns and condition of housing	Local housing office
People or person	Population: number and density	Census data
	Demographic structure of population, such as age, sex, socioeconomic factors, and racial distributions; rural and urban character, and dependency ratio	Census data
		Churches, senior centers
		Civic groups
	Informal groups such as block clubs, service clubs, and friendship networks	Local newspaper
		Telephone directory
		United Way
		Social service agencies
	Formal groups such as schools, churches, businesses, industries, governmental bodies, unions, and health and welfare agencies	Chamber of Commerce
		Tourist bureau
	Linking structures (intercommunity and intracommunity contacts among organizations)	Local or state officials
		Chamber of Commerce
Function	Production, distribution, and consumption of goods and services	State departments
		Business and labor
		Local library
	Socialization of new members	Social and local research reports
	Maintenance of social control	Police station
	Adaptation to ongoing and expected change	Social and local research reports
	Provision of mutual aid	United Way Welfare agencies
		Churches and religious organizations

Nurses in community health practice regularly need to examine how the personal, geographic, and functional dimensions of community shape their nursing practice with individuals, families, and groups. They can use both a conceptual definition and a set of indicators for the concept of *community* in their practice.

In this chapter, the following conceptual definition is used: **community** is a locality-based entity, composed of systems of formal organizations reflecting society's institutions, informal groups, and aggregates. As defined in Chapter 1, an **aggregate** is a collection of individuals who have in common one or more personal or environmental characteristics. The components of community are **interdependent**, and their function is to meet a wide variety of collective needs. This definition of community includes personal, geographic, and functional dimensions and recognizes interaction among the systems within a community. Indicators of the dimensions of this definition are listed in Table 12-1.

The next section describes the community as client and partner of the nurse. The community is first the **setting for practice** for the nurse practicing health-promotion and disease-prevention interventions with individuals, families, and groups. Second, the community is the **target of practice** for the public health nurse whose practice is focused on the broader community rather than on individuals.

COMMUNITY AS CLIENT

Nurses who have a community orientation are often considered unique because of their target of practice. The idea of health-related care being provided within the community is not new. At the turn of the century, most persons stayed at home during illnesses. As a result, the practice environment for nurses was the home rather than the hospital.

As the range of community nursing services expanded, many different kinds of agencies were started and their services often overlapped. For instance, both privately established voluntary agencies and official local health agencies worked to control tuberculosis (TB). The nurses employed by these agencies were called *community health nurses, public health nurses,* or *visiting nurses.* Nurses practiced in clients' homes, not in the hospital. Early public health nursing textbooks included lengthy descriptions of the home environment and tools for assessing the extent to which that environment promoted the health of family members. Health education about the domestic environment was often a major part of home nursing care.

By the 1950s, schools, prisons, industries, and neighborhood health centers, as well as homes, had all become areas of practice for nurses in the community. Many of the new nurses in the community did not consider the environments in which they practiced. Although their practices took place within the community, they focused on the individual client or family seeking care.

When the *location of practice* is the community and the *target of practice* is the individual or family living in the community, the client is the individual or family, not the whole community. Although the clients may be individuals, families or other interacting groups, aggregates, institutions, and communities, the resulting changes are intended to affect the whole community. For example, an occupational health nurse's target might be preventing illness and injury for the individual worker. This would result in maintaining or promoting the health of an entire company workforce. This means that because the nurse works with individuals through health education to teach them safety, the numbers of industry accidents decline from one year to the next. Because of this focus, the nurse not only would help the individual worker seeking service to overcome an injury but also would become involved with promoting vocational rehabilitation and would seek reasonable employment policies for all workers to promote safety.

BRIEFLY NOTED

Many nurses believe that home health nursing is focused on the individual and therefore should not be considered a part of nursing in the community. Other nurses argue that home health nursing focuses on the family, takes place in the community, and should be considered a part of nursing with a community orientation.

THE COMMUNITY AS CLIENT AND PARTNER IN NURSING PRACTICE

The concept of community as client and partner makes direct clinical care an aspect of community health practice (Constance et al, 2002). For instance, direct nursing care may be provided to individuals and family members because their health needs represent common community-related problems rather than problems that are unique to their situations. Changes in their health will affect the health of their communities (Kemsley and Riegle, 2004). In such cases, decisions are made at the individual level because the individual's health is related to the health of the population as a whole and because the individual has an effect on the community's health. Improved health of the community remains the overall goal of nursing intervention. Interventions to stop spouse abuse and elder abuse are two examples of nursing interventions done primarily because of the effects of abuse on society and therefore on the population as a whole.

The concept of community as client and partner also highlights the complexity of the change process. Change for the benefit of the community client often must occur at several levels, ranging from the individual to society as a whole. In his classic work, Ryan (1976) points out that the "victim" cannot always be blamed and expected to correct the problem without changes also being made at the same time in the helping professions and in public policy. For instance, lifestyle-induced health problems, such as smoking, overeating, and lack of exercise cannot be solved simply by asking individuals to choose health-promoting habits. Society must also provide healthy choices. Most individuals cannot change their habits alone; they require the support of family members, friends, community health care systems, and relevant social policies.

A commitment to the health of individuals, families, and groups who make up the community client requires a process of change at each of these levels. Both collaborative practice models involving the community and nurses in joint decision making and specific nursing roles are required for each of the types of clients (Constance et al, 2002). Nursing roles in community health emphasize individual and direct personal care skills and focus on the family as the unit of service. The public health nursing role focuses on the community or the population as the unit of service, especially working with community groups.

Viewing the community client as partner and thus as the target of service means embracing two key concepts: community health and partnership for community health. Together these form not only the goal but also the means of community-oriented practice.

GOALS AND MEANS OF COMMUNITY-ORIENTED PRACTICE

In **community-oriented practice**, the nurse and community seek healthful change together (El Ansari, Phillips, and Zwi, 2004). Their common goal to promote the community's health involves an ongoing series of health-promoting changes. The most effective means of completing healthy changes in the community is through this same partnership.

COMMUNITY HEALTH

Like the concept of community, *community health* has three common characteristics or dimensions: status, structure, and process. Each dimension has a unique effect on a community's health as the goal of community-oriented practice.

Status

Community health in terms of status or outcome is the best known and accepted approach; it involves physical, emotional, and social components. The *physical component* of community health is often measured by traditional morbidity and mortality rates, life-expectancy indices, and risk-factor profiles. *Morbidity and Mortality Weekly Report* published the work of a consensus committee involving representatives from a number of community health-related organizations. This committee identified by consensus 18 community health status indicators, presented in Box 12-3.

The *emotional component* of health status can be measured by client satisfaction and mental health indices. Crime rates and individual and family functional levels reflect the *social component* of community health. Other status measures, such as worker absenteeism and infant mortality rates, reflect the effects of all three components.

Box 12-3	Consensus Set of Indicators* for Assessing Community Health Status

Indicators of Health Status Outcome

1. Race-specific and ethnicity-specific infant mortality, as measured by the rate (per 1000 live births) of deaths among infants less than 1 year of age

Death Rates (per 100,000 Population)† for:

2. Motor vehicle crashes
3. Work-related injury
4. Suicide
5. Lung cancer
6. Breast cancer
7. Cardiovascular disease
8. Homicide
9. All causes

Reported Incidence (per 100,000 Population) of:

10. Acquired immunodeficiency syndrome (AIDS)
11. Measles
12. Tuberculosis
13. Primary and secondary syphilis

Indicators of Risk Factors

14. Incidence of low birth weight, as measured by percentage of total number of live-born infants weighing less than 2500 grams at birth
15. Births to adolescents (females 10 to 17 years of age) as a percentage of total live births
16. Prenatal care, as measured by percentage of mothers delivering live infants who did not receive prenatal care during the first trimester
17. Childhood poverty, as measured by the proportion of children less than 15 years of age living in families at or below the poverty level
18. Proportion of persons living in counties exceeding U.S. Environmental Protection Agency standards for air quality during the previous year

From Consensus set of health status indicators for the general assessment of community health status—United States, *MMWR* 40(27):449, 1991 (updated Aug 2001).
*Position or number of the indicator does not imply priority.
†Age adjusted to the 1940 standard population.

Structure

Community health, when viewed from the structure of the community, is usually defined in terms of community characteristics, as well as *services* and *resources*. Indicators used to measure community health services and resources include service use patterns, treatment data from various health agencies, and provider/client ratios. These data provide information such as the number of available hospital beds or the number of emergency room visits to a particular hospital.

Characteristics of the community structure are commonly identified as social indicators, or correlates, of health. Characteristics of community structure include demographic characteristics, such as age, gender, socioeconomic and racial distributions, and educational levels. Their relationships to health status have been thoroughly documented. For instance, studies have repeatedly shown that health status decreases

with age and improves with higher socioeconomic levels (U.S. Department of Health and Human Services, 2000).

Process

The view of community health as the process of effective community functioning or problem solving is well established. However, it is especially appropriate to nursing because it directs the study of community health to promote effective community action for health promotion.

The term **community health,** as used in this chapter, is defined as the meeting of collective needs by identifying problems and managing interactions within the community itself and between the community and the larger society. This definition emphasizes the process dimension but also includes the dimensions of status and structure. Indicators for all three dimensions are listed in Table 12-2.

The use of status, structure, and process dimensions to define community health is an effort to develop a broad definition of community health, involving indicators that often are not included when discussions focus only on individual and family risk factors as the basis for community health.

There are several different community-oriented health-promotion approaches, but regardless of what approach is taken, specific strategies to improve community health often depend on whether the status, structure, or process dimension of community health is being emphasized, as follows:

- If the emphasis is on the *status dimension,* the best strategy is usually at the levels of primary or secondary prevention at the community level because the objective is either to prevent a disease or to treat it in its early stages. Immunization programs are an example of a nursing intervention at the primary prevention level when the possibility of contracting the disease will likely occur if the immunization is not received.
- Nursing intervention strategies focused on the *structural dimension* are directed to either health services or population demographic characteristics. Intervention aimed at altering health services might include program planning such as developing a new program in occupational health nursing because of all the illnesses and injuries identified through an assessment at a certain industry. Interventions aimed at affecting demographic characteristics might include community development. A group of community leaders may come together because they have recognized that children ages 6 to 17 years do not have adequate health care in the schools. The leaders in partnership with the health departments may be able to plan for school health clinics.
- When the emphasis is on the *process dimension*—usually the level of intervention of the nurse in community health—the best strategy is usually health promotion, which is considered a primary prevention strategy. For example, if family-life education is lacking in a community because of ineffective communication among families, children, school board members, religious leaders, and health professionals, the most effective strategy may be to open discussion among these groups and help community members develop educational programs.

Table 12-2	Concept of Community Health Specified	
Dimensions	**Measures**	**Examples of Data Sources**
Status	Vital statistics (live births, neonatal deaths, infant deaths, maternal deaths)	Census data State health department annual vital statistics
	Incidence and prevalence of leading causes of mortality and morbidity	Census data State health department
	Health risk profiles of selected aggregates	Local health department Support groups Local nonprofit organizations
	Functional ability levels	Census data U.S. Department of Labor
Structure	Health facilities such as hospitals, nursing homes, industrial and school health services, health departments, voluntary health associations, categorical grant programs, and prepaid health plans	Local chamber of commerce United Way
	Health-related planning groups	Local newspapers Local magazines Local government
	Health manpower, such as physicians, dentists, nurses, environmental sanitarians, social workers	Telephone directory State and local labor statistics Professional licensing boards
	Health resource use patterns, such as bed occupancy days and client/provider visits	Medicare and Medicaid databases (federal and state government) Annual reports from hospitals, health maintenance organizations (HMOs), nonprofit agencies
Process	Commitment to community health	Local government Real estate agencies (turnover/vacancy rates, for example)
	Awareness of self and others and clarity of situational definitions	Local history Neighborhood help organizations Local/neighborhood newspapers and radio programs Local government
	Conflict containment and accommodation Participation Management of relationships with society Machinery for facilitating participant interaction and decision making	Social services department Existence of and participation in local organizations Windshield survey—observation of interactions Notices for community organizations and meetings in public places (supermarkets, newspapers, radio)

HEALTHY PEOPLE 2010

One important guideline available for nurses working to improve the health of the community is *Healthy People 2010*, a publication from the U.S. Department of Health and Human Services (2000) that offers a vision of the future for healthy communities and specific objectives to help fulfill that vision. The *Healthy People 2010* vision recognizes the need to work collectively, in community partnerships, to bring about the changes that will be necessary to fulfill this vision. *Healthy People 2010* provides the foundation for a national health promotion and disease prevention strategy built on two goals of increasing the "quality and years of healthy life" and "eliminating health disparities."

BRIEFLY NOTED

A valuable *Healthy People 2010* website can be accessed on the Internet through the WebLinks of this book's website (http://evolve.elsevier.com/stanhope/foundations).

COMMUNITY PARTNERSHIPS

Community partnership is crucial because community members and professionals who are active participants in a collaborative decision-making process have a vested interest in the success of efforts to improve the health of their community. Consequently, successful strategies for improving the community's health must include community partnership as the basic means, or key, for improvement.

Partnership means the active participation and involvement of the community or its representatives in bringing about healthful change (El Ansari, Phillips, and Zwi, 2004). Partnership is defined as the informed, flexible, and negotiated distribution (and redistribution) of power among all participants in the processes of change for improved community health.

As defined here, partnership is a concept that is as essential for nurses to know and use as are the concepts of community, community as client partner, and community health. Experienced nurses know that partnership is important because health is not always a reality but, rather, is generated through new and increasingly effective means

Healthy People 2010

Community as Partner

Healthy People 2010 promotes partnerships with communities, states, and national organizations and suggests the following:

- Taking a multidisciplinary approach to achieving health equity
- Using approaches to improving not only health but also education, housing, labor, justice, transportation, agriculture, and the environment
- Empowering individuals to make informed health care decisions
- Promoting community-wide safety, education, and access to health care
- Tailoring approaches to prevention for the type of community and ensuring community participation in the process

of lay-professional collaboration at the individual, family, group, or community level. For example, polluted air is an issue for many urban neighborhoods. One partnership was developed among parents of asthmatic children, public officials, and other citizens to create a policy about leaf burning in the county. Active efforts by neighborhood residents can make neighborhoods cleaner and healthier places to live (Rowitz, 2001).

Effective partnerships have the following characteristics:

- Equality in decision making
- A shared vision
- Integrity
- Agreement on specific goals
- A plan of action to meet the goals
- A means to evaluate the plan of action

Whether the partnership is between two individuals, a nurse and family, or health, business, political, and educational partners, the characteristics are the same (Rowitz, 2001).

The significance and effectiveness of partnership in improving community health is supported by a growing body of literature. Studies document the use of partnership models involving urban areas and lay advisors (Maurana and Clark, 2000). The roles of these partners-in-health have included listening sympathetically, offering advice, making referrals, and starting programs among a wide range of communities with populations of all ages. They include partnerships with older adults in retirement communities as well as smaller, more rural communities (Lutz, Herrick, and Lehman, 2001; Lyford, Breen, and Grove, 2003). There are also examples of community partnerships for at-risk students at the grade school or middle school level, for promoting policies to strengthen early childhood development, or for the prevention of influenza (Horsley and Ciske, 2005; Kemsley and Riegle, 2004; McMahon, Browning, and Rose-Colley, 2001; Miller et al, 2001). Recent work by El Ansari et al (2004) shows the continuing use of partnership models for improving

health in other countries. In international health, partnership models generally are viewed as empowering people, through their lay leaders, to control their own health destinies and lives. In the United States, partnership models have often involved churches and informal community leaders.

COMMUNITY-FOCUSED NURSING PROCESS: AN OVERVIEW OF THE PROCESS FROM ASSESSMENT TO EVALUATION

Most nurses are familiar with the nursing process as it applies to individually focused nursing care. Using it to promote community health makes this same nursing process community focused (Rosen, 2000). The phases of the nursing process that directly involve the community client as partner begin at the start of the contract or partnership and include assessment, diagnosis, planning, implementation, and evaluation.

ASSESSING COMMUNITY HEALTH

Community assessment is the process of critically thinking about the community and involves getting to know and understand the community client as partner. This helps the nurse in community health to understand individual, family, and group problems and to know what community strengths and resources are available to help the nurse solve the client's problems. The community assessment phase involves a logical, systematic approach to the initial phase of the nursing process. Community assessment helps:

- To identify community needs
- To clarify problems
- To identify strengths and resources

There are different types of community assessment. Community assessments can be short and simple or long and complex. One example of a short and simple community assessment is the **windshield survey**, which is discussed on p. 225. Comprehensive community assessment is the necessary initial phase of the nursing process in community health with the community client as partner.

Assessing community health requires the following three steps:

1. Gathering relevant existing data and generating missing data
2. Developing a composite database
3. Interpreting the composite database to identify community problems and strengths

Data Collection and Interpretation

The primary goal of **data collection** is to get usable information about the community and its health. The systematic collection of data about community health requires the following:

- Gathering or compiling existing data
- Generating missing data

- Interpreting data
- Identifying community health problems and community abilities

DATA GATHERING. **Data gathering** is the process of obtaining existing, readily available data. The following data usually describe the demography of a community:

- Age of the residents
- Gender distribution of the residents
- Socioeconomic characteristics
- Racial distributions
- Vital statistics, including selected mortality and morbidity data
- Community institutions, including health care organizations and the services they provide
- Health personnel characteristics

Often these data have been collected by others via structured interviews, questionnaires, or surveys and are available in published reports at the library or local public health department. These data give the nurse a snapshot of how the clients receiving services fit into the community.

DATA GENERATION. **Data generation** is the process of developing data that do not already exist, through interaction with community members, individuals, families, or groups. This type of information is more difficult to obtain and is generally not statistical in nature. Data that often must be generated include the following:

- Information about a community's knowledge and beliefs
- Values and sentiments
- Goals and perceived needs
- Norms
- Problem-solving processes
- Power
- Leadership
- Influence structures

These data are more likely to be collected by interviews and observation.

COMPOSITE DATABASE ANALYSIS. Combining the gathered and generated data creates a composite database. Data analysis seeks to make sense of the data, as follows:

1. First, data are analyzed and synthesized and themes are noted.
2. **Community health problems,** or needs for action, and **community health strengths,** or abilities, are determined.
3. Next, the resources available to meet the needs are identified.
4. Problems are indicated by differences between the nurse's and community's goals for community health.
5. Strengths, on the other hand, are suggested by similarities between the nurse's and community's concepts of community health and available data.
6. Finally, the resources available to meet the needs are identified.

Data-Collection Methods

Several methods to collect data are needed. Methods that encourage the nurse to consider the community's perception of its health problems and abilities are as important as those

CASE STUDY

Alan Thompson is a nurse in community health and a member of a committee assigned to assess the health care needs of the aging "baby boomers" in Duxbury County. Mr. Thompson and his committee are aware that as the baby-boomer population ages, health care professionals need to prepare for a rapid increase in the number of people older than 65 years. The committee's purpose is to make suggestions to the health department and county officials about how to prepare for the influx in health services that will be needed for these older adults.

Currently, 25% of the population in Duxbury County is older than 65 years. However, in 25 years this percentage is expected to increase to more than 50%. Currently, five primary care providers are in the county, with service waiting lists ranging from 1 to 3 weeks; only one of these providers specializes in geriatric care. One 54-bed long-term nursing care facility is in the northern region of the spacious county. Because of rural roads, there is no public transit system. However, residents may call a hospital shuttle program if they need transportation to a physician's appointment.

methods structured to identify knowledge that the nurse considers essential.

Five useful methods of collecting data follow:

1. Informant interviews
2. Participant observation
3. Windshield surveys
4. Secondary analysis of existing data
5. Surveys

These methods can be grouped into the following two distinct but complementary categories:

1. Methods that rely on what is directly observed by the data collector
2. Methods that rely on what is reported to the data collector

COLLECTION OF DIRECT DATA. *Informant interviews, participant observation,* and *windshield surveys* are three methods of directly collecting data. All three methods require the following:

- Sensitivity
- Openness
- Curiosity
- The ability to listen, taste, touch, and smell
- The ability to see life as it is lived in a community

Informant interviews, which consist of directed talks with selected members of a community about community members or groups and events, are basic to effective data collection. Talking to key informants is a critical part of the community assessment. Key informants are not always people who have a formal title or position; they often have an informal role within the community. Examples of informal key informants are a member of a minority group who is listened to by other members of the group, a church deacon, and a parent who is active and vocal about the school health curriculum.

Also basic is **participant observation**, the deliberate sharing, if conditions permit, in the life of a community. For example, if the nurse lives in the community, activities such as participating in clinical organizations and church life and reading the newspaper give the nurse "observations" of the community's life. Informant interviews and participant observation are good ways to generate information about community beliefs, norms, values, power and influence structures, and problem-solving processes. Such data can seldom be reported in numbers, so they are not often collected. Even worse, conclusions that are based on intuition and are unchecked are sometimes used to replace this type of data. Conclusions from direct data collection methods should be confirmed by those people providing the information.

Informant interviews with social workers and religious leaders can provide data that describe a community that has well-defined clusters of persons with similar problems, such as persons of low income, persons with concerns about adolescent pregnancy, and persons with worries about the health of babies. These data could be difficult to acquire without personal interviews.

Windshield surveys are the motorized equivalent of simple observation. They involve the collection of data that will help define the community, the trends, stability, and changes that will affect the health of the community (Stanhope and Knollmueller, 2000).

BRIEFLY NOTED

If you do a windshield survey as part of your community assessment, go two times: once during the day when people are at work and children are at school, and a second time in the evening after work is done and school is out.

While driving a car or riding public transportation, the nurse can observe many dimensions of a community's life and environment through the windshield, such as the following:
- Common characteristics of people on the street
- Neighborhood gathering places
- The rhythm of community life
- Housing quality
- Geographic boundaries

Windshield surveys can be used by themselves for short and simple assessments. An example of a windshield survey is found in Table 12-3.

COLLECTION OF REPORTED DATA. **Secondary analysis** and **surveys** are two methods of collecting reported data. In secondary analysis, the nurse uses previously gathered data, such as minutes from community meetings. This type of analysis is extremely valuable because it saves time and effort. Many sources of data are readily available and useful for secondary analysis, including the following:
- Public documents
- Health surveys

HOW TO	**Identify a Key Informant for Interviews**

The following may be key informants:
- County health department nurses or church leaders
- Many community members who nurses know and who can identify other key informants
- The president of the parent-teacher organization
- The mayor or other local politicians
- The mother who organized the local chapter of Mothers Against Drunk Driving (informal leader)

HOW TO	**Obtain a Quick Assessment of a Community**

- One way of obtaining a quick, initial sense of the community is to do a windshield assessment using a format like the one provided as an example in Table 12-3.
- Nurses interested in doing a windshield assessment need to either take public transportation, have someone else drive while they take notes, or plan to frequently stop and write down what they see.
- The windshield survey example is organized into 15 elements with specific questions to answer that are related to each element.
- Some of the questions will need to be answered by visiting the library to get secondary data.
- Nurses who use this approach will have an initial descriptive assessment of the community when they are finished.
- Interventions are planned, based on the survey.

- Minutes from meetings
- Statistical data
- Health records

Surveys report data from a sample of persons. They are equally useful, but they take more time and effort than observational methods and secondary analyses because they require time-consuming and costly data collection (see "How To Identify a Key Informant for Interviews"). Thus the nurse does not often use the survey method. However, surveys are necessary for identifying certain community problems (Levine et al, 2003). For example, a lack of accessible personal health services cannot be documented readily and accurately in any other way.

Assessment Issues

Gaining entry or acceptance into the community is perhaps the biggest challenge in assessment. The nurse is usually an outsider and often represents an established health care system that is neither known nor trusted by community members who may therefore react with indifference or even active hostility to the nurse. In addition, nurses may feel insecure about their skills as a community worker and the community may refuse to acknowledge its need for those skills. Because the nurse's success depends largely on the way he or she is viewed, entry into the community is critical. Often the nurse can gain entry by:
- Taking part in community events
- Looking and listening with interest

Table 12-3   Windshield Survey Components

Element	Description
Housing and zoning	What is the age of the houses, architecture? Of what materials are they constructed? Are all neighborhood houses similar in age and in architecture? How would you characterize their differences? Are they detached or connected to others? Do they have space in front or behind? What is their general condition? Are there signs of disrepair—broken doors, windows, leaks, locks missing? Is there central heating, modern plumbing, air conditioning?
Open space	How much open space is there? What is the quality of the space—green parks or rubble-filled lots? What is the lot size of the houses? Lawns? Flower boxes? Do you see trees on the pavements, a green island in the center of the streets? Is the open space public or private? Used by whom?
Boundaries	What signs are there of where this neighborhood begins and ends? Are the boundaries natural—a river, a different terrain; physical—a highway, railroad; economic—difference in real estate or the presence of industrial or commercial units along with residential? Does the neighborhood have an identity, a name? Do you see it displayed? Are there unofficial names?
"Commons"	What are the neighborhood hangouts? For what groups, at what hours (e.g., schoolyard, candy store, bar, restaurant, park, 24-hour drugstore)? Does the "commons" area have a sense of "territoriality," or is it open to the stranger?
Transportation	How do people get in and out of the neighborhood—car, bus, bike, walk, etc.? Are the streets and roads conducive to good transportation and also to community life? Is there a major highway near the neighborhood? Whom does it serve? How frequently is public transportation available?
Service centers	Do you see social agencies, clients, recreation centers, signs of activity at the schools? Are there offices of doctors, dentists; palmists, spiritualists, etc.? Are there parks? Are they in use?
Stores	Where do residents shop—shopping centers, neighborhood stores? How do they travel to shop?
Street people	Whom do you see on the street—an occasional housewife, a mother with a baby? Do you see anyone you would not expect—teenagers, unemployed males? Can you spot a welfare worker, an insurance collector, a door-to-door salesperson? Is the dress of those you see representative or unexpected? Along with people, what animals do you see—stray cats, pedigreed pets, "watchdogs"?
Signs of decay	Is this neighborhood on the way up or down? Is it "alive"? How would you decide? Trash, abandoned cars, political posters, neighborhood-meeting posters, real estate signs, abandoned houses, mixed zoning usage?
Race	Are the residents Caucasian, African-American, or of another minority, or is the area integrated?
Ethnicity	Are there indices of ethnicity—food stores, churches, private schools, information in a language other than English?
Religion	Of what religion are the residents? Do you see evidence of heterogeneity or homogeneity? What denominations are the churches? Do you see evidence of their use other than on Sunday mornings?
Health and morbidity	Do you see evidence of acute or of chronic diseases or conditions? Of accidents, communicable diseases, alcoholism, drug addiction, mental illness, etc.? How far is it to the nearest hospital? Clinic?
Politics	Do you see any political campaign posters? Is there a headquarters present? Do you see evidence of a predominant party affiliation?
Media	Do you see outdoor television antennas? What magazines and newspapers do residents read? Do you see *National Enquirer, Readers' Digest,* publications geared toward African-Americans or seniors in the stores? What media seem most important to the residents—radio, television, print?

Modified from Anderson ET, McFarlane J: *Community-as-partner: theory and practice in nursing,* ed 4, Philadelphia, 2004, Lippincott Williams & Wilkins.

- Visiting people in formal leadership positions
- Employing an assessment guide
- Using a peer group for support
- Keeping appointments
- Clarifying community members' perceptions of health needs
- Respecting an individual's right to choose whether he or she will work with the nurse

Maintaining **confidentiality** is important. Nurses must be very careful to protect the identity of community members who provide sensitive or controversial data. In some cases the nurse may consider withholding data; in other situations the nurse may be legally required to disclose data. For example, nurses are required by law to report child abuse.

IDENTIFYING COMMUNITY PROBLEMS

The windshield assessment activities and the creation of a composite **database** will result in a list of community strengths and health problems. Each problem needs to be identified clearly and stated. The health risk to the community is stated, the person(s) affected are named, and the community factors that led to the problem are defined. This process is an important first step to planning. In the planning phase, priorities are established and interventions are identified.

Each community has its own unique characteristics. Some of these characteristics are strengths on which the nurse can build, but others contribute to the problem identified. An example of a community problem is infant malnutrition. Based on assessment data, the community problem for infant malnutrition using this format would be described as follows:

1. Infant malnutrition problem—children younger than 1 year of age
2. Risk to community—because of children in poor health, new services may have to be provided
3. Persons affected—among families in Jefferson County
4. Community factors:
   - Lack of regular developmental screening for infants in the community
   - No outreach program to identify at-risk infants
   - Families' lack of knowledge about the Women, Infants, and Children (WIC) nutrition program
   - Confusion among community families about WIC program enrollment criteria
   - Community families' lack of infant-related nutritional knowledge

Frequently, a number of community health problems will be identified during the assessment phase. When a number of problems exist, priorities for resolving the problems must be set based on the following (McKenzie, Pinger, and Kotechi, 2008):

- Which problems are important to the community?
- Which segments of the population are most affected?
- What are the benefits to the community?
- What happens to the community or the population if the problem is or is not resolved?
- How much does it cost to implement solutions, in terms of money and resources, to improve the problem and to save lives?

- How do politics, community values, and community priorities affect efforts to solve the problem?
- What does the community expect to happen?

PLANNING FOR COMMUNITY HEALTH

The planning phase includes the following:

- Analyzing the community health problems identified in the community nursing diagnoses
- Establishing priorities among them
- Establishing goals and objectives
- Identifying intervention activities that will accomplish the objectives

Analyzing Problems

Analyzing the problems seeks to clarify the nature of the problem. The nurse identifies the following:

- The origins and effects of the problem
- The points at which intervention might be undertaken
- The parties who have an interest in the problem and its solution

Analysis often requires identifying the following:

- The direct and indirect factors that contribute to the problem
- The outcomes of the problem
- Relationships among the problems (whether one problem causes or is affected by other problems)
- Factors that contribute to the problem

This is important because the nurse can anticipate that several of the same factors that contribute to a problem and affect the outcomes of a problem also cause many other problems.

Problem analysis should be undertaken for each identified problem. It often requires organizing a special group composed of the nurse and the following:

- Persons whose areas of expertise relate to the problem
- Individuals whose organizations are capable of intervening
- Representatives of the community experiencing the problem—the client

Together they can identify the factors contributing to the problem and explain the relationships between each factor and the problem.

This process is seen in Table 12-4 on p. 231 at the end of this chapter as an example of problem analysis. Factors that contribute to the problem and outcomes of the problem for infant malnutrition are listed in the first column. These factors are from all areas of community life. Social or environmental factors are as appropriate as those oriented to the individual. For example, teenage pregnancy is a social factor and high unemployment is an environmental factor; both are related to infant malnutrition. In the second column the relationships between each factor and the problem are noted. The third column contains data from the community and the literature that support the relationship, using the suspected infant malnutrition example.

From the best evidence available, infant malnutrition is thought to be related to inadequate diet, community norms, poverty, disturbed mother–child relationships, and teenage pregnancy.

Problem Priorities

Infant malnutrition represents only one of several community health problems identified by the community assessment. In reality, several community health problems may be identified. They may include lack of clinics, poor housing conditions, a mortality rate from cardiovascular disease that was higher than the national norm, and—as expressed by many residents—a desire to quit smoking.

Each problem identified as part of the assessment process must be put through a ranking process to determine its importance. This is known as **problem prioritizing**.

PROBLEM PRIORITY CRITERIA. Answers to the following questions have been helpful in ranking identified problems:
- How aware is the community of the problem?
- Is the community motivated to resolve or better manage the problem?
- Is the nurse able to influence problem resolution?
- Are there available experts to solve the problem?
- How severe are the outcomes if the problem is unresolved?
- How quickly can the problem be solved?

Using the example of infant malnutrition again, these six questions are listed in the first column of Table 12-5 on p. 231 at the end of this chapter. Note that this one problem is only an example to show how to evaluate each problem using the six criteria.

The members of the partnership answer questions related to their ability to influence and/or change the situation, and the nurse and the community agree on the ability to resolve the problem. One example of the difference between the perceptions of the nurse and community members is smoking in public buildings; the community nurse might identify smoking as a public health problem, but community members might view smoking as an issue of individual choice and personal freedom. For example, recently a midsize community through the local government and the health department passed a regulation to forbid smoking in all public places including restaurants and bars. The outcry from the community residents has been loud. Residents believe their individual rights and freedoms have been taken away by government regulations. It does not matter to the residents that lung cancer rates are high.

This process is repeated separately for each identified problem, and all of the problems are compared. Priorities among the identified problems are established. The problems with the highest priority are the ones selected as the focus for intervention. Table 12-6 on p. 232 at the end of this chapter shows how all problems in the community were prioritized after each one was separately evaluated.

Establishing Goals and Objectives

Once high-priority problems are identified, relevant goals and objectives are developed. **Goals** are generally broad statements of desired outcomes. **Objectives** are the precise statements indicating the means of achieving desired outcomes.

An example of one of the goals and the specific objectives associated with it for the infant malnutrition problem is seen in Table 12-7 on p. 232 at the end of this chapter.

The goal is to reduce the incidence and prevalence of infant malnutrition. The objectives must be *precise, behaviorally stated,* and *measurable* and can be solved in a series of steps implemented over time rather than at once. In this example, the specific objectives pertain to the following:
1. Assessing infant developmental levels
2. Determining WIC program eligibility
3. Implementing an outreach program
4. Enrolling infants in the WIC program
5. Providing supplemental foods in existing diets

As noted, establishing these goals and objectives involves collaboration between the nurse and representatives of the community groups affected by both the problem and the proposed intervention. This often requires a great deal of negotiation among everyone taking part in the planning process. One important advantage offered by the continuous active involvement of people affected by the outcomes is that they have a vested interest in those outcomes and therefore are supportive of and committed to the success of the intervention. Once goals and objectives are chosen, intervention activities to accomplish the objectives can be identified.

Identifying Intervention Activities

Intervention activities, the means by which objectives are met, are as follows:
- The strategies used to meet the objectives
- The ways change will be effected
- The ways the problem cycle will be broken

Because alternative intervention activities do exist, they must be identified and evaluated. Listing possible interventions and selecting the best set of activities to achieve the goal of documenting and reducing infant malnutrition are depicted in Table 12-8 on p. 232 at the end of this chapter.

To achieve the objective related to assessment of infant developmental levels (see Table 12-7, objective 1), five intervention activities are listed in the second column of Table 12-8. Each is relevant to the first objective (developmental levels will be assessed for 80% of infants seen by the health department, neighborhood health center, and private physicians). The first two activities involve WIC program personnel as the principal change agents. The last three involve the nurse, WIC program personnel, and the staff of the health department, neighborhood health center, and private physicians' offices as the change partners.

The expected effect of each of the activities is considered in the second column of Table 12-8. The **value**, or the likelihood that the activity will help meet the objective and finally resolve the problem, is noted in the third column.

Clearly it is more valuable in the long term to educate others in how to assess infant development (activity 4) than to do it for them (activity 1).

It is also necessary to analyze the change process necessary to complete the objective (activity 5). Activity 5 must be done before any other interventions can be considered.

As a result, activities 4 and 5 have higher value scores than does activity 1, in which the professional staff alone carries out the intervention. How is the priority value decided? Answer the questions on p. 233. Read the literature to find evidence about what works best. If five interventions are possible, assign a score between one and five based on the answers to the questions and what the literature says is the best approach.

IMPLEMENTATION IN THE COMMUNITY

Implementation, the fourth phase of the nursing process, involves the work and activities aimed at achieving the goals and objectives. Implementation efforts may be made by the person or group who established the goals and objectives, or they may be shared with or even delegated to others.

Factors Influencing Implementation

Implementation is shaped by the following:
- The nurse's chosen roles
- The type of health problem selected as the focus for intervention
- The community's readiness to take part in problem solving
- Characteristics of the social change process

The nurse taking part in community-oriented intervention has knowledge and skills that the other interveners do not have; the question is how the nurse uses the position, knowledge, and skills.

NURSE'S ROLE. Nurses can act as content experts, helping communities select and attain task-related goals. In the example of infant malnutrition, the nurse can use epidemiologic skills to determine the incidence and prevalence of malnutrition. The nurse can serve as a process expert by increasing the community's ability to document the problem rather than by providing help only as an expert in the area.

Content-focused roles often are considered **change agent** roles, whereas process roles are called **change partner** roles. Change agent roles stress gathering and analyzing facts and implementing programs, whereas change partner roles include those of enabler-catalyst, teacher of problem-solving skills, and activist advocate.

THE PROBLEM AND THE NURSE'S ROLE. The role the nurse chooses depends on the following:
- The nature of the health problem
- The community's decision-making ability
- Professional and personal choices

Some health problems clearly require certain intervention roles, as follows:
- If a community lacks democratic problem-solving abilities, the nurse may select teacher, facilitator, and advocate roles. Problem-solving skills must be explained, and the nurse becomes a role model.
- A problem with determining the health status of the community, on the other hand, usually requires fact-gatherer and analyst roles.
- Some problems require multiple roles. Managing conflict among the involved health care providers, a common problem, demands process skills.

- Collecting and interpreting the data necessary to document a problem require both interpersonal and analytical skills.
- The community's history of taking part in decision making is a critical factor. In a community skilled in identifying and successfully managing its problems, the nurse may best serve as technical expert or advisor.

Different roles may be required if the community lacks problem-solving skills or has a history of unsuccessful change efforts. The nurse may have to focus on developing problem-solving capabilities or on making one successful change so that the community becomes empowered to take on the job of promoting change on its own behalf.

SOCIAL CHANGE PROCESS AND THE NURSE'S ROLE. The nurse's role also depends on the social change process. Not all communities are open to change. The ability to change is often related to the extent to which a community focuses on traditional norms. The more traditional the community, the less likely it is to change. The ability to change is often directly related to the following (Rogers, 2003):
- High socioeconomic status
- A perceived need for change
- The presence of liberal, scientific, and democratic values
- A high level of social participation by community residents

For example, people living in a community might go to an immunization clinic rather than to a private physician if the clinic is nearby and less expensive and if the physician is not always available when needed.

Changes also are easier to accept in the following situations (Rogers, 2003):
- The change is shared in ways that fit in with the community's norms, values, and customs.
- Information is spread by the best communication mode (e.g., mass media for early adopters [people open to change] and face to face for late adopters [people who have more difficulty with change]).

Evidence-Based Practice

The purpose of this intervention was to test the effectiveness of an interdisciplinary team's ability to build community partnerships and implement the core functions of public health nursing. This effort by the local public health department involved a wide variety of different community groups and organizations.
- The outcomes of the intervention supported a practice model built on core public health functions.
- The value of describing and measuring community capacity was apparent, as was the need for a "will to act" within the community—not just having knowledge and skills.
- The organizational climate of the health department shifted to a more participatory collegial model.

   NURSE USE: Evaluation of the interventions indicated that both the agency and the community organizations were affected by this effort.

From Westbrook L, Schultz P: From theory to practice: community health nursing in a public health neighborhood team, *Adv Nurs Sci* 23(2):50–61, 2000.

- Other communities support the change efforts.
- Opinion leaders are identified and used.
- Communication about the change is clear and straightforward.

EVALUATING THE INTERVENTION FOR COMMUNITY HEALTH

Simply defined, **evaluation** is the appraisal of the effects of some organized activity or program. An example of evaluation is provided in the Evidence-Based Practice box. Evaluation may involve the design and conduct of evaluation research, or it may involve the more elementary process of assessing progress by contrasting the objectives and the results (El Ansari et al, 2004). This section deals with the basic approach of contrasting objectives and results.

Evaluation begins in the planning phase, when goals and measurable objectives are established and goal-attaining activities are identified. After implementing the intervention, only the accomplishment of objectives and the effects of intervention activities have to be assessed. Nursing progress notes direct the nurse to perform such appraisals concurrently with implementation. In assessing the data recorded there, the nurse is requested to evaluate whether the objectives were met and whether the intervention activities used were effective. Such an evaluation process is oriented to community health because the intervention goals and objectives come from the nurse's and the community's ideas about health.

Figure 12-1 presents a summary of the complete nursing process with a community client.

Role of Outcomes in the Evaluation Phase

The measurement of outcomes is a particularly important part of the evaluation process. This is one reason for placing emphasis on measurable objectives. El Ansari et al (2001) emphasize outcomes questions about appropriate and effective interventions such as the following:

- Was the appropriate intervention done ineffectively or effectively?
- Were the objectives sensitive enough to measure change?
- Was an inappropriate intervention used?
- Has the health problem been resolved or the risk reduced?

To answer these and other outcomes questions, emphasizing epidemiology and the correct use of rates and numbers are means of evaluating intervention outcomes among defined communities. Often data collected over time can also provide important outcomes information about health trends within the community. As indicated, epidemiologic data and trends do not provide the only measure of success but they do provide important information about the intervention. Nurses need to consider the collection of this type of outcomes data for use as part of the evaluation phase. Outcomes can be measured by looking at changes from before and after the intervention to solve the problems. Changes in the following can be used to see the outcomes of the interventions (Fos and Fine, 2000):

- Demographics
- Socioeconomic factors
- Environmental factors
- Individual and community health status
- Use of health services

In the example of infant malnutrition, it is necessary to look for the number of cases of infant malnutrition in the community before providing education to other health providers about assessment of infant development. A time period for evaluation would be chosen, with follow-up perhaps 1 year later (the time frame). The number of cases of infant malnutrition would be measured to see if a change had occurred and there were fewer cases.

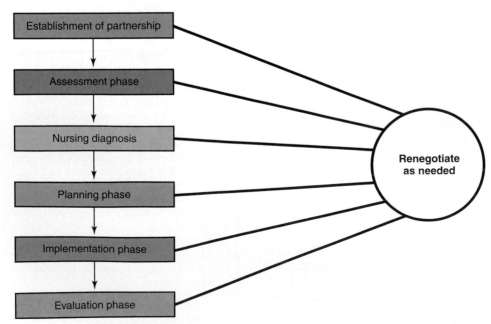

FIGURE 12-1 Summary flow sheet illustrating the nursing process with the community as client.

PERSONAL SAFETY IN COMMUNITY PRACTICE

Personal safety is a prerequisite for effective community-oriented nursing practice, and it should be a consideration throughout the process. An awareness of the community and common sense are the two best guidelines for judgment. For example, common sense suggests not leaving anything valuable on a car seat or leaving the car unlocked. Similar guidelines apply to the use of public transportation. Calling ahead to schedule meetings will help prevent delays or confusion, and it gives the nurse an opportunity to lay the groundwork for the meeting. If there is no telephone or no access to a neighbor's telephone, a time for any future meetings should be established during the initial visit. Regardless of whether telephone contact had been made, rare situations occur that require that the meeting be postponed—for example, if the nurse arrives at a location and is concerned about personal safety because of people unexpectedly loitering by the entrance.

For nurses who are either just beginning their careers in community health or who are just starting a new position,

the following three clear sources of information will help answer any questions about personal safety:

1. *Other nurses, social workers, or health care providers who are familiar with the dynamics of a given community.* They can provide valuable insights into when to visit, how to get there, and what to expect, because they function in the community themselves.
2. *Community members.* The best sources of information about the community are the community members themselves, and one benefit of developing an active partnership with community members is their willingness to share their insight about day-to-day community life.
3. *The nurse's own observations.* Knowledge gained during the data-collection phase of the process should provide a solid basis for an awareness of day-to-day community activity. Nurses with experience practicing in the community generally agree that if they feel uncomfortable in a situation, they should trust their feelings and leave.

Tables 12-4 through 12-8 are specific examples of the assessment of Jefferson County.

Table 12-4   Problem Analysis: Infant Malnutrition

Name of community: Jefferson County
Problem statement: Infant malnutrition in Jefferson County

Factors Contributing to the Problem and Outcomes	Relationship of Factors	Data Supportive to Relationships
1. Inadequate diet	Diets lacking in required nutrients contribute to malnutrition.	All county infants and their mothers seen by public health nurses (PHNs) in 2010 were referred to a nutritionist because of poor diets.
2. Community norms	Bottle-fed babies are less apt to receive adequate amounts of safe milk containing necessary nutrients.	Area general practitioners and nurses agree that 90% of mothers in the county bottle-feed their infants.
3. Poverty	Infant formulas are expensive.	Of new mothers in county, 60% are receiving welfare.
4. Disturbed mother–child relationship	Poor mother–child relationship may result in infant's failure to thrive.	Data from charts of 43 nursing mothers show infants diagnosed with "failure to thrive."
5. Teenage pregnancy	Teenage mothers are most apt to have inadequate diets prenatally, to bottle-feed, to be poor, and to lack parenting skills.	Of births in 2010, 90% were to women 19 years of age or younger.

Table 12-5   Problem Priority: Infant Malnutrition in Jefferson County

Criteria	Rationale for Rating	Problem Priority
1. Community awareness of the problem	Health service providers, teachers, and a variety of leaders have mentioned the problem.	2
2. Community motivation to resolve the problem	Most believable that this problem is not solvable because most of those affected are indigent.	4
3. Nurse's ability to influence problem resolution	Nurses are skilled at raising consciousness and mobilizing support.	3
4. Ready availability of expertise relevant to problem resolution	Women, Infants, and Children (WIC) program and nutritionists are available. A county extension agent is interested.	1
5. Severity of outcomes if the problem is left unresolved	Effects of marginal health services are not well documented.	5
6. Quickness with which problem resolution can be achieved	Time to mobilize a rural community with no history of social action is lengthy.	6

Table 12-6	Problem Priority: All Identified Problems		

Criteria	Problem	Rationale for Rating	Problem Priority
1. Community awareness of the problem	Community's desire to quit smoking	Health service providers, teachers, and a variety of leaders have mentioned the problem.	2
2. Community motivation to resolve the problem	Poor housing standards	Most believe that this problem is not solvable because most of those affected are indigent.	4
3. Nurse's ability to influence problem resolution	Mortality rate from cardiovascular disease	Nurses are skilled at consciousness raising and mobilizing support.	3
4. Ready availability of expertise relevant to problem resolution	Infant malnutrition in Jefferson County	Women, Infants, and Children (WIC) program and nutritionists are available. A county extension agent is interested.	1
5. Severity of outcomes if problem is left unresolved	Lack of primary care clinics	Effects of marginal health services are not well documented.	5
6. Quickness with which problem resolution can be achieved	Teen pregnancy	Time to mobilize a rural community with no history of social action is lengthy.	6

Table 12-7	Goals and Objectives: Infant Malnutrition	

Name of community: Jefferson County
Problem/concern: Infant malnutrition
Goal statement: To reduce the incidence and prevalence of infant malnutrition

Present Date	Objectives (Number and Statement)	Completion Date
2010	1. Developmental levels will be assessed for 80% of infants seen by the health department, the neighborhood health center, and private physicians.	2012
2010	2. Women, Infants, and Children (WIC) program eligibility will be determined for 80% of infants seen by the health department, neighborhood health center, and private physicians.	2012
2010	3. An outreach program will be implemented to identify at-risk infants not now known to health care providers.	2012
2010	4. WIC program eligibility will be determined for 25% of at-risk infants.	2013
2010	5. Of all infants eligible for WIC food supplements, 75% will be enrolled in the program.	2013
2010	6. Of the mothers of infants enrolled in WIC, 50% will demonstrate three ways of incorporating WIC supplements into their infants' diets.	2013

Table 12-8	Plan: Intervention Activities to Assess Infants' Developmental Levels		

Name of community: Jefferson County
Objective number 1 and statement: Developmental levels will be assessed for 80% of infants seen by health department, neighborhood health center, and private physicians

Present Date	Possible Interventions	Intervention Problems/Resources	Completion Date
2010	1. Women, Infants, Children (WIC) program supplies personnel to assess infant developmental levels.	Personnel and time are insufficient; existing community resources (potential) are ignored.	5
2010	2. WIC program provides inservice education to staff on assessment of infant development.	Antipathy between WIC personnel health and other workers is high. The need for education must be assessed first, and enthusiasm for objectives must be created.	4
2010	3. Nurse provides inservice education to staff in the assessment of infant development.	Nurse cannot do it alone.	3
2010	4. Nurse helps WIC personnel identify inservice educational needs of area health care providers about assessment of infant development.	Most likely to build on existing community strengths; nurse skilled in needs assessment and interpersonal techniques is needed to decrease antipathy.	2
2010	5. Nurse helps WIC personnel identify driving and restraining forces relative to the implementation of the objective.	Without this, change effort is likely to fail.	1

CLINICAL APPLICATION

Lily Jones, a nurse in a small city, became aware of the increased incidence of respiratory diseases through contact with families in the community and the local chapter of the American Lung Association. During family visits, Lily noted that many of the parents were smokers. Because most of the families Lily visited had small children, she became concerned about the effects of secondhand smoke on the health of the infants and children among her family caseload.

Further assessment of this community indicated that the community recognized several problems, including school safety and the risk of water pollution, in addition to the smoking problem that Lily had identified during her family

visits. Talks with different community members revealed that they wanted each of these identified problems "fixed," although these same community members also remained uncertain of how to start.

In deciding which of the three identified problems to address first, which criterion would be most important for Lily to consider?
A. The amount of money available
B. The level of community motivation to "fix" one of the three identified problems
C. The number of people in the community who expressed a concern about one of the three identified problems
D. How much control she would have in the process
Answer is in the back of the book.

Checklist for a Community Assessment

Asset Development
- ☐ Land
- ☐ Libraries
- ☐ Parks
- ☐ Police stations
- ☐ Fire stations

Community Organizations
- ☐ Crime Watch
- ☐ Neighborhood Watch
- ☐ Women's clubs
- ☐ Optimist
- ☐ Kiwanis
- ☐ Lions
- ☐ Businesses
- ☐ Schools
- ☐ Colleges

Government Assistance
- ☐ Number of families receiving Aid to Families With Dependent Children
- ☐ Number of persons receiving public assistance
- ☐ Number of persons receiving Medicaid
- ☐ Number of persons receiving food stamps

Health Risk Variables
Population Variables
- ☐ Population
- ☐ Total population density
- ☐ Population age groups (0–4 years of age; 5–17 years of age; 18–64 years of age; 65 and older)

Ethnicity
- ☐ Percentage white
- ☐ Percentage African-American
- ☐ Percentage Hispanic

Socioeconomic Data
- ☐ Percentage of persons below the federal poverty guideline
- ☐ Total number of households
- ☐ Estimated per capita income
- ☐ Estimated average household income

- ☐ Percentage of households with incomes less than $15,000
- ☐ Unemployment rate
- ☐ Occupational status
- ☐ Value of housing
- ☐ Educational level

Birth and Birth-Related Information
- ☐ Fertility rate
- ☐ Percentage of teen births
- ☐ Percentage of low birth weight
- ☐ Percentage of infant mortality

Age-Adjusted Death Rates
- ☐ Accident
- ☐ Cancer
- ☐ Cirrhosis
- ☐ Diabetes
- ☐ Heart disease
- ☐ Human immunodeficiency virus
- ☐ Homicide
- ☐ Pneumonia/flu
- ☐ Respiratory
- ☐ Stroke
- ☐ Suicides

Access to Primary Care
- ☐ Primary care physicians per population (family practice, general practice, pediatrics, internal medicine, and OB/Gyn)
- ☐ Primary care providers per population (nurse midwives, nurse practitioners, and physician assistants)

Inpatient Discharges per 1000 Population
- ☐ Discharges per 1000 population for each service area or the county as a whole excluding newborns
- ☐ Discharges per 1000 population for each service area or the county as a whole for the top five discharges

Survey Data
- ☐ Top five health concerns
- ☐ Insurance status
- ☐ Access to care

From Pickens S, Boumbulian P, Tietz M: Community assessment: strengths, assets, & management, *Inside Prevent Care* 1(6), 1995.

REMEMBER THIS!

- A community is defined as a locality-based entity, composed of systems of formal organizations reflecting societal institutions, informal groups, and aggregates that are interdependent and whose function or expressed intent is to meet a wide variety of collective needs.
- A community practice setting is insufficient reason for saying that practice is oriented toward the community client. When the location of the practice is in the community but the focus of the practice is the individual or family, the nursing client remains the individual or family, not the whole community.
- Community-oriented practice is targeted to the community, the population group in which healthful change is sought.
- *Community health* as used in this chapter is defined as the meeting of collective needs through identifying problems and managing interactions within the community itself and between the community and the larger society.
- Most changes aimed at improving community health involve, of necessity, partnerships among community residents and health workers from a variety of disciplines.
- Assessing community health requires gathering existing data, generating missing data, and interpreting the database.
- Five methods of collecting data useful to the nurse are informant interviews, participant observation, secondary analysis of existing data, surveys, and windshield surveys.
- Gaining entry or acceptance into the community is perhaps the greatest challenge in assessment.
- The nurse is usually an outsider and often represents an established health care system that is neither known nor trusted by community members, who may react with indifference or even active hostility.
- The planning phase includes analyzing and establishing priorities among community health problems already identified, establishing goals and objectives, and identifying intervention activities that will accomplish the objectives.
- Once high-priority problems are identified, broad relevant goals and objectives are developed.
- The goal, generally a broad statement of desired outcome, and objectives, the precise statements of the desired outcome, are carefully selected.
- Intervention activities, the means by which objectives are met, are the strategies that clarify what must be done to achieve the objectives, the ways change will be effected, and the way the problem will be interpreted.
- Implementation, the third phase of the nursing process, is transforming a plan for improved community health into achievement of goals and objectives.
- Simply defined, evaluation is the appraisal of the effects of some organized activity or program.

WHAT WOULD YOU DO?

1. Observe an occupational health nurse, public health nurse, school nurse, family nurse practitioner, or emergency department nurse for several hours. Determine which of the nurse's activities are community oriented, and state the reasons for your judgment.
2. Using your own community as a frame of reference, develop examples illustrating the concepts of community, community client, community health, and partnership for health.
3. Read your local newspaper and identify articles illustrating the concepts of community, community client, community health, and partnership for health.

■ REFERENCES

Anderson ET, McFarlane J: *Community-as-partner: theory and practice in nursing*, ed 4, Philadelphia, 2004, Lippincott Williams & Wilkins.

Blum HL: *Planning for health*, New York, 1974, Human Sciences Press.

Consensus set of health status indicators for the general assessment of community health status—United States, *MMWR* 40(27):449, 1991 (updated Aug 2001).

Constance A et al: MDON: a network of community partnerships. *Fam Com Health* 25:52, 2002.

Council on Linkages between Academia and Public Health Practice: *Core competencies for public health professionals*, Washington, DC, 2001, U.S. Department of Health and Human Services and Public Health Foundation.

El Ansari W, Phillips CJ, Hammick M: Collaboration and partnerships: developing the evidence base, *Health Soc Care Community* 9:215-227, 2001.

El Ansari W, Phillips CJ, Zwi AB: Public health nurses' perspectives on collaborative partnerships in South Africa, *Public Health Nurs* 21:277-286, 2004.

Fos PJ, Fine DJ: *Designing health care for populations*, San Francisco, 2000, Jossey-Bass.

Horsley K, Ciske SJ: From neurons to King County neighborhoods: partnering to promote policies based on the science of early childhood development, *Am J Public Health* 95:562-567, 2005.

Kemsley M, Riegle E: A community-campus partnership: influenza prevention campaign, *Nurse Educ* 29(3):126-129, 2004.

Levine DM et al: The effectiveness of a community/academic health center partnership in decreasing the level of blood pressure in an urban African-American population, *Ethn Dis* 13:354-361, 2003.

Lutz J, Herrick C, Lehman B: Community partnership: a school of nursing creates nursing centers for older adults, *Nurs Health Care Perspect* 22:26-29, 2001.

Lyford J, Breen N, Grove M: Today's educator: diabetes training for schools using a community partnership model in rural Oregon, *Diabetes Educ* 29:564, 2003.

Maurana CA, Clark MA: The health action fund: a community-based approach to enhancing health, *J Health Commun* 5:243-254, 2000.

McKenzie JF, Pinger RR, Kotecki JE: *An introduction to community health*, Jones & Bartlett, 2008.

McMahon B, Browning S, Rose-Colley M: A school-community partnership for at-risk students in Pennsylvania, *J School Health* 71:53-55, 2001.

Miller M et al: Prevention of smoking behaviors in middle school students: student nurse interventions, *Public Health Nurse* 18:77-81, 2001.

Rogers E: *Diffusion of innovations*, ed 4, New York, 2003, Free Press.

Rosen L: Associate and baccalaureate degree final semester students' perceptions of self-efficacy concerning community health nursing competencies, *Public Health Nurse* 17:231-238, 2000.

Rowitz L: *Public health leadership: putting principles into practice*, Gaithersburg, Md, 2001, Aspen.

Ryan W: *Blaming the victim*, New York, 1976, Vintage Books.

Saunders SD, Greaney ML, Lees FD et al: Achieving recruitment goals through community partnerships: the SENIOR project, *Fam Community Health* 26:194, 2003.

Stanhope M, Knollmueller R: *Handbook of community-based and home health nursing practice*, ed 3, St Louis, 2000, Mosby.

U.S. Department of Health and Human Services: *Healthy people 2010*, Washington, DC, 2000, U.S. Department of Health and Human Services.

Westbrook L, Schultz P: From theory to practice: community health nursing in a public health neighborhood team, *Adv Nurse Sci* 23(2):50-61, 2000.

World Health Organization: *Community health nursing: report of a WHO expert committee, tech rep series no 558*, Geneva, Switzerland, 1974, World Health Organization.

Case Management

Ann H. Cary

ADDITIONAL RESOURCES

These related resources are found either in the appendix at the back of this book or on the book's website at http://evolve.elsevier.com/stanhope/foundations.

Evolve Website

- Community Assessment Applied
- Case Study, with questions and answers

- Quiz review questions
- WebLinks, including link to *Healthy People 2010* website

OBJECTIVES

After reading this chapter, the student should be able to:

1. Distinguish between continuity of care, care management, case management, and advocacy.
2. Describe the scope of practice, roles, and functions of a case manager.
3. Compare and contrast the nursing process with the process of case management.
4. Identify methods to manage conflict and the process of achieving collaboration.
5. Define and explain the legal and ethical issues confronting case managers.
6. Identify the relationship between advocacy and case management.

CHAPTER OUTLINE

CONCEPTS OF CASE MANAGEMENT
Definitions of Case Management
Healthy People 2010 **and the Case Management Process**
Case Management and the Nursing Process
Characteristics and Roles
Knowledge and Skill Requirements
Tools of Case Managers
COMMUNITY MODELS OF CASE MANAGEMENT

ADVOCACY, CONFLICT MANAGEMENT, AND COLLABORATION SKILLS FOR CASE MANAGERS
Advocacy
Conflict Management
Collaboration
ISSUES IN CASE MANAGEMENT
Legal Issues
Ethical Issues

KEY TERMS

advocacy: activities for the purpose of protecting the rights of others while supporting the client's responsibility for self-determination; involves informing, supporting, and affirming a client's self-determination in health care decisions.

affirming: ratifying, asserting, or giving strength to the declarations of self or others.
aggregate: populations or defined groups.
assertiveness: the ability to state one's own needs.

autonomy: freedom of action as chosen by an individual.

beneficence: ethical principle stating that one should do good and prevent or avoid doing harm.

care management: a program or process that established systems and monitors the health status of individuals, families, and/or groups. The program or process develops planning and intervention activities, as well as targeted evaluation outcomes for the client and program.

CareMaps: a tool developed by Zander showing cause and effect and identifying expected client/family and staff behaviors against a timeline.

case management: includes the activities implemented with individual clients in the system.

case manager: builds on the basic functions of the traditional role and adapts new competencies for managing the transition from one part of the system to another or to home.

collaboration: mutual sharing and working together to achieve common goals in such a way that all persons or groups are recognized and growth is enhanced.

conflict management: a process of assisting clients in resolving issues between competing needs and resources.

constituency: a group or body that patronizes, supports, or offers representation.

cooperation: working together or associating with others for a common benefit; a common effort.

coordinating: conscious activity of assembling and directing the work efforts of a group of health providers so that they can function harmoniously in the attainment of the objective of client care.

critical paths: a planning technique that focuses on activities, best use of time and resources, and estimated time to complete activities. The technique can be used for planning programs or individual client care as it is related to a specific diagnosis.

demand management: a program that provides to consumers, at the point at which they are deciding how to enter the health care system, information and support to access care.

disease management: a proactive treatment approach, focused on a specific diagnosis, that seeks to manage a chronic health condition and minimize acute episodes in a population.

informing: a communication process in which the nurse interprets facts and shares knowledge with clients.

intercessor: a person who acts on behalf of the client even though the client could act for him or herself.

justice: an ethical principle that claims that equals should be treated equally and those who are unequal should be treated differently according to their differences.

liability: an obligation an individual has incurred or might incur through any act or failure to act, or responsibility for conduct falling below a certain standard that is the cause of client injury.

life care plan: a customized, medically based document that provides assessment of all present and future needs (medical, financial, psychological, vocational, spiritual, physical, and social), including services, equipment, supplies, and living arrangements for a client (Llewellyn and Moreo, 2001).

mediator: a role in which the nurse acts to assist parties to understand each other's concerns and to determine their conclusions concerning the issues. The mediator has no authority to decide on behalf of another.

negotiating: working with others in a formal way to achieve agreement on areas of conflict, using principles of communication, conflict resolution, and assertiveness.

problem-purpose-expansion method: a way to broaden limited thinking that involves restating the problem and expanding the problem statement so that different solutions can be generated.

problem solving: a process of seeking to find solutions to situations that involve difficulty or uncertainty.

promoter: an advocacy role in which the nurse partners with the client and promotes the client's rights to make his or her own decision.

supporting: upholding the client in making decisions about care or about entering the health care system.

telehealth: an organized health care delivery approach to do triage and provide advice, counseling, and referral for a client with a health problem using phones or computers with cameras. The client is usually in the home, and the nurse is at an office, health care facility, or phone bank location.

timelines: landmarks of an episode of health or illness care from initial encounter to the transfer of accountability to the client or another health care agency.

use management: a continual process of evaluating the appropriateness, necessity, and efficiency of health service over a period of time.

CONCEPTS OF CASE MANAGEMENT

Case management is a strategy that is used in an overarching process called **care management.** Care management is an enduring process in which a population manager establishes systems and monitors the health status, resources, and outcomes for an **aggregate**—a targeted segment of the population or a group. Care management strategies were initially developed by health maintenance organizations (HMOs) in the late 1970s to manage the care of different populations while promoting quality of care and ensuring appropriate use and costs. Care management strategies include **use management, critical paths, disease management, demand management,** and **case management** (Box 13-1).

Box 13-1 | **Additional Definitions of Case Management Strategies**

- *Use management* attempts to redirect care and monitors the appropriate use of provider care and treatment services for both acute and community and ambulatory services (Llewellyn and Moreo, 2001).
- *Critical paths* are tools that name activities that can be used in a timely sequence to achieve the desired outcomes for care. The outcomes are measurable, and the critical path tools strive to reduce differences in client care.
- *Disease management* activities target chronic and costly disease conditions that require long-term care interventions (e.g., diabetes). These strategies address the entire cycle of a disease process, typically incorporating primary, secondary, and tertiary care interventions and self-care activities (McClatchy, 2001).
- *Demand management* seeks to control use by providing clients with correct information to empower them to make healthy choices, use healthy and health-seeking behaviors to improve their health status, and make fewer demands on the health care system (Paul, 2000).

The **case manager** is the architect for the target group's health in the care management delivery process. The building blocks used by the manager include the following (Haaag and Kalina, 2005):

- Risk analysis
- Data mapping
- Data monitoring for health processes, indicators, and unexpected illnesses
- Epidemiologic investigation of unexpected illnesses
- Multidisciplinary development of action plans and programs
- Identifying case management triggers or events that promote earlier referrals of high-risk clients when prevention can have dramatic results

Case management, in contrast to care management, involves activities implemented with individual clients in the system. The case manager builds on the basic functions of the traditional role and adapts new competencies for managing the transition from one part of the system to another or to home.

DEFINITIONS OF CASE MANAGEMENT

An historical focus on collaboration is seen in the National Case Management Task Force definition (Mullahy, 2004, p. 9):

A collaborative process which assesses, plans, implements, coordinates, monitors and evaluates the options and services to meet an individual's health needs, using communication and available resources to promote quality, cost effective outcomes.

Case management is defined in public health nursing as the ability to "optimize self-care capabilities of individuals and families and the capacity of systems and communities to coordinate and provide services" (Minnesota Department

of Health, 2003, p. 93). Case management is viewed as only one competency, or skill, that nurses need to have to provide quality care. Case management is identified as one of 17 interventions in the scope of practice of nursing in the community (Minnesota Department of Health, 2003). The following knowledge and skills are required to achieve this competency:

- Knowledge of community resources and financing methods
- Written and oral communication and documentation skills
- Negotiation and conflict-resolution skills
- Critical thinking processes to identify and prioritize problems from the view of the provider and client
- Application of evidence-based practices and outcome measures (Muller and Flarery, 2003)

Case management practice is complex because of the **coordinating** activities of multiple providers, payers, and settings throughout a client's continuum of care. Care by multiple providers (the client, family, significant others, community organizations) must be assessed, planned, implemented, adjusted, and based on mutually agreed-upon goals. The nurse employed and located in one setting will be influencing the selection and monitoring of care provided in other settings by formal and informal care providers. With the use of electronic care delivery through telehealth activities, case management activities are now delivered via telephone, e-mail, fax, and video visits in a client's residence. They may also be delivered to a global network of clients located in different countries.

BRIEFLY NOTED

Although the activities in case management may differ among providers and clients, the goals are as follow:

- To promote quality services provided to clients
- To reduce institutional care while maintaining quality processes and satisfactory outcomes
- To manage resource use through protocols, evidence-based decision making, guideline use, and disease-management programs
- To control expenses by managing care processes and outcomes (Mullahy, 2004)

A particularly challenging problem is the fragmenting of services, which can result in overuse, underuse, gaps in care, and miscommunication. This may ultimately result in costly client outcomes. Case management in rural settings is more complex because of the following:

- Fewer organized community-based systems
- Geographic distance to delivery
- Population density
- Finances
- Pace and lifestyle
- Values
- Social organization differences from the urban setting

HEALTHY PEOPLE 2010 AND THE CASE MANAGEMENT PROCESS

Nurse case managers in their practices have as core values the goals of *Healthy People 2010*. Many of the interventions that nurses use with clients, as well as the design of the health care system and the number of covered lives in those systems, promote further progress in meeting the objectives of *Healthy People 2010*. Case management strategies offer opportunities for nurses to help meet the objectives for specific population targets listed in *Healthy People 2010* (U.S. Department of Health and Human Services, 2000).

The target populations include those who do not have access to health care and those whose lifestyle or health conditions may limit the quality and length of healthy life; variables include ethnicity/race, low income, limited education, gender or sexual orientation, those living in the inner city or rural areas, those without health insurance, and the disabled or those experiencing chronic disease.

This chapter guides the reader through the nature and process of case management for individual and family clients. Case management has had a rich tradition with nursing in the community that dates back to Lillian Wald and the Henry Street Settlement (Tahan, 1998). Nursing has maintained the leadership among health care providers in coordinating resources to achieve health care outcomes based on quality, access, and cost. As health care delivery moves to chronic disease management services with an emphasis on pursuing the most efficient use of services to manage client outcomes, case management emerges to play a strong role.

CASE MANAGEMENT AND THE NURSING PROCESS

Case management activities with individual clients and families will reveal the larger picture of health services and health status of the community. Through a nurse's case management activities, general community weaknesses in quality and quantity of health services often are discovered. For example, the management of a severely disabled child by a nurse case manager may uncover the absence of respite services or parenting support and education resources in a community.

BRIEFLY NOTED

The components of the nursing process are used when implementing the functions of a case manager with clients. The spectrum of case management consists of four activities: assessment, planning, facilitating, and advocacy (Aliotta, 2003; Case Management Society of America, 2002).

While managing the disability and injury claims at an industry, the nurse may discover that referrals for home health visits and physical therapy are generally underused by the acute care providers in the community. Community *assessment, policy development,* and *assurance* activities that frame core functions of public health actions are often the logical next steps for a nurse's practice. When observing lack of care or services at the individual and family intervention levels, the nurse can, through case management, intervene at the community level to make changes (Table 13-1). The case management process involving client and nurse is depicted in Figure 13-1.

CHARACTERISTICS AND ROLES

Case management can be labor intensive, time consuming, and costly. Because of the increasing number of clients with complex problems in nurses' caseloads, the intensity and duration of activities required to support the case management function may soon exceed the demands that the direct caregiver can meet. Managers and clinicians in community health are exploring methods to make case management more efficient.

Llewellyn and Moreo (2001) and Cary (1998) have described the roles that case managers assume in the practice setting (Box 13-2). The roles demanded of the nurse as case manager are vividly influenced by the forces at work in the employing agency. Figure 13-2 presents a case management model.

KNOWLEDGE AND SKILL REQUIREMENTS

Adopting the case management role for a nurse does not happen automatically with an agency position. Knowledge and skills that are developed and refined are essential to success. Stanton and Dunkin (2002), Llewellyn and Moreo (2001), and Cary (1998) suggest knowledge areas useful for nurses

Table 13-1   The Nursing Process and Case Management

Nursing Process	Case Management Process	Activities
Assessment	Case finding	Develop networks with the target population
	Identification of incentives for the target population	Disseminate written materials
		Seek referrals
	Screening and intake	Apply screening tools according to program goals and objectives
	Determination of eligibility	Use written and on-site screens
	Assessment	Apply comprehensive assessment methods (physical, social, emotional, cognitive, economic, self-care capacity)
Diagnosis	Identification of the problem	Hold interdisciplinary, family, and client conferences
		Determine conclusions on the basis of assessment
		Use an interdisciplinary team
Goal Identification/ Planning/outcomes	Problem prioritizing	Validate and prioritize problems with all participants
	Planning to address care needs	Develop activities, time frames, and options
		Gain the client's consent to implement
		Have the client choose options
Implementation	Advocating of clients' interests	Contact providers
		Negotiate services and price
Evaluation	Arrangement of delivery of service	Coordinate service delivery
	Monitoring of clients during service	Monitor for changes in client or service status
	Reassessment	Examine outcomes against goals
		Examine needs against service
		Examine costs
		Examine the satisfaction of client, providers, and the case manager

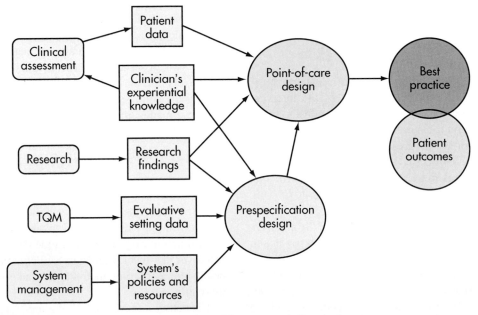

FIGURE 13-1 Factors that require the attention of the nurse and client in the case management process.

and the agency desiring to implement quality case management roles (Box 13-3). If a nurse seeks a case manager position, some of the skills and knowledge areas will need to be developed through academic and continuing education programs, literature reviews, orientation, and mentoring experiences.

Telehealth is a contemporary intervention approach that is used by case managers. It is an organized health care delivery approach to triage and provide advice, counseling, and referral for a client's health problem using phones or computers with cameras. The client is usually in the home, and the nurse is at an office, health care facility, or phone bank location (see the "Evidence-Based Practice" box, p. 242).

TOOLS OF CASE MANAGERS

Case management plans have evolved with a variety of names and methods (e.g., critical paths, critical pathways, CareMaps, multidisciplinary action plans, nursing care plans,

Box 13-2 Case Manager Roles

- *Broker:* Acts as an agent for provider services that are needed by clients to stay within coverage according to the budget and cost limits of health care plan
- *Consultant:* Case manager who works with providers, suppliers, the community, and other case managers to provide case management expertise in programmatic and individual applications
- *Coordinator:* Arranges, regulates, and coordinates needed health care services for clients at all necessary points of services
- *Educator:* Educates client, family, and providers about the case management process, delivery system, community health resources, and benefit coverage so that informed decisions can be made by all parties
- *Facilitator:* Supports all parties in work toward mutual goals
- *Liaison:* Provides a formal communication link among all parties concerning the plan of care management
- *Mentor:* Case manager who counsels and guides the development of the practice of new case managers
- *Monitor/reporter:* Provides information to parties on the status of member and situations affecting patient safety, care quality, and patient outcome and on factors that alter costs and liability
- *Negotiator:* Negotiates the plan of care, services, and payment arrangements with providers; uses effective collaboration and team strategies
- *Patient advocate:* Acts as an advocate, provides information, and supports benefit changes that assist member, family, primary care provider, and capitated systems
- *Researcher:* Case manager who utilizes and applies evidence-based practices for programmatic and individual interventions with clients and communities, participates in the protection of clients in research studies, and initiates and collaborates in research programs and studies
- *Standardization monitor:* Formulates and monitors specific, time-sequenced critical path and care map plans (see pp. 240–241) and disease management protocols that guide the type and timing of care to comply with predicted treatment outcomes for the specific client and conditions; attempts to reduce variation in resource use; targets deviations from standards so adjustments can occur in a timely manner
- *Systems allocator:* Distributes limited health care resources according to a plan or rationale

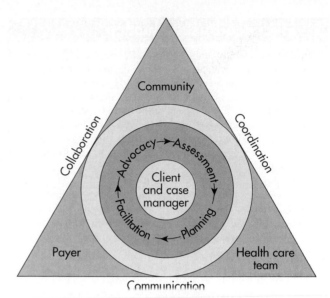

FIGURE 13-2 The Case Management Model.

disease management). Regardless of the term used, standards of client care, standards of nursing practice, and standards of practice for case management serve as a core foundation of case management plans. Likewise, in multidisciplinary action plans, core professional standards of each discipline guide the development of the standards process.

BRIEFLY NOTED

The five "rights" of case management are right care, right time, right provider, right setting, and right price. How does the nurse judge the effectiveness of case management?

A critical path is a case management tool composed of abbreviated versions of processes that are specific to each discipline (e.g., nursing); it is used to achieve a measurable outcome for a specific client "case" (Zander, Etheredge, and Bower, 1987). **CareMaps** became the second generation of critical paths of care. Rather than give definitions, Brown (2001) discusses the various types of evidence that must be accessed, interpreted, and integrated into care design. Brown proposed the Best Practice Health Care Map (BPHM) as a model for providing quality clinical care within a multidisciplinary practice. The Brown BPHM is (1) client centered, (2) scientifically based, (3) population outcomes based, (4) refined through quality assessment and compared to other maps, (5) individualized to each client, and (6) compatible with the larger system or health care agency.

In using CareMaps, it is necessary to be cautious because many are not evidence based (Renholm, Leino-Kilpi, and Suominen, 2002). They are usually developed with expert knowledge from a specific agency and may not be adequate for use in another agency. Adapting the case management care plan is a crucial skill for standardizing the process and outcome of care. It links multiple provider interventions to client responses and offers reasonable predictions for the client's progress. Self-responsibility by clients truly links **autonomy** and self-determination as the core of case management. As a nurse employed to function as a case manager, ample opportunities exist to develop, test, and revise CareMap prototypes for specific client groups experiencing health deficits and to make them evidence based.

Disease management activities target chronic and costly disease conditions that require long-term care interventions (e.g., diabetes, asthma, depression). These strategies are an acceptable approach to organizing services for a specific population across a continuum of primary, secondary, and tertiary prevention interventions. Self-care management activities may involve (McClatchey, 2001):

Evidence-Based Practice

Info-Santé Local Community Service Center (CLSC), the Québec telenursing service, is a telephone health-line nursing service that was implemented in 1995 in 141 community service centers. It operates in continuity with the other resources in the health and social service system. Info-Santé CLSC operates 24 hours a day, 7 days a week, and it received more than 2,260,000 calls in 1997. This report describes the findings from the first province-wide survey of the service, based on a stratified random sample of 4696 callers.

Info-Santé CLSC provides the population of Québec with a first-line response to their physical, psychosocial, and mental health needs. The telenursing protocols used by Info-Santé CLSC are based on a holistic approach to health and have various functions: once nurses have greeted callers and assessed their situation, they provide the relevant information about health, social, and community services; they give professional advice when there is no need for specialized or immediate intervention; and finally, they refer callers to the most appropriate resources when needed.

The descriptive survey evaluation was performed to assess, among other factors, the capacity of the service to develop self-care abilities among users. The services were perceived as useful and effective for solving problems and for helping respondents develop a feeling of self-reliance. It would seem that telenursing leads to two factors that predispose the adoption of health care behaviors: perceived self-efficacy and perceived behavior effectiveness.

NURSE USE: The findings revealed that most respondents were highly satisfied with the service; they followed the nurses' advice and carried out self-care measures as recommended. Nursing interventions helped respondents feel self-reliant and helped them feel that they could solve the same or similar problems should they occur in the future.

From Hagan L, Morin D, Lepine R: Evaluation of telenursing outcomes: satisfaction, self-care practices, and cost savings, *Public Health Nurs* 17(4):305–313, 2000.

Box 13-3 Knowledge Domains for Case Management

- Knowledge of the health care financial environment and the financial dimension of client populations managed by nurses
- Clinical knowledge, skill, and maturity to direct quality-induced timing and sequencing of care activities
- Care resources for clients within institutions and communities: facilitating the development of new resources and systems to meet clients' needs
- Transition planning for ideal timing and sequencing of care
- Management skills: communication, delegation, persuasion, use of power, consultation, problem solving, conflict management, confrontation, negotiation, management of change, marketing, group development, accountability, authority, advocacy, ethical decision making, and profit management
- Teaching, counseling, and education skills
- Program evaluation and research
- Performance improvement techniques
- Peer consultation and evaluation
- Requirements of eligibility and benefit parameters by third-party payers
- Legal issues
- Information systems: clinical and management
- Health care legislation/policy
- Technical information skills
- Outcomes management and applied research

- Case management and risk sharing arrangements between payers and providers
- Programs for monitoring the use of prescriptions and treatment interventions, to assess outcomes and costs
- Protocols for clinical and administrative processes
- Education initiatives to meet the learning needs of both clients and providers about knowledge of cost-effective treatments
- Interventions to modify health behaviors and increase compliance with treatment regimens

Disease management information systems use treatment guidelines to streamline the process, avoid unnecessary care, and act proactively to slow or reduce the effects or complications of the disease process for populations (Llewellyn and Moreo, 2001).

Life care planning is another tool used in case management. It assesses the current and future needs of a client for catastrophic or chronic disease over a life span. The **life care plan** is a customized, medically based document that provides assessment of all present and

future needs (medical, financial, psychological, vocational, spiritual, physical, and social), including services, equipment, supplies, and living arrangements for a client (Llewellyn and Moreo, 2001). These plans may be used by either a plaintiff or defense lawyer to analyze damages. They are also used to set financial rewards, which can be used to pay for care in the future and create a lifetime care plan. Life care plans are typically used for clients experiencing catastrophic illness or adverse events resulting from professional malpractice. Another group of life care planning beneficiaries involves those who have sustained injury when younger and whose care requirements have changed as a result of aging (Demoratz, 2004). A systematic process is used and multidisciplinary input is required. The first phase of the plan is crafted to include a thorough assessment of the client, financial/billing agreements, an information release signed by the client, and a targeted date for report completion. Development of the plan is the second phase. Case management plans are based on a number of factors: social situation, leisure activities, educational and employment status, medical history, physical abilities, current status, and assistance required for completing the activities of daily living.

The plan includes projected costs and resources needed for the frequency and duration of treatments, equipment, and supplies. It also includes plans for future evaluations. The life care plan seeks to portray the needs of a client that are consistent with the changes in a client's life over the predicted life span, taking into account the injury or diagnosis (McCollom, 2002).

COMMUNITY MODELS OF CASE MANAGEMENT

Liberty Mutual Insurance Company has used case management principles for more than 30 years in workers' compensation cases and has expanded services for employees whose conditions were noted to be chronic or catastrophic. Box 13-4 lists examples of case-managed conditions. Case managers coordinate all providers, clients, and services to reduce excessive expenses caused by lack of coordination, failure to use quality alternatives, duplication, and fragmentation. Some states through their Medicaid programs are developing disease management programs for high-cost chronic diseases among their populations, such as asthma and diabetes.

A national study of 2437 people who tested positive for human immunodeficiency virus (HIV) and who had case managers demonstrated that regardless of the model, these clients were more likely to be using life-prolonging HIV medications and meeting the needs for income, health insurance, home care, and supportive emotional counseling than those without case management. Having contact with a case manager was not significantly related to the use of outpatient care, hospital admission, or emergency department visits. Case managers in this study example included social workers, nurses, and AIDS service organization staff (Katz et al, 2001).

Important guidance in developing a community-based case management program can be found in the United States. Case management is a key component of federally financed and many state-financed health delivery options. The experiences of states over the past two decades provide testimony to the importance of case management for populations at risk. For older clients, state-derived case management provides objective advice and assistance with care needs. It also provides access to multidisciplinary providers and services. For payers (federal, state, clients), case management serves as a way to ensure that funds are allocated appropriately to those in greatest need. Case management serves a policy assurance and accountability function for communities.

Within the states, the types of agencies designated to conduct case management are often district offices of state government, area agencies on aging, county social services departments, and private contractors. States maintain the oversight responsibilities for case management agencies to:

1. ensure they are complying with program standards, contracts, reporting, and fiscal controls;
2. identify emerging problems and issues to be resolved by additional state policies; and
3. provide on-site technical assistance and consulting to improve performance. States' payment methods for case management include daily and/or monthly rates, hourly

and/or quarterly rates, capped rates for services, and capped aggregate rates to cover both case management and provider costs (Health Resources and Services Administration [HRSA], 2004).

| Box 13-4 | **Examples of Case-Managed Conditions** |

- Acquired immunodeficiency syndrome (AIDS)
- Amputations
- Cerebrovascular accident (CVA)
- Chronic diseases and disabilities
- Coma
- High-risk neonates
- Multiple fractures
- Severe burns
- Severe head trauma
- Spinal cord injury
- Substance abuse
- Terminal illness
- Transplantation
- Ventilator dependency
- Work-related injuries

ADVOCACY, CONFLICT MANAGEMENT, AND COLLABORATION SKILLS FOR CASE MANAGERS

Three specific skills essential to the role performance of the case manager are discussed: *advocacy, conflict management,* and *collaboration.*

ADVOCACY

For nurses, **advocacy** involves differing activities, ranging from self-reflection to lobbying for health policy. Advocacy is essential for practice with clients and their families, communities, organizations, and colleagues on an interdisciplinary team. The functions of advocacy require scientific knowledge, expert communication, facilitating skills, and problem-solving and affirming techniques. As the Code of Ethics for Nurses (American Nurses Association, 2008) states, "the nurse establishes relationships and delivers nursing services with compassion and respect" (p. 1). The nurse advocate has previously been described as a person who acted on behalf of or interceded for the client. An example of the **intercessor** role is the nurse in community health practice who calls for a well-child appointment for a mother visiting the family planning clinic when the mother is capable of making an appointment on her own. The contemporary goal of advocacy would direct the nurse to move clients toward making the call themselves.

The change over time in the advocacy role to that of **mediator** by the nurse advocate is described as a response to social change, reimbursers, and providers in the health care system. *Mediation* is an activity in which a third

Table 13-2	Nursing Process and Advocacy Process
Nursing Process	**Advocacy Process**
Assessment/diagnosis	Exchange information
	Gather data
	Illuminate values
Goal identification/planning/ outcomes	Generate alternatives and consequences
	Prioritize actions
Implementation	Make decisions
	Support the client
	Assure the client
	Reassure the client
Evaluation	Affirm client decisions
	Evaluate
	Reformulate

Box 13-5	The Information Exchange

Guidelines for exchanging information in the advocacy process include the nurse's responsibility to do the following:
1. Assess the client's present understanding of the situation.
2. Provide correct information.
3. Communicate with the client's literacy level in mind, making the information as understandable as possible.
4. Use a variety of media and sources to increase the client's comprehension.
5. Discuss other factors that affect the decision, such as financial, legal, and ethical issues.
6. Discuss the possible consequences of a decision.

party attempts to provide assistance to those who may be experiencing a conflict in obtaining what they desire. The goal of the nurse advocate as mediator is to help parties understand each other on many levels so that agreement on an action is possible. In the situation of a nurse as case manager for an HMO, mediation activities between an elderly client and the payer (HMO) could accomplish the following results: the client may understand the options for community-based skilled nursing care and the payer may understand the client's desires for a less restrictive environment for care. Although the case manager as mediator does not decide the plan of action (in contrast to the role of arbitrator), he or she facilitates the decision-making processes between the parties so that the desired care can be reimbursed within the range of options available to the client.

In today's practice, the nurse advocate makes the client's rights the priority. The goal of **promoter** for the client's autonomy and self-determination may result in a high degree of client independence in decision making. For example, when a group of young pregnant women is the collective "client," or organization, the nurse advocate's role may be to inform the group of the benefits and consequences of breast-feeding their infants. However, if the new mothers decide on formula feeding, the nurse advocate should support the group and continue to provide parenting, infant, and well-child services.

A different perspective of the nurse advocate as promoter holds that the nurse's role as advocate may demand a variety of functions that are influenced by the client's physical, psychological, social, and environmental abilities. The nurse adapts the advocacy function to the client's dynamic capabilities as the client follows a path to a healthy status. Examples of advocacy in such cases might include promoting a client group's access to onsite physical fitness programs in the occupational setting or supporting parents' and students' concerns about the high fat content of vending machine food in the school system.

BRIEFLY NOTED

For clients who have no health coverage or who do not qualify for other programs, pharmaceutical companies may have a program of free supplies of drugs. Call a pharmaceutical company for information on the eligibility of your client.

Process of Advocacy

The goal of advocacy is to promote self-determination in a **constituency** or client group. It is often critical in promoting a client's self-determination. Table 13-2 compares the nursing process with the advocacy process. The constituency may be a client, family, peer, group, or community. It is often easier for the nurse to inform, support, and affirm another person's decision when the decision matches the values of the nurse. However, when clients make decisions within value systems that are different from those of the nurse, the advocate may feel conflict. Promoting self-determination in others demands a philosophy of free choice. Communication that shows respect, endorses the client's self-determination, and strives to understand and establish the accuracy of clients' knowledge, beliefs, and behaviors is used through both processes. The process of advocacy involves informing, supporting, and affirming.

INFORMING. Knowledge is essential but not sufficient to the outcome of decision making. The interpreting of knowledge is affected by the client's values and the meaning the client assigns to the knowledge. **Informing** clients about the nature of their choices, the content of those choices, and the consequences to the client is not a one-way activity. More active participation of clients in conversations with providers has been linked to better treatment compliance and health outcomes (Johnson et al, 2004). Although the exchange may be initiated at the factual level, it will likely proceed to include the opinions of both parties—the client and the nurse (Box 13-5).

SUPPORTING. Upholding a client's right to make a choice and to act on the choice involves **supporting**. People who become aware of clients' decisions fall into three general groups: supporters, dissenters, and obstructers. *Supporters* approve and support the actions of the clients. *Dissenters* do not approve of and do not support the actions of the clients. *Obstructers* cause difficulties as clients try to implement their decisions. Cary (1998) points to the need for the nurse advocate to assure clients that they have the right and responsibility to make decisions and reassure them that they do not have to change their decisions.

AFFIRMING. Affirming is based on an advocate's belief that a client's decision is consistent with the client's values and goals. The advocate validates that the client's behavior is purposeful and consistent with the choice that was made. The advocate expresses a dedication to the client's wishes; as a result, purposeful exchange of new information may occur so that the client's choice remains viable.

The importance of affirming activities cannot be emphasized strongly enough. It is not the advocate's role in the decision-making process to tell the client which option is "correct" or "right"; instead, the advocate's role involves the following:

- Providing the opportunity for information exchange, thus giving clients the tools that can empower them in making the best decision from their perspective.
- Enabling the client to make an "informed decision." This is a powerful tool for building self-confidence. It gives the client the responsibility for selecting the options and experiencing the success and consequences of the options based on current data.
- Empowering clients in their decision making when they can recognize events that are beyond their control and can link events that occur by chance with predictable events to make decisions they want.

Nurses can promote client decision making by:

- using the information exchange process,
- promoting the use of the nursing process,
- including written techniques (contracts, lists),
- using reflection and prioritizing decisions,
- using role playing to "try on" and determine the "fit" of different options and consequences for the client,
- helping clients recognize the progression of activities they experience as they build their "informed decision-making base," and
- empowering clients with skills that can strengthen their autonomy and confidence in the future.

Advocacy is a process that requires a balance between "doing for" and "promoting autonomy." The process is influenced by the client's physical, emotional, and social abilities. The goal of advocacy is to promote the ultimate degree of self-determination possible for the client given the client's current and potential status; for most clients, this goal can be realized.

Systematic Problem Solving

The nursing process—assessment, diagnosis, goal identification, planning, implementation, and evaluation—constitutes an example of a method of **problem solving** that can be used in the advocacy role. Advocates can be particularly helpful with clients in illuminating values and generating alternatives as described in the following sections.

Box 13-6	**Techniques of Generating Alternatives for Problem Solving**

Brainstorming

1. The nurse, client, professionals, or significant others generate as many alternatives as possible, without critical evaluation.
2. They examine the list for the critical elements the client seeks to preserve (e.g., environmental preferences, degree of control).
3. They analyze the list for consequences, the probability of chance events occurring, and the effect of the alternatives on self and others.

Problem-Purpose-Expansion Method

1. Restate the problem.
2. Expand the problem statement so that different solutions can be generated. For example, if the purpose of the problem statement is to convince the insurance company to approve a longer hospital stay, the nurse and client have narrowed their options. If the purpose of the problem statement is to make the client's convalescence as beneficial and safe as possible, several solutions and options are available, as follows:
   - Obtaining skilled nursing facility placement
   - Obtaining home health skilled services
   - Arranging physician home visits
   - Paying for custodial care
   - Paying for private skilled care
   - Obtaining informal caregiving

ILLUMINATING VALUES. People's values affect their behavior, feelings, and goals. The advocate seeks to understand a client's values. The role of the advocate is to assist clients in discovering their values, which can be particularly demanding in the information exchange and affirming process. One way to help clients state their values is through a process called *clarification*. A simple way to do this is to ask questions such as the following:

- What are 10 things that you enjoy doing?
- What are the most important things to you in life (family, money, happiness, health, comfort, pleasure, recognition)?
- How do you spend a typical day?

GENERATING ALTERNATIVES. Clients and advocates may feel limited in their options if they generate solutions before completely analyzing the problems, needs, desires, and consequences. Several techniques can be used to generate alternatives, including brainstorming and a technique known as the **problem-purpose-expansion method** (Box 13-6).

Impact of Advocacy

Clients are part of larger systems: the family, the work environment, and the community. Each system interacts with the client to shape the available options through resources, needs, and desires. Each system also has both confirming and conflicting goals and processes that need to be understood for client self-determination to be successful. For example, the practice of advocacy among minority groups

Levels of Prevention	Related to Case Management

PRIMARY PREVENTION

Use the information exchange process to increase the client's understanding of how to use the health care system.

SECONDARY PREVENTION

Use case finding to identify existing health problems.

TERTIARY PREVENTION

Monitor the use of prescription medications and adherence to treatment to reduce risk of illness complications.

Modified from Volkema RJ, Bergmann TJ: Conflict styles as indicators of behavioral patterns in interpersonal conflicts, *J Social Psychol* 135:5–15, 2001.

Box 13-7	Categories of Behaviors Used in Conflict Management

- *Competing:* an individual pursues personal concerns at another's expense.
- *Accommodating:* an individual neglects personal concerns to satisfy the concerns of another.
- *Avoiding:* an individual pursues neither personal concerns nor another's concerns.
- *Collaborating:* an individual attempts to work with others toward solutions that satisfy the work of both parties.
- *Compromising:* an individual attempts to find a mutually acceptable solution that partially satisfies both parties.

Modified from Thomas KW, Kilmann RH: *Thomas-Kilmann conflict mode instrument,* NY, 1974, Xicom.

may entail the ability to focus attention on the magnitude of problems caused by diseases affecting minority clients. Whether the client is an individual, family, group, or community, the advocacy function can promote the interest of self-determination that characterizes progressive societies.

Advocacy is not without opposition. Clients and advocates may find barriers to services, vendors, providers, and resources. A community may experience a shortage in nursing home beds, a childcare facility may experience staffing shortages, a family may not have the financial resources to keep a child at home, or a client may find that the school system cannot fund a full-time nurse for its clinic. The reality of scarce resources constitutes a difficult barrier for advocates. However, events such as these often stimulate a community's self-determination to find innovative actions to correct gaps in service (see Levels of Prevention box).

CONFLICT MANAGEMENT

Case managers help clients manage conflicting needs and scarce resources. Mutual benefit with limited loss for everyone is a goal of **conflict management**. Techniques for managing conflict include:

- using a range of active communication skills directed toward learning all parties' needs and desires,
- detecting areas of agreement and disagreement,
- determining abilities to collaborate, and
- assisting in discovering alternatives and valuable activities for reaching a goal.

Negotiating is a strategic process used to move conflicting parties toward an outcome. Parties must see the possibility of achieving an agreement and the costs involved in not achieving an agreement. Preparations must be made as to time, place, and ground rules concerning participants, procedures, and confidentiality. In a conflict situation, parties engage in behaviors that reflect the dimensions of assertiveness and cooperation. **Assertiveness** is the ability to present one's own needs. **Cooperation** is the ability to understand and meet the needs of others. Behaviors seen in conflict management are described in Box 13-7. The Thomas-Kilmann categories

of behaviors noted in this box, although written some time ago, outlines a variety of behaviors that can be valuable in a given situation.

Clearly, flexibility in conflict management behavior can encourage an outcome that meets the client's goals. Helping parties navigate the process of reaching a goal requires effective personal relations, knowledge of the situation and alternatives, and a commitment to the process.

BRIEFLY NOTED

A client's health care benefit plan may omit treatments and services that, according to evidence, improve health outcomes. Other complementary health services (e.g., acupuncture) may be omitted from the benefit plan because the evidence to determine health outcomes is not available. What should be the case manager's role with the client, benefit plan administrator, and the provider when services are not eligible to a client from his or her health plan? Choose the most appropriate roles from Box 13-2.

COLLABORATION

In case management, the activities of many disciplines are needed for success. Clients, the family, significant others, payers, and community organizations contribute to achieving the goal. **Collaboration** is achieved through a developmental process. It occurs in a sequence, yet it is reciprocal between those involved.

The goal of communication in the collaborative development process is to promote respect for, understanding of, and the accuracy of all team members' points of view. Although communication is an essential component in collaboration, it is not sufficient to result in or maintain collaboration. Although the collaboration model recognizes the contributions inherent in joint decision making, one member of the team should be held accountable for the outcome, and the client and the nurse should be responsible for monitoring the entire process.

Teamwork and collaboration clearly demand knowledge and skills about the following:
- Clients
- Health status
- Resources
- Treatments
- Community providers
- Clients' and families' complex needs
- Intrapersonal, interpersonal, medical, nursing, and social dimensions
- Team member and leadership skills

It is unlikely that any single professional has the expertise required in all of these. It is likely, however, that the synergy produced by all involved can result in successful outcomes.

BRIEFLY NOTED

Family caregivers may be poorly prepared to assume high-technology care of the client at home. They often receive inadequate information about the client's illness, likely burdens and benefits of caregiving, financial consequences, and the complex and technical details of a plan of treatment.

CASE STUDY

Through a nurse's case management activities, general community deficiencies in quality and quantity of health services are often discovered. When observing lack of care or services at the individual and family intervention levels, the nurse can, through case management, intervene at the community level to make changes.

George Stone is a nurse in community health practice working as a case manager for the pediatric asthmatic population. He is studying the use of service patterns among children with asthma. Mr. Stone would like to see if the services offered for asthmatic children are being utilized and, if not, the reasons they are underused.

Mr. Stone learns that many families without insurance are not using the free inhalers and spacers that the local Lion's Lodge provides to children without insurance. In fact, the families do not know this service exists. Mr. Stone makes it a priority to educate these families about this service so that they can save money and still receive the necessary medication for their children. Through school nurses, Mr. Stone identifies the current asthmatic students in the area who are eligible for free inhalers and spacers. Flyers are sent to their homes advertising the Lion's Lodge service. Mr. Stone also visits the physicians in the area who specialize in asthma. He educates the physicians and their staff about who is eligible for the free inhalers and spacers and how to get the service for their current and new clients. One year later, Mr. Stone collects new utilization data and compares them with his original findings. He finds a 50% increase in families receiving inhalers and spacers from the Lion's Lodge.

ISSUES IN CASE MANAGEMENT

LEGAL ISSUES

Liability concerns of case managers exist when the following three conditions are met:
1. The provider had a duty to provide reasonable care.
2. A breach occurred through an act or omission to act.
3. The act or omission caused injury or damage to the client.

Case managers must strive to reduce risks, practice wisely within acceptable standards, and limit legal defense costs through professional insurance coverage (Box 13-8).

Legal citings related to case management and managed care include the following:
- Negligent referrals
- Provider liability
- Payer liability
- Breach of contract
- Bad faith

As in any scope of nursing practice, proactive risk-management strategies can lower the provider's exposure to legal liability (Box 13-9). When courts find that cost considerations affect decisions related to medical care, all parties to the decision, such as the nurse, the agency, and all other health providers, will be liable for any resulting damages.

ETHICAL ISSUES

Case managers as nursing professionals are guided in ethical practice by the Code of Ethics for Nursing (American Nurses Association, 2008), by performance indicators for ethics in the Standards of Practice for Case Management (Case Management Society of America, 2002), and by the contract expressed in the Nursing's Social Policy Statement (American Nurses Association, 2008, p. 2):

Nursing is the protection, promotion, and optimization of health and abilities;, prevention of illness and injury, alleviation of suffering through the diagnosis and treatment of human response;, and advocacy in the care of individuals, families, communities and populations.

This contractual philosophy of nursing practice is ideally suited to preserving the principles of autonomy, beneficence, and justice in case management processes. Hendricks and Cesar (2003), Llewellyn and Moreo (2001), and McCollom (2004) describe how case managers may confront dilemmas in each of these areas, as follows:
- Case management may hamper a client's *autonomy* of individual right to choose a provider if a particular provider is not approved by the case management system.
- **Beneficence** can be influenced when excessive attention to cost supersedes or impairs the nurse's duty to provide measures to improve health or relieve suffering.
- **Justice,** as an ethical principle for case managers, considers equal distribution of health care with reasonable quality. Levels of quality and care among provider groups

---

Box 13-8 | Five General Areas of Risk for Case Managers

1. Liability for managing care (Hendricks and Cesar, 2003; Llewellyn and Moreo, 2001):
   - Inappropriate design or implementation of the case management system
   - Failure to obtain all pertinent records on which case management actions are based
   - Failure to have cases evaluated by appropriately experienced and credentialed clinicians
   - Failure to confer directly with the treating provider at the onset of and throughout the client's care
   - Substituting a case manager's clinical judgment for that of the medical provider
   - Requiring the client or his or her provider to accept case management recommendations instead of any other treatment
   - Harassment of clinicians, clients, and family in seeking information and setting unreasonable deadlines for decisions or information
   - Claiming orally or in writing that the case management treatment plan is better than the provider's plan
   - Restricting access to otherwise necessary or appropriate care because of cost
   - Referring clients to treatment furnished by providers who are associated with the case management agency without proper disclosure
   - Connecting case managers' compensation to reduced use and access
2. Negligent referrals (Hendricks and Cesar, 2003; Llewellyn and Moreo, 2001):
   - Referral to a practitioner known to be incompetent
   - Substituting inadequate treatment for an adequate but more costly option
   - Curtailing treatment inappropriately when curtailment caused the injury
   - Referral to a facility or practitioner inappropriate for the client's needs
   - Referral to another facility that lacks care requirements
3. Experimental treatment and technology (Hendricks and Cesar, 2003):
   - Failure to apply the contractual definition of "experimental" treatment found in the client's insurance policy
   - Failure to review sources of information referenced in the client's insurance policy (e.g., Food and Drug Administration [FDA] determination, published medical literature)
   - Failure to review the client's complete medical record
   - Failure to make a timely determination of benefits in light of **timelines** of treatment
   - Failure to communicate to the insured client or participant how coverage was determined
   - Improper financial considerations determining the coverage
4. Confidentiality (Llewellyn and Moreo, 2001):
   - Failure to deny access to sensitive information that is awarded special protection by state law
   - Failure to protect access allowances to computerized medical records
   - Failure to adhere to regulations, such as the Health Insurance Portability and Accountability Act of 1996 (HIPAA) and the Americans with Disabilities Act
5. Fraud and abuse (Llewellyn and Moreo, 2001):
   - Making false statements of claims or causing incorrect claims to be filed
   - Falsifying the adherence to conditions of participation of Medicare and Medicaid
   - Submitting claims for excessive, unnecessary, or poor-quality services
   - Engaging in payment, bribes, kickbacks, or rebates in exchange for referral
   - Coding intervention requirements improperly

Box 13-9 | Elements that Reduce Risk Exposure

1. Clear documentation of the extent of participation in decision making and the reasons for decisions
2. Records demonstrating accurate and complete information on interactions and outcomes
3. Use of reasonable care in selecting referral sources, which may include verification of the provider licensure
4. Written agreements when arrangements are made to modify benefits other than those in the contract
5. Good communication with clients
6. Informing clients of their rights of appeal

can be created when quality providers refuse to accept reimbursement allowances.

- The principle of *nonmaleficence* means "do no harm." When evidence-based plans of care include processes for monitoring care and measuring outcomes, this principle is applied.
- *Veracity,* or truth telling, is absolutely necessary to building a trusting relationship with a client.

Maintaining familiarity with ethical issues published in the case management literature can offer specific assistance for practicing case managers. Table 13-3 lists credentialing and accreditation options and Table 13-4 lists useful resources.

Table 13-3 **Credentialing Resources for Case Managers (Individual Certification Options)**

Organization	Phone Number and Website	Credentials and Initials
American Nurses Credentialing Center	1-800-284-2378 http://www.nursecredentialing.org	Nurses, RNC or RN, BC for Case Management
Professional Testing Corporation	212-356-0660 http://www.ptcny.com	CNLCP-Nurse Life Care Planners CMAC-Case Management Administrators
Certification of Disability Management Specialist Commission	847-944-1330 http://www.cdms.org	Multidisciplinary, CDMS for Certified Disability Management Specialist
Commission for Case Manager Certification	847-944-1330 http://www.ccmcertification.org	Multidisciplinary, CCM for Certified Case Manager
International Commission on Health Care Certification (ICHCC)	804-378-7273 http://www.ichcc.org	CDE for Certified Disability Examiner (specialty certification for life care planners)
National Academy of Certified Case Managers	1-800-962-2260 http://www.naccm.net	Multidisciplinary, CMC for Care Manager Certified
National Board for Certification in Continuity of Care	212-365-0691 http://www.nbccc.net	Multidisciplinary, A-CCC for Continuity of Care Certification–Advanced
Association of Rehabilitation Nurses	1-800-229-7530 http://www.rehabnurse.org	CRRN for Certified Rehabilitation Registered Nurse

Table 13-4 **Websites for Case Management Resources**

Resource	Website	Details
AIDS Education Global Information System	http://www.aegis.com	Contains largest AIDS library
American Accreditation Healthcare Commission (URAC)	http://www.urac.org	Accredits disease management programs and other services
American Nurses Credentialing Center	http://www.nursecredentialing.org	Offers review course materials for case managers preparing for certification examinations by any certifying body
American Medical Association	http://www.ama-assn.org	Includes continuing education unit (CEU) programs
Case Management Society of America	http://www.cmsa.org	Specialty organizations for case managers
Centers for Medicare and Medicaid Services	http://www.cms.hhs.gov	Formerly the Health Care Financing Administration (HCFA); oversees execution of rules and regulations for clients of state and federally funded services
Center Watch Clinical Trial Listing Service	http://www.centerwatch.com	Reviews all clinical trials in the United States
Centers for Disease Control and Prevention	http://www.cdc.gov	Provides education, training, and research for infectious diseases and on appropriate strategies to prevent disease (e.g., asthma, obesity)
The Joint Commission (TJC)	http://www.jointcommission.org	Accredits delivery organizations
Medscape	http://www.medscape.com	Features clinical updates for professionals
National Action Plan on Breast Cancer	http://www.4woman.gov/owh//programs/breasthealth.cfm	Provides information on breast cancer
National Committee for Quality Assurance	http://www.ncqa.org	Publishes HEDIS performance indicators for provider systems and accredits managed care organizations
National Library of Medicine	http://www.nlm.nih.gov	World's largest medical library
Nurseweek	http://www.nurse.com	Provides information links to other sites
Oncolink	http://www.oncolink.upenn.edu	Oncology links
ANA Nursing World Online Journal	http://www.nursingworld.org	Issues in nursing
Commission on Accreditation of Rehabilitation Facilities	http://www.carf.org	Accredits globally the services that may be used by case management clients such as adult day care, assisted living, behavioral health, employment and community services, and medical rehabilitation

CLINICAL APPLICATION

During her visit to the regularly scheduled blood pressure clinic in a local apartment cluster, Mrs. Barnes, a 45-year-old woman, complained of feeling dizzy and forgetful. She could not remember which of her six medications she had taken during the past few days. Her blood pressure readings on reclining, sitting, and standing revealed gross elevation. The nurse and Mrs. Barnes discussed the danger of her present status and the need to seek medical attention. Mrs. Barnes called her physician from her apartment and agreed to be transported to the emergency department.

While in the emergency department, Mrs. Barnes manifested the progressive signs and symptoms of a cerebrovascular accident (CVA, stroke). During hospitalization, she lost her capacity for expressive language and demonstrated hemiparesis and loss of bladder control. Her cognitive function became intermittently confused, and she was slow to recognize her physician and neighbors who came to visit. The utilization management nurse contacted the case manager from the health department to screen and assess for the continuum of care needs as early as possible because she lived alone and family members resided out of town.

It became apparent that family caregiving in the community could be only intermittent because members lived too far away. Mrs. Barnes had residual functional and cognitive deficits that would demand longer-term care.

As the case manager contracted by the plan, place the following actions in the sequence needed to construct a case management plan:
A. *Discuss with the family their schedule of availability to offer care in the client's home.*
B. *Call the client and introduce yourself as a prelude to working with her.*
C. *Obtain information on the scope of services covered by the benefit plan for your client.*
D. *Arrange a skilled nursing facility site visit for the patient and family.*
Answer is in the back of the book.

REMEMBER THIS!

- An important role of the nurse in community health is that of client advocate.
- The goal of advocacy is to promote the client's self-determination.
- When performing in the advocacy role, conflicts may emerge regarding the full disclosure of information, territoriality, accountability to multiple parties, legal challenges to client's decisions, and competition for scarce resources.
- The functions of advocacy and allocation can pose dilemmas in practice.
- Skills important in fulfilling the role of client advocate include the helping relationship, assertiveness, and problem solving.

- Problem solving is a systematic approach that includes understanding the values of each party and generating alternative solutions.
- Brainstorming and the problem-purpose-expansion method are two techniques to enhance the effectiveness of problem-solving skills.
- During conflict, negotiations can move conflicting parties toward an outcome.
- Care management is a strategic program to maintain the health of a population enrolled in a health care delivery system.
- Continuity of care is a goal of community health nursing practice. It requires making linkages with services to improve the client's health status.
- As the structure of the health care system moves toward delivering more services in the community, the achievement of continuity of care will present a greater challenge.
- Case management is typically an interdisciplinary process in which the client is the focus of the plan.
- Documenting case management activities and outcomes is essential to nursing practice in the community.
- Case management is a systematic process of assessment, planning, service coordination, referral, monitoring, and evaluation that meets the multiple service needs of clients.
- Nurses in community health have advocacy and case management functions within their scope of practice.
- Nurses functioning as advocates and case managers need to be aware of the ethical and legal issues confronting their practice.
- Standardization of care for predictable outcomes can be achieved through critical paths, disease management protocols, and multidisciplinary action plans.
- Telehealth application provides new alternatives within resource delivery options but must be customized for clients.

WHAT WOULD YOU DO?

1. Observe a typical workday of a nurse in community health or a public health nurse, noting the types of activities that are done in coordination and case management and the amount of time spent in these areas. Interview several staff members to determine whether they perceive that the amount of their time spent in case management is changing. To what degree are the staff members involved in care management activities?

2. Initiating, monitoring, and evaluating resources are essential components of nursing practice in the community and public health nursing practice. Describe a client situation and the case management process that might occur in the following practices:
   a. School nurse in an elementary school and in a high school
   b. Occupational health nurse in a hospital and in a manufacturing plant
   c. Nurse working in a well-child clinic

3. The values and beliefs held by a nurse in community health influence the nurse's ability to be an advocate for clients. Discuss your values and beliefs about rationing health care and how they may affect your ability to be a client advocate.

■ *REFERENCES*

Aliotta S: Coordination of care, *Case Manager* 14:49–52, 2003.

American Nurses Association: *Code of ethics for nursing*, Washington, DC, 2008, The Association.

American Nurses Association: *Nursing's social policy statement: the essence of the profession-draft*, Silver Spring, Md, December 15, 2008, The Association.

Brown SJ: Managing the complexity of best practice health care, *J Nurs Care Quality* 15:1–8, 2001.

Cary AH: Advocacy or allocation, *Nurs Connection* 11(1):1, 1998.

Case Management Society of America: *Standards of practice for case management*, Little Rock, Ark, 2002, CMSA.

Demoratz MJ: Incorporating life care planning concepts in case management, *Case Manager* 15:48–50, 2004.

Haag AB, Kalina CM: How are community resources used in case management? *AAOHN Offic J Am Assoc Occup Health Nurses* 53:286–287, 2005.

Hagan L, Morin D, Lepine R: Evaluation of telenursing outcomes: satisfaction, self-care practices, and cost savings, *Public Health Nurs* 17(4):305–313, 2000.

Health Resources and Services Administration, Health Systems and Financing Group: *Medicaid case management services by state, 2004*. Archived Webcast (electronic resource:http://www.hrsa.gov/financeMC/webcast-Sept1-Case-Mgmt-by-State-040825.htm).

Hendricks AG, Cesar WJ: How prepared are you? Ethical and legal challenges facing case managers today, *Case Manager* 14:56–62, 2003.

Johnson RL, Roter D, Powe NR et al: Patient race/ethnicity and quality of patient-physician communication during medical visits, *Am J Public Health* 94:2084–2090, 2004.

Katz MH et al: The effects of case management on unmet needs and utilization of medical care and medications among HIV-infected persons, *Ann Intern Med* 135:557–565, 2001.

Llewellyn A, Moreo K: *The essence of case management*, Washington, DC, 2001, American Nurses Credentialing Center.

McClatchey S: Disease management as a performance improvement strategy, *Top Health Inform Manag* 22(2):15–23, 2001.

McCollom P: Guiding the way: the evolution of life care plans, *Contin Care* 21:26–28, 2002.

McCollom P: Advocate versus abdicate, *Case Manager* 15:43–45, 2004.

Minnesota Department of Health: *Public health interventions: applications for public health nursing practice*, St. Paul, Minn, 2003, Minnesota Department of Health.

Mullahy CM: *The case manager's handbook*, Sudbury, Mass, 2004, Jones and Bartlett.

Muller LS, Flarery DL: Defining advanced practice nursing, *Lippincott's Case Manag* 8:230–231, 2003.

Paul KA: Managing the demand for health services by adopting patient-centered programs, *Benefits Q* 16:54–59, 2000.

Renholm M, Leino-Kilpi H, Suominen T: Critical pathways: a systematic review, *J Nurs Adm* 32(4):196–202, 2002.

Stanton MP, Dunkin J: Rural case management: nursing role variations, *Case Manag* 7:48–58, 2002.

Tahan H: Case management: a heritage more than a century old, *Nurs Case Manag* 3(2):55–69, 1998.

Thomas KW, Kilmann RH: *Thomas-Kilmann conflict mode instrument*, NY, 1974, Xicom.

U.S. Department of Health and Human Services: *Healthy People 2010: national health promotion and disease prevention objectives*, Washington, DC, 2000, U.S. Department of Health and Human Services.

Volkema RJ, Bergmann TJ: Conflict styles as indicators of behavioral patterns in interpersonal conflicts, *J Social Psychol* 135:5–15, 2001.

Zander K, Etheredge ML, Bower KA: *Nursing case management: blueprints for transformation*, Waban, Mass, 1987, Winslow Printing Systems.

Disaster Management

Susan B. Hassmiller

ADDITIONAL RESOURCES

These related resources are found either in the appendix at the back of this book or on the book's website at http://evolve.elsevier.com/stanhope/foundations.

Evolve Website

- Community Assessment Applied
- Case Study, with questions and answers
- Quiz review questions
- WebLinks, including link to *Healthy People 2010* website

Real World Community Health Nursing: An Interactive CD-ROM, second edition

If you are using this CD-ROM in your course, you will find the following activities related to this chapter:
- *The Disaster Prevention Drill* in **Disaster Management**
- *Disaster Services Challenge* in **Disaster Management**
- *Preparation for a Disaster* in **Disaster Management**

OBJECTIVES

After reading this chapter, the student should be able to:

1. Define natural and human-made disasters and epidemics.
2. Evaluate the effects of disasters on people and their communities.
3. Describe the disaster management phases of preparedness, response, and recovery and explain the nurse's role in each phase.
4. Describe the steps to take to initiate and maintain a disaster clinic.
5. Identify how community groups and other organizations such as the American Red Cross can work together to prepare for, respond to, and recover from disasters.

CHAPTER OUTLINE

DISASTERS
Healthy People 2010 Objectives
FOUR STAGES OF DISASTER INVOLVEMENT:
PREVENTION, PREPAREDNESS, RESPONSE,
AND RECOVERY
Prevention

Preparedness
Response
Recovery

KEY TERMS

chemical, biological, radiological, nuclear, and explosive (CBRNE): describes the full spectrum of munitions used to create a human-made disaster.
delayed stress reactions: occur after a disaster and can include exhaustion and an inability to adjust to postdisaster routines.

disaster: a human-caused or natural event that causes destruction and devastation that cannot be alleviated without assistance.
disaster medical assistance teams (DMATs): teams of specially trained civilian physicians, nurses, and other health care personnel who are sent to a disaster.

emergency support functions (ESFs): the 15 functions used in a federally declared disaster. Each function is headed by a primary agency.
human-made disasters: destruction or devastation caused by humans.
mitigation: actions or measures to prevent a disaster from occurring or to reduce the severity of its effects.
National Response Framework (NRF): the successor to the national response plan. NRF presents the guiding principles to enable all response partners to prepare for and provide a unified national response to diseases and emergencies.

natural disasters: destruction or devastation caused by natural events.
preparedness: advance preparation to cope with a disaster.
prevention: strengthening a person, family, or community's resources to ensure that a disruption does not occur.
recovery: the last stage in a disaster; when agencies join to restore the economic and civic life of the community.
response: organized actions to deal with a disaster.
triage: process of separating casualties and allocating treatment based on the victim's potential for survival.

Disasters are events that usually occur suddenly and unexpectedly. They seldom can be fully prevented nor can they be adequately prepared for by those who will be affected. They are destructive events that disrupt the normal functioning of a community. Accidents, acts of war or terrorism, or environmental mishaps cause disasters. The most recent disasters in this century are associated with global instability, economic downturns, political upheaval with its often accompanying wars or collapse of governments, famine, mass population displacements, and violence and civil conflicts (Veenema, 2003). The tsunami that devastated areas of Asia in 2004 and the hurricanes in 2005 and 2008 that devastated parts of the United States illustrate the unpredictable nature of disasters. Although disasters are inevitable, there are ways to prevent or manage how people and their communities respond. This chapter describes management techniques to be used in the prevention, preparedness, response, and recovery phases of disaster. The nursing role is discussed for each phase.

DISASTERS

Disasters can affect a single family or a small group, as in a house fire, or they can kill thousands and have economic losses in the millions, as with floods, earthquakes, tornadoes, hurricanes, and bioterrorism. Disasters are expensive in terms of lives affected and/or property lost or damaged. The average cost for a single disaster event is $318 million in developed nations and $28 million in undeveloped nations (International Federation of the Red Cross and Red Crescent Societies, 2004). Hurricanes, earthquakes, and tsunamis escalate the loss of lives, homes, businesses, and even towns and villages. The loss of life can be devastating. Just over 3 million lives were lost in the past decade as a result of conflict (including terrorism) and both natural and technological disasters. In addition to the mortality, billions more people each year are left to deal with the injuries, disease, and homelessness that follow disasters (International Federation of Red Cross and Red Cross Societies, 2004). Hurricane Katrina, the most destructive natural disaster in the history of the United States, made landfall on August 29, 2005 along the coasts of Louisiana, Mississippi, and Alabama. Soon after, on September 23, 2005, Hurricane Rita caused major destruction in Texas and Louisiana (Cary, 2008). Each year there are hurricanes in the United States that batter the coasts and often inland areas.

Unfortunately, developing countries experience a disproportionate burden from natural disasters. These countries are usually poor and have limited resources for dealing with the effects of the disaster. To add to the misery, the governments of some countries thwart the efforts of international aid workers to bring relief to their people. There are political aspects to disasters in addition to the enormous losses to the people. For example, some countries will not accept aid from nations they do not consider their allies or supporters.

The urbanizing and the overcrowding of cities have increased the danger of **natural disasters** because communities have been built in areas that are vulnerable to disasters, such as in known tornado zones or near rivers. Increases in population and developing for habitation of areas vulnerable to natural disasters have led to major increases in insurance payouts in the United States in every decade. Projections suggest that by 2050, at least 46% of the world's population will live in areas vulnerable to natural floods, earthquakes, and severe storms.

BRIEFLY NOTED

Disasters create the most devastation in developing countries, where the death rate is up to 12 times higher than in developed countries. The poor suffer the most, because their houses are less sturdy and they have fewer resources and less means of social security.

Overcrowding and urban development have also increased **human-made disasters**. The stress caused by overcrowding has caused civil unrest and riots. In some parts of the world, modern wars waged over land rights and space have markedly increased the risk of injury and death from disaster. In the United States and other countries, school violence, a human-made disaster, has increased in intensity and magnitude. Disaster recovery efforts are expensive, and the costs are growing because of the number of people involved and the amount of technology that must be restored. People in industrialized countries are becoming less self-sufficient

| Box 14-1 | Types of Disasters |

Natural
- Hurricanes
- Tornadoes
- Hailstorms
- Cyclones
- Blizzards
- Droughts
- Floods
- Mudslides
- Avalanches
- Earthquakes
- Volcanic eruptions
- Communicable disease epidemics
- Lightning-induced forest fires

Human-made
- Conventional warfare
- Nonconventional warfare (e.g., nuclear, chemical)
- Transportation accidents
- Structural collapse
- Explosions/bombing
- Fires
- Toxic materials
- Pollution
- Civil unrest (e.g., riots, demonstrations)

because they rely heavily on technology and social and economic systems within their community. People who live on the brink of disaster every day, physically, emotionally, or economically, are among the first to be affected when disaster strikes. Disasters affect the health of a community in many ways. Disasters may do the following (Veenema, 2003):
- Cause premature deaths, illnesses, and injuries in the affected community
- Destroy the local health care infrastructure and prevent an effective response to the emergency
- Create environmental imbalances, thereby increasing the risk of communicable diseases and environmental hazards
- Affect the psychological, emotional, and social well-being of the people
- Cause shortages of food and water
- Displace populations of people

A **disaster** is any human-made or natural event that causes destruction and devastation that cannot be relieved without assistance. The event need not cause injury or death to be considered a disaster. For example, a hurricane may cause millions of dollars in damage without causing a single death or injury. Box 14-1 lists examples of natural and human-made disasters.

Although natural disasters cannot be prevented, much can be done to prevent further increases in accidents, death, and destruction after impact. A concise, realistic, and well-rehearsed disaster plan is essential. There must also be open, clear, and ongoing communication among involved workers and organizations, Also, many of the human-made disasters listed in Box 14-1 can be prevented (e.g., major transportation accidents and fires resulting from substance abuse).

The United Nations initiated a campaign to educate people on ways to reduce their risk of injury and death caused by national disasters. This campaign led to increased public–private partnering that emphasized **mitigation**, which is what public health experts consider secondary prevention. It is the act of "working to minimize the damage caused by an event that cannot (always) be prevented" (Bissell et al, 2004, p. 195). Mitigation refers to actions or measures that can either prevent the occurrence of a disaster or reduce the severity of its effects (American Red Cross, n.d.a.). For example, we cannot prevent car crashes; however, we can mitigate the results by designing automobiles with seatbelts and airbags and insisting that young children be transported in safety car seats. The following are examples of mitigation activities:
- *Awareness and education:* holding/attending community meetings on disaster preparedness
- *Disaster prevention:* building a retaining wall to divert flood water away from a residence
- *Advocacy:* supporting actions and efforts for effective building codes and proper land use

Dozens of national, state, and local agencies, such as the Institute for Business and Home Safety, American Red Cross (ARC), Centers for Disease Control and Prevention (CDC), and local faith communities partnered during the past decade for disaster reduction to work proactively to save lives and property.

On October 8, 2001, President Bush signed an Executive Order that established the Office of Homeland Security (White House, 2002). In 2003, this became an executive-level department and is now a part of the Cabinet. This department consolidated 22 previous agencies into one unified organization (White House, 2005). The department's mission is to develop and coordinate the implementing of a comprehensive national strategy to secure the United States from terrorist threats or attacks. The department works with executive departments and agencies, state and local governments, and private agencies to ensure adequate strategies for detecting, preparing for, preventing, protecting against, responding to, and recovering from terrorist threats or attacks. Several Presidential directives were also included: developing a National Preparedness Goal (NPG), a National Response Plan (NRP), and a National Incident Management System (NIMS). The goal of these directives was to establish "a unified, all-discipline, and all-hazards approach to domestic incident management" (U.S. Department of Homeland Security, 2005c, p. i). In 2008 the NRP was changed to the **National Response Framework (NRF),** which provides a guide for how communities, tribes, states, the Federal government, and the private sector, as well as nongovernmental organizations, can use a set of guiding principles to prepare for disasters.

HEALTHY PEOPLE 2010 OBJECTIVES

Because disasters affect the health of people in many ways, they have an effect on almost every *Healthy People 2010* objective. Disasters clearly affect the objectives that relate to

Examples of Objectives Developed to Avoid Disasters

8-12   Minimize the risks to human health and the environment posed by hazardous sites

10-1   Reduce infections caused by foodborne pathogens

15-39   Reduce weapon carrying by adolescents on school property

20-5   Reduce deaths by work-related homicides

From U.S. Department of Health and Human Services: *Healthy People 2010: national health promotion and disease prevention objectives,* ed 2, Washington, DC, 2000, U.S. Government Printing Office.

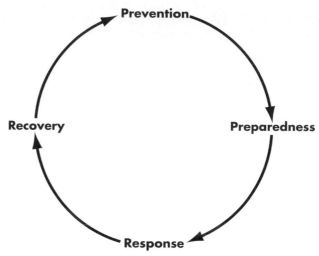

FIGURE 14-1 Disaster management cycle. (Modified from American Red Cross: *Disasters happen,* Washington, DC, 1994, ARC.)

unintentional injuries, occupational safety and health, environmental health, and food and drug safety. In the past few years with the many incidents and scares related to possible bioterrorism, people have become even more aware of the importance of disaster preparedness and how the things they take for granted such as safe food, water, and housing can be threatened. To ensure healthy homes and healthy communities, the following is one objective of the national agenda:

8-21: Ensure that state health departments establish training, plans, and protocols and conduct multiinstitutional exercises to prepare for response to natural and technological disasters.

Other organizations, such as the American Psychological Association and ARC, work with communities in the immediate recovery phase of a disaster and sometimes for years thereafter to effect the *Healthy People 2010* objectives related to mental health. International groups also work to reduce the psychological effects that follow a disaster. The Pan American Health Organization has an educational program set up for emergency response personnel including nurses. The Stress Management in Disaster program is designed to prevent and decrease the psychological dysfunction that occurs in disaster situations (Bryce, 2001).

FOUR STAGES OF DISASTER INVOLVEMENT: PREVENTION, PREPAREDNESS, RESPONSE, AND RECOVERY

The goal of disaster management is to reduce or avoid the potential losses from hazards, assure prompt and appropriate assistance to victims, and achieve rapid and effective recovery. One effective way to consider disaster management is through these four stages of a disaster: prevention, preparedness, response, and recovery. Figure 14-1 shows the disaster management cycle. In disaster preparedness the plan must be both realistic and simple because (1) no plan will ever exactly fit the disaster as it occurs, and (2) all plans must be able to be implemented regardless of which key members of the disaster team are there at the time (Centers for Disease Control and Prevention, 2002; U.S. Department of Health and Human Services, 2001). Since 2001, communities have

become more skilled in developing plans to prepare them for a disaster. They use education, team planning, mock disaster events, and clear assignment of responsibility to health care professionals in the community to design plans to reduce community vulnerability, develop disaster response plans, and provide training before any hazardous event. In February 2005 the Federal Emergency Management Agency (FEMA) released an in-depth citizen guide to preparing for disasters called "Are you ready?". It is available at FEMA's website (www.fema.gov) and provides a step-by-step approach to disaster preparedness. The following discusses all four stages, including the role of the nurse.

PREVENTION

The purpose of **prevention** is to "deter all potential terrorists from attacking America, detect terrorists before they strike, prevent them and their instruments of terror from entering our country, and take decisive action to eliminate the threat they pose" (U.S. Department of Homeland Security, 2005b, p. 21). Prevention "activities may include: heightened inspections; improved surveillance and security operations; public health and agricultural surveillance and testing processes; immunizations, isolation, or quarantine" (U.S. Department of Homeland Security, n.d., p. A-3) and weapons of mass destruction detection: **chemical, biological, radiological, nuclear, and explosive (CBRNE)** (U.S. Department of Homeland Security, 2005a). Since Hurricane Katrina struck in 2005, prevention has included considerable work in strengthening levies and other barriers to prevent water flooding the land.

Within the community, the nurse may be involved in many roles. As community advocates, nurses help maintain a safe environment. Public health nurses in particular will be involved with organizing and participating in mass prophylaxis and vaccination campaigns to prevent, treat, or contain a disease. The nurse should be familiar with the region's local cache of pharmaceuticals and coordination with the

Prepare for Safety in a Disaster: Four Steps

1. Find out what could happen to you:
   a. Determine what types of disasters are most likely to happen.
   b. Learn about warning signals in your community.
   c. Ask about postdisaster pet care (shelters usually will not accept pets).
   d. Review the disaster plans at your workplace, school, and other places where your family spends time.
   e. Determine how to help older adult or disabled family members or neighbors.
2. Create a disaster plan:
   a. Discuss types of disasters that are most likely to happen, and review what to do in each case.
   b. Pick two places to meet, including outside your home and outside your neighborhood.
   c. Choose an out-of-state friend to be your family contact; this person will verify the location of each family member. After a disaster, it may be easier to call long distance than to make local calls.
   d. Review evacuation plans, including care of pets. Identify ahead of time where to go if evacuation is necessary.
3. Complete this checklist:
   a. Post emergency phone numbers next to telephones.
   b. Teach everyone how and when to call 911.
   c. Determine when and how to turn off water, gas, and electricity at the main switches.
   d. Check adequacy of insurance coverage for yourself and your home.
   e. Locate and review the use of fire extinguishers.
   f. Install and maintain smoke detectors.
   g. Conduct a home hazard hunt and fix potential hazards.
   h. Stock emergency supplies and assemble a disaster supplies kit.
   i. Acquire first aid and cardiopulmonary resuscitation (CPR) certification.
   j. Locate all escape routes from your home. Find two ways out of each room.
   k. Find safe spots in your home for each type of disaster.
4. Practice and maintain your plan:
   a. Review the plan every 6 months.
   b. Conduct fire and emergency evacuation drills.
   c. Replace stored water every 3 months and stored food every 6 months.
   d. Test and recharge fire extinguishers according to manufacturer's instructions.
   e. Test your smoke detectors monthly and change the batteries at least once a year.

Strategic National Stockpile (SNS) and how this will be distributed.

Recalling that disasters are not only natural but also human-made, nurses need to assess for and report environmental health hazards including unsafe equipment and faulty structures. They must be aware of high-risk targets and current vulnerabilities and what can be done to eliminate or mitigate the vulnerability. Targets may include military and civilian government facilities, health care facilities, international airports and other transportation systems, large cities, and high-profile landmarks. Terrorists might also target large public gatherings, water and food supplies, banking and finance, information technology, postal and shipping services, utilities, and corporate centers (U.S. Department of Homeland Security, 2005c).

Furthermore, terrorists are capable of spreading fear by sending explosives or chemical and biological agents through the mail. The nurse should also observe for and report any psychological or sociological health hazards such as overcrowding, extreme disrespect, and anger in vulnerable populations that could lead to unrest and violence.

PREPAREDNESS
Personal Preparedness
Nurses who are disaster victims themselves and must provide care to others will experience considerable stress (Gebbie and Qureshi, 2002). Conflicts between family and work-related duties are inevitable. For example, a nurse who is also the mother of a young child will not be able to participate fully, if at all, in disaster relief efforts until she has made arrangements for her child. Advance personal and family preparation can help ease some of the conflicts that arise and allow nurses to attend to client needs sooner. In addition, the nurse assisting in disaster relief efforts must be as healthy as possible, both physically and mentally, to serve clients, families, and other disaster victims.

The ARC and FEMA, two well-known authorities on disaster **preparedness**, **response**, and **recovery,** have devised a personal checklist to help individuals and families prepare for disasters before they strike (Federal Emergency Management Agency, 2005). The "How To" box shows a modified version of FEMA's recommendations entitled Four Steps to Safety. See also www.redcross.org. to get prepared for information on what should be a home kit for disaster.

BRIEFLY NOTED

Emergency supplies needed in case of disaster should be prepared and stored in a sturdy, easy-to-carry container. Important documents should always be kept in a waterproof container. The following are emergency supplies:
- A 3-day supply of water (1 gallon per person per day) and food that will not spoil. Be sure to store a manual can opener and remember that you may not have water, gas or electricity.
- One change of clothing and protective footwear per person, and one blanket or sleeping bag per person
- A first-aid kit that includes a week's supply of your family's prescription medications and over the counter medications that you take. Make a list of your medications and dosages, allergies, physician names.
- Emergency tools including a battery-powered radio, flashlight, and plenty of extra batteries
- Candles and matches
- An extra set of car keys and a credit card, cash, or traveler's checks, picture identification, and proof of address
- Sanitation supplies, including toilet paper, soap, feminine hygiene items, and plastic garbage bags

- Special items for infants, older adults, or disabled family members
- An extra pair of eyeglasses
- Pet supplies if you have animals
- Documents: ID, passport, birth certificate, insurance policies, family contact information, local maps with marked evacuation routes, some money

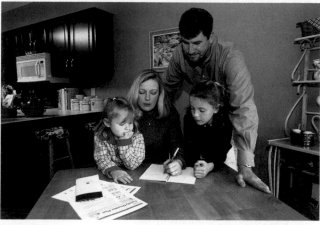

FIGURE 14-2 Understanding the community's disaster plan is a key role for nurses who seek greater involvement in disaster management. (Courtesy of the American Red Cross. All rights reserved in all countries.)

Important documents should always be in waterproof containers. Nurses should consider several contingencies for children and seniors with a plan to seek help from neighbors in the event of being called to a disaster. Many special-needs shelters encourage preregistration for physically or mentally challenged people. Because most shelters do not allow pets other than "pocket" pets, other arrangements will need to be made such as going to a special pet shelter or placing the pet in a bathroom with sufficient food and water. A note should be placed on the front door for emergency personnel as to where the pet might be found. Currently, many local emergency management offices are considering incorporating pets into the local disaster plans.

One way a nurse can ensure that her family is protected is by providing them with the skills and knowledge to help them cope with a disaster. Long-term benefits will come by involving children and/or adolescents in activities such as writing preparedness/response plans, rehearsing the plan, preparing disaster kits, becoming familiar with their school emergency plan and where families should reunite in the event of an emergency, finding out where the evacuation shelters are located and with evacuation routes, and learning about the range of potential hazards in their vicinity. Natural and human-made hazards, including terrorism, should be discussed. Vulnerable types of infrastructure such as dams, chemical plants, bridges, and transportation should be pointed out. Discussion offers children and/or adolescents an opportunity to express their feelings. The ability to control as much as they can during each phase of a disaster provides them with the ability to bounce back (Figure 14-2).

Professional Preparedness

The nurse who is professionally prepared is aware of and understands the disaster plans at the workplace and in the community. These nurses take time to read and understand workplace and community disaster plans and participate in disaster drills and community mock disasters. Adequately prepared nurses can serve as leaders and enable others to have a smoother recovery phase. In a training course for nurses, the ARC recommends that nurses have available these personal items when preparing to help in a disaster (American Red Cross, 1999):

- Copy of professional license
- Official Red Cross identification
- Valid state driver's license
- Materials from pertinent Red Cross training courses
- Disaster Services name badge
- Jacket/sweater

- Inexpensive watch
- First-aid kit
- Flashlight and batteries
- Comfortable shoes
- Raincoat or an all-weather coat
- Washcloth and toilet articles
- Credit card/traveler's checks
- Contact lenses solutions (minimum of 3-week supply)
- Prescriptions/medications (minimum of 3-week supply)
- Battery-operated or wind-up alarm clock
- Leisure materials (e.g., book, exercise clothes, tape deck, music)
- Writing materials, address book, stamps
- Easy-care clothing that meets standards of personal attire (enough for 10 days)

Disaster work is not highly technological. Fieldwork, including shelter management, requires that nurses be creative and willing to improvise in delivering care. All workers should be certified in first aid and cardiopulmonary resuscitation (CPR). In addition, the ARC provides a comprehensive program of disaster training for health professionals, to enable them to provide assistance within their own communities and to other affected communities and countries. The courses teach nurses how to adapt their existing nursing skills to a disaster setting and to the scope of Red Cross disaster nursing. Note that the knowledge the nurse will need for chemical, biological, radiological, nuclear, and explosive (CBRNE) disasters and those involving weapons of mass destruction (WMD) requires a base of specialized information. Box 14-2 describes competencies for all public health workers.

Community Preparedness

The level of community preparedness for a disaster is only as good as the people and organizations in the community make it. Some communities stay prepared for a possible disaster by having a written disaster plan and participating

---

Box 14-2   Bioterrorism and Emergency Readiness: Competencies for all Public Health Workers

1. Describe the role of your agency in emergency response for a wide range of possible emergencies and maintain regular contact with partner professionals.
2. Identify and locate the agency emergency plan.
3. Describe the agency chain of command.
4. Describe and demonstrate in exercises your functional role.
5. Recognize unusual events that might indicate an emergency and describe appropriate action to be taken.
6. Identify limits to your own knowledge, skill, and authority and identify key system resources for referring matters that exceed these limits.
7. Describe communication roles within the agency, the media, and the general public.
8. Demonstrate use of all communication equipment and other pertinent equipment, including the use of personal protective equipment.
9. Participate in continuing education to maintain up-to-date relevant information.
10. Evaluate drills, exercises, or actual events: write after-action reports, update the emergency plan as needed, and implement the changes.
11. Apply creative problem-solving skills.

From The Centers for Disease Control and Prevention: *Bioterrorism and emergency readiness— competencies for all public health workers,* Washington, DC, 2002. Retrieved Aug 16, 2005, from www.nursing.hs.columbia.edu/institutes-centers/chphsr/btcomps.pdf.

Box 14-3   Key Organizations and Professionals in Disaster Management

Health Care Community
- Hospitals
- Mental health professionals
- Pharmacies
- Public health departments
- Rescue personnel

Non-Health Care Community
- Clergy
- Firefighters
- Funeral directors
- The mayor and other municipal or government officials
- Media
- Medical examiners
- Medical supply manufacturers
- Morticians
- Police

---

in yearly disaster drills. Other communities are less prepared and depend on luck and the fact that they are unlikely to experience a disaster. Some organizations within the community may be more prepared than others. For example, most health care facilities have written disaster plans and require employees to perform annual mock drills, but many businesses lack these requirements. In recent years, hospitals and health departments in cities with nursing, medical, and other health professional schools have included their faculty in the disaster planning work so that if a disaster occurs, faculty and students can easily be mobilized to assist.

The Public Health Security and Bioterrorism Preparedness and Response Act of 2002 addressed the need to enhance public health and health care readiness and develop community infrastructures. Public health departments are on the front lines in preparing for and dealing with an emergency or disaster (U.S. Department of Health and Human Services, n.d., p. 1). At the state, country, tribal, and local level, the Office of Emergency Management (OEM) is responsible for developing and coordinating emergency response plans within their defined area. The OEMs are in charge of creating a comprehensive, all-hazard plan. The plan should deal with the four phases of emergency management. It provides planning and training services to local governments, including financial and technical assistance. During an actual emergency or disaster, the state OEM coordinates a state response and recovery program if necessary.

County OEMs are in charge of creating a comprehensive, all-hazard plan that should address realistic dangers to the community and list available resources (Santa Clara County, 2008). The key to disaster preparedness is that the plan must be both realistic and simple with backup contingencies since things will seldom go as planned.

Nurses need to review the disaster history of the community, including how past disasters have affected the health care delivery system, how their particular organizations fit into the plan, and what role they and their organizations are expected to play in a disaster.

Understandings of past disasters and performance in mock disaster drills influence planning for future disasters. For example, real and simulated disaster review may determine that the local community has not appropriately used the county's nurses because of a lack of education about their roles. Health professional students may be assigned to multiple roles rather than having a clear assignment either to the health department or a specific hospital. Many communities are carrying out useful educational programs on what nurses do and what role they can play in a disaster. A solid disaster plan requires the talents, coordination, and cooperation of many different people and organizations, both inside and outside the health profession (Box 14-3).

It is important for all disaster workers to work together cooperatively and with clear role definitions *before* a disaster and to use clear communication to set up and implement their disaster plan. Knowing in advance exactly what is expected of each organization during an emergency or disaster gives the staff the opportunity to acquire necessary knowledge and to practice necessary skills beforehand (Gebbie and Qureshi, 2002).

Finally, the community must have an adequate warning system and a backup evacuation plan to remove those individuals from areas of danger who hesitate to leave. Some people refuse to leave their homes because they are afraid that their possessions will be lost or destroyed by the disaster or from looting after the disaster. Law enforcement personnel or others in authority may have to speak directly to these reluctant residents to convince them to leave their homes and go to safer quarters. Also, some people mistakenly believe that experience with a particular type of disaster is enough preparation for the next one. People must be convinced that predisaster warnings are official, serious, and personally important before they are motivated to take action.

Role of the Nurse in Disaster Preparedness

Nurses have key roles in disaster preparedness to facilitate preparation in the community and place of employment (Figure 14-2). Nurses employed in emergency departments generally know their role in citywide disaster plans for the community. Nurses working in other settings may not have the same preparation, although preparation has greatly increased in recent years.

Nurses can help initiate or update the agency's disaster plan, provide educational programs and materials regarding disasters specific to the area, and organize disaster drills. Nurses also can provide an updated record of vulnerable populations within the community. When calamity strikes, disaster workers must know what kinds of populations they are attempting to assist. For example, if a tornado strikes a retirement village, the needs are quite different from those seen after the tornado hits a church filled with families or a center for the physically challenged. In addition to knowing where special populations exist, the nurse can educate groups about what effect the disaster might have on them. Nurses should review individual strategies, including available specific resources, in the event of an emergency.

One special population that may be overlooked is children in childcare facilities. Children are cared for in many different locations, ranging from freestanding buildings to provider homes. They tend to have little, if any, security against a disaster, and often people come in and out all day. Also, if a disaster occurs, a plan must be in place for how the children can be reunited with their parents. And because of their small size, they may have to be helped to leave the facility. In addition, they are more vulnerable to chemical and biological agents because of their immature physiological and psychological development and they have less fluid reserve than adults and are more susceptible to dehydration. With all populations, review individual strategies, including available specific resources, in the event of an emergency. The following actions are recommended regarding childcare emergency supplies (Gaines and Leary, 2004):

- Put together a family readiness kit and disaster supply kit (see the American Academy of Pediatrics at www. aap.org).
- Gather the supplies recommended by the ARC (www. redcross.org).
- Store things such as first-aid supplies, emergency blankets, medications, ice packs, and nonperishable food in backpacks or rolling containers.

- Put copies of each child's medical information, parent contact information, and local emergency telephone numbers in a portable container.
- Take with you the attendance list of children and some comfort items such as games, toys, blankets, crayons, and paper.

The nurse who leads a preparedness effort can help recruit others within the organization who will help if and when a response is required. Although there is no psychological profile of a disaster leader, try to involve persons in this effort who are flexible, decisive, and emotionally stable and who have physical endurance (Bryce, 2001). The nurse leading the effort should know a great deal about the institution and be familiar with the individuals who work there. Persons with disaster management training, and especially those who have served during real disasters, also make valuable members of any preparedness team.

Nurses serve in many roles in the community. They advocate for a safe environment. They also know that disasters are both natural and human-made, so they assess for and report environmental health hazards. For example, the nurse should be aware of and report unsafe equipment, faulty structures, and the beginning of disease epidemics such as measles or influenza.

Nurses should also understand what the available community resources will be after a disaster strikes, and, most important, how the community will work together. A communitywide disaster plan serves as a roadmap for what "should" occur before, during, and after the response and the role of each participant in the plan. There are a variety of community organizations in which nurses can become involved to assist in a disaster. Two examples are Emergency Medical System/Ambulance Corps and Volunteer Organizations Active in Disasters (VOAD) such as the Salvation Army. The ARC offers classes on disaster health services and disaster mental health services to help participants identify disaster health services preparedness measures that should take place on the local unit level and to become familiar with Red Cross disaster health services procedures and protocols in local disaster operations (American Red Cross, 2000). The Red Cross requires workers to complete the disaster health services or a disaster mental health services course work before assigning an individual to a disaster site as a Red Cross representative. For nurses who choose to volunteer with agencies such as the Red Cross, there are many ways to become involved. After several hours of disaster training, nurses may wish to take the following steps to get actively involved:

- Join a local disaster action team (DAT).
- Act as a liaison with local hospitals.
- Determine health-related appropriateness for shelter sites.
- Plan with pharmacies, opticians, morticians, and other health personnel to facilitate services for disaster victims.
- Plan for needed supplies, and keep them available.
- Teach disaster nursing in the community.

Many community agencies contribute to disaster preparedness. Table 14-1 describes the preparedness responsibilities assumed by the ARC, other voluntary organizations, business and labor organizations, and local government.

Table 14-1 **Disaster Preparedness Responsibilities by Agency**

American Red Cross	Other Voluntary Organizations	Business and Labor Organizations	Local Government
Participates with government in developing and testing a community disaster plan	Collaborate in developing and maintaining a local *Voluntary Organizations Active in Disaster* group to identify roles, resources, and plans for disasters	Develop disaster plans for business locations and integrate their plans with the community disaster plan	Coordinates the development of the community plan and conducts evaluation exercises
Designates persons to serve as representatives at government emergency operations centers and command posts	Identify and train personnel for disaster response	Develop procedures to facilitate continuity of operations in time of disaster	Trains staff to carry out the plan
Develops and tests local Red Cross disaster plans	Identify community issues and special populations for consideration in disaster preparedness	Develop plans for assisting business employees after a disaster	Passes legislation to mitigate the effects of potential disasters
Identifies and trains personnel for disaster response	Make plans to continue to serve regular clients after a disaster	Identify union and business facilities, resources, and people who may be able to support community disaster plans	Designs measures to warn the population of disaster threats
Collaborates with other voluntary agencies in developing and maintaining a local *Voluntary Organizations Active in Disaster* group to promote cooperation and coordinate resources and people for disaster work	Identify facilities, resources, and people to serve in time of disaster	Provide volunteers, financial contributions, and in-kind gifts to the Red Cross and other voluntary organizations to support disaster preparedness	Conducts building safety inspections
Works with business and labor organizations to identify resources and people for disaster work	Educate specific client groups on disaster preparedness	Educate employees and union members about disaster preparedness	Develops procedures to facilitate the continuity of public safety operations in time of disaster
Educates the public about hazards and ways to avoid, prepare for, and cope with their effects			Identifies public facilities, resources, and public employees for disaster work
Acquires material resources needed to ensure effective response			Educates the public about disaster threats in the community and safety procedures

From the American Red Cross: *Disasters happen* (ARC Pub. No. 1570), Washington, DC, 1994, ARC.

Since 2001 the CDC has established a system of Centers for Public Health Preparedness. The goal of these centers is to develop and offer competency-based emergency preparedness training programs to help the public health workforce maintain the essential services of public health while appropriately responding to emergencies (Qureshi et al., 2004).

Mass Casualty Drills or Mock Disasters

Mass casualty drills or mock disasters are key parts of preparedness. Whether the drills are carried out via a computer simulation or enacted in a realistic scenario, the objectives are to
- promote confidence,
- develop skills,
- coordinate activities, and
- coordinate participants. (Gebbie and Qureshi, 2002)

Following the exercise, focus on postaction reports and updating the plan (Hassmiller, 2008). Also, the drill leader needs special skills in disaster management, including the ability to coordinate many organizations at one time. Although a successful disaster drill can allow participants to evaluate the rescue plan and make further recommendations, it should not create a false sense of security (Gebbie et al, 2006).

The terrorist events of September 11, 2001, and the later anthrax cases have increased the awareness of the need to plan for disaster. Considerable information has been compiled on how to specifically plan for human-made disasters, which often occur with no forewarning. Part of planning for a bioterrorism attack is learning the symptoms of illnesses that are likely to be caused by infectious agents. For both natural and human-made disasters, there are often early warning signs. For example, signs of a tornado include hail, strong rain, and a green sky. Signs for a human-made disaster may not be as clear, but being aware of suspicious activities is still important.

CASE STUDY

The Saber city disaster preparedness (DP) team wanted to coordinate a mock terrorist attack to study the effectiveness of its disaster management plan. The goal of the mock attack was to promote confidence, develop skills, coordinate activities, and coordinate participants of the disaster management team. The DP team planned a commonly seen terrorist attack: a bus carrying important politicians would explode outside the federal courthouse in downtown Saber. All participating organizations (including the health department, hospital, police department, and fire department) were notified of the date the mock attack would be held. Volunteers were found to play the victims found on the scene.

After months of planning, the day of the mock attack came. The members of the DP team watched how well the organizations worked together during the events of the mock attack. At noon, reports of an exploded bus in front of the courthouse came across police scanners: "Several people are dead and many more injured." Emergency medical response teams and hazardous material response crews were called to the scene to care for the injured and attend to the potential hazardous exposure. Policemen quickly cleared the area of people and established a barrier around the scene. Firefighters put out the fire on the burning bus.

From the mock attack, the DP team learned that the city of Saber was prepared for a terrorist attack. Communication among organizations flowed smoothly, and the disaster management team was skillful in controlling the situation. Participants in the mock attack stated they were happy to have the practice and felt more confident in their ability to provide care in the case of a major disaster.

RESPONSE

Levels of Disaster and Agency Involvement

The primary objective of disaster responses is to minimize morbidity and mortality. Many small disasters, such as single-family home fires, and even many extensive disasters do not require the assistance of FEMA. In these cases, the ARC and other organizations such as the Salvation Army assist disaster victims. When the President declares a disaster, the Red Cross works with FEMA on the recovery efforts. Table 14-2 describes disaster response responsibilities of ARC, other voluntary organizations, business and labor organizations, and local government.

The level of disaster determines FEMA's response. Levels are not determined by the number of casualties but by the amount of resources needed. According to the American Red Cross (2003), the following are three ways of classifying a disaster:

1. *Disaster Type:* the agent that produced the event, such as a hurricane, a hazardous material accident, or a transportation accident.
2. *Disaster Level:* the anticipated or actual Red Cross disaster response and relief cost required by the event:
   - Level I: costs less than $10,000
   - Level II: costs $10,000 or more, but less than $50,000
   - Level III: costs $50,000 or more, but less than $250,000
   - Level IV: costs $250,000 or more, but less than $2.5 million
   - Level V: costs $2.5 million or more
3. *Disaster Scope:* the basic characteristics of the event's magnitude and the Red Cross unit or units affected and responding to the event:
   - Single-Family Disaster: a disaster that affects an individual or a single-family unit, occurs within the jurisdiction of a single Red Cross chapter, and may require the short-term application of limited human and material resources from that chapter.
   - Local Disaster: a disaster that affects more than one family, occurs within the jurisdiction of a single Red Cross chapter, and generally requires the application of limited human and material resources from the Red Cross chapter.
   - State Disaster: a disaster that affects multiple families, occurs within the jurisdiction of one or more Red Cross chapters within a single state, generally requires the focused commitment of human and material resources from the affected chapter(s), and may require support and assistance from other Red Cross units.
   - Major Disaster: a disaster that generally has one or more of the following characteristics: requires the coordinated response and/or resources of multiple Red Cross units; affects more than a single state; creates national news media attention; is expected to result in an emergency or major disaster declaration by the President of the United States or the mobilization and application of federal government human and/or material resources; involves nuclear power plants and nuclear, chemical, or biological weapons; involves impact of material from space; requires international involvement; has the potential for similar extraordinary or unusual effect; or is expected to require types and/or quantities of services and/or assistance that exceed the combined capacity of the affected Red Cross chapter.
   - Presidentially Declared Disaster: a disaster that requires full or partial implementation of the NRP. Such a disaster generally has one or more of the following characteristics: exceeds the capabilities of a state and its local governments to provide a timely and effective response to meet the needs of the situation; causes or has the potential to cause a substantial number of deaths or injuries; causes or has the potential to cause substantial health and medical problems; or causes or has the potential to cause significant damage, particularly to the economic and physical infrastructure of the state or political subdivisions.

Table 14-2	Disaster Response Responsibilities by Agency		

American Red Cross	Other Voluntary Organizations	Business and Labor Organizations	Local Government
Operates shelters	Provide services that are identified in predisaster planning	Take action to protect employees and ensure the safety of the facility	Provides for the coordination of the overall relief effort
Provides feeding services	Provide regular services to ongoing client groups	Advise public safety forces of hazardous conditions	Advises the public on safety measures such as evacuation
Provides individual and family assistance to meet immediate emergency needs	Identify unanticipated needs and provide resources to meet those needs	Identify resources such as union halls, generators, and heavy equipment to support the disaster response	Provides public health services
Services include providing food, clothing, and shelter	Act as advocate for their client groups	Provide volunteers, financial contributions, and gifts of goods and services to the relief effort	Provides fire and police protection to the affected area
Provides disaster health services, including mental health support	Coordinate services with all other groups involved with the disaster response		Inspects facilities for safety and health codes
Handles inquires from concerned family members outside the area	Seek and accept donations from those wanting to help		Provides ongoing social services for the community
Coordinates relief activities with other agencies, business, labor, and government			Repairs public buildings, sewage and water systems, streets, and highways
Informs the public of available services			
Seeks and accepts contributions from those wanting help			

From the American Red Cross: *Disasters happen* (ARC Pub. No. 1570), Washington, DC, 1994, ARC.

In any large-scale or major national disaster, official agencies respond as do many other concerned citizens, including health care professionals. At times, so many people come "out of the woodwork" to help that role conflict, anger, frustration, and helplessness occur. After the World Trade Center attacks of September 11, 2001, many well-intentioned health care workers attempted to help find victims without being part of the team assigned for that task. In some cases, they risked injuries to themselves and obstructed the assigned rescue teams (Crippen, 2002).

The National Response Framework

Once a federal emergency has been declared, the National Response Framework (NRF) may take effect, depending on the specific needs arising from the disaster. The NRF was released by the Department of Homeland Security in January 2008 as a successor to the National Response Plan. The NRF focuses on response and short-term recovery and is seemingly less cumbersome to use than the NRP had been. This framework "helps define the roles, responsibilities, and relationships critical to effective emergency planning, preparedness, and response to any emergency or disaster" (National Response Framework, 2009).

There are 23 annexes to the NRF that are designed to provide direction in implementing the plan. The Framework

"identifies the key response principles, as well as the roles and structures that organize {a} national response" (National Response Framework, 2009). This framework is meant to be used by government executives, private sector business, nongovernmental leaders and emergency management practitioners. It is built on these five principles: engaged partnerships; tiered response; scalable, flexible, and adaptable operational capabilities; unity of effort through unified command; and readiness to act. See www.fema.gov/nrf for an online resource center with important reference materials.

CASE STUDY

Example of a State Plan for Emergency Preparedness and Response

Due to the national disasters of 9/11/01 in New York City and Washington DC the Virginia Department of Health has added an emergency preparedness and response (EP&R) office at the state, regional, and district levels. These offices are staffed with epidemiologists and emergency planners.

The main functions and duties of the emergency planner in the Virginia Department of Health local districts are to coordinate emergency responses with local agencies for potential public health events or other emergencies due to natural or human-made disasters.

Some of the many functions of the emergency planner include the following:
- Develop and maintain EP&R plans to include smallpox as well as strategic national stockpile (SNS) distribution
- Ensure that the local health department is aware of state plans
- Be a strategic planner
- Be a surge planner
- Partner internally and externally:
  - Liaison to/with other agencies
  - Liaison to/with other districts
  - Emergency Operations Center/director's representative
- District EP&R subject matter expert
- District data manager collects, processes, evaluates, and reports information
- District operations officer
- District SNS Coordinator:
  - Select dispensing sites
  - Recruit, train, assign, and maintain the workforce
  - Site oversight
  - Liaison with all possible involved parties
- District trainer
- Project manager/process team leader
- Unified infielder, e.g., back up epidemiologist on investigations

Prepared by Pamela Burke, BSMT, SM, Emergency Planner for the Thomas Jefferson Health District, Virginia Department of Health, July 2004.

The National Disaster Medical System (NDMS) is part of the ESF of Health and Medical Services. In a presidentially declared disaster, including overseas war, the U.S. Public Health Service can activate **disaster medical assistance teams (DMATs)** to an area to supplement local and state medical care needs. DMATs can also be activated by the Assistant Secretary for Health if requested by a state health officer. Teams of specially trained civilian physicians, nurses, and other health care personnel can be sent to a disaster site within hours of activation. DMATs can provide triage and continuing medical care to victims until they can be evacuated to a national network of hospitals prearranged by the NDMS (U.S. Department of Homeland Security, 2005b). Because of the nature of this country's disasters since the initiation of DMATs, these teams have been used primarily to staff community health outpatient clinics in the affected areas.

Response to Bioterrorism
Biological or chemical terrorist attacks require a very different response. An unannounced dissemination of a biological agent may easily go unnoticed, and the victims may have left the area of exposure long before the act of terrorism is recognized. The first signs that a biological agent has been released may not be apparent for days or weeks, when the

Box 14-4 Chemical and Biological Agent Websites and Resources

- *Health aspects of biological and chemical weapons: report of a WHO group of consultants (2001)* is a standard guide to help countries prepare for emergencies caused by the deliberate use of chemical weapons and 11 potential biological weapons: http://www.who.int/topics/biological-weapons.
- Centers for Disease Control and Prevention: http://www.bt.cdc.gov.
- National Domestic Preparedness Office: http://www.ojp.usdoj.gov/odp/.
- U.S. Public Health Service Office of Emergency Preparedness: http://www.ndms.dhhs.gov.

victims become ill and seek a health evaluation. In this case, the health care professionals, including nurses, are considered the "first on the scene." The five components to a comprehensive public health response to outbreaks of illness are the following (Rotz et al, 2000):
1. Detecting the outbreak
2. Determining the cause
3. Identifying factors that place people at risk
4. Implementing measures to control the outbreak
5. Informing the medical and public communities about treatments, health consequences, and preventive measures

Identifying the chemical or biological agent is the first priority. Rapid identification is vital to protect both the health care workers and any others affected. Box 14-4 lists websites that provide information about specific agents, their signs and symptoms, recommended laboratory tests, and infection control procedures and known antidotes (Veenema, 2002). Nurses need to be familiar with the most likely agents that could be released in a bioterrorism attack. As noted, the time interval between exposure and the onset of symptoms may lag from hours to weeks. The tools of epidemiology are essential in the detection of chemical or biological agents. Veenema (2002) provides a detailed discussion of chemical and biological terrorism.

People who experience or witness a terrorist attack may experience a stress response as well as one or more of the following symptoms (International Council of Nurses, 2009):
- Repeated thoughts about the attack
- Immense fear of everything; this may prevent them from even leaving their homes
- Survivor guilt or questioning why they lived and others did not
- A sense of great loss
- Hesitation to express feelings

Although many of the nursing actions for dealing with terrorism are similar to those in any other disaster, the following list summarizes key actions. The International Council of Nurses Fact Sheet on terrorism and bioterrorism provides useful details on each of the following actions:
- Help people cope with the aftermath of terrorism
- Allay public concerns and fears of bioterrorism

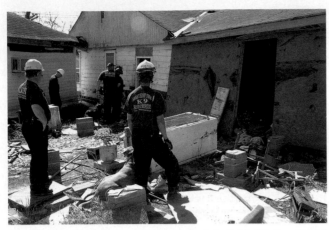

FIGURE 14-3 Ninth Ward, New Orleans, LA, 3-15-06: Special K9 search units and Southeast Louisiana Urban Search and Rescue Team members search for human remains before this house can be demolished. All homes being demolished in the Ninth Ward are searched by a search and recovery team that includes special search recovery dogs so that no human remains are left in houses that are being demolished. (Courtesy of the Marvin Nauman/Federal Emergency Management Agency.)

- Identify the feelings that you and others may be experiencing
- Assist victims to think positively and to move to the future
- Prepare nursing personnel to be effective in a crisis and/or an emergency situation

How Disasters Affect Communities

The physical and emotional effects of disasters on people in a community depend on the following:
- Type, cause, and location of the disaster
- Magnitude and extent of the damage
- Duration
- Amount of warning that was provided

For example, although no one may die in an earthquake, the structural damage to buildings and the continuous aftershocks may last for weeks and cause intense psychological stress. In addition, the longer it takes for structural repairs and other cleanup, the longer the psychological effects can last. The terrorist attacks of September 11, 2001, created extreme anger and grief but also led to a huge increase in compassion and patriotism. Thousands of people helped, from donating blood and money to rescuing victims from the buildings. This same type of commitment was seen following the hurricanes in recent years that displaced so many people from their homes.

Individuals react to the same disaster in different ways, depending on their age, cultural background, health status, social support structure, and general ability to adapt to crises (Figure 14-3).

The sequencing of reactions and level of intensity depend to some extent on the characteristics of the disaster, such as the suddenness of the impact, the duration of the event, and the probability of recurrence (Gerrity and Flynn, 1997). Box 14-5 describes common reactions of adults and children

| Box 14-5 | **Common Reactions to Disasters** |

Adults
- Extreme sense of urgency
- Panic and fear
- Disbelief
- Disorientation and numbing
- Reluctance to abandon property
- Difficulty in making decisions
- Need to help others
- Anger and blaming
- Blaming and scapegoating
- Delayed reactions
- Insomnia
- Headaches
- Apathy and depression
- Sense of powerlessness
- Guilt
- Moodiness and irritability
- Jealousy and resentment
- Domestic violence

Children
- Regressive behaviors (bedwetting, thumb sucking, crying, clinging to parents)
- Fantasies that disaster never occurred
- Nightmares
- School-related problems, including an inability to concentrate and refusal to go back to school

to disasters. Adults typically react first to a disaster with an extreme sense of urgency (Bryce, 2001). Victims become obsessed with personal losses. Other initial reactions include fear, panic, disbelief, reluctance to abandon property, feelings of disorientation and numbness, difficulty in making decisions, a need for information, seeking help for self and family, and offering help to other disaster victims (American Red Cross, 2002). Disturbances in bodily functions, such as gastrointestinal upsets, diarrhea, and nausea and vomiting, are also common (Gerrity and Flynn, 1997).

Anger, especially blaming and scapegoating, is common among victims soon after a disaster (Gerrity and Flynn, 1997). People become angry and begin to blame others as they realize how much they have lost and as they suffer physical fatigue, emotional stress, and a continuing change in personal comfort. Victims being interviewed on television after a disaster often say that FEMA, ARC, and other response organizations simply did not do all that was possible. Later, victims have difficulty sleeping, headaches, apathy and depression, moodiness and irritability, anxiety about the future, domestic violence, feelings of being overwhelmed, feelings of frustration and powerlessness over their future, and guilt over not being able to prevent the disaster or do more to help resolve it (American Red Cross, 2002).

The psychological effects of September 11 were slightly different from those of more contained, single-event disasters. These attacks were totally unexpected and of great magnitude. There was uncertainty and fear about what might

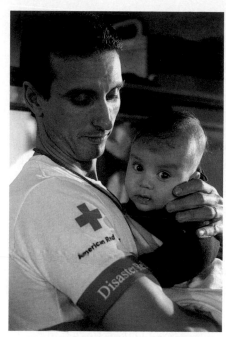

FIGURE 14-4 The effects of a disaster on young children can be especially disruptive. (Courtesy of the American Red Cross. All rights reserved in all countries.)

Box 14-6 lists other populations at risk for severe disruption from a disaster.

Role of the Nurse in Disaster Response

The nurse's role during a disaster depends largely on the nurse's experience, professional role in a community disaster plan, specialty training, and special interest. Flexibility is essential since the only certainty is that there will be continuing changes (American Red Cross, 2002). There may be times when the nurse is the first to arrive on the scene of a disaster. If so, the more usual skills of community assessment, case finding and referring, prevention, health education, surveillance, and working with aggregates will be put aside temporarily so that the nurse can deal with life-threatening problems. Once rescue workers arrive at the scene, plans for triage should immediately begin.

Triage is the process of separating casualties and allocating treatment on the basis of the victims' potentials for survival. Highest priority is always given to victims who have life-threatening injuries but who have a high probability of survival once stabilized (Ciancamerla and Debacker, 2000). Second priority is given to victims with injuries that have systemic complications that are not yet life threatening and could wait 45 to 60 minutes for treatment. Last priority is given to those victims with local injuries without immediate complications and who can wait several hours for medical attention.

Nurses working as members of an assessment team need to provide accurate information to relief managers to facilitate rapid rescue and recovery. Often nurses make home visits to gather needed information. Types of information in initial assessment reports include the following (Noji, 1996):

- Geographic extent of the disaster's impact
- Population at risk or affected
- Presence of continuing hazards
- Injuries and deaths
- Availability of shelter
- Current level of sanitation
- Status of the health care infrastructure

These assessments help match available resources to a population's emergency needs. Also, disaster assessment

happen next (American Red Cross, 2002). When people do not know when or if a next attack will occur, it is hard for them to move beyond their fear and anger. The treatment for terrorism, including military, economic, and other ways to contain the enemy, is all guesswork, and it is essential yet long-term. There is no one right way to handle the situation.

During disasters there may be an exacerbation of an existing chronic disease. For example, the emotional stress of being a disaster victim may make it difficult for people with diabetes to control their blood sugar levels. Grief can have harmful effects on the immune system. It reduces the function of cells that protect against viral infections and tumors. These immunological deficits may lead to more frequent health care visits. Hormones that are produced by the body's flight-or-fight mechanism also play a role in mediating the effects of grief.

The effects on young children can be especially disruptive (Figure 14-4). Children may have heightened sensitivity to sights, sounds, or smells and may experience exaggerated responses to usual activities. In addition, they may have nightmares and fantasies that the disaster never occurred. School-related problems may also develop, including an inability to concentrate or even refusal to go back to school (Gerrity and Flynn, 1997).

Older adults' reactions to disaster depend a great deal on their physical health, chronic illnesses, or functional limitations (Centers for Disease Control and Prevention, n.d.). They react deeply to the loss of personal possessions because of the high sentimental value attached to the items and the limited time left to replace them (Gerrity and Flynn, 1997).

HOW TO	Gather Disaster Information

1. Interview
2. Observation
3. Individual physical examinations
4. Health and illness screening
5. Surveys (sample and special health)
6. Records (census, school, vital statistics, disease reporting)

From Landesman L: *Public health management of disasters: the practice guide*, Washington, DC, 2001, American Public Health Association.

priorities are related to the type of disaster that has occurred (Noji, 1996). For example, assessments in sudden-impact disasters, such as tornadoes and earthquakes, are more concerned with ongoing hazards, injuries and deaths, shelter requirements, and clean water. Assessments in gradual-onset disasters, such as famines, are most concerned with mortality rates, nutritional status, immunization status, and environmental health.

Lack of or inaccurate information regarding the scope of the disaster and its initial effects contributes to the misuse of resources. Often too many volunteers who lack official sponsorship convene at the site of disaster and are disappointed when their help cannot be used. Similarly, well-meaning people may send clothes and food to disaster sites that lack storage and distribution abilities. Contributions that add to the stress of coping with the disaster can be a burden. Local and regional emergency management and public health resources need to be readjusted as assessment reports continue to come in. Establishing a priority of needs that benefit the largest aggregate of affected individuals with the most correctable problems is consistent with the basic tenets of triage.

Ongoing assessments or surveillance reports are just as important as initial assessments. Surveillance reports indicate the continuing status of the affected population and the effectiveness of ongoing relief efforts. They continue to inform relief managers of needed resources. Nurses involved in ongoing surveillance can use the methods listed in the "How To" box to gather information. Surveillance continues into the recovery phase of a disaster.

Shelter Management

Shelters are generally the responsibility of the local Red Cross chapter, although in massive disasters the military may set up "tent cities" or bring in trailers for the masses who need temporary shelter. Nurses, because of their comfort with delivering aggregate health promotion, disease prevention, and emotional support, make ideal shelter managers and team members. Although initially physical health needs are the priority, especially among older adults and the chronically ill, many of the predominant problems in shelters revolve around stress. The shock of the disaster itself, the loss of personal possessions, the fear of the unknown, living in proximity to total strangers, and even boredom can cause stress.

Nurses working in shelters can use the following common-sense approaches to help victims deal with stress (American Red Cross, 2002):

• Listen to victims tell and retell how they feel about the disaster and their current situation.
• Encourage victims to share their feelings with one another if it seems appropriate to do so.
• Help victims make decisions.
• Delegate tasks (reading, crafts, playing games with children) to teenagers and others to help combat boredom.
• Provide the basic necessities (food, clothing, rest).
• Try to recover or get needed items (prescription glasses, medication).
• Provide basic compassion and dignity (e.g., privacy when appropriate and if possible).
• Refer to a mental health counselor if the situation warrants.

The ARC provides specialized training in disaster mental health services. Its objective is to assist workers or clients to understand disaster-related stress and grief reactions, develop adaptive coping and problem-solving skills, and return to a predisaster state of equilibrium or seek recommended further treatment (American Red Cross, 2002). Highly trained mental health counselors, such as psychologists, psychiatrists, clinical social workers, and nurses, are always available in large-scale disasters. They are important members of any disaster team, no matter what the level of disaster, and their services should be used as often as necessary. Working in shelters, nurses are involved in assessment and referral and also perform functions outside the usual scope of care (Cox and Briggs, 2004). The Red Cross provides training for shelter support and using appropriate protocols.

Nurses need to be aware of the surrounding medical facilities and services provided in their area including special needs shelters. Individuals who are medically dependent and not acutely ill but have varied physical, cognitive, and psychological conditions should be directed to a special needs shelter. The federal government provides assistance to special needs shelters through one of the **emergency support functions (ESF 8)** of the National Response Plan, which provides assessment of public health and medical needs, health surveillance, supplies, and medical care personnel, such as teams from the National Disaster Medical System (U.S. Department of Homeland Security, 2005c).

Special needs shelters reduce the surge demands on hospitals and long-term care facilities that often occur during disasters. Although helpful in reducing surge, too many referrals can create a tension between the special needs shelters, the regular shelters, and the health care facilities as roles and responsibilities become blurred and overall resources and personnel are limited. Careful preplanning for a community's special needs populations is essential. In Florida, health department staff preregistered and identified individuals to be placed in special needs shelters well before the series of 2004 hurricanes hit (Association of State and Territorial Health Officials, 2004).

International Relief Efforts

Disasters occur throughout the world, and people suffer from natural disasters and human-made disasters. Civil strife leads to war, famine, and communicable disease outbreaks. Sometimes disaster or relief workers are sent to these international disasters at the request of the affected country's government. At other times, workers are not welcomed but instead may go with the support of the United Nations (UN). When workers are not welcomed, their lives may be in danger, even though they go as peacekeeping agents of the Federation of Red Cross and Red Crescent Societies and the International Committee of Red Cross or as health representatives from the World Health Organization. International disaster or relief workers generally have intense training and preparation before embarking on a mission.

Psychological Stress of Disaster Workers

Both victims and workers experience psychological stress during disasters (Bryce, 2001). Mental health workers often need to assist nurses as well as the public. The degree of workers' stress depends on the nature of the disaster, their role in the disaster, individual stamina, and other environmental factors. Environmental factors include noise, inadequate workspace, physical danger, and stimulus overload, especially exposure to death and trauma. Other sources of stress may emerge from workers thinking they are not doing enough to help, from the burden of making life-and-death decisions, and from the overall change in living patterns (Bryce, 2001).

Disaster nurses who live in the community in which the disaster has struck and who are also victims of the disaster may experience additional stress. Anger and resentment may occur as the job demands time away from their own situation.

Symptoms of early stress and burnout include minor tremors, nausea, inability to concentrate, difficulty thinking, and problems with memory (Bryce, 2001). Suppressing feelings of guilt, powerlessness, anger, and other signs of stress will eventually lead to symptoms such as irritability, fatigue, headaches, and distortions of bodily functions. It is normal to experience stress, but it must be dealt with. The worst thing anyone can do is to deny that it exists.

The American Red Cross (2002) recommends the following strategies for dealing with stress while working at a disaster:

- Get enough sleep.
- Take time away from the disaster (i.e., take breaks).
- Avoid alcohol.
- Eat frequently in small amounts.
- Use humor to break the tension and provide relief.
- Use positive self-talk.
- Take time to defuse or debrief.
- Stay in touch with people at home.
- Keep a journal.
- Provide mutual support.

Delayed stress reactions, or those that occur once the disaster is over, include exhaustion and an inability to adjust to the slower pace of work or home (Bryce, 2001).

Workers may be disappointed if family members and friends do not seem as interested in what they have been through and if coming back home, in general, does not live up to expectations. Also, they may feel frustration and conflict if their needs seem inconsistent with those of their family and co-workers or if they have left the disaster site thinking that so much more could have been done (Bryce, 2001). Issues or problems that once seemed pressing may now seem trivial. Anger may emerge as others present problems that seem trivial compared with those faced by the victims who were left behind. Disaster workers may fantasize about returning to the disaster site if they think that their actions are appreciated more there than at home or the office. Mood swings are common and serve to resolve conflicting feelings. Feelings or actions that persist or that the worker perceives are interfering with daily life should be dealt with by a trained mental health professional (American Red Cross, 2002).

RECOVERY

The recovery period following a disaster includes all involved agencies pulling together to restore the institutions and properly rebuild. For example, the government takes the lead in rebuilding efforts, whereas the business community tries to provide economic support. Many religious organizations help with rebuilding efforts as well. The Internal Revenue Service educates victims as to how to write off losses and the Housing and Urban Development Department provides grants for temporary housing. The CDC provides continuing surveillance and epidemiologic services. Voluntary agencies continue to assess individual and community needs and meet those needs as they are able. When housing is destroyed, groups such as Habitat for Humanity play a valuable role in the rebuilding.

BRIEFLY NOTED

The best time to start thinking about the lessons learned from a recent disaster is during the recovery phase of the disaster cycle.

Role of the Nurse in Disaster Recovery

The role of the nurse in the recovery phase of a disaster is as varied as in the prevention, preparedness, and response phases, and the three levels of prevention are used (Levels of Prevention box). Flexibility is essential in the recovery operation. Community cleanup efforts can cause many physical and psychological problems. For example, the physical stress of moving heavy objects can cause back injury, severe fatigue, and even death from heart attacks. Nurses also must continue to teach proper hygiene and make sure immunization records are current given the threat of disease.

The prolonged effects of disaster intensify acute and chronic illnesses. The psychological stress of cleanup and/or

Levels of Prevention	Related to Disaster Management

PRIMARY PREVENTION

Participate in developing a disaster management plan for the community.

SECONDARY PREVENTION

Assess disaster victims and triage for care.

TERTIARY PREVENTION

Participate in home visits to uncover dangers that may cause additional injury to victims or cause other problems (e.g., house fires from faulty wiring).

moving can cause feelings of severe hopelessness, depression, and grief. These stresses then merge with the long-term results of living in adverse circumstances (Bryce, 2001). In some cases, stress can lead to depression and suicide (Vastag, 2002). Although the majority of people eventually recover from disasters, acute and chronic illness can worsen by their prolonged effects of disaster As a result, referrals to mental health professionals should continue as long as the need exists. See "Evidence-Based Practice" box for a discussion of mental health needs of children after a disaster.

It is important to be alert for environmental health hazards during the recovery phase of a disaster. During home visits, nurses may uncover situations such as a faulty housing structure or lack of water or electricity. Objects that have been blown into the yard by a tornado or that floated in from a flood may be dangerous and must be removed. Also, the nurse should assess the dangers of live or dead animals and rodents that are harmful to a person's health. An example of this would be finding poisonous snakes in and around homes once the waters from a flood start to recede. Case finding and referral are critical during the recovery phase and may continue for a long time. For example, for a full 2 years after the Oklahoma City bombing of the Alfred P. Murrah Federal Building, the ARC supported the Bombing Recovery Project (American Red Cross, 1998). Follow-up home visits were made for all those in need, although the recovery process for some will last for years. In the end, all of the nurses and organizations in the world can only provide partnerships with the victims of a disaster. Ultimately, it is up to individuals to recover on their own.

The hurricanes in the United States over the past several years changed how the health care system prepares for, responds to, and recovers from a disaster. People have learned how critical it is for communities to have a well-organized plan and for key players to know their roles and be flexible and collaborative. The value of an electronic medical record became more apparent in recent years when hospitals, clinics, and health departments lost records during a disaster and when people were relocated for substantial periods of time without access to their medications or their medical records (Cary, 2008).

Evidence-Based Practice

The aftermath of a natural disaster presents many challenges to health care workers. Most epidemiologic investigations after natural disasters have focused on physiological problems and the containment of infectious disease outbreaks. However, these investigations tend to neglect the long-term effects of disasters on affected populations, specifically the long-term mental health effects. Two years after Hurricane Iniki struck the island of Kauai (one of the Hawaiian Islands), the Department of Psychiatry and Pediatrics of Mount Sinai School of Medicine and the National Center for Posttraumatic Stress Disorder studied the effectiveness of public health-inspired, school-based screening and treatment of mental distress following a natural disaster. There were two main objectives of the study. The first was to see if it is possible to identify symptomatic cases in a large population of children, given that few children may be symptomatic and not all symptomatic children outwardly display disordered behavior. The second goal was to determine the efficiency of providing treatment to relatively large numbers of affected children.

The study found that certain children were more likely to experience symptoms of mental health distress. These children included those of the female sex, younger age, and lower socioeconomic status. These children reacted with panic to the hurricane and feared for the physical safety of family and self during the disaster. After being screened, children who were assessed to have high levels of trauma-related symptoms were provided school-based treatment. Children were randomly assigned to group or to individual treatment. Treatment consisted of four weekly sessions. The children were assessed again after treatment was complete, and then again a full year later.

The study found that the levels of mental health distress were significantly lower after treatment and remained at that level a year later without additional treatment. Group and individual treatments did not differ in their effectiveness, but group treatment was associated with higher levels of completion rates. The similarity of clinical ratings and self-report findings as well as control for the passage of time and for the effects of assessment suggest that these results did not merely reflect an immediate response but showed a long-term response to disaster.

NURSE USE: This study suggests that using schools as a natural means to screen and treat children affected by natural disasters is cost effective and valid. This public health-inspired strategy may be useful in other posttraumatic environments. For example, children's psychological recovery in the aftermath of human-made disasters, including community violence and terrorism, may be facilitated in this way.

From Chemtob CM, Nakashima JP, Hamada RS: Psychosocial intervention for postdisaster trauma symptoms in elementary school children, *Arch Pediatr Adolesc Med* 156:211-216, 2002.

CLINICAL APPLICATION

Paula Miller, a nurse in a medium-size public health department in Lincoln, Nebraska, was called to serve on her first national disaster assignment. Her disaster skills were tested when a level I hurricane hit Miami and its surrounding areas. Ms. Miller left Lincoln to help manage a shelter in an elementary school cafeteria in Homestead, Florida, near Miami.

The devastation that she saw en route to the school had a negative effect on her. Assigned to help with client intake, she patiently listened to the disaster victims, referred many of her most distraught clients to the mental health counselor, and set priorities for other needs as they arose. For example, she found that many of her clients had left their medications behind and needed therapy. Other needs included diapers and formulas for infants, prescription eyeglasses, and clothing. By identifying their needs, Ms Miller helped ensure that the master "needs list" was complete.

As the days went on, the stress level in the shelter grew. The crowded living conditions and lack of privacy took its toll on the residents. Around the tenth day of her assignment, Ms Miller began to experience pounding headaches and had difficulty concentrating. She thought she would be fine, but the mental health counselor said that she was experiencing a stress reaction.

Which of the following actions would probably be the most useful for this nurse to take?

A. *Share her feelings with the on-site mental health counselor on a regular basis.*
B. *Call home to share her feelings with family members.*
C. *Meet the needs of her clients to the best of her ability, and accept the fact that stress is a part of the job.*

Answer is in the back of the book.

REMEMBER THIS!

- The number of disasters, both human-made and natural, continues to increase, as does the number of people affected by them.
- The cost to recover from a disaster has risen sharply because of the amount of technology that must be restored.
- Professional preparedness involves an awareness and understanding of the disaster plan at work and in the community.
- Nurses are increasingly getting involved in disaster planning, response, and recovery through their local health department or local government.
- Disaster health and disaster mental health training from an official agency such as the American Red Cross can prepare nurses for the many opportunities that await them in disaster prevention, preparedness, response, and recovery.
- The response to a disaster is determined by its assigned level. Levels are not determined by the number of casualties but by the amount of resources needed.
- Helping clients maintain a safe environment and advocating for environmental safety measures in the community are key roles for the nurse during all phases of disaster management.
- It is important for nurses to know about available community resources, especially for vulnerable populations, during the preparedness stage of disaster management to ensure smoother response and recovery stages.
- People in a community react differently to a disaster depending on the type, cause, and location of the disaster; its magnitude and extent of damage; its duration; and the amount of warning that was provided.

- People react differently to disasters depending on factors such as their age, cultural background, health status, social support structure, and general adaptability to crisis.
- The stress of nurses is compounded if they are both victims and caregivers in a disaster.
- Disaster shelter nurses are exposed to a variety of physical and emotional complaints, including stress. Stress may be instigated by the shock of the disaster, the loss of personal possessions, the fear of the unknown, living in proximity to strangers, and boredom.
- The degree of worker stress during disasters depends on the nature of the disaster, their role in the disaster, individual stamina, noise level, adequacy of workspace, potential for physical danger, stimulus overload, and, especially, being exposed to death and trauma.
- Symptoms of worker stress during disasters include minor tremors, nausea, loss of concentration, difficulty thinking and remembering, irritability, fatigue, and other somatic disorders.
- A key attribute in aiding disaster victims is flexibility.
- The stage of disaster known as recovery occurs as all involved agencies pull together to restore the economic and civic life of the community.

WHAT WOULD YOU DO?

1. If you thought a hurricane might affect your community, what steps would you take to adequately prepare for the possible disaster? What steps would you take to ensure safety and preparedness for your family and for the clients for whom you care? Whose help would you enlist? To whom would you go for advice? Talk with two classmates and compare your answers, and then prepare an action plan.

2. Assume that your community has the potential to be hit by a tornado. List the groups who would be most vulnerable. What steps could you take in advance to reduce their vulnerability? What community resources are available?

3. If you and your classmates saw a tornado moving across the street in a small town as you drove to your clinical site, what steps would you take to determine if people were injured? What would you do first? Who else would you involve? Discuss your replies with a classmate and come up with a consolidated plan.

4. Describe the role of the nurse in the preparedness, response, and recovery stages of disaster. Does all of this make sense to you?

■ *REFERENCES*

American Red Cross: *Disasters happen* (ARC Pub No 1570), Washington, DC, 1994, ARC.

American Red Cross: *Oklahoma City bombing recovery project: answering the call: Roberta Flynn offers encouragement to victims,* Disaster Services News Sheet Feb 27, 1998.

American Red Cross: *Disaster health services: an overview: participants workbook* (ARC Pub No 3076-1A), Washington, DC, 1999, ARC.

American Red Cross: *Disaster health services simulation: instructor manual* (ARC Pub No 3076–2), Washington, DC, 2000, ARC.

American Red Cross: *How do I deal with my feelings?* Washington, DC, 2001, ARC.

American Red Cross: *Disaster mental health services: an overview* (ARC Pub No 3077–2A), Washington, DC, 2002, ARC.

American Red Cross: *Foundations of the disaster services program* (ARC Pub No 3000, p. 12), Washington, DC, 2003, ARC.

American Red Cross: *Committed to helping make families and communities safe from the ravages of natural hazards,* n.d.a. Retrieved Aug 16, 2008, from http://www/redcross.org/services/disaster/0,1082,0-2_00.html.

Association of State and Territorial Health Officials: *Public health emergency preparedness and response to the hurricanes of 2004,* Oct 15, 2004. Retrieved Aug 16, 2005, from http://www.astho.org/pubs/HurricaneCalltranscript.pdf.

Bissell RA et al: Evidence of the effectiveness of health sector preparedness in disaster response: the example of four earthquakes, *Fam Community Health* 27(3):193–204, 2004.

Bryce CP: *Stress management in disasters,* Washington, DC, 2001, Pan American Health Organization.

Cary S: Caring for patients on kidney dialysis in a disaster, *Am J Nurs* 108(1):26–32, 2008.

Centers for Disease Control and Prevention: *Local emergency preparedness and response inventory,* Atlanta, Ga, 2002, Public Health Program Office, available at www.bt.cdc.gov.

Centers for Disease Control and Prevention: *Disaster planning tips for older adults and their families,* Atlanta, Ga, n.d.a. Retrieved Aug 7, 2008, from http://www.cdc.gov/aging/pdf/disaster_planning_tips.pdf.

Chemtob CM, Nakashima JP, Hamada RS: Psychosocial intervention for postdisaster trauma symptoms in elementary school children, *Arch Pediatr Adolesc Med* 156:211–216, 2002.

Ciancamerla G, Debacker M: Triage. In de Boer J, et al: *Handbook of disaster medicine,* Zeist, The Netherlands, 2000, International Society of Disaster Medicine.

Cox E, Briggs S: Disaster Nursing: New frontiers for critical care, *Crit Care Nurse* 24(3):16–22, 2004.

Crippen DW: Disaster management: lessons from September 11, 2001. Presented at 8th World Congress of Intensive and Critical Care Medicine, Sydney, Australia, 2002.

Federal Emergency Management Agency and American Red Cross: *Family disaster planning: 4 steps to safety,* Washington, DC, 1997, FEMA, ARC.

Federal Emergency Management Agency: *Are you ready? An in-depth guide to citizen preparedness,* Washington, DC, 2005.

Gaines SK, Leary J: Public health emergency preparedness in the setting of child care, *Fam Community Health* 27(3):263–268, 2004.

Gebbie KM et al: Role of exercises and drills in the evaluation of public health in emergency response, *Prehosp Disast Med* 21(3):173–182, 2006.

Gebbie KM Qureshi K: Emergency and disaster preparedness: core competencies for nurses—what every nurse should but may not know, *Am J Nurs* 102(1):46–51, 2002.

Gerrity ET, Flynn BW: Mental health consequences of disasters. In Noji EK, editor: *The public health consequences of disasters,* NY, 1997, Oxford University.

Hassmiller SB: Bioterrorism and disaster management. In Stanhope M, Lancaster J, editors: *Public health nursing,* ed 7, St Louis, 2008, Elsevier.

International Council of Nurses: *Fact sheet: terrorism and bioterrorism.* Retrieved Feb 26, 2009, from www.icn.ch/matters_bio.htm.

International Federation of Red Cross and Red Cross Societies: World disaster report, 2004, Chapter 8-disaster data: key trends and statistics, 2004. Retrieved May 29, 2009, from http://www/ofrc/prg/publicat/wdr 2004/index.asp.

Landesman L: *Public health management of disasters: the practice guide,* Washington, DC, 2001, APHA.

National Response Framework Released: January 22, 2008 (www.dhs.gov/xnewreleases). Retrieved Feb 25, 2009, from www.dhs.gov/xnews/releases/pr_1201030569827.shtm.

Noji EK: Disaster epidemiology, *Emerg Med Clin North Am* 14(2):289, 1996.

Qureshi KA et al: Effectiveness of an emergency preparedness training program for public health nurses in New York City, *Fam Community Health* 27(3):244–251, 2004.

Rotz LD et al: Bioterrorism preparedness: planning for the future, *J Public Health Manag Pract* 6(4):45, 2000.

Santa Clara County: *Operational area emergency plan, 2008.* Retrieved Aug 6, 2008, from http:www.sccgov.org/scc/docs%2FEmergency%2c%.

U.S. Department of Health and Human Services: *Interim public health and healthcare supplement to the national preparedness goal* (NPG), n.d. Retrieved June 1, 2005, from http://www.hhs.gov/ophep/npgs.html.

U.S. Department of Health and Human Services: *The public health response to biological and chemical terrorism,* Washington, DC, 2001, available at www.bt.cdc.gov/documents/planning/planningguidance.pdf.

U.S. Department of Homeland Security: *Interim national infrastructure protection plan,* Washington, DC, 2005a. Retrieved Aug 16, 2005, from http://www.dequ.state.mi.us/documents/deq-wb-wws-interim-nipp.pdf.

U.S. Department of Homeland Security: *National disaster medical system-DMAT,* Washington, DC, 2005b. Retrieved Aug 7, 2008, from http://www.ndms.dhhs.gov/dmat.html.

U.S. Department of Homeland Security: *Target capabilities list: version 1.1,* Washington, DC, 2005c. Retrieved Aug 16, 2005, from http://www/.dhs.gov/dhspublic/interapp/press_release/press_release_0639.xml.

U.S. Department of Homeland Security: *Emergencies & disasters: planning and prevention,* n.d.b. Retrieved May 26, 2005, from http://www/dhs.gov/dhspublic/interapp/editorial_0570.xml.

Vastag B: PTSD and depression in NYC, *JAMA* 287(15):1930, 2002.

Veenema TG: Chemical and biological terrorism: current updates for nurse educators, *Nurs Educ Perspect* 23(2), 2002.

Veenema TG: Essentials of disaster planning. In Veenema TG, editor: *Disaster nursing and emergency preparedness for chemical, biological, and radiological terrorism and other hazards,* New York, 2003, Springer.

White House: *President Bush signs Homeland Security Act,* Washington, DC, 2002. Retrieved Aug 16, 2005, from http://www/whitehouse.gov/news.

White House: *President thanks DHS Secretary Chertoff at swearing-in ceremony,* Washington, DC, 2005. Retrieved Aug 16, 2005, from http://www.whitehouse.gov/news/reseases/2005/03/20020202-1.html.

World Health Organization Group of Consultants: *Updated report: health aspects of chemical and biological weapons,* Geneva, Switzerland, 2001, WHO.

Surveillance and Outbreak Investigation

Marcia Stanhope

ADDITIONAL RESOURCES

These related resources are found either in the appendix at the back of this book or on the book's website at http://evolve.elsevier.com/stanhope/foundations.

Evolve Website

• Community Assessment Applied

• Quiz review questions
• WebLinks, including link to *Healthy People 2010* website

OBJECTIVES

After reading this chapter, the student should be able to:
1. Define public health surveillance.
2. List types of surveillance systems.
3. Identify steps in planning, analyzing, interviewing, and evaluating surveillance.

4. Recognize sources of data used when investigating a disease/condition outbreak.
5. Describe role of the nurse in surveillance and outbreak investigation to the national core competencies for public health nurses.

CHAPTER OUTLINE

DISEASE SURVEILLANCE
Definitions and Importance
Uses of Public Health Surveillance
Purposes of Surveillance
Collaboration among Partners
Nurse Competencies
Data Sources for Surveillance
NATIONAL NOTIFIABLE DISEASES
STATE NOTIFIABLE DISEASES
TYPES OF SURVEILLANCE SYSTEMS

Passive System
Active System
Sentinel System
Special Systems
THE INVESTIGATION
Investigation Objectives
Patterns of Occurrence
When to Investigate
INTERVENTIONS AND PROTECTION

KEY TERMS

biological terrorism: an intentional release of viruses, bacteria, or their toxins for the purpose of harming or killing.
chemical terrorism: the intentional release of hazardous chemicals into the environment for the purpose of harming or killing.

common source outbreak: an outbreak in which a group is exposed to a common noxious influence such as the release of noxious gases.
disease surveillance: the ongoing systematic collection, analysis, interpretation, and dissemination of specific health data for use in public health.

endemic: a disease and/or an event that is found to be present (occurring) in a population in which there is a persistent (usual) presence with low to moderate disease/event cases.

epidemic: an occurrence of a disease within an area that is clearly in excess of expected levels (endemic) for a given time period.

event: an occurrence of a phenomenon of health that can be discretely characterized; it can be environmental, occupational, or biological, naturally occurring, or person induced.

holoendemic: a highly prevalent problem found in a population commonly acquired early in life. The prevalence of this problem decreases as age increases.

hyperendemic: a disease/event that is found to have a persistently (usually) high number of cases.

intermittent or continuous source: cases may be exposed periodically or uninterrupted over a period of days or weeks.

mixed outbreak: an outbreak with a common source followed by secondary exposures related to person-to-person contact, as in the spreading of influenza.

National Notifiable Disease Surveillance System (NNDSS): a voluntary system monitored by the Centers for Disease Control and Prevention that includes 52 infectious diseases or conditions with case definitions that are considered important to the public's health.

outbreak: a change (increase) in a disease and/or an event from expected levels to levels that are clearly in excess of expected levels.

outbreak detection: identifying a rise in the frequency of a disease above the usual occurrence of the disease.

pandemic: refers to the epidemic spread of the problem over several countries or continents (such as the SARS outbreak).

point source: a stationary location or fixed facility from which pollutants are discharged; any single identifiable source of pollution, e.g., a pipe, ditch, ship, ore pit, or factory smokestack.

propagated outbreak: an outbreak that does not have a common source and spreads gradually from person to person over more than one incubation period.

sentinel: a surveillance system that monitors key health events when information is not otherwise available or in vulnerable populations to calculate or estimate disease morbidity.

sporadic: problems with an irregular pattern with occasional cases found at irregular intervals.

syndronic surveillance systems: systems developed to monitor illness syndromes or events, such as increased numbers of medication purchases, trips to physicians or emergency departments, or orders for cultures or x-rays, as well as rising levels of school or work absenteeism, which may indicate that an epidemic is developing hours or days before disease clusters are recognized or specific diagnoses are made and reported to public health agencies.

Disease surveillance has been a part of public health protection since the 1200s during the investigations of the bubonic plague in Europe. The Constitution of the United States provides for "police powers" necessary to preserve health safety as well as other events (see Chapter 7). These powers include public health surveillance. State and local "police powers" also provide for surveillance activities. Health departments usually have the legal authority to investigate unusual clusters of illness as well (U.S. Department of Health and Human Services, 2001).

BRIEFLY NOTED

In 1901 the United States began the requirement for reporting cases of cholera, smallpox, and tuberculosis.

DISEASE SURVEILLANCE

DEFINITIONS AND IMPORTANCE

Disease surveillance is "the ongoing systematic collection, analysis, interpretation and dissemination of specific health data for use in public health" (Teutsch and Churchill, 2004). Surveillance provides a means for nurses to monitor disease

trends in order to reduce morbidity and mortality and to improve health (Ching, 2002).

Surveillance is a critical role function for nurses practicing in the community. It is important because it generates knowledge of a disease or **event** outbreak patterns (including timing, geographic distribution, and susceptible populations).

Although surveillance was initially devoted to monitoring and reducing the spread of infectious diseases, it is now used to monitor and reduce chronic diseases and injuries as well as "environmental and occupational exposures" (Ching, 2002) and personal health behaviors. Surveillance systems help nurses and other professionals monitor emerging infections and bioterrorist outbreaks (Pryor and Veenema, 2003). Bioterrorism is one example of an event creating a critical public health concern that involves environmental exposures that must be monitored. This event also requires serious planning in order to be able to respond quickly and effectively. **Biological terrorism** is defined as "an intentional release of viruses, bacteria, or their toxins for the purpose of harming or killing… citizens" (Centers for Disease Control and Prevention, 2001a). **Chemical terrorism** is the intentional release of hazardous chemicals into the environment for the purpose of harming or killing (Centers for Disease Control and Prevention, 2001a). In the event of a bioterrorist attack,

Box 15-1   Features of Surveillance
• Is organized and planned
• Is the principal means by which a population's health status is assessed
• Involves ongoing collection of specific data
• Involves analyzing data on a regular basis
• Requires sharing the results with others
• Requires broad and repeated contact with the public about personal health issues
• Motivates public health action as a result of data analyses to:
• Reduce morbidity
• Reduce mortality
• Improve health

Box 15-2   Purposes of Surveillance
• Assess public health status
• Define public health priorities
• Plan public health programs
• Evaluate interventions and programs
• Stimulate research

From the Centers for Disease Control and Prevention: Updated guidelines for evaluating public health surveillance systems: recommendations from the Guidelines Working Group, *MMWR Morbid Mortal Wkly Rep* 50(RR-13)'1–35, 2001b.

imagine how difficult it would be to control the spread of biological agents such as botulism or anthrax or chemical agents such as sarin or ricin if no data were available about these agents, their resulting diseases or symptoms, and their usual incidence (new cases) patterns in the community. (See Box 15-1 for a summary of the features of surveillance.)

USES OF PUBLIC HEALTH SURVEILLANCE

Public health surveillance can be used to facilitate the following (Centers for Disease Control and Prevention, 2004):
• Estimate the magnitude of a problem (disease or event).
• Determine the geographic distribution of an illness or symptoms.
• Portray the natural history of a disease.
• Detect epidemics and define a problem.
• Generate hypotheses and stimulate research.
• Evaluate control measures.
• Monitor changes in infectious agents.
• Detect changes in health practices.
• Facilitate planning.

PURPOSES OF SURVEILLANCE

Surveillance helps public health departments identify trends and unusual disease patterns, set priorities for using scarce resources, and develop and evaluate programs for commonly occurring and universally occurring diseases or events (Box 15-2).

Surveillance activities can be related to the core functions of public health—assessment, policy development, and assurance. Disease surveillance helps establish baseline (endemic) rates of disease occurrence and patterns of spread. Surveillance makes it possible to initiate a rapid response to an outbreak of a disease or event that can cause a health problem. Surveillance data are assessed and analyzed, and interpretations of these data analyses are used to develop policies that better protect the public from problems such as emerging infections, bioterrorist biological and chemical threats, and injuries from problems such as motor vehicle accidents. Surveillance makes it possible to have ongoing monitoring in place to ensure that disease and event patterns improve rather than deteriorate. It can also make it possible to study whether the clinical protocols and public health policies that are in place can be enhanced based on current science so that disease rates actually decline.

Surveillance data are very helpful in determining whether a program is effective. Such data make it possible to determine whether public health interventions are effective in reducing the spread of disease or the incidence of injuries.

COLLABORATION AMONG PARTNERS

A quality surveillance system requires collaboration among a number of agencies and individuals: federal agencies, state and local public health agencies, hospitals, health care providers, medical examiners, veterinarians, agriculture, pharmaceutical agencies, emergency management, and law enforcement agencies, as well as 911 systems, ambulance services, urgent care and emergency departments, poison control centers, nurse hotlines, school, and industry. Such collaboration promotes the development of a comprehensive plan and a directory of emergency responses and contacts for effective sharing of communication and information. Nurses are often in the forefront of responses to be made in the surveillance process whether working in a small rural agency or a large urban agency; within the health department, school, or urgent care center; or on the telephone performing triage services during a disaster. It is the nurse who sees the event first (Gebbie, Rosenstock, and Hernandez, 2003).

NURSE COMPETENCIES

The national core competencies for public health nurses were developed from the work of the Council on Linkages Between Academia and Public Health Practice (*Core Competencies for Public Health Professionals,* 2000) and by the Quad Council of Public Health Nursing Organizations (2003). These competencies are divided into eight practice domains: analytic assessment skills, policy/program development, communication, cultural competency, community dimensions of practice, basic public health sciences, financial planning/management, and leadership.

To be a participant in surveillance and investigation activities, the staff nurse must have the following knowledge related to the core competencies:
1. Analytic assessment skills:
  • Defining the problem
  • Determining a cause

- Identifying relevant data and information sources
- Partnering with others to give meaning to the data collected
- Identifying risks
2. Communication:
   - Providing effective oral and written reports
   - Soliciting input from others and effectively presenting accurate demographic, statistical, and scientific information to other professionals and the community at large
3. Community dimensions of practice:
   - Establishing and maintaining links during the investigation
   - Collaborating with partners
   - Developing, implementing, and evaluating an assessment to define the problem
4. Basic public health science skills:
   - Identifying individual and organizational responsibilities
   - Identifying and retrieving current relevant scientific evidence
5. Leadership and systems thinking
   - Identifying internal and external issues that have an effect on the investigation
   - Promoting team and organizational efforts
   - Contributing to developing, implementing, and monitoring of the investigation

Although the staff nurse participates in these activities, the advanced practice public health nurse should be proficient in applying these competencies.

The Minnesota Model of Public Health Interventions: Applications for Public Health Nursing Practice (Centers for Public Health Nursing 2001, pp. 15, 16) suggests that surveillance is one of the interventions related to nursing practice in public health. The model provides seven basic steps of surveillance for nurses to follow:

1. Consider whether surveillance as an intervention is appropriate for the situation.
2. Organize the knowledge of the problem, its natural course of history, and its aftermath.
3. Establish clear criteria for what constitutes a case.
4. Collect sufficient data from multiple valid sources.
5. Analyze the data.
6. Interpret and disseminate the data to decision makers.
7. Evaluate the impact of the surveillance system.

DATA SOURCES FOR SURVEILLANCE

Clinicians, health care agencies, and laboratories report cases to state health departments. Data also come from death certificates and administrative data such as discharge reports and billing records (Pryor and Veenema, 2003). The following are select sources of mortality and morbidity data:

1. Mortality data are often the only source of health-related data available for small geographic areas. Examples include the following:
   - Vital statistics reports (e.g., death certificates, medical examiner reports, birth certificates)

2. Morbidity data include the following:
   - Notifiable disease reports
   - Laboratory reports
   - Hospital discharge reports
   - Billing data
   - Outpatient health care data
   - Specialized disease registries
   - Injury surveillance systems
   - Environmental surveys
   - Sentinel surveillance systems

A good example of a process in place to collect morbidity data is the National Program of Cancer Registries. This program provides for monitoring of the types of cancers found in a state and the locations of the cancer risks and health problems in the state.

Each of the data sources has the potential for underreporting or incomplete reporting. However, if there is consistency in the use of surveillance methods, the data collected will show trends in events or disease patterns that may indicate

---

● Healthy People 2010

Surveillance Objectives

1-12 Establish a single toll-free number for access to poison control centers on a 24-hour basis throughout the United States.

3-14 Increase the number of states that have a statewide population-based cancer registry that captures case information on at least 95% of the expected number of reportable cancers.

8-28 Increase the number of local health departments or agencies that use data from surveillance of environmental risk factors as part of their vector control programs.

10-2 Reduce outbreaks of infections caused by key foodborne bacteria.

14-31 Increase the number of persons under active surveillance for vaccine safety via large linked databases.

15-10 Increase the number of states (including the District of Columbia) with statewide emergency department surveillance systems that collect data on external causes of injury.

15-11 Increase the number of states (including the District of Columbia) that collect data on external causes of injury through hospital discharge data systems.

23-2 Increase the proportion of federal, tribal, state, and local health agencies that have made information available to the public in the past year on the Leading Health Indicators, Health Status Indicators, and Priority Data Needs.

23-3 Increase the proportion of all major national, state, and local health data systems that use geocoding to promote nationwide use of geographic information systems (GIS) at all levels.

23-4 Increase the proportion of population-based *Healthy People 2010* objectives for which national data are available for all population groups identified for the objective.

From U.S. Department of Health and Human Services: *Healthy People 2010 objectives,* Washington, DC, 2000, U.S. Department of Health and Human Services.

a change needed in a program or a needed prevention intervention to reduce morbidity or mortality (Centers for Disease Control and Prevention, 2006a).

Mortality data assist in identifying differences in health status among groups, populations, occupations, and communities; monitor preventable deaths; and help to examine cause and effect factors in diseases. Vital statistics can be used to plan programs and to monitor programs to meet *Healthy People 2010* goals.

The **sentinel** surveillance system provides for the monitoring of key health events when information is not otherwise available or in vulnerable populations to calculate or estimate disease morbidity (Centers for Disease Control and Prevention, 2003).

NATIONAL NOTIFIABLE DISEASES

Box 15-3 shows the national notifiable infectious diseases. Reporting of disease data by health care providers, laboratories, and public health workers to state and local health departments is essential if trends are to be accurately monitored. "The data provide the basis for detecting disease outbreaks, for identifying person characteristics, and for calculating incidence, geographic distribution, and temporal trends. They are used to initiate prevention programs, evaluate established prevention and control practices, suggest new intervention strategies, identify areas for research, document the need for disease control funds, and help answer questions from the community" (Cabinet for Human Resources [CHS], 2004).

Box 15-3 Infectious Diseases Designated as Notifiable at the National Level—United States, 2006

Acquired immunodeficiency syndrome (AIDS)
Anthrax
Botulism, foodborne
Botulism, infant
Botulism, other (includes wound and unspecified)
Brucellosis
California serogroup virus neuroinvasive disease
California serogroup virus nonneuroinvasive disease
Chancroid
Chlamydia trachomatis genital infection
Cholera
Coccidioidomycosis
Cryptosporidiosis
Cryptosporiasis
Diphtheria
Eastern equine encephalitis virus neuroinvasive disease
Eastern equine encephalitis virus nonneuroinvasive disease
Ehrlichiosis, human granulocytic (HGE)
Ehrlichiosis, human monocytic (HME)
Ehrlichiosis, human other or unspecified
Giardiasis
Gonorrhea
Haemophilus influenzae, invasive disease
Hansen's disease (leprosy)
Hantavirus pulmonary syndrome
Hemolytic uremic syndrome, postdiarrheal
Hepatitis A, acute
Hepatitis B, acute
Hepatitis B virus infection, chronic
Hepatitis B virus infection, perinatal acute
Hepatitis C virus infection, chronic or resolved
Hepatitis C virus infection, acute
HIV infection, adult
HIV infection, pediatric
Influenza-associated pediatric mortality
Legionellosis
Listeriosis
Lyme disease
Malaria
Measles, total
Meningococcal disease
Mumps

Neurosyphilis
Pertussis
Plague
Poliomyelitis, paralytic
Powassan virus neuroinvasive disease
Powassan virus nonneuroinvasive disease
Psittacosis (Ornithosis)
Q fever
Rabies, animal
Rabies, human
Rocky Mountain spotted fever
Rubella
Rubella, congenital syndrome
Salmonellosis
Severe acute respiratory syndrome-associated coronavirus (SARS-CoV) disease
Shiga toxin-producing *Escherichia coli* (STEC)
Shigellosis
Smallpox
St. Louis encephalitis virus neuroinvasive disease
Streptococcus pneumoniae, drug-resistant
Syphilis, congenital syndrome
Syphilis, early latent
Syphilis, late latent
Syphilis, primary
Syphilis, secondary
Syphilis, total primary and secondary
Syphilis, latent, unknown duration
Tetanus
Toxic shock syndrome (other than streptococcal)
Trichinellosis
Tuberculosis
Tularemia
Typhoid fever
Vancomycin-intermediate *Staphylococcus aureus* (VISA)
Vancomycin-resistant *Staphylococcus aureus* (VRSA)
Varicella
West Nile virus neuroinvasive disease
West Nile virus nonneuroinvasive disease
Western equine encephalitits virus neuroinvasive disease
Western equine encephalitis virus nonneuroinvasive disease
Yellow fever

From the Centers for Disease Control and Prevention: Nationally notifiable infectious diseases—United States, 2004, 2006, available at http://www.cdc.gov/epo/dphsi/phs/infdis2006.htm.

The Centers for Disease Control and Prevention (CDC) and the Council of State and Territorial Epidemiologists have a policy that requires state health departments to report selected diseases to the CDC, **National Notifiable Disease Surveillance System (NNDSS)**. The data for nationally notifiable diseases from 50 states, the U.S. territories, New York City, and the District of Columbia are published weekly in the *Morbidity and Mortality Weekly Report (MMWR)*. Data collection about these diseases and revision of statistics are ongoing. Annual updated final reports are published in the CDC *Summary of Notifiable Diseases—United States* (Centers for Disease Control and Prevention, 2006b).

STATE NOTIFIABLE DISEASES

Requirements for reporting diseases are mandated by law or regulation. Although each state differs in the list of reportable diseases, the usefulness of the data depends on "uniformity, simplicity, and timeliness." Because state requirements differ, not all nationally notifiable diseases are legally mandated for reporting in a state. For legally reportable diseases, states compile disease incidence data (new cases) and transmit the data electronically, weekly, to the CDC through the National Electronic Telecommunications System for Surveillance (NETSS).

BRIEFLY NOTED

To determine which of the national notifiable diseases are reportable in your state, go to your state health department website.

TYPES OF SURVEILLANCE SYSTEMS

Informatics is essential to the mission of protecting the public's health. Surveillance systems are designed to assist public health professionals in the early detection of disease and event outbreaks in order to intervene and reduce the potential for morbidity or mortality, or to improve the public's health status (NEDSS Working Group, 2001; Wagner et al, 2001). Surveillance systems in use today are defined as *passive, active, sentinel,* and *special.*

PASSIVE SYSTEM

In the passive system, case reports are sent to local health departments by health care providers (i.e., physicians, nurses) or laboratory reports of disease occurrence are sent to the local health department. The case reports are summarized and forwarded to the state health department, national government, or organizations responsible for monitoring the problem, such as the CDC or an international organization such as the World Health Organization.

ACTIVE SYSTEM

In the active system, the nurse, as an employee of the health department, may begin a search for cases through contacts with local health providers and health care agencies. In this

---

Box 15-4	**Bioterrorism and Response Networks**

Integrating of training and response preparedness can be supported by the following networks:
- Health Alert Network
- Emergency Preparedness Information Exchange (EPIX)
- The Emerging Infections program
- Epidemiology and Laboratory Capacity program
- Assessment initiative
- Hazardous substances
- Emergency events surveillance
- Influenza surveillance
- Local metropolitan medical response systems

From the Centers for Disease Control and Prevention: Updated guidelines for evaluating public health surveillance systems: recommendations from the Guidelines Working Group, *MMWR Morbid Mortal Wkly Rep* 50(RR-13):1–35, 2001b.

---

system, the nurse names the disease and/or the event and gathers data about existing cases to try to determine the magnitude of the problem (how widespread it is).

SENTINEL SYSTEM

In the sentinel system, trends in commonly occurring diseases or key health indicators are monitored *(Healthy People 2010)*. A disease and/or an event may be the sentinel or a population may be the sentinel. In this system a sample of health providers or agencies is asked to report the problem. The system is useful because it helps monitor trends in commonly occurring diseases and/or events.

SPECIAL SYSTEMS

Special systems are developed for collecting particular types of data; these may be a combination of active, passive, and/or sentinel systems. As a result of bioterrorism, newer systems called **syndronic surveillance systems** are being developed to monitor illness syndromes or events. This approach requires the use of automated data systems to report continued (real time) or daily (near real time) disease outbreaks (Broome et al, 2004) (Box 15-4).

Although all of the systems are important, the nurse is most likely to use the active or passive systems. A passive system may involve the use of the state reportable disease system to complete a community assessment or MAPPS. The active system is used to investigate the possibility of food poisoning, for example, when several school children become ill after eating lunch in the school cafeteria or at the local hot dog stand, or to follow up the contacts of a newly diagnosed client with tuberculosis or a sexually transmitted disease (STD) (Underwood et al, 2003).

THE INVESTIGATION

INVESTIGATION OBJECTIVES

Any unusual increase in disease incidence (new cases) or an unusual event in the community should be investigated. The system used for investigation depends on the intensity

A study was conducted to identify pediatric age groups for influenza vaccination using a real-time regional surveillance system. Evidence has shown that vaccination of school-aged children significantly reduces the transmission of influenza. To explore the possibility of expanding the recommended target population for flu vaccination to include preschool-aged children, the researchers sought to determine which age groups within the pediatric population develop influenza the earliest and are most strongly linked with mortality in the population.

Using a real-time regional surveillance system, patient visits for respiratory illness were monitored in six Massachusetts health care settings. Data from a variety of health-monitoring systems were used: the Automated Epidemiologic Geotemporal Integrated Surveillance system, the National Bioterrorism Syndromic Surveillance Demonstration Project, and the Centers for Disease Control and Prevention U.S. Influenza Sentinel Providers Surveillance Network. Data were retrospectively identified and included patients seen between January 1, 2000 and September 30, 2004.

Study findings indicate that patient age significantly influences the timeliness of presenting at the health care facility with influenza symptoms ($p = 0.026$), with pediatric age groups arriving first ($p < 0.001$); children ages 3 to 4 years are consistently the earliest ($p = 0.0058$). Age also influences the degree of prediction of mortality ($p = 0.036$). Study findings support the strategy to vaccinate preschool-aged children. Furthermore, monitoring respiratory illness in the ambulatory care and pediatric emergency department populations using syndromic surveillance systems was shown to provide even earlier detection and better prediction of influenza activity than the current CDC's sentinel surveillance system.

NURSE USE: It is important to offer the flu vaccine to high-risk populations, such as young children, as recommended by the Centers for Disease Control and Prevention's Advisory Committee on Immunization Practices. Influenza vaccination is the primary method for preventing influenza and its severe complications.

From Brownstein JS, Kleinman KP, Mandl KD: Identifying pediatric age groups for influenza vaccination using a real-time regional surveillance system, *Am J Epidemiol* 162:686–693, 2005.

of the event, the severity of the disease, the number of people and/or communities affected, the potential for harm to the community or the spread of disease, and the effectiveness of available interventions (Sistrom and Hale, 2006). The objectives of an investigation are as follows:

- To control and prevent disease or death
- To identify factors that contribute to the outbreak of the disease and the occurrence of the event
- To implement measures to prevent occurrences

Defining the Magnitude of a Problem and/or an Event

The following definitions provide a way to describe the level of occurrence of a disease and/or an event for purposes of communicating the magnitude of the problem. A disease and/or an event that is found to be present (occurring) in a population is defined as **endemic** if there is a persistent

(usual) presence with a low to moderate number of cases of the disease and/or the event. The endemic levels of a disease and/or an event in a population provide the baseline for establishing a public health problem. For example, foodborne botulism is endemic to Alaska. The baseline must be known to determine the existence of a change or increase in the number of cases from the baseline. If a problem is considered **hyperendemic**, there is a persistently (usually) high number of cases. An example is the high cholera incidence rate among Asians/Pacific Islanders. **Sporadic** problems are those with an irregular pattern with occasional cases found at irregular intervals. **Epidemic** means that the occurrence of a disease within an area is clearly in excess of expected levels (endemic) for a given time period. This is often called the **outbreak**. **Pandemic** refers to the epidemic spread of the problem over several countries or continents (such as severe acute respiratory syndrome [SARS] outbreak). **Holoendemic** implies a highly prevalent problem found in a population that is commonly acquired early in life. The prevalence of this problem decreases as age increases (Chang et al, 2003). **Outbreak detection**, or identifying an increase in frequency of disease above the usual occurrence of the disease, is the function of the investigator (Broome et al, 2004).

PATTERNS OF OCCURRENCE

Patterns of occurrence can be identified when investigating a disease or event. These patterns are used to define the boundaries of a problem to help investigate possible causes or sources of the problem. A **common source outbreak** refers to a group exposed to a common noxious influence such as the release of noxious gases (for example, ricin in the Japanese subway system several years ago). In a **point source** outbreak all persons exposed become ill at the same time, during one incubation period. A **mixed outbreak** (which was described by Gotz et al, [2004] while investigating a foodborne gastroenteritis caused by a Norwalk-like virus) involves a common source followed by secondary exposures related to person-to-person contact, as in the spreading of influenza. **Intermittent or continuous source** cases may be exposed over a period of days or weeks, as in the recent food poisonings at a restaurant chain throughout the United States as a result of the restaurant's purchase of contaminated green onions. A **propagated outbreak** does not have a common source and spreads gradually from person to person over more than one incubation period, such as the spread of tuberculosis from one person to another.

BRIEFLY NOTED

In today's environment of tight budgets, how would nurses know which programs should be developed and continued without good data to indicate what are the most commonly occurring public health problems? How would we know if programs were effective without a source of valid and reliable ongoing data?

Box 15-5   Classification of Agents

- **Infectivity:** Refers to the capacity of an agent to enter a susceptible host and produce infection or disease
- **Pathogenicity:** Measures the proportion of infected people who develop the disease
- **Virulence:** Refers to the proportion of people with clinical disease who become severely ill or die

---

Box 15-6   Types of Agent Factors

1. Biological
   - Bacteria (e.g., tuberculosis, salmonellosis, streptococcal infections)
   - Viruses (e.g., hepatitis A, herpes)
   - Fungi (e.g., tinea capitis, blastomycosis)
   - Parasites (e.g., protozoa causing malaria, giardiasis; helminths [roundworms, pinworms]; arthropods [mosquitoes, ticks, flies, mites])
2. Physical
   - Heat
   - Trauma
3. Chemical
   - Pollutants
   - Medications/drugs
4. Nutrients
   - Absence
   - Excess
5. Psychological
   - Stress
   - Isolation
   - Social support

Box 15-7   Epidemiologic Clues That May Signal a Covert Bioterrorism Attack

- Large number of ill persons with a similar disease or syndrome
- Large number of unexplained disease, syndrome, or deaths
- Unusual illness in a population
- Higher morbidity and mortality than expected with a common disease or syndrome
- Failure of a common disease to respond to usual therapy
- Single case of the disease caused by an uncommon agent
- Multiple unusual or unexplained disease entities coexisting in the same person without any other explanation
- Disease with an unusual geographic or seasonal distribution
- Multiple atypical presentations of disease agents
- Similar genetic type among agents isolated from temporally or spatially distinct sources
- Unusual, atypical, genetically engineered, or antiquated strain of agent
- Endemic disease with an unexplained increase in incidence
- Simultaneous clusters of similar illness in noncontiguous areas, domestic or foreign
- Atypical aerosol, food, or water transmission
- Ill people presenting at about the same time
- Deaths or illness among animals that precedes or accompanies illness or death in humans
- No illness in people not exposed to common ventilation systems, but illness among those people in proximity to the systems

---

HOW TO   Conduct an Investigation

- Confirm the existence of an outbreak.
- Verify the diagnosis and/or define a case.
- Estimate the number of cases.
- Orient the data collected to person, place, and time.
- Develop and evaluate a hypothesis.
- Institute control measures and communicate findings.

Excerpted from Centers for Disease Control and Prevention: Summary of notifiable diseases—United States, 2004, *MMWR Morbid Mortal Wkly Rep* 53:1–5, 2006c.

Causal Factors from the Epidemiologic Triangle

Factors that must be considered as causes of outbreak are categorized as agents, hosts, and environmental factors (see Chapter 9). The belief is that these factors may interact to cause the outbreak and therefore the potential interactions must be examined. Box 15-5 presents definitions used to classify agents in an attack. Box 15-6 lists the type of agent factors that may be present. The host factors associated with cases may be age, sex, race, socioeconomic status, genetics, and lifestyle choices (for example, cigarette smoking, sexual practices, contraception, eating habits). The environmental factors that may be related to a case are physical (for example, weather, temperature, humidity, physical surroundings) or biological (such as insects that transmit the agent). Some of the socioeconomic factors that might affect the development of a disease and/or an event are behavior (could be terrorist behaviors), personality, cultural characteristics of the group, crowding, sanitation, and the availability of health services.

WHEN TO INVESTIGATE

An unusual increase in disease incidence should be investigated. The amount of effort that goes into an investigation depends on the severity or magnitude of the problem, the numbers in the population who are affected, the potential for spreading the disease, and the availability and effectiveness of intervention measures to resolve the problems. Most of the outbreaks of diseases (or increased incidence rates) occur naturally and/or are predictable when compared with the consistent patterns of previous outbreaks of a disease, such as influenza, tuberculosis, or common infectious diseases. When a disease and/or an event outbreak occurs as a result of the purposeful introduction of an agent into the population, then the predictable patterns may not exist. Treadwell et al (2003) provide clues to be used when trying to determine the existence of bioterrorism. These clues are simplified and appear in Box 15-7 (U.S. Department of Health and Human Services, 2001).

The "How To" box provides a brief guide to conducting the investigation.

PRIMARY PREVENTION

Develop a community security plan to reduce the potential for a terrorist attack.

SECONDARY PREVENTION

Investigate an outbreak of food poisoning in a local community.

TERTIARY PREVENTION

Provide health care and treatment for those infected by SARS.

INTERVENTIONS AND PROTECTION

Remember that disease and event surveillance systems exist to help improve the health of the public through the systematic and ongoing collection, distribution, and use of health-related data. A nurse can contribute to such systems and best use the data collected through such systems to help manage endemic health problems and those that are emerging, such as evolving infectious diseases and bioterrorist (human-made) health problems. The functions of surveillance and investigation include detecting cases, estimating the impact of disease or injury, showing the national history of a health condition, determining the distribution and spread of illness, generating hypotheses, evaluating prevention and control measures, and facilitating planning (Broome et al, 2004). Response to bioterrorism or to a large-scale infectious disease outbreak may require the use of emergency public health measures such as quarantine, isolation, closing public places, seizing property, mandatory vaccination, travel restrictions, and disposal of the deceased. Suggestions for protecting health care providers from exposure include the use of standard precautions when coming in contact with broken skin or body fluids, the use of disposable nonsterile gowns and gloves followed by adequate handwashing after removal, and the use of a face shield (U.S. Department of Health and Human Services, 2001).

CLINICAL APPLICATION

As a clinical project the health department asked the public health nursing class at the university to develop a community service message to air on local radio about the potential of a pandemic flu.
What does the message need to contain to help the community prepare?
Answer is in the back of the book.

REMEMBER THIS!

• Disease surveillance has been a part of public health protection since the 1200s during the investigations of the bubonic plague in Europe.
• Surveillance provides a means for nurses to monitor disease trends in order to reduce morbidity and mortality and to improve health.

• Surveillance is a critical role function for nurses practicing in the community.
• Surveillance is important because it generates knowledge of a disease or event outbreak patterns.
• Surveillance focuses on the collection of process and outcome data.
• Although surveillance was initially devoted to monitoring and reducing the spread of infectious diseases, it is now used to monitor and reduce chronic diseases and injuries as well as environmental and occupational exposures.
• Surveillance activities can be related to the core functions of public health assessment, policy development, and assurance.
• A quality surveillance system requires collaboration among a number of agencies and individuals.
• The Minnesota Model of Public Health Interventions: Applications for Public Health Nursing Practice (2001) suggests that surveillance is one of the interventions related to public health nursing practice.
• Clinicians, health care agencies, and laboratories report cases to state health departments. Data also come from death certificates and administrative data such as discharge reports and billing records.
• Each of the data sources has the potential for underreporting or incomplete reporting. However, if there is consistency in the use of surveillance methods, the data collected will show trends in events or disease patterns that may indicate a change needed in a program or a needed prevention intervention to reduce morbidity or mortality.
• The sentinel surveillance system provides for the monitoring of key health events when information is not otherwise available or in vulnerable populations to calculate or estimate disease morbidity.
• Reporting of disease data by health care providers, laboratories, and public health workers to state and local health departments is essential if trends are to be accurately monitored.
• Requirements for reporting diseases are mandated by law or regulation.
• Surveillance systems in use today are defined as passive, active, sentinel, and special.
• Any unusual increase in disease incidence (new cases) or an unusual event in the community should be investigated.
• Patterns of occurrence can be identified when investigating a disease or event. These patterns are used to define the boundaries of a problem to help investigate possible causes or sources of the problem.
• Factors that must be considered as causes of outbreak are categorized as agents, hosts, and environmental factors.
• An unusual increase in disease incidence should be investigated.
• Functions of surveillance and investigation include detecting cases, estimating the impact of disease or injury, showing the national history of a health condition, determining the distribution and spread of illness, generating hypotheses, evaluating prevention and control measures, and facilitating planning.

WHAT WOULD YOU DO?

1. Call the local health department and attend an emergency response team planning meeting. How many agencies are involved? Determine the roles of each agency. Does the nurse have a role on the team? Explain.
2. Go to the Health Hazard Evaluation program website (see WebLinks on the book's website). What is the purpose of this program? How would information from the website be used in a disease investigation?

■ REFERENCES

Broome CV et al: *Framework for evaluating public health surveillance systems for early detection of outbreaks,* CDC Evaluation Working Group on Syndromic Surveillance Systems, 2004.

Brownstein JS, Kleinman KP, Mandl KD: Identifying pediatric age groups for influenza vaccination using a real-time regional surveillance system, *Am J Epidemiol* 162:686–693, 2005.

Cabinet for Human Resources: Surveillance system, 2004, available at http://www.chs.ky.gov/publichealthreportablediseases2002-sum.html.

Center for Public Health Nursing, Office of Public Health Practice: The Minnesota model of public health inter ventions: applications for public health nursing practice, St Paul, Minn, 2001, Minnesota Department of Health.

Centers for Disease Control and Prevention: Update of anthrax associated with intentional exposure and interim public health guidelines, *MMWR Morbid Mortal Wkly Rep* 50(RR-41):889, 2001a.

Centers for Disease Control and Prevention: Updated guidelines for evaluating public health surveillance systems: recommendations from the Guidelines Working Group, *MMWR Morbid Mortal Wkly Rep* 50(RR-13):1–35, 2001b.

Centers for Disease Control and Prevention: Sentinel surveillance method. In *Drug-resistant Streptococcus pneumoniae surveillance manual,* 2003, available at http://www.cdc.gov/drspsurveillancetoolkit/docs/SENTINELMETHOD.pdf.

Centers for Disease Control and Prevention: *Overview of public health surveillance,* 2004, available at http://www.cdc.gov/epo/dphsi/phs/files/overview.ppt.

Centers for Disease Control and Prevention: *An overview of the national electronic disease surveillance system (NEDSS) initiative,* 2006a. Retrieved Sept 2006 from http://www.cdc.gov/nedss/About/overview.html.

Centers for Disease Control and Prevention: *Nationally notifiable infectious diseases—United States,* 2006, 2006b, available at http://www.cdc.gov/epo/dphsi/phs/infdis2006.htm.

Centers for Disease Control and Prevention: Summary of notifiable diseases—United States, 2004, *MMWR Morbid Mortal Wkly Rep* 53:1–5, 2006c.

Chang M et al: Endemic, notifiable bioterrorism-related diseases, United States, 1992-1999, *Emerg Infect Dis* 9:556–564, 2003.

Ching P: *Analysis, reporting and feedback of surveillance data,* Atlanta, Ga, 2002, Centers for Disease Control and Prevention, available at http://www.pitt.edu/~super1/lecture/cdc0271/001.htm.

Gebbie K, Rosenstock L, Hernandez L, editors: *Who will keep the public healthy?* Washington, DC, 2003, Institute of Medicine.

Gotz H et al: Epidemiological investigation of foodborne gastroenteritis outbreak caused by Norwalk-like virus in 30 day care centers, *Scand Infect Dis* 34:115–121, 2002.

NEDSS Working Group: A standards-based approach to connect public health and clinical medicine, *J Public Health Manag Pract* 76:43–50, 2001.

Pryor ER, Veenema TB: Surveillance systems for bioterrorism. In Veenema TG, editor: *Disaster nursing and emergency preparedness for chemical, biological, and radiological terrorism and other hazards,* NY, 2003, Springer, pp 331–353.

Quad Council of Public Health Nursing Organizations: *Core competencies for public health professionals,* 2000, Council on Linkages Between Academic and Public Health Practice, 2003.

Sistrom M, Hale P: Outbreak investigations: community participation and role of community and public health nurses, *Public Health Nurs* 23:256–263, 2006.

Teutsch SM, Churchill RE: *Principles and practices of public health surveillance,* New York, 2004, Oxford University Press.

Treadwell TA et al: Epidemiologic clues to bioterrorism, *Pub health rep* 118:92–98, 2003.

Underwood B et al: Contact tracing and population screening for tuberculosis—who should be assessed? *J Public Health Med* 25:59–61, 2003.

U.S. Department of Health and Human Services: *Healthy People 2010 objectives,* Washington, DC, 2000, U.S. Department of Health and Human Services.

U.S. Department of Health and Human Services: *The public response to biological and chemical terrorism,* Centers for Disease Control and Prevention, 2001. Retrieved Feb 20, 2007, from http://www.bt.cdc.gov/Documents/Planning/PlanningGuidance.pdf.

Wagner M et al: The emergency science of very early detection of disease outbreaks, *J Public Health Manag Pract* 7:51–59, 2001.

evolve http://evolve.elsevier.com/stanhope/foundations

Program Management

Marcia Stanhope
Doris Glick

ADDITIONAL RESOURCES

These related resources are found either in the appendix at the back of this book or on the book's website at http://evolve.elsevier.com/stanhope/foundations.

Evolve Website

- Community Assessment Applied
- Case Study, with questions and answers

- Quiz review questions
- WebLinks, including link to *Healthy People 2010* website

OBJECTIVES

After reading this chapter, the student should be able to:

1. Compare the program management process with the nursing process.
2. Describe the program planning process and its application to nursing in the community.
3. Identify the benefits of program planning.
4. Describe the components of program evaluation and application to nursing practice.
5. Identify an evaluation method.
6. Name the program evaluation sources.
7. Describe the types of program evaluation measures.

CHAPTER OUTLINE

DEFINITIONS AND GOALS

BENEFITS OF PROGRAM PLANNING

PLANNING PROCESS
Basic Program Planning
Program Planning Models for Public Health

PROGRAM EVALUATION
Benefits of Program Evaluation
Evaluation Process
Formulation of Objectives
Sources of Program Evaluation
Aspects of Program Evaluation

KEY TERMS

case registers: systematic registration of acute, chronic, and contagious diseases.

community health index: a summary of the health features of a community that enables us to determine health care delivery needs.

evaluation: provision of information through formal means, such as criteria, measurement, and statistics, for making rational judgments about outcomes of care.

evaluation of program effectiveness: examination of the level of client and provider satisfaction with a program.

formative evaluation: an ongoing evaluation instituted for the purpose of assessing the degree to which objectives are met or activities are being conducted.

health program planning: five-step process of formulating a plan, conceptualizing, detailing, evaluating, and implementing.

needs assessment: systematic appraisal of type, depth, and scope of problems as perceived by clients, health providers, or both.

outcome: a change in client health status as a result of care or program implementation.

planning process: a systematic approach to selecting and carrying out a series of actions to achieve a goal.

program: a health care service designed to meet identified health care needs of clients.

program evaluation: collection of methods, skills, and activities necessary to determine whether a service is needed, likely to be used, conducted as planned, and actually helps people.

strategic planning: a process by which client needs, specific provider strengths, and agency and community resources are successfully matched to offer a service to the community.

summative evaluation: a method used to assess program outcomes or as a follow-up of the results of program activities.

Program management consists of assessing, planning, implementing, and evaluating a program. This chapter focuses primarily on planning and evaluation. Although presented in separate discussions, these factors are related and dependent processes that work together to bring about a successful program. This chapter does not deal with implementing programs, because the majority of the chapters in this book focus on implementation.

The program management process is like the nursing process. One is applied to a program, whereas the other is applied to clients. The process of program management, like the nursing process, consists of a rational decision-making system designed to help nurses determine the following:

• When to make a decision to develop a program
• Where they want to be at the end of the program
• How to decide what to do to have a successful program
• How to develop a plan to go from where they are to where they want to be
• How to know that they are getting there
• What to measure to know whether what they are doing is appropriate

Today, more emphasis is on accountability for nursing actions and client outcomes. The introduction of prospective payment systems, health care reform, managed care, and the new Medicare pay for performance system introduced in 2008 has changed the focus of nursing (Rosenthal, 2007). Planning for nursing care delivery is necessary today if the nurse is to survive in the field of health care delivery. This chapter examines how nurses can *act* instead of *react* by planning programs that can be evaluated for their effectiveness. These programs may be single health-promotion programs for a client group or an ongoing program to provide health care services to a client group.

DEFINITIONS AND GOALS

A **program** is an organized approach to meet the assessed needs of individuals, families, groups, or communities by reducing or eliminating one or more health problems. The following are examples of specific programs in nursing in the community:

• Immunization programs
• Health-risk screening programs for industrial workers
• Family-planning programs

Box 16-1 Two Levels of Evaluation

• *Formative evaluation:* evaluation for the purpose of assessing whether objectives are met or planned activities are completed. This type of evaluation begins with an assessment of the need for a program and is on-going as the program is implemented.
• *Summative evaluation:* evaluation to assess program outcomes or as a follow-up of the results of the program activities and usually occurs when a program is completed or at a specific point in time (e.g., at the end of 1 year or 5 years).

The following are more broadly based group and community programs:

• Community school health programs
• Home health programs
• Occupational health and safety programs
• Environmental health programs
• Community programs directed at specific illnesses through special interest groups (e.g., American Heart Association, American Cancer Society, March of Dimes)

Planning process is defined as the selecting and carrying out of a series of actions to achieve stated goals (Issel, 2004). The goal of planning is to ensure that health care services are acceptable, equal, efficient, and effective. **Evaluation** is defined as the methods used to determine whether a service is needed and likely to be used, whether it is conducted as planned, and whether it actually helps people in need (Posavac and Carey, 2000). The two levels of evaluation are defined in Box 16-1.

BENEFITS OF PROGRAM PLANNING

Systematic planning for meeting client needs does the following:

• Benefits clients, nurses, employing agencies, and the community
• Focuses attention on what the organization and health provider are attempting to do for clients
• Assists in identifying the resources and activities that are needed to meet the objectives of client services
• Reduces role ambiguity (uncertainty) by giving responsibility to specific providers to meet program objectives

- Reduces uncertainty within the program environment
- Increases the abilities of the provider and the agency to cope with the external environment
- Helps the provider and the agency anticipate events
- Allows for quality decision making and better control over the actual program results

Today this type of planning is referred to as **strategic planning** and involves matching client needs, provider strengths and competencies, and agency resources. Everyone involved with the program can anticipate the following:

- What will be needed to implement the program
- What will occur during implementation
- What the program outcomes will be

PLANNING PROCESS

Program planning is required by federal, state, and local governments; by charitable organizations; and by the employing agency. Planning programs and planning for the evaluation of programs are two very important activities, whether the program being planned is a national health insurance program such as Medicare, a state health care program such as early childhood developmental screening programs, a local program such as vision screening for elementary school children, or a health education program on diet and exercise for a group of obese clients. Regardless of the type of program, the planning process is the same.

BASIC PROGRAM PLANNING

Definition of Problem and Need

The initial and most critical step in **health program planning** is defining the problem and assessing client need. The target population, or client, to be served by any program must be identified and involved in designing the program to be developed. Program planners must verify that a current health problem exists and is being ignored or is being unsuccessfully treated in a client group. **Needs assessment** is defined as a systematic appraisal of type, depth, and scope of problems as perceived by clients, health providers, or both (Box 16-2).

Needs assessment includes the steps in Section A,1 of the "How To" box on p. 284. The client may be identified as a community or group, as families, or as individuals. The client should be defined by biological and psychosocial characteristics, by geographic location, and by the problems to be addressed. For example, in a community with

Box 16-2	**Stages Used in Assessing Client Need**

- *Preactive:* projecting a future need.
- *Reactive:* defining the problem based on past needs identified by the client or the agency.
- *Inactive:* defining the problem based on the existing health status of the population to be served.
- *Interactive:* describing the problem using past and present data to project future population needs.

a large number of preschool children who require immunizations to enter school, the client population may be described as all children between 4 and 6 years of age residing in Central County who have not had up-to-date immunizations. This example tells the reader who the client is, what the need is, what the population size is, and where they are located.

A health education program may be necessary to alert the population to the existing need. In the example of the need for immunization of preschool children, public service announcements on television and radio and in newspapers may be used to alert parents to laws requiring immunizations, to the problems of communicable diseases, and to which communicable diseases (e.g., smallpox) have been successfully eradicated by immunization programs. A good example of the use of media to alert the population to a potential health problem caused by terrorism is the 2001 alert about anthrax exposure and symptoms.

Local and national television and newspapers were used to encourage individuals, agencies, and communities to be on the alert for suspicious white powder substances, to indicate who to contact if such substances were identified, and to identify emergency procedures for anyone who may have been exposed.

BRIEFLY NOTED

The needs to be met for the client population must be identified by both the client and the health provider. If the client population does not recognize the need, the program will usually fail.

The size and location of a client population for a program involve more than counting the number of persons in the community who may be eligible for the program. More specifically, they involve defining the number of persons with the problem who are unserved by existing programs and the number of eligible persons who have and have not taken advantage of existing services. For example, consider again the community need for a preschool immunization program. In planning the program, the estimates of numbers of preschool children in the county may be obtained from census data or birth certificates. The nurse then must determine the number of children unserved and the number of children who have not used services for which they are eligible.

Boundaries for the client population are established by defining the size and location of the client population. The boundaries will stipulate who is included and who is excluded in the health program. If the immunization program were designed to serve only preschool children of low-income families, all other preschool children would be excluded.

What people think about the need for a program, or *program feasibility,* might differ among health providers, agency administrators, policymakers, and potential clients.

HOW TO | Develop a Program Plan

A. Describe the problem and need.
  1. Assess client need.
    a. Who is the client?
    b. What is the need to be met?
    c. How large is the client population to be served?
    d. Where are they located?
    e. Are there other programs addressing the same need? (describe)
    f. Why is the need not being met?
  2. Establish program boundaries.
    a. Who will be included in the program?
    b. Who will not be included? Why?
    c. What is the program goal?
  3. Program feasibility.
    a. Who agrees that the program is needed (administrators, providers, clients, funders)?
    b. Who does not agree?
  4. Resources (general).
    a. What personnel are needed? What personnel are available?
    b. What facilities are needed? What facilities are available?
    c. What equipment is needed? What equipment is available?
    d. Is money needed? Is money available?
    e. Are resources (printing, paper, medical supplies) being donated?
      (1) Type
      (2) Amount
  5. Tools used to assess need.
    a. Census data
    b. Key informants
    c. Community forums
    d. Existing program surveys
    e. Surveys of the client population
    f. Statistical indicators (e.g., morbidity/mortality data)
B. Name the problem.
  1. List the potential solutions to the problem.
  2. What are the risks of each solution?
  3. What are the consequences?
  4. What are the outcomes to be gained from the solutions?
  5. Draw a decision tree to show the problem-solving process used.
C. Identify objectives and activities for alternatives.
  1. What are the objectives for each solution to meet the program goal?
  2. What activities will be done to conduct each of the alternative solutions listed under B,1 and based on objectives?
  3. What are the differences in the resources needed for each of the alternative solutions?
  4. Which of the alternative solutions would be chosen if the resources described under A, 4 were the only resources available?
D. Evaluate problem solutions.
  1. Which of the alternative solutions is most acceptable to:
    a. The clients
    b. The agency administrator
    c. You
    d. The community
  2. Which of the alternative solutions appears to have the most benefits to:
    a. The clients
    b. The agency administrator
    c. You
    d. The community
  3. Based on costs, which alternative solution would be chosen by:
    a. The clients
    b. The agency administrator
    c. You
    d. The community
E. Choose the program solution.
  1. Based on the data collected, which of the solutions has been chosen?
  2. Why should the agency administrator approve your request? Give your rationale.
  3. When can the program begin? Give the specific date.

Collecting data on the opinions and attitudes of all persons directly or indirectly involved with the program's success is necessary to determine the program's feasibility, the need to redefine the problem, or the decision to develop a new program or expand an existing program. For example, policymakers in the 1970s decided that neighborhood health clinics were the answer to providing service for low-income residents. They discovered that their opinions were not the same as those of most health providers or clients who were not supportive of developing neighborhood clinics. The neighborhood health clinics failed because the clients would not use them. If the policymakers had explored the ideas of the clients when planning the program, they might have offered another type of service.

Before implementing a health program, *available resources* must be identified. Program resources include personnel, facilities, equipment, and financing. If any one of the four categories of resources is unavailable, the program is likely to be inadequate to meet the needs of the client population.

A number of *needs assessment tools* exist to assist the nurse in the needs assessment process. The major tools used for needs assessment, summarized in Table 16-1, are census data, key informants, community forums, surveys of existing community agencies with similar programs, surveys of residents of the community to be served (client population), and statistical indicators (Rossi, Lipsey, and Freeman, 2004) (see the "Evidence-Based Practice" box).

NAME THE PROBLEM. The need and demand for a program are determined by working with the client. This stage of planning creates options for solving the problem and considers several solutions. Each option for program solution is examined for its uncertainties (risks) and consequences, leading to a set of outcomes.

Table 16-1	**Summary of Needs Assessment Tools**		
Name	**Definition**	**Advantages**	**Disadvantages**
Community forum	Community, group, organization, open meeting	Low cost Learn perspectives of large number of persons	Limited data Limited expression of views Discourages the less powerful Becomes an arena to discuss political issues
Focus groups	Open discussion with small representative groups	Low cost Clients participate in identification of need Initiates community support for the program	Time consuming Allows focus on irrelevant or political issues
Key informant	Identify, select, and question knowledgeable leaders	Provides picture of services needed	Bias of leaders Community characteristics may be incorrectly perceived by informants
Indicators approach	Existing data used to determine the problem	Excellent data on problems and characteristics of client groups	Growth and change in population may make data outdated
Survey of existing agencies	Estimates of client populations via services used at similar community agencies	Easy method to estimate the size of the client group Know the extent of services offered in existing programs	All cases of need may not be reported Exaggeration of services may occur
Surveys	Measurement of total or sample client population by interview or questionnaire	Direct and accurate data on the client population and their problems	Expensive Technically demanding Need many interviews or observations Interviews may be biased

Considering alternative solutions to the problem, some will have more risks or uncertainties than others.

- The nurse must decide between the solution that involves more risk and the solution that is free of risk.
- A "do nothing" decision is always the decision with the least risk to the provider.
- When choosing a solution, the nurse looks at whether the desired outcome can be achieved.
- After careful consideration, the nurse rethinks the solutions.
- Information collected with the tool is used to develop these alternative solutions.
- Decision trees are useful graphic aids that will provide a picture of the solutions and the consequences and risks of each solution.

Figure 16-1 shows the process of using a decision tree.

In the immunization example, the best consequence would be for families to provide for immunizations. The value of this action to the parents, the odds that immunizations will be given if a formal clinic is not available, the cost to the parents versus the taxpayer, and the cost to the community must be considered. Costs to the community include a possible increased incidence of communicable disease or mortality and an increased need for more expensive services to treat the diseases if children are not immunized. If the parents provide the immunizations, costs to the taxpayer and to the community are low.

Identify Objectives and Activities for Alternatives
In this phase the nurse, with client input, considers the possibilities of solving a problem using one of the solutions identified. The nurse considers the costs, resources, and program

Evidence-Based Practice

Community assessment data will help social groups and government understand residents' needs. LexLinc and the University Research Center for Families and Children released results of the first County Self-Assessment, a demographic study of the community. Those involved with the study hope the findings will help local groups more accurately address the needs of the county.

The results are a tool to help community organizations, government, businesses, faith-based organizations, and neighborhood groups make more informed decisions. The survey has data about households, finances, health, crime, and other topics from more than 1500 families. The data show geographic areas with high-service and low-income characteristics.

In the county the average reported income is between $40,000 and $49,000, while the same figure for the targeted areas is $25,000 and $29,000. In nontargeted areas, 97% of those surveyed consider their neighborhood safe, compared with 79% in target sectors.

NURSE USE: The findings are helpful for agencies applying for grants to develop needed programs.

Excerpted from Meredith Kesner, staff writer: Community self-assessment: a demographic study of the community, *Lexington (Kentucky) Herald-Leader,* March 7, 2003, p. B3.

activities needed to choose one of the solutions. For each of the three proposed alternatives in Figure 16-1, the program planner must list activities that would need to be implemented to use each of the alternatives.

To illustrate, consider again the immunization scenario. Using the proposed solution of encouraging the parents to provide the immunizations (the best consequence), examples

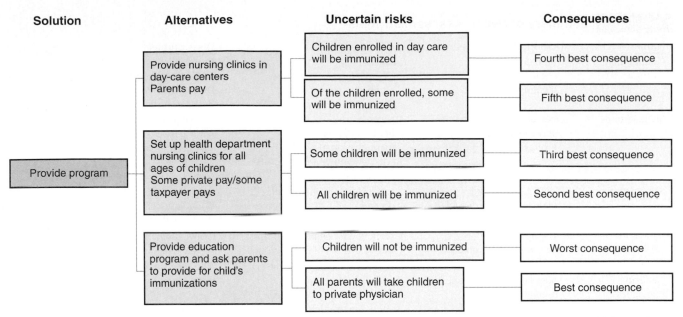

FIGURE 16-1 Ranking of solutions to the problem: providing a preschool immunization program to low-income children using a decision tree.

of activities include developing a script for a health education program and implementing a television program to encourage parents to take children to the physician. If the second, third, or fourth best consequence was chosen, offering a clinic 8 hours per day at the health department and providing a mobile clinic to each day care center for 4 hours each day to provide the immunizations would be possible activities.

For each alternative the nurse lists the resources needed to implement each activity. In the example, personnel could include nurses, volunteers, and clerks; supplies might include handouts, Band-Aids, medications, records, and consent forms; equipment might include syringes, needles, stethoscopes, and blood pressure cuffs; and facilities might include a television studio for a media blitz on the education program and a room with examination tables, chairs, and emergency carts. The costs of each solution must be considered by listing the costs of personnel, supplies, equipment, and facilities for each solution. As indicated, clients should review each solution for acceptance.

Evaluate Problem Solutions

In the evaluation phase of the plan, each alternative is weighed to judge the costs, benefits, and acceptance of the idea to the client, community, and nurse. The information outlined in Section C in the "How To" box on p. 284, would be used to rank the solutions for choice by client and nurse based on cost, benefit, and acceptance. The solution that will provide the desired outcomes must be considered. Looking at available information through literature reviews or interviews might suggest whether each of the options had been tried in

another place or by someone else. The results from other sources would be helpful in deciding whether a chosen solution would be useful.

Choose the Solution

Clients, nurses, and administrators select the best solution. Providing reasons why a particular solution was chosen will help the nurse obtain the approval of the administration for the plan. Involving clients and administrators throughout the planning process helps promote acceptance of the plan. Upon approval, the plan is implemented.

BRIEFLY NOTED

Nurses at all levels of education and preparation can participate in program planning and evaluation.

PROGRAM PLANNING MODELS FOR PUBLIC HEALTH

Program planning began as a public health effort to address health problems (Issel, 2004). The first plans were related to environmental planning for city, water, and sewer services (Rosen, 1958). Population-based program planning began with the need for mass immunizations, such as the program to administer the first polio vaccine. The following are the three models of program planning used in public health today (Box 16-3):

1. PATCH—Planning Approach to Community Health
2. APEXPH—Assessment Protocol for Excellence in Public Health
3. MAPP—Mobilizing for Action Through Planning and Partnership

---

Box 16-3	**Elements of Three Programming Planning Models**

PATCH (Planning Approach to Community Health)	APEXPH (Assessment Protocol for Excellence in Public Health)	MAPP (Mobilizing for Action Through Planning and Partnership)
1. Mobilize the community to act	1. Assess internal organizational capacity	1. Mobilize community members and organizations
2. Collect data	2. Assess priorities for health problems	2. Generate shared visions and common values
3. Choose health priorities	3. Set priorities for health problems	3. Develop a framework for long-range planning
4. Develop a comprehensive intervention plan	4. Implement the plan	4. Conduct needs assessments in four areas: Community strengths Local public health system Community health status Forces of change
5. Evaluate the process		5. Implement plan

From Issel LM: *Health program planning and evaluation,* Sudbury, Mass, 2004, Jones & Bartlett.
Websites: PATCH: www.cdc.org; APEX/MAPP: www.NACHO.org.
PATCH, Planning Approach to Community Health; *APEXPH,* Assessment Protocol for Excellence in Public Health; *MAPP,* Mobilizing for Action Through Planning and Partnership.

The PATCH Model of program planning was developed using Green's PRECEDE model of health education (Green and Krueter, 2005). The PATCH Model does the following (Issel, 2004):

- Considers health education a process that helps people to be more in control of their health
- Provides ways for people to be in control of their health
- Incorporates clients viewed as essential to planning success through the following:
  - Community participation
  - Use of data to develop a comprehensive health promotion strategy
  - Evaluation for improvement
  - Setting long-term goals on increasing community capacity

APEXPH addresses the three core competencies of public health: assessment, assurance, and policy development. This model provides a framework to assess the organization and management of health departments and to work with communities in assessing the health status of the community (Issel, 2004).

MAPP is the newer approach and is a strategic planning model that helps community health workers be facilitators as communities establish priorities in their public health issues and identify resources to address the issues (Issel, 2004).

PROGRAM EVALUATION

BENEFITS OF PROGRAM EVALUATION

The major benefit of **program evaluation** is that it reveals whether the program is meeting its purpose. It should answer the following questions:

- Are the needs for which the program was designed being met?
- Are the problems it was designed to solve being solved?

Quality assurance audits are prime examples of formative program evaluation in health care delivery (see Chapter 17). Evaluation data are used to justify continuing programs in community health. Program records—including client evaluations, community indexes, and **case registers**—serve as the major source of information for program evaluation. Surveys, interviews, observations, and diagnostic tests are ways to assess consumer and client responses to health programs. Planning for the evaluation process is an important part of program planning. When the planning process begins, program evaluation begins with the needs assessment (formative evaluation).

CASE STUDY

Jean Carpenter is the occupational nurse at the regional car factory. She noticed that many of the workers exhibit poor health habits, such as smoking and eating high-fat foods. Through talking with workers who visited the clinic, Ms. Carpenter learned that many of them wanted to take better care of themselves but believed they could not because of the long hours they worked and the high stress of their jobs. She decided to determine if poor health habits were a problem for everyone working in the factory or if they were common only to those who visited the nursing clinic.

Ms. Carpenter sent surveys to all 2000 employees at the factory and received responses from 40% of the employees. From the surveys, she learned that 30% of the workers worked 10 to 12 hours a day each week, 40% smoked one-half to two packs of cigarettes a day, and the most recent meal of 85% did not include any fruits or vegetables.

Ms. Carpenter went to the president of the car factory, shared this information with him, and discussed how poor health could decrease productivity. The president supported her suggestion to implement a health promotion program for the factory employees and offered to provide any space and office materials she needed for the program. Ms. Carpenter is now faced with developing a program plan so she can apply for grant money to fund any other supplies or personnel needed.

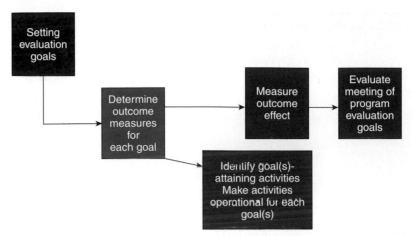

FIGURE 16-2 Using elements of the evaluation process. (From Rossi P, Lipsey M, Freeman H: *Evaluation: a systematic approach*, ed 7, Beverly Hills, Calif, 2004, Sage.)

EVALUATION PROCESS

The evaluation process presented by Rossi, Lipsey, and Freeman (2004) is explained in this section. It is similar to the following steps in the planning process:

1. *Goal setting.* The value and beliefs of the agency, the nurse, and the clients provide the basis for goal setting and should be considered at every step of the evaluation process. In the preschool immunization scenario, the fact that children should not be exposed to early childhood diseases would lead to a program goal to decrease the incidence of early childhood diseases in the county in which the program is planned.
2. *Determining outcome goal measurement.* In the case of the previous goal, disease incidence would be an appropriate goal measurement.
3. *Identifying goal-attaining activities.* This includes activities such as media presentations urging parents to have their children immunized.
4. *Making the activities operational.* This involves the actual administration of the immunizations.
5. *Measuring the goal effect.* Reviewing the records and summarizing the incidence of early childhood disease before and after the program is a measure of goal outcome effect.
6. *Evaluating the program.* This step determines whether the program goal was achieved.

Keep in mind that only one program goal is used in this example. Most programs have multiple goals (Figure 16-2).

FORMULATION OF OBJECTIVES

The *objectives* identified in the planning process set the stage for conducting the program and provide the method for evaluating the activities of the program. The following discussion helps in the development of clear, concise objectives.

Specifying Objectives (Goals)

If the objectives are too general, program evaluation becomes impossible. The objectives must be specific and stated so that anyone reading them could conduct the program without

further instruction. To be truly effective, the program plan should begin with a general program goal and move on to specific objectives that will help meet the program goal. Useful program objectives include the following:

- A statement of the specific behaviors
- Accomplishments
- Success criteria, or expected result, for the program
  Each program objective requires the following:
- A strong, action-oriented verb to specify the behavior
- A statement of a single purpose
- A statement of a single result (**outcome**)
- A time frame for achieving the expected outcome

In this continuing example, a program objective that meets these criteria may be as follows: to decrease (action verb) the incidence of early childhood disease in Center County (outcome) by providing immunization clinics in all schools (purpose) between August and December of 2012 (time frame).

As objectives are developed, an operational indicator for each objective should be considered so the evaluator knows when and if the objective has been met. For instance, an operational indicator for the previous objective would be a 10% to 25% decrease in the incidence rates of the most frequently occurring childhood vaccine-preventable illnesses in Center County. Such indicators provide a target for persons involved with program implementation. A review of *Healthy People 2010* objectives will give the reader examples of objectives that include all the elements just listed.

| Levels of Prevention | Related to Program Planning and Evaluation |

PRIMARY PREVENTION

Plan a community-wide program with the local government and health department to make all public businesses smoke-free to prevent exposure to secondhand smoke.

SECONDARY PREVENTION

Develop screening programs for all workers in businesses to determine the incidence and/or prevalence of respiratory illness, cardiovascular diseases, and lung cancer before implementing the program.

TERTIARY PREVENTION

Evaluate the incidence and/or prevalence of respiratory illness, cardiovascular disease, and lung cancer among nonsmoking workers after the implementation of the program, and provide programs to reduce complications from the diseases.

Levels of Program Objectives

It is customary for objectives to be stated in levels from general to specific. The first level consists of general and broad objectives that are sometimes called *goals.* Their purpose is to focus on the major reason for the program.

A general program objective (goal) may be to reduce the incidence of low-birthweight babies in Center County by 2012 by improving access to prenatal care. The specific objectives, or subgoals, describe the following:

- A measurable behavior
- The circumstances under which the behavior is observed
- The minimal acceptable standard for the performance of the behavior

A specific objective for this program may be to open a prenatal clinic in each health department within the county by January 2011 to serve the population within each census tract of the county. This specific objective is an action-oriented approach to meeting the goal.

Specific program activities are then planned to meet each specific objective, and resources, such as number of nurses, equipment, supplies, and location, are planned for each of the objectives. It is assumed that as each specific objective is met, the general program objective will also be achieved. Remember that several specific objectives are required to meet a general program objective or goal.

SOURCES OF PROGRAM EVALUATION

Major sources of information for program evaluation are program clients, program records, and community indicators. The program participants, or clients, of the service have a unique and valuable role in program evaluation. Whether the clients, for whom the program was designed, accept the services will determine to a large extent whether the program achieves its purpose. Thus their reactions, feelings, and judgments about the program are important to the evaluation.

To assess the response of participants in a program, the evaluator may use the following:
- Written survey in the form of a questionnaire
- Attitude scale
- Interviews
- Observations

Attitude scales are probably used most often, and they are usually phrased in terms of whether the program met its objectives. The client satisfaction survey is an example of an attitude scale often used in the health care delivery system to evaluate the program objectives.

The second major source of information for program evaluation is *program records,* especially clinical records. Clinical records provide the evaluator with information about the care given to the client and the results of that care. Whether a program goal has been met can be determined by summarizing the data from a group of records. For example, if one overall goal is to reduce the incidence of low-birthweight babies through prenatal care, records would be reviewed to obtain the number of mothers who received prenatal care and the number of low-birthweight babies born to them.

A third major source of evaluation is a **community health index**. Health and illness indicators, such as mortality and morbidity data, are probably cited more frequently than any other single index for program evaluation. Incidence and prevalence are valuable indexes used to measure program effectiveness and impact (see Chapter 9 for a further discussion of rates and ratios).

An example of a national program based on a needs assessment of the U.S. population is the national health objectives program called *Healthy People 2010* (U.S. Department of Health and Human Services, 2000). *Healthy People 2010* has two overall goals and 467 specific health objectives, which include an action verb, a result (outcome), and a time frame (10 years) (see Appendix A.1). Each health status objective reflects targets for specific improvements. Many of the objectives focus on interventions designed to reduce or eliminate illness, disability, and premature death among individuals and in communities. Others focus on broader issues such as improving access to quality health care, strengthening public health services, and improving the availability and dissemination of health-related information. The "Levels of Prevention" box shows application examples of program planning and evaluation.

ASPECTS OF PROGRAM EVALUATION

The aspects of program evaluation include the following (Veney and Kaluzny, 2005):
- *Evaluation of relevance:* the need for the program
- *Adequacy:* the program addresses the extent of the need
- *Progress:* tracking of program activities to meet the program objectives
- *Efficiency:* relationship between the program outcomes and the resources spent
- *Effectiveness:* the ability to meet the program objectives and the results of program efforts
- *Impact:* long-term changes in the client population

• *Sustainability:* enough resources (usually money) to continue the program

   See How To box for application of now to do a program evaluation.

BRIEFLY NOTED

Healthy People 2010, the national program to improve the health of all Americans in 10 years, used key informants, census data, statistical indicators, forums, and surveys of existing programs to establish the goals and objectives of the program.

Relevance

Evaluation of *relevance* is an important component of the initial planning phase. As money, providers, facilities, and supplies for delivering health care services are more closely monitored, the needs assessment done by the nurse will determine whether the program is needed.

Adequacy

Evaluation of adequacy looks at the extent to which the program addresses the entire problem defined in the needs assessment. The magnitude of the problem is

---

HOW TO   Do a Program Evaluation

To do a program evaluation, first choose the type of evaluation you wish to do. Second, identify the goal and objectives for evaluation. Third, decide who will be involved in the evaluation. Fourth, answer the questions related to the type of evaluation as follows:

A. Program relevance: needs assessment (formative)
  1. Use answers to all questions listed in Section B of "How To Develop a Program Plan," p. 284.
  2. On the basis of the needs assessment, was the program necessary?

B. Adequacy
  1. Is the program large enough to make a positive difference in the problem and/or need?
  2. Are the boundaries of the services defined so that the problem and/or need can be addressed for the target population?

C. Program progress (formative)
  1. Monitor activities (circle which this reflects: daily, weekly, monthly, annually)
    a. Name the activities provided.
    b. How many hours of service were provided?
    c. How many clients have been served?
    d. How many providers?
    e. What types of clients have been served?
    f. What types of providers were needed?
    g. Where have services been offered (home, clinic, organization)?
    h. How many referrals have been made to community sources?
    i. Which sources have been used to provide support services?
  2. Budget
    a. How much money has been spent to carry out the activities?
    b. Will more or less money be needed to conduct activities as outlined?
    c. Will changes to objectives and activities be needed to keep the program going?
    d. What changes do you recommend and why?

D. Program efficiency (formative and summative)
  1. Costs
    a. How do costs of the program compare with those of a similar program to meet the same goal?
    b. Do the activities outlined in Section C,1 compare with the activities in a similar program?
    c. Although this program costs more/less than expected, is it needed? Why?

2. Productivity (may use national or state averages for comparison)
    a. How many clients does each type of staff see per day (public health nurses, nurses in community health, nurse practitioners)?
    b. How does this compare with similar programs?
    c. Although the productivity level of this program is low/high, is the program needed? Why?
3. Benefits
    a. What are the benefits of the program to the clients served?
    b. What are the benefits to the community?
    c. Are the benefits important enough to continue the program? Why? (Look at cost, productivity, and outcomes of care.)

E. Program effectiveness (summative)
  1. Satisfaction
    a. Is the client satisfied with the program as designed?
    b. Are the providers satisfied with the program outcomes?
    c. Is the community satisfied with the program outcomes?
  2. Goals
    a. Did the program meet its stated goal?
    b. Are the client needs being met?
    c. Was the problem solved for which the program was designed?

F. Impact (summative)
  1. Long-term changes in health status (1 year or more)
    a. Have there been changes in the community's health?
    b. What are the changes seen (e.g., in morbidity or mortality rates, teen pregnancy rates, pregnancy outcomes)?
    c. Have there been changes in individuals' health status?
    d. What are the changes seen?
    e. Has the initial problem been solved or has it returned?
    f. Is new or revised programming needed? Why?
    g. Should the program be discontinued? Why?

G. Sustainability
  1. Was the program funded as a demonstration or by an external agency?
  2. Can money and resources be found to continue the program after the initial funding is gone?

Depending on the answers to the questions, the program can be found to be successful or not.

Developed by Marcia Stanhope using the framework in Veney A, Kaluzny J: *Evaluation and decision making for health services,* Knoxville, Ill, 2005, Beard.

determined by vital statistics, incidence, prevalence, and expert opinion.

Progress

The monitoring of program activities—such as hours of services, number of providers used, number of referrals made, and amount of money spent to meet the program objectives—provides an evaluation of the *progress* of the program. This type of evaluation is an example of **formative evaluation** and occurs on an ongoing basis while the program exists. *Progress evaluation* occurs primarily while implementing the program. The nurse who completes a daily or weekly log of clinical activities (e.g., number of clients seen in the clinic or visited at home, number of phone contacts, number of referrals made, number of community health-promotion activities) is contributing to progress evaluation of the nursing service.

Efficiency

If the reason for the evaluation is to examine the *efficiency* of a program, it may occur on an ongoing basis as a formative evaluation or at the end of the program as a **summative evaluation** that looks at the end result of the program. The evaluator may be able to determine whether the program provides better benefits at a lower cost than a similar program or whether the benefits to the clients or number of clients served justify the costs of the program.

Effectiveness and Impact

An **evaluation of program effectiveness** may help the nurse determine both client and provider satisfaction with the program activities, as well as whether the program met its stated objectives. However, if the evaluation of *impact* is the goal, long-term effects such as changes in morbidity and mortality must be investigated. Both effectiveness and impact evaluations are usually summative evaluation functions primarily performed as end-of-program activities.

Sustainability

A program can be continued if there are resources for the program. Ongoing evaluation of sustainability is important!

BRIEFLY NOTED

The combination of prenatal care programs delivered by nurses and the Women, Infants, and Children (WIC) supplemental nutritional program produces better pregnancy and postnatal outcomes for mothers and babies than does traditional medical care.

CLINICAL APPLICATION

The following is a real-life example of the application of the program management process by an undergraduate nursing student. This activity resulted in the development and implementation of a nurse-managed clinic for the homeless.

This example shows how students as well as providers can make a difference in health care delivery. It also shows that no mystery surrounds the program management process.

Eva was listening to the radio one Sunday afternoon and heard an announcement about the opening of a soup kitchen within the community for the growing homeless population. She was beginning her nursing course in community health and wanted to find a creative clinical experience that would benefit her as well as others. The announcement gave her an idea. Although it mentioned food, clothing, shelter, and social services, nothing was said about health care.

Eva was interested in finding a way to provide nursing and health care services at the soup kitchen. Which of the following should she do?

A. *Talk with key leaders to determine their interest in her idea.*

B. *Review the literature to find out the magnitude of the problem.*

C. *Survey the community to find out if others were providing services.*

D. *Discuss the idea with members of the homeless population.*

E. *Consider potential solutions to the health care problems.*

F. *Consider where she would get the resources to open a clinic.*

G. *Talk with church leaders and nurse faculty members to seek acceptance for her idea.*

Answer is in the back of the book.

REMEMBER THIS!

- Planning and evaluation are essential elements of program management and vital to the survival of the nursing discipline in health care delivery.
- A program is an organized approach to meet the assessed needs of individuals, families, groups, or communities by reducing or eliminating one or more health problems.
- Planning is defined as selecting and carrying out a series of actions to achieve a stated goal.
- Evaluation is defined as the methods used to determine if a service is needed and will be used, whether a program to meet that need is carried out as planned, and whether the service actually helps the people it intended to help.
- To develop quality programs, planning should include four essential elements: problem diagnosis and assessment of need, identification of problem solutions, analysis and comparison of alternative methods, and selection of the best plan and planning methods.
- The initial and most critical step in planning and evaluating a health program is assessment of need.
- Some of the major tools used in needs assessment are census data, community forums, surveys of existing community agencies, surveys of community residents, and statistical indicators.
- The major benefit of program evaluation is to determine whether a program is fulfilling its stated goals.

- Quality assurance programs are prime examples of program evaluation.
- Plans for implementing and evaluating programs should be developed at the same time.
- Program records and community indices serve as major sources of information for program evaluation.
- Planning programs and planning for their evaluation are two of the most important ways in which nurses can ensure successful program implementation.
- The program management process, like the nursing process, is a rational decision-making process.
- Program planning helps nurses and agencies focus attention on services that clients need.
- Planning helps everyone involved understand their role in providing services to clients.
- The assessment of need process provides an evaluation of the relevance that a new service may have to clients.
- A decision tree is a useful tool to choose the best alternative for solving a problem.
- Setting goals and writing objectives to meet the goals are necessary to evaluate program outcomes.
- *Healthy People 2010* is an example of a national program based on needs assessment that has stated goals and objectives on which the program can be evaluated.

WHAT WOULD YOU DO?

1. Choose the definitions that best describe your idea of a program, planning, and evaluation.
2. Apply the program planning process to an identified clinical problem for a client group with whom you are working in the community:
   a. Assess the client need.
   b. Choose tools appropriate to the assessment of needs.
   c. Analyze the overall planning process of arriving at decisions about implementing the program.
   d. Summarize the benefits for program planning that apply to your situation.

3. Given the situation just described, choose three or four of your classmates to work with on the following projects:
   a. Plan for the evaluation of the program in activity 2.
   b. Apply the evaluation process to the situation.
   c. Name the measures you will use to gather data for evaluating your program.
   d. Name the sources you will tap to gain information for program evaluation.
   e. Analyze the benefits of program evaluation that apply to your situation.
   f. Talk with a nurse or administrator in community health about the application of program planning and evaluation processes at the local agency. Compare their answers with your readings.

■ REFERENCES

Green LW, Kreuter M: *Health promotion and planning: an education and ecological approach*, New York, 2005, McGraw-Hill.

Issel LM: *Health program planning and evaluation*, Sudbury, Mass, 2004, Jones & Bartlett.

Kesner M: *Community self-assessment: a demographic study of the community, Lexington (Kentucky) Herald-Leader*, March 7, 2003:B3.

Posavac EJ, Carey RG: *Program evaluation: methods and case studies*, Englewood Cliffs, NJ, 2000, Prentice Hall.

Rosen G: *A history of public health*, Baltimore, 1958, Johns Hopkins University.

Rosenthal M: Nonpayment for performance? Medicare's new reimbursement rule, *New Eng J Med* 16(357):1573-1575, 2007.

Rossi P, Lipsey M, Freeman H: *Evaluation: a systematic approach*, ed 7, Beverly Hills, Calif, 2004, Sage.

U.S. Department of Health and Human Services: *Healthy People 2010: national health promotion and disease prevention objectives*, Washington, DC, 2000, U.S. Department of Health and Human Services.

Veney J, Kaluzny A: *Evaluation and decision making for health services*, Frederick, Md, 2005, Beard.

Chapter 17

Managing Quality

Judith Lupo Wold

ADDITIONAL RESOURCES

These related resources are found either in the appendix at the back of this book or on the book's website at http://evolve.elsevier.com/stanhope/foundations.

Appendix

- Appendix H.3: Quad Council Public Health Nursing Core Competencies and Skill Levels

Evolve Website

- Community Assessment Applied
- Case Study, with questions and answers
- Quiz review questions
- WebLinks, including link to *Healthy People 2010* website

OBJECTIVES

After reading this chapter, the student should be able to:

1. Define quality assurance and explain its role in continuous quality improvement.
2. Discuss at least two general and two specific approaches to quality improvement and examine ways to use them in practice.
3. Plan a model quality assurance program.
4. Identify the purposes for the types of records kept in public health agencies.
5. Evaluate a method for documentation of client care in a community setting.

CHAPTER OUTLINE

HISTORICAL DEVELOPMENTS
QUALITY AND THE CURRENT HEALTH CARE SYSTEM
DEFINITIONS AND GOALS
What Is Quality?
How Does Quality Assurance Relate to Total Quality Management?
APPROACHES TO QUALITY IMPROVEMENT
General Approaches
Specific Approaches

MODEL QUALITY ASSURANCE PROGRAM
Structure
Process
Outcome
Evaluation, Interpretation, and Action
DOCUMENTATION
Records
Community Health Agency Records
Healthy People 2010 and Quality Health Care

KEY TERMS

accountability: being legally, morally, ethically, and socially answerable to someone for something you have done.

accreditation: a credentialing process used to recognize health care agencies or educational programs for provision of quality services and programs.

audit process: a six-step process used to recognize health care agencies or educational programs for provision of quality services and programs.

certification: a mechanism, usually by means of a written examination, that provides an indication of professional competence in a specialized area of practice.

charter: a mechanism by which a state governmental agency grants corporate status to institutions with or without rights to award degrees.

concurrent audit: a method of evaluating the quality of ongoing care through appraisal of the nursing process.

continuous quality improvement (CQI): an approach to managing quality that emphasizes continual improvement in real time, empowering employees to manage quality themselves, including client and family perceptions of quality, and making changes in organizational systems to enable workers to provide high-quality services.

credentialing: a mechanism to produce performance of acceptable quality by individuals or by programs of education and service.

customer: a consumer of products or services.

licensure: legal sanction to practice a profession after attaining the minimum degree of competence to ensure protection of public health and safety.

malpractice litigation: an approach to quality assurance imposed on the health care system by the legal system.

managed care: a health care financing mechanism designed to control costs by influencing the ways, type, and amount of care that clients receive.

outcome: a change in client health status as a result of care or program implementation.

process: the ongoing activities and behavior of health care providers engaged in conducting client care.

professional review organizations (PROs): organizations established by law to monitor the delivery of health care to clients of Medicare, Medicaid, and Maternal and Child Health programs and to monitor the implementation of prospective reimbursement.

quality: continuously striving for excellence while adhering to set specifications or guidelines.

quality assurance (QA): monitoring the activities of client care to determine the degree of excellence attained in the implementation of the activities.

retrospective audit: a method of evaluating the quality of care through appraisal of the nursing process after the client's discharge from the health care system.

risk management: designed to reduce the liability on the part of an agency or individual by assisting employees to act in accordance with set guidelines and procedures.

sentinel method: uses outcome measures to evaluate the quality of care; based on epidemiologic principles.

structure: the component in quality improvement that measures the setting and instruments used to provide care.

total quality management (TQM): an approach to managing the quality of care through appraisal of the nursing process after the client's discharge from the health care system.

tracer method: a way to evaluate the quality of care that measures both process and outcome.

utilization review: a review that is directed toward ensuring that care is actually needed and cost is appropriate for the level of care provided.

Although quality assurance has been a part of the health care arena for a number of years, it is only in the past few years that a major movement to improve health care quality has begun in the United States. The Institute of Medicine (IOM) (2001), not confident in the current health care systems' ability to deliver the quality of care expected, has set forth a series of recommendations to redesign current systems to meet Americans' expectations. Very little is known about the quality of care in this country for the following two reasons:

1. A variety of definitions of *quality* are used.
2. It is difficult to obtain comparable data from all providers and health care agencies.

In a changing health care market, the demand for quality has become a rallying point for health care consumers. All consumers, including private citizens, insurance companies, industry, and the federal government, are concerned about achieving the highest quality outcomes at the lowest possible cost (Wakefield and Wakefield, 2005). In addition to the demand for higher quality and lower cost, the public wants health care to be delivered with greater access and wants health care that is accountable, efficient, and effective.

Moreover, consumers want information about quality. Information is empowering to the consumer. With the expanded use of the Internet, access to information on the quality in health care is readily available on topics ranging from talking to consumers about quality health care (www.talkingquality.gov) to clinical practice guidelines that promise to improve care for all (www.guideline.gov). Total quality management and continuous quality improvement (TQM/CQI), a management style that includes quality assurance, or quality control, is one method used to ensure that the client is obtaining high-quality care at top value for the money spent. Although relatively new in health care, TQM/CQI has been tried and proven in industry.

Both consumers and providers have a vested interest in the quality of the health care system. According to Jonas (2002), the health care provider has three basic reasons to be concerned about health care quality:

1. The principle of nonmaleficence (above all, do no harm) has been a basic ethical principle of the health care system since the writing of the Hippocratic Oath.
2. The principle of beneficence (do good work) is a basic ethical principle of professionalism.

3. The strong social work ethic in the culture places a high value on "doing a good job" (see Chapter 4 for more discussion about ethics).

In health care, a direct link exists between doing a good job and individual and professional survival. Health care providers pride themselves on individual achievement and responsibility for good client outcomes (Kovner and Knickman, 2005). Health care organizations are natural extensions of health care providers and thus can demonstrate their responsibility for optimal outcomes through a rigorous quality improvement process. Leatherman and McCarthy (2002) state that the application of quality improvement strategies in the following six areas of performance could affect both the process and outcomes of health care (p. 12):

1. Consistently providing appropriate and effective care
2. Reducing unjustified geographic variation in care
3. Eliminating avoidable mistakes
4. Lowering access barriers
5. Improving responsiveness to patients
6. Eliminating racial, ethnic, gender, socioeconomic, and other disparities and inequalities in access and treatment

Although the Health Plan Employer Data and Information Set (HEDIS), a data-collection arm of the National Committee for Quality Assurance (NCQA), provides performance information, or report cards, for managed care organizations, no such single report card exists for public health agencies. As a part of a movement to provide quality health care in communities, health departments are examining their place in promoting this quality. McLaughlin and Kaluzny (2006) state that public health and CQI are connected because of the use of systems approaches that public health takes in identifying problems and developing interventions. Aspects of planning, implementing, and evaluating by TQM/CQI fall under each of the core public health functions of assessment, assurance, and policy development. It is, however, with the assurance core function, related to ensuring available access to the health care services that are essential to sustain and improve the health of the population, that TQM/CQI programs must be undertaken. Public health cannot ensure services that improve health if those services lack quality. Public health must maintain quality in its workforce and continually evaluate the effectiveness of its services whether the service is delivered to the individual, the community, or the population. Nurses in community practice are in a perfect position to implement strategies to improve community-oriented health care through the following:

• Community assessments
• Identifying high-risk individuals
• Targeting interventions, case management
• Managing illnesses across a continuum of care (Quad Council of Public Health Organizations, 2004)

These strategies have long been used by nurses. They are gaining attention because they are cost-effective; healthy consumers obviously use fewer health care resources than do sick people. Thus everyone—consumers, providers, and those who pay the health care bills—benefits if people stay healthy. An accepted public health principle of including the recipient of care in the planning of care is increasingly being used as consumers form partnerships in their communities by holding managed care organizations (MCOs) accountable for the quality of health outcomes and for their costs. Partnerships use data-based community assessments to improve health and to ensure that communities do receive quality services (Weisman, Grason, and Strobina, 2000). Consumers are no longer willing to have care just given to them. Instead, they want to be partners in deciding on their care.

In addition, competencies for public health leadership have been developed to ensure the quality and performance of the public health workforce (Wright et al, 2000). (See Appendix H.3 for a list of the competencies.) Records are maintained on all health care system clients to provide complete information about the client and to indicate the quality of care being given to the client within the system. Records are a necessary part of a CQI process, as are the tools and methods for evaluating quality.

HISTORICAL DEVELOPMENTS

Quality management began in nursing with the work of Florence Nightingale, who in 1860 designed a method to collect and present hospital statistics. Nightingale, in her efforts to improve hospital treatment, was also a pioneer in setting standards for nursing care. During the late 1800s, nursing schools were established in the United States. These schools set standards to upgrade nursing care. Licensure for nurses began in 1892, and the first nurse practice acts were established in 1903. By 1903 licensure of nurses was mandatory, and by 1923 all states had either permissive or mandatory laws directing nursing practice. After World War II, the nursing profession began establishing a scientific method of practice that led to the development of the nursing process. Evaluation of nursing activities was added to the assessment, planning, and implementation phases of the nursing process (Maibusch, 1984). The evaluative steps in the nursing process include quality assurance and quality improvement. Tools to measure quality assurance were developed in the 1950s.

In 1966 the American Nurses Association (ANA) created the Divisions on Practice, and in 1972 the Congress for Nursing Practice developed standards for quality assurance programs. In 1973 the Standards for Community Health Nursing Practice were developed. These standards were revised in 1986, in 1999, and in 2007. The name of the standards was also changed to *Public Health Nursing: Scope and Standards of Practice.*

In 1972 the Joint Commission on Accreditation of Hospitals (JCAH) included the responsibilities of nursing in its description of standards for nursing services. The JCAH called on the nursing industry to clearly plan, document, and evaluate nursing care. In the mid-1980s the JCAH became the Joint Commission on Accreditation of Healthcare Organizations (JCAHO) and began developing quality control standards for hospital and home health nursing. Now known simply as The Joint Commission, this organization currently incorporates continuous quality improvement principles in its standards.

Also in 1972 the Social Security Act (PL Law 92-603) was amended to establish the Professional Standards Review Organization (P the SRO) and to mandate the process for the review of the delivery of health care to clients of Medicare, Medicaid, and Maternal and Child Health programs. The PSRO program was modified later to become the **professional review organizations (PROs)** by the 1983 Social Security Amendments. PROs monitor the implementation of the prospective reimbursement system for Medicare clients. The use and effectiveness of PROs in a managed care environment have yet to be determined.

In response to a growing number of malpractice claims in the United States, the National Health Quality Improvement Act of 1986 was established. When funded in 1989, this Act had two major provisions: (1) it encouraged consumers to become informed about their practitioner's practice record, and (2) it created a national clearinghouse of information on provider malpractice records. The Act emphasized the structure rather than the process or outcome of care (National Association for Healthcare Quality, 1993; Dlugacz, Restifo, and Greenwood, 2004).

Efforts to strengthen community-oriented nursing practice have been carried out by several nursing organizations. These include the ANA, the Public Health Nursing Section of the American Public Health Association (APHA), the Association of State and Territorial Directors of Nursing (ASTDN), and the Association of Community Health Nursing Educators (ACHNE). These organizations are now called the *Quad Council.* The quality of nursing education is a major concern of the ACHNE, which was established in 1978. In 1993, 2000, and 2003 four reports published by this organization identified the curriculum content required to prepare nurses for practice in the community (Association of Community Health Nursing Educators, 1993, 2000a,b, 2003). In 2005 the Quad Council reviewed scopes and standards of population-focused (public health) and community-based nursing practice and developed new standards to guide the profession in obtaining the best health outcomes for the populations they served (American Nurses Association, 2007). Quality assurance/quality improvement (QA/QI) programs remain the enforcers of standards of care for many agencies that have not elected to engage in a program of CQI. These activities are called *assurance activities* because they make certain that those policies and procedures are followed so that appropriate quality services are delivered.

QUALITY AND THE CURRENT HEALTH CARE SYSTEM

In the past, it often was accepted that there would be some problems or complications with the production of things or the delivery of services. For example, it was not uncommon for agencies to have a certain number of charting or medication errors. Likewise, if 20 hospital beds were built, two might have errors in their production. What was important

was to keep the number of errors within a reasonable range; "good enough" care or products were tolerated.

Incentives in health care changed with the prospective payment system in 1984 that reimbursed for health care costs according to conditions listed in a standardized list of diagnosis-related groups (DRGs). Before 1984, health care providers were reimbursed on a fee-for-service basis, so the more service provided, the more money received. In contrast, prospective payment set up a fixed rate for payment for procedures and services. For example, removal of the tonsils was reimbursed at the same rate for Joey, who stayed in the hospital for 3 days after surgery because of a postsurgery infection, as it was for Billy, who left the morning after surgery. The amount and quality of services provided became much more important. Doing something only "good enough," if this resulted in complications, would cost more. Quality became important. Today, agencies are financially penalized for medical errors (Centers for Medicare and Medicaid Services, 2005).

Public expectations for good health care have grown. People want easy access to competent, kind, and cost-effective care. They want everything done that money can buy. However, costs keep growing, and in most countries, an unrestricted budget is not available for health care in either the public or private sector. Rather, **managed care** organizations emerged, and they were designed to deliver and monitor health care services within a set budget (Pushwaz, 2007). Likewise, to provide quality health care in communities, health departments are examining their place in promoting community-based health care quality through accreditation standards (National Public Health Performance Standards Program, CDC, 2008). These are not new strategies for nurses. Not only are consumers and providers concerned about the quality of care, but regulatory groups set standards for agencies and have increased their oversight of agency efficiencies.

BRIEFLY NOTED

Although managed care was expected to save money and improve the quality of health care in this country, neither of these expectations has occurred. In fact, for all the money spent on quality improvement, little is known about the quality of health care in America.

DEFINITIONS AND GOALS

WHAT IS QUALITY?

Quality is a hard term to define. To some extent, quality has to be defined in relation to the product and service under consideration. Also, quality is often determined differently by the provider than by the person receiving the product or service. **Quality** is defined by the client as the improvement in health status. It is defined by organizations and providers as accurate intervention, the clinical content of care, and the skill of the provider (Rowitz, 2001). The Institute of Medicine (2001) defines quality health care as "the degree to which health services for individuals and populations increase the likelihood of desired health outcomes and are consistent with current professional knowledge" (p. 1000). Problems with the quality of health care are divided into five groups: variations in services, overuse, underuse, misuse, and disparities in quality (Agency for Healthcare Research and Quality, 2002). The category of misuse is the focus of the IOM's push toward greater client safety. The category of underuse focuses on health disparities as defined in *Healthy People 2010*, and refers to conservative treatment; overuse involves the overordering of unnecessary interventions; disparities relate to differences in quality based on race and socioeconomic issues; and variations in service relate to geographic differences. The term *health services* applies to a wide range of health delivery institutions. Of particular interest to public health are the following:

- The question of access to appropriate and needed services
- A well-prepared workforce
- Improvement in the status of the population's health
- Client satisfaction and well-being
- The processes of client–provider interaction

HOW DOES QUALITY ASSURANCE RELATE TO TOTAL QUALITY MANAGEMENT?

Quality Assurance (QA) has two goals: (1) to ensure the delivery of quality client care, and (2) to demonstrate the efforts of the health care provider to deliver quality care (Jonas, 2002). **Continuous quality improvement (CQI)** builds upon traditional quality assurance by using the analysis methods of the scientific process to look at the work systems and processes of an organization. The "How To" box that follows lists differences between quality assurance and continuous quality improvement. Similarly, **total quality management (TQM)** is a structured, systematic process for planning within the organization. Traditional approaches to quality, such as those used in quality assurance, include the following (Sprague, 2001):

- Focus on assessing or measuring performance
- Ensure that performance conforms to standards
- Take action to bring about change when care does not meet standards

Many agencies now also include TQM strategies in their program of quality evaluation and improvement. It is a process-driven and customer-oriented philosophy of management that embodies the following outcomes (Sprague, 2001):

- Leadership
- Teamwork
- Employee empowerment
- Individual responsibility
- Continuous improvement of system processes that leads to improved outcomes

Customer satisfaction is important in TQM. For example, assume that women have to wait a long time in a Women, Infants, and Children's (WIC) program to be certified as eligible to receive support. Using CQI, all the steps in the appointment process are considered to determine where the

| HOW TO | Differentiate between Quality Assurance and Continuous Quality Improvement |

Quality Assurance	Continuous Quality Improvement
1. External determinants	1. Internal determinants
2. Detects errors	2. Determines requirements and deficiencies and expectations
3. Fixes blame and responsibility	3. Identifies process improvement opportunities
4. Post-event investigation	4. Prevention
5. QA department is responsible	5. All members in the organization are responsible
6. Inspires fear	6. Inspires hope

system's efficiency and effectiveness have stalled and why the women are waiting for a long time.

APPROACHES TO QUALITY IMPROVEMENT

Two basic approaches exist in quality improvement: general and specific. The general approach involves a large governing or official body's evaluation of the ability of a person or an agency to meet specific criteria or standards. General approaches include the licensure of a person or accreditation of a school. Specific quality improvement approaches try to determine whether the care given results in outcomes that are acceptable to the consumer.

GENERAL APPROACHES

General approaches to quality improvement seek to protect the public by ensuring a level of competency among health care professionals. Examples include credentialing, licensure, accreditation, certification, charter, recognition, and academic degrees. Whereas licensure is typically viewed as recognition that a person has met a minimal set of standards to practice his or her trade or profession, **credentialing** is defined as the formal recognition by which individuals or institutions are designated by a qualified agent as having met minimum standards of performance. Credentialing can be mandatory or voluntary. Mandatory credentialing requires statutory laws. State nurse practice acts are examples of mandatory credentialing. Licensing, certification, and accreditation are examples of credentialing, and certification examinations offered by a professional group are examples of voluntary credentialing.

Licensure is one of the oldest general quality assurance approaches. Individual licensure is a contract between the profession and the state whereby the profession is granted control over who can enter into and who exits from the profession. Licensure controls entry into a profession. Exit is generally punitive for some infraction. The licensing process requires that written regulations define the scope and limits of the professional's practice. Job descriptions based on these regulations set minimum and maximum limits on the functions and responsibilities of the practitioner. All 50 states have mandatory nurse licensure, and nurses take the same computerized examination in all 50 states to become licensed to practice nursing. A new approach to interstate practice requires a pact between states so that nurses can practice across state borders. Although reciprocity (which means nurses can have their license accepted through an application process if there is agreement among the states requiring application) exists among states for nursing licensure, interstate practice without approval is an issue for state boards of nursing (National Council of State Boards of Nursing, 2000).

BRIEFLY NOTED

Historically, licensure has protected the public by ensuring at least a beginning level of competence. Nurses are licensed by state government, even though all nurses take the same licensing examination. What do you think about allowing nurses to practice across state lines without registering in each state?

In contrast, **accreditation**, a voluntary approach to quality control, is used for institutions. Both the National League for Nursing (NLN) through the NLN Accrediting Agency and the American Association of Colleges of Nursing (AACN) through the Commission on Collegiate Nursing Education have established separate affiliates to accredit baccalaureate and higher degree nursing programs (Commission on Collegiate Nursing Education, 2008). The NLN also accredits diploma and associate degree programs. In addition, state boards of nursing accredit basic nursing education programs so that their graduates are eligible for the licensing examination.

Although supposedly voluntary, accreditation is considered to be quasi-voluntary, since it is often linked to governmental regulations that encourage programs to participate in the accrediting process to be reimbursed for services. For example, only accredited public health and home health agencies are eligible for reimbursement for Medicare clients. In accreditation, programs do a thorough review of their strengths and limitations in response to a set of criteria that they must address. The program is next reviewed by individuals who are familiar with similar programs; that is, the reviewers may work in comparable programs or agencies. Accreditation processes have evaluated an agency's physical structure, organizational structure, personnel qualifications, and the educational qualifications of its staff. However, beginning in 1990, more emphasis was placed on the evaluation of the outcomes of care and on the educational qualifications of the person providing the care.

Certification, another general and voluntary approach to quality, combines features of licensure and accreditation. Educational achievements, experience, and performance on an examination determine a person's qualifications for functioning in an identified specialty area, such as nursing in the community. The ANA, through its credentialing program, offers certification in several specialty areas. Other professional groups have established examinations to certify practitioners.

Like accreditation, certification can also be a quasi-voluntary process. For example, to function as a nurse practitioner in some states, it is necessary to show proof of educational credentials and take an examination to be "certified" to practice in that state. There are major concerns about certification as a quality assurance mechanism. Certification examinations measure competency by using a written test; however, limited clinical performance has been measured. Today several certification examinations provide for testing by clinical simulation (Commission on Nurse Certification, 2008). Although the nursing profession has recognized the certification process as a means of establishing minimal competence, professional organizations and nurses must communicate the importance of certified nurses to the public.

Charter, recognition, and academic degrees are other general approaches to quality assurance. **Charter** is the mechanism by which a state governmental agency grants corporate status to institutions with or without rights to award degrees (e.g., university-based nursing programs). Recognition is defined as a process whereby one agency accepts the credentialing status of and the credentials conferred by another agency. An example is when state boards of nursing accept nurse practitioner credentials that are awarded by the ANA or by one of the specialty credentialing agencies. A recent approach to recognition is the Magnet nursing services recognition given by the American Nurses Credentialing Center to agency nursing services that, after an extensive review, are considered excellent. This program began with reorganizations of excellent hospital nursing services. The Magnet program has expanded to include nursing home and home health agencies. Reapplication for Magnet status must occur every 4 years to ensure that Magnet organizations stay at the top of their games (American Nurses Credentialing Center, n.d.). Academic degrees are titles awarded by degree-granting institutions to individuals who have completed a predetermined program of studies.

SPECIFIC APPROACHES

Historically, QA programs conducted by health care agencies have measured the performance of individuals and their conformance to standards set forth by accrediting agencies. TQM and CQI are management philosophies and methods that incorporate many tools, including QA, to increase customer satisfaction with quality care (Table 17-1). The goal of TQM and CQI is to eliminate errors in the work process before negative outcomes occur rather than waiting until after the fact to correct individual performance; the focus is on problem prevention and continuous improvement.

According to the Agency for Healthcare Research and Quality (2001), quality health care means doing the right thing, at the right time, in the right way, for the right

Table 17-1	Traditional Management Model Compared with a Total Quality Management Model	

Traditional Management Model	Total Quality Management Model
Legal or professional authority	Collective or managerial responsibility
Specialized accountability	Process accountability
Administrative authority	Participation
Meeting standards	Meeting process and performance expectations
Longer planning horizon	Shorter planning horizon
Quality assurance	Continuous improvement

people—and having the best possible results. To the Institute of Medicine (Institute of Medicine, 2001, p. 3), quality health care is care that is:

- *Effective*—Providing services based on scientific knowledge to all who could benefit and refraining from providing services to those not likely to benefit
- *Safe*—Avoiding injuries to clients from the care that is intended to help them
- *Timely*—Reducing waits and sometimes harmful delays for both those who receive and those who give care
- *Client centered*—Providing care that is respectful of and responsive to individual client preferences, needs, and values and ensuring that client values guide all clinical decisions
- *Equitable*—Providing care that does not vary in quality because of personal characteristics such as gender, ethnicity, geographic location, and socioeconomic status
- *Efficient*—Avoiding waste, including waste of equipment, supplies, ideas, and energy

Total Quality Management/Continuous Quality Improvement (TQM/CQI) in Community and Public Health Settings

In health care, a major group of customers are patients. Health care agencies have only recently begun using TQM.

If an agency uses TQM, it must be focused on the **customer** (client) and everyone in the organization must be "committed to quality" (Rowitz, 2001). There are both internal and external customers. Internal customers are employees in other departments or work units, such as environmental health workers, statisticians, or physicians. External customers are those who pay for the service: regulators, accrediting bodies, clients, and families. The internal customer is often overlooked. Employees forget that their professional colleagues are often customers for their services. For example, nurses working in community settings are often customers of the agency's laboratories or data offices. It is easy to take co-workers for granted and forget that they deserve efficient, effective service just as do clients, families, and other service recipients. Several key determinants that can lead to customer satisfaction are listed in the "How To" box.

HOW TO	Ensure Customer Satisfaction with Services Provided

Tangibles
- Facility attractiveness
- Employee appearance
- Characteristics of other customers

Reliability
- Dependability
- Consistency of service delivery

Responsiveness
- Employee willingness
- Promptness in service delivery

Competence
- Employee knowledge

Understanding the Customer
- Effort to learn customer needs
- Individualized attention

Access
- Distance to facility
- Waiting time
- Hours of operation

Courtesy
- Staff politeness and mannerisms

Communication
- Ability of employees to explain the material in an understandable way
- Openness to questions

Credibility
- Trustworthiness of staff

Security
- Physical safety
- Confidentiality

Customer satisfaction for both internal and external users of services can be assessed through the use of focus groups (of clients or employees), surveys (written or telephone), and response cards. Personnel policies that are motivating and provide continuous training and learning opportunities are important parts of a quality improvement program. In quality improvement, people are not blamed for failures in the system and therefore are supported in their efforts to look for problems and seek ways to improve system performance.

Guidelines provided by the 1991 APHA *Model Standards* linked standards to meeting the health goals for the nation in the year 2000 (McLaughlin and Kaluzny, 2006). *Healthy People 2000* and APHA *Model Standards* (American Public Health Association, 1991) provided not only lists of priority health objectives for the nation and a way for public health to implement TQM/CQI but also the most current statistics and scientific knowledge about health promotion and disease prevention (Durch et al, 1997). Now *Healthy People in Healthy Communities* (U.S. Department of Health and Human Services [USDHHS], 2001) provides the objectives with their stated targets, measurement tools, and reflected intended performance expectations.

Healthy People 2010 builds on *Healthy People 2000* and contains modified and additional objectives for promoting health and preventing disease (U.S. Department of Health and Human Services, 2000). An important part of the framework of *Healthy People 2010* is eliminating health disparities and ensuring access to quality health care for all. Additionally, the *Planned Approach to Community Health* (PATCH) (Centers for Disease Control and Prevention [CDC], 1995); the Assessment Protocol for Excellence in Public Health (APEXPH), APEXPH in Practice (National Association of City and County Health Officials [NACCHO] 1995); and most recently the *Mobilizing for Action through Planning and Partnerships* (MAPP) process (National Association of City and County Health Officials, 2001) provide methods of assessing community needs to see how well health departments are operating to meet existing standards (see Chapter 16).

As health care reform continues, public health agencies face competition and are trying to reform themselves. A promising outcome of reform is the Community Health Improvement Process (CHIP) described by the Institute of Medicine (Durch et al, 1997) in their report *Improving Health in the Community: A Role for Performance Monitoring*. This report describes how private health care and public health can come together in a community-level effort to monitor performance and improve health.

Recognizing the many factors that cause health problems and the fragmenting that continues to exist in the health care system, this public–private collaborative framework involves many stakeholders, including public health, in monitoring the health of entire communities. Performance monitoring is defined as "a continuing community-based process of selecting indicators that can be used to measure the process and outcomes of an intervention strategy for health improvement (making the results available to the community as a whole) to inform assessments of an effective intervention and the contributions of accountable agencies to this" (Durch et al, 1997, p. 418).

Home health care agencies have increasingly adopted quality improvement programs because of the competition that exists. Congruent with the TQM/CQI philosophy, meeting customer expectations is essential for home health care agencies. Models for QA/QI in home health care have been developed to improve the quality of care in TQM/CQI frameworks, emphasizing processes, empowerment, collaboration, consumers, data and measurement, and standards and outcomes (Carmichael, 2005). Datasets of clinical information, such as those developed through the Omaha System and the National Association of Home Care (NAHC) (Clark et al, 2001; National Association of Home Care, 1998), are useful in measuring the quality of care. In 2003 the Home Health Care Quality Initiative (HHQI) was developed by the USDHHS to provide consumers with data on the quality of home health services. *Home Health Compare,* posted on the Medicare website, is a home health report card available to consumers nationwide (U.S. Department of Health and Human Services, n.d.).

Finally, in the area of standards and guidelines, Leatherman and McCarthy (2002) address six areas of performance that need improvement. One of these areas is consistently providing appropriate and effective care. This area is applicable to all health care practitioners including nurses. Evidence-based practice guidelines are one way to deliver consistent, up-to-date care and to improve outcomes for individuals, communities, and populations. In 2001, five Minnesota health plans, covering most of the state's insured population, endorsed standard treatment and prevention guidelines for 50 common diseases (Sprague, 2001). The use of guidelines helps gather data on the effectiveness and outcomes of nurse interventions (Keller et al, 2004a). The Agency for Healthcare Research and Quality (AHRQ), formerly the Agency for Healthcare Policy and Research (AHCPR), has played a major role in developing clinical practice guidelines.

Guidelines are protocols or statements of recommended practice developed by professional organizations; they are based on the distilling of scientific evidence and expert opinion that guide a clinician in decision making (Sprague, 2001). Guidelines provide research-based evidence for interventions and promote improved health outcomes. Using research findings as guidelines or frames of reference can improve nurses' awareness of new or better ways to practice, allow for documentation of nurse interventions, and improve outcomes at all levels of public health nursing practice (Keller et al, 2004b). Keystones of evidence-based practice guidelines arise from client concerns, clinical experience, best practices, and clinical data and research (Malloch and Porter-O'Grady, 2006). Clinical practice guidelines are systematically developed statements to assist practitioner and client decisions about appropriate health care for specific clinical circumstances. See "Evidenced-Based Practice" box for an example.

BRIEFLY NOTED

Total quality management and continuous quality improvement are concepts that give direction for managing a system of care, whereas quality assurance focuses on the care a client receives within the system.

Traditional Quality Assurance

Traditional quality assurance programs are compatible with the quality improvement process. In most health care systems, the overall goal of QA is to monitor the process and outcomes of client care. The following are specific goals:

1. Identify problems between the provider and client
2. Intervene in problem cases
3. Provide feedback regarding interactions between the client and provider
4. Provide documentation of interactions between the provider and client

The specific approaches are often implemented voluntarily by agencies and provider groups interested in the quality of interactions in their setting. However, state and federal governments require mandatory programs within public health agencies. For instance, periodic utilization review, peer reviews (audits), and other quality control measures are required in public health agencies that receive funds from state taxes, Medicaid, Medicare, and other public funding sources. Examples of specific approaches to quality control are agency staff review committees (peer review), utilization review committees, research studies, professional review organization (PRO) monitoring, client satisfaction surveys, risk management, and **malpractice litigation**.

Staff Review Committees

Staff review committees are the most common specific approach to quality assurance in the United States. Staff review (or peer review) committees are designed to monitor the client-specific aspects of certain levels of care. The audit is the major tool used to determine the quality of care.

The **audit process** consists of the following six steps:
1. Selecting a topic for study
2. Selecting explicit criteria for quality care
3. Reviewing records to determine whether the criteria are met
4. Having peer review of all cases that do not meet the criteria
5. Making specific recommendations to correct problems
6. Implementing follow-up to determine whether the problems have been solved

Two types of audits are used in nursing peer review: concurrent and retrospective. The **concurrent audit** is a process audit that evaluates the quality of ongoing care by examining the nursing process. Medicare and Medicaid use concurrent audits to evaluate the care received by public health and/or home health clients. The advantages of the concurrent audit are that it provides the following:
- Identification of problems at the time care is given
- Provision of a mechanism for identifying and meeting client needs during care
- Implementation of measures to fulfill professional responsibilities
- Provision of a mechanism for communicating on behalf of the client

The following are disadvantages of the concurrent audit:
- It is time consuming.
- It is more costly to implement than the retrospective audit.
- Because care is ongoing, it does not present the total picture of care that the client ultimately will receive.

The **retrospective audit**, or outcome audit, evaluates the quality of care through an appraisal of the nursing process after the client's discharge from the health care system. The advantages of the retrospective audit are that it provides the following:
- A comparison of actual practice to standards of care
- Analysis of actual practice findings

Evidence-Based Practice

Home visiting has been a mainstay in the repertoire of the public health nurse for decades. Randomized clinical trials have shown the effectiveness of home visiting, particularly with high-risk clients. Home visiting can be considered as a population-based activity when it meets the criteria that service is rendered to individuals because they are members of an identified population and because those services will improve the health status of that population. Such a finding resulted from an intervention by public health nurses at Lincoln-Lancaster County Health Department. A care pathway tool based on clinical evidence was used to track the milestones of progress by trimester of pregnancy for high-risk antepartal mothers. A review of 55 charts showed that subjects who had from five to nine home visits by the public health nurse during pregnancy had higher average birthweights for babies and higher average hemoglobin levels for mothers than those visited four times or less. Additionally, there was an increased rate of breastfeeding among mothers who had more visits by a public health nurse.

NURSE USE: Such research is important to better describe the population being served and to determine the effect of home visitation on client outcome. The clinical pathway tool described in the article can be used in practice with high-risk pregnant women.

From Fetrick A, Christensen M, Mitchell C: Does public health nurse home health visitation make a difference in the health outcomes of pregnant clients and their offspring?, *Public Health Nurs* 20(3):184–189, 2003.

- A total picture of care given
- More accurate data for planning corrective action

The following are disadvantages of the retrospective audit:
- The focus of evaluation is directed away from ongoing care.
- Client problems are identified after discharge, so corrective action can be used to improve the care only of future clients.

Utilization Review

The purpose of **utilization review** is to ensure that care actually is needed and that the cost is appropriate. The following are the three types of utilization review:
1. *Prospective:* an assessment of the necessity of care before giving service
2. *Concurrent:* a review of the necessity of services while care is being given
3. *Retrospective:* an analysis of the necessity of the services received by the client after the care has been given

Each of these reviews provides an assessment of the appropriateness of the cost of care. Prospectively, care can be denied and money saved. Concurrently, services can be cut if they are not deemed essential. Retrospectively, payment can be denied to the provider if the care was not necessary.

Utilization review began in the middle of the twentieth century because of concerns for increasing health care costs. Insurance companies and professional groups developed the first utilization review committees. These committees became mandatory under the 1965 Medicare law as a way to control hospital costs.

The utilization review process includes development of explicit criteria regarding the need for services and the length of service. Utilization review has been used primarily in hospitals to establish the need for client admission and to determine the length of the hospital stay. In community health, especially home health care, utilization review establishes criteria for admission to agency service, the number of visits a client may receive, the eligibility for client services such as a nursing aide or physical therapist, and discharge.

Advantages of utilization review are that it

* assists clients in avoiding unnecessary care;
* may encourage the consideration of alternative care options, such as home health care, rather than hospitalization;
* can provide guidelines for staff and program development; and
* provides for agency **accountability** to the consumer.

The major disadvantage of utilization review is that not all clients fit the classic picture presented by the criteria used to determine approval or denial of care. For example, an elderly female client was admitted to a home health care agency for care after being discharged from a hospital. The client was hemiplegic as a result of a cerebrovascular accident. After several weeks of physical and speech therapy, the client showed few signs of progress. The utilization review committee considered the client's condition to be stable and did not recognize the continued need for management to prevent future complications; therefore, Medicare payment was denied.

Appeal mechanisms have been built into the utilization review process used by Medicare and Medicaid. The appeal allows providers and clients to present additional data that may help reverse the original decision to deny payment. This is a tedious process and is often difficult for clients to understand and manage.

Risk Management

Risk management committees often are a part of the quality program of a community agency. The goal of risk management is to reduce the liability on the part of the agency and the number of grievances brought against the agency. The risk management committee reviews all risks to which an agency is exposed. It reviews client and personnel safety policies and procedures and determines whether personnel are following the rules. Examples of problems reviewed by a risk management committee are administering an incorrect vaccination dosage, a pediatric client injury caused by a fall from an examining table, or injury to a nurse in community health as a result of an accident while making a home visit. Incident reports are reviewed by the risk management committee for appropriate, accurate, and thorough documentation of any problem that occurs relating to clients or personnel. In addition, patterns are identified that may require changes in policy or staff development to correct the problem. Grievance procedures are established for both clients and personnel as a part of risk management.

Professional Review Organizations

As mentioned, professional standards review organizations (PSROs) were established in 1972 in an amendment to the Social Security Act (PL 92-603) as a publicly mandated utilization and peer review program. This law provided that medical, hospital, and nursing home care under Medicare, Medicaid, and Title V Maternal and Child Health programs would be reviewed for appropriateness and necessity and such care would be reimbursed accordingly. In 1983 Congress passed the Peer Review Improvement Act (PL 97-248), creating PROs. PROs, which replaced PSROs, are directed by the federal government to reduce hospital admissions for procedures that can be performed safely and effectively in an ambulatory surgical setting on an outpatient basis and to reduce inappropriate or unnecessary admissions or invasive procedures by specific practitioners or hospitals. Quality measures include the reduction of unnecessary admissions caused by previous substandard care, avoidable complications and deaths, and unnecessary surgery or invasive procedures (Sprague, 2001).

Institutions contract with PROs for quality reviews. PROs are local (usually state) organizations that establish criteria for care based on local patterns of practice. They can be for-profit or not-for-profit organizations. They have access to physicians or may include physicians in their membership. PROs must define their operational objectives and are required to consult with nurses and other nonphysician health care providers when reviewing the activities of those professionals. PROs monitor access to care and cost of care. Professionals working under the regulation of PROs should develop accurate and complete documentation procedures to ensure compliance with the criteria of the PRO.

There is considerable debate about the limitations and benefits of the federally mandated PRO quality review process. Limitations of the process include jeopardizing professional autonomy, because decision making about care includes professionals, consumers, and government representatives. In addition, control mechanisms may be developed such that the care provided is determined by cost rather than by professional criteria and judgment. On the positive side, the review system develops standards and uses review processes to increase accountability for the care given (Greenberg and Lezzoni, 1995).

In 1985, the authority of PROs was expanded to include the review of services offered by health maintenance organizations (HMOs) and competitive medical plans. In addition, the Medicare Quality Assurance Act was passed to strengthen quality assurance programs and to improve access to care after hospitalization. This act required hospitals receiving Medicare payments to provide to Medicare beneficiaries written discharge plans supervised by registered nurses and social workers.

Evaluative Studies

Evaluative studies for measuring the effectiveness of nursing and health care interventions on client populations increased during the twentieth century. These studies demonstrate

Table 17-2	Quality Assurance Measures	
Structure	**Process**	**Outcome**
Internal Agency	*Peer Review Committees*	*Internal Agency Committees*
Self-study	Prospective audit	Evaluative studies
Review agency documents	Concurrent audit	Survey health status
	Retrospective audit	
External Agency	*Client*	*Client*
Regulatory audit	Satisfaction survey	Malpractice suits
	Utilization review	Satisfaction survey

HOW TO Conduct a Sentinel Evaluation

- Count the cases of unnecessary disease, disability, complications, and death.
- Identify cases of unnecessary disease, disability, and complications. Example: tuberculosis (TB).
- Count the deaths from these causes.
- Examine the circumstances surrounding the unnecessary event (or sentinel) in detail.
- Review morbidity and mortality rates as an index for comparison; determine the critical increase in the untimely event, which may reflect changes in quality of care. Example: compare the incidence and prevalence of TB cases before the increased population occurred.
- Explore health status indicators, such as changes in social, economic, political, and environmental factors that may have an effect on health outcomes. Example: overcrowding in the shelter in which migrant workers stay (environmental) and the inability to follow up on testing because of the transient nature of the population (social).

the effect of nursing and health care interventions on client populations. Three key models have been used to evaluate quality: Donabedian's structure–process–outcome model, the tracer method, and the sentinel method.

Donabedian's (1981, 1985, 1990) model introduced three major components for evaluating quality care. The first component, **structure**, evaluates the setting and instruments used to provide care. Examples of structure are facilities, equipment, characteristics of the administrative organization, client mix, and the qualifications of health providers. The second component is **process**, or evaluating activities as they relate to standards and expectations of health providers in the management of client care. The third component is **outcome**, the net change (or result) that occurs from health care. The three components or methods may be used separately to evaluate a part of care. To obtain an overall picture of the quality of care, the three components should be used together (Table 17-2).

The **tracer method** measures both the process and outcome of care. This method is more effective in evaluating the health care of groups than of individuals. It is also more effective in evaluating care delivered by an institution than care delivered by a person (Kessner and Kalk, 1973). The following are the essential characteristics for implementing the tracer method:

- A tracer, or a problem, that has a definite impact on the client's level of functioning
- Well-defined and easily diagnosed characteristics
- Population prevalence high enough to permit adequate data collection
- A known variation resulting from use of effective health care
- Well-defined management techniques in prevention, diagnosis, treatment, or rehabilitation
- Recognized (documented) effects of nonmedical factors on the tracer

Stevens-Barnum and Kerfoot (1995) provided the following classification system for selecting client groups for tracer outcome studies in nursing:

1. A particular disease
2. Similar treatment
3. Similar needs
4. Similar community
5. Similar lifestyle
6. Similar illness stage

The tracer method provides nurses with data to enable them to show the differences in outcomes as a result of nursing care standards.

The **sentinel method** of quality evaluation is based on epidemiologic principles. This method is an outcome measure for examining specific instances of client care. Changes in the sentinel indicate potential problems. For example, increases in encephalitis in certain communities may result from increases in mosquito populations. New information technologies improve the surveillance of sentinel events and can help identify those sentinels that need to be monitored for quality (Bellin and Dubler, 2001). The characteristics of the sentinel method are described in the "How To" box.

MODEL QUALITY ASSURANCE PROGRAM

The primary purpose of a quality assurance program is to ensure that the results of an organized activity are consistent with the expectations. All personnel affected by a quality assurance program should be involved in its development and implementation. Although administration and management are responsible for the quality of services, the keys to that quality are the knowledge, skills, and attitudes of the personnel who deliver the service.

Figure 17-1 shows a model that identifies seven basic components of a quality assurance program. Based on quality assurance programs, answer the following questions about health care services and nursing care:

- What is being done now?
- Why is it being done?
- Is it being done well?
- Can it be done better?
- Should it be done at all?
- Are there improved ways to deliver the service?
- How much is it costing?
- Should certain activities be abandoned and/or replaced?

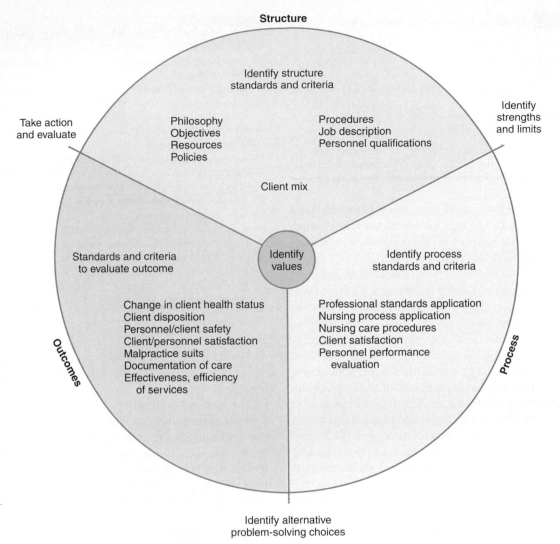

FIGURE 17-1 Model quality assurance programs.

The ANA model and Donabedian's framework for evaluating health care programs using the components of structure, process, and outcome can be used in developing a quality assurance program. Outcome is the most important ingredient of a program, since it is the key to the evaluation of providers and agencies by accrediting bodies, insurance companies, and Medicare and Medicaid through PROs, report cards, and other accrediting agencies.

STRUCTURE

The philosophy and objectives of an agency define its structural standards. In evaluating the structure of an organization, the evaluator determines whether the agency is adhering to the stated philosophy and objectives. Is the agency providing services to populations across the life span? Are primary, secondary, and/or tertiary preventive services offered? Standards of structure are defined by the licensing or accrediting agency, for example, the Community Health Accreditation Program (CHAP)'s standards for accrediting home health agencies.

Identification of standards and criteria for quality assurance begins with writing the philosophy and objectives of the organization. The philosophy includes values identification or the beliefs of the agency about humanity, nursing, the community, and health. The beliefs of the community, the population to be served, and the providers of care are equally important to the agency beliefs, and all need to be considered. Objectives define the intended results of nursing care, descriptions of client behaviors, and/or changes in health status to be demonstrated on discharge. Once objectives are formulated, the required resources are identified to accomplish the objectives. The need for the resources of personnel, supplies and equipment, facilities, and finances is described. Once resources are determined, policies, procedures, and job descriptions are formulated to serve as behavioral guides to the employees of the agency. These documents should reflect the essential nursing and other health provider qualifications needed to implement the services of the agency.

Standards of structure are evaluated internally via a self-study by a committee composed of administrative, management, and staff members. They are also evaluated by a utilization review committee; this committee is often composed of an external advisory group with community representatives for all services offered through an agency, such as a nurse, a physical therapist, a speech pathologist, a physician, a board member, and an administrator from a sister agency. The data from these committees identify the strengths and weaknesses of the agency structure.

BRIEFLY NOTED

Know the standards of care for your agency. Keep your eyes open for recurring practices that are not up to the quality standards of your agency. For example: your clients complain daily about long waits for service. Chances are these same practices may be occurring in other areas of the agency. This knowledge will be valuable in the quality improvement process as your agency strives to improve quality.

PROCESS

An evaluation of process standards is the specific appraisal of the quality of care being given by agency providers such as nurses. Agencies use various methods to determine criteria for evaluating provider activities: conceptual models, such as a developmental model or Neuman's Systems Model; the standards of care of the provider's professional organization, such as the ANA's *Public Health Nursing: Scope and Standards of Practice* (2007); or the nursing process. The activities of the nurse are evaluated to see if they correspond with the nursing care procedures defined by the agency.

The primary approaches used for process evaluation include the peer review committee and the client satisfaction survey. The techniques used for process evaluation are direct observation, questionnaire, interview, written audit, and videotape of client and provider encounters. Once data are collected to evaluate nursing process standards, the peer review committee reviews the data to identify strengths and weaknesses in the quality of care delivered. The peer review committee usually is an internal committee composed of representatives of the nursing staff who are trained to administer audit instruments and conduct client interviews.

OUTCOME

The evaluation of outcome standards, or the result of nursing care, is one of the more difficult tasks facing nursing today. Identifying changes in the client's health status that result from nursing care provides nursing data that demonstrate the contribution of nursing to the health care delivery system. Research studies using the tracer or sentinel method to identify client outcomes and client satisfaction surveys can be used to measure outcome standards. Measures of outcome standards include client admission data about the level of dependence or the acuity of problems and discharge data that may show changes in the levels of dependence and activity.

> **Box 17-1   Types of Problems Studied in a Quality Assurance Program**
>
> - Client death
> - Client injury
> - Personnel and client safety
> - Agency liability
> - Increased costs
> - Denied reimbursement by third-party payers
> - Client complaints
> - Inefficient service
> - Staff noncompliance with standards of structure
> - Lack of resources
> - Unnecessary staff work and overtime
> - Documenting of care
> - Client health status

From these data, strengths and weaknesses in nursing care delivery can be determined. The most common measurement methods are direct physical observations and interviews. Instruments have also been developed to measure general health status indicators in home health. The Omaha System is a classification system that includes nursing diagnosis, protocols of care, and a problem rating scale to measure nursing care outcomes (Clark et al., 2001; O'Brien-Pallas et al, 2001, 2002). In addition, the ANA has developed 10 areas for data collection of outcome criteria in community-based, non-acute care settings, including the following (Rowitz, 2001):

1. Pain management
2. Consistency of communication
3. Staff mix
4. Client satisfaction
5. Prevention of tobacco use
6. Prevention of cardiovascular disease
7. Caregiver activity
8. Identification of the primary caregiver
9. Activities of daily living
10. Psychosocial interactions

Nursing has been involved primarily in evaluating program outcomes to justify program expenses rather than in evaluating client outcomes.

Outcome evaluation assumes that health care has a positive effect on client status. The major problem with outcome evaluation is determining which nursing care activities are primarily responsible for causing changes in client status. In nursing, many uncontrolled factors in the field, such as environment and family relationships, have an effect on client status (Box 17-1). Often it is difficult to determine whether these factors are the cause of changes in client status or whether nursing interventions have the most effect. (See Table 17-2 for a summary of quality assurance measures.)

EVALUATION, INTERPRETATION, AND ACTION

Interpreting the findings of a quality care evaluation is an essential component of the process. It allows for the identification of discrepancies between the quality care standards of the agency and the actual practice of the nurse or other health providers. These patterns reflect the total agency's functioning over time and generate information for decisions to be made about the strengths and limitations of the agency. Regular intervals for evaluation should be established within the agency, and periodic reports should be written so that the combined results of structure, process, and outcome efforts can be analyzed and health care delivery patterns and problems identified. These reports should be used to establish an ongoing picture of changes that occur within an agency to justify community nursing services.

Identification and choices of possible courses of action to correct the weaknesses within the agency should involve both the administration and the staff. The courses of action chosen should be based on their significance, economic benefit, and timeliness. For example, if a nursing problem exists in the recording of client health education, the agency administration and staff may analyze the problem to determine why it is occurring. Reasons that nurses cite for recording inadequacies include a lack of time to do paperwork properly, case overloads that reduce the amount of time spent with clients, and lack of available resources for health education. When such reasons are given, it is not appropriate for managers to deal with the problem by providing a staff development program on the importance of doing and recording health education. Rather, they must determine how to provide the time and resources necessary for the nurses to offer health education to the clients. Economically, it may be more beneficial to provide dictating equipment and clerical assistance so that nurses can dictate notes and other paperwork, giving them more client contact time, or to employ an additional nurse and reduce caseloads.

Taking action is the final step in the quality assurance model. Once the alternative courses of action are chosen to correct problems, actions are implemented to effect a change in the overall operation of the agency. Next, follow-up and evaluation of the actions taken must occur to complete the quality assurance process. Although the performance of nurses is evaluated, remember that the focus of a continuous quality improvement effort is on the process, not the person. It is assumed that nurses and other employees want to provide the best possible care and that problems or variations in a process should not be automatically attributed to their behavior. Because a key to effective quality improvement is continuous learning, staff development is essential for all employees (see "Levels of Prevention" box on p. 307).

CASE STUDY

Ms. Miller is a nurse and the quality assurance director at the Best Care Home Health Agency. Incident report data showed that in the past 3 months, the number of incidents in which a fall resulted in an injury doubled (from 9 falls to 18 falls). Another nurse, Ms. Collins, would like to find out what the agency is currently doing to assess for risk of falls and if it could be done better.

First, Ms. Miller researched the risk factors for falls resulting in injury so that she would know what should be assessed to predict the potential risk for a fall. She found that a history of falls, use of an ambulatory aid, mental status, type of gait, medications, urinary alterations, improper footwear, diagnoses, alcohol abuse, age (older than 65 years), and gender (female) were risk factors for falls, especially falls resulting in an injury such as a fractured hip. Furthermore, in a literature review, Ms. Collins also found several fall assessment tools that were well documented for their effectiveness in predicting the risk for a fall and reducing the occurrences of a fall.

Because an incident report was written for each fall, Ms. Miller was able to backtrack through each client's file to evaluate his or her initial assessment. Looking at the initial assessment, Ms. Collins found that although several risk assessment tools were used for other items, such as the risk for depression, there was no risk assessment tool for falls. Ms. Collins recommended that the agency begin to use one of the fall risk assessment tools to improve their assessment for this incident, with the goal of decreasing the incidence of injuries resulting from falls.

DOCUMENTATION

Documentation is essential to the evaluation of quality care in any organization. The following sections focus on the kinds of documentation that normally occur in a community health agency.

RECORDS

Records are a basic part of the communication structure of organizations. Accurate and complete records are required by law and must be kept by all agencies, both governmental and nongovernmental. In most states, the state departments of health stipulate the kind and content requirements of records for community health agencies. Records provide complete information about the client, indicate the extent and quality of the services provided, resolve legal issues in malpractice suits, and provide information for education and research.

COMMUNITY HEALTH AGENCY RECORDS

Community health agencies keep various types of records to predict population trends in a community, identify health needs and problems, prepare and justify budgets, and make administrative decisions. The kinds of records that the agency keeps can include reports of accidents, births, census, chronic disease, communicable disease, mortality, life expectancy, morbidity, child and spouse abuse, occupational illness and injury, and environmental health.

Agencies also keep records to maintain administrative contact and control of the organization. These records are clinical, service, and financial. The clinical record is the client health record. The provider service records include information about the numbers of clinic clients seen daily, the immunizations given, home visits made daily, transportation

<table>
<tr><td colspan="2">

Levels of Prevention / **Related to Quality Management**

PRIMARY PREVENTION

Implement a staff development program to teach nurses and other providers how to reduce risk by properly documenting interventions.

SECONDARY PREVENTION

Complete an agency evaluation of individual nurse competencies in completing a community assessment on which program decisions will be made.

TERTIARY PREVENTION

Provide a staff development program to teach nurses skills in community assessment when the nurse's competency evaluation indicates that he or she does not have the proper skills.

</td></tr>
</table>

Healthy People 2010

Goal of Improving Access to Comprehensive, High-Quality Health Care, and Examples of Objectives to Eliminate Health Disparities

1-1 Increase the proportion of persons with health insurance
1-4 Increase the proportion of persons who have a specific source of ongoing care
1-6 Reduce the proportion of families that experience difficulties or delays in obtaining health care or do not receive needed care for one or more family members
1-7 Increase the proportion of schools of medicine, schools of nursing, and other health professional training schools whose basic curriculum for health care providers includes the core competencies in health promotion and disease prevention
1-8 In the health professions, allied and associated health profession fields, and the nursing field, increase the proportion of all degrees awarded to members of underrepresented racial and ethnic groups

From U.S. Department of Health and Human Services: *Healthy People 2010: understanding and improving health,* ed 2, Washington, DC, 2000, U.S. Government Printing Office.

and mileage, the provider's time spent with the client, and the amount and kinds of supplies used. The service record is completed on a daily basis by each provider and is summarized monthly and annually to indicate trends in health care activities and costs relative to personnel time, transportation, maintenance, and supplies. The financial records include salaries, overhead, and transportation costs, and they serve as the basis for the cost accounting system. The provider service records are used to correlate with the agency's financial records. These records are basic to peer review and audit.

As an outgrowth of quality assurance efforts in the health care system, comprehensive methods are being designed to document and measure client progress and client outcome from agency admission through discharge. An example of such a method is the client classification system developed at the Visiting Nurses Association of Omaha, Nebraska (Martin, 2005). This comprehensive method for evaluating client care has several components: a classification system for assessing and categorizing client problems, a data base, a nursing problem list, and anticipated outcome criteria for the classified problem. Such schemes are viewed as having the potential to improve the delivery of nursing care, documentation, and the descriptions of client care. Briefly, the implementation of comprehensive documentation methods will enhance the assessment, planning, implementation, and evaluation of client care by nurses and will allow for the organization of pertinent client information for more effective and efficient nurse productivity and communication.

HEALTHY PEOPLE 2010 AND QUALITY HEALTH CARE

One of the two goals of *Healthy People 2010* is to increase the quality and years of healthy life. This will be accomplished by helping individuals of all ages increase their life expectancy and improve their quality of life. According to *Healthy People 2010*, there are substantial differences in life expectancy among population groups within the nation. This is influenced by gender, race, and income. Quality of life reflects a sense of happiness and personal satisfaction. Health-related quality of life reflects a personal sense of physical and mental health and the ability to react to the physical and social environments. Basically, all the objectives are directed toward meeting this goal.

To assess the quality of the outcomes of the objectives related to individuals and communities, several objectives specifically address how the quality assessment will occur, as listed in the *"Healthy People 2010"* box.

CLINICAL APPLICATION

Oscar, a nursing student, has been working in the migrant farmworker clinic and has noted that each practitioner uses a different educational method for teaching good nutrition practices to newly diagnosed diabetic clients. The clinic has seen a substantial increase in the number of new diabetic clients in the Hispanic farmworker population. Oscar knows that practice guidelines for teaching nutrition practices exist in his clinical facility and that charts have an area in which to note nutrition education information. He also knows that for nurses to be most effective and ensure quality client outcomes, research-based practice guidelines should be used by all nurses in the health department.

As part of his course, Oscar must prepare a teaching plan and conduct a class on a health care problem. He obtains permission from his instructor and the director of the clinic to conduct an in-service program. The purpose of Oscar's in-service program is to instruct the nursing staff on how to teach newly diagnosed diabetic clients good nutrition practices. He obtains and studies the guidelines about teaching good nutrition practices, and he researches the methodological background for the development of the guidelines. Oscar's native language is Spanish, so this will help him in determining whether brochures for newly diagnosed diabetic clients regarding good nutrition convey the appropriate message.

As part of his in-service program, Oscar maintains demographic records on attendees and conducts before-and-after tests of knowledge, adding questions about the present use of the guidelines. He plans to follow-up with the nurses in 6 months with a further test and questions about the use of the guidelines. The director will help him determine an outcome measure that can be used with the client population to show effective use of the guidelines.

A. *What outcome measure would be useful in this project?*
B. *How will this help in the overall assessment of quality in the nursing service?*

Answers are in the back of the book.

REMEMBER THIS!

- The health care delivery system is the largest employing industry in the United States; society is demanding increased efficiency and effectiveness from the system.
- Quality control is the tool used to ensure effectiveness and efficiency.
- The managed care industry is changing the face of the American health care delivery system and thus how quality will be defined and measured.
- The objective and systematic evaluation of nursing care is a priority within the profession for several reasons, including the effects of cost on health care accessibility, consumer demands for better quality care, and the increasing involvement of nurses in public and health agency policy formulation.
- Total quality management/continuous quality improvement is a management philosophy used in health care. It is prevention oriented and process evaluation focused.
- The concept of quality includes customer satisfaction.
- Efforts are being made by the public and private sectors to form partnerships to monitor the performance of all players in health care delivery for the purpose of improving the health of communities.
- Quality assurance is the monitoring of the activities of care to determine the degree of excellence attained in the implementation of the activities.
- Quality assurance has been a concern of the profession since the 1860s, when Florence Nightingale called for a uniform format to gather and disseminate hospital statistics.
- Licensure has been a major issue in nursing since 1892.
- Two major categories of approaches exist in quality assurance and improvement today: general approaches and specific approaches.
- Accreditation is an approach to quality control used for institutions, whereas licensure is used primarily for individuals.
- Certification combines features of both licensing and accreditation.
- Three major models have been used to evaluate quality: Donabedian's structure–process–outcome model, the sentinel model, and the tracer model.
- The seven basic components of a quality assurance program are (1) identifying values; (2) identifying structure, process, and outcome standards and criteria; (3) selecting measurement techniques; (4) interpreting the strengths and weaknesses of the care given; (5) identifying alternative courses of action; (6) choosing specific courses of action; and (7) taking action.
- Records are an integral part of the communication structure of a health care organization. Accurate and complete records are required by law of all agencies, whether governmental or nongovernmental.
- Quality assurance and improvement mechanisms in health care delivery are the mechanisms for controlling the system and requesting accountability from individual providers within the system. Records help establish a total picture of the contribution of the agency to the client community.

WHAT WOULD YOU DO?

1. Write your own definition of TQM/CQI; compare your definition with the one given in the text. Are they the same or different? Justify your answer.
2. How does traditional QA fit into the TQM/CQI effort? Explain the relative importance of a continuing QA/QI effort.
3. Interview a nurse who is a coordinator of (or is responsible for) quality assurance and improvement in a local health agency. Ask the following questions and add others you may wish to have answered.
   a. Does the agency subscribe to the TQM/CQI approach to management?
   b. Is a traditional method of QA used to ensure quality?
   c. Describe the components of the quality program.
   d. How are records used in your quality effort?
   e. Discuss the approaches and techniques that are used to implement the quality program.
   f. How has the quality program changed in the health agency over the past 20 years?
   g. What influence has the quality program had on decreasing problems attributable to process? To provider accountability?
   h. List and describe the types of records usually kept in a community health agency. Explain the purpose of each type of record.

■ REFERENCES

Agency for Healthcare Research and Quality: *Your guide to choosing quality health care,* Rockville, Md, 2001, AHRQ available at http://www.ahrq.gov/consumer/qnt/.

Agency for Healthcare Research and Quality: *Improving healthcare quality,* Pub No. 02–P032, 2002, U.S. Department of Health and Human Services.

American Nurses Association: *Public health nursing: scope and standards of practice,* Washington, DC, 2007, ANA.

American Nurses Credentialing Center: *Nursing excellence: your journey—our passion.* Accessed April, 12, 2007 at http://www.nursingworld.org/ancc/magnet.html.

American Public Health Association: *Healthy communities 2000: model standards, guidelines for community attainment of the year 2000 national health objectives*, ed 3, Washington, DC, 1991, APHA.

Association of Community Health Nursing Educators: *Perspectives on doctoral education in community health nursing*, Lexington, Ky, 1993, ACHNE.

Association of Community Health Nursing Educators: *Graduate education for advanced practice education in community/public health nursing*, Chapel Hill, NC, 2000a, ACHNE.

Association of Community Health Nursing Educators: *Essentials of baccalaureate nursing education for entry level community health nursing practice*, Chapel Hill, NC, 2000b, ACHNE.

Association of Community Health Nursing Educators: *Graduate education for advanced practice in community public health nursing*, New York, 2003, ACHNE.

Bellin E, Dubler NN: The quality improvement–research divide and the need for external oversight, *Am J Public Health* 91(9):1512, 2001.

Carmichael S: Total quality management and outcomes based quality improvement: revisiting the basics, *Home Health Care Manag Pract* 17:119–124, 2005.

Centers for Disease Control and Prevention: *Planned approach to community health: guide for local coordinators*, Atlanta, Ga, 1995, CDC, National Center for Chronic Disease Prevention and Health Promotion.

Centers for Disease Control and Prevention: *National public health performance standards program*, Atlanta, Ga, 2008, CDC.

Centers for Medicare and Medicaid Services: *Medicare pay for performance initiatives*, CMS, Baltimore, 2005.

Clark J et al: New methods of documenting health visiting practice, *Community Practitioner* 74(3):108, 2001.

Commission on Collegiate Nursing Education: *Accreditation standards of baccalaureate nursing and graduate degree nursing programs*, Washington, DC, 2008, AACN.

Commission on Nurse Certification: *Clinical Nurse Leader Certification examination handbook*, Washington, DC, 2008, AACN.

Dlugacz YD, Restifo A, Greenwood A: *The quality handbook for health care organizations: a manager's guide to tools and programs*, Hoboken, NJ, 2004, Jossey-Bass.

Donabedian A: *The criteria and standards of quality, vol 2, Exploration in quality assessment and monitoring*, Ann Arbor, Mich, 1981, Health Administration.

Donabedian A: *Explorations in quality assessment and monitoring, vol 3*, Ann Arbor, Mich, 1985, Health Administration.

Donabedian A: The seven pillars of quality, *Arch Pathol Lab Med* 114:1115, 1990.

Durch JS, Bailey LA, Stoto MA, editors: *Improving health in the community: a role for performance monitoring*, Washington, DC, 1997, National Academy.

Greenberg LG, Lezzoni LI: Quality. In Calkins D, Fernandopulle RJ, Marino BS, editors: *Health care policy*, Cambridge, Mass, 1995, Blackwell Science.

Institute of Medicine: *Crossing the quality chasm*, Washington, DC, 2001, National Academy.

Jonas S: Measurement and control of the quality of health care. In Kovner AR, editor: *Health care delivery in the United States*, New York, 2002, Springer.

Keller LO et al: Population-based public health interventions: practice-based and evidence-supported, Part I, *Public Health Nurs* 21:453–468, 2004a.

Keller LO et al: Population-based public health interventions: innovations in practice, teaching and management, Part II, *Public Health Nurs* 21:469–487, 2004b.

Kessner DM, Kalk CE: Assessing health quality—the case for tracers, *New Engl J Med* 288:189, 1973.

Kovner A, Knickman JR, editors: *Jonas and Kovner's health care delivery in the United States*, New York, 2005, Springer.

Leatherman S, McCarthy D: *Quality of health care in the United States: a chartbook*, New York, 2002, Commonwealth Fund.

Maibusch RM: Evolution of quality assurance for nursing in hospitals. In Schrolder PS, Maibusch RM, editors: *Nursing quality assurance*, Rockville, Md, 1984, Aspen.

Malloch K, Porter-O'Grady T: *Evidence-based practice in nursing and health care*, Sudbury, Mass, 2006, Jones and Bartlett.

Martin KS: *The Omaha system: a key to practice, documentation, and information management*, ed 2, St Louis, 2005, Elsevier.

McLaughlin CP, Kaluzny AD, editors: *Continuous quality improvement in healthcare: theory, implementation and applications*, ed 3, Boston, 2006, Jones and Bartlett.

National Association of City and County Health Officials: *APEX-PH in practice*, Washington, DC, 1995, NACCHO.

National Association of City and County Health Officials: *Mobilizing for action through planning and partnerships: web-based tool,* Washington, DC, 2001, NACCHO. Retrieved Sept 25, 2005, from http://mapp.naccho.org.

National Association for Healthcare Quality: *Risk management: NAHQ guide to quality management*, Skokie, Ill, 1993, NAHQ.

National Association of Home Care: *Uniform data set for home care and hospice,* 1998, available at http://www.nahc.org/NAIIC/Research/unidata.html.

National Council of State Boards of Nursing: *Nurse Licensure compact*, Chicago, 2000, NCSBN.

O'Brien-Pallas LL et al: Evaluation of a client care delivery model. I: Variability in nursing utilization in community home nursing, *Nurs Econ* 19(6):267, 2001.

O'Brien-Pallas LL et al: Evaluation of a client care delivery model. II: Variability in nursing utilization in community home nursing, *Nurs Econ* 20(1):13, 2002.

Pushvaz V: Managed care organizations: the next generation, an introduction to medicine, *New Engl J Med* 4(1):November, 2007, Retrieved June 5, 2009, from www.nexgenmd.org.

Quad Council of Public Health Nursing Organizations: Public health nursing competencies, *Public Health Nurs* 219:443–452, 2004.

Rowitz L: *Public health leadership: putting principles into practice*, Gaithersburg, Md, 2001, Aspen.

Sprague L: Quality in the making, *Am J Med* 111(5):422, 2001.

Stevens-Barnum B, Kerfoot K: *The nurse as executive*, Gaithersburg, Md, 1995, Aspen.

Wright K et al: Competency development in public health leadership, *Am J Public Health* 90(8):1202–1207, 2000.

U.S. Department of Health and Human Services: *Healthy People 2010: understanding and improving health*, ed 2, Washington, DC, 2000, U.S. Government Printing Office.

U.S. Department of Health and Human Services: *Healthy people in healthy communities*, Washington, DC, Feb 2001, U.S. Government Printing Office.

Wakefield DS, Wakefield BJ: The complexity of health care quality. In Kovner AR, Knickman JR, editors: *Jonas and Kovner's health care delivery in the United States*, ed 8, New York, 2005, Springer.

Weisman CS, Grason HA, Strobina: Quality management in public and community health: examples from women's health, *Quality Manag Health Care* 10:54–64, 2000.

Wright K et al: Competency development in public health leadership, *Am J Public Health* 90:1202–1207, 2000.

Issues and Approaches in Family and Individual Health Care

Chapter 18

Family Development and Family Nursing Assessment

Joanna Rowe Kaakinen
Linda K. Birenbaum

ADDITIONAL RESOURCES

These related resources are found either in the appendix at the back of this book or on the book's website at http://evolve.elsevier.com/stanhope/foundations.

Appendix

- Appendix G.1: Community-As-Partner Model
- Appendix G.2: Friedman Family Assessment Model (Short Form)

ⓔEvolve Website

- Community Assessment Applied
- Case Study, with questions and answers

- Quiz review questions
- WebLinks, including link to *Healthy People 2010* website

Real World Community Health Nursing: An Interactive CD-ROM, second edition

If you are using this CD-ROM in your course, you will find the following activities related to this chapter:
- *Stages of Family Development* in **Family Health**
- *Friedman Family Assessment Model* in **Family Health**
- *You Conduct the Assessment: Single Parent Family, Aging Family, Multigenerational Family* in **Family Health**

OBJECTIVES

After reading this chapter, the student should be able to:
1. Explain the importance of family nursing in the community setting.
2. Describe family demographics.
3. Define family, family nursing, family health, and healthy/nonhealthy/resilient families.
4. Analyze changes in family function and structure.
5. Compare and contrast the four family social science theoretical frameworks.
6. Explain the various steps of the outcome present-state testing nursing process.
7. Compare and contrast the four ways to view family nursing.
8. Explain one assessment model and approach in detail.
9. Describe the various barriers to family nursing.
10. Share the implications for social and family policy.
11. Discuss issues of families in the future.

CHAPTER OUTLINE

FAMILY NURSING IN THE COMMUNITY
FAMILY DEMOGRAPHICS
DEFINITION OF FAMILY
FAMILY FUNCTIONS
FAMILY STRUCTURE
FAMILY HEALTH
Family Health, Nonhealth, and Resilience
FOUR APPROACHES TO FAMILY NURSING

THEORETICAL FRAMEWORKS FOR FAMILY NURSING
Structure–Function Theory
Systems Theory
Developmental Theory
Interactional Theory
WORKING WITH FAMILIES FOR HEALTHY OUTCOMES
Family Story
Cue Logic

Framing
Present State and Outcome Testing
Intervention and Decision Making
Clinical Judgment
Reflection
FAMILY NURSING ASSESSMENT
Friedman Family Assessment Model

FUTURE IMPLICATIONS FOR SOCIAL
AND FAMILY POLICY
FUTURE OF FAMILIES
BARRIERS TO PRACTICING FAMILY NURSING
HEALTHY PEOPLE 2010 AND FAMILY
IMPLICATIONS

KEY TERMS

dysfunctional families: family units that inhibit clear communication within family relationships and do not provide psychological support for individual members.

family: two or more individuals who depend on one another for emotional, physical, and/or financial support. Members of a family are self-defined.

family demographics: the study of the structure of families and households and the family-related events, such as marriage and divorce, that alter the structure through the number, timing, and sequence of the events.

family functions: behaviors or activities performed to maintain the integrity of the family unit and to meet the family's needs, individual members' needs, and society's expectations.

family health: a dynamic, changing, relative state of well-being that includes the biological, psychological, sociological, cultural, and spiritual factors of the family system.

family nursing: a specialty area that has a strong theory base and consists of nurses and families working together to ensure the success of the family and its members in adapting to responses to health and illness.

family nursing assessment: a comprehensive family data collection process used to identify the major problems facing the family.

family nursing diagnosis: the central issue of concern with the family; this directs the interventions.

family nursing process: a dynamic, organized method of critically thinking about a family.

family nursing theory: a theory whose function is to characterize, explain, or predict phenomena (events) evident within family nursing.

family structure: the characteristics of the individual members (gender, age, number) who constitute the family unit.

functional families: family units that provide autonomy and are responsive to the particular interests and needs of individual family members.

Family nursing is practiced in all settings. The trend in the delivery of health care has been to move health care to community settings; thus family nursing is very pertinent to nurses in community health. **Family nursing** is a specialty area that has a strong theory base and is more than just "common sense" or viewing the family as the context for individual health care. Family nursing consists of nurses and families working together to ensure the success of the family and its members in adapting to responses to health and illness. The purpose of this chapter is to present a current overview of families and family nursing, theoretical frameworks, and strategies for assessing and intervening with families in the community.

FAMILY NURSING IN THE COMMUNITY

Health care decisions are made within the family, the basic social unit of society. Health care occurs in families that are in the larger community and society. Families are responsible for providing or managing the care of family members. In the current health care system, families are significant members of health care teams since they are the ever-present force over the lifetime of care. Families are more responsible than ever for assisting in the health care of ill family members.

Nurses are responsible for the following:
- Helping families promote their health
- Meeting family health needs
- Coping with health problems within the context of the existing family structure and community resources
- Collaborating with families to develop useful interventions

Nurses must be knowledgeable about family structures, functions, processes, and roles. In addition, nurses must be aware of and understand their own values and attitudes pertaining to their own families, as well as being open to different family structures and cultures.

FAMILY DEMOGRAPHICS

Family demographics is the study of the structure of families and households and the family-related events, such as marriage and divorce, that alter the structure through their number, timing, and sequencing.

An important use of family demography by nurses is to forecast stresses and developmental changes experienced by families and to identify possible solutions to family problems. It is important to note that the structure of families has changed over time. The rapid changes that occurred at the close of the twentieth century have implications for family relationships and the ability of families to meet the changing needs of their members.

DEFINITION OF FAMILY

The definition of family is critical to the practice of nursing. Family has traditionally been defined using the legal concepts of relationships such as genetic ties, adoption, guardianship, or marriage. Since the 1980s a broader definition of family has been used that moved beyond the traditional blood, marriage, and legal constrictions.

Family refers to two or more individuals who depend on one another for emotional, physical, and/or financial support. The members of the family are self-defined (Hanson, 2005). Nurses working with families should ask people who they consider to be their family and then include those members in health care planning. The family may range from traditional nuclear and extended family to "postmodern" family structures such as single-parent families, stepfamilies, same-gender families, and families consisting of friends.

BRIEFLY NOTED

Most persons view families and their experiences based on their own family of origin. It is important to be aware of and attempt to understand other family variations.

FAMILY FUNCTIONS

Throughout history, a number of functions have traditionally been performed by families (Hanson, 2005). Six of these **family functions** are summarized in Box 18-1.

Historically, families who performed all of these six functions were considered healthy and good. In contemporary times, the traditional functions of families have been modified and new functions have been added. For example, the financial function of families has changed so that family members do not need each other to stay financially healthy as much as they did in the past. Many married couples are electing to be child-free rather than to reproduce. Families depend on other agencies to provide safety, such as law enforcement, whereas other agencies are involved in the passing of the religious faith (e.g., churches, synagogues). Education (socialization function) is relegated to the schools. Family names are no longer needed to confer status as in the past, when names were very important in a community.

The functions that served families have evolved and changed over time. Some have become more important and others less so (Patterson, 2002). The following new functions are more prominent in modern families:

- The relationship function has become important in contemporary families, thus emphasizing how people get along and their level of satisfaction.
- The health function has become more evident because it is the basis of a lifetime of physical and mental health or the lack thereof.

FAMILY STRUCTURE

Family structure refers to the characteristics and demographics (gender, age, number) of individual members who make up family units. More specifically, the structure of a family defines the roles and the positions of family members (Box 18-2).

Family structures have changed over time. The great speed with which changes in family structure, values, and

---

Box 18-1	Historical Family Functions

1. Families exist to achieve financial survival. Families are economic units to which all members contribute and from which all members benefit.
2. Families exist to reproduce.
3. Families provide protection from hostile forces.
4. Families pass along the culture, including religious faith.
5. Families educate (socialize) their young.
6. Families confer status in society.

Box 18-2	Family and Household Structures

Married Family
- Traditional nuclear family
- Dual-career family
- Spouses reside in the same household
- Commuter marriage
- Husband/father is away from the family
- Stepfamily
- Stepmother family
- Stepfather family
- Adoptive family
- Foster family
- Voluntary childlessness

Single-parent Family
- Never married
- Voluntary singlehood (with children, biological or adopted)
- Involuntary singlehood (with children)
- Formerly married
- Widowed (with children)
- Divorced (with children)
- Custodial parent
- Joint custody of children
- Binuclear family

Multiadult Household (With or Without Children)
- Cohabitating couple
- Communes
- Affiliated family
- Extended family
- New extended family
- Home-sharing individuals
- Same-sex partners

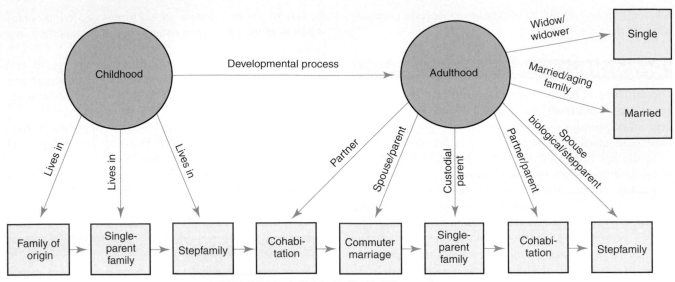

FIGURE 18-1 An individual's family life experiences.

relationships are happening makes working with families at the beginning of the twenty-first century exciting and challenging. As social norms have become more tolerant of a range of choices in relation to managing one's life, there is no longer a general consensus that the traditional nuclear family model is the only "right" model. No "typical family" model exists. As a consequence, the number of family and household types is growing. There is an increasing awareness that more variety exists within and among particular family structures. For example, the single-mother household may be represented by the unmarried teenage mother with an infant (unplanned pregnancy), the divorced mother with one or more children, or the career-oriented woman in her late thirties who elects to have a baby and remain single.

An individual may participate in a number of family life experiences over a lifetime (Figure 18-1).

The following are examples of family life experiences:
- Spending the early, formative years in the family of origin (mother, father, sibling)
- Experiencing some years in a single-parent family because of divorce
- Participating in a stepfamily relationship when the single parent who has custody remarries
- Participating in several additional family types as an adult, building on childhood experience

The following are examples of what an adult may experience:
- Cohabitating while completing a desired education
- Marrying and having a commuter-type marriage while developing a career
- Subsequently divorcing and becoming the custodial parent
- Eventually cohabitating with another partner
- Finally, marrying another partner who also has children

As couples age, they will address issues of the aging family and subsequently the woman may become an elderly single widow. Nurses work with families representing various structures and living arrangements.

Prospects for families for the twenty-first century are numerous. New family structures that currently are experimental will emerge as everyday "natural" families (e.g., families in which the members are not related by blood or marriage but who provide the services, caring, love, intimacy, and interaction needed by all persons to experience a quality life).

FAMILY HEALTH

Despite the focus on family health within nursing, the meaning of family health lacks consensus and is not precise. The term **family health** is often used interchangeably with the concepts of family functioning, healthy families, or familial health. Hanson (2005) defines family health as "a dynamic changing relative state of well-being which includes the biological, psychological, sociological, cultural, and spiritual factors of the family system" (p. 7).

This biopsychosocial/cultural/spiritual approach refers to individual members as well as the family unit as a whole. An individual's health (wellness–illness continuum) affects the entire family's functioning, and in turn the family's functioning affects the health of individuals. Thus assessment of family health involves simultaneous assessment of individual family members and the family system as a whole.

FAMILY HEALTH, NONHEALTH, AND RESILIENCE

Terms related to healthy versus nonhealthy families have varied in the literature. Health professionals have tended to classify clients and their families into two groups: "good families," or **functional families**, and "bad families," or families in need of psychosocial evaluation and intervention (Satariano and Briggs, 1999). The term *family health*

<table>
<tr><td>

Levels of Prevention   **Related to Child Abuse**

PRIMARY PREVENTION

Provide programs in child development for families at risk for child abuse, such as single-parent households.

SECONDARY PREVENTION

Provide programs in child development and behavior management for families that have not yet abused their children but whose children are brought to the attention of social authorities for aggressive behavior problems.

TERTIARY PREVENTION

Provide family therapy for abusive families; remove children from the home.

</td></tr>
</table>

Box 18-3 Characteristics of Healthy Families

1. The family tends to communicate well and listen to all members.
2. The family affirms and supports all of its members.
3. Teaching respect for others is valued by the family.
4. The family members have a sense of trust.
5. The family plays together, and humor is present.
6. All members interact with each other, and a balance in the interactions is noted among the members.
7. The family shares leisure time together.
8. The family has a shared sense of responsibility.
9. The family has traditions and rituals.
10. The family shares a religious core.
11. The privacy of members is honored by the family.
12. The family opens its boundaries to admit and seek help with problems.

Modified from Hanson SMH: *Family health care nursing: theory, practice, and research,* ed 2, Philadelphia, 2001, Davis.

implied mental health rather than physical health. Recently the popular term for nonhealthy families is **dysfunctional families**—also called *noncompliant, resistant,* or *unmotivated;* these phrases denote families that are not functioning well with each other or the world. The label *dysfunctional family* does not allow for family change and intervention and needs to be dropped from the nursing language. Families are neither all good nor all bad; therefore nurses need to view family behavior on a continuum of need for intervention when the family comes in contact with the health care system. All families have both strengths and difficulties. All families have seeds of resilience. The "Levels of Prevention" box shows the levels of prevention for a family experiencing child abuse.

Families with strengths, functional families, and *resilient families* are terms often used to refer to healthy families. Research has been conducted about healthy families, but it is clear that the issues examined all relate to those of relational needs. This means that in healthy families, the basic survival needs are met. The traits ascribed to healthy families are based on attachment and are affectionate in nature (Carter and McGoldrick, 1998).

Studies have reported traits of healthy families as well as family stressors that are useful for nurses to include in their assessment (Boss, 2001; McKenry and Price, 2000; Peterson, 2000). Box 18-3 shows characteristics of families that are healthy and functioning well in society.

The most recent discussions in family literature pertain to family resilience. Family resilience has been defined as the ability to withstand and rebound from adversity (Hawley, 2000; Patterson, 2002; Walsh, 2002). According to Walsh (2002), health care professionals should work with families to find new possibilities in a problem-saturated situation and to help them overcome impasses to change and growth. This is a positive focus on bringing out the best to enhance family functioning and well-being. Family resilience is an important outcome when nurses look at family stressors and assess family strengths. Nurses have a responsibility to help families withstand and rebound from adversity.

FOUR APPROACHES TO FAMILY NURSING

Central to the practice of family nursing is conceptualizing and approaching the family from four perspectives (Hanson, 2005). All have legitimate implications for nursing assessment and intervention (Figures 18-2 and 18-3). Which approach nurses use is determined by many factors, including the health care setting, family circumstances, and nurse resources:

1. *Family as the context, or structure.* This has a traditional focus that places the individual first and the family second. The family as context serves as either a resource or a stressor to individual health and illness. A nurse using this focus might ask an individual client, "How has your diagnosis of insulin-dependent diabetes affected your family?" or "Will your need for medication at night be a problem for your family?"

2. *Family as the client.* The family is first, and individuals are second. The family is seen as the *sum* of individual family members. The focus is concentrated on each individual as he or she affects the family as a whole. From this perspective, a nurse might say to a family member who has just become ill, "Tell me about what has been going on with your own health and how you perceive each family member responding to your mother's recent diagnosis of liver cancer."

3. *Family as a system.* The focus is on the family as client, and the family is viewed as an interacting system in which the whole is more than the sum of its parts. This approach simultaneously focuses on individual members and the family as a whole at the same time. The interactions between family members become the target for nursing interventions (e.g., the direct interactions between the parents, or the indirect interaction between the parents and the child). The systems approach to family always implies that when something happens to one family member, the other members of the family system

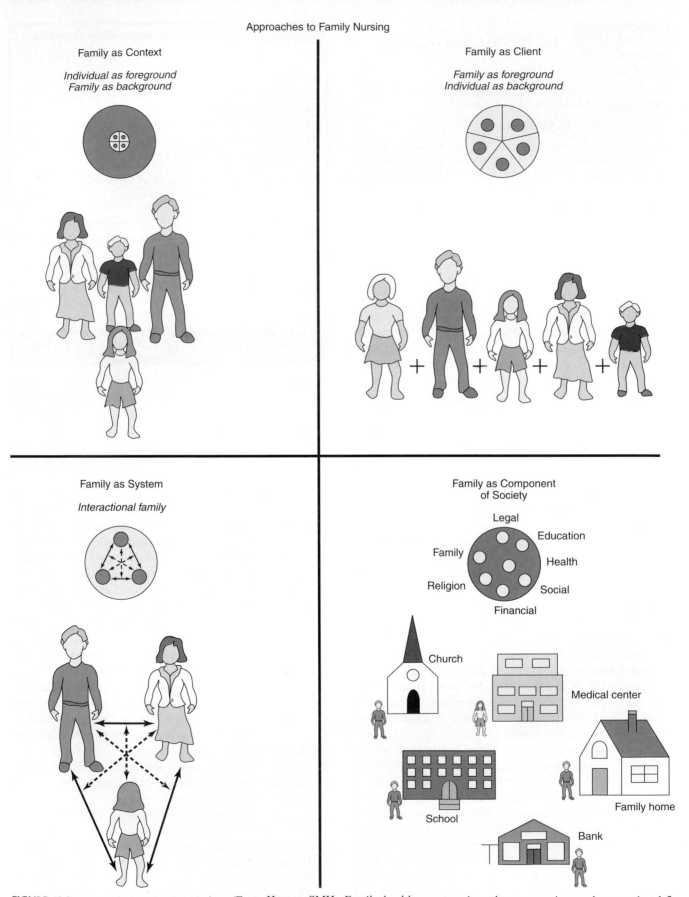

FIGURE 18-2 Approaches to family nursing. (From Hanson SMH: *Family health care nursing: theory, practice, and research,* ed 2, Philadelphia, 2001, Davis.)

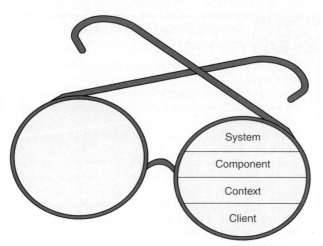

FIGURE 18-3 Four views of the family. (From Hanson SMH: *Family health care nursing: theory, practice, and research,* ed 2, Philadelphia, 2001, Davis.)

are affected. Questions nurses ask when approaching a family as system are, "What has changed between you and your spouse since your child's head injury?" or "How do you feel about the fact that your son's long-term rehabilitation will affect the ways in which the members of your family are functioning and getting along with one another?"

4. *Family as a component of society.* The family is seen as one of many institutions in society, along with health, education, religious, or financial institutions. The family is a basic or primary unit of society, as are all the other units, and they are all a part of the larger system of society. The family as a whole interacts with other institutions to receive, exchange, or give services and communicate. Nurses have drawn many of their tenets from this perspective as they focus on the interface between families and community agencies.

BRIEFLY NOTED

All families have secrets. Some information gleaned from families may be exaggerated, minimized, or withheld from persons outside the family, including health providers.

THEORETICAL FRAMEWORKS FOR FAMILY NURSING

Within the family social science tradition, four conceptual approaches have dominated the field of marriage and family: structure–function theory, systems theory, developmental theory, and interactionist theory (White and Klein, 2002). These theories are constantly evolving and being tested, which helps make this knowledge base stronger and more user-friendly for working with families. The following is a summary of the four major family social theories and what they have contributed to **family nursing theory**.

STRUCTURE–FUNCTION THEORY

The *structure–function framework* from a social science perspective defines families as social systems. Families are examined in terms of their relationship with other major social structures (institutions) such as health care, religion, education, government, and/or the economy. This perspective looks at the arrangement of members within the family, relationships among the members, and the roles and relationships of the members to the whole family (Hanson and Kaakinen, 2005). The primary focus is to determine how family patterns are related to other institutions in society and to consider the family in the overall structure of society. Emphasis is placed on the basic functions of families. With family structure as the focus, the major concern is how well the structure performs its functions. Individuals or family units receive little attention in this approach. Families are studied from the status-role perspective. Family theorists use this approach to understand the social or family system and its relationship to the overall social system. This approach describes the family as open to outside influences yet at the same time maintaining its boundaries. The family is seen as passive in adapting to the system rather than as an agent of change. The framework emphasizes a static societal structure and neglects change as a structural dynamic. Assumptions of the structure–function theory are found in Box 18-4.

This perspective is a useful framework for assessing families and health. Illness of a family member results in alteration of the family structure and function. If a single mother is ill, she cannot carry out her various roles, so grandparents or siblings may have to assume childcare responsibilities. Family power structures and communication patterns are affected when a parent is ill. The family assessment includes determining if changes resulting from the illness influence the family's ability to carry out its functions. Sample assessment questions include the following: "How did the death alter the family structure?" and "What family roles were changed with the onset of the chronic illness?" Interventions become necessary when a change in the family structure alters the family's ability to function. Examples of interventions using this model include helping families use existing support structures and helping families modify the way they are organized so that role responsibilities can be distributed.

The major strength of the structure–function theory to family nursing is its comprehensive approach that views families within the broader community in which they live. The major weakness of this approach is the static picture of the family, which does not allow for dynamic change over time.

SYSTEMS THEORY

The *systems theory* to understanding families was influenced by theory derived from physics and biology. A system is composed of a set of interacting elements; each system can be identified and is distinct from the environment in which it exists. An open system exchanges energy and matter with the environment (negentropy), whereas a closed system is

---

Box 18-4	**Assumptions of Structure–Function Theory**

- A family is a social system with functional requirements.
- A family is a small group that has basic features common to all small groups.
- Social systems, such as families, accomplish functions that serve the individuals in addition to those that serve society.
- Individuals act within a set of internal norms and values that are learned primarily in the family through socialization.

Box 18-5	**Assumptions of the Systems Approach**

- Family systems are greater than and different from the sum of their parts.
- There are many hierarchies within family systems and logical relationships between subsystems (e.g., mother–child, family–community).
- There are boundaries in the family system that can be open, closed, or random.
- Family systems increase in complexity over time, evolving to allow greater adaptability, tolerance to change, and growth by differentiation.
- Family systems change constantly in response to stresses and strains from within and from outside environments. There are structural similarities in different family systems (isomorphism).
- Change in one part of family systems affects the total system.
- Causality is modified by feedback; therefore causality never exists in the real world.
- Family systems patterns are circular rather than linear; change must be directed toward the cycle.
- Family systems are an organized whole; therefore individuals within the family are interdependent.
- Family systems have homeostasis features to maintain stable patterns that can be adaptive or maladaptive.

---

isolated from its environment (entropy). Systems depend on both positive and negative feedback to maintain a steady state (homeostasis). Seeking therapy when the marital relationship is strained is an example of using negative feedback to maintain a steady state. Assumptions of systems theory are found in Box 18-5.

The family system perspective encourages nurses to view clients as participating members of a family. Nurses using this perspective determine the effects of illness or injury on the entire family system. Emphasis is on the whole rather than on individuals. Nursing assessment of family systems includes assessment of the following:

- Individual members
- Subsystems
- Boundaries
- Openness
- Inputs and outputs
- Family interactions
- Family processing
- Adaptation or the ability to change

Assessment questions include the following: "Who is in the family system?" and "How has one member's critical illness affected the entire family system?" Interventions need to assist individual, subsystem, and whole family functioning. Some nursing strategies using this approach include establishing a mechanism for providing families with information about their family members on a regular basis and discussing ways to provide for a normal family life for family members after someone has become ill.

The major strength of the systems framework is that it views families from both a subsystem and a suprasystem approach. That is, it views the interactions within and among family subsystems as well as the interaction among families and the larger supersystems, such as the community, world, and universe. The major weakness of the systems framework is that the focus is on the interaction of the family with other systems rather than on the individual, which is sometimes more important.

DEVELOPMENTAL THEORY

Individual developmental theory has been the core to the nursing of people across the life span. This approach looks at the family system over time through different phases that can be predicted with known family transitions based on norms.

Duvall and Miller (1985) presented the principles of individual development and applied them to the family as a unit. The stages of family development are based on the age of the eldest child. Overall family tasks are identified that need to be accomplished for each stage of family development. Developmental concepts include moving to a different level of functioning, implying progress in a single direction. Family disequilibrium and conflicts are described as occurring during transition periods from one stage to another. The family has a predictable natural history designated by stages, beginning with the simple husband–wife pair. The group becomes more complex with the addition of each new child over time. The group again becomes simple and less complex as the younger generation leaves home. Finally, the group comes full circle to the original husband–wife pair. At each family life-cycle stage, there are developmental needs of the family and tasks that must be performed. These concepts are further refined by Duvall and Miller (1985).

Developmental theory is an attempt to integrate the small-scale (interactive framework) and large-scale (structural framework) analyses of the other two approaches while viewing the family as an open system in relation to structures in society. Developmental theory explains and predicts the changes that occur to humans or groups over time. The achievement of family developmental tasks helps individual members accomplish their tasks. This framework does the following:

- Assists nurses in anticipating clinical problems in families
- Identifies family strengths
- Serves as a guide in assessing the family's developmental stage

Box 18-6	**Assumptions of Developmental Theory**

- In every family there are both individual and family developmental tasks that need to be accomplished for every stage of the individual/family life cycle that are unique to that particular group.
- Families change and develop in different ways because of internal and environmental stimulation.
- Developmental tasks are goals to work toward rather than specific jobs to be completed at once.
- Each family is unique in its composition and complexity of age-role expectations and positions.
- Individuals and families are a function of their history, as well as the current social structure.
- Families have enough in common despite the way they develop over the family life span.
- Families may arrive at similar developmental levels through different processes.

Box 18-7	**Assumptions of Interactional Theory**

- Complex sets of symbols having common meanings are acquired through living in a symbolic environment.
- Individuals distinguish, evaluate, and assign meaning to symbols.
- Behavior is influenced by meanings of symbols or ideas rather than by instincts, needs, or drives; therefore the meaning an individual assigns to symbols is important to understanding behavior.
- The self continues to change and evolve over time through introspection caused by experience and activity.
- The evolving self has several dimensions: the physical body and characteristics and a complex social self. The "me" is a conventional, habitual self that consists of learned, repetitious responses. The "I" is spontaneous to the individual.
- Individuals are actors as well as reactors; they select and interpret the environment to which they respond.
- Individuals are born into a dynamic society.
- The nature of the infant is determined by the environment and responses to the infant rather than by a predisposition to act in a certain way (this is now being challenged).
- Individuals learn from the culture and become the society.
- Individuals' behavior is a product of their history, which is continually being modified by new information.

- Assesses the extent to which the family is fulfilling the tasks associated with its respective stage
- Assesses the family's developmental history
- Assesses the availability of resources essential for performing developmental tasks

In conducting an assessment of a family using the developmental model, several questions can be asked: "Where does this family place on the continuum of the family life cycle?" and "What are the developmental tasks that are not being accomplished?" Typical kinds of nursing intervention strategies using this perspective help the family understand individual and family growth and development stages and deal with the normal transitions between developmental periods (e.g., tasks of the school-age family member versus tasks of the adolescent family member). Assumptions of developmental theory are found in Box 18-6.

The major strength of this approach is that it provides a basis for forecasting what a family will be experiencing at any period in the family life cycle (e.g., role transitions and family structure changes). The major weakness is the fact that the model was developed at a time when the traditional nuclear family was emphasized.

INTERACTIONAL THEORY

Interactional theory views families as units of interacting personalities and examines the symbolic communications by which family members relate to one another. Within the family, each member occupies a position to which a number of roles are assigned. Members define their role expectations in each situation through their perceptions of the role demands. Members judge their own behavior by assessing and interpreting the actions of others toward them. The responses of others in the family serve to challenge or reinforce family members' perceptions of the norms of role expectations (Bomar, 2004). Central to the interaction approach is the process of role taking. Every role exists in relation to some other role, and interaction represents a dynamic process of testing perceptions about one another's roles. The ability to predict other family members' expectations for one's role enables each member to have some knowledge of how to react in the role and indicates how other members will react to performing the role. Assumptions of interactional theory are given in Box 18-7.

Assessment of families using the interactional framework emphasizes interaction between and among family members and family communication patterns about health and illness behaviors appropriate for different roles. Nurses intervene using strategies focused on the following (Bomar, 2004):

- Effectiveness of communication among members
- Ability to establish communication between nurses and families
- Clear and concise messages between members
- Similarities between verbal and nonverbal communication patterns
- Directions of the interaction

Nurses can center their attention on how family members interact with one another, so this approach is useful in explaining family communication, roles, decision making, and problem solving (Friedman, Bowden, and Jones, 2003).

The major strength of this approach is the focus on internal processes within families, such as roles, conflict, status, communication, responses to stress, decision making, and socialization. Processes, rather than end products, of social interactions are the major focus; thus this framework has been used by many nurse scholars. The major weakness is the broadness and lack of agreement about concepts and assumptions of the theory, which has made it difficult to refine. Interactionalists consider families to be comparatively closed units with little relationship to the outside society.

WORKING WITH FAMILIES FOR HEALTHY OUTCOMES

The goal of collaborating with families is to focus care, interventions, and services to achieve the best possible outcome. The Outcome Present-State Testing Model (OPT) **family nursing process** is a dynamic, systematic clinical reasoning process that emphasizes outcome of care (Pesut and Herman, 1999). Building on the traditional nursing process model, OPT emphasizes organizing care around what is called the keystone issue that is challenging family health. By directing care to resolve the keystone family issue, a ripple effect will occur that results in resolving many other problems. The OPT approach is an outcome-driven model of care. Nurses focus on collaborating with the family to achieve the most desirable outcome. Box 18-8 shows the steps of OPT.

FAMILY STORY

Nurses gather information about and from the family to determine the keystone health concerns of the family. Data collection begins when an actual or potential problem is identified by a source, which may be the family, the physician, a school nurse, or a caseworker. The following are examples:

- A family is referred to the home health agency because of the birth of the newest family member. In that district, all births are automatically followed up with a home visit.
- A family calls the Visiting Nurse Association to request assistance in providing care to a family member with a terminal illness.

- A teacher who noticed that a student has frequent absences and demonstrates significant behavior changes in the classroom asks a school nurse to conduct a family assessment.
- A physician requests a family assessment for a child who has failure to thrive.

The assessment process and data collection begin as soon as the referral occurs. Sources of preencounter data the nurse gathers include the following:

- *Referral source.* The information collected from the referral source includes data that lead to identifying a problem for this family. Demographic information and subjective and objective information may be obtained from the referral source.
- *Family.* A family may identify a health care concern and seek help. During the initial intake or screening procedure, valuable information can be collected from the family. Information is collected during phone interactions with the family member, even when calling to set up the initial appointment. This information might include family members' views of the problem, surprise that the referral was made, reluctance to set up the meeting, avoidance in setting up the interview, or recognition that a referral was made or that a probable health care concern exists.
- *Previous records.* Previous records may be available for review before the first meeting between the nurse and the family. Often, a record release for information is necessary to obtain family or individual records.

Before contacting the family to arrange for the initial appointment, the nurse decides the best place to meet with the family, which might be in the home, clinic, or office. Often

---

| Box 18-8 | **Steps of the Outcome Present-State Testing Family Nursing Process Model (OPT)** |

The OPT family nursing process model consists of the following steps, which have been adapted specifically to work with the family as client:

1. *Family story.* The family story provides essential information about individual family members and the family as a whole. Getting the family (client) story represents the data collection process. Nurses collect data about the family via a variety of methods (e.g., interviewing the family client, chart review, process logs, phone logs, phone conversations with other professionals, previous visits with the family, school records).

2. *Cue logic.* The nurse places the data into meaningful clusters of evidence. The clusters of evidence identify problems that are influencing the family's adaptation in the given circumstances. Nurses make connections or see relationships between the sets or clusters of data to identify the "keystone" or foundation problem affecting the family. The keystone issue is specifically stated as a family nursing diagnosis.

3. *Framing.* The role of the nurse is to help the family understand the present state and determine the best possible outcome. It is in this step that nurses think about the family story through the frame of multiple theory-based approaches, some of which were described earlier. By framing the problem from a theory, potential outcomes can be considered given the whole picture of the family client.

4. *Present state and desired outcome.* The keystone issue is stated as the present (priority) problem that needs to be resolved. The outcome is stated in a positive language. By placing side by side the present state with the desired outcome, evaluation criteria become more clear; in OPT, this step is called *testing*. It is these criteria that the nurse will consider to determine if the outcome is being achieved, partially achieved, or not achieved.

5. *Interventions and decision making.* The nurse and family work in a partnership to design and implement a plan of action based on the identified outcome.

6. *Clinical judgment.* Nurses make clinical judgments. If the plan of action results in the achievement of the identified outcome, the nurse may decide to continue with the plan of care or that it is time to put plans in place to terminate the nurse–family partnership. If the outcome is not being achieved or is being partially achieved, it is critical that nurses step outside the situation or event to evaluate and reflect on the whole picture.

7. *Reflection.* Nurses engage in purposeful, deliberate reflection to learn from the experience and build mental patterns of client stories—clusters of evidence, keystone issues, outcomes, and interventions. This requires critical thinking on the part of nurses.

Adapted from Kaakinen JR, Hanson SMH: Family nursing assessment and intervention. In Hanson SMH, Gedaly-Duff V, Kaakinen JR, editors: *Family health care nursing: theory, practice and research*, ed 3, Philadelphia, 2005, FA Davis.

this decision is dictated by the type of agency with which the nurse works (e.g., home health is conducted in the home), or the mental health agency may choose to have the family meet in the neighborhood clinic office.

Advantages to meeting in the family home include the following:

- Meeting in the home makes it possible to view the everyday family environment.
- Family members are likely to feel more relaxed and thereby demonstrate typical family interactions.
- Meeting with a family in their home emphasizes that the problem is the responsibility of the whole family and not one family member.
- Conducting the interview in the home may increase the probability of having more family members present.

The following are two important disadvantages of meeting in the family's home:

1. Their home may be the only sanctuary or safe place for the family or its members to be away from the scrutiny of others.
2. Meeting with a family on their ground requires the nurse to be highly skilled in communication by setting limits and guiding the interaction.

BRIEFLY NOTED

Too much disclosure during the early contacts between the family and nurse may scare the family away. Slow the process down, and take time to build trust.

Conducting the family appointment in the office or clinic allows easier access to other health care providers for consultation. An advantage of using the clinic may be that the family situation is so intense that a more formal, less personal setting may be necessary for the family to begin discussion of emotionally charged issues. A disadvantage of not seeing the everyday family environment is that it may reinforce a possible culture gap between the family and the nurse. See the "How To" box.

After the decision is made regarding where to meet the family, the nurse contacts the family. It is important to remember that the family gathers information about the nurse from this initial phone call to arrange a meeting, so the nurse should be confident and organized. After the introduction, the nurse concisely states the reason for requesting the family visit and encourages all family members to attend the meeting. Several possible times, including late afternoon or evening, for the appointment can be offered, which allows the family to select the most convenient time for all members to be present.

CUE LOGIC

As nurses gather information about the family, they begin to place the information into meaningful datasets that help them see the whole family (as the client), called *cue logic*. Nurses organize information into logical groups (or clusters) to determine the most important keystone issue

---

| HOW TO | Set an Appointment with the Family |

The assessment process starts immediately upon referral. The following are suggestions that will make the process of arranging a meeting with the family easier:

1. Remember that the assessment is reciprocal and the family will be making judgments about you when you call to make the appointment.
2. Introduce yourself, and state the purpose for the contact.
3. Do not apologize for contacting the family. Be clear, direct, and specific about the need for an appointment.
4. Arrange a time that is convenient for the greatest possible number of family members.
5. Confirm the place, time, date, and directions.

---

challenging the family health. One of the most important pieces of information provided by the referral source is the focus, or the cluster of cues or symptoms, that leads them to believe that a problem might exist. However, it is important to view the family with an open approach because the central issue identified by the referral source may not be the actual keystone issue but may be another problem that contributes to the keystone issue. See, for example, the following case study:

> *The Raggs family is referred to the home health clinic by a physician for management of medication. Sam, a 73-year-old husband, has had diabetes for 13 years and has developed insulin-dependent diabetes mellitus. He is being discharged from the hospital. The potential area of concern that prompted the referral was the administration of insulin. After the initial meeting with the family, the nurse finds that administration of the medication is not the central issue for Sam and his wife, Rose. The keystone issue is managing his nutrition. The referral source believed that the family knew how to manage the dietary aspects of diabetes because Sam had had a form of diabetes for 13 years.*

If the keystone family issue is not accurately identified, the family and the nurse will collect data, design interventions, and implement plans of care that do not meet the family's most pressing needs. The importance of identifying the keystone family issue and making an accurate **family nursing diagnosis** is demonstrated by comparing the following two scenarios:

> ***Scenario 1:*** *The hypothesized keystone issue for the Raggs family was identified by the referral source: Is insulin being administered correctly by the Raggs family? On the basis of this keystone issue, the nurse collected only information that pertained to that single problem. The family nursing diagnosis was Lack of Family Knowledge related to the administration of insulin secondary to a new diagnosis of insulin-dependent diabetes as evidenced by the following:*
> - *Verbal statements of concern about giving injections*
> - *Difficulty drawing up the accurate amount of insulin*
> - *Questions about the storage of insulin*

This nursing diagnosis focuses further data collection and plan for interventions on the following:

- *Psychomotor skills of family members necessary to give the insulin injection*
- *Correct amount of insulin to give according to the blood glucose level*
- *Correct storage and handling of the medication and the equipment*

By not looking at the whole family, the nurse based the keystone family nursing diagnosis on a single problem confronting the family—administration of the medication.

Scenario 2: *The nurse conducts the family assessment by focusing on the whole family client story and asks the following keystone question: What is the best way to ensure that the Raggs family understands how to manage the new diagnosis of insulin-dependent diabetes? After collecting and clustering the evidence into logical groupings, the family nursing diagnosis identified was Lack of Family Knowledge related to nutrition management of a family member who has been newly diagnosed with insulin-dependent diabetes. The administration of the medication is only one aspect of the health problem confronting the Raggs family.*

Asking a broader question allows the nurse to view the whole picture of the family dealing with this specific health concern and results in a more comprehensive holistic data-collection process. More evidence was collected in this case scenario because more options for possible interventions were considered concurrently in the clustering of the data. Areas of data collection for this nursing diagnosis included the following:

- *Administration of medication*
- *Nutritional management*
- *Blood glucose monitoring*
- *Activity/exercise*
- *Coping with a changed diagnosis*
- *Knowledge of the pathophysiology of diabetes*

The keystone issue for the family centered on nutritional management, which ultimately affects the administration of medication (Boxes 18-9 and 18-10).

BRIEFLY NOTED

Assessment is interactive. As you are evaluating families, they are evaluating you.

FRAMING

The major difference between these two scenarios was the way the nurse framed the question while listening to the family client story. In the first scenario, the nurse asked a question that allowed only one aspect of the family health to be considered. This type of step-by-step problem-solving process is tedious and time consuming, and it is likely to cause error in identifying the most pressing (or keystone) family nursing diagnosis. In the second

---

Box 18-9 Helpful Reflective Questions in Family Nursing Diagnosis

- Am I continuing to focus on the central issue?
- Am I sure that I am understanding the information correctly?
- Is everyone involved focused on the central issue?
- Have I collected enough information to be drawing inferences or conclusions?
- Have I made any assumptions that might not be true or valid?

Box 18-10 Reflective Critical Thinking Process for the Nurse

1. Is this plan being developed in collaboration with the family?
2. Will the proposed approaches enhance family strengths and increase independence of family members?
3. Is this action within the information and skill level of the family members or their own resources?
4. On a scale of 1 to 10 (with 10 being the highest), how committed and motivated are family members to adhere to the plan?
5. Are there adequate resources available to carry out the plan?
6. How would family members respond to these questions?
7. Will this action diminish or strengthen the coping ability of the family?

From Friedman MM et al: *Family nursing: research, theory and practice,* ed 5, Norwalk, Conn, 2003, Prentice Hall.

HOW TO   Plan for the Assessment Process

Assessment of families requires an organized plan before you see the family. This planning includes the following:

1. Why are you seeing the family?
2. Who will be present during the interview?
3. Where will you see the family, and how will the space be arranged?
4. What are you going to be assessing?
5. How are you going to collect the data?
6. What are you going to do with the information you find?

---

scenario, the nurse asked a question that allowed critical thinking about several options concurrently. The nurse did the following:

- Gathered information from the referral source
- Conducted an assessment of the impact of the new diagnosis on the whole family
- Made a clinical judgment that had a more far-reaching effect on the health outcome of the family

The keystone family issue needs to be stated in a way that matches the nursing classification system used in the agency. Nursing classification systems related to families include the North American Nursing Diagnosis Association system (North American Nursing Diagnosis Association, 2007), the Omaha System (Martin, 2005), the *Diagnostic and Statistical Manual of Mental Disorders* (American Psychiatric Association, 2000), and the *International Classification of*

Diseases (American Medical Association, 2004). After the keystone family diagnosis has been identified and verified with the family, the next steps are as follows:
- Determine the present state
- Determine the outcome
- Test the evaluation criteria determining if the outcome has been achieved

PRESENT STATE AND OUTCOME TESTING

On the basis of the keystone issue, note the following:
- The present state of the health issue challenging the family is clearly identified.
- The nurse works with the family to determine a realistic outcome.
- The outcome depends on the ability of the family to successfully adapt to the health issue.
- The family's strengths, the pattern of family response in similar past situations, and the path of the family health care problem are considered.

The nurse can predict the course of events or the pattern of change expected given information about the family. The types of outcomes possible depend on the focus of the problem for the individual and the family as a whole. The outcome may be directed at the following:
- Preventing a potential problem
- Minimizing the problem
- Stabilizing the problem
- Recognizing that the problem is deteriorating

The outcome is the opposite of the presenting problem and should be stated in positive language. A following case example shows the importance of focusing on the outcome:

> *Scenario 3: The home hospice nurse has been working with the Brush family for 3 weeks. The family consists of the following members: Dylan (the father), Myra (the mother), William (10 years old), Jessica (7 years old), and Beatrice (Myra's 73-year-old mother).*
>
> *Family story: Beatrice was diagnosed with terminal liver cancer 4 weeks ago. The Brush family agreed that Beatrice should live with them and be cared for in their home until her death. Beatrice has other children who live in the same city. The hospice nurse, in collaboration with the Brush family, identified the following keystone family diagnosis:* Family Role Conflict *related to the maternal grandmother moving into her daughter's home after being diagnosed with terminal liver cancer. Myra showed her role conflict by stating, "Sometimes I do not know who I am—daughter, nurse, mother, or wife." The outcome is family role sharing, which will be evaluated by statements that describe minimized role strain and spreading the caregiver role among the extended family members.*
>
> *The nurse, who understands systems theory, knows that what affects one member of the family affects all members of the family. One of the strengths of the family is agreement that caring for the dying grandmother in the home is the right ethical choice for them.*

> *Disrupting the family and their expected roles will be short term because the grandmother will probably not live for more than 4 months. The family has a strong internal and external support system. The extended family is willing to be involved in Beatrice's care. The area of change to be experienced by the family members involves family roles and the expected behaviors of each family member. The course of events is short term, but Myra's role conflict may increase when her caregiver role becomes more intense as her mother gets worse. The type of outcome is to mobilize resources to minimize Myra's role conflict.*
>
> *The Brush family story was viewed through the frame of systems theory, and the following interventions were implemented:*
> - *Assisting the family in the role negotiation of tasks and who performs them*
> - *Educating family members so they can safely care for Beatrice*
> - *Providing respite care for all family members involved in the care process*
> - *Referring the case to home hospice*

INTERVENTION AND DECISION MAKING

During the intervention and decision-making step, nurses need to recognize that the family has the right to make its own health decisions. The role of the nurse is as follows:
- To offer guidance to the family
- To provide information
- To assist in the planning process

The nurse and family work in a partnership to design and implement a plan of action on the basis of the identified outcome. The nurse may assist the family by the following (Friedman, Bowden, and Jones, 2003):
- Providing direct care that the family cannot provide
- Removing barriers to needed services, which helps the family to function
- Improving the capacity of the family to act on its own behalf and to assume responsibility

Decision making can be based on compiling nursing interventions by category (as in the Nursing Intervention Classification [NIC] system), on the Omaha System, or on levels of prevention. See "Evidence-Based Practice" box on p. 324.

CLINICAL JUDGMENT

In making clinical judgments or evaluating the outcome, nurses engage in critical thinking. When an outcome is not achieved, the nurse and the family work together to determine the barriers. Family apathy and indecision are known to be barriers in family nursing (Friedman, Bowden, and Jones, 2003). Friedman et al (2003) also identified the following nurse-related barriers to achieving the outcome:
- Imposing ideas
- Applying negative labels
- Overlooking family strengths
- Neglecting cultural or gender implications

Evidence-Based Practice

Bean, Crane, and Lewis (2002) conducted a content analysis of 440 studies to look at their attention to U.S. ethnic groups. Articles were analyzed according to ethnic population of interest, topic of study, implications for professionals, funding source, and demographic characteristics. Their findings showed an increase in sensitivity and a dedication to ethnic diversity in family science literature. They reported progress in researching African-American and Latino families. However, other ethnic groups are not well researched. Fewer than 16% of the studies focused on other ethnic groups. Only 25% of the studies were found to make specific recommendations.

NURSE USE: These findings raise questions about the ability to generalize nursing interventions to families. This is a serious issue for social and/or family policymakers, because a policy made for families of one culture may not apply to families of another culture.

From Bean RA, Crane DR, Lewis TL: Basic research and implications for practice in family science: a content analysis and status report for U.S. ethnic groups, *Family Relations: Interdisc J Appl Family Stud* 51(1):15–21, 2002.

Family apathy may occur because of value differences between the nurse and the family, because the family is overcome with a sense of hopelessness, because it views the problems as too overwhelming, or because its members have a fear of failure. Additional factors to be considered are that the family may be indecisive because of the following:

- They cannot determine which course of action is better.
- They have an unexpressed fear or concern.
- They have a pattern of making decisions only when faced with a crisis.

An important part of the judgment step in working with families is the decision to terminate the relationship between the nurse and the family. Termination is phasing out the nurse from family involvement. When termination is built into the interventions, the family benefits from a smooth transition process. The family is given credit for the outcomes of the interventions that they helped design. The following strategies are often used in the termination component:

- Decreasing contact with the nurse
- Extending invitations to the family for follow-up
- Making referrals when appropriate

The termination should include a summative evaluation meeting, in which the nurse and family put a formal closure to their relationship.

When termination with a family occurs suddenly, it is important for the nurse to determine the forces bringing about the closure. The family may be initiating the termination prematurely, which requires a renegotiating process. The insurance or agency requirements may be placing a financial constraint on the amount of time the nurse can work with a family. Regardless of how termination comes about, it is an important aspect in working with families.

REFLECTION

The last step in the OPT clinical reasoning model is for nurses to engage in critical, creative, and concurrent reflection about the case. This step has the following three distinct parts:

1. Reflect on the client outcome that is or is not being achieved
2. Reflect on and add the details of this case to the nurse's mental file (or library of knowledge)
3. Engage in self-judgment

By stepping outside the action and viewing the whole picture, including the self, nurses get different perspectives on the problem facing the family (Pesut and Herman, 1999). Seeing the whole picture from outside the action increases the options for action.

CASE STUDY

Marty Belfair, a 55-year-old accountant, is the father of three children and has been married to his wife, Joanne, for the past 25 years. Mr. Belfair's children are Joshua, age 20, Mary, age 17, and Kyle, age 14. Mr. Belfair's mother, Delia, has lived in the Belfair household since her husband, Martin, passed away 4 years ago from lung cancer. A few months ago, Mr. Belfair was diagnosed with bladder cancer. After surgery and chemotherapy, the cancer still has not receded. The family physician estimates Mr. Belfair has only 5 months to live.

Alex Von Bremen is the hospice nurse working with the Belfair family. Mr. Von Bremen explains to the Belfairs that his goal is to work with the whole family in coping with Mr. Belfair's illness. Mr. Von Bremen asks each family member, "How do you feel Mr. Belfair's illness will affect the way in which the members of your family function and interact with one another?"

Joanne Belfair responds, "Right now we do not talk about Marty being sick. It is the elephant in the room. I am afraid that if Marty does not get better, the whole family will fall apart and never see each other."

Delia Belfair shared, "I do not know where I will live. We don't talk about it. I don't know if I'm welcome to stay if Marty's not here."

Mr. Belfair encourages his family: "I know my illness is hard to accept now, but we have been through tough times in the past and the family stayed together then. Remember when I lost my job? We all made sacrifices for the family and were a stronger family as a result."

FAMILY NURSING ASSESSMENT

Family nursing assessment is the cornerstone for family nursing interventions. By using a systematic process, family problem areas are identified and family strengths are emphasized as the building blocks for interventions. Building the interventions with family-identified problems and strengths allows for equal family and provider commitment to the

Box 18-11	Assumptions Underlying Friedman's Family Assessment Model

1. The family is a social system with functional requirements.
2. A family is a small group possessing certain generic features common to all small groups.
3. The family as a social system accomplishes functions that serve the individual and society.
4. Individuals act in accordance with a set of internalized norms and values that are learned primarily in the family through socialization.

From Friedman MM et al: *Family nursing: research theory and practice*, ed 5, Norwalk, Conn, 2003, Prentice Hall.

solutions and ensures more successful interventions. Some family assessment models that are available have been developed by nurses (Hanson, 2005). See "How To" box on p. 322.

The *Family Assessment Intervention Model* and the *Family Systems Stressor Strength Inventory (FS³I)* measure very specific dimensions of stressors and strengths in the family and give a microscopic view of family health. It is a more extensive and specific model that demands in-depth knowledge of family analysis and is useful for doing family research (Hanson and Kaakinen, 2005).

One family assessment model and approach developed by a nurse—the *Friedman Family Assessment Model and Short Form* (Friedman, Bowden, and Jones, 2003)—is presented in Appendix G.2.

FRIEDMAN FAMILY ASSESSMENT MODEL

The Friedman Family Assessment Model (Friedman, Bowden, and Jones, 2003) draws heavily on the structure–function framework and on developmental and systems theory. The model takes a broad approach to family assessment, which views families as a subsystem of society. The family is viewed as an open social system. The family's structure (organization) and functions (activities and purposes) and the family's relationship to other social systems are the focus of this approach.

This assessment approach is important for family nurses because it enables them to assess the family system as a whole, as part of the whole of society, and as an interaction system. The general assumptions for this model are contained in Box 18-11.

The guidelines for the Friedman Family Assessment Model consist of the following six broad categories of interview questions:
1. Identifying data
2. Developmental family stage and history
3. Environmental data
4. Family structure, including communication, power structures, role structures, and family values
5. Family functions, including affective, socialization, and health care
6. Family coping

Each category has several subcategories. There are both long and short forms of this assessment tool. The short form is presented in Appendix G.2.

In summary, this approach was developed to provide guidelines for family nurses who are interviewing a family to gain an overall view of what is going on in the family. The questions are extensive, and it may not be possible to collect all the data at one visit. All the categories may not be pertinent for every family.

FUTURE IMPLICATIONS FOR SOCIAL AND FAMILY POLICY

As a profession, nursing is accountable for participating in the development of legislation and family policy. Government actions that have a direct or indirect effect on families are called *family policy*. All government actions, whether at the local, county, state, or national level, affect the family directly or indirectly, in both negative and positive ways. The range of social policy decisions that affect families is vast, such as health care access and coverage, low-income housing, social security, welfare, food stamps, pension plans, affirmative action, and education. Although all government polices affect families, the United States has no overall, official explicit family policy (Gebbie and Gebbie, 2005).

Most government policies indirectly affect families. Much debate has taken place within government regarding the definition of family. An argument often cited for the lack of more explicit family policies is related to the financial burden that would occur if the definition of family was too broad.

The national health promotion and disease prevention objectives outlined in *Healthy People 2000* (U.S. Department of Health and Human Services, 1990), *Healthy People 2010* (U.S. Department of Health and Human Services, 2000), and *Healthy Communities 2000* (American Public Health Association, 1991) have direct and indirect consequences and outcomes that affect families. The Family Leave legislation passed in the 1990s by the U.S. Congress is an example of a type of family policy that has been positive for families. A family member may take a defined amount of leave for family events (e.g., births, deaths) without fear of losing his or her job. Equally important today is the role that families will be assigned in health care reform. Because families are a primary source for health care beliefs and delivery, it is important that the issues of families and their place in health care reform be obvious.

At the beginning of the twenty-first century, it is natural and wise to look forward and speculate on the future of family nursing, families, and what this might mean for family social policy, especially since threats of bioterrorism and the effects on family stability are changing the world.

FUTURE OF FAMILIES

Each family is an unexplored mystery, unique in the ways in which it meets the needs of its members and of society. Healthy and vital families are essential to the world's future because family members are affected by what their families have invested in them or failed to provide for their growth and well-being. Families will continue to survive and serve as the basic social unit of society.

The following projections and trends for families provide an important lens through which we can reflect on the past and view the future:

- There is a decline in the percentage of nuclear American families: the nuclear family of dad, mom, and biological or adopted children declined from 40% in 1970 to 23% in 2003 (Fields, 2004).
- There is a decline in family households compared with nonfamily households. Family households consist of a householder and one or more people living together related by birth, marriage, or adoption (Simmons and O'Neill, 2001). In the 2000 census, family households made up 68% of the total households, with 76% of those family households composed of married couples (Simmons and O'Neill, 2001).
- The greatest changes in family households have involved married couples with their own children, down from 40% in 1970 to 23% in 2003; other types of family households have grown from 11% in 1970 to 16% in 2003 (Fields, 2004).
- The category of married couples without children has remained relatively stable with only a slight decline (Fields, 2004).
- The average size of all households has declined since 1970 from 3.14 to 2.57 persons per household in 2003 (Fields, 2004).
- More than 90% of Americans marry during their lifetime (Kreider, 2005). In 2001, 53% of men and 59% of women were in first-time marriages, whereas 14% of men and women had been married twice and 3% had been married three or more times (Kreider, 2005).
- Until the 1970s, loss of a spouse was the leading cause of remarriage; this has since been replaced by divorce (Coleman, Ganong, and Fine, 2000). More than 50% of divorced people remarry (Kreider, 2005).
- Whereas gender was previously a leading factor in remarriage rates, recently the person who initiated the divorce has been found to be more a significant factor (Sweeney, 2002). That is, women who initiate divorce are more likely to remarry than women who were the noninitiators. With increasing age, women's (but not men's) opportunities to remarry decline (Sweeney, 2002).
- The length of time between divorce and remarriage is less than 4 years (Coleman, Ganong, and Fine, 2000). Although some persons remarry more than once, remarriages contracted by adults over 40 years of age may be more stable than first marriages (Coleman, Ganong, and Fine, 2000).
- Since the beginning of the twentieth century, the median age for both genders at the time of first marriage has increased steadily. At the beginning of the twenty-first century, the median age of first marriage was 25.1 years for women and 26.8 years for men (Fields, 2004). On the basis of adult and teen attitudes toward family issues, this trend has been projected to continue (Thornton and Young-DeMarco, 2001).

- Between 1970 and 2000, interracial marriages increased from 310,000 to 1,464,000 according to the U.S. Bureau of the Census (World Almanac & Book of Facts, 2002). That is, interracial marriages increased from less than 1% of marriages to 2.6% of the total U.S. marriages in a 30-year period.
- Dual-career marriages, or marriages in which both partners work, have increased as more women enter the labor force.
- Dual employment positively affects children if it includes involvement in parenting, appropriate supervision, and quality childcare.
- Divorce can be said to be increasing, declining, or remaining stable, depending on the time referent. Divorce rates in the 1970s and into the mid-1980s climbed to 5.0/1000, but around 1985 through the 2000s they began to decline to 4.0/1000 (U.S. Bureau of the Census, 2005). In 2001, the median length of a marriage for divorcing couples was 8 years for men and for women (Kreider, 2005).
- The characteristics of people who divorce vary by race, religion, and educational level. The divorce rate for African-Americans is higher than it is for whites, Hispanic Americans, or Asian and Pacific Islander Americans (Kreider and Fields, 2002 Teachman, Tedrow, and Crowder, 2000). Protestants have a higher divorce rate than Catholics. Women and men with at least a bachelor's degree are less likely to divorce than those who have a high school degree or less (Kreider and Fields, 2002).
- One of the most dramatic changes in family structure has been cohabitation, or living together before marriage. Seltzer (2000) suggests that people cohabit for three reasons: some cohabitants would marry but do not do so for economic reasons; others seek a more equalitarian relationship; and others use cohabitation as a trial period to negotiate and assess whether to marry (King and Scott, 2005). The increase in cohabitation crosses all education groups for whites, African-Americans, and Hispanic Americans, but the increase was greater for non-Hispanic whites and for those with a high school degree or less (Seltzer, 2000).
- In the 2000 U.S. Census, 3.8 million households (7.6 million people) reported cohabitation.
- Birthrates in the United States declined during the 1990s, from 4158/1000 women who have children to 4022/1000 (U.S. Bureau of the Census, 2005). In the United States, the trend has been to delay the birth of the first child and to have fewer children. The average age of the mother changed during the past 20 years, with fewer young mothers and more older mothers (U.S. Bureau of the Census, 2005).
- The number of children born to unmarried women continues to climb. In 2002 it is estimated that 34% of all births were to unmarried mothers, compared with 26.6% in 1990 (U.S. Bureau of the Census, 2005). The largest increase has been in unmarried women between 20 and 24 years of age, with data now being reported on women 35 and older (U.S. Bureau of the Census, 2005).

- In 2003 there were approximately 10 million single-mother households and just over 2 million single-father households (Fields, 2004).
- In 2002, 19.8 million children (28% of all children) lived with unmarried parents (Fields, 2004).
- The number of single-parent households varies by ethnicity.
- The most important increase in the number of single-parent families involves single-mother households, which jumped from 11% in 1970 to 26% in 2000; father-only families jumped from 1% to 6% during that same period of time (Fields, 2004).
- Single-parent mothers at the poverty level decreased according to the 2000 U.S. Census, going from 27.8% in 1999 to 24.7% in 2000.
- The number of children who live with a grandparent increased from 3 million in 1970 to 5.6 million in 2002 (Fields, 2004). Of the 5.6 million, 1.3 million live with a grandparent without either of their parents present in the household (Fields, 2003). This change has altered the traditional supportive role of grandparenting to that of primary childrearing.

BARRIERS TO PRACTICING FAMILY NURSING

Many barriers exist that affect the practice of family nursing in a community setting. Two significant barriers to family nursing are the narrow definition of family used by health care providers and social policymakers and the lack of consensus concerning what constitutes a healthy family. Other barriers to practicing family nursing are summarized by Hanson (2005), as follows:

- Until the past decade, most practicing nurses had little exposure to family concepts during their undergraduate education and have continued to practice using the individual focus. Family nursing was viewed as "common sense" and not a theory-based nursing approach.
- Good comprehensive family assessment models, instruments, and strategies in nursing have been lacking.
- Nursing has strong historical ties with the medical model, which views families as structure and not central to individual health care.
- The traditional charting system in health care has been oriented to the individual.
- The medical and nursing diagnosis systems used in health care are disease centered, and diseases are focused on individuals.
- Insurance carriers have traditionally based coverage and reimbursement on the individual, not on the family unit.
- The hours during which health care systems provide services to families are at times of the day when family members cannot accompany one another.

These and other obstacles to family nursing practice are slowly shifting. Nurses must continue to lobby for changes that are more conducive to caring for the family as a whole.

Healthy People 2010

Family Implications
The following objectives directly or indirectly name families as the target for the objective:

1-6 Reduce the proportion of families that experience difficulties or delays in obtaining health care or do not receive needed care for one or more family members
7-7 Increase the proportion of health care organizations that provide patient and family education
8-18 Increase the proportion of persons who live in homes tested for radon concentrations
8-19 Increase the number of new homes constructed to be radon resistant
8-22 Increase the proportion of persons living in pre-1950s housing that have been tested for the presence of lead-based paint
8-23 Reduce the proportion of occupied housing units that are substandard
9-12 Reduce the proportion of married couples whose ability to conceive or maintain a pregnancy is impaired
11-1 Increase the proportion of households with access to the Internet at home
15-4 Reduce the proportion of persons living in homes with firearms that are loaded and unlocked
15-25 Reduce residential fire deaths
19-18 Increase food security among U.S. households and in so doing reduce hunger
29-9 Increase the use of appropriate personal protective eyewear in recreational activities and hazardous situations around the home

From U.S. Department of Health and Human Services: *Healthy People 2010*, Washington, DC, 2000, U.S. Government Printing Office.

HEALTHY PEOPLE 2010 AND FAMILY IMPLICATIONS

Although *Healthy People 2010* emphasizes individual and community issues, some objectives relate specifically to families or homes, as shown in the *Healthy People 2010* box.

CLINICAL APPLICATION

The idealized family portrayed in the media during the twentieth century consists of a working father, a mother who stays home, and their children. Many families today compare their turbulent, hectic lives with those of the fictionalized past and find their situations wanting.

A. *Did the idealized version of the traditional family ever really exist?*
B. *Some people believe that American families are in decline, whereas others believe that families are healthy. What do you think?*
C. *What seems to be happening with the definition of American families?*
D. *How does a definition of family influence our care and society's support of families?*
Answers are in the back of the book.

REMEMBER THIS!

- Families are the context within which health care decisions are made. Nurses are responsible for assisting families in meeting health care needs.
- Family nursing is practiced in all settings.
- Family nursing is a specialty area that has a strong theoretical base and is more than just common sense.
- Family demographics is the study of structures of families and households, as well as events that alter the family such as marriage, divorce, births, cohabitation, and dual careers.
- Demographic trends affecting the family include the age of individuals when they marry, an increase in interracial marriages with subsequent children, an increase in the number of divorced people remarrying, an increase in dual-career marriages, an increase in the number of children from families in which marriage is disrupted, a large increase in the divorce rate, a dramatic increase in cohabitation, an increase in the number of children who spend time in a single-parent family, a delay of childbirth, an increase in the number of children born to women who are single or who have never married, and an increase in the number of children who live with grandparents.
- Traditionally, families have been defined as a nuclear family: mother, father, and young children. A variety of family definitions exist, such as a group of two or more, a unique social group, and two or more persons joined together by emotional bonds.
- The six historical functions performed by families are economic survival, reproduction, protection, cultural heritage, socialization of young, and conferring status. Contemporary functions involve relationships and health.
- Family structure refers to the characteristics, gender, age, and number of the individual members who make up the family unit.
- Family health is difficult to define, but it includes the biological, psychological, sociological, cultural, and spiritual factors of the family system.
- The four approaches to viewing families are family as context, family as client, family as a system, and family as a component of society.
- Structure–function theory views the family as a social system with members who have specific roles and functions.
- Systems theory describes families as a unit of the whole, composed of members whose interactional patterns are the focus of attention.
- Family developmental theory is one theoretical framework used to study families. This approach emphasizes how families change over time and focuses on interactions and relationships among family members.
- Interactional theory focuses on the family as a unit of interacting personalities and examines the communication processes by which family members relate to one another.
- Nurses should ask clients whom they consider to be family and then include those members in the health care plan.
- The OPT family nursing process is a dynamic, systematic, organized method of critically thinking about the family.
- The purpose of the initial family interview is based on the keystone issue.
- It is important for the nurse to recognize that the family has the right to make its own health decisions.
- The nurse, in working with families, must evaluate the family outcomes and response to the plan, not the success of the interventions.
- The Friedman Family Assessment Model takes a macroscopic approach to family assessment, which views the family as a subsystem of society.
- The future of family, health care, and nursing is not an exact science. However, all areas are changing and many challenges are to be understood and overcome in this new century.

WHAT WOULD YOU DO?

1. Select six or more health professionals and ask them to define *family*. Analyze the responses for commonalities and differences. Write your definition of family.
2. From the chapter, define *family nursing*. Does this match your definition? Why? Why not? State your definition, and explain why yours is different from the one in the chapter.
3. Form small groups and discuss the implications of family demography and demographic trends for nursing.
4. Develop a typology of the different family structures and household arrangements representative of your community. This information may be available from various sources, such as the health department, schools, other social and welfare agencies, and census data.
5. Describe how a family assessment is different from an individual client assessment process.
6. What kind of difficulties could you experience when arranging for a family assessment interview?
7. Break into small groups and discuss the family from the point of view of each of the four family social science theories. Which theory would you choose to apply in your practice and why?

■ REFERENCES

American Medical Association: *International classification of diseases: clinical modifications (ICD-9-CM), vols 1 and 2, rev 9*, Dover, Del, 2004, AMA.

American Psychiatric Association: *Diagnostic & statistical manual of mental disorders (DSM-IV-TR)*, ed 4, Washington, DC, 2000, APA.

American Public Health Association: *Healthy Communities 2000: model standards: guidelines for community attainment of year 2000 national health objectives*, Washington, DC, 1991, The Association.

Bean RA, Crane DR, Lewis TL: Basic research and implications for practice in family science: a content analysis and status report for US ethnic groups, *Family Relations: Interdisc J Appl Family Stud* 51:15–21, 2002.

Bomar P: *Nurses and family health promotion: concepts, assessment, and interventions*, ed 3, Philadelphia, 2004, Saunders.

Boss P: *Family stress management*, ed 2, Newbury Park, Calif, 2001, Sage.

Carter B, McGoldrick M: The family life cycle and family therapy: an overview. In Carter B, McGoldrick M, editors: *The changing family life cycle: a framework for family therapy*, New York, 1998, Gardner Press.

Coleman M, Ganong L, Fine M: Reinvestigating remarriage: another decade of progress, *J Marriage Fam* 62:1288–1307, 2000.

Duvall EM, Miller BL: *Marriage and family development*, ed 6, New York, 1985, Harper & Row.

Fields J: *Children's living arrangements and characteristics: March 2002. Current population reports, P20–547*, Washington, DC, 2003, U.S. Census Bureau.

Fields J: *American's families and living arrangements: 2003. Current population reports, P20–553*, Washington, DC, 2004, U.S. Census Bureau.

Friedman MM, Bowden VR, Jones EG: *Family nursing: research, theory and practice*, ed 5, Upper Saddle River, NJ, 2003, Prentice Hall.

Gebbie K, Gebbie E: Families, nursing and social policy. In Hanson SMH, Gedaly-Duff V, Kaakinen JR, editors: *Family health care nursing*, ed 3, Philadelphia, 2005, FA Davis.

Hanson SMH: Family health care nursing: an overview. In Hanson SMH, Gedaly-Duff V, Kaakinen JR, editors: *Family health care nursing: theory, practice and research*, ed 3, Philadelphia, 2005, FA Davis.

Hanson SMH, Kaakinen JR: Theoretical foundations for family nursing. In Hanson SMH, Gedaly-Duff V, Kaakinen JR, editors: *Family health care nursing: theory, practice and research*, Philadelphia, 2005, FA Davis.

Hawley DR: Clinical implications of family resilience, *Am J Fam Ther* 28:101–116, 2000.

King V, Scott ME: A comparison of cohabiting relationships among older and younger adults, *J Marriage Fam* 67:271–285, 2005.

Kreider RM, Fields JM: *Number, timing and duration of marriages and divorces: 1996*, U.S. Census Bureau, Department of Commerce, 2002, U.S. Government Printing Office, pp 1–20.

Kreider RM: *Number, timing and duration of marriages and divorces: 2001. Current Population Reports, P70–97*, Washington, DC, 2005, U.S. Census Bureau.

Martin KS: *The Omaha System: a key to practice, documentation, and information management*, ed 2, St Louis, 2005, Elsevier.

McKenry PC, Price SJ, editors: *Families and change: coping with stressful events and transitions*, ed 2, Newbury Park, Calif, 2000, Sage.

North American Nursing Diagnosis Association: *Nursing diagnoses: definitions and classifications, 2007–2008*, Philadelphia, 2007, NANDA.

Patterson JM: Integrating family resilience and family stress theory, *J Marriage Fam* 64(5):349–360, 2002.

Peterson GH: *Making healthy families*, Berkeley, Calif, 2000, Shadow and Light.

Pesut D, Herman J: *Clinical reasoning: the art and science of critical and creative thinking*, Boston, 1999, Delmar.

Satariano HJ, Briggs NJ: The good family syndrome. In Wegner GD, Alexander RJ, editors: *Readings in family nursing*, ed 2, Philadelphia, 1999, Lippincott, Williams & Wilkins.

Seltzer JA: Families formed outside of marriage, *J Marriage Fam* 62:1247–1268, 2000.

Simmons R, O'Neill G: *Households and families: 2000*, U.S. Census Bureau, Department of Commerce, 2001, U.S. Government Printing Office, pp 1–8.

Sweeney MM: Remarriage and the nature of divorce, *J Fam Issues* 33(3):410–440, 2002.

Teachman JD, Tedrow LM, Crowder KD: The changing demography of America's families, *J Marriage Fam* 62:1234–1246, 2000.

Thornton A, Young-DeMarco L: Four decades of trends in attitudes toward family issues in the United States: the 1960s through the 1990s, *J Marriage Fam* 63:1009–1037, 2001.

U.S. Bureau of the Census: *Statistical abstract of the United States, section 2, Vital statistics*, p. 57–88, 2005.

U.S. Department of Health and Human Services: *Healthy People 2000: national health promotion and disease prevention objectives*, Washington, DC, 1990, U.S. Department of Health and Human Services.

U.S. Department of Health and Human Services: *Healthy People 2010*, Washington, DC, 2000, U.S. Government Printing Office.

Walsh F: A family resilience framework: innovative practice applications, *Fam Relat* 51:130–137, 2002.

White JM, Klein DN: *Family theories: an introduction*, ed 2, Thousand Oaks, Calif, 2002, Sage.

World Almanac & Book of Facts: *Interracial married couples in the U.S., 1960–2000*, New York, 2002, World Almanac Books.

evolve   http://evolve.elsevier.com/stanhope/foundations

Family Health Risks

Debra Gay Anderson
Heather Ward
Diane C. Hatton

ADDITIONAL RESOURCES

These related resources are found either in the appendix at the back of this book or on the book's website at http://evolve.elsevier.com/stanhope/foundations.

Evolve Website

- Community Assessment Applied
- Case Study, with questions and answers
- Quiz review questions
- WebLinks, including link to *Healthy People 2010* website

Real World Community Health Nursing: An Interactive CD-ROM, second edition

If you are using this CD-ROM in your course, you will find the following activities related to this chapter:
- *Stages of Family Development* in **Family Health**
- *Friedman Family Assessment Model* in **Family Health**
- *You Conduct the Assessment: Single Parent Family, Aging Family, Multigenerational Family* in **Family Health**

OBJECTIVES

After reading this chapter, the student should be able to:

1. Analyze the various approaches to defining and conceptualizing family health.
2. Determine the major risks to family health.
3. Study the interrelationships among individual health, family health, and community health.
4. Explain the relevance of knowledge about family structures, roles, and functions for family-focused, community-oriented nursing.
5. Discuss the implications of policy and policy decisions, at all government levels, on families.
6. Explain the application of the nursing process (assessment, planning, implementation, evaluation) to reducing family health risks and promoting family health.

CHAPTER OUTLINE

EARLY APPROACHES TO FAMILY HEALTH RISKS
Health of Families
Health of the Nation
CONCEPTS IN FAMILY HEALTH RISK
Family Health
Health Risk

Health Risk Appraisal
Health Risk Reduction
Life Events
Family Crisis
MAJOR FAMILY HEALTH RISKS AND NURSING INTERVENTIONS
Family Health Risk Appraisal

The authors acknowledge the contribution of Carol Loveland-Cherry to the content of this chapter.

COMMUNITY-ORIENTED NURSING APPROACHES TO FAMILY HEALTH RISK REDUCTION
Home Visits

Contracting with Families
Empowering Families
COMMUNITY RESOURCES

KEY TERMS

behavioral risk: personal health habits and behaviors (e.g., diet patterns) that contribute to individual and family health status.

biological risk: a potential health danger for a person who may be prone to certain illnesses because of inherited genetics or family lifestyle patterns.

contracting: making an agreement between two or more parties involving a shift in responsibility and control toward a shared effort by client and professional as opposed to an effort by the professional alone.

economic risk: a possible danger to a family's health determined by the relationship between family financial resources and the demands on those resources.

empowerment: helping people acquire the skills and information necessary for informed decision making and ensuring that they have the authority to make decisions that affect them.

family crisis: a situation in which the demands of the situation exceed the resources and coping capacity of the family.

family health: a condition including the promotion and maintenance of physical, mental, spiritual, and social health for the family unit and for individual family members.

health risk appraisal: the process of identifying and analyzing an individual's prognostic characteristics of health and comparing them with those of a standard age group, thereby making it possible to predict a person's likelihood of prematurely developing the health problems that have high morbidity and mortality in this country.

health risk reduction: application of selected interventions to control or reduce risk factors and minimize the incidence of associated disease and premature mortality. Risk reduction is reflected in greater congruity between appraised and achievable ages.

health risks: the factors that determine or influence whether disease or other unhealthy results occur.

home visits: provision of community health nursing care where the individual resides.

in-home phase: the actual visit of the nurse to the home; it gives the nurse the opportunity to assess the family's neighborhood and community resources, as well as the home and family interactions.

initiation phase: the first contact between the nurse and the family. It provides the foundation for an effective therapeutic relationship.

life-event risks: age-related risks to a person's health that often occur during transitions from one developmental stage to another.

policy: a settled course of action to be followed by a government or institution to obtain a desired end.

postvisit phase: after a home visit is concluded, the nurse documents the visit and the services provided.

previsit phase: contact between the nurse and the family before an actual home visit is made.

risk: the probability of some event or outcome occurring within a specified period of time.

social risks: risky social situations that can contribute to the stressors experienced by families. If adequate resources and coping processes are not available, breakdowns in health can occur.

termination phase: when the purpose of a home visit has been accomplished, the nurse reviews with the family what has occurred and what has been accomplished. This provides a basis for planning further home visits.

transitions: movement from one developmental or health stage or condition to another that may be a time of potential risk for families.

A focus on the family is vital in promoting the health of individuals as well as the health of the community (Friedman, 2002; Nightingale et al, 1978). The family as a client unit is basic to the practice of community-oriented nursing, and nurses are responsible for promoting healthy families in society. Families in the twenty-first century continue to be more diverse. The purpose of this chapter is to note the influences, both individual and in society, that place families at risk for poor health outcomes and to discuss how positive outcomes for families can be accomplished.

It is important to place the family in the context of the twenty-first century. Americans tend to idealize *family* and wish for a return to family values and a golden past. Instead

of looking into the past and wishing for a time when families were more cohesive, a look at the future is needed to recognize and to build on families' strengths. Rather than arguing for a return to the traditional family (male breadwinner and woman at home), serious discussions are needed about how to make today's diverse families succeed. Building support for families within society will lead to healthier families. Therefore nurses should be involved in community assessment, planning, development, and evaluation activities that emphasize family issues and how to sustain families.

The family is both an important environment affecting the health of individuals and a social unit whose health is basic to that of the community and the larger population.

It is within the family that health values, health habits, and health risk perceptions are developed, organized, and performed. Individuals' health behaviors are affected by and acted out within the family environment, the larger community, and society. In the same manner, it is in the context of community norms and values that family health habits are developed. For example, in a television commercial for an over-the-counter stimulant, a man is featured who is able to coach his child's basketball team, work at a rehabilitation center, and work as a borough inspector for the city, all done while he is pursuing a college degree at night. The commercial credits the drug for providing the man with the energy needed to be successful in all of these areas. The message is clear: you can, and must, do it all, and taking drugs to succeed is a viable option. The risks to individual and family health are affected by the social norms—in this example, the norm is increasing productivity through drugs.

To intervene effectively and appropriately with families to reduce their health risk and thereby promote their health, it is necessary to understand family structure and functioning, family theory, nursing theory, and models of health risk. However, it is necessary to go beyond the individual and the family and understand the complex environment in which the family exists. Increasing evidence of the effects of social, biological, economic, and life events on health requires a broader approach to addressing health risks for families. Pender et al (2005) identified the following six categories of risk factors:

1. Genetics
2. Age
3. Biological characteristics
4. Personal health habits
5. Lifestyle
6. Environment

In this chapter, family health risks in these six categories are identified and analyzed, and approaches to reducing these risks are discussed. Options for structuring nursing interventions with families to decrease health risks and to promote health and well-being are explored.

EARLY APPROACHES TO FAMILY HEALTH RISKS

HEALTH OF FAMILIES

Historically, studies of the family in health and illness focused on the following three major areas:

1. The effect of illness on families
2. The role of the family in the cause of disease
3. The role of the family in its use of services

In his classic review of the family as an important unit, Litman (1974) pointed out the important role that the family (as a primary unit of health care) plays in health and illness and emphasized that the relationship between health, health behavior, and family "is a highly dynamic one in which each may have a dramatic effect on the other" (Litman, 1974, p. 495). Mauksch (1974) proposed the idea of distinguishing between family health and individual health. Pratt's (1976)

examination of the role of the family in health and illness included the role of family health in promoting behavior. Pratt proposed the *energized family* as being an ideal family type that was most effective in meeting health needs. The energized family is characterized by the following:

- Promotion of freedom and change
- Active contact with a variety of other groups and organizations
- Flexible role relationships
- Equal power structure
- A high degree of autonomy in family members

Doherty and McCubbin (1985) proposed a family health and illness cycle with the following six phases:

1. Family health promotion
2. Family risk reduction
3. The family's vulnerability to illness
4. Their illness response
5. Their interaction with the health care system
6. Their ways of adapting to illness

HEALTH OF THE NATION

Increased attention has been given to improving the health of everyone in the United States. As a result of major public health and scientific advances, the leading causes of morbidity and mortality shifted from infectious diseases to chronic diseases, accidents, and violence, all of which have strong lifestyle and environmental components. A population-focused study in Alameda County, California (Belloc and Breslow, 1972) demonstrated relationships between the following seven lifestyle habits and decreased morbidity and mortality:

1. Sleeping 7 to 8 hours daily
2. Eating breakfast almost every day
3. Never or rarely eating between meals
4. Being at or near the recommended height-adjusted weight
5. Never smoking cigarettes
6. Using no or only a moderate amount of alcohol
7. Engaging in physical activity regularly

These lifestyle health habits are still important today for improved health in the twenty-first century.

A growing body of literature supports the notion that lifestyle and the environment interact with heredity to cause disease. In response to these findings and the limited effect of medical interventions on the growing numbers of injuries and chronic disease, the government launched a major effort to study the health status of the population. Part of this effort was a report by the Division of Health Promotion and Disease Prevention of the Institute of Medicine that examined how the physical, socioeconomic, and family environments related to decreasing risk and promoting health (Nightingale et al, 1978). The Surgeon General's Report on Health Promotion and Disease Prevention (Califano, 1979) described the risks to good health. Health objectives for the nation were established and then evaluated and restated for the year 2000 and again for 2010 (U.S. Department of Health and Human Services, 2000).

From U.S. Department of Health and Human Services: *Healthy People 2010: national health promotion and disease prevention objectives*, ed 2, Washington, DC, 2000, U.S. Government Printing Office.

Healthy People 2010

Objectives Related to Family and Home Health

1-6 Reduce the proportion of families that experience difficulties or delays in obtaining health care or do not receive needed care for one or more family members

7-7 Increase the proportion of health care organizations that provide patient and family education

8-16 Reduce indoor allergen levels

8-18 Increase the proportion of persons who live in homes tested for radon concentration

9-12 Reduce the proportion of married couples whose ability to conceive or maintain a pregnancy is impaired

19-18 Increase food security among U.S. households, and in so doing reduce hunger

27-9 Reduce the proportion of children who are regularly exposed to tobacco smoke at home

The notion of **risk**, a factor predisposing or increasing the likelihood of ill health, takes on increased importance. Specific attention is paid to those environmental and behavioral factors that lead to ill health with or without the influence of heredity. Reducing health risks is a major step toward improving the health of the nation. Although the family is considered an important environment related to achieving important health objectives, limited attention has been given to (or research done on) family health risk and the role of society in promoting healthy families. The *Healthy People 2010* box shows objectives that relate to families.

CONCEPTS IN FAMILY HEALTH RISK

Two things motivate individuals to participate in health behaviors:

1. A desire to promote our own health using "behaviors directed toward increasing the level of well-being and actualizing the health potential of individuals, families, communities and society" (Pender et al, 2005).
2. A desire to protect our health using those behaviors "directed toward decreasing the chances of a specific illness or dysfunction in individuals, families, and communities, including active protection against unnecessary stressors" (Pender et al, 2005).

An individual can reduce health risk by engaging in health-protecting and health-promoting behaviors. Understanding family health risk requires an examination of several related concepts:

- Family health
- Family health risk
- Risk appraisal
- Risk reduction
- Life events
- Lifestyle
- Family crisis

These concepts will be defined and discussed. It is important to remember that *health* can be defined in a number of ways and that it is defined by individuals based on their own culture and value system.

FAMILY HEALTH

Family theorists refer to healthy families but generally do not define family health. Based on the variety of perspectives of family (see Chapter 18), definitions of healthy families can be seen within the guidelines of any one of the frameworks. For example, within the developmental framework, **family health** can be defined as possessing the abilities and resources to accomplish family developmental tasks. Thus the accomplishment of stage-specific tasks is one indicator of family health.

The Neuman Systems Model (Neuman and Fawcett, 2002) defines family health in terms of system stability as characterized by the following five interacting sets of factors:

1. Physiological
2. Psychological
3. Sociocultural
4. Developmental
5. Spiritual

Neuman's Systems Model is a wellness-oriented model in which the nurse uses strengths and resources to keep the family healthy in the face of change. In this model, the client family is seen as a whole system with the five interacting factors that were just listed. Nurses can use preventive health care both to reduce the possibility that a family encounters a life stress and to help strengthen the family's ability to adapt to the stress. The following clinical example applies the Neuman Systems Model to one family's situation:

The Harris family consists of Ms. Harris (Gloria), 12-year-old Kevin, 8-year-old Leisha, and Ms. Harris's mother, 75-year-old Betty. Kevin was recently diagnosed with insulin-dependent diabetes mellitus, and the family was referred by the endocrinology clinic to the local health department to work with the family in adjusting to the diagnosis.

The focus of Neuman's Systems Model would be to assess the family's ability to adapt to this stressful change and then focus on their strengths to stabilize the family reaction. The answer to questions about the following *five interacting variables* would be an important component of the assessment:

1. Physiological:
   Is the Harris family physically able to deal with Kevin's illness?
   Is everyone else in the family currently healthy?
   Are there current health stressors?
2. Psychological:
   How well will the family be able to deal with the illness psychologically?
   Are their relationships stable and healthy?
   Are there any memories of other family members with diabetes?

3. Sociocultural:
   How will the sociocultural variable come into play in Kevin's illness?
   Does the family have social support?
   Are the treatment and diagnosis culturally sensitive?
   Can family members support each other?
4. Developmental:
   How will Kevin's development as a preadolescent be affected by diabetes?
   How will the family's development change?
   How will Kevin's diagnosis affect Leisha?
5. Spiritual:
   How will the family's spiritual beliefs be affected by the diagnosis?
   What effect will they have on Kevin's treatment and willingness to adhere to therapy?

HEALTH RISK

Several factors contribute to the development of healthy or unhealthy outcomes. Clearly, not everyone exposed to the same event will have the same outcome. The factors that determine or influence whether disease or other unhealthy results occur are called **health risks**. Controlling health risks is done through disease prevention and health promotion efforts. Health risks can be classified into general categories. *Healthy People 2010* (U.S. Department of Health and Human Services, 2000) identifies the following major categories:

- Inherited biological risk, including age-related risks
- Social and physical environmental risk
- Behavioral risk

Although single risk factors can influence outcomes, the combined effect of several risks has greater influence. For example, a family history of cardiovascular disease is a single biological risk factor that is affected by smoking (a behavioral risk that is more likely to occur if other family members also smoke) and by diet and exercise. Diet and exercise are influenced by family and society's norms. For example, people in the Northwest and West are more likely to eat heart-healthy diets and to exercise than are people who live in the Midwest and South; thus communities in the Northwest and West are often more supportive of exercise and bicycle paths and diets lower in fat than are communities in other parts of the United States. Therefore the health outcomes for the Northwest and West should be more positive because they support healthy diet and exercise. The combined effect of a family history, family behavioral risks, and society's influences is greater than each of the three individual risk factors (smoking, diet, and exercise).

HEALTH RISK APPRAISAL

Health risk appraisal refers to the process of assessing for the presence of specific factors in each of the categories that have been identified as being associated with an increased likelihood of an illness, such as cancer, or *an unhealthy event,* such as an automobile accident. Several techniques have been developed to accomplish health risk appraisal, including computer software programs and paper-and-pencil instruments. One technique is the Youth Risk Behavior Surveillance System instrument of the Centers for Disease Control and Prevention (2005). The general approach is to determine whether a risk factor is present and to what degree. On the basis of scientific evidence, each factor is weighted and a total score is derived. This appraisal method provides an individual score that can be examined as a whole within the family, thus appraising the health risks that are likely to be experienced by other members of the family.

HEALTH RISK REDUCTION

Health risk reduction is based on the assumption that decreasing the number or the magnitude of risks will decrease the probability of an undesired event. For example, to decrease the likelihood of adolescent substance abuse, family behaviors such as parents not drinking, alcohol not available in the home, and family contracts related to alcohol and drug use may be useful. Health risks can be reduced through a variety of approaches, such as those just described. It is important to note the specific risk and the family's tolerance of it. Pender, Murdaugh, and Parsons (2005) provide the following examples of different kinds of risks:

- Voluntarily assumed risks, such as overeating, are tolerated better than those imposed by others.
- Risks about which scientists debate and are uncertain are more feared than risks about which scientists agree, such as the causes of colon cancer.
- Risks of natural origin, such as hurricanes, are often considered less threatening than those created by humans.

Thus risk reduction is a complex process that requires knowledge of the specific risk and the family's perceptions of the nature of the risk.

BRIEFLY NOTED

Government priority for funding health risk reduction and health promotion programs, including assistance programs, would have greater benefit to the population's health than funding for illness activities.

LIFE EVENTS

Life events can increase the risk for illness and disability. These events can be categorized as either normative or nonnormative. *Normative events* are those that are generally expected to occur at a particular stage of development or of the life span. Normative events can be identified from the stages of the family life cycle (Carter and McGoldrick, 1999; Wright, 2000) (Table 19-1).

The following are examples of normative events:

- A child leaving home to go to college
- Retirement from work
- Starting a first job

Table 19-1 Family Life Cycle Stages

Family Life Cycle Stages	Key Principles for Emotional Transition Process	Second-Order Changes in Family Status Required to Proceed Developmentally
Leaving home; single young adults	Accepting emotional and financial responsibility for yourself	Differentiation of self in relation to the family of origin Development of intimate peer relationships Establishment of self as related to work and financial independence
The joining of families through marriage; the new couple	Commitment to a new system	Formation of marital system Realignment of relationships with extended families and friends to include spouse
Families with young children	Accepting new members into the system	Adjusting the marital system to make space for child(ren) Joining in child-rearing, financial, and household tasks Realignment of relationships with an extended family to include parenting and grandparenting roles
Families with adolescents	Increasing the flexibility of family boundaries to include children's independence and grandparents' frailties	Shifting of parent–child relationships to permit adolescent to move in and out of the system Refocus on midlife marital and career issues Beginning the shift toward caring for the older generation
Launching children and moving on	Accepting a multitude of exits from and entries into the family system	Renegotiation of the marital system as a dyad Development of an adult-to-adult relationship between grown children and their parents Realignment of relationships to include in-laws and grandchildren Dealing with disabilities and death of parents (grandparents)
Families in later life	Accepting the shifting of generational roles	Maintaining your own and couple functioning and interests in the face of physiological decline; exploration of new familial and social role options Support for a more central role of the middle generation Making room in the system for the wisdom and experience of the older generation, and supporting them without overfunctioning for them Dealing with the loss of a spouse, siblings, and other peers and preparing for your own death Life review and integration

From Carter B. *Expanded family life cycle:* Indiv Family & Soc, Table "Family Life Cycle Stages," © 1999. Reproduced by permission of Pearson Education, Inc.

Nonnormative events, in contrast, are those that are unpredictable, such as the following:

- A family move related to the job market
- Divorce
- Death of a child

Furthermore, life events, especially when more than one event occurs, can result in a family crisis under certain conditions.

FAMILY CRISIS

A **family crisis** occurs when the family is not able to cope with an event and becomes disorganized or dysfunctional. McKenry and Price (2005) differentiate between family resources and family coping strategies. When the demands of the situation exceed the resources of the family, a family crisis exists. When families experience a crisis or a crisis-producing event, they attempt to gather their resources to deal with the demands created by the situation. Examples of family resources are money and extended family members. Families cope by using known processes and behaviors to help them manage or adapt to the problem. Thus if a family were to experience an unexpected illness in the main wage earner, family resources might include financial assistance from relatives or emotional support. Family coping

strategies, in contrast, would include being able to ask a relative to loan them emergency funds or being able to talk with relatives about the worries they were experiencing.

On the basis of the existing literature, it is important to note that the amount of support available to families in times of crisis from government and nongovernment agencies varies in different locales. In addition, the rules and conditions of support often differ and may inhibit families from seeking support, particularly if the conditions are demeaning.

MAJOR FAMILY HEALTH RISKS AND NURSING INTERVENTIONS

As mentioned, risks to a family's health arise in three major areas:

1. Biological and age-related risks
2. Environmental risks
3. Behavioral risks

In most instances, a risk in one of these areas may not be enough to threaten family health, but a combination of risks from two or more categories could be. For example, there may be a family history of cardiovascular disease, but often the health risk is increased by an unhealthy lifestyle. An understanding of each of these categories provides the

---

- **Determinants of health:** An individual's biological makeup influences health through interactions with social and physical environments as well as behavior.
- **Behaviors:** These may be learned from other family members.
- **Social environment:** This includes the family; it is where culture, language, and personal and spiritual beliefs are learned.
- **Physical environment:** Hazards in the home may affect health negatively, and a clean and safe home has a positive influence on health.

---

basis for a comprehensive approach to family health risk assessment and intervention. The interrelationships among the various groups of risk are clear when the objectives for the nation are considered as described in *Healthy People 2010* (U.S. Department of Health and Human Services, 2000). Most of the national health objectives are based on individual risk factors; some relate to families, work, school, and communities.

FAMILY HEALTH RISK APPRAISAL

Assessment of family health risk requires many approaches. As in any assessment, the first and most important task is to get to know the family, their strengths, and their needs (see Chapter 18). This section focuses on appraisal of family health risks in the areas of biological and age-related risk, social and physical environmental risk, and behavioral risk. *Healthy People 2010* (U.S. Department of Health and Human Services, 2000) defines health and the risk categories. Box 19-1 includes several definitions related to family health.

Biological and Age-Related Risk

The family plays an important role in both the development and the management of a disease or condition. Some illnesses can be related to either genetics or lifestyle patterns. These factors contribute to the **biological risk** for certain conditions. Patterns of cardiovascular disease, for example, can often be traced through several generations of a family. Such families are said to be at risk for cardiovascular disease. How or whether cardiovascular disease is found in a family is often influenced by the lifestyle of the family. Consistent research evidence supports the positive effects of diet, exercise, and stress management on preventing or delaying cardiovascular disease. The development of hypertension can be managed by the following:

- Following a low-sodium diet
- Maintaining a normal weight
- Exercising regularly
- Employing effective stress management techniques, such as meditation

Diabetes mellitus is another disease with a strong genetic pattern, and the family plays a major role in the management of the condition. Family patterns of obesity increase individuals' risks for the following conditions (U.S. Department of Health and Human Services, 2000):

- Heart disease
- Hypertension
- Diabetes
- Some types of cancer
- Gallbladder disease

It is often difficult to separate biological risks from individual lifestyle factors.

Transitions (movement from one stage or condition to another) are times of potential risk for families. Age-related or **life-event risks** often occur during transitions from one developmental stage to another. Transitions present new situations and demands for families. These experiences often require families to do the following:

- Change behaviors, schedules, and patterns of communication
- Make new decisions
- Reallocate family roles
- Learn new skills
- Identify and learn to use new resources

The demands that transitions place on families have implications for the health of the family unit and individual family members and can be considered as life-event risks. How prepared families are to deal with a transition depends on the nature of the event. If the event is normative, or anticipated, it is possible for families to do the following:

- Identify needed resources
- Make plans
- Learn new skills
- Otherwise prepare for the event and its consequences

This kind of anticipatory preparation can increase the family's coping ability and decrease stress and negative outcomes. If, on the other hand, the event is nonnormative, or unexpected, families have little or no time to prepare and the outcome can be increased stress, crisis, or even dysfunction.

Several normative events have been identified for families. The developmental model organizes these events into stages and identifies important transition points. It provides a useful framework for identifying normative events and preparing families to cope successfully with related demands. The developmental tasks associated with each stage identify the types of skills families need. The kinds of normative events families experience are usually related to the addition or loss of a family member, such as the following:

- The birth or adoption of a child
- The death of a grandparent
- A child moving out of the home to go to school or take a job
- The marriage of a child

Health-related responsibilities are associated with each of these tasks. For example, the birth or adoption of a child requires that families learn about human growth and development, parenting, immunizations, management of childhood illnesses, normal childhood nutrition, and safety issues.

Nonnormative events present different kinds of issues for families. Unexpected events can be either positive or negative. A job promotion or inheriting a substantial sum of money may be unexpected but is usually a positive event.

More often, nonnormative events are unpleasant, such as the following:
- A major illness
- Divorce
- The death of a child
- The loss of the main family income

Lorenz, Wickrama, and Conger (2004) advocated a systems-oriented concept of family stress. They pointed out that families develop a series of processes to manage or transform inputs to the system (e.g., energy, time) to outputs (e.g., cohesion, growth, love), known as *rules of transformation*. Over time, families develop these patterns in enough quantity and variety to handle most changes and challenges. However, when families do not have an adequate variety of rules to allow them to respond to an event, the event becomes stressful. Rather than being able to deal with the situation, they fall into a pattern of trying to figure out what they need to do, and the usual tasks of the family are not adequately addressed. Rules that were implicit in the family are now reconsidered and redefined.

Furthermore, the family stress theory of Lorenz et al (2004) proposes three levels of stress:
- Level I is change "in the fairly specific patterns of behavior and transforming processes" (e.g., change in who does which household chores).
- Level II is change "in processes that are at a higher level of abstraction" (e.g., change in what are defined as family chores).
- Level III is change in highly abstract processes (e.g., family values).

Coping strategies can be identified to address each level of stress that families go through in sequence, if necessary.

CASE STUDY

The Mitchell family consists of Mr. Mitchell (Harry), Mrs. Mitchell (Shirley), 18-year-old Annie, 15-year-old Michelle, 13-year-old Sean, and 7-year-old Bobby. Mr. Mitchell is the pastor of Faith Baptist Church, where he has served the past 15 years. Mrs. Mitchell is a housemother and primary caretaker for the children.

For the past year, Mrs. Mitchell has felt tired and "rundown." At her annual physical, she describes her symptoms to her physician. After several tests, Mrs. Mitchell is diagnosed with stomach cancer. She starts to cry and says, "How will I tell my family?"

Mrs. Mitchell's primary physician refers the family to Trisha Farewell, a nurse in community health. Ms. Farewell calls the household and speaks with Mrs. Mitchell. Ms. Farewell tells Mrs. Mitchell that she was referred by the physician and she can help Mrs. Mitchell cope with the diagnosis. Mrs. Mitchell confides in Ms. Farewell that it has been 2 weeks since she received the diagnosis but she has yet to tell her husband and children. Mrs. Mitchell asks Ms. Farewell if she can help her tell her family and explain what it all means. Ms. Farewell makes an appointment to go to the Mitchell household and facilitate the family meeting.

Biological Health Risk Assessment

One of the most effective techniques for assessing the patterns of health and illness in families is the genogram. Briefly, a genogram is a drawing that shows the family unit of immediate interest and includes several generations using a series of circles, squares, and connecting lines. Basic information about the family, relationships in the family, and patterns of health and illness can be obtained by completing the genogram with the family. The following is shown in Figure 19-1:
- A square indicates a male.
- A circle indicates a female.
- An *X* through either a square or a circle indicates a death.
- Marriage is indicated by a solid horizontal line.
- Offspring/children are noted by a solid vertical line.
- A broken horizontal line indicates a divorce or separation.
- Dates of birth, marriage, death, and other important events can be indicated where appropriate.
- Major illness or conditions can be listed for each individual family member.

Patterns can be quickly assessed and provide a guide for the health interviewer about health areas that need further exploring.

The genogram in Figure 19-1 was completed for the fictional Graham family. Some of the interesting health patterns that can be seen from the genogram are the repetition of the following:
- Hypertension
- Adult onset diabetes
- Cancer
- Hypercholesterolemia

Completing a genogram requires interviews with as many family members as possible. It is suggested that a family chronology, a timeline of family events over three generations, be completed to extend the genogram for a better description of family patterns.

A more intensive and quantitative assessment of a family's biological risk can be achieved through the use of a standard family risk assessment. Because such assessments involve other areas in addition to biological risk, one will be described later, after the description of the assessment of other types of risk.

Both normative and nonnormative life events pose potential risks to the health of families. Even events that are generally viewed as being positive require changes and can place stress on a family. The normative event of the birth of a child, for example, requires considerable changes in family structures and roles. Furthermore, family functions are expanded from previous levels, requiring families to add new skills and establish additional resources. These changes can in turn result in strain and, if adequate resources are not available, stress. Therefore, to adequately assess life risks, both normative and nonnormative events occurring in the family need to be considered. Community-level support groups have been successful in assisting families in dealing with a variety of stressful situations and crises (e.g., Families Anonymous, Bereaved Parents, Parents and Friends of Lesbian and Gay

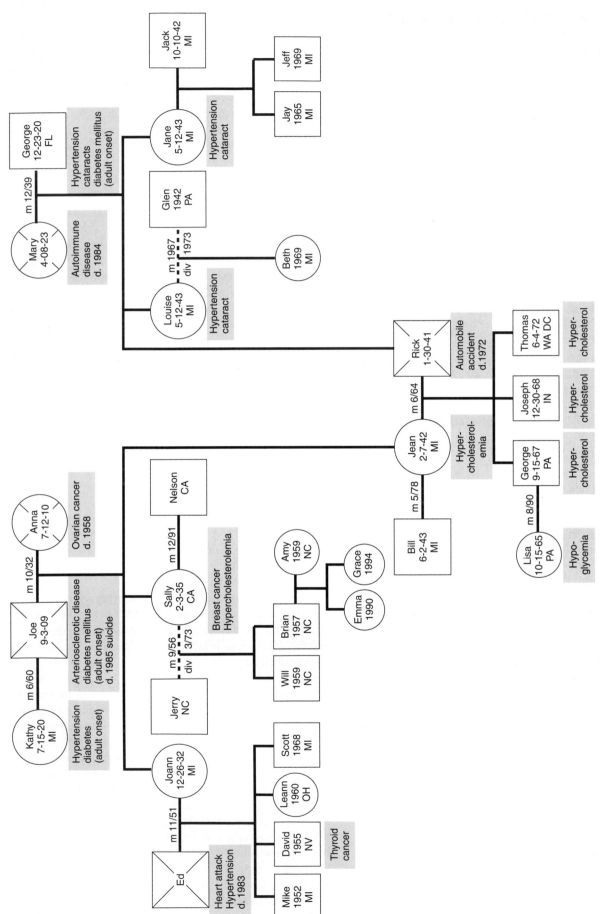

FIGURE 19-1 Family genogram of the Graham family. (Developed by Carol Loveland-Cherry. In Stanhope M, Lancaster J: *Public health nursing*, ed 7, St Louis, 2008, Mosby.)

Whitley et al. (2001) examined the physical and mental health status and health-related behaviors of 100 African-American grandmothers who were the primary caregivers for their grandchildren (n = 2.5 grandchildren). The study assessed the grandmothers' physical health conditions using two standardized instruments: the Short Form-36 General Health Survey (SF-36) (Ware and Sherbourne, 1992) and the Healthier People, Health Risk Appraisal (HRA) (Hutchins, 1991). To obtain additional physical health data, registered nurses (RNs) gathered the following information from each grandmother: blood pressure, weight, cholesterol count, and glucose levels.

The results of the study indicated that the grandmothers experienced only moderate interference with their many activities of daily living as a result of health or emotional factors. However, serious health risks were identified. The health data from the RNs revealed that 23% of the grandmothers had diabetes, 54% had hypertension, 22% had high cholesterol, and 80% were at least 20% overweight. Fifty-two percent of the grandmothers said that they had experienced one or more serious personal losses during the year, and 45% perceived their health as being fair or poor. In contrast, a lack of emotional support was found to be a problem with only 18% of the sample and the grandmothers reported that their emotional health was equal to or better than that of the general population.

The findings of this study suggest that African-American grandmothers may have difficulty meeting the demands of parenting on a long-term basis without the support of others, specifically in relation to their physical health. With the health risks identified, longevity and quality of life will be in jeopardy if health habits are not changed.

It is important that culturally sensitive educational interventions are developed for population groups. Even though these grandmothers have a strong desire to fulfill the parental role in the children's lives, a potential exists for these grandmothers to develop serious health problems in later years.

NURSE USE: Health problems could disrupt the secure home environment that the grandmothers have worked to establish for the children. The onset of many of these problems may be avoided or at least delayed with interventions from the community that would provide needed health and social services to support these families.

From Hutchins EB: *Health risk appraisal,* Decatur, Ga, 1991, The Healthier People Network; Whitley DM, Kelley SJ, Sipe TA: Grandmothers raising grandchildren: are they at increased risk of health problems?, *Health Soc Work* 26:105–114, 2001.

Persons, Single Parents) that arise from both life events and age-related events. Nurses have been instrumental in developing and moderating such groups.

Environmental Risk

The importance of **social risks** to family health is gaining increased recognition. A family's health risk increases if they are living in the following:
- High-crime neighborhoods
- Communities without adequate recreation or health resources
- Communities that have major noise pollution or chemical pollution
- Other high-stress environments

One social stress is discrimination, whether racial, cultural, or other. The psychological burden resulting from discrimination is itself a stressor, and it adds to the effects of other stressors. The implication of these examples of risky social situations is that they contribute to the stressors experienced by the families. If adequate resources and coping processes are not available, breakdowns in health can occur.

The poor are at greater risk for health problems. **Economic risk**, which is related to social risk, is determined by the relationship between the financial resources of a family and the demands on those resources. Having adequate financial resources means that a family is able to purchase the following necessary services and goods related to health:
- Adequate housing
- Clothing
- Food
- Education
- Health or illness care

The amount of money that a family has available is related to situational, cultural, and social factors. A family may have an income well above the poverty level, but because of a devastating illness of a family member, it may not be able to meet current financial demands. Likewise, families from ethnic populations or families with same-sex parents frequently experience discrimination in finding housing. Even if they find housing, they may not be welcome and may be harassed, resulting in increased stress.

Unfortunately, not all families have access to health care insurance. For families at the poverty level, programs such as Medicaid are available to pay for health and illness care. Families in the upper income brackets usually have health insurance through an employer, or they can afford to either purchase health insurance or pay for health care out of pocket. An increasing number of middle-income families have major wage earners in jobs that do not have health benefits. These people often do not have enough income to purchase health care but earn too much money to qualify for public assistance programs. Consequently, many families have financial resources that allow them to maintain themselves but that limit the quality of their purchasing power, such as the following:
- Illness care may be available but not preventive care.
- Food high in fat and calories may be affordable, whereas fresh fruit and vegetables may not be.

Nutritious diets are important in preventing illness and promoting health. Buescher et al (2003) studied the relationship of participation in Women, Infants, and Children (WIC) to Medicaid costs and use of health care services and found that children who participated in WIC were more linked to the health care system and were more likely to receive both preventive and curative care than children not participating in WIC.

Environmental Risk Assessment

Assessment of environmental health risk is less defined and developed. Information on relationships that the family has with others such as relatives and neighbors; their connections

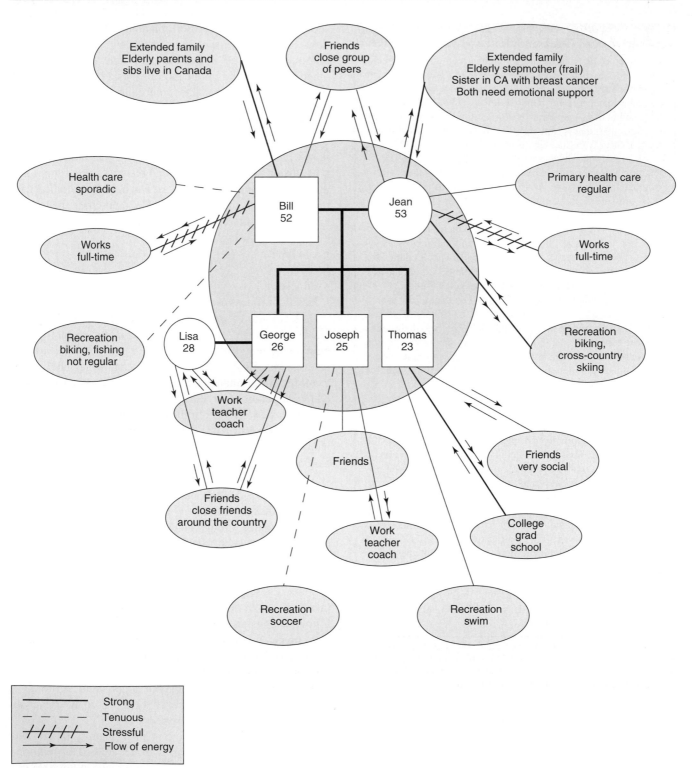

FIGURE 19-2 Ecomap of the Graham family. (Developed by Carol Loveland-Cherry. In Stanhope M, Lancaster J: *Public health nursing,* ed 7, St. Louis, 2008, Mosby.)

with other social units—church, school, work, clubs, and organizations; and the flow of energy, positive or negative, can be assessed through the use of an ecomap.

An ecomap represents the family's interactions with other groups and organizations, accomplished by using a series of circles and lines. Consider the family of interest (the Graham family in Figure 19-2), as follows:

- It is represented by a circle in the middle of the page.
- Other groups and organizations are then indicated by other circles.

- Lines, representing the flow of energy, are drawn between the family circle and the circles representing other groups and organizations.
- An arrowhead at the end of each line indicates the direction of the flow of energy (into or out of the family).
- The weight of the line indicates the intensity of the energy.

The Graham family ecomap indicates that much of the family energy goes into work (also a source of stress for the parents). Major sources of energy for the Grahams are their immediate and extended families and friends.

In addition to the support network shown by the ecomap, other aspects of social risk include characteristics of the neighborhood and community in which the family lives. A nurse who has worked in the general geographic area may already have done a community assessment and have a working knowledge of the neighborhood and community. To understand their perceptions of the community it is important for the nurse to obtain certain information from the family.

- Information about the origins of the family is useful to understand other social resources and stressors.
- Information about how long the family has lived in their current location and the immigration patterns of the family and their ancestors provides insight into the pressures they experience.

Economic risk is one of the foremost predictors of health. Families often consider financial information private, and both the nurse and the family may be uncomfortable when discussing finances. It is not necessary for the nurse to know actual family income except in instances in which it is needed to determine whether families are eligible for programs or benefits.

- It is useful to know whether the family's resources are adequate to meet their needs.
- It is important to understand that the family may be quite comfortable with their finances and standard of living, which may be different from those of the health care provider.
- The provider should not try to push financial values onto the family.
- In terms of health risk, it is important to understand the resources that families have to obtain health and/or illness care; adequate shelter, clothing, and food; and access to recreation.
- Families with limited resources may qualify for programs such as Medicaid, Aid to Dependent Families, WIC, or Maternal Support Systems/Infant Support Systems.
- Families with wage earners with medical benefits and those with enough income are usually able to afford adequate health care.

Unfortunately, in a growing number of families, the main wage earner is employed but receives no medical benefits and the salary is not sufficient for health promotion or illness-related care. This is a **policy** issue for which nurses are very capable of drafting legislation and providing testimony related to the stories of families in their caseloads.

Behavioral (Lifestyle) Risk

Personal health habits continue to contribute to the major causes of morbidity and mortality in the United States. The pattern of personal health habits and **behavioral risk** defines individual and family lifestyle risk. The family is the basic unit within which health behavior—including health values, health habits, and health risk perceptions—is developed, organized, and performed. Families maintain major responsibility for the following:

- Determining what food is purchased and prepared
- Setting sleep patterns
- Planning family activities
- Setting and monitoring norms about health and health risk behaviors
- Determining when a family member is ill
- Determining when health care should be obtained
- Carrying out treatment regimens

In 2002, more than half of all deaths in the United States were attributed to heart disease or cancer, both of which identify diet as a major cause (National Center for Health Statistics, 2005). General guidelines from the U.S. Department of Health and Human Services (USDHHS) and the U.S. Department of Agriculture (USDA) include the following:

- Eating a variety of foods
- Maintaining a healthy weight
- Choosing a diet low in fat and cholesterol
- Choosing a diet that includes plenty of vegetables, fruits, and grain products
- Limiting the use of sugars, salt, and sodium
- Consuming alcohol only in moderation

Regular physical exercise is effective in promoting and maintaining health and preventing disease. The following are among the benefits of regular physical activity (U.S. Department of Health and Human Services, 2000):

- Increased muscle strength
- Increased endurance
- Increased flexibility
- Management of weight
- Prevention of colon cancer, stroke, and back injury
- Prevention and management of coronary heart disease, hypertension, diabetes, osteoporosis, and depression

Families can structure time and activities for family members. It is helpful when the community in which they live promotes exercise by having accessible parks and walking or biking paths that help families select activities that provide moderate, regular physical exercise, rather than sedentary activities in the home setting.

BRIEFLY NOTED

Adolescents from families who have close, supportive interactions, have clearly set and enforced rules, and have parents who are involved with their children are at decreased risk for alcohol use or misuse. These family patterns can be enhanced through family-focused intervention sessions in the home.

Substance use and abuse are major contributors to morbidity and mortality in the United States. Tobacco use has been identified as the single most preventable cause of death. It has been associated with the following:

- Several types of cancer
- Coronary heart disease
- Low birthweight
- Premature births
- Sudden infant death syndrome
- Chronic obstructive pulmonary disease

Furthermore, passive smoke has been linked to disease in nonsmokers and children. Drug use, including alcohol, is a major social and health problem. In 2001, 41% of traffic deaths were alcohol related (National Cancer Institute, 2001; National Highway Traffic Safety Administration, 2002). Drug use is associated with the following:

- Transmission of human immunodeficiency virus (HIV)
- Fetal alcohol syndrome
- Liver disease
- Unwanted pregnancy
- Delinquency
- School failure
- Violence
- Crime

The literature consistently identifies the following family factors that decrease the risk of substance use in children:

- Family closeness
- Families doing activities together
- Behavior modeled in the family

Although violence and abusive behavior are not limited to families, the amount of intrafamilial violence is thought to be underestimated. It is difficult to collect data and obtain accurate statistics on family violence because the issue is so sensitive for families. Evidence supports the intergenerational nature of violence and abuse—that is, abusers were often abused as children.

Behavioral (Lifestyle) Health Risk Assessment

Families are the major source of factors that can promote or inhibit positive lifestyles. They regulate time and energy and the boundaries of the system. A number of tools exist for assessing individuals' lifestyle risks, but few are available for assessing family lifestyle patterns. Although assessment of individual lifestyles contributes to determining the lifestyle risk of a family, it is important to look at risks for the family as a unit. One approach is to identify family patterns for each of the lifestyle components included in *Healthy People 2010*. In the areas of health promotion, health protection, and preventive services, lifestyle can be assessed in several dimensions. From the literature on health behavior research, the critical dimensions include the following:

- Value placed on the behavior
- Knowledge of the behavior and its consequences
- Effect of the behavior on the family
- Effect of the behavior on the individual
- Barriers to performing the behavior
- Benefits of the behavior

It is important to assess the frequency, intensity, and regularity of specific behaviors. It is also important to evaluate the resources available to the family for implementing the behaviors. Thus items for assessment of physical activity include the following:

- The value that a family places on physical activity
- The hours that a family spends in exercise
- The kinds of exercise the family does
- The resources available for exercise

COMMUNITY-ORIENTED NURSING APPROACHES TO FAMILY HEALTH RISK REDUCTION

HOME VISITS

Nurses work with families in a variety of settings, including clinics, schools, support groups, and offices. However, an important aspect of the community-oriented nurse's role in reducing health risks and promoting the health of populations has been the tradition of providing services to families in their homes.

Purpose

Home visits give a more accurate assessment of the following than do clinical visits:

- The family structure
- The natural or home environment
- Behavior in that environment

Home visits also provide opportunities to identify both barriers and supports for reaching family health promotion goals. The nurse can work with the client directly to adapt interventions to match resources. Visiting the family in its home may also contribute to the family's sense of control and active participation in meeting its health needs.

Home visiting programs are receiving increased attention and provide a broad range of services to achieve a variety of health-related goals. In a long-term follow-up project of current adolescents whose unmarried mothers received prenatal and postnatal nursing visits at home (Drummand, Weir, and Kysela, 2002), researchers found that these teens had the following:

- Fewer instances of running away
- Fewer arrests
- Fewer convictions and violations of probation
- Fewer sexual partners over a lifetime
- Fewer cigarettes smoked per day
- Fewer days having consumed alcohol in the previous 6 months, when compared with a group of teens whose mothers had not received the nurse visits

In addition, the parents of the nurse-visited children reported fewer behavioral problems related to the use of alcohol and drugs. Long-term effects of home visits are positive and are shown to be cost-effective for society. As a result, several states have reinstituted home visits for high-risk families. If the home visit is to be a valuable and effective intervention, careful and systematic planning must occur.

Advantages and Disadvantages

The effectiveness of health promotion services in the home has been critically reexamined by agencies such as health departments and visiting nurses associations (Drummond et al, 2002). Advantages include the following:

- Client convenience
- Client control of the setting
- Provision of an option for those clients unwilling or unable to travel
- The ability to individualize services
- A natural, relaxed environment for the discussion of concerns and needs

Costs are a major disadvantage. The cost is high for the following:

- Previsit preparation
- Travel to and from the home
- Time spent with one client
- Postvisit preparation

Many agencies have actively explored alternative modes of providing service to families, particularly group interventions. The important issue is determining which families would benefit the most and how home visits can most effectively be structured and scheduled. With increasing demands for home health care, the home visit is again becoming a prominent mode for delivery of nursing services.

Process

The components of a home visit are summarized in Table 19-2. Building a trusting relationship with the family client is the cornerstone of successful home visits. The following five skills are fundamental to effective home visits:

Table 19-2	Phases and Activities of a Home Visit
Phase	**Activity**
I. Initiation	Clarify the source of referral for the visit
	Clarify the purpose for the home visit
	Share information on the reason and purpose of the home visit with the family
II. Previsit	Initiate contact with the family
	Establish a shared perception of purpose with the family
	Determine the family's willingness for a home visit
	Schedule the home visit
	Review the referral and/or family record
III. In-home	Introduce self and professional identity
	Interact socially to establish rapport
	Establish the nurse–client relationship
	Implement the nursing process
IV. Termination	Review the visit with the family
	Plan for future visits
V. Postvisit	Record the visit
	Plan for the next visit

From Whitley DM, Kelley SJ, Sipe TA: Grandmothers raising grandchildren: are they at increased risk of health problems?, *Health Soc Work* 26:105–114, 2001.

1. Observing
2. Listening
3. Questioning
4. Probing
5. Prompting

The need for these skills is evident in all phases of the home visit process.

INITIATION PHASE. Usually, a home visit is initiated as the result of a referral from a health or social agency. However, a family may request services, or the nurse may initiate the home visit as a result of case finding activities. The **initiation phase** is the first contact between the nurse and the family. It provides the foundation for an effective therapeutic relationship. Subsequent home visits should be based on need and mutual agreement between the nurse and the family. Frequently, nurses are not sure of the reason for the visit. As a result, the visit may be compromised and come aimlessly or abruptly to a premature halt. The nurse must be

HOW TO	**Prepare for the Home Visit: Previsit Phase**

- First, if at all possible, nurses should contact the family by telephone before the home visit to introduce themselves, to identify the reason for the contact, and to schedule the home visit. A first telephone contact should be a maximum of 15 minutes. Nurses should give their name and professional identity—for example, "This is Karen Smith. I'm a nurse from the Fayette County Health Department."
- The family should be informed of how they came to the attention of the nurse—for example, as the result of a referral or a contact from observations or records in the school setting. If a referral has been received, it is important and useful to ascertain whether the family is aware of the referral.
- A brief summary of the nurse's knowledge about the family's situation will allow the family to clarify their needs. For example, the nurse might say, "I understand that your baby was discharged from the hospital yesterday and that you requested some assistance with learning more about how to care for your baby at home."
- A visit should be scheduled as soon as possible. Letting the family know agency hours available for visits, the approximate length of the visit, and the purpose of the visit is helpful to the family in determining when to set the visit. Although the length of the visit may vary, depending on circumstances, approximately 30 minutes to 1 hour is usual.
- If possible, the visit should be arranged when as many family members as possible will be available for the entire visit. It is also important for the nurse to tell the client about any fee for the visit and subsequent visits and possible methods for payment.
- The telephone call can terminate with a review by the nurse of the time, place, and purpose for the visit and a means for the family to contact the nurse in case they need to verify or change the time for the visit or to ask questions. If the family does not have a telephone, another method for setting up the visit can be used. A note can be dropped off at the family home or sent by mail informing the family of when and why the home visit will occur and providing a way for the family to contact the nurse if necessary.

clear about the purpose of the home visit and this purpose or understanding must be shared with the family.

PREVISIT PHASE. The **previsit phase** has several components. For the most part, these are best accomplished in order, as presented in the "How To" box.

The family may refuse a home visit. Less experienced nurses or students may mistakenly interpret this as a personal rejection. Families make decisions about when and which outsiders are allowed entry into their homes. The nurse needs to explore the reasons for the refusal, considering the following:

- There may be a misunderstanding about the reason for a visit
- There may be a lack of information about services

The contact may be terminated as requested (1) if the nurse determines that either the situation has been resolved or services have been obtained from another source, and (2) if the family understands that services are available and how to contact the agency if desired. However, the nurse should leave open the possibility of future contact. There are instances in which the nurse will be mandated to persist in requesting a home visit because of legal obligations, such as follow-up of certain communicable diseases.

Before visiting a family, the nurse should review the referral or, if this is not the first visit, the family record. If time has lapsed between the contact and the visit, a brief telephone call to confirm the time often ensures that someone will be at home.

Personal safety is an issue that may arise either in approaching the family home or once the family has opened the door to the nurse.

- Nurses need to examine personal fears and objective threats to determine if safety is indeed an issue.
- Certain precautions can be taken in known high-risk situations.
- Agencies may provide escorts for nurses or have them visit in pairs.
- Readily identifiable uniforms may be required.
- A sign-out process indicating the timing and location of home visits may be used routinely.

Home visits are generally very safe; however, as with all worksites, the possibility of violence exists. Therefore the nurse needs to use caution. If a reasonable question exists about the safety of making a visit, the nurse should not make the visit.

The nurse should be aware that families may feel that they are being checked up on, that they are seen as being inadequate or dysfunctional, or that their privacy is being impinged on. Nursing services, especially those from health departments, have been identified by the public as being "public services" for needy families or those with inadequate funds to pay for care. These potential areas of concern underlie the need for sensitivity on the part of the nurse, the need for clarity in information regarding the reason for the visits, and the need to establish collaborative, trusting relationships with the family.

Another factor that may affect the nature of the home visit is whether the visit is viewed as voluntary or required (Wasick and Bryant, 2000). A *voluntary* home visit (a visit requested by the client) is characterized by the following:

- Easier entry for the nurse
- Client-controlled interaction
- An informal tone
- Mutual discussion of the frequency of future visits

In contrast, the client may feel little need for *required* home visits (often legally mandated), which may contribute to the following:

- Difficult entry for the nurse
- Interaction that is nurse controlled
- A more formal, investigatory tone to the visit with distorted nurse–client communication
- No mutual discussion of the frequency of future visits

IN-HOME PHASE. The actual visit to the home constitutes the **in-home phase** and affords the nurse the opportunity to assess the family's neighborhood and community resources, as well as the home and family interactions. The actual home visit includes several of the following components:

- The nurse provides personal and professional identification and tells the client the location of the agency.
- A brief social period allows the client to assess the nurse and establish rapport.
- The nurse describes his or her role, responsibilities, and limitations.
- Finally, it is important that the nurse determine the client's expectations.

The major portion of the home visit involves establishing the relationship and implementing the nursing process. Assessment, intervention, and evaluation are ongoing. The reason for the visit then determines what then occurs in the home visit. Keller et al (2004a,b) recommend using the Intervention Wheel to guide nursing practice during home visits. The Intervention Wheel provides guidelines for the purpose of home visits. Some reasons for visits are listed in Box 19-2.

It is important that the nurse be realistic about what can be accomplished in a home visit. In some situations, one visit may be all that is possible or appropriate. In this instance, needs and the resources available to meet them are explored with the family and it is determined whether further services are desired or indicated. If further services are indicated and the nurse's agency is not appropriate, the nurse can assist the family in identifying other services available in the community and can help in initiating referrals. Although it is not unusual to have only one home visit with a family, often multiple visits are made. The frequency and intensity of home visits vary not only with the needs of the family but also with the eligibility of the family for services as defined by agency policies and priorities. It is realistic to expect an initial assessment and at least the beginning of building a relationship on a first visit.

Families may or may not be able to control interruptions during the visit. Telephones ring, pets join in the visit, people come and go, and televisions are left on. The nurse can ask that, for a limited time, televisions be turned off or that other disruptive activities be limited. Families may be so used to the background noises and routine activities that they do not recognize them as being potentially disruptive.

| Box 19-2 | **Reasons for the Home Visit** |

Nursing interventions may include some or all of the 17 resources identified by the Minnesota Department of Health, Section of Public Health Nursing:
- Advocacy
- Case management
- Coalition building
- Collaboration
- Community organizing
- Consultation
- Counseling
- Delegated medical treatment and observations
- Disease and other health investigation
- Health teaching
- Outreach
- Policy development and enforcement
- Case finding
- Referral and follow-up
- Screening
- Social marketing
- Surveillance

From Keller LO et al: Population-based public health interventions: practice-based and evidence-supported. Part I, *Publ Health Nurs* 21:453–468, 2004.

TERMINATION PHASE. When the purpose of the visit has been accomplished, the nurse reviews with the family what has occurred and what has been accomplished. This is the major focus of the **termination phase**, and it provides a basis for planning further home visits.
- Ideally, termination of the visit and, ultimately, termination of service begin at the first contact with the establishment of a goal or purpose.
- If communication has been clear to this point, the family and nurse can now plan for future visits, specifically the next visit.
- Planning for future visits is part of another issue: setting goals and planning service.
- Contracting is a constructive approach to working with clients and is receiving increasing attention by health professionals.
- The purpose and components of contracting with clients are discussed on p. 346.

POSTVISIT PHASE. Even though the nurse has now concluded the home visit and left the client's home, responsibility for the visit is not complete until the interaction has been recorded. A major task of the **postvisit phase** is documenting the visit and services provided.
- Agencies may organize their records by families.
- The basic record may be a "family" folder with all members included. However, often this does not occur, although it is useful for the family history and background.
- Each family member often has a separate record, and other family members' records are cross-referenced. This is because the focus often shifts from the family to the individual.

- Consequently, nursing diagnoses, goals, and interventions are directed toward individual family members rather than the family unit.
- Record systems and formats vary from agency to agency.
- The nurse needs to become familiar with the particular system used in the agency.

All systems should include the following:
- A database
- A nursing diagnosis and problem list
- A plan, including specific goals
- Actual actions and interventions
- Evaluation

These are the basic elements needed for legal and clinical purposes. The format may consist of the following:
- Narratives
- Flow sheets
- Problem-oriented medical records (POMR)
- Subjective, objective, assessment plans (SOAP)
- A combination of formats

It is important that recording be current, dated, and signed.

The nurse should use theoretical frameworks that are appropriate to the family-centered nursing process. For example, a nursing diagnosis of *ineffective mothering skill* related to lack of knowledge of normal growth and development is an individual-focused nursing diagnosis. *Inability of a family to accomplish the stage-appropriate task of providing a safe environment for a preschooler* related to lack of knowledge and resources is a family-focused nursing diagnosis based on knowledge of the developmental approach to families. At times, it may be necessary to present information for a specific family member. However, the emphasis should be on the individual as a member of and within the structure of the family.

BRIEFLY NOTED

A home visit is more than just an alternative setting for service; it is an intervention.

CONTRACTING WITH FAMILIES

Increasingly, health professionals look at working with clients in an interactive, collaborative style. This approach is consistent with a more knowledgeable public and the recent self-care movement in the United States. However, it may not be consistent with other cultures that look to health care providers for more direct guidance; therefore, it is important to determine the family's value system before assuming that contracting will work.

Contracting, which is making an agreement between two or more parties, involves a shift in responsibility and control toward a shared effort by the client and professional as opposed to an effort by the professional alone. The premise of contracting is family control. It is assumed that when the family has legitimate control, its ability to make healthful choices is increased. This active involvement of the client is reflected in several nursing models—for example, that of Orem (1995). Contracting is a strategy aimed at formally involving the family in the nursing process and jointly defining the roles of both the family members and the health professional.

Purposes

The nursing contract is a working agreement that is continuously renegotiable and may or may not be written. It may be either a contingency or a noncontingency contract, as follows:

- A *contingency contract* states a specific reward for the client after completion of the client's portion of the contract.
- A *noncontingency contract* does not specify rewards.

The implied rewards are the positive consequences of reaching the goals specified in the contract.

For family health risk reduction, it is essential that the contract be made with all responsible and appropriate members of the family. Involving only one individual is not sufficient if the goal is family health risk reduction, which requires a total family system effort and change. Scheduling a visit with all family members present may require extra effort; if meeting with the entire family is not possible, each family member can review a contract, give input, and sign it. This allows active participation by all family members without the necessity of finding a time when everyone involved can be present.

Process of Contracting

Contracting is a learned skill on the part of both the nurse and the family. All persons involved need to know the purpose and process of contracting. The three general phases are *beginning, working,* and *termination.* The three phases can be further divided into eight sets of activities, as summarized in Table 19-3.

The first activity is collection and analysis of data, and it involves both the family and the nurse. An important aspect of this step is obtaining the family's view of the situation and its needs and problems. The nurse can do the following:

- Present his or her observations
- Validate them with the family
- Obtain the family's view

Table 19-3   Phases and Activities in Contracting

Phase	Activity
I. Beginning phase	Mutual data collection and exploration of needs and problems
	Mutual establishment of goals
	Mutual development of a plan
II. Working phase	Mutual division of responsibilities
	Mutual setting of time limits
	Mutual implementation of a plan
	Mutual evaluation and renegotiation
III. Termination	Mutual termination of a contract

It is important that goals be mutually set and realistic. A pitfall for nurses and clients who are new to contracting is to set overly ambitious goals. The nurse should recognize that there may be discrepancies between professional priorities and those of the client and determine whether negotiating is required. Because contracting is a process characterized by renegotiating, the goals are not static.

Throughout the process, the nurse and family continually learn and recognize what each can contribute to meeting the health needs. The exploring of resources allows both parties to become aware of their own and one another's strengths and requires a review of the nurse's skills and knowledge, the family support systems, and community resources.

Developing a plan to meet the goals involves the following:

- Specifying activities
- Prioritizing goals
- Selecting a starting point
- The nurse and the family deciding who will be responsible for which activities
- Setting time limits that involve deciding on a deadline for accomplishing (or evaluating progress toward accomplishing) a goal and the frequency of contacts

At the agreed-on time, the nurse and family together evaluate the progress in both process and outcome. The contract can be modified, renegotiated, or terminated on the basis of the evaluation.

Advantages and Disadvantages of Contracting

Contracting takes time and effort and may require the family and nurse to reorient their roles. Increased control on the part of the family also means increased responsibility. Some nurses may have difficulty relinquishing the role of the controlling expert professional. Contracts are not always successful, and contracting is neither appropriate nor possible in some cases. Some clients do not want to have this kind of involvement; they prefer to defer to the "authority" of the professional. The following are included in this group:

- Individuals with minimal cognitive skills
- Those who are involved in an emergency situation
- Those who are unwilling to be more active in their care
- Those who do not see control or authority for health concerns as being within their domain

Some of these clients may learn to contract; others never will.

The nursing process does not necessarily provide an active role for the family as a client; the assumption that a need exists is based on professional judgment only, and it is also assumed that changes can and should be made within the family unit. Contracting is one alternative approach that depends on the following:

- The value of input from both the nurse and family
- The competency of the family
- The family's ability to be responsible
- The dynamic nature of the process

This not only allows for but also requires continual renegotiating. Although it may not be appropriate in all situations or with all families, contracting can provide direction and structure to health risk reduction and health promotion in families.

EMPOWERING FAMILIES

Approaches for helping individuals and families assume an active role in their health care should focus on **empowerment** rather than enabling or help giving (Herandez et al, 2005). Help-giving interventions do not always have positive outcomes for clients. If families do not perceive a situation as a problem or need, offers of help may cause resentment. Help giving also may have negative consequences if there is not a match between what is expected and what is offered. A nurse's failure to recognize a family's competencies and to define an active role for them can lead to the family's dependency and lack of growth. This can be frustrating for both the nurse and the family. For families to become active participants, they need to feel a sense of personal competence and a desire for and willingness to take action. Definitions of empowerment reflect the following three characteristics of the empowered family seeking help:

• Access and control over needed resources
• Decision-making and problem-solving abilities
• The ability to communicate and to obtain needed resources

The last characteristic refers to the fact that families may need to learn how to do the following:

• Identify sources of help
• Contact agencies
• Ask critical questions
• Negotiate with agencies to have family needs met

These characteristics generally reflect a process by which people (individuals, families, organizations, or communities) take control of their own lives. The following are the outcomes of empowerment:

• Positive self-esteem
• The ability to set and reach goals
• A sense of control over life and change processes
• A sense of hope for the future (Koelen and Linstrom, 2005; Powers and Bendall, 2003; Wolfe et al, 2003)

The "Levels of Prevention" box shows prevention strategies applied to families.

Levels of Prevention — Related to Families

PRIMARY PREVENTION

Complete a family genogram and assess health risks with the family to contract for family health activities to prevent diseases from developing.

SECONDARY PREVENTION

Use a behavioral health risk survey and identify the factors leading to obesity in the family.

TERTIARY PREVENTION

Develop a contract with the family to change nutritional patterns to reduce further complications from obesity.

Empowerment requires a viewpoint that often conflicts with the views of many helping professions, including nursing. Empowerment's underlying assumption is one of a partnership between the professional and the client as opposed to one in which the professional is dominant. Families are assumed to be either competent or capable of becoming competent. This implies that the professional is not an unchallenged authority who is in control. Empowerment promotes an environment that creates opportunities for competencies to be used. Finally, families need to determine that their actions result in behavior change. A nursing intervention that incorporates the principles of empowerment meets the following requirements:

• It is directed toward the building of nurse–family partnerships.
• It emphasizes health risk reduction and health promotion.

The nurse's approach to the family should be positive and focused on competencies rather than on problems or deficits. The interventions need to be consistent with family cultural norms and the family's perception of the problem. Rather than making decisions for the family, the nurse supports the family in primary decision making and bolsters their self-esteem by recognizing and using family strengths and support networks. Interventions that promote desired family behaviors increase family competency, decrease the need for outside help, and result in families seeing themselves as being actively responsible for bringing about desired changes.

The goal of an empowering approach is to create a partnership between the nurse and the family characterized by cooperation and shared responsibility.

COMMUNITY RESOURCES

Families have varied and complex needs and problems. The nurse is often involved in mobilizing several resources to effectively and appropriately meet family health promotion needs. Although the specific resources vary from community to community, general types can be identified as follows:

• Government resources such as Medicare and Medicaid
• Aid to Families With Dependent Children
• Supplementary Security Income, Food Stamps, and WIC, available in most communities

These programs primarily provide support for basic needs (e.g., illness and/or health care, nutrition, funds for housing and clothing), and funds are based on meeting eligibility criteria.

In addition to government agencies providing health-related services to families, most communities have voluntary (nongovernment) programs. Local chapters of such organizations provide education, support services, and some direct services to individuals and families, such as the following:

• American Cancer Society
• American Heart Association
• American Lung Association
• Muscular Dystrophy Association

These agencies provide primary prevention and health promotion services as well as screening programs and assistance after the disease or condition is diagnosed. Local social service agencies (e.g., Catholic Social Services) provide direct services such as counseling to families. Other voluntary organizations provide direct service (e.g., shelters for homeless or battered individuals, substance abuse counseling and treatment, Meals on Wheels, transportation, clothing, food, furniture).

Health resources in the community may be *proprietary, voluntary,* or *public.*

In addition to private health care providers, nurses should be aware of voluntary and public clinics, screening programs, and health promotion programs.

Identifying resources in a community requires time and effort. One valuable source is the telephone book. Often community service organizations, such as the local chamber of commerce and health department, publish community resource listings. Regardless of how the resource is identified, the nurse must be familiar with the types of services offered and any requirements or costs involved. If this information is not available, the nurse can contact the resource.

Locating and using these systems often requires skills and patience that many families lack. Nurses work with families to identify community resources, and as client advocates they help families learn to use resources. This may involve the following:
• Sharing information with families
• Rehearsing with families what questions to ask
• Preparing required materials
• Making the initial contact
• Arranging transportation

The appropriateness and effectiveness of resources should be evaluated with families afterward. It is important to remember that navigating the maze of resources is often difficult for the nurse. If a family is in crisis or does not have a phone or a home base from which to call or receive return calls, this process is even more difficult and their sense of helplessness may be increased. Therefore the nurse's assistance, while promoting the family's sense of empowerment, is both necessary and complex.

CLINICAL APPLICATION

The initial contact between a community-oriented nursing service and a family provides limited information, and the situation that develops may be much more complex than anticipated. The following example, based on an actual case, illustrates the issues and approaches outlined in this chapter.

The Fayette County Health Department was notified that Amy Cress, age 16 years, had been referred by the school counselor at the local high school for prenatal supervision. Amy was 4 months pregnant, in apparently good health, in the tenth grade, and living at home with her mother, stepfather, and younger sister. The family lived in a rural area outside of a small farming community. The father of the baby also lived in the community and continued to see Amy on a regular basis. The referral information provided

the nurse with a beginning, but limited, assessment of the family situation.
A. *What would you do first as the nurse assigned to this family?*
B. *How would you help this family empower itself to take responsibility for this situation?*
C. *After the initial contact, how would you extend the assessment to the entire family system?*
D. *Would you contract with this family? How? On what terms?*

Answers are in the back of the book.

REMEMBER THIS!

• The importance of the family as a major client system for community-oriented nurses in reducing health risks and promoting the health of individuals and populations is well documented.
• The family system is a basic unit within which health behavior, including health values, health habits, and health risk perceptions, is developed, organized, and performed.
• Knowledge of family structure and functioning is fundamental to implementing the nursing process with families in the community.
• Nurses need to go beyond the individual and family and to understand the complex environment in which the family functions to be effective in reducing family health risks. Categories of risk factors that are important to family health are biological risk, environmental risk (including economic factors), and behavioral risk.
• Several factors contribute to the experience of healthy or unhealthy outcomes. Not everyone exposed to the same event will have the same outcome. The factors that influence whether disease or other unhealthy results occur are called *health risks.* The accumulated risks are synergistic; their combined effect is more important than individual effects.
• An important aspect of nursing's role in reducing health risk and promoting the health of populations has been the tradition of providing services to individual families in their homes.
• Home visits afford the opportunity to gain a more accurate assessment of the family structure and behavior in the natural environment. They also provide opportunities to observe the home environment and to identify both barriers and supports to reducing health risks and reaching family health goals.
• Increasingly, health professionals have come to look toward working with clients in a more interactive, collaborative style.
• Contracting, which is making an agreement between two or more parties, involves a shift in responsibility and control from the professional alone to a shared effort by client and professional.
• Families have varied and complex needs and problems. The nurse often mobilizes several resources to effectively and appropriately meet family health needs.

WHAT WOULD YOU DO?

1. Select one of the *Healthy People 2010* objectives and identify how biological risk (including age-related risk), environmental risk (including economic risk), and behavioral risk contribute to family health risks for that objective. Give examples.
2. Select three to four families (hypothetically or from actual situations) who represent different ethnic and socioeconomic backgrounds. Complete a family genogram and ecomap for each family, and identify and compare major health risks. Summarize your findings.
3. Select one or more agencies in which community-oriented nurses work, and examine the agency and nursing philosophies and objectives with emphasis on individual care, family care, illness care, risk reduction, and health promotion. If you were to accept a position with this agency, what approach to family risk reduction would you be required to use? Is there a better way?
4. Identify three public health problems in your community, and discuss the implications of these problems for the health of families. How did you arrive at your conclusions?

■ *REFERENCES*

Belloc NB, Breslow L: Relationship of physical health in a general population survey, *Am J Epidemiol* 93:329, 1972.

Buescher PA et al: Child participation in WIC: Medicaid costs and use of health care services, *Am J Public Health* 93:145-150, 2003.

Califano JA Jr: *Healthy people: the surgeon general's report on health promotion and disease prevention*, Washington, DC, 1979, U.S. Government Printing Office.

Carter B, McGoldrick M: *The expanded family life cycle*, ed 3, Boston, 1999, Allyn & Bacon.

Centers for Disease Control and Prevention: *Youth Risk Behavior Surveillance System, 2005*, available at http://www.cdc.gov/HealthyYouth/yrbs/index.htm.

Doherty WJ, McCubbin HI: Family and health care: an emerging arena of theory, research and clinical intervention, *Family Relat* 34(1):5, 1985.

Drummond JE, Weir AE, Kysela GM: Home visitation practice: models, documentation, and evaluation, *Public Health Nurs* 19:21-29, 2002.

Friedman M: *Family nursing theory and practice*, East Norwalk, Conn, 2002, Appleton & Lange.

Hernandez P, Almeida R, Dolan-Del-Vecchio K: Critical consciousness, accountability, and empowerment: key processes for helping families heal, *Family Process* 44:105-119, 2005.

Keller LO et al: Population-based public health interventions: practice-based and evidence- supported. Part I, *Public Health Nurs* 21:453-468, 2004a.

Keller LO et al: Population-based public health interventions: innovations in practice, teaching, and management. Part II, *Public Health Nurs* 21: 469-487, 2004b.

Koelen MA, Linstrom B: Making healthy choices easy choices: the role of empowerment, *Eur J Clin Nutr* 59:10-15, 2005.

Litman TJ: The family as a basic unit in health and medical care: a social behavioral overview, *Soc Sci Med* 8:495, 1974.

Lorenz F, Wickrama KAS, Conger R, editors: *Family Research Consortium Summer Institute (1996), continuity and change in family relations: theory, methods, and empirical findings (Advances in Family Research)*, Mahwah, NJ, 2004, Lawrence Erlbaum Associates, Inc.

Mauksch HO: A social science basis for conceptualizing family health, *Soc Sci Med* 8:521, 1974.

McKenry P, Price S: *Families and change: coping with stressful situations and transitions*, ed 3, Thousand Oaks, Calif, 2005, Sage.

National Cancer Institute: *Cancer facts: environmental tobacco smoke*, 2001, available at http://cis.nci.nih.gov/fact/3_9.htm.

National Center for Health Statistics: Health United States 2004, Washington DC, 2005, U.S. Government Printing Office.

National Center for Health Statistics: *Health, United States, 2005. With chartbook on trends in the health of Americans*, Hyattsville, Md, 2005, National Center for Health Statistics.

National Conference of State Legislatures: *State family and medical leave laws*, 2002. Available at www.ncsl.org.

National Highway Traffic Safety Administration, U.S. Department of Transportation: *Traffic safety facts 2001: alcohol*, Washington, DC, 2002, NHTSA, available at http://www-nrd.nhtsa.gov.

Neuman B, Fawcett J: *The Neuman Systems Model*, ed 5, Upper Saddle River, NJ, 2002, Prentice Hall.

Nightingale EO et al: *Perspectives on health promotion and disease prevention in the United States*, Washington, DC, 1978, Institute of Medicine, National Academy of Sciences.

Orem DE: *Nursing: concepts of practice*, ed 5, St. Louis, 1995, Mosby.

Pender NJ, Murdaugh C, Parsons MA: *Health promotion in nursing practice*, ed 5, Stamford, Conn, 2005, Appleton & Lange.

Powers TL, Bendall D: Improving health outcomes through patient empowerment, *J Hosp Market Publ Relat* 15:45-59, 2003.

Pratt L: *Family structure and effective health behavior*, Boston, 1976, Houghton-Mifflin.

U.S. Department of Health and Human Services: *Healthy People 2010: understanding and improving health*, ed 2, Washington, DC, 2000, U.S. Government Printing Office.

Ware JE, Sherbourne CD: The MOS 36-item short-form health survey (SF-36) I: conceptual framework and item selection, *Med Care* 30:473-483, 1992.

Wasick BH, Bryant DM: *Home visiting: procedures for helping families*, ed 2, Newbury Park, Calif, 2000, Sage Publications.

Whitley DM, Kelley SJ, Sipe TA: Grandmothers raising grandchildren: are they at increased risk of health problems? *Health Soc Work* 26:105-114, 2001.

Wolfe M et al: Patient empowerment strategies for a safety net, *Nurs Econ* 21:219-225, 207, 2003.

Wright LM: *Nursing and families: a guide to family assessment and intervention*, ed 3, Philadelphia, 2000, Davis.

Chapter 20

Health Risks across the Life Span

Marcia K. Cowan
Monty Gross
Lisa M. Kaiser
Diane C. Hatton
Cynthia Westley
Kathleen Ryan Fletcher

ADDITIONAL RESOURCES

These related resources are found either in the appendix at the back of this book or on the book's website at http://evolve.elsevier.com/stanhope/foundations.

Appendix

- Appendix A.2: Schedule of Clinical Prevention Services
- Appendix D.1: Recommended immunization schedule for persons aged 0 through 6 years, United States, 2009
- Appendix D.2: Recommended immunization schedule for persons aged 7 through 18 years, United States, 2009
- Appendix D.3: Catch-up immunization schedule for persons aged 4 months through 18 years who start late or who are more than one month behind, United States, 2009
- Appendix D.4: Summary of Recommendations for Childhood and Adolescent Immunization
- Appendix D.5: Summary of Recommendations for Adult Immunization
- Appendix D.6: Recommendations for Preventive Pediatric Health Care
- Appendix E.2: Accident Prevention in Children
- Appendix F.1: Screening for Common Orthopedic Problems

- Appendix F.2: Vision and Hearing Screening Procedures
- Appendix F.3: Tanner Stages of Puberty
- Appendix G.1: Community-As-Partner Model
- Appendix G.2: Friedman Family Assessment Model (Short Form)

⊝ Evolve Website

- Community Assessment Applied
- Quiz review questions
- WebLinks, including link to *Healthy People 2010* website

Real World Community Health Nursing: An Interactive CD-ROM, second edition

If you are using this CD-ROM in your course, you will find the following activities related to this chapter:
- *You Conduct the Assessment: Single-Parent Family, Aging Family, Multigenerational Family* in **Family Health**

OBJECTIVES

After reading this chapter, the student should be able to:
1. Discuss major health problems of children and adolescents.
2. Evaluate the role of the nurse in community health with specific at-risk populations in the community.

3. Describe ways to promote child and adolescent health within the community.
4. Define men's health and women's health.
5. Describe the women's health movement in the United States.

6. Describe the health status of women in the United States.
7. Discuss risk factors and their consequences on men's health and women's health.
8. Explain how men's lifestyles affect their health
9. Define terms commonly used to refer to elders.
10. Identify the multidimensional influences on aging and how these affect the health status of an elder.
11. List chronic health problems often experienced by elders.
12. Describe several community-based models for gerontology nursing practice.

CHAPTER OUTLINE

CHILDREN'S HEALTH
Major Public Health Problems
Nutrition
Immunizations
Environmental Health Hazards
Homeless Families and Children
ADULT HEALTH
Women's Health
Men's Health
Women's Health Concerns

Men's Health Concerns
Shared Health Concerns
OLDER ADULTS' HEALTH
Health of Older Adults
Demographics
Definitions Related to the Health of Older Adults
Multidimensional Influences on Aging
Chronic Health Concerns of Older Adults
Community Resources

KEY TERMS

advance directives: written or oral statements by which a competent person makes known his or her treatment preferences and/or designates a surrogate decision maker.

ageism: prejudice toward older people, similar to racism or sexism.

aging: the sum total of all changes that occur in a person with the passing of time.

anorexia nervosa: an intense fear of becoming obese, with disturbance in body image, resulting in strict dieting and excessive weight loss.

attention deficit disorder with or without hyperactivity (ADD/ADHD): inappropriate degree of inattention, impulsiveness, and hyperactivity for age and development.

basic activities of daily living (ADLs): basic personal care activities that include eating, toileting, dressing, bathing, transferring, walking, and getting outside.

body maintenance: maintaining optimal functioning, performance, and capacity to do things.

bulimia: persistent concern with body shape and weight. Recurrent episodes of binge eating followed by extreme methods to prevent weight gain such as purging, fasting, or vigorous exercise.

caregiver burden: the physical, psychological, emotional, social, and financial problems that can be experienced by those who provide care for impaired others.

chronic illness: an illness in which a cure is not expected and nursing activities address function, wellness, and psychosocial issues.

durable power of attorney: a legal way for a client to designate someone else to make health care decisions when he or she is unable to do so.

five I's: five conditions believed to adversely affect the aging experience: intellectual impairment, immobility, instability, incontinence, and iatrogenic drug reactions.

geriatrics: the study of disease in old age.

gerontological nursing: the specialty of nursing concerned with the assessment of the health and functional status of older adults, planning and implementing health care and services to meet the identified needs, and evaluating the effectiveness of such care.

gerontology: the specialized study of the process of growing old.

homeless child syndrome: the combination of the effects of homelessness on children resulting in health problems, environmental dangers, and stress.

hormone replacement therapy (HRT): a hormone combination of estrogen and progesterone used for postmenopausal women who have not had a hysterectomy.

immunization: a process of protecting an individual from a disease through introduction of a live, killed, or partial component of the invading organism into the individual's system.

instrumental activities of daily living (IADLs): those activities of daily living that help individuals manage their lives, such as cooking, shopping, paying bills, cleaning house, and using the telephone.

living will: a document that allows a client to express wishes regarding the use of medical treatments in the event of a terminal illness.

long-term care: care that is delivered to individuals who depend on others for assistance with basic tasks over a sustained period.

menopause: permanent cessation of menstruation resulting from loss of ovarian follicular activity.

neglect: failure to act as an ordinary, prudent person; conduct contrary to that of a reasonable person under a specific circumstance.

osteoporosis: condition characterized by increased bone brittleness.

Patient Self-Determination Act:: a law that requires providers who receive Medicare and Medicaid payments to give their clients written information regarding their legal options for treatment choices if they become incapacitated.

perimenopausal: the period immediately before menopause when endocrinological, biological, and clinical features of approaching menopause commence, continuing for at least the first year after permanent cessation of menstruation.

prostate cancer: the second most common cancer among men in the United States; sometimes hard to diagnose because of a lack of symptoms.

testicular cancer: a commonly found solid malignant mass (tumor) that is found in the testicles of men.

testicular self-examination (TSE): a procedure performed by men to assess the condition of their testicles and detect abnormalities.

three D's: types of intellectual impairment: progressive intellectual impairment (dementia), mood disorder (depression), and acute confusion (delirium).

women's health: women's life span that involves health promotion, maintenance, and restoration.

This chapter examines the health status of individuals across the life span. Emphasis is on the history, health status, leading causes of death and disease, and health risks of five distinct groups: children, adolescents, women, men, and older adults. Major public health problems of populations across the life span as identified in *Healthy People 2010* are addressed (USDHHS, 2000), and strategies that nurses in the community can use to meet health needs throughout the life span are emphasized. The pivotal role of individuals in ensuring the family's and community's health is highlighted in the discussion of programs to ensure a healthy environment for its children and adolescents. Factors influencing access to health services, including unequal services, financial and employment issues, gender-power issues, family considerations, health behaviors, and health care providers' attitudes, are considered. Health policy, including major legislation affecting health services, and future directions for health are discussed.

CHILDREN'S HEALTH

The future of the United States depends on how the children are cared for. Focusing on the health needs of children increases the chances of future adults who value and practice healthy lifestyles. Nurses in the community have the following two major roles in the area of child and adolescent health:

1. The nurse provides direct services to children and their families: assessment, management of care, education, and counseling (see Appendixes D.1–D.6, E.2, and F.1–F.3).
2. Nurses are involved in the assessment of the community and the establishment of programs to ensure a healthy environment for its children.

The roles of the nurse offer the opportunity to teach healthy lifestyles to children and caregivers and to provide family-centered care in the community.

Ongoing growth and development make the pediatric population unique. Physical, cognitive, and emotional changes occur more rapidly during childhood and adolescence than any other time in the life span. Health visits are scheduled at key ages to monitor these changes. Recommendations for

Box 20-1	**Nursing Assessment for Child Health**

- Physical assessment
- Nutritional needs
- Elimination patterns
- Sleep behaviors
- Development and behavior
- Safety issues
- Parenting concerns

well-child care are found in Appendix D.6 and Appendix A.2. Nursing assessments include growth and health status, development, quality of the parent–child relationship, and family support systems (Box 20-1).

BRIEFLY NOTED

There were 73 million children through age 18 years in the United States in 2003, representing almost 25% of the population. More than one-third of them live in low-income families, with one out of six living below poverty levels. Minority children are overrepresented in the statistics.

MAJOR PUBLIC HEALTH PROBLEMS

OBESITY

Obesity among the youth of the nation has reached epidemic proportions. *Healthy People* objectives have addressed youth fitness and obesity since 1990, yet the numbers of obese youth continue to rise (Table 20-1).

Overweight is defined by using the body mass index (BMI), which is a ratio of weight to height. The National Health and Nutrition Examination Survey (NHANES) indicates that about two-thirds of U.S. adults are overweight, which is 16% higher than the data from a 1994 survey. One-third of all U.S. adults are obese, with BMIs greater than 30 (National Center for Health Statistics, 2005). The risks for childhood obesity are related to obesity in the parents. If both parents are obese, the child has an 80% chance of being obese. The numbers of obese children and teenagers

Table 20-1	Prevalence of Overweight among U.S. Youth				
Age	**1963–1980**	**1988–1994**	**1999**	**2002**	**2004**
6 to 19 years	4% to 7%	11%	13% to 14%	16%	33%

From National Center for Health Statistics: *FASTATS,* Washington, DC, 2005, U.S. Government Printing Office, available at www.cdc.gov/nchs/fastats/adolescents_health.htm; U.S. Department of Health and Human Services: *Health United States 2004,* USDHHS pub. no. CPHS 24-1232, Washington, DC, 2004, U.S. Government Printing Office; U.S. Department of Health and Human Services: *Healthy People 2010: national health promotion and disease prevention objectives,* ed 2, Washington, DC, 2000, U.S. Government Printing Office.

remained at 4% to 7% for years. This number more than doubled between 1980 and 2002. It was estimated in 2006 that obesity among children ages 2–5 years was at 12.4%, and about 17% among children ages 6–19 years, with BMIs greater than 95% (Ogden et al., 2008). At least 70% of overweight children will become overweight adults. The obesity rates are even higher in Native American, Hispanic, and African-American groups. Lower socioeconomic groups and urban settings have been associated with higher rates of obesity (Greger and Edwin, 2001; U.S. Department of Health and Human Services, 2004).

The medical consequences of obesity vary. Obese children and teens have an increased prevalence of the following:
- Hypertension
- Respiratory problems
- Hyperlipidemia
- Bone and joint difficulties
- Hyperinsulinemia
- Menstrual problems

The psychosocial disadvantages of overweight in the young may include the following:
- Teasing
- Scholastic discrimination
- Low self-esteem
- Negative body image

There is a downward spiral of overweight, poor self-image, increasing isolation, and decreasing activity, which together lead to increasing overweight. Long-term risks include cardiovascular disease, diabetes, and cancer.

High-fat diets and inactivity are the major contributors to obesity. The American diet in general tends to be high in fat, calories, and sugar, with generous serving sizes. School lunches and "fast-food" meals tend to be oversized and nutritionally poor. Vending machines with "junk food" choices are common in schools. Colas and sugary fruit punch add "empty calories." Snacking on high-sugar and high-fat foods is a problem pattern. Advertising directed at children glorifies poor food choices.

Television and computer time contribute to a sedentary lifestyle. NHANES II showed that 20% of American children participate in fewer than three sessions of vigorous activity per week. More than 60% of teenagers do not exercise regularly. Only one-third of schools offer daily physical education. Typically, very little time in physical education classes is devoted to exercise (U.S. Department of Health and Human Services, 2000).

Box 20-2	Guidelines for Managing Childhood Obesity

- Set goals related to healthier lifestyle, not dieting.
- Keep objectives realistic and obtainable.
- Modify family eating habits to include low-fat food choices. Serve calorie-dense foods that incorporate the Food Guide Pyramid: whole grains, fruits, vegetables, lean protein foods, and low-fat dairy products.
- Encourage family members to stop eating when they are satisfied. Encourage recognizing hunger and satiation cues.
- Schedule regular times for meals and snacks. Include breakfast, and do not skip meals.
- Have low-calorie, nutritious snacks ready and available. Avoid having empty-calorie junk foods in the home.
- Encourage keeping food intake and activity diaries.
- Promote physical activity. Make daily exercise a priority. Encourage family participation. Find ways to make the activity fun. Include peers.
- Limit television viewing. Do not allow snacking while watching television.
- Scale back computer time. Replace sedentary time with hobbies, activities, and chores.
- Recognize healthier food choices when eating out. Order broiled, roasted, grilled, or baked items. Split orders, or take home "doggie bags."
- Praise and reward children for the progress they make in reaching nutrition and activity goals. Emphasize the unique positive qualities of each child.
- Understand the genetic features of the child's/adolescent's body type. Acceptance of the "rounder" child may be a part of reaching health goals.

Interventions need to be based on goals of lifestyle changes for the entire family. The goal is to modify the way the family eats, exercises, and plans daily activities. Strategies for working with families are discussed in Box 20-2. The goal of managing weight in children and adolescents is to normalize weight. This may involve the following:
- Just slowing the rate of weight gain
- Allowing children to "grow" into their weight
- Improving dietary habits
- Increasing physical activity
- Improving self-esteem
- Improving parent relationships

Healthy People 2010 objectives include improving the nutritional status and physical activity patterns of the nation's youth. Nurses in community health can use the interventions

Table 20-2	Leading Cause of Injury by Age Group* 2002–2005			
1 year	**1 to 4 years**	**5 to 9 years**	**10 to 14 years**	**15 to 24 years**
Suffocation	Motor vehicle accident	Motor vehicle accident/pedestrian	Motor vehicle accident	Motor vehicle accident
Motor vehicle accident	Drowning	Drowning	Drowning	Poisoning
Drowning	Fires/burns	Fires/burns	Poisoning	Drowning

From National Center of Injury Prevention Control: Centers for Disease Control and Prevention: childhood injury report, 2008, available at www.cdc.gov/ncipc.
*Listed in order of frequency.

in the *Healthy People 2010* box (p. 379) to accomplish these goals in the community.

INJURIES AND ACCIDENTS

Injuries and accidents are the most important causes of preventable disease, disability, and death among children. Each year, 20% to 25% of all children will have a serious health problem related to accidents or injuries. Most are preventable. The key to changing behaviors is teaching age-appropriate safety. Injuries are the number-one cause of death for children up to age 21 years in the United States. Some progress is being made in reducing the number of accidents and injuries (U.S. Department of Health and Human Services, 2004a).

Motor vehicle accidents are the leading cause of death among children and teenagers. One fourth of those deaths involve drunk drivers. One half of the children who are killed in motor vehicle accidents are unrestrained. Surveys show that 20% of infants and 40% of children and teenagers are unrestrained in cars. As many as 80% of children who are using seatbelts or car seats are restrained incorrectly (National Center for Injury Prevention and Control, 2002, 2008). Motor vehicle accidents include not only automobile collisions but also pedestrian injuries. Drowning and burns account for most of the other deaths; poisons and falls also contribute heavily (National Center for Injury Prevention and Control, 2008). Age-related development is an important issue in identifying risks to children. Table 20-2 lists the three leading injury-related causes of death by age.

Infants

Infants sustain injuries for the following reasons:
- Their small size increases the possibility of injury.
- Their small airway may be easily occluded.
- Their small body fits through places in which the head may be entrapped.
- Infants are handled on high surfaces for the convenience of the caregiver, placing them at great risk for falls.
- In motor vehicle accidents, the small size of an infant's body increases the risk of being crushed or being propelled into surfaces.
- Immature motor skills do not allow infants to escape from injury, placing them at risk for drowning, suffocation, and burns.
- Homicide is increasing in this age group, especially during the first week of life. Baby-shaken syndrome and blunt trauma are the leading causes of trauma to the head.

Toddlers and Preschoolers

This population experiences a large number of falls, poisonings, and motor vehicle accidents. These children are active, and their increasing motor skills make supervision difficult. They are inquisitive and have relatively immature cognitive abilities.

School-Age Children

This age group has difficulty judging speed and distance, placing them at risk for pedestrian and bicycle accidents. The use of bicycle helmets would prevent deaths. Peer pressure often inhibits the use of protective devices such as helmets and limb pads. Sports and athletic injuries are increased in this age group (National Center for Injury Prevention and Control, 2008).

Adolescents

Injury during adolescence is often due to risk-taking, which becomes more conscious at this time, especially among males.
- The death and serious injury rates for males are higher than for females.
- Adolescents are at the highest risk of any age group for motor vehicle deaths, drowning, and intentional injuries.
- Use of weapons and drug and alcohol abuse play an important role in injuries in this age group.
- Youth gangs are more violent than in the past and seem to be increasing in prevalence.
- Suicide is the second leading cause of death among youths between the ages of 15 and 24 years (National Center for Injury Prevention and Control, 2008).
- Poor social adjustment, psychiatric problems, and family disorganization increase the risk for suicide.
- Suicide is the third leading cause of death among youths between the ages of 10 and 24 years (National Center for Injury Prevention and Control, 2008).

BRIEFLY NOTED

Most states have enacted laws allowing health care providers to treat adolescents in certain situations without parental consent. These include emergency care, substance abuse, pregnancy, and birth control. All 50 states recognize the "mature minors doctrine." This allows youths 15 years of age and older to give informed medical consent if it is apparent that they are capable of understanding the risks and benefits and if the procedure is medically indicated.

Box 20-3 Injury-Prevention Topics

- Car restraints, seatbelts, airbag safety
- Preventing fires, burns
- Poison prevention
- Preventing falls
- Preventing drowning, water safety
- Bicycle safety
- Safe driving practices
- Sports safety
- Pedestrian safety
- Gun control
- Decreasing gang activities
- Substance abuse prevention

Box 20-4 Guidelines for Playground Safety

- Playgrounds should be surrounded by a barrier to protect children from traffic.
- Activity centers should be distributed to avoid crowding in one area.
- Surfaces should be finished with substances that meet Consumer Product Safety Commission (CPSC) regulations for lead.
- Durable materials should be used.
- Sand, gravel, wood chips, and wood mulch are acceptable surfaces for limiting the shock of falls.
- Equipment should be inspected regularly for protrusions that could puncture skin or entangle clothes.
- Multiple-occupancy swings, animal swings, rope swings, and trampolines are not recommended.

Data from Swartz MK: Playground safety, *J Pediatr Health Care* 6:161, 1992.

Abuse and Neglect

In 2001, 3.1 million children were reported to have been abused or neglected. This is a number that is often underreported because it is difficult to prove. Abuse occurs in all income, racial, and ethnic groups. Children under 6 years of age represented 85% of the fatalities; children younger than 1 year old accounted for 41% of the fatalities. Some children suffer multiple types of maltreatment (U.S. Department of Health and Human Services, 2003a).

Injury and Accident Prevention

The nurse has a responsibility in the prevention of accidents and injuries. The nurse is responsible for identification of risk factors by assessing the characteristics of the child, family, and environment. Interventions include anticipatory guidance, environmental modification, and safety education.

Education should focus on age-appropriate interventions based on a knowledge of the leading causes of death and the leading risk factors. Topics to consider are listed in Box 20-3.

Health care provider offices, schools, and day-care facilities provide opportunities to teach children, adolescents, and their families how to prevent injuries. Safety can be incorporated into required health education courses. The *Healthy People 2010* objectives target head injuries, motor vehicle injuries, fires/smoke alarms, falls, drowning, and poisonings. Community-sponsored car seat and seatbelt safety checks and safety fairs are another way to educate families. Injury prevention should be addressed at all health visits. Schools, day-care centers, and community groups often need guidance toward developing safe places for children to play. One child is injured on a playground every 2½ minutes. Each year, more than 66,000 children sustain severe injuries.

The U.S. Consumer Product Safety Commission has published guidelines for playground safety that cover structure, materials, surfaces, and maintenance of equipment (Box 20-4). The developmental skills of specific ages are incorporated, as well as recommendations for physically

challenged children. Nurses can use these guidelines to help the community establish standards for play areas.

ALTERATIONS IN BEHAVIOR

Behavioral problems in the child and adolescent are highly variable and may include the following:
- Eating disorders
- Attention problems
- Substance abuse
- Elimination problems
- Conduct disorders and delinquency
- Sleep disorders
- School maladaptation

A healthy self-concept is supported by positive interactions with others. Problem behaviors may provide negative feedback, which may generate low self-esteem. A child's coping mechanisms are influenced by the individual developmental level, temperament, previous stress experiences, role models, and support of parents and peers. Maladaptive coping mechanisms present as problem behaviors. Inappropriate behaviors may lead to further physical or developmental problems.

Attention deficit disorder with or without hyperactivity (ADD/ADHD) is a combination of inattention and impulsiveness, and it may include hyperactivity not appropriate for the age. ADD/ADHD frequently includes low self-esteem, labile mood, low frustration tolerance, temper outbursts, and poor academic skills (National Institute of Mental Health, 2008).
- The evaluation is based on symptoms.
- The diagnosis is made by excluding other disorders.
- Symptoms vary with the severity of the problem, and interventions range from simple to complex.
- A familial tendency exists; several members of a family may be affected.
- Treatment involves a family focus and includes health professionals and educators.

Population-focused interventions include programs to improve stress management skills, problem-solving skills, impulse control, and interpersonal relationships. Strategies include the following:

- Self-help programs and guides
- Intensive summer camps
- Parent workshops
- Behavior counseling through mental health centers
- School-based intervention programs

TOBACCO USE

Smoking has been identified as the most important preventable cause of morbidity and mortality in the United States, yet 45 million Americans smoke. Smoking is associated with cardiovascular disease, cancer, and lung disease. Secondhand smoke, smoke exhaled or given off by a burning cigarette, is toxic. Approximately 3000 nonsmokers die each year of lung cancer as a result of secondhand smoke (American Lung Association, 2008a,b). Parents often do not understand or believe the effects of smoking on children. Children exposed to secondhand smoke experience increased episodes of ear and upper respiratory tract infections. Children of smokers are more likely to smoke. Teenagers who become smokers are rarely able to quit (Brown, 2002). About half of all teenagers who smoke regularly will die from smoking-related disease (National Center for Health Statistics, 2002).

The number of teenagers who smoke has been decreasing since 1997, but they are starting younger. Currently, almost 20% of high school students and 10% of middle school students smoke on a daily basis (American Lung Association, 2008). Tobacco industry advertising has increased through the use of advertisements in the media, on billboards, and in sponsorship of sporting events. Cigarette advertisements appear in "teen" magazines, and companies offer logo products that appeal to children.

BRIEFLY NOTED

Although many states have laws prohibiting the sale of cigarettes to minors, restrictions are not enforced. Minors continue to be able to purchase tobacco products.

Interventions to discourage smoking focus on the parent, the child or adolescent, and public policy. Parents should be offered the following:

- Educational programs dealing with the negative effects of smoking on children
- Interventions to stop smoking
- Ways to create a smoke-free environment
- Behavior-modification techniques

Antismoking programs directed toward children and teenagers are more successful if the focus is on short-term effects rather than on long-term effects. Developmentally, children and teenagers cannot visualize the future consequences of smoking. The immediate health risks and the cosmetic effects should be emphasized. Teaching should include how advertising puts pressure on people to smoke. Music, sports, and other activities, including stress-reducing techniques,

should be encouraged. Teaching social skills to resist peer pressure is critical.

Nurses should become politically active in the following areas:

- Banning tobacco advertising
- Enforcing restrictions of the sale of tobacco to minors
- Increasing funds for antismoking education
- Restricting public smoking to reduce the incidence of smoking
- Encouraging insurers to reimburse smoking cessation therapies

ASTHMA

There are 8.9 million children up to age 18 with asthma, representing an increase of greater than 75% from 1980 to 2003 (Federal Interagency Forum on Child and Family Statistics, 2005). Preschool children are increasingly among the newly diagnosed cases. Low-income and minority groups, especially Hispanic and African-American youth, are more likely to be hospitalized or to die from asthma. Box 20-5 lists nursing guidelines for asthmatic children. Population-focused strategies for asthma management include the following:

- Education programs for families of children and adolescents who have asthma
- The development of home and environmental assessment guides to identify triggers
- Education and outreach efforts in high-risk populations to aid in case finding (e.g., in areas with low income, high unemployment, and substandard housing, where there is exposure to secondhand smoke)
- Development of clean air policies within the community (e.g., no burning of leaves, use of smoke-free zones)
- Improved access to care for asthmatic patients (e.g., developing clinic services with consistent health care providers to decrease emergency department use)
- Assessment of schools and day-care centers for asthma "friendliness" (Box 20-6)

Box 20-5	**Nursing Guide: Asthma in Children**

Family teaching includes the following:
- Disease process and complications
- Warning signs
- Medications: purpose and administration techniques
- Equipment: cleaning and use
- Trigger avoidance
- Exercise planning: type (intensity, duration), monitoring, coordination with family patterns and school activity
- Smoking prevention: additive effects to disease
- Action plan review
- Emergency plan review
- Coordination of services: primary care provider, school staff, pharmacy, provider of durable medical equipment
- Referral to support groups, camps for psychosocial needs, community education groups, educational websites
- Referral for qualification for state or federal programs (e.g., Children's Specialty Services)

Box 20-6	School Survey for Asthma "Friendliness"

- Is the school free from tobacco smoke?
- How is the air quality? Reduce or eliminate allergens or irritants (mold, dust mites, roaches, strong chemical odors)
- Is a school nurse available?
- How are medications administered to students?
- Are emergency plans in place for taking care of students with asthma?
- Have the staff and students been taught about asthma and how to help a student with asthma?
- Are good options available for safe participation in physical education class?

NUTRITION

Promoting good nutrition and dietary habits is one of the most important parts of maintaining child health. The first 6 years are the most important for developing sound lifetime eating habits. The quality of nutrition has been widely accepted as an important influence on growth and development. It is now becoming recognized that it plays an important role in disease prevention.

Atherosclerosis begins during childhood. Other diseases, such as obesity, diabetes, **osteoporosis**, and cancer, may also have early beginnings. Low-income and minority families are at increased risk for poor nutrition, but all groups show poor dietary habits.

FACTORS INFLUENCING NUTRITION

The child and family both provide a range of variables that influence nutritional habits. Ethnic, racial, cultural, and socioeconomic factors influence what the parents eat and how they feed their children. The child brings the following individual issues to the nutritional arena:

- Slow eating
- Picky patterns
- Food preferences
- Allergies
- Acute or chronic health problems
- Changes with acceleration and deceleration of growth

Parents often have unrealistic expectations of what children should eat. Table 20-3 offers guidelines to daily requirements for all ages.

NUTRITIONAL ASSESSMENT

Physical growth serves as an excellent measure of adequacy of the diet. Height, weight, and head circumference of children younger than 3 years are plotted on appropriate growth curves at regular intervals to allow assessment of growth patterns. Good nutritional intake supports physical growth at a steady rate.

A 24-hour diet recall by the parent is a helpful screening tool to assess the amount and variety of food intake. If the recall is fairly typical for the child, the nurse can compare the intake with basic recommendations for the child's age.

Nurses will want to ask about the family's and child's concerns regarding diet and look at the family's meal patterns. A key area of nutrition assessment includes the child's and family's amount of exercise. Behavior problems that occur during meals may also be an issue.

NUTRITION DURING INFANCY

The first year of life is critical for growth of all major organ systems of the body. Nutrition during this time influences how an infant will grow and thrive. Most of the brain growth that occurs during the life span occurs during infancy. The digestive and renal systems are immature at birth and during early infancy. Certain nutrients are not handled well, and energy needs are high.

Types of Infant Feeding

Breastfeeding is the preferred method of infant feeding. Breast milk provides appropriate nutrients and antibodies for the infant. Breastfed infants have fewer illnesses and allergies. If breastfeeding is not chosen, commercially prepared formulas are an acceptable alternative. Although evaporated milk with added sugar has been used in the past as a low-cost alternative to breast milk, it is now discouraged. Errors in mixing and the lack of vitamins and minerals have been common problems.

NUTRITION DURING CHILDHOOD

The skill and desire to self-feed begins at approximately 1 year of age. The parental role begins to shift at this time to providing a balanced, healthy range of foods as the child assumes more independence. Growth rate and caloric needs decrease during this time. Nurses can best assist parents by offering information on daily needs and healthy food choices. Suggestions for children might include the following:

- Try offering frequent, small meals.
- Offer a balanced diet incorporating variety and foods that the child likes.
- Limit milk intake to the recommendations for age.
- Consider the child's developmental level and safety; avoid nuts, popcorn, grapes, and similar foods to decrease the risk of aspiration in young children.
- Encourage children to help with food selection and preparation based on developmental skills.
- Do not give vitamin and iron supplements unless directed by a physician or nurse practitioner.
- Avoid using food as a punishment or reward.

ADOLESCENT NUTRITIONAL NEEDS

The preadolescent and adolescent years are a time of increased growth that is accompanied by increases in appetite and nutritional requirements. Caloric and protein requirements increase for boys 11 to 18 years of age. Girls have an increased protein need but a decreased caloric need during the same age span. The amount of iron needed by the adolescent is nearly double the amount needed by adults.

| Table 20-3 | Daily Dietary Guidelines: Childhood and Adolescence |

Food Group	1 to 3 Years		4 to 6 Years		7 to 12 Years		Adolescent	
	Servings/Day	Serving Size	Servings/Day	Serving Size	Servings/Day	Serving Size	Servings/Day	Serving Size

Dairy
1 serving =
  Milk ½ c
  Cheese ½ oz
  Yogurt ⅓ c
  Pudding ½ c
	2–3	½ c	2	¾ c	2–3	1 c	2–3	1 c

Protein
1 oz lean meat =
  1 egg or
  1 oz cheese or
  2 T peanut
    butter or
  ¼ c cottage
    cheese
  ½ c dried peas
    or beans
	2	1 oz	2	2 oz	2	2 oz	2–3	2 oz

Vegetables/fruits
1 small fruit =
  ½ c juice or
  ½ cut fruit
	4–5	3–4 T (¼ c)	4–5	4–6 T (½ c)	At least 5	⅓–½ c	At least 5	½ c

Breads/cereals
1 slice =
  ½ c cereal or
  1 oz cold cereal
    or
  ½ c pasta or
  2–3 crackers
	3–4	½ slice	4	½ slice	6–11	1 slice	6–11	1 slice

Adolescent nutritional needs are influenced by physical alterations and psychosocial adjustments. Teenagers are often free to eat when and where they choose. Eating habits acquired from the family are abandoned. Most food is consumed away from the home. Fad foods and diets are prominent. Accelerated growth and poor eating habits put the adolescent at risk for poor nutritional health. Adolescents have the most unsatisfactory nutritional status of all age groups. Deficiencies in iron, vitamins, calcium, riboflavin, and thiamine are most common (American Academy of Pediatrics Committee on Nutrition, 2004).

Nurses initiate activities that promote improved nutritional status by doing the following:

• Providing information on good nutrition in individual or group sessions
• Providing diet assessment
• Offering educational activities that focus on the effects of fad foods and diets
• Supplying the deficient nutrients
• Providing a daily food guide (see Table 20-3)
• Suggesting snacks and quick foods that supply essential nutrients
• Explaining relationship of good nutrition to healthy appearance
• Assessing the risks for eating disorders

IMMUNIZATIONS

Routine **immunization** of children has been very successful in preventing selected diseases. The ultimate challenge is making sure that children receive immunizations.

Pediatric providers are reporting increasing parental resistance to vaccinating their children. The NIS survey for 2007 shows 8% of children 19 to 35 months were not immunized for MMR (Centers for Disease Control and Prevention, 2008), which is an alarming development. Parents do not appreciate the seriousness of vaccine preventable diseases because the prevalence is low in the world. They are confused by media misinformation about the consequences of vaccines, including autism. They have concerns about the data showing the safety of vaccines. They doubt the agencies making recommendations and the companies who manufacture vaccines. It is important to understand their concerns and to educate them about vaccine safety.

• The goal of immunization is to protect the individual by using immunizing agents to stimulate antibody formation.
• Cost and convenience are two critical issues in determining whether children are immunized.
• Successful programs combine low-cost or free immunizations provided at convenient times and locations.

- Repeatedly urging parents to obtain immunizations for their children is important.

IMMUNIZATION RECOMMENDATIONS

Pediatric providers are reporting increasing parental resistance to vaccinating their children. The NIS survey for 2007 shows 8% of children 19 to 35 months were not immunized for MMR (MMWR, 2008), which is an alarming development. Parents do not appreciate the seriousness of vaccine preventable diseases because prevalence is so low in the world. They are confused by media misinformation about the consequences of vaccines, including autism. They have concerns about the data showing the safety of vaccines. They doubt the agencies making recommendations and the companies who manufacture vaccines. It is important to understand their concerns but to educate them about vaccine safety.

Immunization recommendations rapidly change as new information and products are available. Two major organizations are responsible for guidelines: the American Academy of Pediatrics (AAP) and the U.S. Public Health Service's Advisory Committee on Immunization Practices (ACIP). Appendixes D.1–D.3 list current recommendations from the Centers for Disease Control and Prevention (CDC). The main goal of the guidelines is to provide flexibility to ensure that the largest number of children will be immunized. All health care providers are urged to access immunization status at every encounter with children and to update immunizations whenever possible. See Appendixes D.1 –D.5 for immunizing agents, contraindications, and side effects.

CONTRAINDICATIONS

There are relatively few contraindications to giving immunizations. Minor acute illness is not a contraindication. Immunizations should be deferred with moderate or acute febrile illnesses because the reactions may mask the symptoms of the illness or the side effects of the immunization may be accentuated by the illness.

People of all ages are immunized, but those with the following conditions are not routinely immunized and require medical consultation:

- Pregnancy
- Generalized malignancy
- Immunosuppressive therapy or immunodeficiency disease
- Sensitivity to components of the agent
- Recent immune serum globulin, plasma, or blood administration

ENVIRONMENTAL HEALTH HAZARDS

The environment directly affects the health of children. Growth, size, and behaviors place the pediatric population at greater risk for damage from toxins. Lead poisoning is the most common environmental health hazard. Pesticides and poor air quality also pose serious risks. Indoor air pollutants increased as houses were built "tightly" to conserve energy,

---

Box 20-7 Environmental Hazard Assessment

- Home and other buildings visited regularly, including schools and day-care centers
- Age
- Basement
- Mobile home
- Remodeling or renovation
- Heat source
- Pesticide use
- Hobbies involving toxic substances
- Parental or adolescent occupational exposure
- Reside near industry, waste areas, highways, or polluted areas
- Smoke exposure
- Dietary sources of toxins
- Breastfeeding
- Water source
- Dietary supplements or ethnic remedies

---

and as more chemicals were used in production (American Academy of Pediatrics, 2003).

Growing tissues absorb toxins readily. Developing organ systems are more susceptible to damage. Smaller size means an increased concentration of toxins per pound of body weight. The fact that children are short exposes them to lower air spaces, where heavy chemicals tend to concentrate. Outdoor play, especially during summer months, increases the opportunity for exposure to air pollutants. The type of play involves running and breathing hard, which increases the volumes of pollutants inhaled. Chewing and mouthing behaviors offer contact to toxins such as lead. Playing on the floor increases exposure to chemicals in rugs and flooring. Rolling in grass results in exposure to pesticides. Playground materials may be treated with chemicals. Exposure risks for adolescents are similar to those for adults and are primarily through work, school, and hobbies.

Populations at greatest risk include children with respiratory diseases and children from low-income families. Children with asthma and other respiratory problems are at risk from poor air quality and chemical irritants. The problems increase in urban and industrialized areas, where pollutant levels are high. Low-income populations are more likely to have substandard housing. Poor nutritional status increases the risk of complications. Screening and treatment may be delayed if there is limited access to health care. Low-income neighborhoods have been shown to have higher levels of contaminants in the water source than the general population. They are also likely to be located closer to waste areas (American Academy of Pediatrics, 2003).

It is critical to assess environmental health hazards during health care visits (Box 20-7). Referral for treatment may be necessary. Counseling families on risk reduction is important.

Population-focused nurses identify environmental problems within the community. They target at-risk populations and participate in community interventions. Bringing screening programs into neighborhoods at risk may facilitate early case finding and interventions. Lobbying efforts and education can effect public policy changes to make the environment healthier.

HOMELESS FAMILIES AND CHILDREN

The actual numbers of homeless children and adolescents are difficult to determine. Estimates vary from 200,000 to 800,000. Families make up the fastest growing segment of the homeless population; 25% to 40% of the homeless are families, often a single mother with two or three children (National Center for Health Statistics, 2002). The length of the duration of disruptions in support systems and the amount of disruption determine the effects of homelessness on health. Children in homeless situations are often not immunized and suffer from poor nutrition. They have limited or no access to health care. Often there is increased exposure to environmental hazards, violence, and substance abuse (**homeless child syndrome**).

Children experience the following:

- Chronic illness, such as tuberculosis, asthma, anemia, and chronic otitis media
- More frequent hospitalizations
- Behavioral problems such as sleep disorders, withdrawal, aggression, or depression
- School performance problems that may be caused by lack of regular attendance
- Developmental delays as a result of the lack of an appropriate environment to foster development

The nurse may be involved in outreach programs combining health care workers and community members to take the health care services to the homeless.

- Identifying a consistent team to provide continuity of care on a regular basis is important.
- The family is often removed from its network of neighbors, friends, relatives, and the usual health care providers.
- Emphasis should be placed on preventive and follow-up care and immediate problems.

Services include physical examinations, behavioral and developmental assessments, nutritional support, screening tests, and immunizations.

BRIEFLY NOTED

The number of children with health insurance is decreasing in spite of the introduction of the state child health insurance plans.

ADULT HEALTH

This part of the chapter examines the health of men and women in the United States. Definitions of women's health, men's health, historical perspectives (including the women's health movement), relevant legislation, health policy, and *Healthy People 2010* objectives that target women and men are considered. Trends in programs and services as well as access to health care are analyzed. Women's health is embedded in their communities, not just in their individual bodies (Goldman and Hatch, 2000). "*Recognizing and preventing men's health*

Box 20-8 **U.S. Preventive Health Service Recommendations for Primary Prevention Strategies for Women**

- Regular dental examinations
- Regular physical examinations, including Papanicolaou (Pap) test and mammography
- Adequate calcium intake
- Regular physical activity, including weight-bearing activities
- Diet with less than 30% fat, limit cholesterol intake, increase intake of high-fiber foods
- Limit alcohol and tobacco use; encourage smoking-cessation programs
- Hormone replacement therapy for **perimenopausal** and postmenopausal women
- Family planning and contraceptive counseling
- Home smoke detectors and security systems
- Daily dental care: floss and brush with fluoride toothpaste
- Set home water temperature at 120° to 130° F
- Appropriate immunizations: pneumococcal, influenza, and tetanus/diphtheria boosters
- Use of lap/shoulder belts
- Sexually transmitted disease prevention: consistent and correct use of barrier protection

From U.S. Preventive Services Task Force, Agency for Healthcare Research and Quality: *Guide to clinical preventive services*, ed 3, 2000, available at http:www.ahcpr.gov/clinic/cps3dix.htm.

---

problems is not just a man's issue, due to its impact on wives, mothers, daughters, and sisters—it is truly a family issue" (Frank Murkowski, Former U.S. Senator and Governor of Alaska). However, men and their families live in communities that form the environment for major public health issues.

WOMEN'S HEALTH

To understand women's health issues, it is first necessary to understand the term **women's health**. Over a decade ago, the American Academy of Nursing's 1996 Expert Panel on Women's Health said that women's health includes their entire life span and involves health promotion, maintenance, and restoration. This term recognizes that the health of women is related to the biological, social, and cultural dimensions of women's lives. Moreover, women's normal life events or rites of passage, such as menstruation, childbirth, and menopause, are considered part of normal female development rather than syndromes or diseases requiring medical treatment only. This broad emphasis on women's health is in contrast to the view of women solely in terms of their reproductive health or their role in parenting children. Box 20-8 offers illness-prevention strategies for women that reflect the new emphasis on women's health.

HISTORY OF THE WOMEN'S HEALTH MOVEMENT

The women's health movement had its seeds in the women's movement. The first Women's Rights Convention, organized by Elizabeth Cady Stanton, was held in Seneca Falls, New York, in 1848, and the participants called it one of the most courageous acts on record (National Women's History Project, 2002). After women won the right to vote in 1920, the organized women's movement took several directions. A visiting nurse, Margaret Sanger, initiated one of the most influential movements in women's health. She led the birth control movement endorsing a woman's right to be educated about family planning. In 1921 Sanger organized the American Birth Control League, which later evolved into the Federation of Planned Parenthood in 1942. Despite Sanger's work with women and birth control, it was not until the landmark Supreme Court decision, *Griswold v. Connecticut,* in 1965 that the U.S. Supreme Court made birth control legal for married couples. Fortunately, Sanger lived to see this historic turn of events. She died a few months later in 1966 (Katz, 2001).

The woman's movement enjoyed a resurgence in the 1960s—a second wave of activism. Several events highlighted this era: President John Kennedy's establishment of the President's Commission on the Status of Women in 1961, the publishing by Betty Friedan in 1963 of *The Feminist Mystique,* the passage of title VII of the 1964 Civil Rights Act that banned sexual discrimination in the workplace, and the development of the National Organization for Women (NOW) in 1966 (National Women's History Project, 2002).

In 1973 a powerful Supreme Court made a decision that came to be commonly known as *Roe v. Wade.* This landmark case addressed a woman's right to have an abortion. In 1976 Congress passed the Hyde Amendment, which excluded payment for abortions for low-income women through Medicaid; however, in cases of rape or incest, federal funding is allowed for the termination of pregnancy (Center for Reproductive Rights, 2005). Unintended pregnancies remain a major problem for U.S. women. Consequently, a campaign to reduce unintended pregnancies was mounted (U.S. Department of Health and Human Services, 2000).

In 1974 the National Women's Health Network began to monitor national health policy. This organization serves as a clearinghouse and advocate for women's health, and it has played an important role in the development of policy and legislation (National Women's Health Network, 2005). Thus the women's movement that began in Seneca Falls many years ago has evolved today into a national movement that encompasses women's health.

BRIEFLY NOTED

The Office on Women's Health in the Department of Health and Human Services was established in 1991 to improve the health of American women by advancing and coordinating a comprehensive women's health agenda throughout the U.S. Department of Health and Human Services. Almost a decade and a half later, the Men's Health Act of 2005, which would amend the Public Health Service Act to establish an Office of Men's Health within the Department of Health and Human Services, was introduced in both the U.S. House (HR 457) and Senate (S 228) in February 2005.

MEN'S HEALTH

Porche and Willis (2004) define men's health as "a holistic, comprehensive approach that addresses the physical, mental, emotional, social, and spiritual life experiences and health needs of men throughout their lifespan." (pp. 251-252) These authors expect this definition to evolve as the men's health agenda and movement mature. To design a comprehensive population-based plan that includes men, it is important to view the aspects of the male gender from various perspectives, such as personal growth, development, healing, and health within existing physical, psychological, and social contexts that form men's intrapersonal and environmental conditions.

Historically, men have dominated professions including medicine and research. As a result, the majority of clinical research focused more on male than female subjects (Simon, 2002). Although more research has been conducted on males, men still are not as healthy as women.

An important obstacle to improving men's health is their apparent reluctance to consult their primary care provider. In the United States, masculinity emphasizes physical strength, proneness to violence, the suppression of emotional expression, and competitiveness that can be detrimental to men's health (Sabo, 2000). In general, men are reluctant to seek care and are not well connected to the health care system. In one study, men have been found to be three times less likely than women to visit a physician; 33% of men did not have a primary care physician to call upon when needed and delayed seeking care despite adverse signs and symptoms (Galdas et al, 2004; Sandman et al, 2000). African-American men and Latino men are even less likely than white men to consult their physicians (Brown et al, 2000). This behavior increases their risk for and the severity of illness. Not only does this behavior limit the opportunity to prevent disease through screening, health education, and counseling, but also once they are diagnosed management and treatment will be less effective.

The lack of health insurance is also an obstacle to access to health care for men that decreases the use of preventive services and medical treatments that could reduce disease and improve health status. Sandman et al (2000) reported that one in five working-aged men were uninsured. Ethnic minorities are more likely than white males to be uninsured (Brown, 2000). Employer-based insurance programs and the Medicaid program provide some support, but a wide gap in coverage still exists.

Obstacles such as these provide opportunities and challenges for the nurse. The nurse must develop strategies to get men involved in lifestyle changes that prevent illness. All health care providers must do a better job at reaching out to men and offer the guidance and knowledge to improve men's health. The nurse must take an active role in public policy development and implementation.

An Ingenta search of journals shows numerous publications focused on women's health, women's nutrition, and women's health policy issues. In comparison, the *Journal of Men's Health,* the *International Journal of Men's Health,* and the *Journal of Men's Health and Gender* are some of the few devoted to men's health. *Harvard Men's Health Watch* is a newsletter established in 1996 that is a resource on men's health issues. There are also valuable government-managed sources for information on men's health.

Large numbers of men do not receive the health screenings intended to prevent and identify disease. Nurses play a key role in encouraging men to identify primary care providers and obtain a physical examination and the recommended screening tests appropriate to that individual.

Men who can establish a working relationship with their health care provider and participate in the recommended screening tests may live healthier, happier, and longer lives. Some health screenings clearly are beneficial while health care providers and researchers debate the benefit of other screening procedures. As a health care professional, it is important to keep up to date on current research and the literature to identify the appropriate screenings for the specific population served.

The nurse can assume many roles to fulfill responsibilities to improve the health of men in the community. As an educator, the nurse provides the knowledge and skill for replacing unhealthy behaviors with a healthy lifestyle. As a client advocate, the nurse supports and interacts with those agencies to obtain the needed resources. The nurse acts as a change agent to assess needs and system influences, identify and set priorities, plan and implement programs, and evaluate results. Working within groups and communities, nurses can identify needs and priorities and develop interventions to reduce health risks and improve the health status not only of men but also of their wives, mothers, daughters, and sisters and the communities in which they live.

WOMEN'S HEALTH CONCERNS

REPRODUCTIVE HEALTH

Women often use health care services for reproductive issues or problems, and nurses are frequently the health professionals they encounter. Nurses in the community are in a unique position to advocate for policies that increase women's access to services for reproductive health. In addition, many nurses discuss contraception with women of childbearing age. Contraceptive counseling requires accurate knowledge of current contraceptive choices and a nonjudgmental approach. The goal of contraceptive counseling is to ensure that women have appropriate instruction to make informed choices about reproduction. The choice of method depends on many factors including the woman's health, frequency of sexual activity, number of partners, and plans to have future children. No method provides a 100% guarantee against pregnancy or disease. The only 100% guarantee is not having intercourse, or abstinence (U.S. Food and Drug Administration, 2003).

The problem of unintended pregnancy exists among adolescents as well as adult women. Nurses must use caution and not assume that any woman is fully informed about contraception and that the method is used correctly and consistently. Because of the efforts of women's advocates such as

Margaret Sanger, U.S. women have a wide array of contraceptives from which to choose today.

Many women's health advocates have argued for expanding prenatal care to include preconceptual counseling (Gottesman, 2004; Kirkam et al, 2005; Maloni and Damato, 2004; Moos, 2004). Preconceptual counseling addresses risks before conception and includes education, assessment, diagnosis, and interventions. The purpose is to reduce or eliminate health risks for women and infants. For example, estimates are that 4000 pregnancies in the United States each year result in an infant born with spina bifida or anencephaly. Research has shown that intake of folic acid can significantly reduce the occurrence of these very serious and often fatal neural tube defects by 50% to 70%. However, research shows a continuing lack of awareness about the importance of taking folic acid supplements among women in low socioeconomic groups.

BRIEFLY NOTED

The Centers for Disease Control and Prevention (CDC) has launched a national campaign to educate women of reproductive age about the importance of folic acid intake before conception.

Nurses can promote increased awareness of folic acid intake among targeted women in their communities and they can educate health care professionals who serve these women as well (Ahluwalia and Daniel, 2001; Centers for Disease Control and Prevention, 2005c).

Another concern critical to preconception awareness is exposure to substances including alcohol. A major preventable cause of birth defects, mental retardation, and neurodevelopmental disorders is fetal exposure to alcohol during pregnancy. The American Academy of Pediatrics (AAP) (2000) noted that exposure to alcohol *in utero* is linked to a number of neurodevelopmental problems called *alcohol-related neurodevelopmental disorder* and *alcohol-related birth defects*. Children with these health problems can have lifelong disabilities. The recommendation of the AAP is abstinence from alcohol for women who plan to become pregnant or who are pregnant. Nurses can participate in campaigns that print and broadcast advertisements informing women of childbearing age that drinking during pregnancy can cause birth defects.

In addition, it is critical for nurses to work toward eliminating factors associated with an increased incidence of substance use during pregnancy. For example, research shows that since 1995, the rates of alcohol use during pregnancy have decreased; however, binge drinking and frequent drinking have not declined and exceed the *Healthy People 2010* targets (Centers for Disease Control and Prevention, 2002; National Center for Health Statistics, 2002). To adequately address substance use during pregnancy, therefore, nursing interventions also need to address intimate-partner violence.

Also related to women's reproductive health is access to prenatal care. Many argue that prenatal care is associated with improved birth outcomes. In the United States, estimates for the year 2000 indicated that, in general, 83.2% of women receive prenatal care in their first trimester. Four percent received late or no care. Only 69% of mothers ages 15 to 19 years received first-trimester care, and 4% of these teen mothers received late or no care (Centers for Disease Control and Prevention, National Center for Health Statistics, 2002). For many women, barriers to prenatal care include the following:

- Lack of transportation
- Cumbersome bureaucratic systems
- Health professionals who refuse to treat Medicaid patients
- Crowded clinics
- Lack of childcare

Again, nurses can serve as advocates not only to encourage their clients to utilize prenatal care services but also to work toward the establishment of services that are accessible, affordable, and available to all pregnant women.

MENOPAUSE

Menopause, also referred to as *the change* or *change of life,* is the time at which the levels of the hormones *estrogen* and *progesterone* change in a woman's body. This change leads to the stopping of menstruation. The decline in these hormone levels affects a variety of functions. These effects can be seen in changes in the following (U.S. Department of Health and Human Services, National Institute on Aging, 2003):

- Vaginal and urinary tract
- Cardiovascular system
- Bone density
- Libido
- Sleep patterns
- Memory
- Emotions

A common complaint from women is the phenomenon known as *hot flashes.*

Women's attitudes toward menopause vary greatly and are influenced by culture, age, support, and the recounted experiences of other women. Menopause has been viewed on a continuum from a normal progression of aging to a disease state or time of imbalance or ill health.

Treatment for the unpleasant side effects of menopause has traditionally been with **hormone replacement therapy (HRT)**. However, researchers have found increases in the rates of coronary heart disease, stroke, and pulmonary embolism in women taking HRT compared to those taking a placebo. The use of HRT remains controversial (National Institutes of Health, 2005).

BRIEFLY NOTED

Recently, the National Institutes of Health (NIH) announced that it has stopped a major clinical trial examining the benefits of hormone replacement therapy for healthy menopausal women because of the increased risk for invasive breast cancer (National Institutes of Health, 2002).

OSTEOPOROSIS

It is estimated that one in every two American women older than 50 years of age will experience an osteoporosis-related fracture in her lifetime (National Institute of Arthritis and Musculoskeletal and Skin Diseases, 2005). It is thought that the falling level of estrogen contributes to the loss of bone. Now, with the changes in beliefs about the risks involved in HRT, other measures designed to thwart the progression of osteoporosis will receive more attention. Primary prevention activities aimed at women need to include the following:

- Diets that are rich in calcium and vitamin D
- Exposure to sunlight for 20 minutes a day, recommended as an alternative source of vitamin D
- Exercise, especially weight-bearing activities such as walking, running, stair climbing, and weight lifting, to improve bone density
- Limiting alcohol consumption and avoiding smoking (National Institute of Arthritis and Musculoskeletal and Skin Diseases, 2005)

BREAST CANCER

Breast cancer is the second leading cause of cancer deaths among all women (National Center for Health Statistics, 2008). Although the incidence of breast cancer is higher in white women than in African-American women, the death rate for African-American women is higher. Secondary prevention that includes screening activities, such as mammography, clinical breast examination, and self-breast examination, make a difference in death rates. Early detection can promote a cure whereas late detection typically ensures a poor prognosis. The differences in the outcomes between women of color and white women point to issues associated with early detection, access to health care, and follow-up by a regular care provider (Schulz et al, 2002).

FEMALE GENITAL MUTILATION

Common in many African countries and certain Asian and Middle Eastern countries, female genital mutilation (FGM) is a practice that is centuries old. Banned in the early 1990s in Somalia, FGM is now at an all-time high in that country because of that country's preoccupation with civil war. According to the World Health Organization (WHO), the rate of genital cutting in Somalia today is approximately 98%. Justification for FGM is related to tradition, inequities in power, and the compliance of women to community norms or law (World Health Organization, 2005). This practice is considered an important part of a woman's access to marriage and childbearing.

FGM can take several forms, ranging from the excision of the clitoris with partial or total removal of the labia minora, to the severe form in which the labia majora are fused following the removal of the clitoris and labia minora (Bosch, 2001). These procedures are associated with

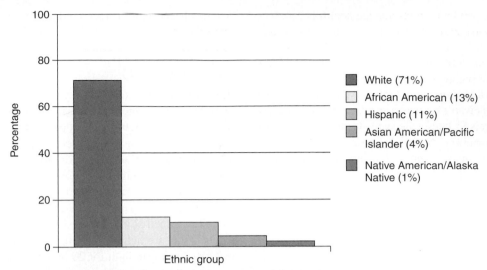

FIGURE 20-I Distribution of U.S. women in racial and ethnic groups.

morbidity related to substantial complications such as hemorrhage, infection, tetanus, and septicemia. Long-term effects of FGM include impaired urinary and menstrual functioning, chronic genital pain, cysts, neuromas, ulcers, urinary incontinence, and infertility (Ford, 2001). Increasingly, women who have been mutilated are immigrating to the United States. Thus nurses need to be familiar with the practices of immigrants in their communities and with state statutes related to FGM.

HEALTH DISPARITIES AMONG SPECIAL GROUPS OF WOMEN

Women of color represent approximately 29% of all women in the United States (USDHHS, Office of Women's Health, 2003). These women come from the five major ethnic and racial groups depicted in Figure 20-1.

However, using the major groups of women as shown in Figure 20-1 excludes many of the subgroups of women in U.S. society. For example, subgroups include recent immigrants, who may not view themselves as being part of these racial and ethnic groups and can even be undercounted in the census (Stover, 2002). Rural women are another unique subgroup not captured by the five major groups. Rural women of color have special health-related problems including geographic and informational isolation, few services, limited transportation, and poverty (Hargraves, 2002).

Women of color experience many of the same health problems as their white counterparts. However, as a group they experience the following (Cornelius, Smith, and Simpson, 2002; Satcher, 2001):

- Poorer health
- Access to fewer health care services
- A disproportionate rate of earlier deaths
- Fewer preventive health services
- Inadequate insurance

The process of addressing these disparities is daunting. The intent is to close the gap in health disparities while preserving the richness and unique influences of various cultures. Evidence suggests that ensuring access to a regular health care provider is the key to meeting the preventive health care needs of women of color (Cornelius, Smith, and Simpson, 2002). Many providers do not incorporate preventive screenings into their practice; therefore nurses can target interventions designed to address preventive health issues. In particular, culturally sensitive and gender-sensitive programs are needed for communities with women of color. Nurses are well positioned to advocate for these types of programs necessary for communities with women of color.

BRIEFLY NOTED

Because of the known health disparities experienced by women of color, preventive services should target diversity and cultural awareness throughout the entire program planning process.

Incarcerated women represent an increasing issue for nurses in the United States. Although female incarceration rates are lower than male rates at all ages, both rates reveal considerable racial and ethnic disparities. African-American and non-Hispanic women had a prison and jail rate that is three times higher than that of Hispanic women and six times higher than that of white women. Although the rate of incarceration for men exceeds that of women, from 1995 to 2004 the annual rate increase among women was 4.8%; for men, it was 3.1%. At the end of 2004 women constituted 7% of all state and federal prisoners (U.S. Department of Justice, Bureau of Justice Statistics, 2005).

Lesbians have been considered a hidden but special population in many ways, partly because of the social stigma associated with lesbianism coupled with the fear of discrimination. The social environments that lesbians share may influence their behaviors and produce patterns of both negative and positive health habits that influence their health status (Aaron, 2001).

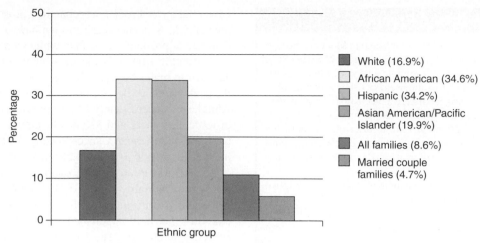

FIGURE 20-2 Poverty rate of families headed by women.

Findings indicate that lesbians and bisexual women in the United States are found to have a higher prevalence of several risk factors than their heterosexual counterparts with regard to smoking, alcohol use, and lack of preventive cancer screening (Rosenberg, 2001). To improve the health of lesbian women, services that address their unique needs are warranted. Safe places in which these women are able to voice their concerns and receive effective health promotion, disease prevention, and treatment are critical. Nurses can work as advocates to reduce stereotypes and discrimination toward lesbian women.

According to the Office on Women's Health (OWH), 26 million American women live with some type of disability (U.S. Department of Health and Human Services, 2005b). The varying conditions that comprise disability make women's roles more challenging. Many disabling conditions and diseases disproportionately affect women. Many issues surround women with disabilities. Concerns associated with health, aging, civil rights, abuse, and independent living are examples of the types of problems facing them.

Persistent stereotyping and treatment of disabled women as asexual and dependent are major barriers to addressing their needs. Physical problems impose many barriers to sexual activity in women with disabilities; this is compounded by the reluctance of health care providers to address the topic. Older women with disabilities may have had inadequate information about sexual issues, and they may be too embarrassed to ask questions related to their specific concerns.

Although all women are subjected to violence and abuse, women with disabilities are thought to endure abuse for longer periods than their nondisabled counterparts and are also more likely to suffer abuse at the hands of caregivers and personal assistants (Curry, Hassouneh-Phillips, and Johnston-Silverberg, 2001).

Nurses can develop an awareness of the many health-related issues facing disabled women in society. Care should be taken to recognize the physical barriers that prevent women from accessing health care, such as structures that are not accessible despite the recommendations of the Americans with Disabilities Act (ADA). Some women are physically unable to position themselves on examination tables, posing a challenge in providing routine gynecological examinations.

Nurses are positioned to act in a variety of roles such as an advocate, educator, and case manager. Having knowledge about appropriate community resources is the key in identifying services geared toward meeting these women's needs. Developing health-promotion programs targeted at this vulnerable, high-risk group will assist in promoting health and well-being among this growing population.

Unfortunately, many U.S. women do not have the resources to achieve a basic level of health. Although poverty rates dropped in 2000, many in the United States, particularly women, remain poor (U.S. Department of Labor, 2001). Women who subsist below the poverty line are at great risk for becoming homeless. Poverty is a special problem for *head-of-household* women. Poverty among head-of-household women also reflects the disparities that exist in the United States between various ethnic and racial groups, as female-headed African-American and Hispanic families suffer disproportionately higher rates of poverty than other families (Figure 20-2).

Some U.S. politicians have proposed that unless women marry, they will remain poor (Dionne, 2002). Many factors make it difficult for these women to rise out of poverty.

In addition to increasing the incomes of U.S. workers, public services need to include the following:

- Adequate health insurance
- Childcare
- Housing
- Efficient public transportation

To support the interests of low-income women, nurses can effect change in these services by participating in debates with health policymakers at local, state, and national levels (Ehrenreich, 2002).

Older Women

Women make up the largest proportion of the older population in the United States. In 2003, 58% of those aged 65 years and older and 70% of those aged 85 years and older were women; these numbers are expected to double (U.S. Bureau of the Census, 2003).

Older women, especially women of color and women from lower socioeconomic groups, experience higher rates of chronic illness and disability than their white and more affluent counterparts. Women with lower levels of education, with lower incomes, and who are enrolled in Medicare programs are more likely to report fair or poor health than women from higher socioeconomic groups. Low-income and less-educated women report not only more chronic illness but also more symptoms, including severe pain from arthritis, than their white and more affluent counterparts (Bierman and Clancy, 2001).

To improve the health of older women, nursing programs in community health need to address these racial, ethnic, and socioeconomic disparities. The improvement of preventive services and the management of chronic conditions are imperative. However, it will also be necessary to consider older women's socioeconomic status, educational levels, and racial and ethnic backgrounds to adequately address their health needs (see "Evidence-Based Practice" box).

MEN'S HEALTH CONCERNS

Prostate cancer is the most frequently diagnosed cancer in men, with 218,890 cases estimated to have occurred in 2007 (National Cancer Institute, 2009). Approximately one in six men will be diagnosed with prostate cancer, making it the second leading cause of cancer deaths in men (American Cancer Society, 2006; Stotts, 2004). There is no clear evidence about what causes this or how to prevent prostate cancer. Although all men are at risk for developing prostate cancer, men who

have a father or brother who has had prostate cancer are at greater risk. African-American men have a 51% higher incident rate of prostate cancer than white men (Stotts, 2004).

Testicular cancer is the most common solid tumor diagnosed in males between the ages of 15 and 40 years with the peak incidence between the ages of 18 and 40 years. The American Cancer Society (ACS) predicted 8250 new cases of testicular cancer and 370 deaths due to cancer of the testis in 2006 (American Cancer Society, 2006). Age-adjusted incidence shows 6.3/100,000 of white men and 1.5/100,000 of African-American men are diagnosed with testicular cancer with a mortality rate of 0.3/100,000 and 0.2/100,000, respectively. Unfortunately, the cause of testicular cancer is unknown. The only established relationship to testicular cancer is cryptorchidism. The good news is that testicular cancer is rare, and the 5-year survival rate by race was reported to be 96.3% for white men and 87.8% for African-American men.

Because painless testicular enlargement is commonly the first sign of testicular cancer, the testicular self-examination has traditionally been recommended for men. However, in 2004 the U.S. Preventive Services Task Force (USPSTF) updated previously published guidelines that significantly altered that tradition (U.S. Preventive Services Task Force, 2004). The new guidelines state:

The USPSTF found no new evidence that screening with clinical examination or **testicular self-examination (TSE)** *is effective in reducing mortality from testicular cancer. Even in the absence of screening, the current treatment interventions provided very favorable health outcomes. Given the low prevalence of testicular cancer, limited accuracy of screening tests, and no evidence for the incremental benefits of screening, the USPSTF concluded that the harms of screening exceed any potential benefits.*

SHARED HEALTH CONCERNS

MORTALITY

Ranking the causes of death from most frequent to least serves as a useful indicator for illustrating the relative burden of cause-specific mortality. Diseases of the heart are the number one cause of death for both males and females followed by various cancers. Keep in mind that the ranking may not reflect the most important cause of death for a specific population. When establishing community priorities, it is vital to identify and define the community of interest. Community priorities will change as adults age.

- Before the age of 45 years, accidents followed by assaults and intentional self-harm have been identified as the leading causes of death for men.
- Between the ages of 45 and 54 years, diseases of the heart ranked first.
- However, cancer ranks first in males age 55 to 64 years.
- In the 65 years and older age group, this changes again as diseases of the heart return to first place followed by cancer.
- Between the ages of 55 and 84 years, chronic lower respiratory diseases hold the number three ranking.

- In men 85 years of age and older, cerebrovascular disease is ranked third, moving chronic lower respiratory diseases down to fourth.

CARDIOVASCULAR DISEASE

One in eight American men and one in five women reported having cardiovascular disease in 2005 (Neyer et al, 2007). Heart disease is one of the most significant public health problems in the United States, resulting in an enormous increase in premature mortality and disability (Barnett et al, 2001). Cardiovascular disease (CVD) is the leading cause of death in the United States. Within CVD, coronary heart disease (CHD) is the major category that is responsible for the majority of deaths. Diagnoses of the CHD category predominantly include myocardial infarction, acute ischemic heart disease, angina pectoris, and atherosclerosis.

Barnett et al (2001) reported that many community-based public health programs to reduce heart disease and prevent its onset have had limited effectiveness, which created a renewed sense of urgency to develop and implement more effective programs and policies to reduce the burden of heart disease on society. The American Heart Association has identified factors that increase the risk of coronary artery disease (Khot et al, 2003). The degree to which each risk factor is present also should be considered (Greenland et al, 2003). Some of the risk factors can be modified by the person; other factors cannot. The major risk factors that cannot be changed include increasing age, male gender, and heredity. The major risk factors that can be modified, treated, or controlled by lifestyle changes include smoking, high blood cholesterol, high blood pressure, lack of physical activity, diabetes, and poor dietary habits.

Risk Factors for Coronary Heart Disease

Cigarette smoking has been declining since 1964; however, it is currently declining at a slower rate (National Center for Health Statistics, 2005). Cigarette smoking has a synergistic effect on the other risk factors that greatly increases the likelihood of developing CHD. Of clients with premature CHD, 85% to 90% had at least one risk factor, which was most commonly cigarette smoking (Khot et al, 2003). Smoking is strongly linked to chronic lower respiratory diseases, which are the fourth leading cause of death in women and the fifth leading cause of death in men. Eliminating cigarette smoking could significantly delay the onset of CHD and prevent many lung diseases. Therefore smoking cessation is a major public health focus.

A high blood cholesterol (HBC) level is a major risk factor for cardiovascular disease. Higher levels of cholesterol are correlated with a high risk of coronary artery disease and hypertension. Cholesterol levels may be lowered through dietary modification, physical activity, weight control, and/or drug treatment.

Public screening for cholesterol levels has the potential to detect large numbers of people with elevated levels of cholesterol and raise awareness of HBC as a risk factor for CHD. The public health community must increase public education and awareness about the risks of HBC and must promote lifestyle changes.

High blood pressure or hypertension is estimated to occur in one in three U.S. adults and, because hypertension does not have symptoms, one-third of these people do not know they have the disease. Uncontrolled hypertension leads to heart attack, stroke, kidney damage, and a host of other complications. Therefore hypertension is called "the silent killer" and is not being adequately managed (American Heart Association, 2006).

According to Khot et al (2003), it is clear that the majority of these risk factors for CHD are largely preventable by living a healthy lifestyle and that focusing efforts to improve these lifestyles has great potential in reducing the "epidemic" of CHD. Men and women have significantly different survival rates from myocardial infarctions: 42% of women die within the first year following a myocardial infarction compared to 24% of men. Some explain this difference by noting that women typically develop their disease almost 10 years after men and have more co-occurring morbidities that contribute to their poor outcomes. Others argue that women are not diagnosed and treated as aggressively as men and that medications traditionally used for men can have adverse effects on women (Agency for Healthcare Research and Quality, 2005).

As with men, many factors predispose women to CVD. Physical factors contributing to the development of CVD include smoking, high blood cholesterol levels, diabetes mellitus, obesity, hypertension, diets high in fat and low in fiber, and physical inactivity (Gerhard-Herman, 2002; Oliver-McNeil and Artinian, 2002). Although it was thought that hormone replacement therapy had a positive effect on the incidence of CVD, as noted earlier research has not supported this claim (Writing Group for the Women's Health Initiative Investigators, 2002).

Sociocultural factors that influence CVD in women include lack of knowledge about health, limited preventive care, and decreased access to care. Identifying women at risk through a careful family history can alert the nurse to situations that might place women at high risk for CVD. In addition, the U.S. Preventive Services Task Force *Guide to Clinical Preventive Services* recommends routine screening for hypertension for adults, including women, 18 years of age and older and screening for lipid disorders among women 45 years of age and older (Agency for Healthcare Research and Quality, U.S. Preventive Services Task Force, 2005).

STROKE

Strokes and cardiovascular diseases affect different areas of the body, but they share the same risk factors that cause damage to the vascular system that supplies needed oxygen to the body. The death rate from strokes has fallen (National Center for Chronic Disease Prevention and Promotion, 2005). Still, more than 700,000 strokes still occur every year, resulting in major life changes. Strokes tend to run in families, and men are 1.25 times more likely than women to experience a stroke (American Heart Association, 2006). African-American males have almost twice the stroke incidence as white males. There have been various community-based programs that have been effective and beneficial

| Box 20-9 | **Community-Based Intervention for Men with Diabetes** |

A nurse may consider a roadmap tailored to a men's health perspective. *Roadmaps* are a form of the population-based care model for the delivery of planned care. Group Health Co-operative (GHC) implemented the Diabetes Roadmap (Wagner et al, 2002). The Diabetes Roadmap contained guidelines for diabetes care, patient education, self-management, primary care practice redesign, access to expert support, a diabetes registry, and organizational leadership. Published results indicate that the program increased adherence to guidelines.

in reducing the impact strokes have on a community (Jiang et al, 2004; Morgenstern et al, 2002). These programs often include health education and management to reduce risk factors. Collaboration between health care institutions, community leaders, emergency medical services, and support groups within the community is needed for these programs to be effective.

DIABETES MELLITUS

Diabetes is a serious public health challenge for the United States. Of the 20.8 million people with diabetes, 10.9 million, or 10.5% of all men 20 years of age and older, have diabetes (National Center for Chronic Disease Prevention and Promotion, 2005). In the United States, diabetes is an epidemic; 1 in 12 adults reportedly has diabetes. It is also estimated that for every two people who have diabetes, there is another person who does not know that he or she has it. Mortality rates from diabetes continue to rise for all ethnic and socioeconomic groups, but evidence suggests that complications and mortality rates are highest among low-income and minority groups (Bassett, 2005). For example, research suggests African-Americans and Hispanics have higher rates of complications and readmissions after hospital stays (Jiang et al, 2005), and estimates indicate that one of two Latinas will develop diabetes (Bassett, 2005). The many complications associated with diabetes include heart disease, stroke, hypertension, retinopathy, kidney disease, neuropathies, amputations, and dental disease (National Institute of Diabetes and Digestive and Kidney Diseases [NIDDK], National Diabetes Information Clearinghouse, 2005).

This disease is expected to worsen before improving. There is a tremendous need to strive to limit the toll this disease takes on the person and the community. Community-based education programs (Box 20-9) have been shown to be effective in helping clients manage the disease better and become more aware of the test results used to monitor diabetes (Polonsky et al, 2005).

The socioeconomic status of women with diabetes is lower than that of women without diabetes. In the year 2000, 25% of women with diabetes over the age of 25 years also had a low level of formal education. Women with higher education may have opportunities to make decisions differently, have greater access to health care, and have a higher

standard of living, all which greatly impact health and health outcomes (Beckles and Thompson-Reid, 2002).

Addressing the diabetes epidemic involves more than a focus on individual factors. Recent research supports the importance of also addressing social and economic factors related to health and well-being when tackling the diabetes epidemic. These social determinants of health include the characteristics of communities, such as income distribution and segregation. This broader perspective also includes attention to policies that affect the availability of healthy foods (Schulz et al, 2005).

Gestational diabetes mellitus (GDM) is a condition characterized by carbohydrate intolerance that is first identified or develops during pregnancy. The incidence of gestational diabetes is increasing in the United States.

During pregnancy, women with gestational diabetes have a greater risk for preeclampsia, cesarean section, and infection. "Women are more likely to develop gestational diabetes if they are older, have a higher pre-pregnancy weight, high body mass index, or weight gain in young adulthood, have a high parity or history of a previous adverse pregnancy, or have preexisting hypertension, or a family history of diabetes" (Rowley et al, 2001, p. 73).

Reducing the morbidity and mortality of diabetes along with enhancing the quality of life for women with diabetes is a key area of focus for nurses. Two approaches involve (1) health care system interventions optimizing diabetic care, and (2) community-based diabetes self-management education interventions (Centers for Disease Control and Prevention, 2001).

- Primary prevention includes educating adults about nutrition and the risks of obesity, smoking, and physical inactivity. Community interventions addressing healthy eating, exercise, and weight reduction also can benefit adults at risk for diabetes.
- Secondary prevention includes screening for diabetes with finger-stick blood glucose tests or glucose tolerance tests. Screening is also accomplished by a thorough history and physical examination.
- Tertiary prevention targets activities aimed at reducing the complications of the disease. Examples are intense monitoring of blood glucose levels, modification of diet and/or medications, and efforts to prevent long-term complications.

MENTAL HEALTH

Although both men and women suffer from the burden of mental illness, women experience certain conditions more often than men. In the United States, for example, depression and anxiety disorders are twice as likely to affect women as men, and women experience eating disorders nine times as often as men (National Institute of Mental Health [NIMH], 2002).

A number of factors contribute to depression in women. Researchers are exploring how biological factors, including genetics and sex hormones, affect women's increased risk for depression. Other scientists are focusing on how psychosocial factors such as life stress, trauma, and interpersonal relationships contribute to women's depression (Mazure et al, 2002).

Nursing scholars also have documented the conditions under which women experience depression. For example, the long-term consequences of intimate partner violence often involve depression and posttraumatic stress disorder (Campbell, 2002). Campbell argues that the global incidence of depression could be attributable to the experiences of women as a result of domestic violence, but this premise remains to be tested. Some researchers examining this problem have reported that college women with histories of intimate partner violence have a higher incidence of depression, anxiety, and other measures of psychiatric symptomatology than non-abused women (Amar and Gennaro, 2005). Other researchers have found traumatic life events and sexual orientation to be risk factors for depression (Matthews et al., 2002). Still others argue that health professionals must use caution not to medicalize all the unhappiness in the lives of women but to also explore the possibility that women's restrictive social roles can lead to depression (Wright and Owen, 2001).

Noting women's increased risk for depression, the U.S. Preventive Services Task Force (Agency for Healthcare Research and Quality, U.S. Preventive Services Task Force, 2005b) recommends screening for depression in adults when there are adequate systems in place to make an accurate diagnosis as well as provide effective treatment and follow-up. Risk factors for depression include female sex, a family history of depression, unemployment, and chronic disease. The U.S. Preventive Services Task Force (USPSTF) recommends the following two screening questions: (1) "Over the past two weeks have you felt down, depressed, or hopeless?" (2) "Over the past two weeks have you felt little interest or pleasure in doing things?" Nurses can encourage health professionals in their communities to screen and treat depression among women and to work for health services to address stress and generally improve the mental well-being of women.

Because adverse working conditions and numerous pathological conditions clearly are detrimental to men's health, there is a great need to focus on the mental health of men. Twenty-six percent of adult men reported high levels of depressive symptoms and one-third reported a moderate level of depressive symptoms (Sandman et al, 2000). Both men with poor health and less-educated men are more depressed. Men between 25 and 54 years of age are at greatest risk for suicide (Knox and Caine, 2005). Suicide, one of the leading causes of death in men, is preventable.

Poor mental states adversely affect men's physical health directly by depressing the immune system and indirectly by motivating the men to participate in unhealthy behaviors, such as increased alcohol consumption, smoking, poor eating habits, and avoiding health care interventions (Thomas, 2004) (see "Evidence-Based Practice" box).

Establishing support groups for men in the community may be an avenue to reduce symptoms of depression. However, men are not known to use traditional support groups.

Evidence-Based Practice

A population-based alcohol reduction intervention can reduce men's deaths. Holder et al. (2000) demonstrated that a coordinated, comprehensive, population-based intervention can reduce patterns of high-risk alcohol consumption by young men (e.g., binge drinking, drinking and driving, and underage drinking), which are linked to vehicular accidents and homicides. The community interventions consisted of five prevention strategies: (1) to mobilize the community to support the project through community coalitions and media advocacy, (2) to advise alcohol distributors and retailers to develop policies to reduce intoxication and drunk driving, (3) to reduce underage access by advising retailers to stop selling alcohol to men younger than 21 years, (4) to increase the actual and perceived risk of arrest for drunk driving, and (5) to assist the community in developing local restriction of alcohol through zoning laws.

NURSE USE: Nurses in community health can plan interventions targeted to reduce high-risk drinking and alcohol-related injuries and assaults.

Other strategies that the nurse can work with the community to implement include (1) buying state-of-the-art breath-testing technology, (2) encouraging police to conduct roadside checks to detect drinking and driving, and (3) encouraging police to conduct sting operations to enforce responsible beverage distribution.

Modified from Holder HD et al: Effect of community-based interventions on high-risk drinking and alcohol-related injuries, *JAMA* 284(18):2341–2347, 2000.

More innovative approaches such as online chat rooms may be used as a possible venue for support groups where men may feel more comfortable expressing their emotional needs. The nurse must be knowledgeable and sensitive to men's mental health care needs to tailor effective interventions.

CANCER

Cancers of all types are a serious public health concern. Cancers are the second leading cause of death in the United States. Cancer rates declined, however, during the 1990s, and for the first time, rates for lung cancer among women remained level between 1995 and 2001 (National Cancer Institute [NCI], 2005). Researchers speculate that cancer rates among women are high because of the aging population, with a larger number of women aged 50 to 74 years (Edwards et al., 2002).

Following heart disease, cancer is the second leading cause of death in the United States. Men have a 46% lifetime probability of developing cancer, compared to a 38% lifetime probability for women (Jemal et al, 2005). African-American men have a 40% higher death rate from all cancers combined than white men. The three leading causes of cancer death for males are cancer of the lung and bronchus, colon and rectum, and prostate (American Cancer Society, 2006). Lung cancer is the leading cause of cancer deaths in women followed by cancer of the breast and colorectal cancers (Centers for Disease Control and Prevention, National Center for Health Statistics, 2005).

Overall, white women have a higher incidence rate for all cancers while African-American women have a higher mortality rate for all cancers (Edwards et al., 2002). A diagnosis of cancer is a life-changing event that often forces women to make many decisions that leave them with feelings of being overwhelmed and out of control. A diagnosis of cancer can change how a woman feels about her body and how she relates to and interacts with others (Spira and Kenemore, 2001).

Lung cancer is the leading cause of cancer death in both men and women. What is tragic about lung cancer is that it, in most cases, could have been prevented by living a healthier lifestyle. Helping men stop smoking will lower their risk of developing cancer, as well as the risk for heart attack and stroke. Primary prevention aimed at young girls that highlights the harmful effects of tobacco is one strategy for nurses to employ to reduce smoking.

BRIEFLY NOTED

It is clear that tobacco use in any form has detrimental effects on personal health. Current legislation has limited or banned smoking in public places. These policies have been criticized by smokers who cite the "common courtesy approach" as being effective.

Colorectal cancer is the third most prevalent form of cancer in both men and women (American Cancer Society, 2006). However, mortality rates for both men and women have declined over the past 20 years, due primarily to increased screening and improved treatments. Obesity, physical inactivity, smoking, heavy alcohol consumption, a diet high in red or processed meats, and insufficient intake of fruits and vegetables are risk factors for colorectal cancer. Reducing these risk factors will reduce the incidence of the disease.

Women more than 75 years of age are at increased risk for this cancer, and the 5-year relative survival rate is about 60%. African-American women have the highest incidence and death rates attributable to colorectal cancer (Edwards et al, 2002). Primary prevention and early detection are critical to the survival of people with colorectal cancer. Nurses can inform adults of their risks, the signs and symptoms of the disease, and screening opportunities in their communities.

HIV/AIDS/STDs

Sexually transmitted diseases (STDs) are a major public health problem. The Centers for Disease Control and Prevention (2005a,b) estimates that 19 million new infections occur each year (see "How To" box).

HIV/AIDS in Women

The proportion of all AIDS cases among adult and adolescent women has more than tripled in the United States since 1985. Female adults and adolescents comprised only 7% of all AIDS cases reported in 1985, but by 2003 the percentage

| **HOW TO** | **Prevent Sexually Transmitted Diseases (STDs)** |

Nurses play a vital role in preventing STDs. Five key concepts provide the foundation for the prevention and control of STDs:
1. Education and counseling of persons at risk on ways to adopt safer sexual behavior
2. Identification of asymptomatically infected persons and of symptomatic persons unlikely to seek diagnostic and treatment services
3. Effective diagnosis and treatment of infected persons
4. Evaluation, treatment, and counseling of sex partners of persons who are infected with an STD
5. Preexposure vaccination of persons at risk for vaccine-preventable STDs

From Centers for Disease Control and Prevention: *CDC HIV-AIDS fact sheet,* 2006, CDC.

had grown to 27% (Centers for Disease Control and Prevention, National Center for HIV, STD, and TB Prevention [NCHSTBP], 2005a). Research shows profound differences in the ethnic and racial distribution of HIV/AIDS in U.S. women. Generally, the most common way that HIV/AIDS is transmitted to U.S. women is through heterosexual contact, which accounted for 71% of cases in 2003. Twenty-seven percent of the cases were contracted through injection drug use and 2% were from other or unidentified risk factors (Centers for Disease Control and Prevention, National Center for HIV, STD, and TB Prevention, 2005b). Regional differences, however, do exist. For example, in 2003 most of the AIDS cases among female adults and adolescents were in the northeastern and southern regions of the United States. In addition, in the northeastern United States, slightly more women reported injection drug use rather than heterosexual contact as the source of their exposure. In the midwestern and western regions, statistics were nearly equally distributed between these two sources of exposure, with heterosexual contact being in the majority. In the southern region, women typically reported heterosexual contact rather than injection drug use as the source of infection (Centers for Disease Control and Prevention, National Center for HIV, STD, and TB Prevention, 2005b).

When women acquire HIV/AIDS via heterosexual transmission, their partners are usually injection drug users. Women who have used injection drugs themselves are certainly at risk for infection too. Women who use noninjection drugs, such as methamphetamines and crack cocaine, and are trading sex for money and/or drugs are also at high risk (Centers for Disease Control and Prevention, National Center for HIV, STD, and TB Prevention, 2005a).

Alarming statistics regarding the prevalence of HIV/AIDS among women of childbearing age have prompted the CDC to recommend HIV screening for all pregnant women. Testing based on a risk basis misses many women who are HIV positive. The health of HIV-positive women, moreover, can improve with antiretroviral therapy. Therapy can also reduce the chances of HIV transmission to the infant before, during, or after birth (Centers for Disease Control and Prevention, National Center for HIV, STD, and TB Prevention, 2005c).

Women with HIV/AIDS require specific health and social services to reduce the burden of their disease. These include services that integrate both prevention and treatment of HIV/AIDS as well as comorbidities such as other sexually transmitted diseases and problematic substance use (Centers for Disease Control and Prevention, National Center for HIV, STD, and TB Prevention, 2005a). Nurses serve as advocates by focusing on the high-risk behaviors of individual women, and also on the factors in their communities that lead to injection drug use and sexual exposure to HIV. Interventions to improve education, employment opportunities, and adequate housing, as well as to decrease drug use, isolation, and poverty, can have a critical impact on this epidemic.

HIV/AIDS in Men

Men represent the largest proportion of all HIV/AIDS cases among adults and adolescents in the United States (men, 73%; women, 27%) (Centers for Disease Control and Prevention, 2005b). The estimated number of AIDS cases increased by 7% in men from 2000 to 2004 (Centers for Disease Control and Prevention, 2005b). The number of deaths from AIDS among all persons with AIDS decreased by 8% from 2000 to 2004 (Centers for Disease Control and Prevention, 2005b). The reduction in deaths from AIDS included a decrease of estimated deaths among men who have sex with men (MSM) and intravenous drug users (IDUs). As the numbers of deaths from AIDS decreased, the prevalence of persons living with AIDS increased (Centers for Disease Control and Prevention, 2005b).

Of the male adults and adolescents living with HIV/AIDS, 60% were MSM, 19% were IDUs, 13% were exposed through heterosexual contact, and 7% were MSM who were also IDUs (Centers for Disease Control and Prevention, 2005b). Survival after AIDS diagnosis varies by mode of transmission. It is greatest among MSM, followed by men with heterosexual contact, and lowest among men who were IDUs (Centers for Disease Control and Prevention, 2005b).

Racial and ethnic disparities exist in the diagnoses of HIV/AIDS. In 2003 half of the population living with HIV/AIDS were African-American (Centers for Disease Control and Prevention, HIV/AIDS Fact Sheets, 2006a). More than half of new AIDS cases reported to the CDC are among African-American and Hispanic persons (Centers for Disease Control and Prevention, Office of Minority Health, 2006). HIV infection is the leading cause of death for African-American men ages 35 to 44 years (Centers for Disease Control and Prevention, Office of Minority Health, 2006). In 2001 HIV/AIDS was the third leading cause of death among Hispanic men ages 35 to 44 years (Centers for Disease Control and Prevention, HIV/AIDS Fact Sheets, 2006b). Regional disparities exist as well. From 2000 to 2004, the estimated number of AIDS cases increased the most in the southern United States, followed by the midwest, the northeast, and the west (Centers for Disease Control and Prevention, 2005b). African-Americans accounted for the majority of diagnoses in the south and northeast, with African-American males accounting for more HIV/AIDS diagnoses than any other racial and ethnic populations in these regions (Centers for Disease Control and Prevention, 2006).

HIV/AIDS prevention efforts have been effective in slowing the rate of the epidemic as evidenced by the decline of new HIV infections in the United States (Centers for Disease Control and Prevention, 2006c). Current recommendations of HIV prevention strategies include the following:
- HIV prevention counseling
- Testing, and referral services
- Partner notification
- Prevention for high-risk populations
- Health education and risk reduction activities
- Perinatal transmission prevention
- School-based HIV prevention (Centers for Disease Control and Prevention, 2006c)

BRIEFLY NOTED

If a person with HIV or AIDS knowingly infects another person, it may be considered a criminal offense.

ACCIDENTS AND INJURIES

The age-adjusted fatal rate of injury was 2.6 times higher for men than for women. The nonintentional injury rate for men was 1.3 times higher than that for women. Unintentional injuries are the leading cause of death in men of all races below the age of 45 years. From ages 45 to 54 years, it is still ranked the third cause of death, and between the ages of 55 and 64 years, it is the fourth leading cause of death. In women unintentional injuries are the seventh leading cause of death. Motor vehicle accidents were the leading cause of unintentional fatal injuries, followed by falls and poisoning. Young males between the ages of 19 and 29 years are the least likely to wear a seat belt while driving or riding in a car (Agency for Healthcare Research and Quality, 2004). Although public safety programs exist that focus on the prevention of specific types of injuries, more programs are needed aimed specifically at men.

WEIGHT CONTROL

American women spend a great deal of time, energy, and money in the never-ending pursuit of the body beautiful. In 1998 the National Institutes of Health (NIH) began using the calculation of BMI to define overweight and obesity in individuals. BMI is the relationship of body weight and height. A BMI of 25 to 29.9 is defined as overweight, while a BMI of 30 and above is considered obese (U.S. Department of Health and Human Services, National Women's Health Information Center, 2004; U.S. Department of Health and Human Services, 2005b). Table 20-4 shows how to calculate BMI. The number of overweight and obese women in the United States continues to rise, and, as with other health statistics, reflects health disparities. Among females aged 20 to 74 years, data indicate that 78% of African-American women are overweight and 50.8% are obese, 71.8% of Hispanic women are overweight and 40.1% are obese, and

Table 20-4	BMI Determination and Interpretation*
BMI†	**Category**
<18.5–24.9	Normal weight
25.0–29.9	Overweight
30.0–39.9	Obesity
>40	Extreme obesity

*From National Institutes of Health: Do you know the health risks of being overweight?, Rockville, Md, 2004.
†Body mass index is a method used to determine optimal weight for height and is an indicator for obesity or malnutrition. Two formulas may be used for its calculation:
BMI = Weight (in kilograms)/Height (in meters squared)
BMI = [Weight (in pounds)/Height (in inches squared)] × 703

Box 20-10	Risks Associated with Overweight and Obesity
Type 2 diabetes	Poor female reproductive
High blood pressure	health
High cholesterol levels	Complications of pregnancy
Coronary heart disease	Menstrual irregularities
Congestive heart failure	Infertility
Angina pectoris	Irregular ovulation
Stroke	Cancers
Asthma	Uterus
Osteoarthritis	Breast
Musculoskeletal disorders	Kidney
Gallbladder disorders	Liver
Sleep apnea and	Pancreas
respiratory problems	Esophagus
Gout	Colon and rectum
Bladder control problems	

From Centers for Disease Control and Prevention: *Overweight and obesity: health consequences,* 2006. (last updated March 22, 2006). Retrieved May 4, 2006, from http://www.cdc.gov/nccdphp/dnpa/obesity/consequences.htm.

57.5% of white women are overweight and 30.6% are obese (U.S. Department of Health and Human Services, National Women's Health Information Center, 2004).

Obesity is a major health concern among women as it is linked to the development of a number of health problems (Box 20-10). Nurses can provide education regarding the risks of obesity to health. The educational offerings can be fashioned after a community health model using the levels of prevention to establish effective interventions for women at risk for weight control issues.

In addition to obesity, other eating disorders have increased among U.S. women. These include anorexia nervosa and bulimia. **Anorexia nervosa** is defined as a fear of gaining weight coupled with disturbances in perceptions of the body. Excessive weight loss is the most noticeable clue. Individuals with anorexia rarely complain of weight loss because they view themselves as normal or overweight. Many of these women also struggle with psychological problems, including depression, obsessive symptoms, and social phobias. **Bulimia** is characterized by a persistent concern with the shape of the body along with body weight, recurrent episodes of binge eating, a loss of control during these binges, and use of extreme methods to prevent weight gain, such as purging, strict dieting, fasting, use of laxatives or diuretics, or vigorous exercise (National Institute of Mental Health, 2001).

Through comprehensive physical and psychosocial assessments, as well as histories of dietary practice, nurses identify women with eating disorders and provide appropriate referrals. Weight control strategies include promoting healthy eating habits and regular physical activity. At a population level, nurses advocate against advertising that promotes exceptionally thin bodies for women. They also promote community-wide exercise and healthy eating programs.

By looking at men's magazines, it seems as if the ultimate definition of physical fitness is the firm "six-pack" abdomen. Well-toned men are pictured climbing steep rock formations, skillfully navigating a ski slope, or running along the beach. Nutrition tips are often included to help the man fight fat and achieve this shape. Are men following the tips and matching this magazine image of men? It seems they are not.

In 2003 only 35.4% of adult males 18 years of age and older engaged in regular leisure-time activity, defined as three or more sessions per week of vigorous activity lasting at least 20 minutes or five or more sessions per week of light to moderate activity lasting at least 30 minutes. Men engage less in regular leisure-time activity as they age. It peaks at 39.6% for the 18- to 44-year-old age group. For men 75 years of age and older, only 23% report regular leisure-time activity (U.S. Department of Health and Human Services, 2005).

Regular physical activity throughout life decreases risk factors for hypertension, cardiovascular diseases, and diabetes, and is associated with lower death rates.

Most communities have fitness clubs, sports complexes, and community centers that provide a safe environment and guidance for exercise programs. A lack of physical activity often leads to being overweight or to obesity.

Being overweight or obese not only increases the risk of heart disease, diabetes, and some forms of cancer, it increases the severity of diseases associated with hypertension, arthritis, and other musculoskeletal problems. An increasing number of men are overweight and obese (U.S. Department of Health and Human Services, 2005b).

The average height of adult men and women is approximately 1 inch taller than it was in 1962, but they weigh proportionally much more. The average weight for men has increased from 166 pounds in 1962 to 191 pounds in 2002. The trend of adults being overweight or obese appears to be continuing (Flegal et al, 2002).

The large number of overweight adults is a major public health concern. In 2001 the U.S. Surgeon General announced a call to action for individuals, families, communities, schools, worksites, health care, media, industry, organizations, and government to take action to decrease the number of people who are overweight and obese (U.S. Department of Health and Human Services, 2001).

Men and women both have unquestionable biological and physiological needs for rest, exercise, and food consumption to maintain health. When asked, men and women differ on the most important needs to maintain health. Women listed food first, then exercise, and then rest. Men rate exercise first, then sleep, and food last. Men emphasized the nutrient quality of food; women focused on the food's calories rather than its nutrient value. Men perceived **body maintenance** activities as essential to producing health and emphasized sports and outdoor activities as influencing better body maintenance. In addition, men viewed the body as a medium of action; function and capacity were of major importance.

The concept of body maintenance images has two components: inner and outer. Inner refers to optimal functioning, performance, and the capacity to do things. Outer refers to appearance, movement within social space, and having the potential to be heard and touched. Men discern the inner phenomenon as a function and capacity more than the outer body phenomenon of appearance. Men would rather look at how they went through the day, what they accomplished, and what kind of physical shape they are in so they can perform their tasks and life activities. Less attention is given to having good color and skin tones.

Men need to take an individual conscious look at themselves and develop a plan to stay healthy and free of illness by becoming knowledgeable about health and their own individual bodies. Along with knowledge comes the desire to be healthy. In addition, men need to set health-related goals and develop an action plan. With the support of the nursing profession, men can take responsibility for changing and for maintaining healthier lifestyles. Table 20-5 outlines some health care needs for men.

OLDER ADULTS' HEALTH

HEALTH OF OLDER ADULTS

The number of people ages 65 years and older in the United States has steadily increased since the turn of the century. Since most health care for older adults is delivered outside of the acute care setting, nurses in the community in particular have been providing nursing care to an increased proportion of this population, which calls for specialized knowledge, skills, and abilities in gerontology.

DEMOGRAPHICS

An individual born in 1900 could expect to live to be about 47 years of age. A newborn in 2002 can expect to live to be about 77 years of age (U.S. Bureau of the Census, 2001). The oldest old (those older than 85 years) are the fastest growing subgroup of older adults. The longer an individual lives, the more likely that person will live even longer.

Persons reaching the age of 65 years have an average life expectancy of an additional 18 years. Future growth projections reveal that by the year 2030, when the baby boom generation reaches age 65 years, there will be about 71 million older adults. That number represents more than twice the number in society today.

A closer look at the demographics today reveals a sex ratio of 145 women for every 100 men. Women outlive men by about 7 years, an advantage that is suspected to be biological. Minority populations today represent about 18% of all older adults, with projections that the minority composition will double by the year 2030 (U.S. Bureau of the Census, 2001). Most older adults live in a noninstitutional community setting, and a majority of them live with someone else. About 4.5% live in a nursing home, a likelihood that increases significantly as one ages. Older adults as a whole are not an affluent group. Chronological age is an arbitrary way to project health care needs because the state of health differs widely among this population. The age of 65 years has been used as a benchmark since 1935, when Franklin Delano Roosevelt used this age in eligibility criteria for Social Security. This seemed to be a reasonable criterion at the time, since most individuals did not live long enough to collect Social Security. As life expectancy has grown, the age at which a person becomes eligible for Social Security has changed and is based on birth date. Although chronological age is limiting, some projections in the area of physical function and prevalence of chronic illness can be made. One-fourth of older adults report having difficulty in carrying out **basic activities of daily living (ADLs)** such as bathing, dressing, and eating and **instrumental activities of daily living (IADLs)** such as preparing meals, taking medications, and managing money, with a disproportionate share of individuals with disability in the higher age group (National Center for Health Statistics, 2004).

The last few years of life are often characterized by a decline in physical functioning. A goal for nurses is to help maximize functional status and minimize functional decline. Health promotion and disease prevention strategies must be emphasized in the older adult.

BRIEFLY NOTED

Surveys documenting the functional status rating of an individual by the nurse, the caregiver, and the clients themselves often differ. Many factors can cause the different perspectives in measuring and noting functional status.

DEFINITIONS RELATED TO THE HEALTH OF OLDER ADULTS

Aging, if defined purely from a physiological perspective, has been described as a process of deterioration of body systems. This definition is obviously inadequate to describe the multidimensional aging process in elders. *Aging* can be more

Table 20-5   **Men's Health Care Needs**

	Biological	Psychosocial	Combination
Expression		Desire to communicate with others about health care concerns	
Support		Support from others about certain sex roles and lifestyles that influence their physical and mental health	
Respect and dignity			Attention from professionals regarding factors that may cause illness or affect a man's expression of illness, including occupational factors, leisure patterns, and interpersonal relationships
Health-seeking knowledge and behaviors	Information about their body's functions, what is normal and abnormal, what action to take, and the contributions of proper nutrition and exercise Self-care instruction including testicular and genital self-examinations Physical examination and history taking, including sexual and reproductive health and illness across the life span		
Holistic medical care and availability		Adjustment of the health care system to men's occupational constraints related to time and location of health care	Treatment for problems of couples, including interpersonal problems, infertility, family planning, sexual concerns, and sexually transmitted diseases
Parental guidance		Help with fathering (e.g., being included as a parent in the care of children) Help with fathering as a single parent—in particular, with a child of the opposite sex, in addressing the child's sexual development and concerns	
Coping		Recognition that feelings of confusion and uncertainty in a time of rapid social change are normal and may mark the onset of a healthy adaptation to change	
Fiduciary		Financial ways to obtain the preceding needs	

appropriately defined as the total of all changes that occur in a person with the passing of time. Influences on how one ages come from several domains, including physiological as well as psychological, sociological, and spiritual processes. The physiological declines associated with aging have been easier to understand than aging as a process of growth and development.

Myths associated with aging have evolved over time. Some of the common myths involve the perception that all older adults are infirm and senile and cannot adapt to change and learn new behaviors or skills.

These myths are easily debunked by older adults who run marathons, learn to use the Internet, and are vibrant members of society. **Ageism** is the term used for prejudice toward older people. Prejudice may be obvious or subtle. Ageism fosters a stereotype that does not allow older adults to be viewed realistically.

Gerontology is the specialized study of the processes of growing old. **Geriatrics** is the study of disease in old age. **Gerontological nursing** is the specialty of nursing concerned with the assessment of the health and functional status of older adults, planning and implementing health care and services to meet the identified needs, and evaluating the effectiveness of such care (Meinor and Lueckenotte, 2006).

MULTIDIMENSIONAL INFLUENCES ON AGING

The client experiences aging in many ways: physiologically, psychologically, sociologically, and spiritually. Physiological changes occur in all body systems with the passing of time. How and when these processes occur between individuals vary widely, as well as the degree of aging within the various body systems in the same individual. Table 20-6 highlights physiological changes with the aging of body systems and the nursing implications of these changes. The effect of these physiological changes overall result in a diminished physiological reserve, a decrease in homeostatic mechanisms, and a decline in immunological response.

No known intrinsic psychological changes occur with aging. The influences of the environment and culture on personal development and maturation are substantial and further limit the ability of the nurse to predict how an individual psychologically ages.

Some known and some disputed changes in brain function over time may influence cognition and behavior. Reaction speed and psychomotor response are somewhat slower, which can be related to the neurological changes with aging. This is demonstrated particularly during timed tests of performance in which speed is an influencing variable. It has also been demonstrated in simulated tests of driving skills where speed of response, perception, and attention slow with age. Typically older individuals can learn and perform as well as younger individuals, although they may be slower and it may take them longer to accomplish a specific task.

Intellectual capacity does not decline with age as was previously thought. An age-associated memory impairment, benign senescent forgetfulness, involves very minor memory loss. This is not progressive and does not cause dysfunction in daily living. Reassurance is important for the older adult and families since anxiety often exacerbates the problem of mild memory impairment. Memory aids (e.g., mnemonics, signs, notes) may help the elder compensate for this type of impairment.

Many external factors affect mental health and aging, particularly those associated with loss and change. Adapting and coping responses of even the most resilient individuals will be challenged when successive losses and changes occur within a relatively short period.

The later years for many older adults mark a period of changing social dynamics. Social networks provide the structure for social support. Most older people continue to respond to life situations as they did earlier in their lives. Old age does not bring about radical changes in beliefs and values but may bring about abrupt changes over which they have little control. How individuals stay involved in activities and with people who bring their lives meaning and support

Table 20-6	Physiologic Age-Related Changes in Body Systems	
System	**Age-Related Change**	**Implication for Nursing**
Skin	Skin thins	Skin breakdown and injury
	Atrophy of sweat glands	Increased risk of heat stroke
	Decrease in vascularity	Frequent pruritus, dry skin
Respiratory	Decreased elasticity of lung tissue	Reduced efficiency of ventilation
	Decreased respiratory muscle strength	Atelectasis and infection
Cardiovascular	Decrease in baroreceptor sensitivity	Orthostatic hypotension and falls
	Decrease in the number of pacemaker cells	Increased prevalence of dysrhythmias
Gastrointestinal	Dental enamel thins; loss of teeth/caries	Periodontal disease
	Gums recede	Swallowing dysfunction
	Delay in esophageal emptying	Constipation
	Decreased muscle tone	
	Altered peristalsis	
Genitourinary	Decreased number of functioning nephrons	Modifications in drug dosing may be required
	Reduced bladder tone and capacity	Incontinence more common
	Prostate enlargement	May compromise urinary function
Neuromuscular	Decrease in muscle mass	Decrease in muscle strength
	Decrease in bone mass	Osteoporosis, increased risk of fracture
Sensory	Loss of neurons/nerve fibers	Altered sensitivity to pain
	Decreased visual acuity, depth perception, adaptation to light changes	May pose safety issues
	Loss of auditory neurons	Hearing loss may cause limitation in activities
	Altered taste sensation	May change food preferences and intake
Immune	Decrease in T cell function	Increased incidence of infection
	Appearance of autoantibodies	Increased prevalence of autoimmune disorders

is a major factor that can contribute to ongoing health and vitality.

Higher socioeconomic status, income, and education tend to be reflected in large and differing social networks (Ebersole, Hess, and Luggen, 2004). Families typically remain involved with aging parents, with estimates that more than 5 million are involved in some type of parent care. Not all individuals do remain in their own home or in the home of another. As people age, social role and status may change and elders are more vulnerable to social isolation.

Although most of the multidimensional influences of aging are marked by decline and loss, some have suggested that an increased spiritual awareness and consciousness accompany aging and that religion is a powerful cultural force in the lives of older clients. Spirituality refers to the need to transcend physical, psychological, and social identities to experience love, hope, and meaning in life. Religious affiliations and religious rituals are two aspects of spirituality that can include other activities and relationships. Caring for pets and plants or experiencing nature through a walk in the woods can also foster spiritual growth. Physical and functional impairments and fear of death may challenge our spiritual integrity. Having a strong sense of spirituality enables individuals who are physically and functionally dependent on others to avoid despair by appreciating that they are still capable of giving and deserving of receiving love, respect, and dignity.

CHRONIC HEALTH CONCERNS OF OLDER ADULTS

Chronic illnesses occur over a long period with occasional acute exacerbations and remissions. They can affect multiple systems and be expensive and discouraging. The prevalence of chronic disease rises with lengthening of life span and highly technical medical care. Not only do chronic conditions cause disability and activity restriction, they often require frequent hospitalizations for exacerbations.

Health care in general is oriented toward acute illness. In **chronic illness**, cure is not expected, so nursing activities need to be more holistic, addressing function, wellness, and psychosocial issues. With chronic illness, the focus is on healing (a unique process resulting in a shift in the body/mind/spirit system) rather than curing (elimination of the signs and symptoms of disease). Eliopoulos (2001) lists the following goals for chronic care:
• Maintain or improve self-care capacity
• Manage the disease effectively
• Boost the body's healing abilities
• Prevent complications
• Delay deterioration and decline
• Achieve the highest possible quality of life
• Die with comfort, peace, and dignity

Chronic illness requires a shift in perspective compared with the rapid onset and focus on curing of an acute problem. The focus is on the development of self-management skills. The nurse is in partnership with the client, paying attention

to the client's self-concept and self-esteem as well as to the resources that are needed to manage the disease outside the medical system. Goals for care are structured to help clients adjust their day-to-day choices to maintain the highest level of functional ability possible within the limits of their conditions. The motivation to make lifestyle changes necessary to cope with chronic illness stems from the fear of death; disability; pain; and negative effects on work, family, or activity.

Tierney, McPhee, and Papadakis (2002) outline chronic conditions called the **five I's** that can adversely affect the aging experience, as follows:
1. **I**ntellectual impairment
2. **I**mmobility
3. **I**nstability
4. **I**ncontinence
5. **I**atrogenic drug reactions

In addition, Tierney named the **three D's** of intellectual impairment, as follows:
1. **D**ementia (progressive intellectual impairment)
2. **D**epression (mood disorder)
3. **D**elirium (acute confusion)

Immobility is most often caused by degenerative joint disease and results in pain, stiffness, loss of balance, and psychological problems. Fear of falling is a major cause of immobility. This is related to instability, which results in falls in 30% of elders each year.

Urinary incontinence often contributes to institutional care and social isolation. For that reason it is difficult to estimate the numbers of individuals involved and the cost of incontinence. It is important to address continence routinely in the assessment process, identify the type of incontinence, and intervene appropriately.

Iatrogenic drug reactions result from changes in the older individual's absorption, metabolism, and excretion process that lead to altered responses to drugs. Many elderly people take numerous medicines, increasing the chance of drug reactions.

BRIEFLY NOTED

The average older adult in the community has 11 different prescriptions filled each year. Hazards of this situation include drug interactions, side effects, and overmedication, which lead to chemically induced impairment.

One often overlooked concern of elders is that of abuse. *Elder abuse* encompasses physical, psychological, financial, and social abuse or violation of an individual's rights. Abuse consists of the following:
• The willful infliction of physical pain or injury
• Debilitating mental anguish and fear
• Theft or mismanagement of money or resources
• Unreasonable confinement or the deprivation of services

Neglect refers to a lack of services that are necessary for the physical and mental health of an individual by the individual or a caregiver. Older persons can make independent choices with which others may disagree. Their right to self-determination can be taken from them if they are declared incompetent. Exploitation is the illegal or improper use of a person or their resources for another's profit or advantage. During the assessment process, nurses need to be aware of conflicts between injuries and explanation of cause, dependency issues between client and caregiver, and substance abuse by the caregiver. Nearly all 50 states have enacted mandatory reporting laws and have instituted protective service programs. The local social services agency or area agency on aging can help with information on reporting requirements.

The **Patient Self-Determination Act** of 1991 requires those providers receiving Medicare and Medicaid funds to give clients written information regarding their legal options for treatment choices if they become incapacitated. A routine discussion of advance medical directives can help ease the difficult discussions faced by health care professionals, family, and clients. The nurse can assist an individual to complete a values history instrument. These instruments ask questions about specific wishes regarding different medical situations.

This clarifying process then leads to completion of **advance directives** to document these preferences in writing. There are two parts to the advance directives. The **living will** allows the client to express wishes regarding the use of medical treatments in the event of a terminal illness. A **durable power of attorney** is the legal way for the client to designate someone else to make health care decisions when he or she is unable to do so. A do-not-resuscitate (DNR) order is a specific order from a physician not to use cardiopulmonary resuscitation. State laws vary widely regarding the implementing of these tools, so it is important to consult a knowledgeable source of information. It is also important to involve the family, and especially the designated decision maker or agent, in these discussions so that everyone understands the client's choices.

BRIEFLY NOTED

Legislated rights of the elderly include the following:
- Individualized care
- Freedom from discrimination
- Privacy
- Freedom from neglect and abuse
- Control of one's own funds
- Ability to sue
- Freedom from physical and chemical restraint
- Involvement in decision making
- Voting
- Access to community services
- Raise grievances
- Obtain a will
- Enter into contracts
- Practice the religion of one's choice
- Dispose of one's own personal property

FAMILY CAREGIVING

Eighty-five percent of all elderly people live in homes alone, with spouses or other family or friends. Female spouses represent the largest group of family caregivers. *Stress, strain,* and *burnout* are words that are used to reflect the negative effects of the family **caregiver burden**. Issues involve the work itself, past and present relationships, effect on others, and the caregivers' lifestyle and well-being. It is estimated that at least 5 million adults are providing direct care to an elderly relative at any given time, with another 44 to 45 million assuming some type of responsibility for an elderly relative. For many families the caregiving experience is a positive, rewarding, and fulfilling one. Nursing intervention can facilitate good health for older persons and their caregivers and contribute to meaningful family relationships during this period. Eliopoulos (2001) uses the acronym *TLC* to represent these interventions, as follows:

T = training in care techniques, safe medication use, recognition of abnormalities, and available resources

L = leaving the care situation periodically to obtain respite and relaxation and maintain their normal living needs

C = care for themselves (the caregiver) through adequate sleep, rest, exercise, nutrition, socialization, solitude, support, financial aid, and health management

BRIEFLY NOTED

Older adults are at increased risk for infection. Prevention in the community includes encouraging routine handwashing and adapting Universal Precautions specifically to the practice setting.

COMMUNITY RESOURCES

STRATEGIES FOR CHILD HEALTH CARE IN THE COMMUNITY

Nurses are in a position to work with groups of families or individuals through programs targeting the health care needs of those at risk. Three strategies for common pediatric concerns are identified to model nursing interventions in the community. Strategies include programs based in the home, targeted at the needs of homeless persons, or centered in day care or school settings. Community resources for children are given in Box 20-11.

PROGRAMS AND SERVICES FOR WOMEN

Changes in the health care delivery system have a profound effect on women. Women are the gatekeepers of their families' health care. They make 75% of the health care decisions in American households. In addition, women make more physician visits and purchase more prescription drugs. Because of women's greater involvement with health services, they can play a major role in family health promotion.

Traditional centers of care for women such as Planned Parenthood, feminist women's health centers, and local

Levels of Prevention Across the Life Span

PRIMARY PREVENTION

- Provide community education about the benefits of breast-feeding and the need for dietary supplementation with vitamin D to prevent childhood rickets.
- Collaborate with a variety of organizations such as the American Heart Association to design and implement interventions aimed at reducing women's risk for cardiovascular disease.
- In group and individual counseling about HIV, caution male clients that they should not share needles, syringes, razors, or toothbrushes.

SECONDARY PREVENTION

- Target high-risk groups such as infants who live in sunshine-deprived areas (northern climates, urban areas) for alkaline phosphatase levels or serum assays of 25-hydroxyvitamin D.
- Provide screening activities such as blood cholesterol and blood pressure monitoring as examples of secondary prevention for women.
- Advise a man who had unprotected sex to be tested with a standard enzyme-linked immunosorbent assay (ELISA), followed by a confirmatory Western blot test.
- Provide a comprehensive geriatric assessment at a health fair. Invite all older clients to participate, and screen blood pressure and cholesterol and for signs and symptoms of coronary artery disease and stroke.

TERTIARY PREVENTION

- Offer counseling regarding vitamin D and calcium supplements and nutrition to reduce complications from childhood rickets.
- Develop a community-based exercise program for a group of women who have cardiovascular disease.
- Teach men who are newly diagnosed with HIV to exercise regularly, eat a balanced nutritious diet, sleep at least 8 hours a day, and stop or limit alcohol consumption.
- Provide a diabetes clinic targeted to older clients with diabetes to teach them how to identify and prevent foot complications and about lifestyle changes to cope with this chronic illness.

Box 20-11 Community Resources for Children's Health Care

- Children's service clinics
- Well-child clinics
- Immunization clinics
- Infectious disease clinics
- Children's specialty services
- Family violence and child abuse centers
- School health programs
- Head Start
- Parents Anonymous
- Crisis hotlines
- Community education classes
- Early intervention/developmental services
- Childbirth education classes
- Breastfeeding support groups
- Parent support groups
- Family planning clinics
- Women, Infants, and Children (WIC) programs
- Medicaid
- Youth employment and training program

---

community health centers can serve as models for women-centered health care delivery. More women's health clinics are being made available since the Office of Women's Health with USDHHS opened in 2001 to address the need for more women's health services (U.S. Department of Health and Human Services, Office on Women's Health, 2003).

Community Care Settings for Elders

Senior centers were developed in the early 1940s to provide social and recreational activities. Now many centers are multipurpose, offering recreation, education, counseling, therapies, hot meals, and case management, as well as health screening and education. Some offer primary care services.

Adult day health is for individuals whose mental and/or physical function requires additional health care and supervision. It serves as more of a medical model than the senior center, and often individuals return home to their caregivers at night.

Home health can be provided by working in multidisciplinary teams. Nurses provide individual and environmental assessments, direct skilled care and treatment, and provide short-term guidance and instruction. They work closely with the family and other caregivers to provide necessary communication and continuity of care.

Hospice represents a philosophy of caring for and supporting life to its fullest until death occurs. The hospice team encourages the client and family to jointly make decisions to meet physical, emotional, spiritual, and comfort needs.

Assisted living covers a wide variety of choices, from a single shared room to opulent independent living accommodations in a full-service, life care community.

Nursing homes or **long-term care** *facilities,* as they are often called, house only 4.5% of the elderly population at a given time; however, 25% of those older than 65 years will spend some time in a nursing home. Nursing homes provide a safe environment, special diets and activities, routine personal care, and the treatment and management of health care needs for those needing rehabilitation, as well as those needing a permanent supportive residence.

Healthy People 2010

Objectives across the Life Span

Children

8-22 Increase the proportion of persons living in pre-1950s housing that have been tested for the presence of lead-based paint to eliminate elevated blood lead levels in children

14-24 Increase the proportion of young children who receive all vaccines that have been recommended for universal administration for at least 5 years

15-20 Increase the use of child restraints in cars

19-3 Reduce the proportion of children and adolescents who are overweight or obese

22-8 Increase the proportion of the nation's public and private schools that require daily physical education for all students

24-7 Increase the proportion of children with asthma who receive appropriate asthma care according to the National Asthma Education and Prevention Program guidelines

27-9 Reduce the proportion of children who are regularly exposed to tobacco smoke at home

Women

2-9 Reduce the overall number of cases of osteoporosis among adults age 50 years and older from 10% to 8%

3-3 Reduce the breast cancer death rate from 27.7 deaths per 100,000 to 22.2 per 100,000

9-1 Increase the proportion of intended pregnancies from 51% to 70%

15-35 Reduce the annual rate of rape or attempted rape from 0.9 per 1000 to 0.7 per 1000

16-6 Increase the proportion of pregnant women who receive early and adequate prenatal care

16-18 Increase the proportion of mothers who breastfeed their babies

Men

3-7 Reduce the death rate from prostate cancer

9-6 Increase male involvement in pregnancy prevention and family planning efforts

12-2 Increase the proportion of adults age 20 years and older who are aware of the early warning symptoms and signs of a heart attack and the importance of accessing rapid emergency care by calling 911

13-2 Reduce the number of new AIDS cases among adolescent and adult men who have sex with men

26-7 Reduce intentional injuries resulting from alcohol- and illicit-drug-related violence

Older Adults

2-3 Reduce the proportion of all adults with chronic joint symptoms who have difficulty in performing two or more personal care activities, thereby preserving their independence

2-10 Reduce the proportion of adults who are hospitalized for vertebral fractures associated with osteoporosis

6-3 Reduce the proportion of adults with disabilities who report feelings such as sadness, unhappiness, or depression that prevent them from being active

12-6 Reduce hospitalizations of older adults with heart failure as the principal diagnosis

17-3 Increase the proportion of primary care providers, pharmacists, and other health care professionals who routinely review with their patients with chronic illnesses or disabilities all new prescribed and over-the-counter medicines

22-4 Increase the proportion of adults who perform physical activities that enhance and maintain muscular strength and endurance

27-1 Reduce tobacco use by older adults

28-7 Reduce visual impairment due to cataract

From U.S. Department of Health and Human Services: *Healthy People 2010: understanding and improving health,* ed 2, Washington, DC, 2000, U.S. Government Printing Office.

CLINICAL APPLICATION

Neighbors and the administrator of the senior high-rise residence where Mrs. Eldridge, a 79-year-old widow, lives reported her to the nurse who visited residents there. Mrs. Eldridge lives alone, and no one had been observed coming or going from her apartment recently. When Mrs. Eldridge was seen by her neighbors, she appeared self-neglected and did not appear to recognize her neighbors.

When the nurse made a visit to the apartment, Mrs. Eldridge answered the door. She was pleasant but there was an odor of stale urine. The nurse validated the unkempt appearance of both Mrs. Eldridge and the apartment. Even though Mrs. Eldridge was hesitant and unsure in her answers, the history revealed medical problems. A son and daughter-in-law lived in the next county and phoned at least once a week; their number was taped to the table by the phone.

However, the son is an alcoholic and the daughter-in-law has beginning symptoms of cardiovascular disease (CVD). Mrs. Eldridge's greatgrandchild has asthma and is cared for by the son and daughter-in-law. Several pill bottles were observed on the kitchen counter with the names of a local physician and pharmacist.

The nurse noted that both Mrs. Eldridge and her clothes were dirty and that she moved without aids and appeared steady on her feet. The kitchen was littered with unwashed dishes and empty frozen-food boxes, which Mrs. Eldridge could not recall being bought or having been delivered. A billfold with several bills was lying open on the kitchen counter, as well as an uncashed Social Security check.

A. *What should the nurse do about the situation she found?*

1. *Call adult protective services and get an emergency order to put Mrs. Eldridge in a nursing home.*

2. *Call Mrs. Eldridge's son and see if his mother can move in with him since she cannot take care of herself.*

3. *Complete a physical and mental examination to first determine the cause of Mrs. Eldridge's situation.*

4. *Call Mrs. Eldridge's pharmacist to see what medications she is taking.*
5. *Call Mrs. Eldridge's son to discuss the situation with him and to make plans with him and his mother for her future.*

B. *What factors make this a difficult situation?*

Answers are in the back of the book.

REMEMBER THIS!

- Good nutrition is essential for healthy growth and development and influences disease prevention in later life. The adolescent population is at greatest risk for poor nutritional health.
- Immunizations are successful in prevention of selected diseases. Barriers to immunizing children are cost and inconvenience.
- The family is critical to the growth and development of the child. Social support is one of the most powerful influences on successful parenting.
- Accidents and injuries are the major cause of health problems in the child and adolescent population. Most are preventable. Nurses have a major role in anticipatory guidance and prevention.
- Nurses are involved in strategies to meet the needs of the pediatric population in the community. Home-based service programs have been successful in providing care for at-risk populations. Children of homeless families are at risk for health problems, environmental dangers, and stress. Community programs to provide health care for the homeless may decrease those risks.
- The women's health movement was pivotal in bringing national recognition to women's health issues.
- Women have a longer life expectancy than men. However, women are more likely to have acute and chronic conditions that require them to use health services more than men.
- Relationships are crucial to the development of female identity.
- Women are known as the gatekeepers of health. Women make 75% of the health care decisions in American households.
- Women of color are statistically more likely to have poor health outcomes because of a poor understanding of health, lack of access to health care, and lifestyle practices.
- Smoking is a risk factor for a number of major health problems, including lung cancer, heart disease, osteoporosis, and poor reproductive outcomes.
- The failure to include women in medical research has resulted in a lack of understanding about the distinctive issues surrounding the diagnosis and treatment of the major diseases for women.
- Heart disease is the leading cause of death among women older than 50 years and the second leading cause of death among women ages 35 to 39 years.
- Cancer is the second leading cause of death for women.

- In response to the past lack of equality in health-related research and the provision of clinical care, there is now a major national focus on women's health issues.
- Men are physiologically the more vulnerable gender, demonstrated by shorter life spans and a higher infant mortality.
- Life expectancy of men in the United States is one of the lowest in developed countries.
- Men engage in more risk-taking behaviors, such as physical challenges and illegal behaviors, than do women.
- The most significant death rate differences between men and women are for AIDS, suicides, homicides, and accidents.
- Men tend to avoid diagnosis and treatment of illnesses that may result in serious health problems.
- The population ages 65 years and older in the United States is steadily growing, accompanied by an increase in chronic conditions, a greater demand for services, and strained health care budgets.
- Most older adults live in the community. The last few years of life often represent functional decline. Nurses strive to help elders maximize functional status and minimize costs through direct care and appropriate referral to community resources.
- Nurses address the chronic health concerns of elders with a focus on maintaining or improving self-care and preventing complications to maintain the highest possible quality of life.
- Assessing the elder incorporates physical, psychological, social, and spiritual domains. Individual and community-focused interventions involve all three levels of prevention through collaborative practice.

WHAT WOULD YOU DO?

1. Develop a plan of nursing care for a family that has experienced a sudden infant death syndrome (SIDS) death.
2. Develop a nutritional program for (1) mothers who are breastfeeding their infants, (2) a group of 5 year olds in a kindergarten class, and (3) a group of high school sophomores. What factors do these programs have in common? How do they differ?
3. Design a teaching plan for a middle-aged woman that reflects a maximum level of health promotion for her and her family.
4. Analyze mortality and morbidity data in your county and rank the order of the 10 most prevalent health problems for women. Compare these with men's health problems.
5. Interview an elder within your family and ask him or her to list any health problems, how your relative would rate his or her health on a scale of 1 to 10 (with 10 being the highest), and what is included in a typical day's activities. Also, ask the elder to provide a 24-hour dietary recall.
6. Describe what you can do to aid in overcoming the myths and examples of ageism that are pervasive in society.

■ *REFERENCES*_____

Aaron DJ: Behavioral risk factors for disease and preventive health practices among lesbians, *Am J Publ Health* 91:972–975, 2001.

Agency for Healthcare Research and Quality: *Young men are least likely to use seat belts, but almost 90 percent of American adults wear them regularly,* Rockville, Md, 2004, available at www.ahrq.gov/news/press/pr2004/menseatpr.htm.

Agency for Healthcare Research and Quality: *Research on cardiovascular disease in women,* 2005, available at http://www.ahrq.gov/research/womheart.pdf.

Agency for Healthcare Research and Quality, U.S. Preventive Services Task Force: *The guide to clinical preventive services,* 2005, available at http://www.ahrq.gov/clinic/pocketgd.pdf.

Ahluwalia IB, Daniel KL: Are women with recent live births aware of the benefits of folic acid? *MMWR Morbid Mortal Wkly Rep* 50 (RR–6):3, 2001.

Amar AF, Gennaro S: Dating violence in college women: associated physical injury, healthcare usage, and mental health symptoms, *Nurs Res* 54:235–242, 2005.

American Academy of Nursing: Women's health and women's health care: recommendations of the 1996 AAN Expert Writing Panel on Women's Health, *Nurs Outlook* 45:7–15, 1996.

American Academy of Pediatrics: Fetal alcohol syndrome and alcohol-related neurodevelopmental disorders, *Pediatrics* 106:358, 2000.

American Academy of Pediatrics: *Red book: 2003 report of the committee on infectious diseases,* ed 26, Elk Grove Village, Ill, 2003, AAP.

American Academy of Pediatrics Committee on Nutrition: *Pediatric nutrition handbook,* ed 5, Elk Grove Village, Ill, 2004, AAP.

American Cancer Society: *Cancer facts and figures, 2006,* Atlanta, Ga, 2006, ACS, available at www.cancer.org/downloads/STT/CAFF2006PWSecured.pdf.

American Heart Association: *2002 heart and stroke statistical update,* Dallas, Tex, 2006, AHA, available at www.americanheart.org/downloadable/heart/.

American Lung Association: *Trends in lung cancer morbidity and mortality,* 2008a, available at www.lungusa.org.

American Lung Association: *Trends in tobacco use,* 2008b, available at www.lungusa.org.

Barnett E et al: *Men and heart disease: an atlas of racial and ethnic disparities in mortality,* ed 1, Morgantown, WV, 2001, West Virginia University, Office for Social Environment and Health Research, available at www.cdc.gov/cvh/maps/cvdatlas/=atlas_mens/mens_download.htm.

Bassett MT: Diabetes is epidemic, *Am J Publ Health* 95:1496, 2005.

Beckles GLA, Thompson-Reid PE: Socioeconomic status of women with diabetes—United States, 2000, *JAMA* 287:2496, 2002.

Bierman AS, Clancy CM: Health disparities among older women: identifying opportunities to improve quality of care and functional health outcomes, *J Am Med Womens Assoc* 56:155–160, 2001, available at http://jamwa.=amwa-doc.org/vol56/56_4_1a.htm.

Bosch X: Female genital mutilation in developed countries, *Lancet* 358:1177–1178, 2001.

Brown ML: The effects of environmental tobacco smoke on children: information and implications for PNPs, *J Pediatr Health Care* 15:6, 2002.

Campbell JC: Health consequences of intimate partner violence, *Lancet* 359:1331, 2002.

Center for Reproductive Rights: *Abortion coverage under the Medicaid program,* 2005, available at http://www.crlp.org/pub_fac_portrait.html.

Centers for Disease Control and Prevention: Alcohol use among women of childbearing age: United States, 1991–1999, *MMWR Morbid Mortal Wkly Rep* 51:273, 2002.

Centers for Disease Control and Prevention: Strategies for reducing morbidity and mortality from diabetes through health-care interventions and diabetes self-management education in community settings: a report on recommendations of the Task Force on Community Preventive Services, *MMWR Morbid Mortal Wkly Rep* 50(RR–15):1–15, 2001.

Centers for Disease Control and Prevention: *HIV/AIDS surveillance report: 2004,* Vol 16, Atlanta, 2005a, U.S. Department of Health and Human Services, Centers for Disease Control and Prevention, available at http://www.cdc.gov/hiv/stats/hasrlink.htm.

Centers for Disease Control and Prevention: *Trends in reportable sexually transmitted diseases in the United States, 2004,* Atlanta, 2005b, USDHHS.

Centers for Disease Control and Prevention: *Folic acid, professional resources,* 2005c, available at http://www.cdc.gov/ncbddd/folicacid/health_overview.htm.

Centers for Disease Control and Prevention: *CDC HIV/AIDS fact sheets* (last updated April 14, 2006). *HIV/AIDS among African Americans,* 2006a. Retrieved April 29, 2006, from http://www.cdc.gov/hiv/topics/aa/resources/factsheets/pdf/aa.pdf.

Centers for Disease Control and Prevention: *CDC HIV/AIDS fact sheets* (last updated April 14, 2006). *HIV/AIDS among Hispanics,* 2006b. Retrieved April 29, 2006, from http://www.cdc.gov/hiv/pubs/facts/hispanic.pdf.

Centers for Disease Control and Prevention: *Comprehensive HIV prevention: essential components of a comprehensive strategy to prevent domestic HIV,* Atlanta, 2006c, U.S. Department of Health and Human Services, Centers for Disease Control and Prevention, available at http://www.cdc.gov/hiv/resources/reports/comp_hiv_prev/pdf/comp_hiv_prev.pdf.

Centers for Disease Control and Prevention: *Overweight and obesity: health consequences* (last updated March 22, 2006), 2006d. Retrieved May 4, 2006, from http://www.cdc.gov/nccdphp/dnpa/obesity/consequences.htm.

Centers for Disease Control and Prevention, Morbidity and Mortality Weekly Report: national, state, and local area vaccination coverage among children aged 19–35 months—United States, 2007, *MMWR Morbid Mortal Wkly Rep* 57(35):961-966, 2008.

Centers for Disease Control and Prevention, Morbidity and Mortality Weekly Report: Racial/ethnic disparities in diagnoses of HIV/AIDS—33 states, 2001–2004, *MMWR Morbid Mortal Wkly Rep* 55(5):121–125, 2006, available at http://www.cdc.gov/mmwr/preview/mmwrhtml/mm5505a1.htm.

Centers for Disease Control and Prevention, National Center for Health Statistics: *Health, United States, 2005. With chartbook on trends in the health of Americans,* Hyattsville, Md, 2005, available at http://www.cdc.gov/nchs/hus.htm.

Centers for Disease Control and Prevention, National Center for Health Statistics: *Prenatal care, 2002,* available at http://www.cdc.gov/nchs/fastats/prenatal.htm.

Centers for Disease Control and Prevention, National Center for HIV, STD, and TB Prevention: *HIV/AIDS 2003 surveillance report, table 5,* 2005a, available at http://www.cdc.gov/hiv/stats/2003SurveillanceReport/table5.htm.

Centers for Disease Control and Prevention, National Center for HIV, STD, and TB Prevention: *HIV/AIDS surveillance in women. Slide series through 2003,* 2005b, available at http://www.cdc.gov/hiv/graphics/women.htm.

Centers for Disease Control and Prevention, National Center for HIV, STD, and TB Prevention: *Why does CDC recommend HIV screening for all pregnant women?* 2005c, available at http://www.cdc.gov/hiv/pubs/faq/faq14.htm.

Centers for Disease Control and Prevention, Office of Minority Health: *Eliminate disparities in HIV and AIDS* (last updated April 4, 2006), 2006. Retrieved April 29, 2006, from http://www.cdc.gov/omh/AMH/factsheets/hiv.htm.

Cornelius LJ, Smith PL, Simpson GM: What factors hinder women of color from obtaining preventive health care? *Am J Publ Health* 92:535–539, 2002.

Curry MA, Hassouneh-Phillips D, Johnston-Silverberg A: Abuse of women with disabilities: an ecological model and review, *Violence Against Women* 7:50–79, 2001.

Dionne EJ: The welfare-marriage wars, *The Washington Post*, Feb 6, 2002, available at http://proquest.umi.com/pqdweb?Ts=…=1&Did=000000109681459&Mtd=1&Fmt=3.

Ebersole P, Hess P, Luggen A: *Toward healthy aging: human needs and nursing responses*, St. Louis, Mo, 2004, Mosby.

Edwards BK et al: Annual report to the nation on the status of cancer, 1973–1999: featuring implications of age and aging on U.S. cancer burden, *Cancer* 94:2766–2792, 2002.

Ehrenreich B: *Nickel and dimed*, New York, 2002, Holt.

Eliopoulos C: *Gerontological nursing*, ed 5, Philadelphia, 2001, Lippincott, Williams & Wilkins.

Federal Interagency Forum on Aging Related Statistics: *Older Americans 2000: key indicators of well-being*, 2000, available at http://www.agingstats.gov/chartbook2000/Population1-9.pdf.

Federal Interagency Forum on Child and Family Statistics (FIFOCFS): *America's children: key national indicators of well-being*, Washington, DC, 2005, U.S. Government Printing Office.

Flegal KM et al: Prevalence and trends in obesity among US adults, 1999–2000, *JAMA* 228:1723–1727, 2002.

Ford N: Tackling female genital cutting in Somolia, *Lancet* 358:1179, 2001.

Galdas PM et al: Men and health help-seeking behavior: literature review, *J Adv Nurs* 49:616–623, 2004.

Gerhard-Herman M: Cardiovascular disease in women, *Female Patient* 27:25–29, 2002.

Greger N, Edwin CM: Obesity: a pediatric epidemic, *Pediatr Ann* 30:11, 2001.

Goldman B, Hatch MC: *Women and health*, San Diego, Calif, 2000, Academic Press.

Gottesman MM: Patient education: preconception education: caring for the future, *J Pediatr Health Care* 18:40–44, 2004.

Greenland P et al: Major risk factors as antecedents of fatal and nonfatal coronary heart disease events, *JAMA* 290:891–897, 2003.

Hargraves M: Elevating the voices of rural minority women, *Am J Publ Health* 92:514–515, 2002.

Jemal A et al: Cancer statistics, 2005, *CA Cancer J Clin* 55:10–30, 2005.

Jiang B et al: Effects of urban community intervention on 3-year survival and recurrence after first-ever stroke, *Stroke: J Am Heart Assoc* 35:1242–1247, 2004.

Jiang HJ et al: Racial/ethnic disparities in potentially preventable readmissions: the case of diabetes, *Am J Public Health* 95:1561–1567, 2005.

Katz E: *Margaret Sanger: biographical sketch*, 2001, available at http://www.nyu.edu/projects/sanger/ms-bio.htm.

Khot UN et al: Prevalence of conventional risk factors in patients with coronary heart disease, *JAMA* 290:898–904, 2003.

Kirkam C, Harris S, Grzybowski S: Evidence-based prenatal care: part I. General prenatal care and counseling issues, *Am Fam Physician* 71:1307–1316,1321–1322, 1257–1259, 2005.

Knox K, Caine E: Establishing priorities for reducing suicide and its antecedents in the United States, *Am J Publ Health* 95:1898–1903, 2005.

Maloni JA, Damato EG: Reducing the risk for preterm birth: evidence and implications for neonatal nurses, *Adv Neonatal Care* 4:166–174, 2004.

Matthews AK et al: Prediction of depressive distress in a community sample of women: the role of sexual orientation, *Am J Public Health* 92:1131, 2002.

Mazure CM, Keita GP, Blehar MC: *Summit on women and depression: proceedings and recommendations*, Washington, DC, 2002, American Psychological Association, available at www.apa.org/pi/wpo/women&;depression.pdf.

Meinor S, Lueckenotte A: *Gerontological nursing*, ed 3, St. Louis, 2006, Mosby.

Moos M: Preconceptional health promotion: progress in changing a prevention paradigm, *J Perinatal Neonatal Nurs* 18:2–13, 2004.

Morgenstern L et al: Improving delivery of acute stroke therapy: the TLL Temple Foundation stroke project, *Stroke* 33:160–166, 2002.

National Cancer Institute: *Women's health report fiscal years 2003-2004*, 2005, available at http://women.cancer.gov/planning/whr0304/whr0304.pdf.

National Cancer Institute: *Prostate cancer*, Bethesda, Md, 2009, National Institutes of Health.

National Center for Chronic Disease Prevention and Promotion: *National diabetes fact sheet*, 2005, available at www.cdc.gov/diabetes/pubs/estimates05.htm.

National Center for Health Statistics: *Health, United States, 2005. With chartbook on trends in the health of Americans*, Hyattsville, Md, 2005, available at http://www.cdc.gov/nchs/data/hus/hus05.pdf.

National Center for Health Statistics: *FASTATS*, Washington, DC, 2002, U.S. Government Printing Office.

National Center for Health Statistics: *FASTATS*, Washington, DC, 2004, U.S. Government Printing Office.

National Center for Health Statistics: *FASTATS*, Washington, DC, 2005, U.S. Government Printing Office.

National Center for Health Statistics: *FASTATS*, Washington, DC, 2008, U.S. Government Printing Office.

National Center for Injury Prevention and Control: *Fact sheet*, 2002, available at www.cdc.gov/ncipc.

National Center for Injury Prevention and Control: *Fact sheet*, 2008, available at www.cdc.gov/ncipc.

National Institute of Arthritis and Musculoskeletal and Skin Diseases (NIAMSD): *Osteoporosis overview*, 2005, available at http://www.osteo.org/newfile.asp?doc=r106i&doctitle=Osteoporosis+Overview+%2D+HTML+Version&doctype=HTML+Fact+Sheet.

National Institute of Diabetes and Digestive and Kidney Diseases, National Diabetes Information Clearinghouse: *General information and national estimates on diabetes in the United States, 2003*, 2005, available at http://diabetes.niddk.nih.gov/dm/pubs/statistics/.

National Institute of Mental Health: *Eating disorders: facts about eating disorders and the search for solutions*, 2001, available at www.nimh.nih.gov/publicat/eatingdisorder.cfm#ed2.

National Institute of Mental Health: *Women's mental health consortium*, 2002, available at http://www.nimh.nih.gov/wmhc/index.cfm.

National Institute of Mental Health: *Attention deficit and hyperactivity disorder*, Bethesda, Md, 2008, NIMH.

National Institutes of Health; National Heart, Lung, and Blood Pressure Institute: *NHLBI stops trial of estrogen plus progestin due to increased breast cancer risk, lack of overall benefit*, 2002, available at http://www.nhlbi.nih.gov/new/press/02-07-09.htm.

National Institutes of Health; National Heart, Lung, and Blood Institute: *Questions and answers about the WHI postmenopausal hormone therapy trials*, 2005, available at http://www.nhlbi.nih.gov/whi/whi_faq.htm#q1.

National Women's Health Network: *About NWHN*, 2005, available at http://www.womenshealthnetwork.org/about/index.php.

National Women's History Project: *Living the legacy: the women's rights movement 1848–1998*, 2002, available at http://www.legacy98.org/move-hist.html.

Neyer JR et al: Prevalence of Heart Disease U.S., 2005, *JAMA* 297:12, 2007.

Ogden CL, Carroll MD, Flegal KM: High body mass index for age among U.S. children and adolescents, 2005–2006, *JAMA,* 299:2401–2405, 2008.

Oliver-McNeil S, Artinian NT: Women's perceptions of personal cardiovascular risk and their risk-reducing behaviors, *Am J Crit Care* 11:221–227, 2002.

Polonsky W et al: A community-based program to encourage patients' attention to their own diabetes care: pilot development and evaluation, *Diabetes Educ* 31:691–699, 2005.

Porche D, Willis D: Men's health, *Nurs Clin North Am* 39:251–258, 2004.

Rosenberg J: Lesbians are more likely than U.S. women overall to have risk factors for gynecologic and breast cancer, *Fam Plan Perspect* 33:183–184, 2001.

Rowley DL et al: The reproductive years. In Beckles GLA, Thompson-Reid PE, editors: *Diabetes and women's health across the life span: a public health perspective,* Atlanta, 2001, U.S. Department of Health and Human Services, Centers for Disease Control and Prevention, National Center for Chronic Disease Prevention and Health Promotion, Division of Diabetes Translation, available at http://www.cdc.gov/diabetes/pubs/pdf/women.pdf.

Sabo D: Men's health studies: origins and trends, *J Am College Health* 49:133–142, 2000.

Sandman D et al: *Out of touch: American men and the health care system,* New York, 2000, Commonwealth Fund.

Satcher D: American women and health disparities, *J Am Med Womens Assoc* 56:131–133, 2001.

Schulz AJ et al: Healthy eating and exercising to reduce diabetes: exploring the potential of social determinants of health frameworks within the context of community-based participatory diabetes prevention, *Am J Publ Health* 95:645–651, 2005.

Schulz MA et al: Outcomes of a community-based three-year breast and cervical cancer screening program for medically underserved, low income women, *J Am Acad Nurse Pract* 14:219, 2002.

Simon H: *The Harvard Medical School guide to men's health,* New York, 2002, Free Press.

Spira M, Kenemore E: Cancer as a life transition: a relational approach to cancer wellness in women, *Clin Social Work J* 30:173, 2001.

Stotts R: Cancers of the prostate, penis, and testicles: epidemiology, prevention, and treatment, *Nurs Clin North Am* 39: 327–340, 2004.

Stover GN: Colorful communities: toward a language of inclusion, *Am J Publ Health* 92:512–514, 2002.

Tierney LM, McPhee SJ, Papadakis MA: *Current medical diagnosis and treatment,* ed 41, East Norwalk, Conn, 2002, Appleton & Lange.

Thomas S: Men's health and psychological issues affecting men, *Nurs Clin North Am* 39:259–270, 2004.

U.S. Bureau of the Census: *2003 American community survey summary tables, Table 1: general demographics,* 2003, available at http:www.census.gov/acs/www/Products/Profiles/Single/2003/ACS/Tabular/010/01000US1.htm.

U.S. Bureau of the Census, Population Estimates Program, Population Division: *Resident population estimates of the United States by sex, race, and Hispanic origin,* 2001, available at http://eire.census.gov/popest/archives/national/nation3/intfile3-1.txt.

U.S. Department of Health and Human Services, Health Resources and Services Administration, Maternal and Child Health Bureau: *Child Health USA 2003,* Rockville, Md, 2003, USDHHS.

U.S. Department of Health and Human Services: *Progress review,* Washington, DC, 2004a, USDHHS.

U.S. Department of Health and Human Services: *Health United States, 2004,* USDHHS pub no CPHS 24-1232, Washington, DC, 2004b, U.S. Government Printing Office.

U.S. Department of Health and Human Services: *The surgeon general's call to action to prevent and decrease overweight and obesity in 2001,* 2001, available at www.surgeongeneral.gov/library.

U.S. Department of Health and Human Services: *Healthy People 2010: national health promotion and disease prevention objectives,* Washington, DC, 2000, U.S. Department of Health and Human Services.

U.S. Department of Health and Human Services, National Institute on Aging: *Menopause: one woman's story, every woman's story: a resource for making healthy choices,* 2003, available at http://www.nia.nih.gov/health/pubs/menopause/menopause.pdf.

U.S. Department of Health and Human Services: *The surgeon general's call to action to prevent and decrease overweight and obesity,* 2001, available at www.surgeongeneral.gov/topics/obesity/calltoaction/factsheet01.pdf.

U.S. Department of Health and Human Services: *Health, United States, 2005. With chartbook on trends in health of Americans,* 2005, available at www.cdc.gov/nchs/hus.htm.

U.S. Department of Health and Human Services, National Women's Health Information Center: *Obesity,* 2004, available at http://www.4woman.gov/pub/steps/Obesity.htm.

U.S. Department of Health and Human Services, Office on Women's Health: *The health of minority women,* 2003. Retrieved 2005 from http://www.womenshealth.gov/owh/minority.htm.

U.S. Department of Health and Human Services, Office on Women's Health: *History,* 2005a, available at http://www.womenshealth.gov/owh/about/history.htm.

U.S. Department of Health and Human Services, Office on Women's Health: *The Office on Women's Health, women with disabilities,* 2005b, available at http://www.4women.gov/wwd/index.htm.

U.S. Department of Justice, Bureau of Justice Statistics: *Prisoners in 2004. Bureau of Justice Statistics.* Retrieved Oct 24, 2005, from http://www.ojp.usdoj.gov/bjs/pub/pdf/p04.pdf.

U.S. Department of Labor, Bureau of Labor Statistics: Women's earnings 76 percent of men's in 2000, *Monthly labor review, 2001,* available at http://www.bls.gov/opub/ted/2001/sept/wk1/art02.htm.

U.S. Food and Drug Administration: *Birth control guide,* updated 2003, available at http://www.fda.gov/fdac/features/1997/babytabl.html.

U.S. Preventive Services Task Force: *Screening for testicular cancer: recommendation statement,* 2004, available at www.guideline.gov/summary/summary.aspx?doc_id=4777&nbr=003456&string=testicular+AND+examination.

Wagner E et al: A survey of leading chronic disease management programs: are they consistent with the literature? *J Nurs Care Quality* 16:67–80, 2002.

World Health Organization: Genital and sexual mutilation of females, *Womens Int Network News* 28:61, 2005.

Wright N, Owen S: Feminist conceptualizations of women's madness: a review of the literature, *J Adv Nurs* 36:143, 2001.

Writing Group for the Women's Health Initiative Investigators: Risks and benefits of estrogen plus progestin in healthy postmenopausal women, *JAMA* 288, 2002.

PART VI

Vulnerability: Predisposing Factors

Chapter 21

Vulnerability and Vulnerable Populations: An Overview

Juliann G. Sebastian

ADDITIONAL RESOURCES

These related resources are found either in the appendix at the back of this book or on the book's website at http://evolve.elsevier.com/stanhope/foundations.

Evolve Website

- Community Assessment Applied
- Case Study, with questions and answers
- Quiz review questions
- WebLinks, including link to *Healthy People 2010* website

Real World Community Health Nursing: An Interactive CD-ROM, second edition

If you are using this CD-ROM in your course, you will find the following activities related to this chapter:
- *The Vulnerability Challenge* in **Vulnerability**
- *Vulnerability: You're in Charge* in **Vulnerability**

OBJECTIVES

After reading this chapter, the student should be able to:
1. Define the term vulnerable populations and describe selected groups who fall into this category.
2. Describe factors that led to the development of vulnerability in certain populations.
3. Examine ways in which public policies affect vulnerable populations and can reduce health disparities in these groups.
4. Examine the individual and social factors that contribute to vulnerability.
5. Describe strategies that nurses can use to improve the health status and eliminate health disparities of vulnerable populations.

CHAPTER OUTLINE

VULNERABILITY: DEFINITION AND INFLUENCING FACTORS

PREDISPOSING FACTORS

OUTCOMES OF VULNERABILITY

PUBLIC POLICIES AFFECTING VULNERABLE POPULATIONS
Ways in Which Managed Care and Insurance Affect Vulnerable Populations

NURSING INTERVENTION
Levels of Prevention
Assessment Issues
Planning and Implementing Care for Vulnerable Populations

KEY TERMS

advocacy: a set of actions undertaken on behalf of another while supporting the other's right to self-determination. Nurses may function as advocates for vulnerable populations by working for the passage and implementation of policies that will result in improved public health services for these populations. An example would be a nurse who serves on a local coalition for uninsured people and works toward development of a plan for sharing the provision of free or low-cost health care by local health care organizations and providers.

case management: interchangeable term with care management. Used to describe a service given to clients that contains the following activities: screening, assessment, care planning, arranging for, and coordinating service delivery, monitoring, reassessment, evaluation, and discharge. Case management is a process that enhances continuity and appropriateness of care. It is most often used with clients whose health problems are actually or potentially chronic and complex.

comprehensive services: health services focusing on more than one health problem or concern.

cumulative risks: the additive effects of multiple risk factors.

disadvantaged: people who lack adequate resources that other people may take for granted.

disenfranchisement: a sense of social isolation; a feeling of isolation from mainstream society.

federal poverty level: income level for a certain family size that the federal government uses to define poverty.

health disparities: refers to the wide variations in health services and health status among certain population groups.

human capital: the combined human potential of the people living in a community.

linguistically appropriate health care: communicating health-related assessment and information in the recipient's primary language when possible and always in a language the recipient can understand.

poverty: lacking resources to meet basic living expenses for food, shelter, clothing, transportation, and medical care.

resilience: the ability to withstand many forms of stress and deal with several problems simultaneously without developing health problems.

risk: the likelihood that some event or outcome will occur in a given time frame.

social justice: providing humane care and social supports for the most disadvantaged members of society (Linhorst, 2002).

vulnerability: results from the interaction of internal and external factors that cause a person to be susceptible to poor health.

vulnerable populations: those with increased risk of developing poor health outcomes.

wrap-around services: social and economic services provided, either directly or through referrals, in addition to available comprehensive health services. In this way, social and economic services that will help ensure the effectiveness of health services are "wrapped around" health services.

The old saying, "All men [and women] are created equal" is really not true. People have different genetic compositions, social and environmental resources, skills, support systems, and access to health services. People with lower incomes and less education tend to be at higher risk for health problems. A goal in the United States is to eliminate health disparities by expanding access to health care for vulnerable or at-risk populations. This chapter details the nurse's use of the nursing process with vulnerable population groups and presents case examples to clarify these ideas.

VULNERABILITY: DEFINITION AND INFLUENCING FACTORS

Vulnerability is defined as susceptibility to actual or potential stressors that may lead to an adverse effect. Vulnerability to poor health does not mean that some people have personal deficiencies. Rather, it results from the interacting effects of many internal and external factors over which people have little or no control. For example, a person may have some biological limitations that are made more severe by pollution, lead-based paint, excessive noise, or other external factors.

Vulnerable populations are those groups who have an increased risk of developing adverse health outcomes.

As discussed in Chapter 9, **risk** is an epidemiologic term that means some people have a higher probability of illness than others do. In the epidemiologic triangle, the agent, host, and environment interact to produce illness or poor health. The natural history of a disease model explains how certain aspects of physiology and the environment, including personal habits, social environment, and physical environment, make it more likely that a person will develop particular health problems. For example, a smoker is at risk for developing lung cancer because cellular changes occur with smoking. However, not everyone who is at risk develops health problems. Some individuals are more likely than others to develop the health problems for which they are at risk. These people are more *vulnerable* than others. The web of causation model better explains what happens in these situations. A vulnerable population group is a subgroup of the population that is more likely to develop health problems as a result of exposure to risk or to have worse outcomes from these health problems than the rest of the population. That is, the interaction among many variables creates a more powerful combination of factors that predispose the person to illness. Vulnerable populations often experience multiple **cumulative risks**, and they are particularly sensitive to the effects of those risks. Risks come from environmental hazards (e.g., lead exposure from lead-based paint from peeling walls or that which has been used in toy manufacturing or melamine added to milk supplies), social hazards (e.g., crime, violence), personal behavior (e.g., diet, exercise habits, smoking), or biological or genetic makeup (e.g., congenital addiction, compromised immune status). Members of vulnerable populations often have multiple illnesses, with each affecting the other. Some members of vulnerable populations do not succumb to the health risks that impinge on them. It is important to learn what factors help these people to resist, or have **resilience** to, the effects of vulnerability.

Vulnerable individuals and families often have many risk factors. For example, nurses work with pregnant adolescents who are poor, have been abused, and are substance abusers. Nurses also work with substance abusers who test positive for human immunodeficiency virus (HIV) and for hepatitis B virus (HBV), as well as those who are severely mentally ill. Nurses in community health work with homeless and marginally housed individuals and families. They also provide care for migrant workers and immigrants. Any of these groups may be victimized by abuse and violence. Box 21-1 lists vulnerable population groups. Each of these groups is discussed in detail in Chapters 22 through 27. This chapter highlights some of the problems that the vulnerable populations just described have with access to care, quality and appropriateness of care, and health outcomes.

Vulnerable populations are more likely than the general population to suffer from health disparities. **Health disparities** refer to the wide variations in health services and health status among certain population groups. Both *Healthy People 2010* (U.S. Department of Health and Human Services, 2001a) and *Healthy People in Healthy Communities* (U.S. Department of Health and Human Services, 2001b) discuss vulnerable population groups and illness prevention and health promotion objectives for them. Because of the continuing disparities in health status between certain demographic subgroups of people living in the United States and those who have adequate care, a major effort is underway to eliminate the less-than-adequate care experienced by some groups as defined by "age, gender, race or ethnicity, education or income, disability, geographic location or sexual orientation" (U.S. Department of Health and Human Services, 2001a, p. 11).

One of the two overarching goals of *Healthy People 2010* (U.S. Department of Health and Human Services, 2001a) is the elimination of health disparities. Twenty-eight focal areas in *Healthy People 2010* emphasize access, chronic health problems, injury and violence prevention, environmental health, food safety, health communication, health educational programming, and individual health-related behaviors. *Healthy People 2010* objectives seek to establish realistic targets for improvement.

As discussed in other chapters, *Healthy People 2010* is an implementation guide for all federal and most state health initiatives. It is especially relevant to a discussion of vulnerable populations, since these underserved and disadvantaged populations have fewer resources for promoting health and treating illness than does the average person in the United States. For example, a family or individual below the federal poverty line is considered **disadvantaged** in terms of access to economic resources. These groups are thought to be vulnerable because of the combination of risk factors, health status, and lack of the resources needed to access health care and reduce risk factors (Flaskerud et al, 2002).

Areas that show health disparities across population groups include infant mortality, childhood immunization rates, and disease-specific mortality rates. Statistics from the Centers for Disease Control and Prevention (CDC) showed that infant mortality rates reached an historic low in the United States in 2000 with 6.9 deaths per 1000 live births overall. This is largely due to the increased rates of mothers receiving early prenatal care and the declining rate

---

Box 21-1	**Vulnerable Population Groups of Special Concern to Nurses**

- Poor and homeless persons
- Pregnant adolescents
- Migrant workers and immigrants
- Severely mentally ill individuals
- Substance abusers
- Abused individuals and victims of violence
- Persons with communicable disease and those at risk
- Persons who are human immunodeficiency virus (HIV) positive or have hepatitis B virus (HBV) or sexually transmitted disease

---

● **Healthy People 2010**

Goals for Vulnerable Populations

The following are examples of objectives that nurses in community health who work with vulnerable populations should note:

1-5	Increase the proportion of persons with a usual primary care provider
18-7	Increase the proportion of children with mental health problems who receive treatment
18-9	Increase the proportion of adults with mental disorders who receive treatment
18-13	Increase the number of states, territories, and the District of Columbia with an operational mental health plan that addresses cultural competence
24-1	Reduce asthma deaths
25-11	Increase the proportion of adolescents who abstain from sexual intercourse or use condoms if currently sexually active

From U.S. Department of Health and Human Services: *Healthy People 2010: understanding and improving health*, ed 2, Washington, DC, 2000, U.S. Government Printing Office.

of cigarette smoking among pregnant women. Despite this success, the United States continues to rank 27th among industrialized countries in the rate of infant mortality. Sweden reports the lowest rates of 3.5 deaths per 1000 infants. Infant mortality rates vary by race. The U.S. infant mortality rate did not drop from 2000 to 2005. However, preliminary data indicate a 2% drop from 2005 to 2006. This rate continues to be higher than in other developed countries. Rates in the United States are 2.4% higher for non-Hispanic black women than for non-Hispanic white women. Rates are also elevated for Puerto Rican, American Indian, and Alaska Native women. Overall in the United States in 2005, there were 6.86 infant deaths per 1000 live births (Centers for Disease Control and Prevention, 2006, 2008; MacDorman and Mathews, 2008). African-Americans have significantly higher death rates from prostate and breast cancer and from heart disease than non-Hispanic whites living in the United States. Hispanics have higher mortality rates from diabetes than non-Hispanic whites living in the United States. Race and ethnicity are not thought to be the causes of these disparities, although research is underway to determine biological susceptibilities by race, ethnicity, and gender. Rather, poverty and low educational levels are more likely to contribute to social conditions in which disparities develop. People who are poor often live in unsafe areas, work in stressful environments, have less access to healthful foods and opportunities for exercise, and are more likely to be uninsured or underinsured.

Vulnerability results from the combined effects of limited resources. Limitations in physical resources, environmental resources, personal resources (or human capital), and biopsychosocial resources (e.g., the presence of illness, genetic predispositions) combine to cause vulnerability (Aday, 2001). **Poverty**, limited social support, and working in a hazardous environment are examples of limitations in physical and environmental resources. People with preexisting illnesses, such as those with communicable or infectious diseases or those with chronic illnesses such as cancer, heart disease, or chronic airway disease, have less physical ability to cope with stress than those without such physical problems. **Human capital** refers to all of the strengths, knowledge, and skills that enable a person to live a productive, happy life. People with little education have less human capital because their choices are more limited than are those of people with higher levels of education.

There are many aspects to vulnerability. Vulnerability often comes from a feeling of lack of power, limited control, victimization, disadvantaged status, disenfranchisement, and health risks. Vulnerability can be reversed by obtaining resources to increase resilience. Useful nursing interventions to increase resilience include case finding, health education, care coordination, and policy making related to improving health for vulnerable populations.

One aspect of vulnerability, **disenfranchisement**, refers to a feeling of separation from mainstream society. The person does not seem to have an emotional connection with any group in particular or with the larger society. Some groups such as the poor, the homeless, and migrant workers are "invisible" to society as a whole and tend to be forgotten in health and social planning. Vulnerable populations are at risk for disenfranchisement, since their social supports are often weak as are their linkages to formal community organizations such as churches, schools, and other types of social organizations. They may also have few informal sources of support, such as family, friends, and neighbors. In many ways, vulnerable groups have limited control over potential and actual health needs. In many communities, these groups are in the minority and disadvantaged, since typical health planning focuses on the majority. Disadvantage also results from lack of resources that others may take for granted. Vulnerable population groups have limited social and economic resources with which to manage their health care. For example, women may endure domestic violence rather than risk losing a place for themselves and their children to live. Women who are among the working poor are more likely to become homeless when they leave an abusive partner. They may not be able to pay for a place to live when they lose their partner's income.

PREDISPOSING FACTORS

Social and economic factors predispose people to vulnerability. Poverty is a primary cause of vulnerability, and it is a growing problem in the United States. Poverty is a relative state. In 2007 the official poverty rate was 12.5%. During that year 37.3 million people lived in poverty. The poverty rate is at the following levels for these groups:

8.2% for non-Hispanic whites
24.5% for blacks
10.2% for Asians
21.55 for Hispanics (U.S. Census Bureau, 2008).

The poverty rate increased from 17.4 in 2006 to 18.0 in 2007 for children under 18 years of age. Other age groups remained unchanged. In 2007 the **federal poverty level** for a family of four was $21,203 (U.S. Bureau of the Census, 2007). However, many people who earn just a little more than the federal poverty level are unable to pay for their living expenses but are ineligible for assistance programs.

People who do not have the financial resources to pay for medical care are considered medically indigent. They may be self-employed or work in small businesses and cannot afford health benefits. Other people have inadequate health insurance coverage. This may be either because the deductibles or copayments for their insurance are so high that they have to pay for most expenses or because few conditions or services are covered. In these situations, poverty in its relative sense causes vulnerability because uninsured and underinsured people are less likely to seek preventive health services due to the cost. They are then more likely to suffer the consequences of preventable illnesses.

Age is related to vulnerability, since people at both ends of the age continuum are often less able physiologically to adapt to stressors. For example, infants of substance-abusing mothers risk being born addicted and having severe physiological problems and developmental delays. Elderly individuals are more likely to develop active infections from communicable diseases such as the flu or pneumonia and generally have more difficulty recovering from infectious processes than younger people because of their less effective immune systems. Older people also may be more vulnerable to safety threats and loss of independence because of their age, multiple chronic illnesses, as well as impaired mobility. Chapter 24 discusses substance abuse and Chapter 26 describes communicable disease risk.

Also, changes in normal physiology can predispose people to vulnerability. This may result from disease processes, such as in someone with single or multiple chronic diseases. As discussed in Chapter 27, human immunodeficiency virus (HIV) is a pathophysiological situation that increases vulnerability to opportunistic infections.

A person's life experiences, especially those early in life, influence vulnerability or resilience. For example, children who survive disasters may experience difficulties in later life if they do not receive adequate counseling. Higher levels of confidence in one's ability or internal locus of control appears to protect children (particularly adolescents) from the negative effects of disaster and trauma. A person with an internal locus of control can control his or her behavior and not depend entirely on external people, events, or forces to control behavior. Vulnerable population groups often develop an external locus of control. They may believe that events are outside their control and result from bad luck or fate. People with an external locus of control have more difficulty taking action or seeking care for health problems. They may minimize the value of health promotion or illness prevention because they do not think they have control over their health destinies. Also, people who have been abused or have experienced chronic stress may have used up a lot of the reserves that others would normally have for coping with new forms of stress. A study by investigators at the Centers for Disease Control and Prevention (Middlebrooks and Audage, 2008) looked retrospectively at the link between childhood stressors and adult health. This study was referred to as the Adverse Childhood Experiences study. In particular, the investigators looked at the stress caused by child abuse, neglect, and repeated exposure to intimate partner violence. They discussed three kinds of stress: (1) positive stress, which comes from short-lived adverse events and which children can manage with the help of supportive adults; (2) tolerable stress, which is more intense but still short-lived, such as stress arising from a natural disaster or frightening accident; or (3) toxic stress, which results from intense adverse experiences that are sustained over time. Children cannot handle toxic stress alone. When the stress response is activated for a length of time, it can lead to permanent developmental changes in the brain. The support of helping adults can enable the child's stress response to return to normal. As will be discussed in Chapter 25, child maltreatment can be a source of toxic stress. The "Evidence-Based Practice" box describes this study in more detail and provides actions that all health professionals can take to reduce toxic stress in the community with its untoward effect on children and their growth and development.

OUTCOMES OF VULNERABILITY

Outcomes of vulnerability may be negative, such as a lower health status than the rest of the population, or they may be positive with effective interventions. Vulnerable populations often have worse health outcomes than other people in terms of morbidity and mortality. These groups have a high prevalence of chronic illnesses, such as hypertension, and high levels of communicable diseases including tuberculosis (TB), hepatitis B, and sexually transmitted diseases (STDs), as well as upper respiratory infections including influenza. They also have higher mortality rates than the general population because of factors such as poor living conditions, diet, and health status, as well as crime and violence, including domestic violence.

There is often a cycle to vulnerability. That is, poor health creates stress as individuals and families try to manage health problems with inadequate resources. For example, if someone with acquired immunodeficiency syndrome (AIDS) develops one or more opportunistic infections and is either uninsured or underinsured, that person and the family and caregivers will have more difficulty managing than if the person had adequate insurance. Vulnerable populations often suffer many forms of stress. Sometimes when one problem is solved, another quickly emerges. This can lead to feelings of hopelessness, which result from an overwhelming sense of powerlessness and social isolation. For example, substance abusers who feel powerless over their addiction and who have isolated themselves from the people they care about may see no way to change their situation.

PUBLIC POLICIES AFFECTING VULNERABLE POPULATIONS

Three pieces of legislation have provided direct and indirect financial subsidies to certain vulnerable groups. The Social Security Act of 1935 created the largest federal support program for elderly and poor Americans in history. This act was intended to ensure a minimal level of support for people at risk for problems resulting from inadequate financial resources. This was accomplished by direct payments to eligible individuals. Later, the Social Security Act Amendments of 1965, Medicare and Medicaid, provided for the health care needs of elderly, poor, and disabled people who might be vulnerable to impoverishment resulting from high medical bills or to poor health status from inadequate access to health care. These acts created third-party health care payers at the federal and state levels. Title XXI of the Social Security Act, enacted in 1998, created the State Children's Health Insurance Program (SCHIP), which provides funds to insure currently uninsured children. The SCHIP program is jointly funded by the Federal and State governments and administered by the states. Using broad Federal guidelines, each state designs its own program, determines who is eligible for benefits, sets the payment levels, and decides upon the administrative and operating procedures. The program is subject to change when states undergo budget reductions (Centers for Medicare and Medicaid Services, 2008). There

Evidence-Based Practice

Researchers at the Centers for Disease Control and Prevention examined retrospectively the effects of childhood stress on health when the children became adults. They were interested in looking particularly at how child abuse and neglect and the witnessing of repeated family violence lead to toxic stress. They described toxic stress as resulting from "adverse experiences that may be sustained for a long period of time" and can disrupt early brain development, affect the functioning of important biological systems, and lead to long-term health problems (p. 3). The researchers were especially interested in the adult participants' exposure to abuse (emotional, physical, and sexual), neglect (emotional and physical), and household dysfunction (a mother treated violently, household substance abuse or mental illness, parental separation or divorce, or an incarcerated household member). They found associations between higher adverse childhood experiences and many negative behaviors: those with higher numbers of adverse childhood experiences were at greater risk for alcoholism and were more likely to marry an alcoholic, to initiate drug use and experience addiction, to have 30 or more sexual partners, and to have a higher percentage of both lifetime and recent depression. They recommended the use of the social ecological model that the Centers for Disease Control and Prevention uses. This model looks at the complex interplay between individual, relationship, community, and societal factors. They recommend individual, relationship and community, organizational, and social level strategies. Many of their strategies can easily be used in nursing.

NURSE USE: Nurses can conduct group educational sessions for parents that teach them skills in parenting and in which they can learn the skill and ask questions in a nonthreatening setting. Nurses also can screen for child maltreatment, especially if they work in schools, work in community clinics, and make home visits. A relationship strategy is to have nurses visit families in their homes over time to teach them skills, provide support, and make referrals if needed. A community and social level strategy would be to initiate or be part of a public awareness campaign related to a variety of health issues, including child maltreatment.

From Middlebrook JS, Audage NC: *The effects of childhood stress on health across the lifespan*, Atlanta, Ga, 2008, Centers for Disease Control and Prevention, National Center for Injury Prevention. Retrieved Oct 4, 2008, from www.cdc.gov/ncip/pub-res/pdf/childhood_stress.pdf.

Box 21-2   Nursing Roles When Working with Vulnerable Population Groups

- Case finder
- Health educator
- Counselor
- Direct care provider
- Population health advocate
- Community assessor and developer
- Monitor and evaluator of care
- Case manager
- Advocate
- Health program planner
- Participant in developing health policies

---

difficult for vulnerable populations to improve their health. Nurses can identify areas in which they can work with vulnerable populations to break the cycle. The nursing process guides nurses in assessing vulnerable individuals, families, groups, and communities; developing nursing diagnoses of their strengths and needs; planning and implementing appropriate therapeutic nursing interventions in partnership with vulnerable clients; and evaluating the effectiveness of interventions.

In some situations, the nurse works with individual clients. The nurse also develops programs and policies for populations of vulnerable persons. In both examples, planning and implementing care for members of vulnerable populations involve partnerships between the nurse and client. Nurses who direct and control the client's care cannot establish a trusting relationship and may inadvertently foster a cycle of dependency and lack of personal health control. In fact, the most important initial step is for nurses to establish that they are trustworthy and dependable. For example, nurses who work in a community clinic for substance abusers must overcome any suspicion that clients may have of them and eliminate any fears clients may have of being manipulated.

Nurses working with vulnerable populations may fill numerous roles, including those listed in Box 21-2. They identify vulnerable individuals and families through outreach and case finding. They encourage vulnerable groups to obtain health services, and they develop programs that respond to their needs. Nurses teach vulnerable individuals, families, and groups strategies to prevent illness and promote health. They counsel clients about ways to increase their sense of personal power and help them identify strengths and resources. They provide direct care to clients and families in a variety of settings, including storefront clinics, mobile clinics, shelters, homes, neighborhoods, worksites, churches, and schools.

Some examples of care to clients, families, and groups are as follows: (1) a nurse in a mobile migrant clinic might administer a tetanus booster to a client who has been injured by a piece of farm machinery and may also check that client's blood pressure and cholesterol level during the same visit; (2) a home-health nurse seeing a family referred by the courts for child abuse may weigh the child, conduct a nutritional assessment, and help the family learn how to manage anger and disciplinary problems; (3) a nurse working in a school-based clinic may lead a support group for pregnant adolescents and conduct a birthing class; and (4) nurses working with people being treated for TB monitor drug treatment compliance to ensure that they complete their full course of therapy.

Public health nurses and nurses in community health serve also as population health advocates and work with local, state, or national groups to develop and implement healthy public policy. They also collaborate with other community members and serve as community assessors and developers, and they monitor and evaluate care and health programs. *Healthy People in Healthy Communities* describes one approach for working collaboratively with communities to develop healthy communities and eliminate health disparities (U.S. Department of Health and Human Services, 2001b). Nurses often function as case managers for vulnerable clients, making referrals and linking them to community services. **Case management** services are especially important for vulnerable persons since they often do not have the ability or resources to make their own arrangements. They may not be able to speak the language or they may be unable to navigate the complex telephone systems that many agencies establish. They also serve as advocates when they refer clients to other agencies, work with others to develop health programs, and influence legislation and health policies that affect vulnerable populations.

The nature of nurses' roles varies depending on whether the client is a single person, a family, or a group. For example, a nurse might teach an HIV-positive client about the need for prevention of opportunistic infections, may help a family with an HIV-positive member understand myths about transmission of HIV, or may work with a community group concerned about HIV transmission among students in the schools. In each case, the nurse teaches individuals how to prevent infectious and communicable disease. The size of the group and the teaching method for each group differ.

Health education is often used in working with vulnerable populations. The nurse should teach members of populations with low educational levels what they need to do to promote health and prevent illness rather than directing health education to groups that the nurse *thinks* might be at high risk even though there is no evidence to support the perception. For example, in a study of cardiovascular disease risk for rural Southern women, Appel, Harrell, and Deng (2002) found that only body mass index and educational level predicted risk for cardiovascular disease within this population. They recommended health education for all low-income rural southern women and not just for particular racial groups. A new concern for nurses in public and community health is whether the populations with whom they work have adequate health literacy to benefit from health education. It may be necessary to collaborate with an educator, an interpreter, or an expert in health communications to design messages that vulnerable individuals and groups can understand and use.

LEVELS OF PREVENTION

Healthy People 2010 (U.S. Department of Health and Human Services, 2001a) objectives emphasize improving health by modifying the individual, social, and environmental determinants of health. One way to do this is for vulnerable individuals to have a primary care provider who both coordinates health services for them and provides their preventive services. This primary care provider may be an advanced practice nurse or a primary care physician (e.g., a family practice physician). Another approach is for a nurse

---

Levels of Prevention	Related to Vulnerable Populations

PRIMARY PREVENTION

- Provide culturally and economically sensitive health teaching about balanced diet and exercise.
- Develop a portable immunization chart, such as a wallet card, that mobile population groups such as the homeless and migrant workers can carry with them.

SECONDARY PREVENTION

- Conduct screening clinics to assess for things such as obesity, diabetes, heart disease, or tuberculosis (TB).
- Develop a way for homeless individuals to read their TB skin test, if necessary, and to transfer the results back to the facility at which the skin test was administered.

TERTIARY PREVENTION

- Develop community-based exercise programs for people identified as obese or who have increased blood pressure or increased blood sugar.
- Provide directly observed medication therapy for people with active TB.

---

to serve as a case manager for vulnerable clients and, again, coordinate services and provide illness prevention and health promotion services.

One example of primary prevention is to give influenza vaccinations to vulnerable populations who are immunocompromised (unless contraindicated). Secondary prevention is seen in conducting screening clinics for vulnerable populations. For example, nurses who work in homeless shelters, prisons, migrant camps, and substance abuse treatment facilities should know that these groups are at high risk for acquiring communicable diseases. Both clients and staff need routine screening for TB. Screening homeless adults and providing isoniazid to those who test positive for TB are examples of secondary prevention. An example of tertiary prevention is conducting a therapy group with the residents of a group home for severely mentally ill adults. Nurses who work with abused women to help them enhance their levels of self-esteem are also providing tertiary preventive activities.

ASSESSMENT ISSUES

Nurses who work with vulnerable populations need good assessment skills, current knowledge of available resources, and the ability to plan care based on client needs and receptivity to help. They also need to be able to show respect for the client. The "How To" box lists guidelines for assessing members of vulnerable population groups.

Because members of vulnerable populations often experience multiple stressors, assessment must balance the need to be comprehensive while focusing only on information that the nurse needs and the client is willing to provide. Remember to ask questions about the client's perceptions of his or her *socioeconomic resources,* including identifying people

Setting the Stage
- Create a comfortable, nonthreatening environment.
- Learn as much as you can about the culture of the clients you work with so that you will understand cultural practices and values that may influence their health care practices.
- Provide a culturally competent assessment by understanding the meaning of language and nonverbal behavior in the client's culture.
- Be sensitive to the fact that the individual or family you are assessing may have other priorities that are more important to them. These might include financial or legal problems. You may need to give them some tangible help with their most pressing priority before you will be able to address issues that are more traditionally thought of as health concerns.
- Collaborate with others as appropriate; you should not provide financial or legal advice. However, you should make sure to connect your client with someone who can and will help them.

Nursing History of an Individual or Family
- You may have only one opportunity to work with a vulnerable person or family. Try to complete a history that will provide all the essential information you need to help the individual or family on that day. This means that you will have to organize in your mind exactly what you need to ask, and no more, and why the data are necessary.
- It will help to use a comprehensive assessment form that has been modified to focus on the special needs of the vulnerable population group with whom you work. However, be flexible. With some clients, it will be both impractical and unethical to cover all questions on a comprehensive form. If you know that

you are likely to see the client again, ask the less-pressing questions at the next visit.
- Be sure to include questions about social support, economic status, resources for health care, developmental issues, current health problems, medications, and how the person or family manages their health status. Your goal is to obtain information that will enable you to provide family-centered care.
- Determine if the individual has any condition that compromises his or her immune status, such as AIDS, or if the individual is undergoing therapy that would result in immunodeficiency, such as cancer chemotherapy.

Physical Examination or Home Assessment
- Again, complete as thorough a physical examination (on an individual) or home assessment as you can. Keep in mind that you should collect only data for which you have a use.
- Be alert for indications of physical abuse, substance use (e.g., needle marks, nasal abnormalities), or neglect (e.g., underweight, inadequate clothing).
- You can assess a family's living environment using good observational skills. Does the family live in an insect- or rat-infested environment? Do they have running water, functioning plumbing, electricity, and a telephone?
- Is perishable food (e.g., mayonnaise) left sitting out on tables and countertops? Are bed linens reasonably clean? Is paint peeling on the walls and ceilings? Is ventilation adequate? Is the temperature of the home adequate? Is the family exposed to raw sewage or animal waste? Is the home adjacent to a busy highway, possibly exposing the family to high noise levels and automobile exhaust?

who can provide support and financial resources. Support from other people may include information, caregiving, emotional support, and help with instrumental activities of daily living, such as transportation, shopping, and babysitting. Financial resources may include the extent to which the client can pay for health services and medications, as well as questions about eligibility for third-party payment. The nurse should ask the client about the perceived adequacy of both formal and informal support networks.

When possible, assessment should include an evaluation of clients' *preventive health needs,* including age-appropriate screening tests, such as immunization status, blood pressure, weight, serum cholesterol, Papanicolaou (Pap) smears, breast examinations, mammograms, prostate examinations, glaucoma screening, and dental evaluations. It may be necessary to make referrals to have some of these tests done for clients. Assessment should also include preventive screening for physical health problems, for which certain vulnerable groups are at a particularly high risk. For example, people who are HIV positive should be evaluated regularly for their T4 cell counts and for common opportunistic infections, including TB and pneumonia. Intravenous drug users should be evaluated for HBV, including liver palpation and serum antigen tests as necessary. Alcoholic clients should also be asked about symptoms of liver disease and should be

evaluated for jaundice and liver enlargement. Severely mentally ill clients should be assessed for the presence of tardive dyskinesia, indicating possible toxicity from their antipsychotic medications.

Vulnerable populations should be assessed for *congenital* and *genetic predisposition* to illness and either receive education and counseling as appropriate or be referred to other health professionals as necessary. For example, pregnant adolescents who are substance abusers should be referred to programs to help them quit using addictive substances during their pregnancies and, ideally, after delivery of their infants as well. Pregnant women older than 35 years should receive amniocentesis testing to determine if genetic abnormalities exist in the fetus.

The nurse should also assess the amount of *stress* the person or family is having. Does the family have healthy coping skills and healthy family interaction? Are some family members able and willing to care for others? What is the level of mental health in each member? Also, are diet, exercise, and rest and sleep patterns conducive to good health?

The nurse should assess the *living environment* and *neighborhood surroundings* of vulnerable families and groups for environmental hazards such as lead-based paint, asbestos, water and air quality, industrial wastes, and the incidence of crime.

CASE STUDY

Felicia is a 22-year-old single mother of three children whose primary source of income is Aid to Families with Dependent Children. She is worried about the future because she will no longer be eligible for welfare by the end of the year. She has been unable to find a job that will pay enough for her to afford childcare. Her friend, Maria, said that Felicia and her children could stay in Maria's trailer for a short time, but Felicia is afraid that her only choice after that will be a shelter.

Felicia recently took all three children with her to the health department because 15-month-old Hector needed immunizations. Felicia was also concerned about 5-year-old Martina, who had had a fever of 100° to 101° F on and off for the past month. Felicia and her friends in the trailer park think that some type of hazardous waste from the chemical plant next door to the park is making their children sick. Now that Martina was not feeling well, Felicia was particularly concerned. However, the health department nurse told her that no appointments were available that day and that she would need to bring Martina back to the clinic on the next day. Felicia left discouraged because it was so difficult for her to get all three children ready and on the bus to go to the health department, not to mention the expense. She thought maybe Martina just had a cold and she would wait a little longer before bringing her back. However, she wanted to take care of Martina's problem before losing her medical card. Felicia is desperate to find a way to manage her money problems and take care of her children.

PLANNING AND IMPLEMENTING CARE FOR VULNERABLE POPULATIONS

Nurses who work in community settings typically have considerable involvement with vulnerable populations. The relationship with the client will depend on the nature of the contact (see the "How To" box on p. 396). Some will be seen in clinics and others in homes, schools, and at work. Regardless of the setting, the following key nursing actions need to be used:

- *Create a trusting environment.* Trust is essential, since many of these individuals have previously been disappointed in their interactions with health care and social systems. It is important to follow through and do what you say you are going to do. If you do not know the answer to a question, the best reply is "I do not know, but I will try to find out."
- *Show respect, compassion, and concern.* Vulnerable people have been defeated again and again by life's circumstances. They may have reached a point at which they question if they even deserve to get care. Listen carefully, since listening is a form of respect as well as a way to gather information to plan care.
- *Do not make assumptions.* Assess each person and family. No two people or groups are alike.
- *Coordinate services and providers.* Getting health and social services is not always easy. Often people feel like they are traveling through a maze. In most communities a large number of useful services exist. People who need them simply may not know how to find them. For example, people may need help finding a food bank or a free clinic or obtaining low-cost or free clothing through churches or in second-hand stores. Clients often need help in determining if they meet the eligibility requirements. If gaps in service are found, nurses can work with others to try to get the needed services established.
- *Advocate for accessible health care services.* Vulnerable people have trouble getting access to services. Neighborhood clinics, mobile vans, and home visits can be valuable for them. Also, coordinating services at a central location is helpful. These multiservice centers can provide health care, social services, day care, drug and alcohol recovery programs, and case management. When working with vulnerable populations, it is a good idea to arrange to have as many services as possible available in a single location and at convenient times. This "one-stop shopping" approach to care delivery is very helpful for populations experiencing multiple social, economic, and health-related stresses. Although it may seem difficult and costly to provide comprehensive services in one location, it may save money in the long run by preventing illness.
- *Focus on prevention.* Use every opportunity to teach about preventive health care. Primary prevention may include child and adult immunization and education about nutrition, foot care, safe sex, contraception, and the prevention of injuries or chronic illness. It also includes providing prophylactic antituberculosis drug therapy for HIV-positive people who live in homeless shelters or giving flu vaccine to people who are immunocompromised or older than 65 years. Secondary prevention would include screening for health problems such as TB, diabetes, hypertension, foot problems, anemia, drug use, or abuse.

BRIEFLY NOTED

People who spend time in homeless shelters, substance abuse treatment facilities, and prisons often get communicable diseases such as influenza, TB, and methicillin-resistant *Staphylococcus aureus* (MRSA). Nurses who work in these facilities should plan regular influenza vaccination clinics and TB screening clinics. When planning these clinics, nurses should work with local physicians to develop signed protocols and should plan ahead for problems related to the transient nature of the population. For example, nurses should develop a way for homeless individuals to read their TB skin test if necessary and transfer the results back to the facility where the skin test was administered. It is helpful to develop a portable immunization chart, such as a wallet card, that mobile population groups such as the homeless and migrant workers can carry with them.

HOW TO | Intervene with Vulnerable Populations

Goals

- Set reasonable goals that are based on the baseline data you collected. Focus on reducing disparities in health status among vulnerable populations.
- Work toward setting manageable goals with the client. Goals that seem unattainable may be discouraging.
- Set goals collaboratively with the client as a first step toward client empowerment.
- Set family-centered, culturally sensitive goals.

Interventions

- Set up outreach and case-finding programs to help increase access to health services by vulnerable populations.
- Do everything you can to minimize the "hassle factor" connected with the interventions you plan. Vulnerable groups do not have the extra energy, money, or time to cope with unnecessary waits, complicated treatment plans, or confusion. As your client's advocate, you should identify what hassles may occur and develop ways to avoid them. For example, this may include providing comprehensive services during a single encounter, rather than asking the client to return for multiple visits. Multiple visits for more specialized aspects of the client's needs, whether individual or family group, reinforce a perception that

health care is fragmented and organized for the professional's convenience rather than the client's.

- Work with clients to ensure that interventions are culturally sensitive and competent.
- Focus on teaching clients skills in health promotion and disease prevention. Also, teach them how to be effective health care consumers. For example, role-play asking questions in a physician's office with a client.
- Help clients learn what to do if they cannot keep an appointment with a health care or social service professional.

Evaluating Outcomes

- It is often difficult for vulnerable clients to return for follow-up care. Help your client develop self-care strategies for evaluating outcomes. For example, teach homeless individuals how to read their own tuberculosis (TB) skin test, and give them a self-addressed, stamped card they can return by mail with the results.
- Remember to evaluate outcomes in terms of the goals you have mutually agreed on with the client. For example, one outcome for a homeless person receiving isoniazid therapy for TB might be that the person return to the clinic daily for direct observation of compliance with the drug therapy.

- *Know when to "walk beside" the client and when to encourage the client to "walk ahead."* At times it is hard to know when to do something for people and when to teach or encourage them to do for themselves. Nursing actions range from providing encouragement and support to providing information and active intervention. It is important to assess for the presence of strength and the ability to problem solve, cope, and access services. For example, a local hospital might provide free mammograms for women who cannot pay. The nurse would need to decide whether to schedule the appointments for clients or to give them the information and encourage them to do the scheduling.
- *Know what resources are available.* Be familiar with community agencies that offer health and social services to vulnerable populations. Also follow up after you make a referral to make sure the client was able to obtain the needed help. Examples of agencies found in most communities are health departments, community mental health centers, voluntary organizations such as the American Red Cross, missions, shelters, soup kitchens, food banks, nurse-managed or free clinics, social service agencies such as the Salvation Army or Travelers' Aid, and church-sponsored health and social services.
- *Develop your own support network.* Working with vulnerable populations can be challenging, rewarding, and at times exhausting. Nurses need to find sources of support and strength. This can come from friends, colleagues, hobbies, exercise, poetry, music, and other sources.

In addition to the nursing actions described, the "How To" box summarizes goals and interventions and evaluates outcomes with vulnerable populations.

In general, more agencies are needed that provide comprehensive services with nonrestrictive eligibility requirements. Communities often have many agencies that restrict eligibility to make it possible for more people to receive services. For example, shelters may prohibit people who have been drinking alcohol from staying overnight and sometimes limit the number of sequential nights a person can stay. Food banks usually limit the number of times a person can receive free food. Agencies are often very specialized as well. For vulnerable individuals and families, this means that they must go to several agencies to obtain services for which they qualify and that meet their health needs. This is tiring and discouraging, and people may forgo help because of these difficulties.

Nurses need to know about community agencies that offer various health and social services (see the "How To" box on p. 397). It is important also to follow up with the client after a referral to ensure that the desired outcomes were achieved. Sometimes, excellent community resources may be available but impractical because of transportation or reimbursement issues. Nurses can identify these potential problems by following through with referrals, and they can also work with other team members to make referrals as convenient and realistic as possible. Although clients with social problems such as financial needs should be referred to social workers, it is useful for nurses to understand the close connections between health and social problems and know how to work effectively with other professionals. A list of community resources can often be found in the telephone directory, and many communities publish these lists. The following are examples of agency resources found in most communities:

HOW TO Coordinate Health and Social Services for Members of Vulnerable Populations

Nurses who work with vulnerable populations often need to coordinate services across multiple agencies for members of these groups. It is helpful to have a strong professional network of people who work in other agencies. Effective professional networks make it easier to coordinate care smoothly and in ways that do not add to clients' stress. Nurses can develop strong networks by participating in community coalitions and attending professional meetings. When making referrals to other agencies, a phone call can be a helpful way to obtain information that the client will need for the visit. When possible, having an interdisciplinary, interagency team plan care for clients at high risk for health problems can be quite effective. It is crucial to obtain the clients' written and informed consent before engaging in this kind of planning because of confidentiality issues. The following list of tips can be helpful:

- Be sure to involve clients in making decisions about the kinds of services they will find beneficial and can use.
- Work with community coalitions to develop plans for service coordination for targeted vulnerable populations.
- Collaborate with legal counsel from the agencies involved in the coalitions to ensure that legal and ethical issues related to care coordination have been properly addressed. Examples of issues to address include privacy and security of clinical data and ensuring compliance with the Health Insurance Portability and Accountability Act (HIPAA), contractual provisions for coordinating care across agencies, and consent to treatment from multiple agencies.
- Develop policies and protocols for making referrals, following up on referrals, and ensuring that clients receiving care from multiple agencies experience the process as smooth and seamless.

HOW TO Use Case Management in Working with Vulnerable Populations

- Know available services and resources.
- Find out what is missing; look for creative solutions.
- Use your clinical skills.
- Develop long-term relationships with the families you serve.
- Strengthen the family's coping and survival skills and resourcefulness.
- Be the roadmap that guides the family to services, and help them get the services.
- Communicate with the family and the agencies who can help them.
- Work to change the environment and the policies that affect your clients.

- Health departments
- Community mental health centers
- American Red Cross and other voluntary organizations
- Food and clothing banks
- Missions and shelters
- Nurse-managed neighborhood clinics

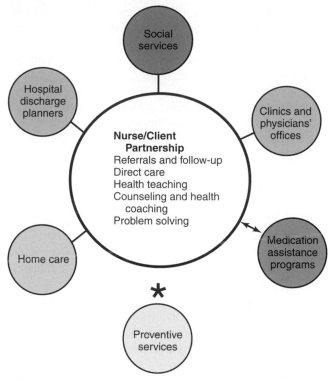

FIGURE 21-1 The nurse as case manager for vulnerable populations.

- Social service agencies such as Traveler's Aid and the Salvation Army
- Church-sponsored health and service assistance

Two other important categories of resources for vulnerable people are their own personal coping skills and social supports (Aday, 2001). These groups are often resourceful and creative in managing multiple stressors. Nurses can work with clients to help them identify their own strengths and draw on those strengths when managing their health needs. Also, clients may be able to depend on informal support networks. Even though social isolation is a problem for many vulnerable clients, nurses should not assume that they have no one who can or will help them. Case management involves linking clients with services and providing direct nursing services to them including teaching, counseling, screening, and immunizing. Lillian Wald was the first case manager. She linked vulnerable families with various services to help them stay healthy (Buhler-Wilkerson, 1993). Nurses are often the link between personal health services and population-based health care. Linking, or brokering, health services is accomplished by making appropriate referrals and by following up with clients to ensure that the desired outcomes from the referral were achieved. Nurses are effective case managers in community nursing clinics, health departments, hospitals, and various other health care agencies. Nurse case managers emphasize health promotion and illness prevention with vulnerable clients and focus on helping them avoid unnecessary hospitalization. Figure 21-1 illustrates the coordination and brokering aspect of the nurse's role as case manager for vulnerable populations.

As can be seen, many of these nursing actions are in the realm of case management in which the nurse makes referrals and links clients with other community services. In the case manager role, the nurse often is an advocate for the client or family. The nurse serves as an advocate when referring clients to other agencies, when working with others to develop health programs, and when trying to influence legislation and health policies that affect vulnerable population groups.

CLINICAL APPLICATION

Ms. Green, a 46-year-old farm worker pregnant with her fifth child, has come to the clinic requesting treatment for swollen ankles. During your assessment, you learned that she had seen the nurse practitioner (NP) at the local health department 2 months ago. The NP gave her some sample vitamins, but Ms. Green lost them. She has not received regular prenatal care and has no plans to do so. Her previous pregnancies were essentially normal, although she said she was "toxic" with her last child. She also said that her middle child was "not quite right." He is in the seventh grade at age 15. Ms. Green is 5 feet 2 inches tall, weighs 180 pounds, and has a blood pressure of 160/90. She has pitting edema of the ankles and a mild headache.

Ms. Green says that she usually takes chlorpromazine hydrochloride (Thorazine) but has run out of it and cannot afford to have her prescription refilled. She says that she has been in several mental hospitals in the past and that she has been more agitated and now has problems managing her daily activities. As her agitation grows, she says that she usually hears voices and this really makes her aggressive.

None of her children lives with her, and she has no plans for taking care of the infant. She thinks she will ask the child's father, a race track worker, to help her, since she usually travels around the country with him.

A. *What additional information do you need to help you adequately assess Ms. Green's health status and current needs?*

B. *What nursing activities are suggested by her history, physical, and psychological descriptions?*

Answers are in the back of the book.

REMEMBER THIS!

- All countries have population subgroups who are more vulnerable to health threats than the general population.
- Vulnerable populations are more likely to develop health problems as a result of exposure to risk or to have worse outcomes from those health problems than the population as a whole.
- Vulnerable populations are more sensitive to risk factors than those who are more resilient, since they are often exposed to cumulative risk factors. These populations include poor or homeless persons, pregnant adolescents, migrant workers, severely mentally ill individuals, substance abusers, abused individuals, people with communicable diseases, and people with sexually transmitted diseases.

- Factors leading to the growing number of poor people in the United States include reduced earnings, decreased availability of low-cost housing, more households headed by women, inadequate education, lack of marketable skills, welfare reform, and reduced Social Security payments to children.

- Poverty has a direct effect on health and well-being across the life span. Poor people have higher rates of chronic illness and infant morbidity and mortality, shorter life expectancy, and more complex health problems.

- Child poverty rates are twice as high as those for adults. Children who live in single-parent homes are twice as likely to be poor than those who live with both parents.

- The complex health problems of homeless people include the inability to obtain adequate rest, sleep, exercise, nutrition, and medication; exposure; infectious diseases; acute and chronic illness; infestations; and trauma and mental health problems.

- Health care is increasingly moving into the community. This began with deinstitutionalization of the severely mentally ill population and is continuing today as hospitals reduce inpatient stays. Vulnerable populations need a wide variety of services, and because these are often provided by multiple community agencies, nurses coordinate and manage the service needs of vulnerable groups.

- Socioeconomic problems, including poverty and social isolation, physiological and developmental aspects of age, poor health status, and highly stressful life experiences, predispose people to vulnerability. Vulnerability can become a cycle, with the predisposing factors leading to poor health outcomes, chronic stress, and hopelessness. These outcomes increase vulnerability.

- Nurses assess vulnerable individuals, families, and groups to determine which socioeconomic, physical, biological, psychological, and environmental factors are problematic for clients. They work as partners with vulnerable clients to identify client strengths and needs and develop intervention strategies designed to break the cycle of vulnerability.

WHAT WOULD YOU DO?

1. Examine health statistics and demographic data in your geographic area to determine which vulnerable groups are predominant. Look through your phone book or on the web for examples of agencies that you think provide services to these vulnerable groups. If the agency has a web page, read about the target populations they serve, the types of services they provide, and how they are reimbursed for services. Learn about different agencies and share results during class. Based on your findings, identify gaps or overlaps in services provided to vulnerable groups in your community. How could you deal with these gaps and overlaps to help clients receive needed services?

2. Identify nurses in your community who work with vulnerable groups. Invite these nurses to come to class and talk about their experiences. What is their typical day? What are the rewards? What are the challenges? How do they deal with frustration, competing demands, and stress?

3. Discuss welfare reform with your classmates. How does the U.S. welfare system work? Who gets welfare? What should be done to improve the system? Is your state a leader in welfare reform?

4. Suppose you are making a home visit to a person whose home is not clean. Food is everywhere, and roaches are crawling around the house. What do you do if the person asks you to sit down? What if you are offered food?

■ *REFERENCES*

Aday LA: *At risk in America: the health and health care needs of vulnerable populations in the United States*, San Francisco, 2001, Jossey Bass.

Aiken LH, Salmon ME: Health care workforce priorities: what nursing should do now, *Inquiry* 31(3):318–329, 1994.

American Association of Retired Persons (AARP): *What is Medicare drug coverage?* Retrieved Sept 23, 2008, from www.aarp.org/health/medicare/drug_coverage/what_is_medicare_drug_coverage.htm.

Appel SJ, Harrell JS, Deng S: Racial and socioeconomic differences in risk factors for cardiovascular disease among southern rural women, *Nurs Res* 51(3):140–147, 2002.

Buhler-Wilkerson K: Bringing care to the people: Lillian Wald's legacy to public health nursing, *Am J Publ Health* 83(12):1778–1786, 1993.

Centers for Disease Control and Prevention: *Infant mortality rates,* 2008. Retrieved Oct 4, 2008, from www.cdc/gov.infant mortality.

Centers for Disease Control and Prevention: *U.S. Mortality drops sharply in 2006 latest data show*. Retrieved June 11, 2008, from Cdc.gov.nchs/pressroom/08/newsreleases/mortality2006/htm.

Centers for Medicare and Medicaid Services: *Low cost health insurance for families and children, 2008*. Retrieved Sept 23, 2008, from www.cms.hhs.gov/LowCostHealthInsFamChild.

Flaskerud JH et al: Health disparities among vulnerable populations: evolution of knowledge over five decades in nursing research publications, *Nurs Res* 51(2):74–85, 2002.

Hargraves JL: *The insurance gap and minority health care, 1997-2001,* Center for Studying Health System Change Tracking Report 2:1–4, 2002.

Linhorst DM: Federalism and social justice: implications for social work, *Soc Work* 47(3):201–208, 2002.

MacDorman MF, Mathews TJ: *Recent trends in infant mortality in the U.S.,* NCHS Data Brief #9, Hyattsville Md, October 2008, National Center for Health Statistics.

Middlebrooks JS, Audage NC: *The effects of childhood stress on health across the lifespan,* Atlanta, 2008, Centers for Disease Control and Prevention, National Center for Injury Prevention and Control.

U.S. Census Bureau: *Poverty: 2007 highlights*. Retrieved Sept 23, 2008, www.census/gov/hhes/wwwpoverty/poverty06/pov07hi/html.

U.S. Department of Health and Human Services: *Healthy People 2010: understanding and improving health,* Washington, DC, 2001a, U.S. Government Printing Office.

U.S. Department of Health and Human Services: *Healthy People in Healthy Communities: a community planning guide using Healthy People 2010,* Washington, DC, 2001b, U.S. Government Printing Office.

Woodward A, Kawachi I: Why reduce health inequalities? *J Epidemiol Community Health* 54:923–929, 2000.

Rural Health and Migrant Health

Angeline Bushy
Marie Napolitano

ADDITIONAL RESOURCES

These related resources are found either in the appendix at the back of this book or on the book's website at http://evolve.elsevier.com/stanhope/foundations.

e Evolve Website

- Community Assessment Applied
- Case Study, with questions and answers
- Quiz review questions
- WebLinks, including link to *Healthy People 2010* website

Real World Community Health Nursing: An Interactive CD-ROM, second edition

If you are using this CD-ROM in your course, you will find the following activity related to this chapter:
- *Vulnerability: You're in Charge* in **Vulnerability**

OBJECTIVES

After reading this chapter, the student should be able to:
1. Compare and contrast definitions for rural and urban.
2. Describe the health status of rural and urban populations on selected health measures.
3. Discuss access to service issues of rural underserved populations.

4. Define "migrant farm worker" and discuss common health problems of this group and their families and barriers they experience when seeking health care.
5. Explain the nursing role for serving persons in rural and urban areas, including migrant farmworkers.

CHAPTER OUTLINE

DIFFERENCES IN RURAL VERSUS URBAN

POPULATION CHARACTERISTICS AND CULTURAL CONSIDERATIONS

HEALTH STATUS OF RURAL RESIDENTS
Women's Health Including Maternal and Infant Health
Health of Children
Mental Health
Health of Minorities, in Particular, Migrant Farmworkers
CULTURAL CONSIDERATIONS IN MIGRANT HEALTH CARE
Nurse–Client Relationship

Health Values
Health Beliefs and Practices
OCCUPATIONAL AND ENVIRONMENTAL HEALTH PROBLEMS IN RURAL AREAS
Pesticide Exposure
RURAL HEALTH CARE DELIVERY ISSUES AND BARRIERS TO CARE
NURSING CARE IN RURAL ENVIRONMENTS
HEALTHY PEOPLE 2010 NATIONAL HEALTH OBJECTIVES RELATED TO RURAL HEALTH

KEY TERMS

central: counties in large (1 million or more population) metro areas that contain all or part of the largest central city.

farm residency: residency outside the area zoned as "city limits"; usually infers involvement in agriculture.

fringe: remaining counties in large (1 million or more population) metro areas.

frontier: regions having fewer than six persons per square mile.

Health Professional Shortage Areas (HPSAs): geographic areas that have insufficient numbers of health professionals according to criteria established by the federal government. It often consists of rural areas in which a physician, nurse practitioner, or nurse in community health provides services to residents who live in several counties.

medium: counties in metropolitan areas with less than 250,000 people.

migrant farmworker: a person whose primary employment is in agriculture on a seasonal basis, who has been employed in that work within the past 2 years, and who has a temporary abode.

Migrant Health Act: legislation passed in the United States in 1962 that provides support for clinics serving agricultural workers. Grants were given to community-based and state organizations in the United States and its territories to enable them to provide culturally sensitive, comprehensive medical services to migrant and seasonal farmworkers and their families. In 2002, 670,000 people received services from the funds from the Migrant Health Act.

nonfarm residency: residence within an area zoned as "city limits."

pesticide exposure: health risk to farmworkers who work in fields that have been treated with pesticides. Residue from pesticides also enters farmworkers' homes and their food. Risks include mild psychological and behavioral deficits and acute severe poisoning that can result in death.

rural: communities having fewer than 20,000 residents or fewer than 99 persons per square mile.

rural–urban continuum: residence ranging from living on a remote farm, to a village or small town, to a larger town or city, to a large metropolitan area with a "core inner city."

small: counties in metro areas with fewer than 1 million people.

suburbs: areas adjacent to a highly populated city.

urban: geographic areas described as nonrural and having a higher population density, more than 99 persons per square mile; cities with a population of at least 20,000, but fewer than 50,000.

Access to health care is a national priority that remains unsolved. Access is a problem in rural areas, including farms that rely on migrant workers to harvest their crops, and in urban inner cities. This chapter discusses major issues surrounding health care delivery in rural environments. These issues may differ from those experienced by people living in **urban** or more populated areas. One particular environment, that of the migrant worker, is discussed in detail because of the growing number of migrant workers and their often unique health needs.

Formal rural nursing began with the Red Cross Rural Nursing Service, which was organized in November 1912 (Bigbee and Crowder, 1985). Before that time, care of the sick in a small community was provided by informal social support systems. When self-care and family care were not effective in bringing about healing, healing women who had skills in helping others heal and who lived in the community provided care. Over time, rural people have had many health needs. Although these needs are not all unique, they are different from those of urban populations. Scarcity of health professionals, poverty, limited access to services, lack of knowledge, and social isolation have plagued many rural communities for generations. For migrant workers, a language barrier and cultural differences often exist between them and the farm owners and other area residents.

DIFFERENCES IN RURAL VERSUS URBAN

Each of us has an idea as to what constitutes a rural as opposed to an urban residence. However, the distinctions are becoming blurred as people move further away from cities and towns into less-developed areas. **Rural** is defined generally either in terms of the geographic location and population density or the distance from (e.g., 20 miles) or the time needed (e.g., 30 minutes) to commute to an urban center. Other definitions link rural with **farm residency** and urban with **nonfarm residency**. Some consider *rural* to be a state of mind. For the more affluent, rural may bring to mind a recreational, retirement, or resort community located in the mountains or in lake country where people can relax and participate in outdoor activities, such as skiing, fishing, hiking, or hunting. For people with limited resources, rural may imply poor and/or crowded housing with lack of adequate facilities for water and sewage.

Just as each city has its own unique features, there is no "typical rural town." For example, rural towns in Florida, Oregon, Alaska, Hawaii, and Idaho are different from one another and quite different from those in Vermont, Texas, Tennessee, Alabama, and California. Descriptions and definitions for *rural* areas are more subjective and relative in nature than for *urban* areas.

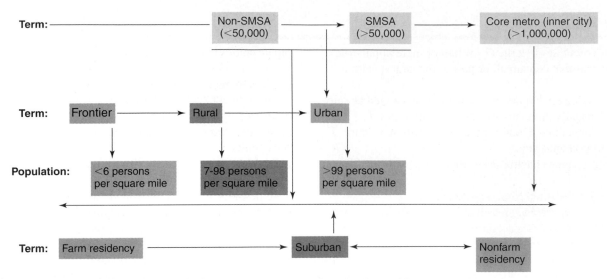

FIGURE 22-1 The continuum of rural–urban residency.

For example, "small" communities with populations of more than 20,000 have some features that are found in cities. A person who lives in a community with fewer than 2000 people may consider a community with a population of 5000 to 10,000 to be a city. Although some communities may seem geographically remote on a map, the people who live there may not feel isolated. They may think they are within easy reach of services through telecommunication and dependable transportation, although extensive shopping facilities may be 50 to 100 miles from the family home, obstetric care may be 150 miles away, and nursing services in the district health department in an adjacent county may be 75 or more miles away.

Frequently used definitions to describe rural and urban and to differentiate between them are provided by several federal agencies (U.S. Bureau of the Census, 2001; U.S. Department of Agriculture, 2001-2002). These definitions often fail to take into account the relative nature of ruralness. Rural and urban residencies are not opposing lifestyles. Rather, they are on a **rural–urban continuum** ranging from living on a remote farm, to a village or small town, to a larger town or city, to a large metropolitan area with a core inner city (Figure 22-1).

The *2006 NCHS Urban-Rural Classification Schemes for Counties,* a publication of the National Center for Health Statistics, classifies counties into six levels of urbanization, from the most urban to the most rural (Ingram and Franco, 2006). Four subclassifications are listed for metropolitan (metro) counties and two subclassifications are listed for nonmetropolitan (nonmetro) counties. Metropolitan subclassifications involve the following:

1. **Central**: counties in large (1 million or more population) metro areas that contain all or part of the largest central city
2. **Fringe**: the remaining counties in large (1 million or more population) metro areas
3. **Medium**: counties in metro areas with less than 1 million population

4. **Small**: counties in metro areas with less than 250,000 residents

Nonmetropolitan subclassifications include *micropolitan* and *noncore.* These nonmetropolitan counties are subdivided based on the size of their population and their adjacency to metropolitan or micropolitan areas (U.S. Bureau of the Census, 2004). The population has shifted significantly from urban to less-populated regions of the United States. The fastest-growing rural counties are located in rural areas and along the edges of larger metropolitan counties. This so-called "doughnut effect" refers to people moving away from highly populated areas to **suburbs** of urban centers. Most of the population growth has been in counties with a booming economy, with room to grow, and in western and southern states. People often move to more rural areas in order to purchase affordable homes. Of the 10 fastest-growing counties with 10,000 persons or more, three were located in western states, six in southern states, and one in a midwestern state (U.S. Bureau of the Census, 2004). Although data are collected differently, accounting for some differences, in general, about 25% of all U.S. residents live in rural settings. In this chapter, rural refers to areas having fewer than 99 persons per square mile and communities having 20,000 or fewer inhabitants.

POPULATION CHARACTERISTICS AND CULTURAL CONSIDERATIONS

Although regional variations exist, in general there is a higher proportion of whites in rural areas (about 82%) than in core metropolitan areas (about 62%). Of the total rural population in the United States, nearly 5 million are African-American, almost 4 million are Hispanic, 1 million are Native American, and half a million are Asian-Pacific Islanders. Lifestyle, health status, and health needs vary greatly among rural populations (Probst et al, 2002). The *U.S. Census 2000* data reveal that rural communities are demographically bipolar. In respect to age distribution, there are higher-than-average numbers of younger (ages 6–17 years) and older residents (older than 65 years) in rural settings. Persons 18 years of age and older living in rural areas are more likely to be or to have been married than are adults in the three urban categories. As a group, rural people also are more likely to be widowed. Adults in rural areas tend to have fewer years of formal schooling than urban adults have (U.S. Bureau of the Census, 2001).

Although there are regional variations, rural families tend to be poorer than their urban counterparts. Comparing annual incomes with the standardized index established by the U.S. Bureau of the Census, more than 25% of rural Americans live at or near the poverty level and nearly 40% of all rural children are impoverished (Centers for Disease Control and Prevention, 2001). Compared with those in metropolitan settings, a substantially smaller percentage of families living in nonmetropolitan areas are at the high end of the income scale. They are also more likely to have public rather than private health insurance or to be uninsured.

The working poor in rural areas are particularly at risk for being underinsured or uninsured. In working poor families, one or more of the adults are employed but still cannot afford private health insurance. Furthermore, their annual income is such that it disqualifies the family from obtaining public insurance. Several reasons help explain this (Gamm and Hutchinson, 2004):

- Individuals are self-employed in a family business, such as ranching or farming, or they work in small enterprises, such as a service station, restaurant, or grocery store, that do not provide group health insurance.
- A person may be employed in part-time or in seasonal occupations, such as farm laborer and construction, and health insurance is often not an employee benefit.
- A family member may have a preexisting health condition that makes the cost of insurance prohibitive, if it is even available to them.
- A few rural families fall through the cracks and cannot get any type of public assistance because of other deterrents, such as language barriers, being physically compromised, the geographic location of an agency, lack of transportation, or having undocumented-worker status. Insurance, or the lack of it, has serious implications for the overall health status of rural residents and for the nurses who provide services to them.

HEALTH STATUS OF RURAL RESIDENTS

Despite the significant number of people who live in rural areas, their health problems and health behaviors are not fully understood. This section summarizes what is known about the overall health status of rural adults and children. The health status measures that are addressed are perceived health status, diagnosed chronic conditions, physical limitations, frequency of seeking medical treatment, usual source of care, maternal and infant health, children's health, mental health, minorities' health, and environmental and occupational health risks (Centers for Disease Control and Prevention, 2001).

BRIEFLY NOTED

Compared with urban Americans, rural residents have:
- Higher infant and maternal morbidity rates
- Higher rates of chronic illness, including heart disease, chronic obstructive pulmonary disease, unintentional motor vehicle traffic-related injuries, suicide, hypertension, cancer, and diabetes
- Unique health risks associated with occupations and the environment, such as machinery accidents, skin cancer from sun exposure, and respiratory problems associated with exposure to chemicals and pesticides
- Stress-related health problems and mental illness (although the incidence is not known)

In general, people in rural areas have a poorer perception of their overall health and functional status than their urban counterparts. Rural residents older than 18 years assess their health status less favorably than do urban residents. Studies show that rural adults are less likely to engage in preventive behavior, which increases their exposure to risk. Specifically, they are more likely to smoke and report higher rates of alcohol use and obesity. They are less likely to engage in physical activity during leisure time, wear seatbelts, have regular blood pressure checks, have Papanicolaou (Pap) smears, and do breast self-examinations. These behaviors then influence their overall health (Centers for Disease Control and Prevention, 2001).

Compared with their urban counterparts, rural adults are more likely to have one or more of the following chronic conditions: heart disease, chronic obstructive pulmonary disease, hypertension, arthritis and rheumatism, diabetes, cardiovascular disease, and cancer. Nearly 50% of all rural adults have been diagnosed with at least one of these chronic conditions, compared with about 25% of nonrural adults. Also, the rate of acquired immunodeficiency syndrome (AIDS) is increasing in rural areas (Centers for Disease Control and Prevention, 2001).

The percentage of rural adults who receive medical treatment for both life-threatening illness and degenerative or chronic conditions is higher than that of urban adults. Life-threatening conditions include malignant neoplasms, heart disease, cardiovascular problems, and liver disorders. Degenerative or chronic diseases include diabetes, kidney disease, arthritis and rheumatism, and chronic diseases of the circulatory, nervous, respiratory, and digestive systems. In essence, chronic health conditions, coupled with their poor health status, limit the physical activities of a larger proportion of rural residents than of their urban counterparts (Gamm and Hutchinson, 2004).

Rural adults tend to have an overall poorer health status and are less likely to seek medical care than urban adults. Not only are they less likely to see medical care, but also there are simply fewer physicians from whom care can be sought. Ten percent of the U.S. physicians work in rural areas, whereas 25% of the population lives there. In addition, rural people are less likely to have employer-sponsored health insurance or prescription drug coverage. People living in rural areas have a greater risk than do their urban counterparts in being involved in an accident. Specifically, one third of motor vehicle accidents and two thirds of all deaths due to motor vehicle accidents occur on rural roads. Likewise, rural people are twice as likely to die of unintentional injuries, and they have a significantly higher risk for gunshot deaths (National Rural Health Association, 2009). Nurses can teach them how to prevent accidents, engage in safer and more healthful lifestyle behaviors, and reduce the risk of chronic health problems, and they can help them more effectively manage existing chronic conditions.

BRIEFLY NOTED

- Americans who live in the suburbs are significantly better by many key health measures than those who live in the most rural and most urban areas of the nation.
- Death rates for working-aged adults are higher in the most rural and the most highly populated urban areas. The highest death rates for children and young adults occur in the most rural counties.
- Residents of rural areas have the highest death rates due to unintentional injuries in general and motor vehicle injuries in particular.
- Homicide rates are highest in the central counties of large metropolitan areas. Suicide rates are highest in the most rural areas.
- Suburban residents are more likely to exercise during leisure time and more likely to have health insurance. Suburban women are the least likely to be obese.
- Both the most rural and the most urban areas have a high percentage of residents without health insurance. Residents in the most rural communities have the fewest dental visits.
- Teenagers and adults in rural counties are more likely to smoke.
- The AIDS rates are increasing more quickly in rural areas (30%) than in metropolitan areas (25.8%). Rural communities have the highest rates of increase in AIDS cases, representing 6.7% of all cases in the United States, with heterosexual contact accounting for most cases in many areas.
- In rural areas, gay men often are not openly gay and tend to engage in unprotected sex with strangers. Homophobia, racism, sexism, and AIDS stigma make human immunodeficiency virus (HIV) prevention efforts nearly impossible in some rural areas. The migration of people from urban to rural areas is cited as one possible contributor to the increased rates in rural areas. Among HIV-infected persons, more interstate than intrastate migration takes place from the time of diagnosis until death (Centers for Disease Control and Prevention, 2001).

In general, a person who has a usual source of care is more likely to seek care when ill and is more likely to follow prescribed regimens. Rural adults are more likely than urban adults to identify a particular medical provider as their usual source of care. The providers most often seen by rural adults are general practitioners and advanced practice registered nurses (APRNs). In contrast, urban adults are more likely to seek care from a medical specialist. This trend may change as managed care expands and more plans require primary care providers to serve as gatekeepers (Health Resources

Evidence-Based Practice

The health issues facing rural communities are vast and are often complex. To meet the needs of rural populations, community agencies must collaborate with rural residents in the effort to impact research, policy, and service delivery if they are to enact any lasting change. As Moulton et al. (2007) note, one way to explore the needs of rural communities is to meet with them in informal settings in which they can make their needs and issues known. In this article, the Center for Rural Health at the University of North Dakota School of Medicine and Health Sciences conducted a series of meeting with organizations serving rural citizens to expand their understanding of barriers to the provision of health services in the rural setting. Through this effort, the Center has been able to establish on-going collaborations with rural agencies that continue to influence both communication and service.

In an effort to truly determine the health issues facing rural North Dakota, the Center organized 13 rural community meetings in 2003. Of the 13 communities asked to participate, five were Native American. As noted, the meetings were designed to "determine how the Center could assist community health care practitioners and organizational leaders in negotiating the many barriers present in rural health care" (Moulton et al, 2007, p. 93). As a result of this outreach, the authors have designed this particular article as a how-to of sorts for community health care outreach, laying out a very convenient road map for replication.

Nine themes were extracted from the 13 meeting transcripts. These themes reflect the most pressing threats to health care in North Dakota and the most significant issues faced by participating organizations related to health care and the role the Center might play in addressing those concerns. Of the selected themes, health care workforce recruitment and retention, adequate reimbursement, access, and prevention were cited as the most pressing barriers to health care in North Dakota's rural communities. Given the breadth of these themes, nine work groups were formed to address the issues pertaining to each theme and to make recommendations to the Center for improvement.

NURSE USE: Concerning lessons learned, the authors note that making the process as convenient as possible for participants, accurate information concerning agency involvement, respect for cultural differences, and a focused purpose were elements that others who might replicate such a structure should keep in mind. In summation, this effort proved that in order to meet the needs of rural communities, enlisting rural people and agencies is a must. Not only can collegiality and good will flourish, but pragmatic and efficient services depend on knowing the issues that truly confront rural people and their health care.

From Moulton et al: Identifying rural health care needs using community conversations, *J Rural Health* 23(1): 92–96, 2007.

Services Administration, 2003; Bureau of Health Professions, 2005a, b).

BRIEFLY NOTED

Nurses must be especially thorough in their health assessment of rural and migrant clients who may not receive regular care for chronic health conditions.

Traveling time and/or distance to ambulatory care services affect access to care for both rural and urban residents. For the rural people it may be the distance they must travel, and for the urban people it may be not so much the distance but the amount of traffic they encounter. Both groups tend to wait the same amount of time once they arrive at the clinic or physician's office.

Often rural health professionals live and practice in a particular community for decades, and they may provide care to people who live in several counties. One or two nurses in a county health department may offer a full range of services for all residents in a specified area, which may span more than 100 miles from one end of a county to the other. Consequently, rural physicians and nurses frequently report, "I provide care to individuals and families with all kinds of conditions, in all stages of life, and across several generations." It should not come as a surprise that rural respondents who participate in national surveys are able to identify a usual source and a usual provider of health care (Bushy, 2000, 2002a; Bushy and Bushy, 2001) (see "Evidence-Based Practice" box on p. 404).

WOMEN'S HEALTH INCLUDING MATERNAL AND INFANT HEALTH

Despite conflicting reports, it seems that overall rural populations have higher infant and maternal morbidity rates, especially counties designated as **Health Professional Shortage Areas (HPSAs)**. These areas tend to have a high proportion of racial minorities and fewer specialists, such as pediatricians, obstetricians, and gynecologists, are available to provide care to at-risk populations. There are extreme variations in pregnancy outcomes from one part of the country to another, and even within states. For example, in several counties located in the north-central and intermountain states, the pregnancy outcome is among the finest in the United States. However, in several other counties within those same states, the pregnancy outcome is among the worst. Particularly at risk are women who live on or near Indian reservations, women who are migrant workers, and women who are of African-American descent and live in rural counties of states located in the deep south (Bushy, 2002b; Probst et al, 2002; Gamm and Hutchinson, 2004).

Most nurses understand the effects of socioeconomic factors, such as income level (poverty), education level, age, employment/unemployment patterns, and use of prenatal services, on pregnancy outcomes. There are other, less-known determinants, such as environmental hazards, occupational risks, and the cultural meaning placed on childbearing and childrearing practices by a community. The effects of these multifaceted factors vary.

HEALTH OF CHILDREN

A comparison of rural and urban children younger than 6 years of age with respect to access to providers and use of services shows the following (Jolk, 2003):
• Urban children are less likely to have a usual provider but are more likely to see a pediatrician when they are ill.
• Both rural adults and children are more likely to have a general practitioner as their regular caregiver.

School nurses play an important role in the overall health status of children in the United States. The availability of school nurses in rural communities varies from region to region. They tend to be scarce in **frontier** and rural areas of the United States due to (1) a shortage of health care professionals in the area and (2) fewer tax payers, thus less income to support school nurses.

However, some creative approaches have enabled counties to provide better health care and school nursing services. For example, two or more counties may enter into a partnership in which they share the cost of a "district" health nurse. Other counties have forged partnerships with an agency in an urban setting and contracted for specific health care services. In both of these situations, it is not unusual for the nurse to provide services to all children attending schools in the participating counties. In some frontier states, schools may be more than 100 miles apart and as many miles or more from the district health office. Because of the number of schools and distances between them, the county nurse may be able to visit each school only once, maybe twice, in a school term. Usually the nurse's visit is to update immunizations and perhaps to teach maturation classes to students in the upper grades.

MENTAL HEALTH

Stress, stress-related conditions, and mental illness are prevalent among populations that have economic difficulties. When the economy in an area is depressed due to slowdowns in mining or lumbering, manufacturing, plant reductions or closings, adverse weather that affects crops, job losses follow. Economic recession contributes to a family's not having insurance or being underinsured or to their losing their home due to mortgage foreclosure. Often, even if mental health services are available and accessible, rural residents delay seeking care when they have an emotional problem until an emergency or a crisis arises. There appears to be a more persistent, endemic level of depression among rural residents. This prevalence may be related to the high rate of poverty, geographic isolation, and an insufficient number of mental health services. Depression may also contribute to the escalating incidence of accidents and suicides, especially among rural male adolescents and young men. The incidence has increased dramatically over the past decade and continues to rise in this group, to the point of being epidemic in some small communities (Beeson, 2003).

Like many of the indicators in the previous sections, reports on the incidence of domestic violence and alcohol

work, 8 weeks traveling, and 10 weeks unemployed, often returning to their country of origin, usually Mexico, during this period of time (Guasasco, Heuer, and Lausch, 2002).

BRIEFLY NOTED

Substandard wages paid to migrant farmworkers allow Americans to pay less for their fruits and vegetables. Also many migrant farmworkers often send part of their salaries to family members who live in their country of origin.

Housing

When migrant workers reach a worksite, housing may not be available, it may be too expensive, or it may be in poor condition. Housing conditions vary among states and localities. Housing for migrant farmworkers may be in camps with cabins, trailers, or houses. Some even live in cars or tents if necessary. National data about the type and quality of housing occupied by farmworkers are limited; however, data do indicate that the housing is generally crowded by federal standards (Culp and Umbarger, 2004). When housing costs are high as many as 50 men may live in one house. In some cases three or more families may share one house or mobile home. Much of the housing is substandard and lacks adequate sanitation and working appliances or may have severe structural defects (National Center for Farmworker Health, Inc., 2005a). Many also support a home and family in their country of origin.

Housing may be located next to fields that have been sprayed by pesticides or where farm machinery is a danger to children. Poor quality and crowded places of residence can contribute to health problems such as tuberculosis (TB), gastroenteritis, and hepatitis and to exposure to high levels of lead. Renting housing in rural areas is nearly impossible because of barriers such as high rent, substantial rental deposits, long-term leases, lack of credit, discrimination, and a lack of rental units. Federal programs provide some funds for farmworker housing, but they are insufficient to meet the demand. Increased funding and better coordination among agencies are needed as is an increase in the availability of safe public housing.

Issues in Migrant Health

Poor and unsanitary working and housing conditions make farmworkers susceptible to health problems no longer seen as dangers to the general public or seen at a much lower rate (such as tuberculosis, pesticide poisoning) or a high infant mortality rate (National Center for Farmworker Health, Inc., 2005d). In general, migrant workers have identified diabetes, poor dental health, obesity, and depression as major health problems (Cason, Snyder, and Jensen, 2004). Also, despite the fact that the **Migrant Health Act** provides primary and supplemental health services to migrant workers and their families and that migrant health centers serve more than 600,000 individuals at more than 360 sites across the country, these clinics serve fewer than 20% of

this population (National Center for Farmworker Health, Inc., 2005a). These workers and their families tend to use hospital emergency rooms and private physicians more often than migrant health clinics (Napolitano, 2008). The factors that interfere with their ability to seek care are finances, culture, transportation, mobility, language, inability to get off work, and fear of immigration (Perilla et al, 1998). Specifically, the following factors limit adequate provision of health care services:

- *Lack of knowledge about services.* Because of their isolation and lack of fluency in English, migrant farmworkers lack usual sources for information about available services, especially if they are not receiving public benefits.

- *Inability to afford care.* The Medicaid program, which is intended to serve the poor, is often not available to migrant farmworkers, especially undocumented workers. Workers may not remain in a geographic area long enough to be considered for benefits or may lose benefits when they relocate to a state with different eligibility standards. Their salaries may fluctuate monthly, making them ineligible for periods of time. If they do not work, they are not paid, so many avoid taking time off to get care.

- *Availability of services.* The Welfare Reform legislation of 1996 changed the availability of federal services accessible to certain immigrants to this country (Mines, Gabbard, and Steinman, 1997). Immigrants are treated differently depending on whether they were in the United States before August 22, 1996, and the category of immigrant to which they are designated. As a result of this legislation, each state determined whether it would fill any or part of the services gap to immigrants. Many legal immigrants and undocumented immigrants are ineligible for services such as Supplemental Security Income (SSI) and food stamps.

- *Transportation.* Health care services may be located far from work or home. Transportation can be unavailable, unreliable, or expensive. Many migrant farmworkers do not have access to vehicles. Privacy is compromised when migrant workers depend on employers to provide transportation to clinics (Napolitano, 2008).

- *Hours of services.* Many health services are available only during work hours; therefore seeking health care leads to lost earnings.

- *Mobility and tracking.* While migrant families move from job to job, their health care records typically do not go with them. This leads to fragmented services in areas such as treatment for TB, chronic illness management, and immunizations. For example, health departments are known to dispense medications for TB on a monthly basis. Adequate treatment for TB requires 6 to 12 months of medication. When migrant farmworkers move, they must independently seek out new health services to continue their medications. Also, people with TB may forfeit treatment because they are afraid of immigration authorities (National Center for Farmworker Health, Inc., 2005e).

Evidence-Based Practice

In their study of the health care status and patterns of children in U.S. immigrant families, Huang, Yu, and Ledsky (2006) found that parent's citizenship can play a significant role in the health care of children. The authors note that children of immigrant families are the fastest growing and most diverse cross section of the U.S. child population, and despite their overall low morbidity and mortality rates, they were significantly less likely to have visited a health care provider in the past year. Using a representative national survey (National Survey of America's Families), the authors note that immigrant families are more likely to live in poverty, have less access to healthcare, and are less likely to be insured.

As noted, one of the greatest obstacles to appropriate health care for immigrant families and their children is the limited access to public health programs and services as a result of their citizen status. Even for those children who are eligible, the authors suggest that many immigrant families do not participate for fear that this will lead to trouble with authorities, impacting their ability to return or remain in the country. Additional limitations include a lack of understanding concerning health care resources and language barriers. Taken together, these factors distance immigrant families from the health care system.

The authors note that recent reforms in welfare and immigration have become increasingly restrictive, and in some instances have made services for even legal immigrants cumbersome and bureaucratic. In effect, this narrowing of services signals to many immigrant families that they should avoid these public services altogether. Paired with decreases in work-related insurance, these restrictions create a large population of families without access to or knowledge of appropriate health services.

NURSE USE: Informing and encouraging eligible immigrant families to enroll their children in available programs and services is the first step in connecting them to the health care system. However, these programs must be culturally and linguistically competent if they are to attract and support immigrant families and their children. Lastly, greater advocacy on behalf of immigrant families will be a must if the current tide of restrictive policies and legislation is to be stemmed.

From Huang ZJ, Yu SM, Ledsky R: Health status and health service access and use among children in U.S. immigrant families, *Am J Pub Health* 96(4):634–640, 2006.

- *Discrimination.* Although migrant farmworkers and their families bring revenue into the community, they are often perceived as poor, uneducated, transient, and ethnically different. These perceptions foster acts of discrimination against them.
- *Documentation.* Many farmworkers and their families are legal residents of the United States. However, some workers are undocumented and not in compliance with Immigration and Naturalization Service regulations. Some illegal workers fear that securing services in a federally funded or state-funded clinic may lead to discovery and deportation. Consequently, the person may use various names when accessing health care services. This then makes it difficult to maintain accurate health records or track usage of services.
- *Language.* Because the majority of seasonal farmworkers are primarily Spanish speakers, the recruitment and retention of bicultural/bilingual health care provider staff are important priorities.
- *Cultural aspects of health care.* See the section, "Cultural Considerations in Migrant Health Care."

Other Specific Health Problems

Dental disease ranks as one of the top five health problems for farmworkers ages 5 to 19 years. Farmworkers of all ages consistently have more dental disease than the general population. A California Agricultural Worker Health Survey reported high rates of untreated caries, missing or broken teeth, and gingivitis (National Center for Farmworker Health, Inc., 2005f). Inadequate knowledge of oral health and lack of access to care (and the resources to pay) were prevalent among those surveyed. Often because they lack insurance or money to pay the dental bill, farmworkers delay getting dental care until they have an oral emergency. This means that they do not get regular dental education or preventive care. Migrant health centers with dental care have a high rate of utilization (Lombardi, 2001).

The incidence of TB is estimated to be higher among migrant farmworkers than the general population. Seasonal farmwork has significant occupational threats to health since many farmworkers constantly stoop or climb, work with soil, and carry heavy loads. They also may have direct contact with plants and soil treated with chemical fertilizers and pesticides. Often their drinking and bathing water may be unsafe. The Occupational Safety and Health Administration (OSHA) requires that employers with 11 or more agricultural workers provide drinking water, hand washing facilities, and toilets. Compliance with OSHA regulations is poor, and OSHA can inspect only a small percentage of farms (National Center for Farmworker Health, Inc., 2005d). TB is more common among immigrants from countries with higher rates of the disease (National Center for Farmworker Health, 2005e) including migrants from Mexico, Haiti, and Southeast Asia. Frequently, the disease is resistant to commonly used antituberculosis drugs. Restricted mobility and lack of resources for the migrant population make it difficult to screen, treat, and monitor individuals and families. Also, the transient nature of migrant work and the prolonged treatment of TB make it difficult to ensure patient compliance with screening and treatment (National Center for Farmworker Health, Inc., 2005e, 2005g).

Studies have found higher rates of seropositive HIV among certain migrant groups compared with persons born in the United States, including women farmworkers who have been infected from heterosexual contact with men who use drugs or men who have sex with other men (National Center for Farmworker Health, Inc., n.d.). Migrant farmworkers are at high risk for HIV due to lack of education, low use of condoms, and social isolation, which can lead to drug abuse and multiple sexual contacts.

Like other people in rural areas, migrant farmworkers experience high levels of depression that are associated with the stress of adjusting to a new culture, low self-esteem, and discrimination. They may also be at risk for developing anxiety-related disorders (Hovey and Magana, 2002). A study of migrant children in North Carolina (Kupersmidt and Martin, 1997) found elevated levels of mental health problems. These included phobias, different types of anxiety, avoidance, and depression.

Migrant women are at risk for significant anxiety caused by their duties and responsibilities. In addition to working all day under the same conditions as the men, the women then return home to cook, clean, and take care of the children (Hovey and Magana, 2002). Unfortunately, an unknown number of these women experience domestic violence, which is a major health problem with significant physical, emotional, and psychological consequences. Because of lack of access to care and information, migrant women may not receive prenatal care early or at all (National Center for Farmworker Health, Inc., 2005a).

Children of Migrant Workers

Migrant farmworker parents want a better future for their children. In fact, this strong desire was the catalyst that caused many farmworkers to leave their country of origin. These children often appear to the outsider as happy, outgoing, and inquisitive. On the surface, they may look like children from any other aggregate. However, they often suffer from health care deficits including malnutrition (vitamin A, iron), infectious diseases (upper respiratory infection, gastroenteritis), dental caries (caused by prolonged use of the bottle, bottle propping, limited access to fluoride or dental care), inadequate immunization status, pesticide exposure, injuries, overcrowding and exposure to lead in poor housing conditions, and disruption of their social and school life (see the "Evidence-Based Practice" box on p. 409).

In many instances it is difficult to determine the exact age of children in migrant communities. Children as young as 12 years of age may need to work for the family's economic survival. The Fair Labor Standards Act states that the minimum age that a child can work in agriculture is 14 years; the age is 16 years in other industries. Children 12 to 13 years of age can work on a farm with the parents' consent or if the parent works on the same farm. Children younger than 12 years can work on a farm with fewer than seven full-time workers (Davis, 2001). Some additional protections are provided to children by the majority of states, such as limiting the number of hours they can work per day and week. These children have particularly difficult lives and lifestyles that are hard to break out of due to their mobility, which affects their ability to complete their education. Children who move often are two and a half times more likely to repeat a school grade than are those who do not move (National Center for Farmworker Health, Inc., 2005a). The Migrant Head Start program, though not able to meet all needs, clearly helps the children it serves.

BRIEFLY NOTED

Children of migrant farmworkers experience many hardships. They may have to help with the agricultural work while trying to maintain their schoolwork and to fit into two different cultures. These can be challenging expectations, especially if the children have to move a lot or are sick frequently.

Some adolescent farmworkers accompany their parents to work; however, others come either alone or with an uncle, cousin, or friend. These children are vulnerable to low wages; no education; social isolation; alcohol, drug, and HIV risks; and occupational hazards. Machinery related accidents, drowning, and firearms and explosives were the three leading causes of deaths for farmworker children (Rivara, 1997).

Federal law does not protect children from overworking or from the time of day they work outside of school. Therefore children may work until late in the evenings or very early in the mornings every day of the week if not protected by state law or if inadequately monitored. Adolescent farmworkers are often too tired after working to do homework and to attend classes. Child farmworkers may attend three to five schools a year, which disrupts both school performance and social integration (National Center for Farmworker Health, Inc., 2009). Frequent change in schools and constant fatigue set these children up for failure. It has been reported that only 55% of migrant children graduate from high school nationwide (National Center for Farmworker Health, Inc., 2001).

Some migrant children, as young as 8 years of age, stay home to care for younger children. The Migrant Head Start Program is a safe, healthy, and educative option for children ages 6 months to 5 years. However, inadequate funding results in lack of services for all migrant children. The Migrant Education Program is a state and nationally sponsored summer school program for farmworkers' children older than 5 years. However, this program is not available to all eligible migrant youth.

Nurses can play an important role in the lives of migrant children as portrayed in the words of migrant children in southern Georgia. During focus groups, these children talked about the importance of nurses in their health and health care (Wilson, Pittman, and Wold, 2000). For example, one child stated, "the nurses teach you how to stay healthy, like good things to eat, how to stay safe, and how to learn in school." Another child said "the nurse also told us how to stay safe in our neighborhood, like staying away from people who drink and take drugs" (Wilson, Pittman, and Wold, 2000, p. 143).

CULTURAL CONSIDERATIONS IN MIGRANT HEALTH CARE

As discussed in Chapter 5, to provide culturally competent care to migrant farmworkers, nurses need to appreciate and understand the cultural backgrounds of these individuals.

Because the majority of migrant farmworkers are of Mexican descent, this section focuses on Mexican cultures. Although certain health beliefs and practices have been identified with the Mexican culture, the nurse must remember that beliefs and practices differ among regions and localities of a country and among individuals. Mexico is a multicultural country; therefore the cultural backgrounds of Mexican immigrants vary, depending on their place of origin. Many indigenous groups in Mexico speak their regional dialect. Mexican immigrants may or may not be able to read, understand or speak Spanish. Mexican immigrants who are less educated, with fewer economic resources, and from the rural areas tend to possess more traditional beliefs and practices.

NURSE–CLIENT RELATIONSHIP

The nurse is considered an authority figure who should respect (*respeto*) the individual, be able to relate to the individual (*personalismo*), and maintain the individual's dignity (*dignidad*). Mexican individuals prefer polite, nonconfrontational relationships with others (*simpatia*). At times, because of *simpatia,* individuals and families may appear to understand what is being said to them (by nodding their heads) when in actuality they do not understand. The nurse should take measures to validate the understanding of these individuals. The Mexican individual expects to talk about personal matters (chit-chat) for the first few minutes of an encounter. They expect the nurse not to appear rushed and to be a good listener. Humor is appreciated, and touching as a caring gesture is seen as a positive behavior.

Mexican clients may not seek care with health professionals first. Rather, they may have consulted with knowledgeable individuals in their family or community (the popular arena of care) or with folk healers (the traditional arena of care). Examples of the members of the popular arena are the "senora" or wise, older woman living in the community, one's grandmother (la abuela), and the local parish priest.

HEALTH VALUES

Family, in general, is a significant component of a Mexican individual's health care and social support system. The female in the household is considered to be the caretaker, whereas the male is considered to be the major decision maker. However, Mexican females in certain families have significant influence over most matters, including health decisions. Grandmothers and sisters are highly significant to the wife (female) in the immediate family. They provide advice, care, and support. Even though they communicate regularly with their family in Mexico, they may not have a support system in the United States.

Love of their children, rather than concern for their own health, may encourage migrant parents to adopt healthier lifestyles. One example is when the parents of a child with asthma choose to stop smoking (Napolitano, 2008). In Oregon, when asked if they protected themselves from pesticide exposure, Mexican migrant parents responded negatively in general. However, they were willing to change their behaviors if, as a result, their children would be protected from pesticides (Napolitano et al, 2002).

The Mexican client may be more willing to follow the advice of another Mexican individual with a similar health problem rather than the advice of the health professional. When health care providers fail to take into account the client's culture and ways of living, the client is likely to ignore the information and turn to their friends and family for information. Although the majority of Mexican immigrants may identify themselves as Catholics, many Mexican individuals belong to other churches. The individual's religion may influence his or her health practices such as birth control; however, the nurse cannot assume that a Catholic, for example, will not use some method of birth control.

HEALTH BELIEFS AND PRACTICES

In the Mexican culture, health may be considered a gift from God. Another common perception of health is that a healthy person is one who can continue to work and maintain daily activities independent of symptoms or diagnosed diseases. A person may miss a clinic appointment if he or she is able to work that day. Mexican immigrants may believe that illness is a punishment from God and think this is why therapies have not cured them. This more commonly occurs with chronic illnesses. Four more common folk illnesses that a nurse may encounter with the Mexican client are (1) *mal de ojo* (evil eye), (2) *susto* (fright), (3) *empacho* (indigestion), and (4) *caida de mollera* (fallen fontanel). Symptoms and treatments may vary depending on the individual's or family's origin in Mexico. Other cultural beliefs relate to hot–cold balance, pregnancy, and postpartum behaviors (*cuarentena*). When experiencing a folk illness, the traditional Mexican individual would prefer to seek care with a folk healer. The more common healers are the *curanderos, herbalistas,* and *espiritualistas.* The most commonly used herbs are *manzanilla* (chamomile), *yerba buena* (peppermint), *aloe vera, nopales* (cactus), and *epazote.*

OCCUPATIONAL AND ENVIRONMENTAL HEALTH PROBLEMS IN RURAL AREAS

Four high-risk industries that are found primarily in rural areas are forestry, mining, fishing, and agriculture. Each day, over 200 agricultural workers suffer lost-work-time injuries, and almost 5% result in permanent impairment (National Institute for Occupational Safety and Health, 2008). Farming and ranching do not often fall under OSHA guidelines, because they are considered small enterprises. Therefore safety standards are not enforceable. Nor is Workers' Compensation insurance usually available for the agriculture industry.

BRIEFLY NOTED

In many states, Workers' Compensation benefits are not available to migrants for on-the- job injuries because these tend to be small, often family operations.

Runovers from tractor falls and trailing equipment are the most common unintentional injuries in farming (National Safety Council, 2008a). Other reported injuries have included fractures or sprains from falls from ladders or equipment; strains and sprains from prolonged stooping, heavy lifting, and carrying; amputations, deaths, and crush injuries from tractors, trucks, and other machinery; pesticide poisoning; electrical injuries; and drowning in ditches.

The physical demands of harvesting crops 12 to 14 hours a day take their toll on the musculoskeletal system. Think about the pain that ensues from stooping over to pick strawberries all day, reaching overhead while on a ladder to pick pears, or lifting heavy crates of produce. Back and neck pain were the most common types of chronic pain reported with many workers leaving or changing their jobs (National Center for Farmworker Health, 2005d; Villarejo et al, 2000).

Naturally occurring plant substances or applied chemicals can cause irritation to the skin (contact dermatitis) or to the eyes (allergic or chemical conjunctivitis). Green tobacco sickness (dermal exposure to wet tobacco) was experienced by 50% of tobacco workers interviewed in North Carolina (Quandt et al, 2000). Eye problems are often caused by exposure to chemicals, dust, and pollen (Mines, Mullinax, and Saca, 2001; Villarejo et al, 2000), and the lack of eye care because of unavailability of resources can lead to chronic eye problems and loss of vision for these individuals. Cancer is another cited, but not well-documented, health problem for migrant farmworkers, mainly because of their exposure to chemicals. A high prevalence of breast cancer, brain tumors, non-Hodgkin's lymphoma, and leukemia has been found in agricultural communities (Larson, 2001; Ray and Richards, 2001; Mills and Yang, 2005).

PESTICIDE EXPOSURE

Most of the North American food supply is treated with agricultural chemicals (i.e., pesticides), with the largest group being the organophosphate pesticides. These pesticides are known to be potential hazards (Villarejo et al, 2000; Von Essen, 1998). Farmworkers are exposed not only to the immediate effects of working in fields that are foggy or wet with pesticides but also to the unknown long-term effects of chronic exposure to agricultural chemicals. The farmworker's clothing and dwelling also can be major sources of cross-contamination for both the worker and his or her family. The Environmental Protection Agency (EPA) and OSHA require that farmworkers be given information about pesticide safety. However, migrant farmworkers may not receive this information or may get ineffectual training or may not be able to read the educational information (Napolitano et al, 2002).

How to Recognize the Symptoms of Pesticide Exposure

Acute health effects of **pesticide exposure** include mild psychological and behavioral deficits such as memory loss, difficulty with concentration, mood changes, abdominal pain, nausea, vomiting, diarrhea, headache, malaise, skin rashes, and eye irritation. Acute severe pesticide poisoning can result in death. More chronic exposure may lead to long-term damage to the central nervous system and the liver (National Safety Council, 2008b) (see the "How To" box).

RURAL HEALTH CARE DELIVERY ISSUES AND BARRIERS TO CARE

Although each rural community is unique, the experience of living in a rural area has several common characteristics (Ramsbottom-Lucier et al, 1996; Schwartz, 2002) (see Box 22-2). Barriers to health care may be associated with whether services and professionals are available, affordable, accessible, or acceptable to rural consumers. Availability implies that health services exist and have the necessary personnel to provide essential services. Sparseness of population limits the number and array of health care services in a given geographic region. Therefore the cost of providing special services to a few people often is prohibitive, particularly in frontier states, where the number of physicians, nurses, and

---

HOW TO | **Recognize the Signs and Symptoms of Pesticide Exposure**

Signs and symptoms of pesticide exposure vary according to the amount and length of time of the exposure. The majority of body systems can be affected by pesticide exposure.
- Symptoms of acute poisoning include neuromuscular (headache, dizziness, confusion, irritability, twitching muscles, muscle weakness), respiratory (shortness of breath, difficulty breathing, nasal and pharyngeal irritation), and gastrointestinal (nausea, vomiting, diarrhea, stomach cramps).
- Symptoms of chronic exposure can be related to illnesses and conditions such as cancers, Parkinson's like symptoms, infertility or sterility, liver damage, and polyneuropathy and neurobehavioral problems.
- If symptoms of pesticide exposure are suspected, the nurse should develop a pesticide exposure history. A good example of an exposure form can be found at http://pesticide.umd.edu.

Box 22-2 Barriers to Health Care in Rural Areas
- Great distances to obtain services
- Lack of personal transportation
- Unavailable public transportation
- Lack of telephone services
- Unavailable outreach services
- Inequitable reimbursement policies for providers
- Unpredictable weather and/or travel conditions
- Inability to pay for care
- Lack of "know-how" to procure entitlements and services
- Inadequate provider attitudes and understanding about rural populations
- Language barriers (caregivers are not linguistically competent)
- Care and services not culturally appropriate

other types of health care providers is insufficient. Consequently, where services and personnel are scarce, they must be allocated wisely. Accessibility implies that a person has logistical access to, as well as the ability to purchase, needed services. Affordability is associated with both the availability and accessibility of care. It infers that services are of reasonable cost and that a family has sufficient resources to purchase them when they are needed. Acceptability of care means that a particular service is appropriate and offered in a manner that is congruent with the values of a target population. This can be hampered by both the client's cultural preference and the urban orientation of health professions.

Providers' attitudes, insights, and knowledge about rural populations are important. A demeaning attitude, lack of accurate knowledge about rural populations, or insensitivity about the rural lifestyle on the part of a nurse can cause difficulties in relating to those clients. Moreover, insensitivity generates mistrust, causing rural clients to view professionals as outsiders to the community. On the other hand, some professionals in rural practice express feelings of professional isolation and lack of community acceptance. To resolve these conflicting views, nursing faculty members can expose students to the rural environment with clinical experiences that include opportunities to provide care to clients in their natural (e.g., rural) setting to gain accurate insight about that particular community.

To develop community health programs that are available, accessible, affordable, and appropriate, nurses must design strategies and implement interventions that mesh with a client's belief system. This implies that a family and a community are actively involved in planning and delivering care for a member who needs it. Nurses must have an accurate perspective of rural clients. Although the importance of forming partnerships and ensuring mutual exchange seems obvious, most research about rural communities has been for policy or reimbursement purposes. Little empirical data are available about rural family systems in terms of their health beliefs, values, perceptions of illness, health care-seeking behaviors, and what constitutes appropriate care. Therefore nurses must be actively involved in conducting and implementing research on the nursing needs of rural populations to expand the profession's knowledge of this population and to provide services that are based on evidence.

NURSING CARE IN RURAL ENVIRONMENTS

Rural people often develop independent and creative ways to cope because of the distance, isolation, and sparse resources they encounter. They may prefer to seek help first through their informal networks, such as neighbors, extended family, church, and civic clubs, before seeking a professional's care. Nurses describe some interesting differences when they work in rural areas versus urban ones. The boundaries between one's home and work roles may blur in that the nurse may go to the same church, shop at the same stores, and have children in the same schools as their clients. Thus many, if not all, clients are personally known as neighbors, as friends

of an immediate family member, or perhaps part of one's extended family. There are, then, both social informality and a corresponding lack of anonymity in a small town. Some rural nurses say, "I never really feel like I am off duty because everybody in the county knows me through my work." In part, this may be because nurses are highly regarded by the community and viewed by local people as experts on health and illness. Residents may ask health-related questions and recommendations about physicians when they see the nurse (who may be a neighbor, friend, or relative) in a grocery store, at a service station, during a basketball game, or at church functions. Nurses in rural areas may also be expected to, in general, know something about everything, and this can be a demanding expectation. Some of the challenges of rural practice are professional isolation, limited opportunities for continuing education, lack of other kinds of health personnel or professionals with whom one can interact, heavy workloads, the ability to function well in several clinical areas, lack of anonymity, and for some, a restricted social life (Bushy, 2002b; Bushy and Bushy, 2001). Many nurses value the close relationships with clients and co-workers along with the diverse clinical experiences that evolve from caring for clients of all ages who have a variety of health problems, caring for clients for long periods (in some cases, across several generations), opportunities for professional development, greater autonomy, and the pleasures of living in a rural area. The nurse can often keep a finger on the pulse of the community by staying active in local political, social, religious, and employment activities that affect their clients. The nurse can be a catalyst for change, act as a community educator, and know how to find resources and services (Box 22-3).

Box 22-3   Characteristics of Nursing Practice in Rural Environments

- Variety and/or diversity in clinical experiences
- Broader and expanding scope of practice
- Generalist skills
- Flexibility and creativity in delivering care
- Sparse resources (materials, professionals, equipment, fiscal)
- Professional and/or personal isolation
- Greater independence and autonomy
- Role overlap with other disciplines
- Slower pace
- Lack of anonymity
- Increased opportunity for informal interactions with clients and co-workers
- Opportunity for client follow-up upon discharge in informal community settings
- Discharge planning allowing for integration of formal and informal resources
- Care for clients across the life span
- Exposure to clients with a full range of conditions and diagnoses
- Status in the community (viewed as prestigious)
- Viewed as a professional role model
- Opportunity for community involvement and informal health education

---

| Box 22-4 | Comparison of U.S. Urban (Metro) and Rural (Nonmetro) Residents' Health Status |

Residents of Fringe Counties of Large Metro Areas Have the Following:

- Lowest levels of premature mortality, partly reflecting lower death rates for unintentional injuries, homicide, and suicide
- Lowest levels of smoking, alcohol consumption, and child-bearing among adolescents
- Lowest prevalence of physical inactivity during leisure time among women
- Lowest levels of obesity among adults
- Greatest number of physician specialists and dentists per capita
- Lowest percentage of the population without health insurance
- Lowest percentage of the population who had no dental visits

Residents in the Most Rural (Nonmetro) Areas Have the Following:

- Highest death rates for children and young adults
- Highest death rates for unintentional and motor vehicle traffic-related injuries
- Highest mortality rates among adults for ischemic heart disease and suicide
- Highest levels of smoking among adolescents
- Highest levels of physical activity during leisure time among men
- Highest levels of obesity among adults
- Highest percentage of adults with activity limitations caused by chronic health conditions
- Fewest physician specialists and dentists per capita
- Least likely to have seen a dentist
- Highest percentage of the population without health insurance

From Centers for Disease Control and Prevention: *United States, 2001: urban and rural health chartbook,* Washington, DC. Retrieved Aug 2001 from http://www.cdc.gov/nchs/data/hus/hus01.pdf.

Nurses working in rural areas, including those working with migrant farmworkers, can use many community health nursing skills. One of the first and most important is that of prevention. Given the barriers to receiving health care in rural areas, the ideal situation is to prevent health disruptions whenever possible. Case management and community health primary health care (COPHC) are two effective models to use to address some of those deficits and resolve rural health disparities (Box 22-4). The "Clinical Application" section demonstrates how nursing case management can allow an older adult resident to stay at home in a rural environment if adequate supports can be provided. Outcomes are often remarkably different when case management is used. Additional information on case management is found in Chapter 13. Chapter 3 provides information about COPHC. See Box 22-5 for a brief description of COPHC steps.

The need for nursing services in the community varies by community. However, there is a prevailing need in most rural areas for the following:

- School nurses
- Family planning services

| Box 22-5 | Community Health Primary Health Care (COPHC): A Partnership Process |

The steps in the COPHC process include the following:
1. Define and characterize the community.
2. Identify the community's health problems.
3. Develop or modify health care services in response to the community's identified needs.
4. Monitor and evaluate program process and client outcomes.

| Levels of Prevention | Related to Rural Health Including Migrant Farmworkers |

PRIMARY PREVENTION

Teach workers how to reduce exposure to pesticides.

SECONDARY PREVENTION

Conduct screening, such as urine testing for pesticide exposure.

TERTIARY PREVENTION

Initiate treatment for the symptoms of pesticide exposure such as nausea, vomiting, and skin irritation.

- Prenatal care
- Care for individuals with AIDS and their families
- Emergency care services
- Children with special needs, including those who are physically and mentally challenged
- Mental health services
- Services for older adults (especially frail older adults and those with Alzheimer's disease), such as adult day care, hospice, respite care, homemaker services, and meal deliveries to older adults who remain at home

Providing a continuum of care has been hindered by the closure of many small hospitals in the past two decades and the possible continuation of this trend.

HEALTHY PEOPLE 2010 NATIONAL HEALTH OBJECTIVES RELATED TO RURAL HEALTH

The goals of *Healthy People 2010* have important implications for nurses who work with rural and migrant populations. Many objectives are relevant to these groups. The following components need to be integrated to make the national health objectives relevant to rural populations:

- Health statistics must be meaningful and understandable, and they must include appropriate process objectives that can be measured readily.
- Strategies must be designed that involve the public, private, and voluntary sectors of the community to achieve agreed-upon local objectives.
- Coordinated efforts are needed to ensure that the community works together to achieve the goals.

Healthy People 2010

Selected Objectives* for Migrant Farmworker Populations

Environmental Health

8-13 Reduce pesticide exposures that result in visits to a health care facility

8-24 Reduce exposure to pesticides as measured by urine concentrations of metabolites

Immunizations and Infectious Diseases

14-1 Reduce or eliminate indigenous cases of vaccine preventable diseases

14-11 Reduce tuberculosis

14-12 Increase the proportion of all tuberculosis patients who complete curative therapy within 12 months

Maternal Infant and Child Health

16-6 Increase the proportion of pregnant women who receive early and adequate prenatal care

Occupational Safety and Health

20-1 Reduce deaths from work-related injuries

20-2 Reduce work-related injuries resulting in medical treatment, lost time from work, or restricted work activity

20-8 Reduce occupational skin diseases or disorders among full-time workers

Oral Health

21-10 Increase the proportion of children and adults who use the oral health care system each year

21-12 Increase the proportion of low-income children and adolescents who received any preventative dental service during the past year

Sexually Transmitted Diseases

25-8 Reduce HIV infections in adolescent and young adult females age 13–24 years that are associated with heterosexual contact

From the U.S. Department of Health and Human Services: *Healthy People 2010: national health promotion and disease prevention objectives,* ed 2, Washington, DC, 2000, U.S. Government Printing Office.
*These fit many other rural workers.

HOW TO Build Professional, Community, and Client Partnerships

1. Gain the local perspective.
2. Assess the degree of public awareness and support for the cause.
3. Identify special interest groups.
4. List existing services to avoid duplication of programs.
5. Note real and potential barriers to existing resources and services.
6. Generate a list of potential community volunteers and professionals who are willing to assist with the project.
7. Create awareness among target groups of a particular program (e.g., individuals, families, seniors, church and recreation groups, health care professionals, law enforcement personnel, and members of other religious, service, and civic clubs).
8. Identify potential funding sources to implement the program.
9. Establish the community's health care priority list and involve large numbers of community members in considering and selecting their health care options.
10. Incorporate business principles in marketing the program.
11. Measure the health system's local economic impact.
12. Educate residents about the important role the local health care system plays in the economic infrastructure of the community and the consequences of a system failure.
13. Develop local leadership and support for the community's health system through training and providing experience in decision making.

developing health-promoting programs to prevent chronic health problems and establishing community programs to meet the needs of those having chronic illness, specifically cardiovascular disease, diabetes, hypertension, and accident-related disabilities. The *Healthy People 2010* box illustrates selected objectives pertinent to migrant workers and many other rural people.

When implementing community-focused health plans that flow from *Healthy People in Healthy Communities 2010,* always consider rural factors, such as sparse population, geographic remoteness, scarce resources, personnel shortages, and physical, emotional, and social isolation. Remember that members of the community must be involved in developing the plan and assume some ownership for it. The "How To" box describes ways to build community partnerships.

CLINICAL APPLICATION

Ethyl Lewis, a 73-year-old widow, was diagnosed more than 10 years ago with progressive Parkinson's disease. Her husband of more than 40 years died suddenly 3 years ago after a serious stroke. Her two married daughters live in California and Illinois. Her small Midwestern town has 1000 residents, and the nearest health care is 100 miles away. Her 75-year-old widowed sister, Suzanna Ames, also lives in town. Their brother Bill Jones (age 71) has recently entered the county nursing home located in a town 20 miles

For example, consider the following components in developing a health plan for a rural county having a large population of young people: objectives for women of childbearing age, children, and adolescents. Priority objectives should include offering accessible prenatal care programs, improving immunization levels, providing preventive dental care instructions, implementing vehicular accident prevention and firearm safety programs, and educating teachers and health professionals for early identification of cases of domestic violence. On the other hand, consider a rural county that has a higher number than the national average of individuals older than 65 years. Priority objectives in the health plan should target the health risks and problems of older adults in that community. Specific objectives might include away. Despite her physical rigidity and ataxia, Ms Lewis manages to live alone in her two-bedroom home with her dog and cat. She insists that she will not relinquish her private, independent lifestyle as her brother has. Yet within this past year she has been hospitalized three times: for a bad chest cold, for a bladder infection, and after a neighbor found her lying unconscious in the garden. Her doctor says that this last episode was related to "a heart problem."

After discharge, a home-health nurse, Liz Moore, was assigned as her case manager. Ms. Moore's office is based at the County Senior Center near the nursing home where her brother is a resident. He is also one of the clients whom the nurse checks on weekly. She provides outreach services to all the residents in the county who are referred by a large home-health agency in the city. As a case manager, she works closely with the hospital's discharge planners to arrange a continuum of care for clients in the two-county area. Her activities include coordinating formal and informal services for clients, including nutrition, hydration, pharmacological care, personal care, homemaker services, and routine activities, such as writing checks, home maintenance, and emergency backup services.

A. *Describe the nursing roles that the nurse assumes in coordinating a continuum of care for Ethyl in terms of nutrition, transportation, and health care.*
B. *Identify formal health care and support resources that can be accessed for Ms. Lewis.*
C. *Identify informal support resources that can be used to ensure that Ms. Lewis is safe.*
D. *Identify three outcomes that have been achieved by using nursing care management.*
E. *Select a rural community in your geographic area. Create hypothetical situations, or select real clients with real health problems (e.g., an older adult with Alzheimer's disease, a middle-aged person with cancer requiring end-of-life care, a child who is dependent on technology as a result of a farm accident). Prepare a list of services and referral agencies in that community that could be used to develop a continuum of care for each of these cases. How are these the same as or different from the case described in this chapter?*

Answers are in the back of the book.

REMEMBER THIS!

- Rural environments are diverse and different from those in urban areas.
- The health status of rural populations varies, depending on genetic, social, environmental, economic, and political factors.
- The incidence of working poor in rural America is higher than in more populated areas.
- Rural adults 18 years and older are in poorer health than their urban counterparts; nearly 50% have been diagnosed with at least one major chronic condition. However, they average one less physician visit each year than healthier urban counterparts.

- About 26% of rural families are below the poverty level; more than 40% of all rural children younger than 18 years of age live in poverty.
- A migrant farmworker is a laborer whose principal employment involves traveling from place to place planting or harvesting agricultural products and living in temporary housing situations.
- An estimated 3 to 5 million migrant farmworkers are in the United States. These numbers are controversial because of the inconsistency in defining farmworkers and limitations in obtaining data.
- The life expectancy of the migrant farmworker is 49 years, compared with 75 years for other U.S. residents.
- Health problems of migrant farmworkers are linked to their work environment, limited access to health services and education, and lack of economic opportunities.
- Migrant farmworkers are faced with uncertainty regarding work and housing, inadequate wages, unsafe working conditions, and lack of enforcement regarding legislation for field sanitation and safety regulations.
- Farmworkers are exposed not only to the immediate effects in the fields (foggy or wet with pesticides) but also to unknown long-term effects of chronic exposure to pesticides.
- When harvesting is completed, the migrant farmworker becomes simultaneously homeless and unemployed. Forced migration to find employment leaves little time or energy to seek out and improve living standards. Many of them return to their country of origin after the growing season ends.
- Children of migrant farmworkers may need to work for the family's economic survival.
- Nurses must consider the belief systems and lifestyles of a rural population when assessing, planning, implementing, and evaluating community services.
- Barriers to rural health care include the lack of availability, affordability, accessibility, and acceptability of services.
- Partnership models, in particular COPHC, are effective models to provide a comprehensive continuum of care in environments with scarce resources.

WHAT WOULD YOU DO?

1. Think about a rural community with which you are familiar:
   - Discuss the economic, social, and cultural factors that affect the lifestyle in this rural area. What do you think are the health care-seeking behaviors of residents who live there?
   - Identify barriers that affect accessibility, affordability, availability, and acceptability of services in the health care delivery system for that rural community.
   - What do you think are or would be the challenges, opportunities, and benefits of living and practicing as a nurse in this rural environment?
2. Outreach workers are personnel generally hired by an agency, such as a health department, who provide education to migrant persons. Lay health promoters are often from a community of migrant peoples who also provide

community-based education. Find out if both of these roles exist in your community. Interview these people, or work with them for a few hours. Compare and contrast their roles. How are they complementary? How are they duplicative? How can they work together to maximize health? How are their approaches to education different (e.g., does one use a protocol or template, whereas the other is led by community concerns)?

3. Interview community leaders to determine the presence of migrant or seasonal farmworkers in your area. Compare and contrast information about migrant and seasonal farmworkers by interviewing teachers, clergy, and politicians versus migrant outreach workers, wage and hour personnel, Department of Labor personnel, and Migrant Head Start program employees.

4. In some areas of the United States, placement agencies specialize in helping businesses hire migrant workers. Determine whether an agency of this type exists in your area. If it does, interview a key person and ask questions that would enable you to access information such as how they recruit workers, how long workers typically stay in one location, what health screening they do, and who provides health services to the workers they place.

■ *REFERENCES*

Beeson P: *Some notes and data on rural suicide,* 2003, National Association for Rural Mental Health. Retrieved July 13, 2008, from http://www.narmh.org/pages/resnotes.html.

Bigbee J, Crowder E: The Red Cross Rural Nursing Service: an innovation of public health nursing delivery, *Public Health Nurs* 2(2):109, 1985.

Bureau of Health Professions: *Health professional shortage areas,* Washington, DC, 2005a, U.S. Department of Health and Human Services.

Bureau of Health Professions: *Nurse shortage counties,* Washington, DC, 2005b, U.S. Department of Health and Human Services.

Bushy A: *Orientation to nursing in the rural community,* Thousand Oaks, Calif, 2000, Sage.

Bushy A: International perspectives on rural nursing: Australia, Canada, United States, *Aust J Rural Health* 10(2):104–111, 2002a.

Bushy A: *Resource manual: rural minorities, their health issues and resources,* Kansas City, Mo, 2002b, National Rural Health Association.

Bushy A, Bushy A: Critical access hospitals: rural nursing issues, *J Nurs Adm* 31(6):301–310, 2001.

Cason K, Synder A, Jensen L: *The health and nutrition of Hispanic and seasonal farm worker,* Harrisburg, Penn, 2004, The Center for Rural Pennsylvania.

Centers for Disease Control and Prevention: United States, 2001: urban and rural health chartbook, Washington, DC. Retrieved Aug 2001 from http://www.cdc.gov/nchs/data/hus01.pdf.

Culp K, Umbarger M: Seasonal and migrant agricultural workers, *AAOHN J* 52:383–390, 2004.

Davis S: *Child labor, migrant health issues,* Monograph Series, National Center for Farmworker Health, Oct 2001.

Gamm LD, Hutchinson LL, editors: *Rural healthy people 2010: a companion document to Healthy People 2010,* vol 3, College Station, Tex, 2004, Texas A & M University System Health Science Center, School of Rural Public Health, Southwest Rural Health Research Center.

Guasasco C, Heuer LF, Lausch C: Providing health care and education to migrant farmworkers: nurse-managed centers: a qualitative study, *J Community Health Nurs* 23(4):166–171, 2002.

Health Resources Services Administration: *United States personnel fact book,* Rockville, Md, 2003.

Hovey J, Magana C: Cognitive, affective, and physiological expressions of anxiety symptomatology among Mexican migrant farmworkers: predictors and generational differences, *Community Ment Health J* 38(3):223–237, 2002.

Ingram DD, Franco S: *2006 NCHS urban-rural classification scheme for counties,* Washington, DC, 2006, National Center for Health Statistics.

Jolk D: *Comparison of metropolitan-nonmetropolitan poverty during the 1990s,* Washington, DC, 2003, U.S. Department of Agriculture.

Kupersmidt J, Martin S: Mental health problems of children of migrant and seasonal farm workers: a pilot study, *J Am Acad Child Adolesc Psychiatry* 36:224–232, 1997.

Larson A: *Environmental/occupational safety and health: migrant health issues, monograph series,* Oct 2001, National Center for Farmworker Health.

Lombardi G: *Dental/oral health services: migrant health issues, monograph series,* Oct 2001, National Center for Farmworker Health.

Mills P, Yang R: Breast cancer risk in Hispanic agricultural workers in California, *Int J Occup Health* 80:123–131, 2005.

Mines R, Gabbard S, Steinman A: *A profile of U.S. farm workers, demographics, household composition, income and use of services,* U.S. Department of Labor, Office of the Assistant Secretary for Policy, Commission on Immigration Reform, April 1997.

Mines R, Mullinax N, Saca L: *The Binational Farmworker Health Survey: an in-depth study of agricultural worker health in Mexico and the United States,* Davis, Calif, 2001, California Institute for Rural Studies.

Napolitano M, et al: Un Lugar Seguro Para Sus Ninos: Development and evaluation of a Pesticide Education Video, *J Immigr Health* 4:135–145, 2002.

Napolitano M: Migrant health issues, In Stanhope M, Lancaster J, editors: *Public health nursing: population-centered health care in the community,* St. Louis, 2008, Mosby.

National Center for Farmworker Health, Inc: *Child labor: Fact sheet about farmworkers,* 2009. Retrieved July 9, 2009. from www.ncfh.org.

National Center for Farmworker Health, Inc: *Overview of America's farmworkers: the agricultural economy.* Retrieved Feb 21, 2005a, from www.ncfh.org/aaf_01.php.

National Center for Farmworker Health, Inc: *Migrant and season farmworker demographics fact sheet.* Retrieved Feb 21, 2005b, from www.ncfh.org.

National Center for Farmworker Health, Inc: *Facts about farmworkers.* Retrieved Feb 21, 2005c, from www.ncfh.org.

National Center for Farmworker Health, Inc: *Overview of America's farmworkers: occupational safety and health.* Retrieved Feb 21, 2005d, from www.ncfh.org/aaf_03.php.

National Center for Farmworker Health, Inc: *Overview of America's farmworkers: insurance and assistance programs.* Retrieved Feb 21, 2005e, www.ncfh.org/aaf_04.php.

National Center for Farmworker Health, Inc: *Oral health,* 2005f, National Center for Farmworker Health. Retrieved July 1, 2008, from http://www.ncfh.org.factsheets.php.

National Center for Farmworker Health, Inc: *Tuberculosis,* 2005g, National Center for Farmworker Health. Retrieved July 3, 2008, from http://www.ncfh.org/factsheets.php.

National Center for Farmworker Health, Inc: *HIV/AIDS,* n.d. National Center for Farmworker Health. Retrieved July 8, 2008, from hyyp://www.ncfh.org/docs/fs-hiv_aids.pdf.

National Center for Farmworker Health, Inc: *Migrant health issues: introduction,* monograph series, 2001.

National Institute for Occupational Safety and Health: *Agricultural safety, 2008,* Centers for Disease Control and Prevention. Retrieved July 8, 2008, from http://www.cdc.gov/niosh/topics/aginjury/default/html.

National Rural Health Association: What's different about rural health? Retrieved March 9, 2009, from www.ruralhealthweb. org. 2007–2009.

National Safety Council: *Falls from tractors and trailing equipment,* 2008a. Retrieved July 8, 2008, from http:www.nsc.org/ resources/factsheets/ag/falls.aspx.

National Safety Council: *Pesticides,* 2008b. Retrieved July 8, 2008, from http://www.nsc.org/resources/factsheets/environment/ pesticides.aspx.

Office of the Federal Registrar: *Code of Federal Regulations: Public Health Title 42, Chapter 1, Section 56.102,* 1994.

Perilla J et al: Listening to migrant voices: focus groups on health issues in South Georgia, *J Community Health Nurs* 15(4): 251–263, 1998.

Probst JC et al: *Minorities in rural America: an overview of population characteristics,* Columbia SC, 2002, South Carolina Rural Health Research Center.

Quandt S et al: Migrant farmworkers and green tobacco sickness: new issues for an understudied disease, *Am J Ind Med* 37: 307–315, 2000.

Ramsbottom-Lucier M et al: Hills, ridges, mountains and roads: geographical factors and access to care in a rural state, *J Rural Health* 12(5):386, 1996.

Ray D, Richards P: The potential for toxic effects of chronic, low-dose exposure to organophosphates, *Toxicol Lett* 120:343–351, 2001.

Rivara F: Fatal and non-fatal injuries to children and adolescents in the United States, 1990–1993, *Inj Prev* 3(3):190–194, 1997.

Schwartz T: Making it safer down on the farm, *Am J Nurs* 102(3):114–115, 2002.

U.S. Bureau of the Census: *Resident population of the United States by sex, race, and Hispanic origin: 2000.* Retrieved April 2, 2001, from www.census.gov/population/estimates/nation.

U.S. Bureau of the Census: *100 fastest growing counties.* Retrieved July 6, 2008, from http://www/census/gove/popest/counties/ co-est 2004.09.html.

U.S. Department of Agriculture: *Agriculture fact book,* Washington, DC, 2001–2002, USDA.

Villarejo D et al: *Suffering in silence: a report on the health of California's agricultural workers,* Woodland Hills, Calif, 2000, The California Endowment.

Von Essen S: Health and safety risks in production agriculture, *West J Med* 169:214–220, 1998.

Wilson A, Pittman K, Wold J: Listening to the quiet voices of Hispanic migrant children about health, *J Pediatr Nurs* 15(3):137–147, 2000.

Homelessness, Poverty, Mental Illness, and Teen Pregnancy

Dyan A. Aretakis
Christine Di Martile Bolla
Anita Thompson-Heisterman

ADDITIONAL RESOURCES

These related resources are found either in the appendix at the back of this book or on the book's website at http://evolve.elsevier.com/stanhope/foundations.

Evolve Website

- Community Assessment Applied
- Case Study, with questions and answers
- Quiz review questions
- WebLinks, including link to *Healthy People 2010* website

Real World Community Health Nursing: An Interactive CD-ROM, second edition

If you are using this CD-ROM in your course, you will find the following activity related to this chapter:
- *Vulnerability: You're in Charge* in **Vulnerability**

OBJECTIVES

After reading this chapter, the student should be able to:
1. Describe the social, political, cultural, and environmental factors that influence poverty.
2. Discuss the effects of poverty on the health and well-being of individuals, families, and communities.
3. Discuss how being homeless affects the health and well-being of individuals, families, and communities.
4. Describe the ways in which teen pregnancies affect the baby, the parents, and their families.

5. Develop nursing interventions for the prevention of pregnancy problems that at-risk adolescents might experience.
6. Explain the extent of the problem of patients who have mental illness or who are at risk for mental illness.
7. Explain nursing interventions for poor and homeless people, pregnant teens and their significant others, and individuals who are mentally ill or at risk for mental illness.

CHAPTER OUTLINE

SCOPE OF MENTAL ILLNESS IN THE UNITED STATES
Deinstitutionalization
At-Risk Populations for Mental Illness

LEVELS OF PREVENTION AND THE NURSE IN COMMUNITY HEALTH
ROLE OF THE NURSE

KEY TERMS

abortion: termination of a pregnancy by spontaneous or induced expulsion of a human fetus during the first 12 weeks of gestation.

adoption: the action of taking a child by choice into a relationship; to take voluntarily as one's own child.

consumer price index (CPI): the basic indicator of inflation—a measurement of inflation by comparison of prices overall and of categories of consumed goods and services purchased by urban wage earners and their families over a certain period.

crisis poverty: a situation of hardship and struggle; it may be transient or episodic and can result from lack of employment, lack of education, domestic violence, or similar issues. These issues can lead to persistent poverty.

cultural attitudes: the beliefs and perspectives that a society values.

deinstitutionalization: effort to move long-term psychiatric patients out of the hospital and back into their own community.

Federal Income Poverty Guidelines: a definition of poverty drafted by the Social Security Administration in 1964. The federal government defines poverty in terms of income, family size, the age of the head of household, and the number of children younger than 18 years. The guidelines change annually to be consistent with the consumer price index.

gynecological age: number of years from menarche.

homeless persons: the federal government defines a homeless person as one who lacks a fixed, regular, and adequate address or has a primary nighttime residence in a supervised publicly or privately operated shelter for temporary accommodations.

low birthweight: birthweight of less than 5½ pounds.

mental health: ability to engage in productive activities and positive relationships and to adapt to change and cope with adversity.

mental illness: refers to all diagnosable mental disorders; it can affect persons of all ages, races, cultures, socioeconomic levels, and educational levels and persons of both genders.

neighborhood poverty: refers to spatially defined areas of high poverty, characterized by dilapidated housing and high levels of unemployment.

paternity: fatherhood.

persistent poverty: refers to individuals and families who remain poor for long periods.

poverty: refers to having insufficient financial resources to meet basic living expenses. These expenses include cost of food, shelter, clothing, transportation, and medical care.

sexual debut: first intercourse.

sexual victimization: suffering from a destructive or injurious sexual action.

Stewart B. McKinney Homeless Assistance Act of 1994: Public Law 100-77 passed in 1987 officially involved the federal government in meeting the needs of homeless persons. It was intended to respond to the range of emergency needs facing homeless Americans, such as food, shelter, and health care.

Temporary Assistance to Needy Families (TANF): formerly called Aid to Families with Dependent Children (AFDC), a federal and state program to provide financial assistance to needy children deprived of parental support because of death, disability, absence from the home, or in some states, unemployment. This program mandates that women heads-of-household find employment to retain their benefits.

Women, Infants, and Children (WIC): a special supplemental food program administered by the Department of Agriculture through the state health departments; it provides nutritious foods that add to the diets of pregnant and nursing women, infants, and children younger than 5 years. Eligibility is based on income and nutritional risk as determined by a health professional.

Four groups of people who represent members of vulnerable populations—the poor, the homeless, pregnant teens, and those who are mentally ill—present complex nursing needs. In a society that values self-reliance, individual responsibility, and personal accountability, members of these vulnerable groups may not get the respect they deserve. It is important for nurses to understand their own beliefs about these groups and to understand the issues surrounding such client's illness and/or personal situation. To be able to

interact effectively with these groups it is important for the nurse to identify health care needs, barriers to care, and essential health care services for each of these groups, and in some instances for their families as well.

This chapter describes the many ways that poverty, homelessness, mental illness, and teen pregnancy affect the health status of individuals, families, and communities and contains effective nursing intervention strategies for these groups.

ATTITUDES, BELIEFS, AND MEDIA COMMUNICATION ABOUT VULNERABLE GROUPS

Cultural attitudes are the beliefs and perspectives that a society values. Perspectives about individual responsibility for health and well-being are influenced by prevailing cultural attitudes. The media communicate thoughts and attitudes through literature, film, art, television, and newspapers. Media images of persons on welfare or who are homeless, pregnant, or mentally ill are influenced by cultural attitudes and values. For example, criminals in films and television programs are often portrayed as poor, desperate persons whereas some are shown as being seriously mentally ill or drug users.

Nurses can examine their beliefs, values, and knowledge about these vulnerable groups by considering the following clinical situations and questions:

- You are doing health screening at a homeless shelter and one of the clients asks you for money for bus fare. Do you give it to her?
- You are in the home of an older adult client whose kitchen is covered with roaches. What are your obligations in terms of the client's home environment? Where do you sit if the client offers you a chair?
- You are making a visit to an especially unclean home. What do you do if the client offers you some food?
- What interventions would you initiate for a group of poor or homeless families in a local shelter?
- You are asked to develop a health promotion program for a group of pregnant teens. What do you do if you have trouble capturing their attention?
- How could you effectively advocate for a group of seriously mentally ill people who need treatment that is not being adequately provided in the community?

There are no easy answers to these questions. However, nurses' behaviors in these situations influence their

HOW TO	Test Values and Beliefs about Poverty

In order to clarify their own values and perspectives about poverty, nurses should ask themselves the following questions about poverty and persons living in poverty:
- What do I believe to be true about being poor?
- What do I personally know about poverty?
- How have family and friends influenced my ideas about being poor?
- Have I ever personally been poor?
- How have media images of poor persons helped shape our images of poverty and poor persons?
- What do I feel when I see a hungry child? A hungry adult?
- Do I believe that people are poor because they just don't want to work? Or do I believe that society has a significant influence on one's becoming poor?
- What really causes poverty?
- What do I really think can be done to prevent poverty and homelessness?

relationships with their clients. Nurses are expected to value individuals, promote health, respect and restore human dignity, and improve the quality of life of individuals, families, and aggregates (Jacobs, 2001). Conflicts in values, beliefs, and perceptions may arise when nurses work with persons from different social, cultural, and economic backgrounds. A lack of agreement between the professional's and the client's perceptions of need can lead to conflict. As a result of this conflict, clients may fail to follow the prescribed treatment protocol; the nurse may then inaccurately interpret the client's behavior as resistance, lack of cooperation, or noncompliance.

DEFINING AND UNDERSTANDING POVERTY

In 2007, 37.3 million people had incomes below the federal poverty level. Approximately 18% of persons living in poverty were under 18 years of age. The overall poverty rate for all age groups is 12.5% of the population (U.S. Bureau of the Census, 2007). The number of people living in poverty increases during times of economic stress when unemployment increases. People who live in poverty are not a homogeneous group, therefore, be sure to listen to and learn about each person. In general, **poverty** refers to having insufficient financial resources to meet basic living expenses. These expenses include food, shelter, clothing, transportation, and health care. People who are poor are more likely to live in dangerous environments, to be unemployed, underemployed or work at high-risk jobs, to eat less nutritious foods, and to have multiple stressors.

For years, income level has been used as the criterion that determines whether someone is poor. Although income continues to be the measurement of choice, the federal *poverty* guidelines have been renamed the federal *income* guidelines. Income is also a qualifying factor for a variety of programs, such as federal housing subsidies; **Temporary Assistance to Needy Families (TANF)**, formerly called *Aid to Families with Dependent Children (AFDC)*; medical assistance; food stamps; **Women, Infants, and Children (WIC);** and Head Start.

The federal government uses two terms to discuss poverty: poverty thresholds and poverty guidelines. The Poverty Threshold Guidelines are issued by the U.S. Bureau of the Census and are used primarily for statistical purposes. The **Federal Income Poverty Guidelines** are issued by the U.S. Department of Health and Human Services (USDHHS) and are used to determine whether a person or family is financially eligible for assistance or services under a particular federal program. The federal income guidelines are updated annually to be consistent with the **consumer price index (CPI)**. The CPI is a measure of the average change over time in the prices paid by urban consumers for a fixed market basket of consumer goods and services (Blau, 2004).

Many people who earn slightly more than the government-defined income levels (Table 23-1) are unable to meet their living expenses and are not eligible for government

Table 23-1	Poverty Thresholds for 2007, by Size of Family (Including Related Children under 18 Years of Age)

Size of Family Unit	Income Guideline ($)
1	10,590
2	13,540
3	13,853
4	18,267
5	22,029
6	25,337
7	29,154
8	32,606
9 or more	39,223

From U.S. Bureau of the Census: *Current population survey,* Washington, DC, 2002, U.S. Government Printing Office.

assistance programs. In a family of four, for example, whose annual income is considered above the defined income level of $19,223, the adult family members would not qualify for Medicaid in some states (U.S. Bureau of the Census, 2005). The terms *persistent poverty* and *neighborhood poverty* are used to describe types of poverty. **Persistent poverty** refers to individuals and families who remain poor for long periods and who pass poverty on to their descendants. **Neighborhood poverty** refers to geographically defined areas of high poverty, characterized by dilapidated housing and high levels of unemployment. For nurses, the most significant factor is being able to accept and respect clients and attempt to understand how their life situations influence their health and well-being. Being poor is one variable that must be measured against the presence of other variables that may increase or decrease the negative effects of poverty.

It was not until 1964 that the Social Security Administration established the income level of the official poverty line. Individuals and families with incomes below the federal poverty line were considered to be living in poverty. In 1965 the Medicare amendments to the Social Security Act were passed. Policy changes during the 1980s led to an emphasis on defense spending rather than on social programs. A series of events in the 1980s, such as the visibility of the homeless and the media attention on an underclass of individuals, seemed to blame the person for being poor. During the 1990s, record numbers of people received welfare benefits. In 1996 a bill creating the TANF program was enacted. This welfare reform legislation replaced the AFDC program with a program of temporary welfare benefits. Under TANF, people are provided with benefits for a limited time and are required to find jobs and/or to enroll in job-training programs. Overall poverty has declined following welfare reform. Unfortunately, the economic status of many families on welfare who were forced to work has declined. Because persons working full-time for minimum wage do not receive other types of government compensation, they have incomes below the federal poverty level (Zedlewski, Chaudry, and

Simms, 2008). The economic downturn in the first decade of the twenty-first century has sent even more people into poverty and resulted in more people losing their homes, and many retirees having their anticipated retirement income reduced or lost.

The causes of poverty are complex and interrelated. The following factors affect the growing number of poor persons in the United States:

- Decreased earnings
- Increased unemployment rates
- Changes in retirement benefits, particularly when companies close or file for bankruptcy protection and eliminate or reduce retirement benefits
- Changes in the labor force
- Increase in female-headed households
- Inadequate education and job skills
- Inadequate antipoverty programs
- Inadequate welfare benefits
- Weak enforcement of child support statutes
- Dwindling Social Security payments to children
- Increased numbers of children born to single women

As the fiscal characteristics of most industrialized nations have changed from industrial economies to service economies, job opportunities have increasingly excluded workers who do not have at least a high school education. Many manufacturing jobs do not pay sufficient salary to support a family. Also, many jobs at the lower end of the pay scale do not include health care or retirement benefits.

POVERTY AND HEALTH: EFFECTS ACROSS THE LIFE SPAN

Poverty directly affects health and well-being, resulting in
- higher rates of chronic illness;
- higher infant morbidity and mortality;
- shorter life expectancy;
- more complex health problems;
- more significant complications and physical limitations resulting from the higher incidence of chronic disease, such as asthma, diabetes, and hypertension; and
- hospitalization rates greater than those for persons with higher incomes.

These poor health outcomes are often secondary to barriers that impede access to health care, such as an inability to pay for health care, lack of insurance, geographic location, language, an inability to find a health care provider, transportation difficulties, inconvenient clinic hours, and negative attitudes of health care providers toward poor clients. Access to health care is especially difficult for the working poor. Many employers, especially those paying low or minimum wage, do not provide health care insurance for their employees. Persons working for these employers are ineligible for most public health insurance programs, and they are often unable to obtain affordable health care.

Poverty, while presenting a significant obstacle to health across the life span, has an especially negative effect on *women of childbearing age.* Women living in poverty have lower levels of physical functioning and higher reported

| Box 23-1 | The Effects of Poverty on the Health of Children |

- Higher rates of prematurity, low birthweight, and birth defects
- Higher infant mortality rates
- Increased incidence of chronic disease
- Increased incidence of traumatic death and injuries
- Increased incidence of nutritional deficits
- Increased incidence of growth retardation and developmental delays
- Increased incidence of iron deficiency anemia
- Increased incidence of elevated blood lead levels
- Increased incidence of infections
- Increased risk for homelessness
- Decreased opportunities for education, income, and occupation

levels of bodily discomfort than women in higher socioeconomic groups. Prevalence rates for ulcer disease, asthma, and anemia are significantly higher in this group. Poor women also report significantly more risk behaviors for infection with human immunodeficiency virus (HIV) than more affluent women (Ellen et al, 2004).

Poverty has significant effects on *adolescent women.* Poor teens are four times more likely than nonpoor teens to have below-average academic skills. Regardless of their race, poor teens are nearly three times more likely to drop out of school as their nonpoor counterparts. Teenage women who are poor and who have below-average skills are more likely to have children than nonpoor teenage women. Poor pregnant women are more likely than other women to receive late or no prenatal care and to deliver low-birthweight babies, premature babies, or babies with birth defects (Fowles, Hendricks, and Walker, 2005).

Many American *children* are members of the "5H" club. They are hungry, homeless, hugless, hopeless, and without health care (Elders, 1994). The 2007 poverty rate of 18% for children is higher than that for any other age group (U.S. Bureau of the Census, 2007). Moreover, poverty among young African-American and Hispanic children is more than three times that of white, non-Hispanic children. Poverty among children (newborn to age 5 years of age) has increased in all racial and ethnic groups, as well as in all urban, suburban, and rural geographic areas. Under current federal law, noncustodial parents are required to provide financial support to their children. Current child support policies are designed to provide financial security to children, prevent single-parent families from entering the welfare system, help single-parent families get off welfare as quickly as possible, and decrease welfare expenditures. Individual states are responsible for locating nonsupporting custodial parents, establishing paternity, and enforcing financial responsibility. In most states, government involvement in locating noncustodial parents begins when the custodial parent applies for TANF.

Although the term *deadbeat dad* was created for fathers who do not contribute to the financial support of their

children, noncustodial mothers are equally responsible under the law to provide for the economic well-being of their children. Thus the term *deadbeat parent* is more gender-sensitive and appropriate.

Young children (newborn to age 5 years) are at highest risk for the most harmful effects of poverty, especially lack of adequate nutrition and brain development. Other risk factors include maternal substance abuse or depression, exposure to environmental toxins, trauma and abuse, and poor-quality daily care (Evans, Boxhill, and Pinkava, 2008). Selected effects of poverty on the health of children are shown in Box 23-1. Poverty also increases the likelihood of chronic disease, injuries, traumatic death, developmental delays, poor nutrition, inadequate immunization levels, iron deficiency anemia, and elevated blood lead levels. These children may also be hungry and fatigued and experience dizziness, irritability, headaches, ear infections, frequent colds, weight loss, inability to concentrate, and increased school absenteeism (Emerson, 2004).

In 2007 an estimated 9.7% of *older adults* (65 years and older) lived in poverty (U.S. Bureau of the Census, 2007). This represents a decrease in the poverty rate for this age group, largely because of improvements in Social Security and the Supplemental Security Income program. However, poor elders are at greater risk for chronic illness, which leads to complications, poor dental health, and an overall higher mortality rate than older adults in general. Certain groups of older adults, such as African-Americans, remain vulnerable to the effects of poverty. They are, for example, at greater risk for chronic and nutrition-related diseases than older white adults (Kelley-Moore and Ferraro, 2004). Risk increases for older adults who are alone and unable to manage their personal affairs. Many older adults are eligible for benefits but do not know how to access them.

BRIEFLY NOTED

A client's advice to nurses who care for the poor is as follows:
- Treat the poor like everyone else.
- Do not be condescending.
- Do not make it obvious that someone is poor.
- Do not prejudge; ask if someone wants to pay on their bill.
- Remember that people can't always pay for their medicine.
- Suggest programs that might help, such as food banks, churches, and clothing centers.
- Poor people need a lot of support.
- Many poor people need help to learn how to promote their own health given a paucity of resources.

Poverty affects both *urban* and *rural communities.* Several characteristics describe poor communities. For example, poorer neighborhoods may have more minority residents and single-parent families, higher rates of unemployment, and lower wage rates. These residents are also more likely to be victims of crime, substance abuse, racial discrimination, and police brutality. Differences in quality and level of education also exist. Health care is less available to residents of poor neighborhoods. Housing conditions in some areas are deplorable, with many families living in run-down shacks or condemned apartment buildings. People who live in poverty are often exposed to environmental hazards, such as inadequate heating and cooling, exposure to rain and snow, inadequate water and plumbing, and the presence of pests and other vermin.

UNDERSTANDING THE CONCEPT OF HOMELESSNESS

Poverty can lead to homelessness. Homelessness, like poverty, is a complex concept. Although people who have never been homeless cannot truly understand what it means to be homeless, nurses can increase their sensitivity toward homeless clients and aggregates by examining their own personal beliefs, values, and knowledge of homelessness. The questions in the "How To" box can aid in reflection and value clarification. Some homeless people find lodging in shelters or with family or friends. Others are less fortunate and live inside only sporadically; at other times they live on the streets.

BRIEFLY NOTED

Poverty and homelessness are affected by the employment rate. When companies close, downsize, or relocate, workers often go long periods without a steady income.

People who live on the street are the poorest of the poor, and they may be viewed as faceless, nameless, invisible, and inaudible entities. It is important for nurses to respect the individuality of all clients including those who are homeless. People become homeless for many reasons and there is no one set of circumstances or patterns that leads to and sustains homelessness.

HOW TO	**Evaluate the Concept of Homelessness**

- What is it like to live on the streets?
- What issues might confront a young mother and her children inside a homeless shelter?
- How is it that people are so poor that they have no place to go?
- What really causes homelessness?
- How do you respond to the person on the street asking for money to buy a sandwich or catch a bus?
- How is your response different (or not) when a young mother with children asks you for money?
- How do you react to the smell of urine in a stairwell or elevator?

According to the **Stewart B. McKinney Homeless Assistance Act of 1994**, a person is considered homeless who (National Coalition for the Homeless, 2008a, p. 1)

lacks a fixed, regular, and adequate night-time residence and… has a primary night-time residency that is:
A. *a supervised publicly or privately operated shelter designed to provide temporary living accommodation;*
B. *an institution that provides a temporary residence for individuals intended to be institutionalized; or*
C. *a public or private place not designed for, or ordinarily used as, a regular sleeping accommodation for human beings.*

This definition generally refers to persons who are homeless on the streets or in shelters or who face eviction within 1 week. There are two common ways to determine the number of people who are homeless: (1) point-in-time-counts, counting the number of persons who are homeless on a given day or during a given week, or (2) period prevalence counts, which examines the number of people who are homeless over a given period of time (National Coalition for the Homeless, 2008b). It is hard to know exactly how many people are homeless. Accuracy is complicated by several factors:

- **Homeless persons** are often hard to locate, since many sleep in boxcars, on roofs of buildings, in doorways, or under freeways. Others stay temporarily with relatives.
- Once located, many homeless persons refuse to be interviewed or deliberately hide the fact that they are homeless.
- Some persons experience short intervals of homelessness or have intermittent homeless episodes. They are harder to identify at any specific time.
- It is difficult to generalize from one location to another. For example, the patterns of homelessness differ in large versus small cities and in urban versus rural areas.

The concept of homelessness includes the following two broad categories:

1. **Crisis poverty**
   - Lives are generally marked by hardship and struggle.
   - Homelessness is often transient or episodic.
   - The homeless person may resort to brief stays in shelters or other temporary accommodations.
   - Homelessness may result from lack of education or employment, obsolete job skills, or domestic violence.
   - These issues lead to persistent poverty and need to be addressed along with efforts to find stable housing.
2. Persistent poverty
   - These men and women are chronically homeless, and many of them have mental or physical disabilities.
   - This group is most frequently identified with homelessness in the United States.
   - Physical and mental disabilities often coexist with alcohol and other drug abuse, severe mental illness, other chronic health problems, and/or chronic family difficulties.
   - These people lack money and family support.
   - This group often ends up living on the streets, and they need economic assistance, rehabilitation, and ongoing support.

Box 23-2	Who Are America's Homeless?

- Persons living in poverty
- Families
- Children
- Single adults, especially males
- Female heads of household
- Victims of domestic violence
- People who abuse alcohol or other substances
- Adolescent runaways
- Older adults with no place to go and no one to care for them
- Persons who are mentally ill
- Veterans

From National Coalition for the Homeless: *Who is homeless?*, Fact Sheet #3, Washington, DC, 2008, National Coalition for the Homeless.

Many homeless people previously had homes and managed to survive on limited incomes. Today's homeless include people of every age, sex, ethnic group, and family type. They are both rural and urban people. Surprisingly, the single homeless tend to be younger and better educated than stereotypes would suggest. Many are longstanding residents of their communities and have some history of job success. Two trends have influenced homelessness over the past 25 years: a growing shortage of affordable rental homes and a simultaneous increase in poverty (National Coalition for the Homeless, 2008a). More single men are homeless than women. Families with children are the fastest growing segment of the homeless population, with the numbers higher in rural areas. Approximately 16% of the single adult homeless population have some form of serious mental illness (U.S. Conference of Mayors, 2005). Box 23-2 summarizes the characteristics of America's homeless.

Many homeless sleep at night in shelters but must leave during the day. This means that during the day, they sit or stand on the street, in parks, alleys, shopping centers, libraries, and in places such as trash bins or cardboard boxes or under loading docks at industrial sites. They may also seek shelter in public buildings, such as train and bus stations. Those who do not sleep in shelters may sleep in single-room-occupancy hotels, all-night movie theaters, abandoned buildings, and vehicles.

BRIEFLY NOTED

The Substance Abuse and Mental Health Services Administration (SAMHSA) has launched a Homelessness Resource Center Web site. The site is designed to support persons working to improve the lives of individuals who are homeless and also have mental health conditions, substance use disorders, and histories of trauma. The site is http://www.homeless.samhsa.gov.

CAUSES OF HOMELESSNESS

Most people move into homelessness gradually. Once they give up their own dwellings, they move in with family or friends. Only when all other options are exhausted do people go to shelters or seek refuge on the streets. Many factors contribute to the increasing numbers of homeless persons:

- More people living in poverty
- A decrease in the number of affordable housing units, the gentrification of neighborhoods, and the consequent increased costs for housing
- Loss of single-room-occupancy buildings in which people could rent a room on a long-term basis
- Emergency demands on income
- Alcohol and drug addiction
- Limited numbers of transitional treatment facilities for deinstitutionalized mentally ill individuals; this is important, since a sizable number of homeless people suffer from significant mental illness

EFFECTS OF HOMELESSNESS ON HEALTH

Homelessness is correlated with acute and chronic illness, acquired immunodeficiency syndrome (AIDS), trauma (O'Connell et al, 2005), and with difficulty accessing health care services. Health care is usually crisis oriented and sought in emergency departments, and those who access health care have a hard time following prescribed regimens. For example, an insulin-dependent diabetic man who lives on the street may sleep in a shelter. His ability to get adequate rest, exercise, take insulin on a schedule, eat regular meals, or follow a prescribed diet is virtually impossible. How does someone purchase an antibiotic without money? How is a child treated for scabies and lice when there are no bathing facilities? How does an older adult with peripheral vascular disease elevate his legs when he must be out of the shelter at 7 am and on the streets all day? These health problems are often directly related to poor access to preventive health care services. Homeless people devote a large portion of their time trying to survive. Health promotion activities are a luxury for them not a part of their daily lives. *Healthy People 2010* has goals to increase awareness and use of preventive health services (see *Healthy People 2010* box), but this is very hard for the homeless.

Homeless people often have the following health problems:
- Hypothermia and heat-related illnesses
- Infestations and poor skin integrity
- Peripheral vascular disease and hypertension
- Diabetes and nutritional deficits
- Respiratory infections and chronic obstructive pulmonary diseases
- Tuberculosis (TB)
- HIV/AIDS
- Trauma
- Mental illness
- Use and abuse of tobacco, alcohol, and illicit drugs

Homeless persons are on their feet for many hours and often sleep in positions that compromise their peripheral circulation. Hypertension is exacerbated by high rates of alcohol abuse and the high sodium content of foods served in fast-food restaurants, shelters, and other meal sites. Crowded living conditions put homeless persons at risk for exposure

● Healthy People 2010

Objectives Related to Poor and Homeless People, Adolescent Reproductive Health, and Mental Illness

1-1	Increase the proportion of persons with health insurance
1-4	Increase the proportion of persons who have a specific source of ongoing care
1-6	Reduce the proportion of families that experience difficulties or delays in obtaining health care, or who do not receive needed care for one or more family members
9-7	Reduce pregnancies among adolescents
9-10	Increase the proportion of sexually active, unmarried adolescents aged 15 to 17 years who use contraception that both effectively prevents pregnancy and provides barrier protection against disease
18-3	Reduce the proportion of homeless adults who have serious mental illness (SMI) to 19% from 25%
18-4	Increase employment of persons with SMI from 43% to 51%
18-14	Increase the number of states from 24 to 50 that have screening, crisis intervention, and treatment services for older adults

From U.S. Department of Health and Human Services: *Healthy People 2010: national health promotion and disease prevention objectives,* ed 2, Washington, DC, 2000, U.S. Government Printing Office.

to viruses and bacteria that cause pneumonia and TB. AIDS is also a growing concern among the homeless population. The seroprevalence of HIV infection in the homeless is estimated to be at least double that found in the general population. The use of intravenous drugs and the risk for sexual assault are other factors. Homeless persons with AIDS tend to develop more virulent forms of infectious diseases, to have longer hospitalizations, and to have less access to treatment (Lopez-Zetina et al, 2001). Trauma is a major cause of death and disability for homeless people. Major trauma includes gunshot or stab wounds, head trauma, suicide attempts, and fractures. Minor trauma includes bruises, abrasions, concussions, sprains, puncture wounds, eye injuries, and cellulitis.

In addition to its effects on physical health, homelessness also affects psychological, social, and spiritual well-being. Becoming homeless means more than losing a home or a regular place to sleep and eat; it also means losing friends, personal possessions, and familiar surroundings. Homeless persons live in chaos, confusion, and fear. Many describe experiencing loss of dignity, low self-esteem, lack of social support, and generalized despair.

HOMELESSNESS AND AT-RISK POPULATIONS

Being homeless affects health across the life span. Imagine the effect of homelessness on pregnancy, childhood, adolescence, or older adulthood; each group has different needs. Nurses must be aware of the unique needs of homeless clients at every age.

Homeless pregnant women are at high risk for complex health problems. Outcomes for homeless pregnant women

are significantly poorer than for pregnant women in the general population. Pregnant homeless women present several challenges. They have higher rates of sexually transmitted diseases, higher incidences of addiction to drugs and alcohol, poorer nutritional status, and a higher incidence of poor birth outcomes (e.g., lower birthweight and lower Apgar scores). Although homeless women who are pregnant are at increased risk for complications of pregnancy, they have less access to prenatal care. The severity of homelessness has been shown to significantly predict lower birthweight and preterm births, even for homeless women receiving regular prenatal care (Bloom et al, 2004).

The health problems of homeless children, although similar to those of poor children, often have more serious consequences. Homeless children have poorer health than children in the general population, and they experience more symptoms of acute illness, such as fever, ear infection, diarrhea, and asthma, than their housed counterparts (Craft-Rosenberg, Powel, and Culp, 2000). Homeless children living on the streets in urban areas are at greatest risk of poor health due to poor nutrition, inconsistent health care, high levels of anxiety, and an inability to practice good health behaviors. Homeless children also experience higher rates of school absenteeism, academic failure, and emotional and behavioral maladjustments. The stress of homelessness can be manifested in behaviors such as withdrawal, depression, anxiety, aggression, regression, and self-mutilation. Homeless children may have delayed communication, more mental health problems, and histories of abuse. Also, they are less likely to have attended school than their housed counterparts (Craft-Rosenberg et al, 2000).

Homeless adolescents living on the streets exhibit greater risk-taking behaviors including earlier onset of sexual activity. They also have poorer health status and decreased access to health care than do teens in the general population. Furthermore, homeless adolescents are at high risk of contracting serious communicable diseases, such as AIDS and hepatitis B, and are more likely to use alcohol and illicit substances. Homeless teens often have histories of runaway behavior, physical abuse, and sexual abuse. Once on the streets, many homeless adolescents exchange sex for food, clothing, and shelter. In addition to the increased risk of sexually transmitted diseases and other serious communicable diseases, homeless adolescent girls who exchange sex for survival are at high risk for unintended pregnancy (Rew, 2002) (see the "Evidence-Practice box").

Homeless older adults are the most vulnerable of the impoverished older-adult population. They have lived in long-standing poverty, have fewer supportive relationships, and are likely to have become homeless as a result of catastrophic events. Life expectancy for homeless older adults is significantly lower than for older housed adults. Permanent physical deformities, often secondary to poor or absent medical care, are common among homeless older adults. They often suffer from untreated chronic conditions, including TB, hypertension, arthritis, cardiovascular disease, injuries, malnutrition, poor oral health, and hypothermia (Sterigiopoulos and Herrmann, 2003). As with younger homeless persons,

Evidence-Based Practice

Rew et al (2008) examined the effects of the duration of homelessness and gender on personal and social resources, cognitive and perceptual factors, and sexual health behaviors among homeless youth. Their data were gathered at a large drop-in center for runaway and homeless youth in central Texas. A sample of 805 youth between the ages of 16 and 23 years was recruited for the study. The investigators gathered demographic data and the history of homelessness from surveys they developed. Other valid scales were used to measure each of the conceptual variables. Their findings demonstrated that both duration of homelessness and gender have both direct and interaction effects on self-reports of personal and social resources, AIDS knowledge, and sexual risk behaviors. They found that chronically homeless youth in their sample reported higher levels of sexual risk-taking behaviors. Young women, regardless of the length of time as homeless, reported similar levels of social connectedness, while newly homeless young men had greater connectedness than those who were chronically homeless.

NURSE USE: Nurses working in the community may have opportunities to work directly with homeless youth and provide interventions to promote sexual health and decrease risk-taking behavior.

From Rew L et al: Interaction of duration of homelessness and gender on adolescent sexual health indicators, *J Nurs Schol* 4(2):109–115, 2008.

older adults who are homeless must focus their energy on survival, leaving little time for health promotion activities.

Homelessness has a negative effect on the health of persons across the life span. Nurses need to identify the precursors to homelessness, anticipate the effects of homelessness on physical, emotional, and spiritual well-being, and become knowledgeable about resources to assist the homeless.

TRENDS IN ADOLESCENT SEXUAL BEHAVIOR AND PREGNANCY

Teen pregnancy is an area of public health concern because of its significant effect on communities. Many teens who become pregnant get caught in a cycle of poverty, school failure, and limited life options, and some become homeless. Each year 800,000 to 900,000 teens become pregnant, and more than half of them go on to have babies. Births to teenagers make up 10% of all births in the United States (Franzetta et al, 2005). Teen birthrates increase by age, with the highest rates occurring among teens 19 years of age. The U.S. teen birth rate increased in 2006 for the first time in 15 years and remains higher than that of any other developed nation (Moore, 2008). The rate of increase was 3%, and it is not known if this is the beginning of a trend or a 1 year fluctuation. There was a small decline in contraceptive use among sexually active high school age females between 2003 and 2005, which may explain some of the increase. Prior to 2006, the decreases were attributed to stabilization of the numbers of teens becoming sexually active, increased condom use, and increased use of more effective

and long-acting hormonal methods of birth control (Centers for Disease Control and Prevention, 2008). More than 82% of teens are unmarried at the time of their child's birth and fewer than 8% of these unmarried mothers will marry the baby's father in the year following the birth (Franzetta et al, 2005). *Healthy People 2010* (U.S. Department of Health and Human Services, 2000) identified goals to reduce teen pregnancy and birthrates.

In 2000, 29% of pregnancies to teenagers were ended by elective abortion (Franzetta et al, 2005). There has been a decreasing rate of elective abortions in recent years. This decrease was caused in part by decreases in the pregnancy rate, but may also have resulted from laws that required parental notification or consent for minors requesting abortion services in some states. African-American and white teens choose abortion at similar rates. Adolescents who terminate their pregnancies by abortion differ from those who give birth in the following ways: they are more likely to complete high school, are more successful in school, have higher educational aspirations, and are more likely to come from a family of a higher socioeconomic status (Fergusson, Boden, and Horwood, 2007).

BACKGROUND FACTORS

Many adults have difficulty understanding why young people would jeopardize their careers and personal potential by becoming pregnant during the teen years. Adolescents, however, do not view the world in the same way adults do. Teens often feel invincible and may not recognize the risk related to their behaviors or anticipate the consequences. That is, they may not believe that sexual activity will lead to pregnancy. When teens become pregnant, many do not think they will experience any negative effects on their lives. Many think they are unique and different and that everything will work out fine. The developmental changes of adolescence, coupled with potential background disadvantages, can magnify the problems facing the pregnant and parenting teen. Pregnant teens often express the unrealistic attitude that they can do it all: school, work, parenting, and socializing.

The characteristics of the teens who are giving birth are changing. A disproportionate number of them are poor (more than 75%), have limited educational achievements, and see few advantages in delaying pregnancy as they do not expect that their circumstances will improve at a later time (Whitman et al, 2001). Most teens report that their pregnancy was unplanned. They typically say they think a pregnancy should be delayed until people are older, have completed their education, and are employed and married. Their behaviors, however, do not support their opinions. In fact, some teens actually seem eager to become pregnant. Several factors that often contribute to pregnancy are discussed next.

SEXUAL ACTIVITY, USE OF BIRTH CONTROL, AND PEER AND PARTNER PRESSURE

The **sexual debut**, or first experience with intercourse, for a teen affects pregnancy risk. Although the percentage of sexually active teens today is much greater than it was in the

1970s, there have been decreases in recent years. The Youth Risk Behavior Surveillance System monitors six categories of health-risk behaviors among youth and young adults. One of these categories relates to sexual behaviors that contribute to unintended pregnancy and sexually transmitted diseases. During the 30 days before the 2007 survey was conducted, results indicated that 47.8% of the high school students who were surveyed had ever had sexual intercourse. Of that percent, 35.0% were currently sexually active, and 38.5% of the currently sexually active teens had not used a condom during the last sexual intercourse (Centers for Disease Control and Prevention, 2008). In the ninth grade, 32.8% of students are sexually active, 43.8% by the tenth grade, 55.5% by the eleventh grade, and 64.6% by the twelfth grade. Male students (10.1%) and African-American students (26.2%) were more likely than white, Hispanic/Latino, or female students to initiate sexual activity before age 13. African-American students (72.6%) are more likely to report a history of sexual activity, followed by Hispanic/Latino (58.2%) and white students (43.6%) (Centers for Disease Control and Prevention, 2008). The *Healthy People 2010* goal is to increase the proportion of adolescents who have never engaged in sexual intercourse to 88% by age 15 and to 75% by age 17 (baselines of 81% girls and 79% boys by age 15 years; 62% girls and 57% boys by age 17 years) (U.S. Department of Health and Human Services, 2000). Clearly, this goal set in 2000 is not being met.

Although more teens have begun using birth control in the past 10 years, there still is concern. In the survey mentioned above, of the 35.0% of sexually active high school students, 61.5% said that they or their partner had used a condom during the last sexual intercourse, and 16.0% reported that they or their partner had used birth control pills (Centers for Disease Control and Prevention, 2008).

Half of all first-time pregnancies occur within 6 months of initiating intercourse. Teens have many myths that contribute to poor use of birth control, such as believing you cannot get pregnant the first time, and some teens have incorrect knowledge about a woman's fertile time. Failure to use birth control can also reflect teens' embarrassment in discussing this practice with partners, friends, parents, and health care providers and the obstacles they encounter finding facilities that provide confidential and affordable birth control.

The earlier the sexual debut, the less likely a birth control method will be used, because younger teens have less knowledge and skill related to sexuality and birth control. School-based sex education can come too late or not at all. Birth control is usually discussed in the secondary-school curriculum, but this could be eighth grade in one school district and tenth grade in another; school curricula are not standardized. Younger teens may falsely believe that they are too young to purchase birth control methods such as condoms. Confidential reproductive health care services may be available for teens, but problems are still associated with transportation, school absences, and costs of care that ultimately restrict access to these services.

Teens can be influenced by peers, partners, and parents. They are more likely to be sexually active if their friends are sexually active (Bearman and Bruckner, 1999). Both young men and young women may think that allowing a pregnancy to happen verifies one's love and commitment for the other. In addition, young men from socioeconomically disadvantaged backgrounds may be more likely to say that fathering a child would make them feel more manly, and they are less likely to use an effective contraceptive (Marsiglio, 1993). Onetoughjob.org, an on-line support for parents, offers the following tips on talking about sex with children.

- By talking to your child about sex, you are reinforcing established family values.
- You are letting your child know she can talk to you about anything, nothing is taboo.
- Have the conversation more than once to make it more comfortable and normal to talk about.
- The first time you discuss sex with your child talk through the embarrassment.
- Find a conversation starter—don't wait for your child to ask a direct question.
- Inquire about what the culture at school is, what kids are doing, and what your child thinks about that.
- Tell your own stories, use humor, and show that this was once new to you too.
- Encourage questions and let your child know you want her to be safe and healthy.

Nurses can teach, coach, and support parents in learning how to talk with their children directly and providing useful, factual information.

OTHER FACTORS

A history of **sexual victimization**, family structure, and parental behaviors can influence teen pregnancy. These teens are more likely to have been sexually abused during their lifetime, with rates recorded as high as 67% (Klein and the Committee on Adolescence, 2005). Adolescent girls with a history of sexual abuse are at risk for earlier initiation of voluntary sexual intercourse, are less likely to use birth control, are more likely to use drugs and alcohol at first intercourse, and are more likely to have older sexual partners. The youngest women are more likely to experience coercive sex (65% of women who had intercourse before age 14 reported that it was involuntary) (Child Trends, 2005). Young women may also become pregnant as a result of forced sexual intercourse. A history of sexual victimization will influence a young woman's ability to exert control over future sexual experiences, which will affect the use of birth control and rejection of unwanted sexual experiences. All these factors contribute to an increased risk for becoming pregnant (Osborne and Rhodes, 2001). Also, young women who have experienced a lifetime of economic, social, and psychological deprivation may think that a baby will bring joy into an otherwise bleak existence. Some mistakenly think that a baby can provide the love and attention that her family has not provided.

Family structure can influence adolescent sexual behavior and pregnancy. Adolescents raised in single-parent families are more likely to have intercourse and to give birth than those raised in two-parent families. Parenting styles can influence a young woman's risk for early sexual experiences and pregnancy. Parents who are extremely demanding and controlling or neglectful and who have low expectations are least successful in instilling parental values in their children. Parents who have high demands for their children to act maturely and who offer warmth and understanding with parental rules have children more likely to exhibit appropriate social behavior and to delay early sexual experiences and pregnancy. Children of parents who are neglectful are the most sexually experienced, followed by children of parents who are very strict. Furthermore, parents who discuss birth control, sexuality, and pregnancy with their children can positively influence delay of sexual initiation and effective birth control use. Parents who do not communicate about sexuality with their teens may find them more at risk for sexual permissiveness and pregnancy (Kirby, 2001b).

YOUNG MEN AND PATERNITY

While there have been declines in the number of pregnant female teens in recent years, there are few data about the numbers for teen males. Approximately 14% of adolescent teens have made a female partner pregnant and 2% to 7% became fathers during the teen years (Marcell, Raine, and Eyre, 2003). Teen fathers face special challenges because of their own social problems including delinquency, alcohol or substance use, school problems, and limited future plans or ability to provide support. **Paternity**, or fatherhood, is legally established at the time of the birth for a married teen. It is more difficult to establish paternity among nonmarried couples. Some of the difficulty lies in the complexity of the specific state system for young men to acknowledge paternity. In some states, a young man may have to work with the judicial system outside of the hospital after the birth, and if he is younger than 18 years, he may need to involve his parents.

Some young couples do not attempt to establish paternity and prefer a verbal promise of assistance for the teen mother and child. Although a verbal commitment may be acceptable when the child is born, the mother may become more inclined to pursue the establishment of paternity later when the relationship ends or for reasons related to financial, social, or emotional needs of the child. Young women who receive state or federal assistance (e.g., Aid for Dependent Children, Medicaid) may be asked to name the child's father so the judicial process can be used to establish paternity.

Young men's reactions to learning that their partner is pregnant vary. The reaction often depends on the nature of the relationship before the pregnancy. Many young men will accompany the young woman to a health care center for pregnancy diagnosis and counseling and prenatal visits and will attend the delivery. They may also choose to be involved with their children regardless of changes in their relationships with the teen mother. It is not unusual for a young man

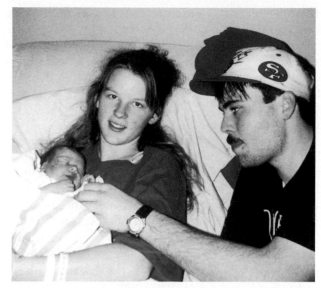

FIGURE 23-1 It is important to include both the teen mother and the father in teaching about child development.

to be excluded or even rejected by the young woman's family (usually her mother). He may then begin to act as though he is disinterested when he may really feel that he cannot provide resources for his child or know how to take care of him or her (Krishnakumar and Black, 2003) (Figure 23-1).

Nurses can acknowledge and support the young man as he develops in the role of father. His involvement can positively affect his child's development and provide greater personal satisfaction for himself and greater role satisfaction for the young mother. Mothers who report less social support from their baby's father are more apt to be unhappy and distressed in the parenting role and consequently more at risk for abuse of their child (Zelenko et al, 2001). The immediate concerns revolve around his financial responsibility, living arrangements, relationship issues, school, and work. The families of both teen parents can help to clarify these issues and identify roles and responsibilities.

EARLY IDENTIFICATION OF THE PREGNANT TEEN

Some teens delay seeking pregnancy services because they do not recognize signs such as breast tenderness and a late period. Most young women, however, suspect pregnancy as soon as a period is late. These young women may still delay seeking care since they falsely hope that the pregnancy will just go away. A teen also may delay seeking care to keep the pregnancy a secret from family members, who may pressure her to terminate the pregnancy, or because they do not want to have a gynecological examination.

Pay attention to subtle cues that a teenager may offer about sexuality and pregnancy concerns, such as questions about fertile periods or requests for confirmation that you need not miss a period to be pregnant. Once the nurse identifies the specific concern, information can be provided about how and when to obtain pregnancy testing. The nurse should determine how a teenager would react to the possible pregnancy before completing the test. If the test is negative, the nurse should assess whether the young woman would consider birth control counseling to prevent pregnancy. A follow-up visit is important after a negative test to determine if retesting is necessary or if another problem exists.

If the pregnancy test is positive, the next step is to perform a physical examination and pregnancy counseling. It is useful to do both at the same time so that the counseling is consistent with the findings of the examination. The purpose of the examination is to assess the duration and well-being of the pregnancy, as well as to test for sexually transmitted infection. Pregnancy counseling should include the following:

- Information on adoption, abortion, and childrearing
- Assessment of support systems for the young woman
- Identification of the immediate concerns she might have

The availability of affordable **abortion** services up to 13 weeks of gestation varies from community to community. Similarly, second-trimester services may be available locally or involve extensive travel and cost. The nurse should be knowledgeable about abortion services and provide information or refer the pregnant teenager to a pregnancy counseling service that can assist.

The pregnant teenager needs information about **adoption,** such as current policies among agencies that allow continued contact with the adopting family. Also, church organizations, private attorneys, and social service agencies provide a variety of adoption services with which the nurse should be familiar. Box 23-3 lists guidelines for adoption counseling. About 8% of adolescent women ages 17 years and younger relinquish custody of their infants (American College of Obstetricians and Gynecologists, 2007).

Pregnancy counseling requires that the nurse and young woman explore strengths and weaknesses for personal care and responsibility during a pregnancy and parenting. Young women vary in their interest in including the partner or their parents in this discussion. Issues to raise include education and career plans, family finances and qualifications for outside assistance, and personal values about pregnancy and parenting at this time in their life. Often it is difficult to focus on counseling in any depth at the time of the initial pregnancy testing results. A follow-up visit is usually more productive and should be arranged as soon as possible.

As decisions are made about the course of the pregnancy, the nurse is instrumental in referral to appropriate programs such as WIC (a supplemental food program for women, infants, and children), Medicaid, and prenatal services. The young woman and her family also need to know about expected costs of care and, if there is a family insurance policy, whether it will cover the pregnancy-related expenses of a dependent child. For those without insurance, the family can apply for Medicaid or determine whether local facilities offer indigent care programs (e.g., Hill-Burton programs for assistance with hospital expenses). The nurse can also begin prenatal education and counseling on nutrition, substance abuse and use, exercise, and special medical concerns.

Box 23-3 Guidelines for Adoption Counseling

1. Assess your own thoughts and feelings on adoption. Do not impose your opinion on the decision-making process of teen mothers.
2. Be knowledgeable about state laws, local resources, and various types of adoption services.
3. Choose language sensitively. Examples follow:
   a. Avoid saying "giving away a child" or "putting up for adoption." It is more appropriate and positive to say "releasing a child for adoption," "placing for adoption," or "making an adoption plan."
   b. Avoid saying "unwanted child" or "unwanted pregnancy." A more appropriate term may be *unplanned pregnancy.*
   c. Avoid saying "natural parents" or "natural child," because the adopted parents would then seem to be "unnatural." The terms *biological parents* and *adopted parents* are more appropriate.
4. Assess when a discussion of adoption is appropriate. It can be helpful to begin with information on adoption and then explore feelings and concerns over time. Individuals will vary in how much they may have already considered adoption, and this will influence the counseling session.
5. Assess the relationship between the pregnant teen and her partner and what role she expects him to play. Discuss the reality of this.
6. It may be helpful for a pregnant teen to talk with other teens who have been pregnant, are raising a child, have released a child for adoption, or have been adopted themselves.
7. A young woman can be encouraged to begin writing letters to her baby. These can be saved or given to the child when released to the adoptive family.

Modified from Brandsen CK: *A case for adoption,* Grand Rapids, Mich, 1991, Bethany.

SPECIAL ISSUES IN CARING FOR THE PREGNANT TEEN

Pregnant teenagers are considered high-risk obstetric clients. Pregnancy complications can result from poverty, late entry into prenatal care, sporadic prenatal care, and limited self-care knowledge. Teens are more likely to get no prenatal care or to begin the care later in the pregnancy than their older counterparts. Barriers are the real or perceived costs of care, denial of the pregnancy, fear of telling their parents, transportation, dislike of the care provided, or the attitude of the providers (Bensussen-Walls and Saewye, 2001; Hock-Long et al, 2003). Teens are more likely than adult women to deliver infants weighing less than 5½ pounds or to deliver before 37 weeks of gestation. These low-birthweight and premature infants are at greater risk for death in the first year of life and are more at risk for long-term physical, emotional, and cognitive problems including autism (Schendel and Bhasin, 2008). For example, low-birthweight and premature infants can be more difficult to feed and soothe. This challenges the limited skills of the young mother and can further strain relations with other members of the household, who may not know how to offer support or assistance. The risk for low-birthweight infants and premature births can

Table 23-2	Adolescent Nutritional Needs during Pregnancy	
Nutrient	**Daily Requirement during Pregnancy***	**Food Source**
Calcium	1300 mg (decrease to 1000 mg for 19 year olds)	Macaroni and cheese; Taco Bell chili cheese burrito; pizza; McDonald's Big Mac; puddings, milk, yogurt; also fortified juices, water, breakfast bars
Iron	30 mg (recommendation is for 30 mg elemental iron as daily supplement)	Meats, dried beans and peas, dark green leafy vegetables, whole grains, fortified cereal; absorption of iron from plant foods improved by vitamin C sources taken simultaneously
Zinc	15 mg	Seafood, meats, eggs, legumes, whole grains
Folate (folic acid)	0.6 mg (prenatal vitamins contain 0.4 to 1.0 mg of folic acid)	Green leafy vegetables, liver, breakfast cereals
Vitamin A	800 mcg	Dark yellow and green vegetables, fruits
Vitamin B_6	2.2 mg	Chicken, fish, liver, pork, eggs
Vitamin D	5 mcg	Fortified milk products and cereals

*Higher ranges are especially important for the younger pregnant teen.

be reduced if the teen gets early and regular prenatal care. After the pregnancy, nursing supervision is important to ensure that the mother and infant care is appropriate and that everyone in the home is coping adequately with the strain of a small infant. Nursing interventions through education and early identification of problems may dramatically alter the course of the pregnancy and the birth outcome.

Violence

Teens are more likely to experience violence during their pregnancies than adult women. Age may be a factor in their greater vulnerability to potential perpetrators who include partners, family members, and other acquaintances. Violence in pregnancy has been associated with an increased risk for substance abuse, poor compliance with prenatal care, and poor birth outcome. In the case of partner violence, young women may be protective of their partners because of fear or helplessness. Eliciting this history from an adolescent is not easy. The nurse must ask about violence at each visit. Frequent routine assessments are more revealing than a single inquiry at the first prenatal visit. Violence that begins in pregnancy may continue for several years after, with increasing severity. Variations by ethnicity have also been observed during this postpartum period; intimate partner violence may peak at 3 months postpartum among African-American and Hispanic/Latino new mothers and at 18 months for white mothers (Harrykissoon, Rickert, and Wiemann, 2002). The nurse should look for physical signs of abuse, as well as for controlling or intrusive partner behavior.

Nutrition

The nutritional needs of a pregnant teenager are especially important. First, the teen lifestyle does not lend itself to overall good nutrition. Fast foods, frequent snacking, and hectic social schedules limit nutritious food choices. Snacks, which account for approximately a third of a teen's daily caloric intake, tend to be high in fat, sugar, and sodium and limited in essential vitamins and minerals. Second, the nutritive needs of both pregnancy and the concurrent adolescent growth spurt

require the adolescent to change her diet substantially. The growing teen must increase caloric nutrients to meet individual growth needs as well as allow for adequate fetal growth. Third, poor eating patterns of the teen and her current growth requirement may leave her with limited reserves of essential vitamins and minerals when the pregnancy begins. The nurse can assess the pregnant teenager's current eating pattern and provide creative guidance. For example, protein can be increased at fast-food establishments by ordering milkshakes instead of soft drinks and cheeseburgers or broiled chicken sandwiches instead of hamburgers. Healthy eating is very important during pregnancy (Ward, 2006).

The recommended nutritional needs of the adolescent may depend on the **gynecological age** of the teen—that is, the number of years between her chronological age and her age at menarche as well as her chronological age. Young women with a gynecological age of 2 or less years or those younger than 16 years may have increased nutrient requirements because of their own growth. Furthermore, the younger and still-growing teen may compete nutritionally with the fetus. Fetuses may show evidence of slower growth in young women (Stang, Story, and Feldman, 2005). The nurse, in collaboration with a nutritionist, can determine the nutritional needs of the pregnant teenager so that education can be tailored appropriately. Table 23-2 describes adolescent nutritional needs in pregnancy.

Weight gain during pregnancy is one of the strongest predictors of infant birthweight. Although precise weight gain goals in adolescence are controversial, pregnant adolescents who gain 25 to 35 pounds have the lowest incidence of low-birthweight babies. Younger teen mothers (ages 13 to 16 years), because of their own growth demands, may need to gain more weight then older teen mothers (ages 17 years and older) to have the same-birthweight baby. Teenagers who begin the pregnancy at a normal weight should be counseled to begin weight gain in the first trimester and to average gains of 1 pound per week for the second and third trimesters (Stang, Story, and Feldman, 2005). Be alert to the teens' views about weight gain. Family support of the pregnant teen can influence adequate weight gain and good nutrition during the pregnancy. Nutrition education should emphasize what causes weight gain and how fetal growth will benefit.

Iron deficiency is the most common nutritional problem among both pregnant and nonpregnant adolescent females. The adolescent may begin a pregnancy with low or absent iron stores due to heavy menstrual periods, a previous pregnancy, growth demands, poor iron intake, or substance abuse. The increased maternal plasma volume and increased fetal demands for iron (especially in the third trimester) can further compromise the adolescent. Iron deficiency in pregnancy may contribute to increased prematurity, **low birthweight**, postpartum hemorrhage, maternal headaches, dizziness, shortness of breath, and so on (Stang et al, 2005). The nurse can reinforce the need for the teen to take prenatal vitamins during pregnancy and after the baby's birth. Vitamins should contain 30 to 60 mg elemental iron daily. The nurse should educate the teen about iron-rich foods and foods that promote iron absorption, such as those containing vitamin C.

Infant Care

Many adolescents have cared for babies and small children and feel confident and competent. Few teens are ever prepared, however, for the reality of 24-hour care of an infant. The nurse can help prepare the teen for the transition to motherhood while she is still pregnant. The trend toward early discharge from the hospital has made prenatal preparation even more important. The nurse can enlist the support of the teen's parents in education about infant care and stimulation. Young fathers-to-be would benefit from this education as well. Adolescents may not know how to communicate with an infant or know about their growth and development, or they may have unrealistic expectations about their children's development (Andreozzi et al, 2002); for example, they may expect their children to feed themselves at an early age or think that their children's behavior is more difficult than an adult mother might think. These skills can be taught and may prevent the child from later developing academic or behavioral problems.

Abusive parenting is more likely to occur when the parents have limited knowledge about normal child development or when they cannot adequately empathize with a child's needs. Younger teens are at risk for being unable to understand what their infant or child needs. This frustration may be exhibited as abusive behavior toward the child. Teens who exhibit more psychological distress or lack social supports should also be continuously assessed for risk of child abuse (Zelenko et al, 2001).

After the birth of the baby, the nurse should observe how the mother responds to infant cues for basic needs and distress. Specific techniques that the new mother can be instructed to use in early childcare are listed in the "How To" box. Parenting education should begin as early as possible. Adolescents who feel competent as parents have higher self-esteem, which in turn positively influences their relationship

---

| HOW TO | **Promote Interactions between the Teen Mother and Her Baby** |

The nurse can make the following suggestions to the teen mother:

- Make eye contact with your baby. Position your face 8 to 10 inches from your baby's face, and smile.
- Talk to your baby often. Use simple sentences, but try to avoid baby talk. Allow time for your baby to "answer." This will help your baby acquire language and communication skills.
- Babies often enjoy when you sing to them, and this may help soothe them during a difficult time or help them fall asleep. Experiment with different songs and melodies to see which your baby seems to like.
- Babies at this age cannot be spoiled. Instead, when babies are held and cuddled, they feel secure and loved.
- Babies cry for many reasons and for no reason at all. If your baby has a clean diaper, has recently been fed, and is safe and secure, he or she may just need to cry for a few minutes. What works to calm your baby may be different from other babies you have known. You can try rocking, gentle reassuring words, soft music, or quiet.
- Make feeding times pleasant for both of you. Do not prop the bottle in your baby's mouth. Instead, you should sit comfortably, hold your baby in your arms, and offer the bottle or breast.
- When babies are awake, they love to play. They enjoy taking walks and looking at brightly colored objects or pictures and toys that make noises, such as rattles and musical toys.

---

with their child (Koniak-Griffin and Turner-Pluta, 2001). Recognizing these good parenting skills and providing positive feedback help a young mother gain confidence in her role.

Schooling and Educational Needs

Teen parents may have had limited school success before the pregnancy. In addition, the demands of pregnancy and parenting may make completing high school difficult or impossible (Johnson, 2008). Returning to school may reduce the possibility of a closely spaced second birth, which would pose both physical and emotional stresses for the teen. Federal legislation passed in 1975 prohibits schools from excluding students because they are pregnant. Instead it is important to keep the pregnant adolescent in school during the pregnancy and to have her return as soon as possible after the birth. Several factors may positively influence a young woman's return to school. These include her parents' level of education and their marital stability, small family size, whether there have been reading materials at home, whether her mother is employed, and whether the young woman is African-American. It may be hard to find affordable quality childcare. Young women who have pregnancy complications may choose home instruction. The availability of home education depends on state board of education regulations. If the teen returns to school, be sure to discuss these needs: (1) using the bathroom frequently, (2) carrying and drinking more fluids or snacks to relieve nausea, (3) climbing stairs and carrying heavy bookbags, and (4) fitting comfortably behind stationary desks. Schools that are committed to keeping students enrolled are generally helpful and will assist in accommodating special needs.

A useful example of a program to reduce teenage pregnancy has been implemented in New Britain, Connecticut as part of the National Campaign to Prevent Teen Pregnancy. This program has applicability for nurses who work with youth in the community. Its goal is to keep young people in school rather than focusing on sex education. Since it began in 1993, only three of about 200 boys and girls who have participated in the multiyear, intensive after-school program have become pregnant or fathered a child. The motto of the program is displayed on the walls and on T-shirts and is "Diplomas Before Diapers." Students spend time developing basic work skills and academics. The philosophy of the program is that college is the only sure way to achieve success in their community, which has lost many of its decent paying factory jobs (Isaacs and Colby, 2008). They spend 1 hour per week only on discussions about sex education.

SCOPE OF MENTAL ILLNESS IN THE UNITED STATES

Mental health and illness can be viewed as a continuum. **Mental health** is defined in *Healthy People 2010* (U.S. Department of Health and Human Services, 2000) as being able to engage in productive activities and fulfilling relationships with other people, to adapt to change, and to cope with adversity. Mental health is an integral part of personal well-being, of both family and interpersonal relationships, and of contributions to community or society. Mental disorders are conditions that are characterized by alterations in thinking, mood, or behavior, which are associated with distress and/or impaired functioning (U.S. Department of Health and Human Services, 2000). **Mental illness** refers collectively to all diagnosable mental disorders. Severe mental disorders are determined by diagnoses and criteria that include the degree of functional disability (American Psychiatric Association, 2000).

Mental disorders occur across the life span and affect persons of all races, cultures, sexes, and educational and socioeconomic groups. They are common in the United States and internationally. In any given year it is estimated that about 26.2% of Americans 18 years and older suffer from a diagnosable mental disorder. This is about one in four adults. When these percentages were applied to the 2004 Census, the estimate was that 57.7 million people were affected. However, the main burden comes from those who suffer from a serious mental illness. At least one in five children and adolescents between ages 9 and 17 years has a diagnosable mental disorder, and about 5% of children and adolescents are extremely impaired by mental, behavioral, and emotional disorders. An estimated 25% of older people experience specific mental disorders that are not part of normal aging, such as depression, anxiety, substance abuse, and dementia. Alzheimer's disease, the primary cause of dementia, affects

about 4.5 million Americans, and this number has more than doubled since 1980. One in 10 people over age 65 years and nearly half of those over age 85 years are affected. Affective disorders include major depression and manic-depressive or bipolar illness. Approximately 20.9 million adults (9.5%) of the U.S. population 18 years and older in a given year have a mood disorder, and the median age of onset is 30 years. Major depressive disorder is the leading cause of disability in Americans between the ages of 15 and 44 years and affects 14.8 million adults 18 years and older. More women than men are affected. Anxiety disorders, including panic disorder, obsessive-compulsive disorder, posttraumatic stress disorder (PTSD), generalized anxiety disorder, and phobias affect as many as 40 million (18.1%) people in the United States annually (National Institute of Mental Health, 2008). Schizophrenia affects about 2.2 million adults a year in the United States with an equal distribution between men and women. Mental disorders can also be a secondary problem among people with other disabilities. Depression and anxiety, for example, occur more frequently among people with disabilities (U.S. Department of Health and Human Services, 2000).

The effect of mental illness on overall health and productivity is often underestimated. In the United States, mental illness is on a par with heart disease and cancer as a cause of disability. Despite the prevalence of mental illness, only 25% of persons with a mental disorder obtain help for their illness in any part of the health care system, and the majority of persons with mental disorders receive no specialty mental health services. In comparison, between 60% and 80% of persons with heart disease seek and receive care. Of those ages 18 years and older getting help, about 15% receive help from mental health specialists. Of young people ages 9 to 17 years who have a mental disorder, 27% receive treatment in the health sector and an additional 20% of children and adolescents use mental health services only in their schools (U.S. Department of Health and Human Services, 2000). Given this information, it is critical that nurses recognize and provide health services for those with mental disorders in nontraditional community settings, such as schools.

BRIEFLY NOTED

Managed care programs tend to reduce coverage for inpatient hospital stays for people with mental illness. However, community survival for those with serious mental illness requires a broad range of well-coordinated services, including mental and physical health, housing assistance, substance abuse treatment for some, and social and vocational rehabilitation.

In addition to diagnosable mental conditions, awareness and concern are increasing regarding the public health burden of stress including the level of global stressors. Strengthening the public health sector to respond to terrorism involves developing mental health responses as well as other defenses. Nurses play an important role in identifying stressful events, assessing stress responses, educating communities, and intervening to prevent or alleviate disability and disease resulting from stress.

Although all of us are vulnerable to stressful life events and may develop mental health problems, persons with chronic and persistent mental illness have many problems. They may not have access to adequate health services or suitable housing. Many accessible and coordinated services are needed to enable people with chronic mental illness to stay in the community, yet these are not always available. The following descriptions of several key issues and populations at high risk for mental illness illustrate the scope of this public health concern.

DEINSTITUTIONALIZATION

Deinstitutionalization involved moving many people from state psychiatric hospitals to communities. The cost of institutional care was perhaps the main reason for the movement; other influences included the discovery of psychotropic medications and civil rights activism (Boyd, 2005; Lamb, 2001). The goal of deinstitutionalization was to improve the quality of life for people with mental disorders by providing services in the communities in which they lived rather than in large institutions. To change the locus of care, large hospital wards were closed and persons with severe mental disorders were returned to the community to live. Many were discharged to the care of family members; others went to nursing homes. Still others were placed in apartments or other types of adult housing; some of these were supervised settings and others were not.

Not surprisingly, the community-based services were not often in place when persons were released to the community, and continuity of care became a problem. According to Mowbry, Grazier, and Holter (2002), although deinstitutionalization was noble in conception, it was bankrupt in implementation. For example, families were not prepared for the treatment responsibilities they had to assume and few mental health systems offered them education and support programs. Although many older adult clients were admitted to nursing homes and personal care settings, education programs were seldom available for staff. The staff often lacked the skills necessary to treat persons with mental disorders. In addition, some clients found themselves in independent settings such as rooming houses and single-room occupancy hotels with little or no supervision and others were placed in jails and prisons (Boardman, 2006). These types of issues prompted additional legislation and advocacy efforts.

The development of community mental health centers (CMHCs) was based partially on the principle that persons with mental disorders had a right to treatment in the least restrictive environment (Boyd, 2005). Although CMHCs did prove less restrictive than institutions, they lacked necessary services. For example, people with severe mental disorders require daily monitoring or hospitalization during acute episodes of illness. Even though hospital services were available, many individuals expressed their rights to refuse treatment and resisted admission. Also, transitional care after discharge

for those who were admitted to hospitals was not available in most communities (Lamb, 2001). With the repeal of the Mental Health Systems Act in 1980, federal leadership was reduced and costs were shifted back to the states from the federal government. This further impeded the implementation and provision of community mental health services. State systems of mental health services developed in varied ways and were often inadequate. In 1990 the Americans with Disabilities Act (ADA) was passed. The ADA mandated that individuals with mental and physical disabilities not be discriminated against and be brought into the mainstream of American life through access to employment and public services (Boyd, 2005). History reveals that past legislation promoted the rights of persons with mental disorders, but litigation was also responsible for the lack of growth, if not the decline, in community mental health services.

AT-RISK POPULATIONS FOR MENTAL ILLNESS
Children and Adolescents

Healthy People 2010 objectives aim to increase the number of children screened and treated for mental health problems. Children are at risk for disruption of normal development by biological, environmental, and psychosocial factors that impair their mental health, interfere with education and social interactions, and keep them from realizing their full potential as adults (U.S. Department of Health and Human Services, 2000). For example, children may become depressed after a loss or may develop behavior problems from abuse or neglect. Examples of environmental factors include crowded living conditions, violence, separation from parents, and lack of consistent caregivers. Ruchkin et al (2007) found that exposure to community violence was related to significant stress and depression in children. Depression, anxiety, and attention deficit disorders are often diagnosed in children, and mental retardation, Down syndrome, and autism are examples of chronic disorders. These problems affect growth and development and influence mental health during adolescence.

Suicide is a significant cause of death in young persons between ages 15 and 24 years. In the Youth Risk Behavior Survey, 6.9% of the respondents had attempted suicide in the 12 months before the survey. Females had a rate of 9.3% compared to males 4.6% (National Institute of Mental Health, 2008). A *Healthy People 2010* objective is to reduce the rate of suicide attempts by adolescents. Some of the risk factors for both adolescents and adults include prior suicide attempts, stressful life events, and access to lethal methods. In addition to depression and substance abuse, adolescent problems include conduct disorders and eating disorders.

Effective service for children, particularly for those with serious emotional disturbances, depends on promoting collaboration across critical areas of support including schools, families, social services, health, mental health, and juvenile justice. Better services and collaboration for children with serious emotional disturbance and their families will result in greater school retention, decreased contact with the juvenile justice system, increased stability of living arrangements, and

HOW TO	Prevent a Culture of Youth Violence

Yearwood (2001) asked Dr. Bell, a nationally known community mental health psychiatrist, how youth violence could be prevented. He suggested that community mental health providers work to do the following:

- Reestablish the village through the creation of coalitions and partnerships.
- Provide access to health care and mental health care to treat conditions associated with violent behavior.
- Improve bonding, attachment, and connectedness by supporting mothers and families.
- Improve self-esteem among youths by recognizing and building on strengths.
- Increase social skills by helping children learn to stop, think, and act.
- Reestablish the adult protective shield by educating and supporting parents.
- Minimize the effects of trauma through early intervention.

From Yearwood E: Is there a culture of youth violence?, *J Child Adolesc Psychiatr Nurs* 15(1):35, 2001.

improved educational, emotional, and behavioral development. One of the objectives of *Healthy People 2010* is to ensure that children in the juvenile justice system receive access to mental health assessment and treatment (U.S. Department of Health and Human Services, 2000). Children and adolescents require a variety of mental health services, including crisis intervention and both short-term and long-term counseling. Nurses working in community settings, well-child clinics, and home health can help offset this problem through prevention and education and by including parents in program planning. Because many children and adolescents lack services or access to them, community mental health assessment activities are essential. Assessment activities include identifying types of programs available or lacking in places in which children and adolescents spend time. Assessments should be performed in schools and in homes of clients, as well as in day-care centers, churches, and organizations that plan and guide age-specific play and entertainment programs. Assessment data are essential for planning and developing programs that address mental health problems prevalent from the prenatal period through adolescence. Preventing problems during these developmental periods can reduce mental health problems in adulthood. Further interventions can be found in the "How To" box on youth violence.

Adults

Stress contributes to adult's mental health status. Sources of stress include multiple-role responsibilities, job insecurity, lack of or diminishing resources, and unstable relationships. These and other conditions can undermine mental health and contribute to serious mental illness, depression, anxiety disorders, and substance abuse. Objectives of *Healthy People 2010* are aimed at helping adults access treatment in order to decrease associated human and economic costs and to reduce rates of suicide.

At some time or another, almost all adults will experience a tragic or unexpected loss, a serious setback, or a time of profound sadness, grief, or distress. Major depressive disorder, however, differs both in intensity and duration from normal sadness or grief. Depression disrupts relationships and the ability to function and can be fatal. In 2004, 32,439 or about 11 per 100,000 people committed suicide in the United States. More than 90% of those who kill themselves have a mental or substance abuse disorder. The diagnosable mental disorder is most likely to be depression. Other risk factors include prior suicide attempts, stressful life events, and access to lethal methods. Four times as many men as women die by suicide, and the highest rate is in white men over age 85. However, women attempt suicide two to three times more often than men (National Institute of Mental Health, 2008). Also domestic violence can lead to posttraumatic stress disorder (PTSD) and major depression among women. Available medications and psychological treatment can help 80% of those with depression, yet only a few seek help. Those with depression are more likely to visit a physician for some other reason, and the mental health condition may not be noted. Therefore it is important that nurses in all settings recognize and screen for depression.

Anxiety disorders are common both in the United States and elsewhere. An alarming 24% of the population will experience an anxiety disorder, many with overlapping substance abuse disorders. Anxiety disorders may have an early onset and are characterized by recurrent episodes of illness and periods of disability.

The lifetime rates of cooccurrence of mental disorders and addictive disorders are high. About one in four persons in the United States experiences a mental disorder in the course of a year (National Institute of Mental Health, 2008). Individuals with cooccurring disorders are more likely to experience a chronic course and to use services than are those with either type of disorder alone, yet the services are often fragmented and treatment occurs in different segments of the system.

How can nurses intervene? The general medical sector, including primary care clinics, hospitals, and nursing homes, has long been identified as the initial point of contact for many adults with mental disorders; for some, these providers may be the only source of mental health services. Early detection and intervention for mental health problems can be increased if persons presenting in primary care are assessed for mental health problems. Nurses are in an ideal position to assess and detect mental health problems. They conduct comprehensive biopsychosocial assessments and are often the professionals most trusted with sensitive information by clients. The use of screening tools for depression, anxiety, substance abuse, and cognitive impairment can assist in early detection and intervention for mental health problems. Suicide can be prevented in many cases by early recognition and treatment of mental disorders and by preventive interventions that focus on risk factors. Thus reduction in access to lethal methods and recognition and treatment of mental and substance abuse disorders are among the most promising approaches to suicide prevention. Nurses, long respected as community health providers, can work with legislators to develop measures to limit access to weapons such as handguns.

Adults with Serious Mental Illness

Objectives of *Healthy People 2010* that address tertiary prevention and are targeted to persons with serious mental illness are to reduce the proportion of homeless adults who have serious mental illness, to increase their employment, and to decrease the number of adults with mental disorders who are incarcerated. Brief hospital stays and inadequate community resources have resulted in an increased number of persons with serious mental illness living on the streets or in jail. It is estimated that 7% of those in jail suffer from a mental illness (U.S. Department of Health and Human Services, 2000). Some people arrested for nonviolent crimes could be better served if diverted from the jail system to a community-based mental health treatment program with linkage to mental health services. Overall about 6% of American adults suffer from serious mental illness. This equates to 1 in 17 people (National Institute of Mental Health, 2008). Approximately 25% of homeless persons in the United States have a serious mental illness, and only 41% of persons with serious mental illness have any form of employment (U.S. Department of Health and Human Services, 2000). Many people with severe mental disorders live in poverty because they lack the ability to earn or maintain a suitable standard of living. Even people who live with family caregivers or in supervised housing are at risk for inadequate services, because the long-term care they require frequently depletes human and fiscal resources. Rehabilitation services, intensive case management, and persistent patient outreach and engagement strategies have been shown to be effective in helping persons with serious mental illness (Schaedle et al, 2002; Ziguras and Stewart, 2000) and in lowering rates of hospitalization.

CASE STUDY

Although not even 2 years old, twins Reba and Tracy have had an eventful childhood. Their 16-year-old mother, Sheri, started prenatal care late in her pregnancy and delivered them at 35 weeks of gestation; they were small for gestational age. Sheri and the baby's father, Jeb, who was 21, had dropped out of high school; he used illegal drugs. The twins left the hospital at 2 weeks of age to live with Sheri at the Salvation Army apartments. Sheri's erratic and hostile behavior was impossible for her parents to tolerate. Her father was on disability compensation for extreme hypertension, and his elderly, bedridden mother lived in the mobile home as well.

Sheri, Jeb, and the twins were evicted from the Salvation Army when Sheri was found to be using drugs, so they moved in with some other young friends. By the time the twins were 15 months old, they showed clear signs of developmental delay. Tracy seemed not to see well, and Reba did not walk yet. Neither spoke an intelligible word and neither

was up to date on immunizations. With Sheri's permission, public health nurse Gina Smith talked with Sheri's parents about taking custody of the twins so that they might get the stability and care they needed. The grandparents agreed, and Sheri looked relieved when she moved the girls in with her parents. Sheri returned to living with friends.

Ms. Smith assessed the safety of the grandparents' mobile home for toddlers. She reviewed the normal milestones the girls should be attaining and taught the grandparents games they could play that would help the girls progress in their speech. She brought children's books from the local Book Buddies program for them to look at together. Normal nutritional needs for toddlers were reviewed. Within months the girls started talking and gaining weight. Tracy got glasses, and Reba got physical therapy to help her learn to walk. With the help of the nurse and their grandparents, the twins began to thrive.

Created by Deborah C. Conway. Assistant Professor, School of Nursing, University of Virginia

Nurses can provide important case management services, coordinate resources for consumers, and function as important members of assertive community treatment (ACT) programs, which provide continuous assistance to persons with mental illness. Nurses by philosophy and training promote independent living and provide support and encouragement for persons to achieve a maximal level of wellness and function. Nurses recognize the importance of the mental health benefits of meaningful work that improves self-esteem and independence. Nursing interventions can be provided in shelters, soup kitchens, and other places in which homeless persons receive food and protection.

Older Adults

In the United States, the population older than 65 years has steadily increased since the year 2000. As the life expectancy of individuals continues to grow, the number experiencing mental disorders in later life will increase. This trend will be expensive and will challenge us to deliver the needed mental health services for older adults. Although many older people maintain highly functional lives, others have mental health deficits associated with normal sensory losses related to aging, failing physical health, difficulty performing activities of daily living, and social deprivation or isolation. Life changes related to work roles and retirement often result in reduced social contacts and support. Other losses are associated with the death of a spouse, other family members, or friends. Reduced social networks and contacts brought about by these life events can influence mood and contribute to serious states of depression. However, depression is not a normal part of aging.

The depression rate among older adults is half that of younger people, but the presence of a physical or chronic illness increases rates of depression. Depression rates for older adults in nursing homes range from 15% to 25%. As previously mentioned, in the United States, men over age 85

Box 23-4	Examples of Sources of Information and Help for People with Mental Illness and Mental Health Problems

- Alcoholics Anonymous
- Al-Anon
- American Anorexia/Bulimia Association
- American Association of Suicidology
- Anxiety Disorders Association of America
- Attention Deficit Information Network
- Children and Adults with Attention Deficit Disorder
- Depressive/Manic Depressive Association
- Gamblers Anonymous
- National Center for Post-Traumatic Stress Disorder
- National Center for Learning Disabilities
- Obsessive-Compulsive Foundation
- Overeaters Anonymous
- Schizophrenics Anonymous

See this book's Evolve website at http://evolve.elsevier.com/stanhope/ foundations for more information about these organizations.

years are in the highest risk category for suicide. Alzheimer's disease and vascular conditions can cause a severe loss of mental abilities with behavioral manifestations. Twenty-five percent of those older than 85 years have some form of dementia. All these conditions affect the mental health status of individuals and their family caregivers.

Older adults, because they may depend on others for care, are at risk for abuse and neglect. Healthy aging activities such as physical activity and establishing social networks improve the mental health of older adults. Older adults underutilize the mental health system and are more likely to be seen in primary care or to be recipients of care in institutions (Robertson and Mosler-Ashley, 2002). The nurse can reach them by organizing health promotion programs through senior centers or other community-based settings. Home health care nurses can assess and intervene to protect those at risk for abuse and neglect, and mental health nurses can provide stress management education for nursing home staff. Stress management for caregivers and respite day-care programs for an older adult family member can increase coping and prevent abuse. Nurses can advocate with health authorities and localities to increase awareness of the importance of meeting the mental health needs of this growing population.

Most family caregivers are women who care for a spouse, an aging parent, or a child with a long-term disabling illness. These caregivers are also at risk for health disruption. The impact of caregiving has been studied with persons who care for those with chronic illness and with fathers of persons with schizophrenia. Caregivers of persons with severely disabling mental disorders often have their mental health threatened by lack of social support (Doornbas, 2002), the stigma of the disease, and chronic strain (Czuchta and McCay, 2001). During stressful life events such as these, it is important for caregivers to know how to manage the many competing demands in their lives.

Activities to improve the mental health status of adults include public education programs, prevention approaches,

and providing mental health services in primary care. Specific approaches to reduce stress include use of community support groups, education about lifestyle management, and worksite programs. Nevertheless, most programs currently available for adults, families, and caregivers with health problems primarily monitor or restore health rather than prevent problems. Therefore the nurse can refer family caregivers and others to organizations such as the local Alliance for the Mentally Ill for group support services. In addition, many national organizations designed for groups with specific problems have local chapters or information that can be accessed on the Internet (Box 23-4). Some state activities expand mental health services to include older adults, and *Healthy People 2010* aims to increase cultural competence within the mental health system.

Cultural Diversity

As discussed in Chapter 5, health care providers need to understand the cultural differences among the various populations they serve. In particular, nurses need to know how various groups in the United States perceive mental health and mental illness and treatment services. These factors affect whether people seek mental health care, how they describe their symptoms, the duration of care, and the outcomes of the care received. Research has shown that various populations use mental health services differently. They may not seek mental health services in the formal system, they may drop out of care, or they may seek care at much later stages of illness, driving the service costs higher. Although all socioeconomic and cultural groups have mental health problems, low-income groups are at greater risk because they often lack minimal resources for meeting basic physical and mental health needs.

The predominant minority populations in the United States are Hispanics, African-Americans, Asian and Pacific Islander Americans, and Native Americans including Native Alaskans. There is a great deal of diversity among these groups as well as within each of these groups because they comprise subgroups with unique cultural differences. Therefore it is important to avoid simplification and overgeneralization in discussions about the characteristics and problems of minorities. Rather, it is critical to conduct community assessments to determine unique characteristics and factors that contribute to mental health needs within specific aggregates of the population. The information presented here is intended to stimulate thinking and awareness for developing nursing activities in individual communities. Community assessments that include data about specific populations from organized agencies such as the Indian Health Service are important because assessment data guide the nurses' activities during all steps of the nursing process. Nurses working within broad-based coalitions of consumers, families, other providers, and community leaders can help achieve the goals of accessible, culturally sensitive, and quality mental health services for all of our people.

LEVELS OF PREVENTION AND THE NURSE IN COMMUNITY HEALTH

It is important for nurses to understand levels of prevention related to poverty, homelessness, mental illness, and teen pregnancy. Nurses can influence political and social policies and programs such as for affordable housing, community outreach services, preventive health services, and other assistance programs for their clients. It is difficult to separate services for these high-risk groups into primary, secondary, and tertiary levels of prevention because interventions can be assigned to more than one level. Affordable housing, for example, may qualify as primary prevention, but it could also be an important secondary or tertiary preventive intervention.

Examples of primary preventive services include affordable housing, housing subsidies, effective job-training programs, employer incentives, preventive health care services, multisystem case management, birth control services, safe-sex education, needle-exchange programs, parent education, and counseling programs. As a primary prevention for mental health problems, nurses can provide education about stress reduction techniques to seniors attending a health fair. They also can form networks with other health professionals to educate policymakers and the public about the value of these preventive services. These programs could provide health education and other forms of care to strengthen community residents and consequently prevent many devastating sequelae.

Secondary preventive activities are aimed at reducing the prevalence or pathological nature of a condition. They involve early diagnosis, prompt treatment, and limitation of disability. For example, these services might target persons on the verge of becoming high risk because of the threat of homelessness, as well as those who are newly homeless.

Examples include supportive and emergency housing, targeted case management, housing subsidies, soup kitchens and meal sites, and comprehensive physical and mental health services. Nurses can work with homeless and near-homeless aggregates to provide education about existing services and strategies for influencing public policy that will provide more comprehensive services for homeless and near-homeless persons. Screening members of a community for depression during National Depression Screening Day is an example of secondary prevention.

Tertiary prevention efforts attempt to restore and enhance functioning. On a community level, these might include support of affordable housing, promotion of psychosocial rehabilitation programs, and involvement in advocacy groups for the mentally ill or homeless population. Tertiary prevention of homelessness includes comprehensive case management, physical and mental health services, emergency-shelter housing, needle-exchange programs, and drug and alcohol treatment. It is important to know about the social and political environment in which problems occur. Nurses can influence politicians and other policymakers at the federal, state, and local levels about the plight of vulnerable populations in their community.

ROLE OF THE NURSE

Nurses have a critical role in the delivery of health care to poor, homeless, mentally ill, and other high-risk people. To be effective, nurses need strong physical and psychosocial assessment skills, current knowledge of available resources, and an ability to convey respect, dignity, and value to each person. Nurses need to be able to work with their clients to promote, maintain, and restore health. Nurses must be prepared to look at the whole picture: the person, the family, and the community interacting with the environment. The assessment may take place in the home or in a community site. Visiting in the home provides a great deal of useful information about the family, their resources, support systems, and knowledge of common housekeeping and health issues. For example, the nurse should assess for the adequacy of heating and cooling, water, cleanliness, cooking facilities, food storage, sleeping arrangements, and safety issues such as loose rugs, fire extinguishers, and fire alarms. The following strategies are important to consider when working with at-risk individuals, families, and aggregates:

- *Create a trusting environment.* Trust is essential to the development of a therapeutic relationship. Many clients and families have been disappointed by their interactions with health care and social systems; they are now mistrustful and see little hope for change. By following through and doing what they say they will do, nurses can establish trusting relationships with clients. If the answer to a question is unknown, an appropriate response might be, "I don't know the answer, but I will try to find out. Let me make a few phone calls and I will let you know Friday." Reliability helps build the foundation for a trusting relationship.

Levels of Prevention	Related to Community Mental Health

PRIMARY PREVENTION: PREVENT DISABILITY

- Educate populations about mental health issues.
- Teach stress reduction techniques.
- Support and provide prenatal education.
- Provide parenting classes.
- Provide support to caregivers.
- Provide bereavement support.

SECONDARY PREVENTION: LIMIT DISABILITY

- Conduct screenings to detect mental health disorders.
- Provide mental health interventions after stressful events.

TERTIARY PREVENTION: REDUCE DISABILITY

- Provide health promotion activities to persons with serious and persistent mental illness.
- Promote support group participation for those with mental health disabilities.
- Advocate for rehabilitation and recovery services.

- *Show respect, compassion, and concern.* High-risk clients are defeated so often by life's circumstances that they may feel that they do not deserve attention. Listen carefully, and empathize with clients so that they believe that they are worthy of care. Clients may not always be treated with respect and dignity by health and social services workers. Because clients respond well to nursing interactions that demonstrate respect, it is helpful to use reflective statements that convey acceptance and understanding of their situation.

- *Do not make assumptions.* A comprehensive and holistic assessment is crucial to identifying underlying needs. Just because a young mother with three preschool children misses a clinic appointment does not mean that she does not care about the health of her children; she may not have transportation, one child may be sick, or she may be sick. Find out the reason for the absence, and help solve the problem.

- *Coordinate a network of services and providers.* The multiple and complex needs of high-risk clients make working with them challenging. Many services exist, but often the people who could benefit are unaware of their existence. Developing a coordinated network of providers involves conducting a thorough assessment of the service area to identify available federal, state, and local services. Where are the food banks? Where can you get clothing? What programs are available in the local churches and schools? How do people access these services? What are the eligibility requirements? How helpful are the people who work at the service agencies? What service is provided to eligible individuals and families? Specifically, four types of programs in the community have the strongest evidence of encouraging pregnancy prevention: HIV and sexuality education programs with a life skills component; clinic-based programs with a focus on sexual behavior; service learning programs that include both volunteer work and classroom discussions about the service; and programs that are multifaceted and have youth development components, health care services, and close relationships with staff (Kirby, 2001a). Nurses can identify these services and help link families with appropriate resources (see "How To" box). In addition, a thorough assessment of available services in a nurse's service area can identify significant gaps in essential services. Once these gaps are identified, nurses serving as case managers can work with other health care providers and with community members to advocate for necessary services.

- *Advocate for accessible health care services.* Poverty, homelessness, mental illness, and teen pregnancy can create a number of barriers that prevent access to health care services. Nurses can advocate for accessible and convenient locations of health care services. Neighborhood clinics, mobile vans, and home visits can bring health care to people unable to access care. Coordinating services at a central location often improves client compliance because it reduces the stress of getting to multiple places. Many shelters and transitional housing units have clinics on site.

HOW TO	Apply Case Management Strategies

- Determine available services and resources.
- Determine missing resources, and develop creative solutions for service deficiencies.
- Integrate and use clinical skills.
- Establish long-term therapeutic relationships with families.
- Enhance the family's personal coping skills, survival skills, and resourcefulness.
- Facilitate service delivery on behalf of the family.
- Guide the family toward the use of appropriate community resources.
- Communicate and collaborate with professionals from multiple service systems.
- Advocate for the development of creative solutions.
- Participate in policy analysis and political activism.
- Manipulate and modify the environment as needed.
- Connect with local, state, and federal legislators.

These multiservice centers provide health care, social services, day care, drug and alcohol recovery programs, and comprehensive case management.

- *Focus on prevention.* Nurses can use every opportunity to provide preventive care and health teaching. Important health promotion (primary prevention) topics include child and adult immunization, education regarding sound nutrition, foot care, safe sex, contraception, and prevention of chronic illness. Screening for health problems such as TB, diabetes, hypertension, foot problems, and anemia is an important form of secondary prevention. Know what other screening and health promotion services are available in the target area, such as nutrition programs, job-training programs, educational programs, housing programs, and legal services. All these services may be included in a comprehensive plan of care. Younger sisters of pregnant teens are twice as likely to become pregnant themselves. Thus health teaching about sexuality issues when seeing the teens in the home or clinic can increase their knowledge and awareness.

- *Know when to walk beside the client and when to encourage the client to walk ahead.* This area is often difficult for the nurse to implement. Nursing interventions range from extensive care activities to minimal support. At times, nursing actions include providing encouragement and support or providing information. At other times, nurses may actually call a pediatrician to set up an appointment for a sick child and may call again to see that the appointment was kept. Nurses assess for the presence of strengths, problem-solving ability, and coping ability of an individual or family while providing information on where and how to gain access to services. For example, a local hospital may provide free mammograms for uninsured women. Women who qualify for this free service may not take advantage of it because they are afraid that they may have breast cancer. Nurses can find out about this important service, inform the women of the service, teach them about the importance of preventive care, and assess and deal with fear and anxiety. The challenge for the nurse becomes choosing whether to schedule the appointments for the women or to simply provide them with a referral sheet, knowing that many will not follow through. The choice is not clear, but the goal is to make a needed screening intervention available without taking away the woman's right to decide what to do for herself.

- *Develop a network of support for yourself.* Caring for high-risk populations is challenging, rewarding, and at times exhausting. It is important to find a source of personal strength, renewal, and hope. The people you encounter are often looking to you to maintain hope and provide encouragement. Discover for yourself what restores and encourages you. For some nurses it is poetry, music, painting, or weaving. For others it is a walk in a peaceful place, a weekend retreat, a good run, a workout at the gym, or meeting with other nurses who are engaged in the same work. Be attentive to your own needs, and create the time and space to restore your spirit.

CLINICAL APPLICATION

A local youth-serving agency requested the assistance of a nurse in community health, Kristen, in the implementation of a new high school-based program for pregnant and parenting teen girls. The primary goal of the program is to keep these teens in school through graduation. The secondary goal is to provide knowledge and skills about healthy pregnancy, labor and delivery, and parenting. After delivery, students enrolled in this program were paid for school attendance and this money could be used to defray the costs of childcare.

A nurse in community health was the ideal choice to conduct the educational sessions. The group met weekly during the lunch hour. The curriculum that was developed had topics ranging from early pregnancy through the toddler years. Occasionally, Kristen brought in outside speakers such as a labor and delivery nurse or an early intervention specialist.

She also met individually with each enrolled student to provide case management services. Ideally, she would ensure that each student had a health care provider for prenatal care, that each was visited at home by a nurse in community health, that each had enrolled in WIC and Medicaid if eligible, and that both the pregnant teen and her partner knew about other parenting and support groups.

One educational session that was particularly interesting was the discussion about the postpartum course—the 6 weeks after delivery. There were many lively discussions about labor experiences, as well as some emotional discussions about the reality of coming home with a baby and changes in the relationship with their male partner. Many girls benefited from understanding the normalcy of postpartum blues, but one young woman recognized that she had a more serious and persistent depression and privately approached the nurse for assistance.

At the end of the first school year, the dropout rate for pregnant and parenting teens had been reduced by half and preterm labor rates had also declined. The local school board and a local youth-serving agency joined together to provide financial support to continue this program for an additional 2 years. Kristen was asked to expand the educational programs and interventions she had developed.
What are some directions in which Kristen might expand the program? List four.
Answers are in the back of the book.

REMEMBER THIS!

- Poverty and homelessness affect the health status of people.
- To understand poverty, homelessness, mental illness, and teen pregnancy, consider your personal beliefs and attitudes, clients' perceptions of their condition, and the social, political, cultural, and environmental factors that influence the client's situation.
- The definition of poverty varies depending on the source consulted. The federal government defines poverty on the basis of income, family size, age of the head of household, and number of children younger than 18 years. Those who are poor insist that poverty has less to do with income and more to do with a lack of family, friends, love, and support.
- Factors leading to the growing number of poor persons in the United States include decreased earnings, diminishing availability of low-cost housing, increases in the number of households headed by women (women's incomes are traditionally lower than men's), inadequate education, lack of marketable job skills, welfare reform, and reduced Social Security payments to children.
- Poverty has a direct effect on health and well-being across the life span. Poor persons have higher rates of chronic illness, higher infant morbidity and mortality, shorter life expectancy, and more complex health problems.
- At present, the following groups often constitute the homeless in both rural and urban areas: families, single mothers, single women, recently unemployed persons, substance abusers, adolescent runaways, mentally ill individuals, and single men.
- Factors contributing to homelessness include an increase in the number of persons living in poverty, diminishing availability of low-cost housing, increased unemployment, substance abuse, lack of treatment facilities for mentally ill persons, domestic violence, and family situations causing children to run away.
- The complex health problems of homeless persons include an inability to get adequate rest, exercise, and nutrition; exposure; infectious diseases; acute and chronic illness; infestations; trauma; and mental health problems.
- The provision of reproductive health care services to teens requires sensitivity to the special needs of this age group including knowing about state laws concerning confidentiality and services for birth control, pregnancy, abortion, and adoption.

- Factors such as a history of sexual victimization, family dysfunction, substance use, and failure to use birth control can influence whether a young woman becomes pregnant.
- Adolescents, especially those who become pregnant, have special nutritional needs.
- The pregnant teen will need support during and after the pregnancy from the family and friends and from the father of the baby.
- Prevalence rates for mental health problems are high, and people are at risk for threats to mental health at all ages across the life span.
- Low income and minority groups are often at increased risk for mental illness because they may lack access to services.
- Nurses have a critical role in the delivery of care to persons who are high risk. Nurses bring to each client encounter the ability to assess the client in context, and to intervene in ways that restore, maintain, or promote health.

WHAT WOULD YOU DO?

1. Examine health statistics and demographic data to identify the rate of poverty and homelessness in your geographic area. What resources and agencies are available in your area to support homeless persons? What services are available from federal, state, and local sources? Identify a specific geographic region and assess this target area in terms of services for poor and homeless persons. Do a literature search to identify recommended state-of-the-art interventions for poor and homeless persons. Compare the recommended programs and interventions with those available in your target area. How does your area measure up? Give some specific recommendations about how you would fill the gaps.

2. Examine the specific programs identified in the preceding assessment. How do those who need services access them? Working with other students, make appointments with key persons in the agencies identified to find out what each agency offers, which particular aggregate is served, how clients access the services, who is eligible, how the agency receives funding, and what methods are used to evaluate the agency's ability to meet the needs of its targeted aggregates. Give some examples.

3. Identify nurses in your community who work with the homeless or with other vulnerable groups. Invite these nurses to come to a class meeting to share their experiences. What constitutes a typical workday? What are the rewards and challenges of working with vulnerable populations? How do they deal with the frustrations and challenges of their work? What advice might they offer to students working with vulnerable aggregates? What programs do they recommend? How would you advocate for vulnerable aggregates in your practice?

4. Design and offer a childbirth preparation class for pregnant teens and their support persons. Include a plan for identifying potential participants, select a site that is accessible, and develop an evaluation method.

5. For 1 week, keep a list of incidents related to mental health problems that you learn about in the local media. Categorize the incidents according to age, sex, and socioeconomic, ethnic, or minority status.

6. Visit with representatives of your local self-help organizations for consumers to determine their adequacy of resources for the populations discussed in this chapter.

■ REFERENCES

American College of Obstetricians and Gynecologists: *Adolescent facts: pregnancy and STDs*, Washington, DC, 2007, ACOG.

American Psychiatric Association: *Diagnostic and statistical manual of mental disorders,* ed 4-TR, Washington, DC, 2000, APA.

Andreozzi L et al: Attachment classifications among 18-month-old children of adolescent mothers, *Arch Pediatr Adolesc Med* 156:20, 2002.

Bearman P, Bruckner H: *Power in numbers: peer effects on adolescent girls' sexual debut and pregnancy*, Washington, DC, 1999, National Campaign to Prevent Preteen Pregnancy.

Bensussen-Walls W, Saewye EM: Teen-focused care versus adult-focused care for the high risk pregnant adolescent: an outcomes evaluation, *Pub Health Nurs* 18:424–435, 2001.

Blau JM: Economic indicators provide future market insights, *Urol Times* 32:32–36, 2004.

Bloom KC et al: Barriers to prenatal care for homeless pregnant females, *J Obstet Gynecol Neonat Nurs* 33(4):428–435, 2004.

Boardman JB: Health access and integration for adults with serious and persistent mental illness, *Fam Syst Health* 24(1):3–18, 2006.

Boyd MA: Social change and mental health. In Boyd MA, editor: *Psychiatric nursing: contemporary practice*, ed 3, Philadelphia, 2005, Lippincott Williams & Wilkins.

Centers for Disease Control and Prevention: Youth risk behavior surveillance—United States, 2007, *MMWR Morb Mortal Wkly Rep* 57(SS-4):1, 21, 2008.

Child trends: a demographic portrait of statutory rape, Washington, DC, 2005, The Office of Population Affairs, USDHHS.

Craft-Rosenberg M, Powel SR, Culp K: Health status and resources of rural homeless women and children, *West J Nurs Res* 22:863–878, 2000.

Czuchta DM, McCay E: Help seeking for parents of individuals experiencing a first episode of schizophrenia, *Arch Psychiatr Nurs* 15(4):159, 2001.

Doornbas MM: Family caregivers and the mental health system: reality and dreams, *Arch Psychiatr Nurs* 16(1):39, 2002.

Elders J: "An urban health crisis," Keynote address presented at Mothers and Children 1994, Washington, DC, 1994.

Ellen JM et al: Perceived social cohesion and prevalence of sexually transmitted diseases, *Sex Transm Dis* 31:117–123, 2004.

Emerson E: Poverty and children with intellectual disabilities in the world's richer countries, *J Intellect Dev Disabil* 20:319–339, 2004.

Evans GW, Boxhill L, Pinkava M: Poverty and maternal responsiveness: the role of maternal stress and social resources, *Int J Behav Develop* 32(3):232–237, 2008.

Fergusson DM, Boden JM, Horwood LJ: Abortion among young females and subsequent life outcomes, *Perspect Sex Reprod Health* 39(1):6–12, 2007.

Fowles ER, Hendricks JA, Walker LO: Identifying healthy eating strategies in low-income pregnant women: applying a positive deviance model, *Health Care Women Int* 26:807–820, 2005.

Franzetta H et al: *Facts at a glance: child trends*, 2005. Sponsored by the William and Flora Hewlett Foundation, Washington, DC. Retrieved Oct 5, 2008, from http://www.childtrends.org.

Harrykissoon SD, Rickert VI, Wiemann CW: Prevalence and patterns of intimate partner violence among adolescent mothers during the postpartum period, *Arch Pediatr Adolesc Med* 156:325, 2002.

Hock-Long L et al: Access to adolescent reproductive health services: financial and structural barriers to care, *Perspect Sex Reprod Health* 35:144–147, 2003.

Isaacs SL and Colby DC, editors: To improve health and health care. Volume XI. *The Robert Wod Johnson Foundation anthology,* San Francisco, Jossey-Bass, 2008:59–82.

Jacobs BB: Respect for human dignity: a central phenomenon to philosophically unite nursing theory and practice through consilience of knowledge, *ANS Adv Nurs Sci* 24(1):17–35, 2001.

Johnson P: *Reduce teen pregnancy to reduce the dropout rate,* 2008. Retrieved Sept 15, 2008, from http://carborocitizen.com/main/2008/05/08/reduce-teen-pregnacies-to-reduce-the-dropout-rate/.

Kelley-Moore JA, Ferraro KF: The black/white disability gap in later life? *J Gerontol, Ser B: Psychol Serv Social Sci* 59: S34–S43, 2004.

Kirby D: *Emerging answers: research findings on programs to reduce teen pregnancy,* Washington, DC, 2001a, National Campaign to Prevent Teen Pregnancy.

Kirby D: Understanding what works and what doesn't in reducing adolescent sexual risk-taking, *Fam Plann Perspect* 33(6):276, 2001b.

Klein JD and the Committee on Adolescence: Adolescent pregnancy: current trends and issues, *Pediatrics* 116:281, 2005.

Koniak-Griffin D, Turner-Pluta C: Health risks and psychosocial outcomes of early childbearing: a review of the literature, *J Perinat Neonat Nurs* 15:1–17, 2001.

Krishnakumar A, Black M: Family processes within three-generation households and adolescent mothers' satisfaction with father involvement, *J Fam Psychol* 17:488–498, 2003.

Lamb HR: Deinstitutionalization at the beginning of the new millennium. In Lamb HR, Wienberger LE, editors: *Deinstitutionalization: promise and problems—new directions for mental health services,* San Francisco, 2001, Jossey-Bass.

Lopez-Zetina J et al: Prevalence of HIV and hepatitis B and self-reported injection risk behavior during detention among street-recruited injection drug users in Los Angeles County, 1994-1996, *Addiction* 96:589–596, 2001.

Marcell AV, Raine T, Eyre SL: Where does reproductive health fit into the lives of adolescent males? *Perspect Sex Reprod Health* 35:180–186, 2003.

Marsiglio W: Adolescent males' orientation toward paternity and contraception, *Fam Plann Perspect* 25(1):22, 1993.

Moore KA: *Teen births: examining the recent increase.* The National Campaign to Prevent Teen and Unplanned Pregnancy, October 2008. Retrieved Oct 8, 2008, from http://TheNationalcampaign.org/resources/pdf/TeenBirths_Examineincrease.pdf.

Mowbry CT, Grazier WL, Holter M: Managed behavioral health care in the public sector: will it become the third shame of the states? *Psychiatr Serv* 53(2):157, 2002.

National Coalition for the Homeless: *How many people experience homelessness?* Fact sheet #2, Washington, DC, June 2008a, Author. Retrieved Oct 9, 2008, from http://www.nationalhomeless.org/publications/facts.html.

National Coalition for the Homeless: *Who is homeless?* Fact sheet #3, Washington, DC, June 2008b, Author. Retrieved Oct 9, 2008, from http://www.nationalhomeless.org/publications/facts.html.

National Institute of Mental Health: *The numbers count: mental disorders in America.* Retrieved Oct 6, 2008, from http://www.nimh.nih.gov/health/publications/the=numbers=count-mental-disorders-in-america.

O'Connell JJ et al: A public health approach to reducing morbidity and mortality among homeless people in Boston, *J Public Health Manag Pract* 11:311–317, 2005.

One tough job.org. *Tips on talking about sex,* 2008. Retrieved Oct 9, 2008, from www.onetoughjob.org.

Osborne LN, Rhodes JE: The role of life stress and social support in the adjustment of sexually victimized pregnant and parenting adolescents, *Am J Community Psychol* 29(6):833, 2001.

Rew S: Relationships of sexual abuse, connectedness, and loneliness to perceived well-being in homeless youth, *J Specialists Pediatr Nurs* 7:51–74, 2002.

Rew L et al: Interaction of duration of homelessness and gender on adolescent sexual health indicators, *J Nurs Schol* 4(2): 109–115, 2008.

Robertson S, Mosler-Ashley P: Patterns of confiding and factors influencing mental health service use in older adults, *Clin Gerontol* 26(1-2):101–116, 2002.

Ruchkin V et al: Violence exposure and psychopathology in urban youth: the mediating role of posttraumatic stress, *J Abnormal Psychol* 35(4):578–593, 2007.

Schaedle R et al: A comparison of expert's perspectives on assertive community treatment and intensive case management, *Psychiatr Serv* 53(2):207, 2002.

Schendel D, Bhasin TK: Birth weight and gestational age characteristics of children with autism, including a comparison with other developmental disabilities, *Pediatrics* 121:1155–1161, 2008.

Stang J, Story M, Feldman S: Nutrition in adolescent pregnancy, *Int J Childbirth Educ* 20(2):4–11, 2005.

Sterigiopoulos V, Herrmann N: Old and homeless: a review and survey of older adults who use shelters in an urban setting, *Canadian J Psychiatry* 48:374–380, 2003.

U.S. Bureau of the Census: *Poverty: 2007 highlights.* Retrieved Sept 23, 2008, from www.census/gov/hhes/www/poverty/poverty07/pov07hi.html.

U.S. Bureau of the Census: *Current population survey,* Washington, DC, 2005, U.S. Government Printing Office.

U.S. Conference of Mayors: *A status report on hunger and homelessness in America's cities: 2004,* available from the U.S. Conference of Mayors, 2005. 1620 Eye St. NW, 4th Floor, Washington, DC, 20006–4005.

U.S. Department of Health and Human Services: *Healthy People 2010: understanding and improving health,* ed 2, Washington, DC, 2000, U.S. Government Printing Office.

Ward E: *Top tips for pregnancy nutrition,* 2006. Retrieved Aug 20, 2008, from http://webmd.com/solutions/infant-nutrition/nutrition-tips.

Whitman RL et al: *Interwoven lives,* Mahwah, NJ, 2001, Lawrence Erlbaum.

Zedlewski SR, Chaudry A, Simms M: *A new safety net for low-income families,* Washington, DC, 2008, The Urban Institute.

Zelenko MA et al: The child abuse potential inventory and pregnancy outcome in expectant adolescent mothers, *Child Abuse Negl* 25:1481, 2001.

Ziguras SJ, Stewart GW: A meta-analysis of the effectiveness of mental health case management over 20 years, *Psychiatr Serv* 51(11):1410, 2000.

Alcohol, Tobacco, and Other Drug Problems in the Community

Mary Lynn Mathre

ADDITIONAL RESOURCES

These related resources are found either in the appendix at the back of this book or on the book's website at http://evolve.elsevier.com/stanhope/foundations.

@ Evolve Website

• Community Assessment Applied

• Case Study, with questions and answers
• Quiz review questions
• WebLinks, including link to *Healthy People 2010* website

OBJECTIVES

After reading this chapter, the student should be able to:
1. Describe attitudes about alcohol, tobacco, and other drug problems.
2. Differentiate among these terms: substance use, abuse, dependence, and addiction.
3. Discuss the differences among the major psychoactive drug categories of depressants, stimulants, marijuana, hallucinogens, and inhalants.

4. Explain the role of the nurse in primary, secondary, and tertiary prevention of alcohol, tobacco, and other drug problems as it relates to individual clients and their families.
5. Explain the effect of substance abuse on the community and on people within the community.

CHAPTER OUTLINE

SCOPE OF THE PROBLEM
Definitions
PSYCHOACTIVE DRUGS
Depressants
Stimulants
Marijuana
Hallucinogens
Inhalants
PREDISPOSING AND CONTRIBUTING
FACTORS FOR SUBSTANCE ABUSE
PRIMARY PREVENTION AND THE
ROLE OF THE NURSE
Drug Education

SECONDARY PREVENTION AND THE
ROLE OF THE NURSE
Assessing for ATOD Problems
Drug Testing
High-Risk Groups
Codependency and Family Involvement
TERTIARY PREVENTION AND THE
ROLE OF THE NURSE
Detoxification
Addiction Treatment
Smoking Cessation Programs
Support Groups
NURSE'S ROLE

KEY TERMS

addiction treatment: focuses on the addiction process by helping clients view addiction as a chronic disease and assisting them in making lifestyle changes to halt the progression of the disease.

Alcoholics Anonymous (AA): lay, self-help group that practices a 12-step approach to recovery for persons suffering from alcoholism.

alcoholism: addiction to alcohol.

blood alcohol concentration (BAC): also called blood alcohol level (BAL); the amount of alcohol in the blood, commonly expressed as grams of alcohol per 100 milliliters of blood. Most state legal limits of intoxication while driving are 0.08% or 0.1%.

brief interventions: interventions that are sometimes made by health care professionals who are not treatment experts and that have been found to be effective in helping alcohol, tobacco, and other drug abusers and addicts reduce their consumption or follow through with treatment referrals. They can have six parts: feedback, responsibility, advice, menu of options, empathy, and self-efficacy.

codependency: a condition characterized by preoccupation and extreme dependency (emotionally, socially, and sometimes physically) on a person. Eventually this dependence on another person becomes a pathological condition that affects the person in all of his or her relationships.

cross-tolerance: condition in which tolerance to one drug results in a decreased response to another drug in the same general category.

denial: a primary symptom of addiction. The person may lie about use, play down use, and blame; may also use anger or humor to avoid acknowledging the problem to self and to others.

depressants: drugs that reduce the activity of the central nervous system.

detoxification: the process of allowing time for the body to metabolize and/or excrete accumulations of a drug. It is often called social detoxification if the withdrawal symptoms are not life-threatening and do not require medication, or medical detoxification if the symptoms require medical management.

drug addiction: a pattern of abuse characterized by an overwhelming preoccupation with the use (compulsive use) of a drug and securing its supply, and a high tendency for relapse if the drug is removed.

drug dependence: physiological change in the central nervous system as a result of chronic drug use.

enabling: the act of shielding or preventing the addict from experiencing the consequences of the addiction. It also applies to shielding individuals from the consequences of their actions more generally.

fetal alcohol syndrome (FAS): a condition that may occur when a woman has consumed alcohol regularly during pregnancy (about six drinks per day). Infants tend to be of low birthweight and mentally retarded and may have behavioral, facial, limb, genital, cardiac, or neurological impairments.

hallucinogens: (also known as psychedelics): drugs that stimulate the nervous system and produce varied changes in perception and mood.

harm reduction: (also called harm minimization): a public health approach to substance abuse problems. This approach acknowledges, without judgment, that licit and illicit drug use is a reality, and the focus of interventions is to minimize these drugs' harmful effects rather than to simply ignore or condemn them; also to facilitate responsible use of substances.

inhalants: substances, often common household chemicals, that are inhaled by drug users. Inhalants fall into four categories: volatile organic solvents, aerosols, volatile nitrites, and gases; they are inhaled from bottles, aerosol cans, or soaked cloth.

injection drug users (IDUs): includes intravenous and subcutaneous drug injection, with the latter usually being over the abdominal area and called "popping." The sharing of paraphernalia to prepare or inject the drug can result in transmission of blood-borne pathogens, such as human immunodeficiency virus (HIV).

mainstream smoke: smoke inhaled and exhaled by the smoker.

MDMA (Ecstasy): semisynthetic drug classified as a mood elevator that produces feelings of empathy, openness, and well-being.

polysubstance use or abuse: drugs from different categories used together or at different times to regulate how the person feels.

psychoactive drugs: drugs that affect mood, perception, and thought.

set: expectation, including unconscious expectation, as a variable determining a person's reaction to a drug.

setting: the environment—physical, social, and cultural—as a variable determining a person's reaction to a drug.

sidestream smoke: smoke that comes off a cigarette from the outside rather than being drawn through the cigarette.

stimulants: drugs that increase the activity of the central nervous system, causing wakefulness.

substance abuse: use of any substance that threatens a person's health or impairs his or her social or economic functioning.

tolerance: in pharmacology, the need for increasing doses of a drug over time to maintain the same effect.

withdrawal: physical and psychological symptoms that occur when a drug upon which a person is dependent is removed.

Substance abuse is the number one national health problem, causing more deaths, illnesses, and disabilities than any other health condition. Considerable death and disability are caused by the use of alcohol, tobacco, and illicit drugs. The substance abuser is not only at risk for personal health problems but also may be a threat to the health and safety of family members, co-workers, and other members of the community. Substance abuse and addiction affect all ages, races, sexes, and segments of society. As seen in the WebLinks at http://evolve.elsevier.com/stanhope/foundations; *Healthy People 2010* (U.S. Department of Health and Human Services, 2000) lists tobacco as the third priority area and alcohol and other drugs as the fourth priority area, with a total of 46 objectives, as well as related objectives in other priority areas. The newer phrase, *alcohol, tobacco, and other drug (ATOD) problems,* rather than *substance abuse,* reminds us that alcohol and tobacco represent the major drugs of abuse when discussing substance abuse, drug addiction, or chemical dependency.

SCOPE OF THE PROBLEM

ATOD abuse and addiction can cause multiple health problems for individuals. Heavy ATOD use is associated with many problems, including low-birth-weight neonates and congenital abnormalities; accidents, homicides, and suicides; chronic diseases, such as cardiovascular diseases, cancer, and lung disease; violence; and family disruption. Factors that contribute to the substance abuse problem include lack of knowledge about the use of drugs; the labeling of certain drugs (alcohol, nicotine, and caffeine) as nondrugs; lack of quality control of illegal drugs; and drug laws that label certain drug users as criminals.

Every culture has beliefs and attitudes toward ATOD. These attitudes are influenced by the way society categorizes drugs as either "good" or "bad." In the United States, good drugs are over-the-counter (OTC) drugs or drugs prescribed by a health care provider, although this makes them no less problematic or addictive. Bad drugs are the illegal drugs, and persons who use these drugs are considered criminals regardless of whether the drug has caused any problems. Americans rely heavily on prescription and OTC drugs to relieve (or mask) anxiety, tension, fatigue, and physical or emotional pain. Rather than learning nonmedicinal methods of coping, many people choose the "quick fix" and take pills to deal with their problems or negative feelings. Addicts are often viewed as immoral, weak-willed, or irresponsible persons who should try harder to help themselves. Although alcoholism was recognized as a disease by the American Medical Association in 1954, and drug addiction was recognized as a disease some years later, much of the public and many health care professionals have failed to change their attitudes and accept alcoholics and addicts as ill persons in need of health care.

In many cultures, people with ATOD problems are treated through the criminal justice system. However, a new approach, the harm reduction model, is a health care approach to ATOD problems. This approach was first used in Great Britain, the Netherlands, Germany, Switzerland, and Australia. Increased interest and momentum are spreading throughout Europe and Canada. This new public health model recognizes the following:
- Addiction is a health problem.
- Any psychoactive drug can be abused.
- Accurate information can help people make responsible decisions about drug use.
- People who have ATOD problems can be helped.

This approach accepts that psychoactive drug use is endemic, and it focuses on pragmatic interventions, especially education, to reduce the adverse consequences of drug use and get treatment for addicts. The United States has already taken a **harm reduction** approach with tobacco and alcohol. Educational campaigns are used to inform the public about the health risks of tobacco use. Warnings have appeared on tobacco product labels since 1967 as a result of the surgeon general's 1966 report on the dangers of smoking. In 1971 a ban on television and radio cigarette advertising was imposed. Cigarette smoking has decreased since that time. Smoking is on the decline among eighth and twelfth graders. According to the report, 4% of eighth graders smoked in 2006, down from 5.5% in 2001. For the twelfth graders, in 2006, 12% smoked compared to 19% in 2001 (Johnson, O'Malley, and Bachman 2007). Education is continuing to address the dangers of alcohol abuse and to establish guidelines for safe alcohol use.

Nurses need to identify the causes of various health problems and plan realistic, nonjudgmental, holistic, and positive actions. One approach is the harm reduction model for ATOD problems. To develop a therapeutic attitude, the nurse must realize that any drug can be abused, that anyone may develop drug dependence, and that drug addiction can be successfully treated.

DEFINITIONS

The terms *drug use* and *drug abuse* have virtually lost their usefulness because the public and government have narrowed the term *drug* to include only illegal drugs rather than including prescription, OTC, and legal recreational drugs. The current phrase *alcohol, tobacco, and other drugs* (ATOD) is a reminder that the leading drug problems involve alcohol and tobacco. The term *substance* broadens the scope to include alcohol, tobacco, legal drugs, and even foods. **Substance abuse** is the use of any substance that threatens a person's health or impairs social or economic functioning. This definition is more objective and universal than the government's definition of drug abuse, which is the use of a drug without a prescription or any use of an illegal drug. Although any drug or food can be abused, this chapter focuses on psychoactive drugs—drugs that affect mood, perception, and thought.

Drug dependence and drug addiction are often used interchangeably, but they are not synonymous. **Drug dependence** is a state of neuroadaptation (a physiologic change in the central nervous system [CNS] and alterations in other systems caused by the chronic, regular administration of a drug).

People who are dependent on drugs must continue using them to prevent symptoms of withdrawal (Introduction, *Merck Manual,* 2008). For example, when a person is given an opiate such as morphine on a regular basis for pain management, the morphine needs to be gradually tapered rather than abruptly stopped to prevent symptoms of **withdrawal**. Drug dependence is both psychological and physical. Psychological dependence includes feelings of satisfaction and a desire to repeat the drug experience or to avoid the discomfort of not having the drug. Craving and compulsion are part of this dependence. Physical dependence is seen when there is an abstinence effect. This effect results in physical changes that are uncomfortable (Introduction, *Merck Manual,* 2008).

Drug addiction is a pattern of abuse characterized by an overwhelming preoccupation with the use (compulsive use) of a drug and securing its supply and a high tendency to relapse if the drug is removed. Addicts may be both physically and psychologically dependent on a drug and there may be a risk of harm and the need to stop drug use (Introduction, *Merck Manual,* 2008).

Alcoholism is addiction to the drug called *alcohol*. Alcoholism and drug addiction are recognized as illnesses under a biopsychosocial model. Simply stated, the disease concept of addiction and alcoholism identifies them as chronic and progressive diseases in which a person's use of a drug or drugs continues despite problems it causes in any area of life—physical, emotional, social, economic, or spiritual.

PSYCHOACTIVE DRUGS

Although any drug can be abused, ATOD abuse and addiction problems generally involve **psychoactive drugs**. These drugs, which can alter emotions, are used for enjoyment in social and recreational settings and for personal use to self-medicate physical or emotional discomfort. Psychoactive drugs are divided into categories according to their effect on the CNS and the general feelings or experiences the drugs may induce. The Internet or a pharmacology text can provide detailed information on these drug categories (e.g., depressants, stimulants, hallucinogens). Often, if persons cannot obtain their drug of choice, another drug from the same category will be substituted. For example, a person who cannot drink alcohol may begin using a benzodiazepine as an alternative because both are CNS depressants.

DEPRESSANTS

Depressants lower the body's overall energy level, reduce sensitivity to outside stimulation, and, in high doses, induce sleep. Low doses of depressants may produce a feeling of stimulation caused by initial sedation of the inhibitory centers in the brain. In general, depressants decrease heart rate, respiration rate, muscular coordination, and energy while dulling the senses. Higher doses lead to coma and, if the vital functions shut down, death. Major categories include alcohol, barbiturates, benzodiazepines, and the opioids. This chapter discusses alcohol and heroin.

Alcohol

Alcohol (ethyl alcohol, or ethanol) is the oldest and most widely used psychoactive drug in the world. Roughly 45 to 50% of adults are current drinkers; 20% are former drinkers, and 30 to 35% are lifetime abstainers. Between seven and 10% of adults meet the criteria for having an alcohol disorder in any given year (Alcohol, *Merck Manual,* 2008). In 2006 a national survey found that young people between the ages of 12 and 20 are more likely to use alcohol than use tobacco or illicit drugs, including marijuana. Youth tend to drink less often than adults, but they consume more alcohol per occasion. On average, youth report consuming five drinks per occasion, and they increasingly binge drink. Specifically, 80% of college students indicate that they drink alcohol, about 40% binge drink, and around 20% say they binge drink three or more times in a 2-week time period (National Institute on Alcohol Abuse and Alcoholism, 2007). Alcohol abuse costs billions of dollars in lost productivity, property damage, medical expenses from alcohol-related illnesses and accidents, family disruptions, alcohol-related violence, and neglect or abuse of children.

Chronic alcohol abuse has multiple metabolic and physiological effects on all organ systems. Gastrointestinal (GI) disturbances include inflammation of the GI tract, malabsorption, ulcers, liver problems, and cancers. Cardiovascular disturbances include cardiac dysrhythmias, cardiomyopathy, hypertension, atherosclerosis, and blood dyscrasias. CNS problems include depression, sleep disturbances, memory loss, organic brain syndrome, Wernicke-Korsakoff syndrome, and alcohol withdrawal syndrome. Neuromuscular problems include myopathy and peripheral neuropathy. Males may experience testicular atrophy, sterility, impotence, or gynecomastia, and females who consume alcohol during pregnancy may produce neonates with fetal alcohol syndrome (FAS) or fetal alcohol effects (FAE). Some of the metabolic disturbances include hypokalemia, hypomagnesemia, and ketoacidosis. Also, endocrine disturbances may result in pancreatitis or diabetes (Alcohol, *Merck Manual,* 2008). The National Institute on Alcohol Abuse and Alcoholism reported that research has shown conclusively that familial transmission of alcoholism is at least in part genetic and not just the result of family environment. Studies in recent years have confirmed that identical twins, who share the same genes, are about twice as likely as fraternal twins, who share on average 50% of their genes, to resemble each other in terms of the presence of alcoholism. Recent research also reports that 50% to 60% of the risk for alcoholism is genetically determined, for both men and women. Genes alone do not preordain that someone will be an alcoholic; features in the environment along with gene–environment interactions account for the remainder of the risk (Alcohol, *Merck Manual,* 2008).

Blood alcohol concentration (BAC) is determined by the concentration of alcohol in the drink, the rate of drinking, the rate of absorption (slower in the presence of food), the rate of metabolism, and a person's weight and sex. The amount of alcohol the liver can metabolize per hour is equal to about ¾-ounce of whiskey, 4 ounces of wine, or 12 ounces of beer. **Tolerance** will develop with chronic consumption, and a person can reach a high BAC with minimal CNS effects. Women are more affected by alcohol than men, since women have less alcohol dehydrogenase activity than men (except for males with chronic alcoholism). Because this enzyme detoxifies alcohol, a deficiency results in a higher bioavailability of alcohol. Consequently, females suffer the long-term effects of alcohol intake at much lower doses in a shorter time span (Gordon, 2002). Alcohol use in moderation may provide health benefits by providing mild relaxation and lowering the serum cholesterol (Abramson et al, 2001). Stott et al (2008) found that of in their study of 3000 women between the ages of 70 and 82 years, the moderate consumption of alcohol resulted in better mental acuity and slower cognitive decline. Controlled drinking organizations such as Moderation Management (see.www.moderation.org) provide guidelines for persons who want to have alcohol in their lives.

Heroin

Heroin is one of the opioids. Opiates include the natural drugs found in the opium poppy, namely, *opium*, *morphine*, and *codeine*. Opioids are synthetic drugs, such as heroin (semisynthetic), meperidine, methadone, oxycodone, and propoxyphene; they mimic the effects of the natural opiates. Opiates are by far the most effective drugs for pain relief. When used for pain control, only about 0.1% of patients will develop addiction; thus fear of addiction is not a reason to undertreat pain.

Dependence on opioids is increasing, and chronic use can lead to dependence. Heroin is the most often frequent recreationally used opioid although abuse of prescription opioids is increasing (Opioids, *Merck Manual,* 2008). The demographics of the typical heroin user have changed over time. Its use is growing among younger middle-class and Hispanic Americans, who are often snorting or smoking a purer product. A Caron Foundation study found that 90% of their admissions for heroin addiction were white, more than 50% were employed full-time, and almost 89% had a high school diploma or higher level of education. Also, more than 70% of their adolescent admissions lived in suburban or rural locales (Gordon, 2001). Tolerance develops readily with opioids and can reach striking levels. There is cross-tolerance with opioids: tolerance to one opioid extends to other opioids. Physical dependence also develops quickly. A therapeutic dose taken regularly over 2 to 3 days can lead to some tolerance and dependence. Then when the drug is stopped, the user may have mild flu-like withdrawal symptoms. Less than 2 weeks of continuous use can cause withdrawal symptoms if the drug is not tapered. While the effects of withdrawal are not life threatening they generally include CNS hyperactivity with flu-like symptoms, anxiety, and drug craving. The more serious complications come from contaminants, the unsanitary administration of the drug, and complications due to overdose or the intoxication it can cause (Opioids, *Merck Manual,* 2008**).**

Evidence-Based Practice

The widespread use of alcohol and other drugs poses particular problems during hospitalization. Although nurses have been identified as an appropriate group to screen patients and provide acute and ongoing management to people with drug and alcohol-related problems, rates of screening are low. The aims of this study were to identify current practices for screening by nurses working in medical and surgical wards, determine their knowledge relating to problems associated with substance use, and identify their self-reported skills in managing patients with drug- and alcohol-related problems.

A chart audit of medical records was completed and a survey was distributed to nurses working in the study wards. Screening for alcohol and drug use was documented on only 22 of 79 medical records, and detailed information about quantity and duration of use was recorded in only nine. Overall, the nurses reported that they had little knowledge about substance use problems, and felt that they lacked skills to care adequately for these patients.

NURSE USE: The results of this study suggest a need for comprehensive training and education to ensure that nurses are familiar with policies and protocols for the management of patients and to assist nurses to provide evidence-based care and make appropriate referrals to specialist services.

Griffiths RD et al: Drink a little; take a few drugs: do nurses have knowledge to identify and manage in-patients at risk of drugs and alcohol?, *Drug Alcohol Rev* 26:545–552, 2007.

Evidence-Based Practice

The exploratory study of Courbasson et al (2007) examined the benefits of adding auricular acupuncture to a 21-day outpatient treatment program for women with concurrent substance abuse problems, anxiety, and depression. The structured treatment program was psychoeducational in nature and sought to determine if the acupuncture could be a viable alternative option to treatment as usual (TAU). The researchers also wanted to explore whether the addition of acupuncture would reduce the dropout rate of the treatment program.

The 185 women who received the acupuncture reported less physiological cravings for substances, felt significantly less depressed and anxious, and were better able to reflect on and resolve difficulties than the women in the control group. Because of these findings, the study concluded that auricular acupuncture showed promise as an adjunct therapy for addicted women in psychoeducational treatment programs.

NURSE USE: The use of auricular acupuncture seems to be an easily administered and cost-effective treatment alternative to medications for preventing substance abuse relapse and for improving overall health and well being. The increased emergence of clinical studies recommending the use of acupuncture shows that such an alternative therapy could outweigh Western skepticism about such a practice. Further research is recommended in order to continue to explore the issue.

From Courbasson CMA, de Sorkin AA, Dullerud B: Acupuncture treatment for women with substance use and anxiety/depression: an effective alternative therapy?, *Fam Commun Health* 30:112–120, 2007.

STIMULANTS

People use **stimulants** to feel more alert or energetic. These drugs activate or excite the nervous system. An increase in alertness and energy results as the stimulant causes the nerve fibers to release noradrenaline and other stimulating neurotransmitters. However, these drugs do not give the person more energy; they only make the body expend its own energy sooner and in greater quantities than it normally would. Stimulants can be useful and have few negative effects if used carefully and appropriately. The body must be allowed time to replenish itself after use of a stimulant. The cost for the "high" is the "down" state after the use of a stimulant—a feeling of sleepiness, laziness, mental fatigue, and possibly depression. Many persons abusing stimulants begin a vicious cycle of avoiding the down feeling by taking another dose. They then become physically dependent on the stimulant to function. Common stimulants include nicotine, cocaine, caffeine, and amphetamines.

Nicotine

Smoking is the foremost preventable cause of death in the United States (Centers for Disease Control and Prevention, 2004). One in five deaths in the United States is attributed to cigarettes. Table 24-1 highlights cigarette smoking-related mortality in the United States. The Centers for Disease Control and Prevention (CDC) estimates an average of 438,000 deaths per year are caused by complications of cigarette smoking (Centers for Disease Control and Prevention, 2006). From 1985 to 2003 the prevalence of adult smoking in the United States declined from 29.5% to 18.6% and remained constant at 20.8% from 2004 to 2005 (Farrelly et al, 2008). Nicotine, the active ingredient in the tobacco plant, is a toxic drug. To protect itself, the body quickly develops tolerance to the nicotine. If a person smokes regularly, tolerance to nicotine develops within hours, compared with days for heroin or months for alcohol. Pipes and cigars are less hazardous than cigarettes because the harsher smoke discourages deep inhalation. However, pipes and cigars increase the risk of cancer of the lips, mouth, and throat.

Smoke can be inhaled directly by the smoker (**mainstream smoke**), or it can enter the atmosphere from the lighted end of the cigarette and be inhaled by others in the vicinity (**sidestream smoke**). Sidestream smoke contains higher concentrations of toxic and carcinogenic compounds than mainstream smoke. An estimated 3000 annual lung cancer deaths and over one million illnesses in children are attributed to sidestream smoke (Barry, 2007). Smoking bans are being adopted to reduce the discomfort and health hazards among nonsmokers.

Nicotine is also used as chewing tobacco or snuff. Marketed as "smokeless tobacco," a wad is put in the mouth and the nicotine is absorbed sublingually. Higher doses of nicotine are delivered in the smokeless forms because the nicotine is not destroyed by heat. Nevertheless, this form is less addictive because nicotine enters the bloodstream less directly.

Table 24-1	**Cigarette Smoking-Related Mortality**		
Disease	**Men**	**Women**	**Overall**
Cancers			
Lung	82,234	97,686	119,920
Other	21,659	9,743	31,402
Total	**103,893**	**47,429**	**151,322**
Cardiovascular Diseases			
Hypertension	3,233	2,151	5,450
Heart disease	88,644	45,591	134,235
Stroke	14,978	8,303	23,281
Other	11,682	5,172	16,854
Total	**118,603**	**61,117**	**179,820**
Respiratory Diseases			
Pneumonia	11,292	7,881	19,173
Bronchitis/ emphysema	9,234	5,541	14,865
Chronic airway obstruction	30,385	18,579	48,982
Other	787	668	1,455
Total	**51,788**	**32,689**	**84,475**

Modified from Centers for Disease Control and Prevention: *Tobacco information and prevention source (TIPS)*, 2005, available at http://www.cdc.gov/tobacco/research_data/health_consequences/mortali.htm.

Cocaine

Cocaine comes from the coca shrub found on the eastern slopes of the Andes mountains and has been cultivated by South American Indians for thousands of years. The Indians chew a mixture of the coca leaf and lime to get a mild stimulant effect similar to coffee. By 1860 cocaine was isolated from the plant as a hydrochloride salt. It could be dissolved in water and used intravenously or orally when mixed in soft drinks. By the early 1900s, the common route of administration of the white powder was intranasal "snorting" (Weil and Rosen, 1998). At present in the United States most cocaine is snorted, although smoking crack cocaine is widely discussed. In the latter, cocaine is dissolved in water, mixed with baking soda (hydrochloride salt), and then heated to form rocks, or "crack."

The effects of cocaine vary with the mode of use. Injected or smoked cocaine produces hyperstimulation, alertness, euphoria, and feelings of competence and power (Cocaine, *Merck Manual,* 2008). Smoking cocaine gives intense effects because the drug quickly reaches the brain through the blood vessels in the lungs. Cocaine's interaction with dopamine seems to be the basis for the addictive patterns. The extreme euphoria is believed to be caused by cocaine's effect of dopaminergic stimulation. Chronic administration can lead to neurotransmitter depletion (especially of dopamine), which results in an extreme dysphoria characterized by apathy, sadness, and anhedonia (lack of joy). Thus a cocaine user can get caught up in a dangerous cycle of gaining an extreme high followed by an extreme low. To avoid that low the person consumes more cocaine. Crack addiction develops rapidly and is expensive, with addicts needing between $100

Table 24-2	**Caffeine Content in Commonly Consumed Substances**

Substance	Caffeine Content (mg)
Coffee (5 oz)	
Brewed	60–180
Instant	30–120
Decaffeinated	1–5
Chocolate	
Cocoa (5 oz)	2–20
Semisweet (1 oz)	5–35
Tea (5 oz)	
Brewed	20–90
Iced	67–76
Soft drinks (12 oz)	
Colas	40–45
Mountain Dew	53
Orange soda, ginger ale, Sprite, 7 Up, and several fruit-flavored drinks	0
Prescription Drugs	
Propoxyphene (Darvon Compound-65)	32.4
Fiorinal	40
Ergotamine (Cafegot)	100
Over-the-Counter Drugs	
Anacin	32
Excedrin	65
No-doze	100
Vivarin	200

and $1000 per day. Addicts who soon are overwhelmed by their cravings may engage in criminal activities such as theft or prostitution to get drug money.

Street cocaine ranges in purity from 50% to 60% and may be cut with other drugs, such as procaine or amphetamine, or any white powder, such as sugar or baby powder. High doses can cause extreme agitation, paranoid delusions, hyperthermia, hallucinations, cardiac dysrhythmias, pulmonary complications, convulsions, and possibly death (Cocaine, *Merck Manual,* 2008).

Caffeine

Caffeine is one of the most widely used psychoactive drugs in the world. Caffeine is found in coffee, tea, chocolate, soft drinks, and various medications (Table 24-2). Moderate doses of caffeine from 100 to 300 mg per day increase mental alertness and probably have little negative effect on health. Higher doses can lead to insomnia, irritability, tremulousness, anxiety, cardiac dysrhythmias, GI disturbances, and headaches. Regular use of high doses can lead to physical dependence, and the withdrawal symptoms may include headaches, slowness, and occasional depression (Juliano and Griffiths, 2004). Treating afternoon headaches with analgesics containing caffeine may in reality be preventing a withdrawal symptom from heavy morning coffee consumption.

Amphetamines

Amphetamines are a class of stimulants similar to cocaine, but the effects last longer and the drugs are cheaper. Amphetamines have a chemical structure similar to adrenaline and noradrenaline and are generally used to decrease fatigue, increase mental alertness, suppress appetite, and create a sense of well-being. Historically, amphetamines have been issued to American soldiers and pilots to decrease fatigue and increase mental alertness. They are popular among people who need to stay awake for long hours to work or study. They can be taken as pills, injected, snorted, or smoked (Amphetamines, *Merck Manual,* 2008). When taken intravenously, they quickly induce an intense euphoric feeling (a "rush"). The user may speed for several days (go on a "speed run") and then fall into a deep sleep for 18 or more hours ("crash"). They cause an elevation in mood, increased wakefulness, alertness, concentration, intensified physical performance, and a feeling of well-being; they typically cause erectile dysfunction in men while enhancing sexual desire. Use is often associated with unsafe sexual practices including exposure to sexually transmitted diseases and HIV (Amphetamines, *Merck Manual,* 2008). Users are prone to accidents since the drug produces a state of excitement and grandiosity, and their usual danger warning signals do not work effectively.

BRIEFLY NOTED

Other drugs containing caffeine, ephedrine, or phenylpropanolamine (singly or in combination) are referred to as "look-alikes." These drugs gained market attention after access to amphetamines was controlled by prescription. These chemicals are often found in OTC cold remedies as a nasal decongestant and in diet pills (e.g., Dexatrim).

MARIJUANA

Marijuana (*Cannabis sativa* or *C. indica*) is the most widely used illicit drug in the United States. Compared with the other psychoactive drugs, marijuana has little toxicity and is one of the safest therapeutic agents known (Marijuana, *Merck Manual,* 2008). Psychological dependence can occur with chronic use, but little is known about any potential physical dependence. However, because of its illegal status, there is no quality control, and a user may consume contaminated marijuana. Users enjoy a mild euphoria, a relaxed feeling, and an intensity of sensory perceptions. Some call the effect a dreamy state of consciousness in which ideas seem disconnected, unanticipated, and free-flowing. Time, color, and spatial perceptions may be altered (Marijuana, *Merck Manual,* 2008). Side effects include dry and reddened eyes, increased appetite, dry mouth, drowsiness, and mild tachycardia. Adverse reactions include anxiety, disorientation, and paranoia.

The greatest physical concern for chronic users is possible damage to the respiratory tract from smoking the drug. For chronic users tolerance can develop, as well as physical dependence; however, the withdrawal symptoms are benign.

Addiction can occur for some chronic users and is difficult to treat because the progression tends to be subtle. Despite its beneficial effects, especially in treating pain, the only legal access to this medicine was through the U.S. Food and Drug Administration's (FDA's) Compassionate Investigational New Drug Program. This program was closed in 1992. In response to this complete prohibition, some health care organizations support access to this medication through formal resolutions, including several state nurses' associations, the American Nurse's Association, and the American Public Health Association. Thirteen states have passed laws allowing patients to use marijuana as medicine under the recommendation of their physician, but the federal government continues its total prohibition efforts. See www.medicalcannibis.com for a full list of supporting organizations.

HALLUCINOGENS

Also called *psychedelics* ("mind vision"), **hallucinogens** can produce hallucinations, cause intoxication, and lead to altered perception and impaired judgment. Responses to these drugs is related to the user's mood, basic emotional makeup, and expectations (**set**), including the ability to cope with perceptual distortions, expectations, and the immediate surroundings (**setting**). The physical effects are more constant and consist of CNS stimulation. Chronic use can lead to psychological effects and impaired judgment, which can then lead to dangerous decisions or accidents (Hallucinogens, *Merck Manual,* 2008).

The two broad chemical families of hallucinogen are the indole hallucinogens and those that resemble adrenaline and amphetamines. The indoles are related to hormones (serotonin) made in the brain by the pineal gland and include drugs such as lysergic acid diethylamide (LSD), psilocybin, mushrooms, and morning glory seeds. The second group, which lacks the chemical structure called the *indole ring*, includes peyote, mescaline, and 3,4-methylenedioxymethamphetamine (MDMA [Ecstasy]). Phencyclidine (PCP) is in a class by itself. It is a potent anesthetic and analgesic with CNS stimulant, depressant, and hallucinogenic properties; its use was especially high in the 1980s. LSD is the best-known drug in the hallucinogen category, but MDMA will be discussed because it is currently a popular drug.

MDMA (Ecstasy)

MDMA (Ecstasy or Adam or "E") is an amphetamine analog commonly taken as a pill. This semisynthetic drug was first patented by Merck Pharmaceuticals in 1914. It was not widely used until the late 1970s and early 1980s, when psychiatrists and psychotherapists began using it to facilitate psychotherapy. It is classified as a mood elevator that produces feelings of empathy, openness, and well-being. Taken orally, its effects are experienced in 20 to 40 minutes, with the peak effect at 60 to 90 minutes, ending after about 3 to 5 hours. Ecstasy has gained current popularity as a "club" drug used at all-night "rave" dances. Deaths have occurred at these rave parties secondary to overheating. Some of these deaths have been listed as overdoses of Ecstasy, because it raises the body's temperature, pulse rate, and blood pressure. Harm reduction strategies such as having free water available and rooms for people to relax could help prevent such overdoses. An additional risk to illicit Ecstasy use is adulteration of the drug by other more toxic drugs. See www.DanceSafe.org for additional information.

INHALANTS

Inhalants are often among the first drugs that young children use. The primary abusers of most inhalants are adolescents who are 12 to 17 years of age. Use often ends in late adolescence.

Inhalants, which include gases and solvents, do not fit neatly into other categories. The four categories of inhalants are volatile organic solvents, aerosols, volatile nitrites, and gases. These substances are inhaled ("huffed") from bottles, aerosol cans, or soaked cloth or put into bags or balloons to increase the concentration of the inhaled fumes and decrease the inhalation of other substances in the vapor (e.g., paint particles). See www.inhalants.org for examples of products in these categories and specific drug information. Inhalant users can get high several times in a short period since the inhalants are short-acting and have a rapid onset. Users are predominately white. Experimental use is about equal for males and females, but males are more likely to engage in chronic use. Depending on the dose, the user may feel a slight stimulation, less inhibition, or even lose consciousness. There is a link between school performance and use of an inhalant. Other signs include paint or stains on clothes or the body; spots or sores around the mouth; red or runny eyes or nose; chemic breath odor; a drunk, dazed, or dizzy appearance; nausea and loss of appetite; and finally anxiety, excitability, and irritability. Chronic users may have poor school attendance or be delinquent and involved in theft and burglary (National Institute on Drug Abuse, 2008). Users can die from "Sudden sniffing death" syndrome, and this can occur from the first to the hundredth time he or she uses the inhalant. This death appears to be related to acute cardiac dysrhythmia. Dangers with administration of gases increase when inhaling directly from pressurized tanks because the gas is very cold and can cause frostbite to the nose, lips, and vocal cords. Also, if a gas such as nitrous oxide is not mixed with oxygen, the user may die from asphyxiation (National Institute on Drug Abuse, 2008).

PREDISPOSING AND CONTRIBUTING FACTORS FOR SUBSTANCE ABUSE

In addition to the specific drug being used, two other major variables influence the particular drug experience: set and setting (Weil and Rosen, 1998). To understand various patterns of drug use and abuse by individuals, all three factors (drug, set, and setting) should be considered.

Set refers to the individual using the drug, as well as that person's expectations, including unconscious expectations, about the drug being used. A person's current health may alter a drug's effects from one day to the next. Some people are genetically predisposed to alcoholism or other drug addiction, and their chemical makeup is such that simply consuming the drug triggers the disease process. Persons with underlying mood disorders or other mental illness may try to self-medicate with psychoactive drugs. Sometimes their choice of drug exacerbates their symptoms; for example, a depressed person might consume alcohol and become more depressed.

Setting is the influence of the physical, social, and cultural environment within which the use occurs. Social conditions influence the use of drugs. The fast pace of life, competition at school or in the workplace, and the pressure to accumulate material possessions are daily stressors. Pharmaceutical, alcohol, and tobacco companies are continuously bombarding the public with enticing advertisements pushing their products as a means of feeling better, sleeping better, or having more energy, or just as a "treat." People grow up believing that most of life's problems can be solved quickly and easily through the use of a drug. For persons of a lower socioeconomic background and with minimal education or employment possibilities, many of life's opportunities may seem out of reach. Rather than seeking relief through medical care, the use of psychoactive drugs may offer a way to numb the pain or escape from a hopeless reality. They also rely on alcohol or illicit drugs, which are more readily available. For some, dealing in illicit drugs may appear to be the only way to avoid a future of poverty and unemployment.

PRIMARY PREVENTION AND THE ROLE OF THE NURSE

The harm reduction approach to substance abuse focuses on health promotion and disease prevention. Primary prevention for ATOD problems includes (1) the promotion of healthy lifestyles and resiliency factors and (2) education about drugs and guidelines for their use. Nurses can be effective in teaching, promoting, and facilitating people in choosing healthy options rather than reliance on drugs. This may entail adding these health-promoting actions to the use of prescription drugs or complementary remedies if the latter are consistent with the recommendations of the health care provider.

Specifically, you can teach clients to be assertive in their relationships with others and how to make more beneficial decisions by looking carefully at the pros and cons of each option and the related consequences. People may turn to medications, especially psychoactive drugs, when they experience persistent health problems such as difficulty sleeping, muscle tension, lack of energy, chronic stress, and mood swings. Nurses can help clients understand that medications may mask problems rather than solve them. Stress reduction and relaxation techniques along with a balanced lifestyle can address these problems more directly than medications can. Lack of sleep, improper diet, and lack of exercise contribute to many health complaints. Assisting clients to balance their need for rest, nutrition, and exercise on a daily basis can reduce these complaints. Nurses can provide useful

---

HOW TO | Set Up Community-Based Activities Aimed at Substance Abuse Prevention

- Increase involvement and pride in school activities.
- Organize student assistant programs (students helping students).
- Organize a Students Against Drunk Driving (SADD) chapter.
- Mobilize parental awareness and action groups (e.g., Mothers Against Drunk Driving [MADD]).
- Increase the availability of recreational facilities.
- Encourage parental commitment to nondrinking parties.
- Encourage religious institutions to convey nonuse messages and provide activities associated with nonuse.
- Curtail media messages that glamorize drug and alcohol use.
- Support and reinforce antidrug use peer-pressure skills.
- Provide general health screenings, including alcohol, tobacco, and other drug (ATOD) use.
- Collaborate with community leaders to solve problems related to crime, housing, jobs, and access to health care.

---

information to groups, assisting in the development of community recreational resources or facilitating stress reduction, relaxation, or exercise groups. Nurses can help people learn about drug-free community activities. The "How To" box lists community activities in which the nurse may become involved.

Lack of educational opportunities, job training, or both can contribute to socioeconomic stress and poor self-esteem, which can lead to drug use to escape the situation. Nurses can help clients identify community resources and solve problems to meet basic needs rather than avoid them. In addition to decreasing risk factors associated with ATOD problems, it is important to increase protective or resiliency factors. Prevention guidelines to teach parents and teachers how to increase resiliency in youths include the following strategies:

- Help them develop an increased sense of responsibility for their own success.
- Help them identify their talents.
- Motivate them to dedicate their lives to helping society rather than believing that their only purpose in life is to be consumers.
- Provide realistic appraisals and feedback, stress multicultural competence, and encourage and value education and skills training.
- Increase cooperative solutions to problems rather than competitive or aggressive solutions.

These skills also apply to adults. The objectives in *Healthy People 2010* provide guidance for ways to decrease the reliance on alcohol, drugs, and tobacco (U.S. Department of Health and Human Services, 2000) (see the "Levels of Prevention" box on p. 453).

DRUG EDUCATION

ATOD problems include more than abuse of psychoactive drugs. Today more than 450,000 different drugs and drug combinations are available, and prescription drugs are involved in almost 60% of all drug-related emergency room visits and 70% of all drug-related deaths. Nurses know about medication administration, the possible dangers of indiscriminant drug use, and the inability of drugs to cure all problems. Nurses can influence the health of clients by destroying the myth of good drugs versus bad drugs. This means (1) teaching clients that no drug is completely safe and that any drug can be abused, (2) helping persons learn how to make informed decisions about their drug use to minimize potential harm, and (3) teaching them to always tell their health care provider what supplements they are taking.

Drug technology is growing, yet the public receives little information about how to safely use this technology. Harm reduction as a goal recognizes that people consume drugs and that they need to know about the use of drugs and risks involved to make decisions about their drug use. Drug education should begin on an individual basis by reviewing the client's prescription medications. Because a physician or nurse practitioner has prescribed the medication, clients often presume little risk is involved.

Is the client aware of any untoward interactions this drug may have with other drugs being used or with food? A common occurrence with drug users is taking drugs from different categories together or at different times to regulate how they feel, known as **polysubstance use or abuse**. For example, a person may drink alcohol when snorting cocaine to "take the edge off"; or some intravenous drug users combine cocaine with heroin (speedball) for similar reasons. Polysubstance use can cause drug interactions that can have additive, synergistic, or antagonistic effects. Indiscriminant polysubstance abuse may lead to serious physiological consequences and can be complicated for the health care professional to assess and treat. It is important to encourage clients to ask questions about their drug use. The "How To" box lists seven key pieces of information that clients should obtain before taking a drug or medication to decrease the possible harm from unsafe medication consumption.

HOW TO	**Determine the Relative Safety of a Drug for Personal or Client Use**

Before using a drug or medication, always determine the following:
- The chemical being taken
- How and where the drug works in the body
- The correct dosage
- Whether there will be drug interactions, including interactions with herbal remedies
- If there are potential allergic reactions
- If there will be drug tolerance
- If the drug will produce physical dependence*

From Miller M: *Drug consumer safety rules,* Mosier, Ore, 2002; Mothers Against Misuse and Abuse, available at www.mamas.org.
*Caution: Approximately 10% of the population may suffer from the disease of addiction. For them, responsible use of psychoactive drugs is limited because of their disease. They need to notify their physician of the addiction if the use of psychoactive medicines is being considered as treatment.

Nurses can identify references and community resources available to provide the necessary information, and they can clarify the information. User-friendly reference texts and on line resources are available that describe drug interactions among medications, other drugs (including alcohol, tobacco, marijuana, and cocaine), and other substances (food and beverages), and that serve as excellent guides for nurses and their clients. See www.drugdigest.org for more information. Clients should learn about and ask questions about their prescription medications, self-administered over-the-counter, including supplement and herbal remedies and recreational drugs. This does not mean that nurses should encourage other drug use but, rather, that the potential harm from self-medication can be reduced if clients have the necessary information to make more informed decisions.

Parents should seek information about their use of medications so they can act as role models for their children. It can be confusing for children and adolescents to be told to "just say no" to drugs when they see their parents or drug advertisements try to "quick fix" every health complaint, feeling of stress, anxiety, or depression with a medication. The simple "just say no" approach does not help young people for several reasons. First, children are naturally curious, and drug experimentation is often a part of normal development. Second, children from dysfunctional homes may use drugs to get attention or to escape an intolerable environment. And finally, the "just say no" approach does not address the powerful influence of peer pressure (Substance Use in Children and Adolescents, *Merck Manual,* 2008).

Drug education has moved into the school curriculum with Project DARE (Drug Abuse Resistance Education), the most widely used school-based drug-use prevention program in the United States. This program uses law enforcement officers to teach the material, but recent studies find that it is less effective than other interactive prevention programs and may even result in increased drug use (West and O'Neal, 2004). Basic ATOD prevention programs for young people should combine efforts to increase resiliency factors with drug education. Nurses can serve as educators or as advisors to the school systems or community groups to ensure that all of these areas are addressed. Role playing is useful in teaching many of these skills.

SECONDARY PREVENTION AND THE ROLE OF THE NURSE

To identify substance abuse and plan appropriate interventions, nurses must assess each client individually. When drug abuse, dependence, or addiction is identified, the nurse should assist clients to understand the connection between their drug-use patterns and the negative consequences on their health, their families, and the community.

ASSESSING FOR ATOD PROBLEMS

During health assessment, the nurse should assess for substance abuse problems including both self-medication practices and recreational drug use. Thus all relevant drug-use history is collected and aids in the assessment of drug-use patterns. Note any changes in drug-use patterns over time. After obtaining a medication history, follow-up questions can determine if problems exist. The following are examples:

- If using a prescription drug, is the client following the directions correctly?
- Has the client increased the dosage or frequency above the prescription level?
- Is the person using any prescribed psychoactive drugs?
- If so, for how long and what is the dosage?

BRIEFLY NOTED

Think of the "4 H's" to remember what to ask when assessing drug-use patterns: How taken (route), How much, How often, and How long.

When assessing self-medication and recreational or social drug-use patterns, determine the reason the person uses the drug. Some underlying health problems (e.g., pain, stress, weight, insomnia) may be relieved by nonpharmaceutical interventions. The amount, frequency, and duration of use and the route of administration of each drug should be determined. To establish the presence of a substance abuse problem, it is necessary to determine if the drug use is causing any negative health consequences or problems with relationships, employment, finances, or the legal system. The "How To" box lists examples of questions to ask to determine the presence of socioeconomic problems that are often secondary to substance abuse. If a pattern of chronic, regular, and frequent use of a drug exists, nurses should assess for a history of withdrawal symptoms to determine if there is physical dependence on the drug. A progression in drug-use patterns and related problems warns about the possibility of addiction. **Denial** is a primary symptom of addiction. Methods of denial include the following:

- Lying about use
- Minimizing use patterns
- Blaming or rationalizing

Levels of Prevention   Related to Substance Abuse

PRIMARY PREVENTION

Provide community education to teach healthy lifestyles; focus on how to resist getting involved in substance abuse.

SECONDARY PREVENTION

Institute early detection programs in schools, the workplace, and other areas in which people gather to determine the presence of substance abuse.

TERTIARY PREVENTION

Develop programs to help people reduce or end substance abuse.

- Intellectualizing
- Changing the subject
- Using anger or humor
- "Going with the flow" (agreeing that a problem exists, stating the behavior will change, but not demonstrating any behavior changes)

A problem should be suspected if the client becomes defensive or exhibits other behavior indicating denial when asked about alcohol or other drug use.

DRUG TESTING

During the 1980s, preemployment or random drug testing in the workplace gained popularity. Drug testing can be done by examining a person's urine, blood, saliva, breath (alcohol), or hair. The most common method of drug screening is urine testing. Urine testing indicates only past use of certain drugs, not intoxication. Thus persons can be identified as having used a certain drug in the recent past, but the degree of intoxication and extent of performance impairment cannot be determined with urine testing. Also, most drug-related problems in the workplace are related to alcohol, and alcohol is not always included in a urine drug screen. When is drug testing appropriate? Drug testing that follows documented impairment may help substantiate the cause of the impairment, and thus it serves as a backup rather than the primary screening method. It is also useful for recovering addicts. Part of their treatment is to abstain from psychoactive drug use; therefore, a urine test yielding positive results for a drug indicates a relapse.

Blood, breath, and saliva drug tests can indicate current use and amount. Any of these tests can help determine

HOW TO   Assess Socioeconomic Problems Resulting from Substance Abuse

If the client admits to use of alcohol, tobacco, or other drugs, ask the following questions:

- Do your parents, spouse, or friends worry or complain about your drinking or using drugs?
- Has a family member gone for help about your drinking or using drugs?
- Have you neglected family obligations as a result of drinking or using drugs?
- Have you missed work because of your drinking or using drugs?
- Does your boss complain about your drinking or using drugs?
- Do you drink or use drugs before or during work?
- Have you ever been fired or quit a job because of drinking or using drugs?
- Have you ever been charged with driving under the influence (DUI) or being drunk in public (DIP)?
- Have you ever had any other legal problems related to drinking and using drugs, such as assault and battery, breaking and entering, or theft?
- Have you had any accidents while intoxicated, such as falls, burns, or motor vehicle accidents?
- Have you spent your money on alcohol or other drugs instead of paying your bills (e.g., telephone, electricity, rent)?

alcohol intoxication, and they are often used to substantiate suspected impairment. A serum drug screen can be useful when overdose is suspected to determine the specific drug ingested. The testing of hair is gaining attention because the results can provide a long history of drug-use patterns.

Alcohol and other drug testing should be used as a clinical and public health tool but not for harassment and punishment. For example, approximately 40% to 50% of people who are seen in trauma centers were drinking at the time of their injuries. Hence, it is recommended that breath alcohol testing should be routinely done for patients admitted to the emergency department for traumatic injuries (Physicians and Lawyers for National Drug Policy, 2008).

Employee assistance programs (EAPs) are a beneficial service in many work settings. Often a sizable number of EAP clients have substance use problems since most adults with these problems are employed. Recent research estimated that 29% of full-time workers engaged in binge drinking in the past month, while 8% engaged in heavy drinking; an additional 8% reported the use of illicit drugs (Substance Abuse and Mental Health Services Administration, 2006). EAP programs can identify health problems among employees and offer counseling or referral to other health care providers as necessary. Such programs provide early identification of and intervention for substance abuse problems; they also offer services to employees to reduce stress and provide health care or counseling so that they may prevent substance abuse problems from developing. Nurses frequently develop and run these programs.

HIGH-RISK GROUPS

Identifying high-risk groups helps nurses design programs to meet specific needs and to mobilize community resources.

Adolescents

The younger a person is when beginning intensive experimentation with drugs, the more likely dependence will develop. Underage drinking is seen as the most serious drug problem for youth in the United States. Almost one in five eighth graders and almost half of high school seniors report recent use of alcohol, compared with 21% of seniors reporting recent use of marijuana. In fact, the rate of illicit drug use has been declining, including drinking and the use of marijuana, cocaine, and heroin. The proportion of youths ages 12 to 17 years who indicated a greater risk from smoking one or more packs of cigarettes per day increased from 63.1% in 2002 to 68.7% in 2006 (Substance Abuse and Mental Health Services Administration, 2007). There is more work to be done in the area of prevention since studies indicate that the younger the age at which youth begin substance abuse, the greater likelihood that the abuse will continue into adulthood.

Heavy drug use during adolescence can interfere with normal development. Note that *Healthy People 2010* objectives 27-4 and 26-9 refer to delay of the initiation of the use of tobacco, alcohol, and marijuana (see *Healthy People 2010* box). Family-related factors (genetics, family

Healthy People 2010

Objectives Related to ATOD Use

26-9	Increase the age and proportion of adolescents who remain alcohol and drug free
26-10	Reduce past-month use of illicit substances
26-11	Reduce the proportion of persons engaging in binge drinking of alcoholic beverages
26-12	Reduce the average annual alcohol consumption
26-13	Reduce the proportion of adults who exceed guidelines for low-risk drinking
26-14	Reduce steroid use among adolescents
26-15	Reduce the proportion of adolescents who use inhalants
26-16	Increase the proportion of adolescents who disapprove of substance use
26-17	Increase the proportion of adolescents who perceive great risk associated with substance abuse
27-1	Reduce tobacco use by adults
27-2	Reduce tobacco use by adolescents
27-3	Reduce initiation of tobacco use among children and adolescents
27-4	Increase the average age of first use of tobacco products by adolescents and young adults
27-5	Increase smoking cessation attempts by adult smokers
27-6	Increase smoking cessation during pregnancy
27-7	Increase smoking cessation attempts by adolescent smokers
27-8	Increase insurance coverage of evidence-based treatment for nicotine dependency
27-9	Reduce the proportion of children who are regularly exposed to tobacco smoke at home
27-10	Reduce the proportion of nonsmokers exposed to environmental tobacco smoke
27-11	Increase smoke-free and tobacco-free environments in schools, including all school facilities, property, vehicles, and events
27-12	Increase the proportion of worksites with formal smoking policies that prohibit smoking or limit it to separately ventilated areas
27-13	Establish laws on smoke-free indoor air that prohibit smoking or limit it to separately ventilated areas in public places and worksites

From U.S. Department of Health and Human Services: *Healthy People 2010: national health promotion and disease prevention objectives,* Washington, DC, 2000, U.S. Government Printing Office.

stress, parenting styles, child victimization) appear to be the greatest variable that influences substance abuse among adolescents. The cooccurrence with psychiatric disorders (especially mood disorders) and behavioral problems is also associated with substance abuse among adolescents, leaving peer pressure as a less-influential factor. Research suggests that successful social influence-based prevention programs may be driven by their ability to foster social norms that reduce an adolescent's social motivation to begin using ATOD. One particularly effective treatment approach for adolescents is the use of family-oriented therapy (Substance Abuse and Mental Health Services Administration, 2008).

Older Adults

Older adults (65 years of age and older) represent 13% of the U.S. population and are the fastest growing segment of U.S. society. This group is expected to represent 21% of the population by the year 2030. They consume more prescribed and OTC medications than any other age group. Alcohol and prescription drug misuse affects as many as 17% of adults ages 60 years and older. Problems with alcohol consumption, including interactions with prescribed and OTC drugs, far outnumber any other substance abuse problem among older adults (Office of Applied Studies, 2005). The increased use of prescription drugs and alcohol by older adults may be related to coping problems. Problems of relocation, possible loss of independence, retirement, illness, death of friends, and lower levels of achievement contribute to feelings of sadness, boredom, anxiety, and loneliness. Factors such as slowed metabolic turnover of drugs, age-related organ changes, enhanced drug sensitivities, a tendency to use drugs over long periods, and a more frequent use of multiple drugs all contribute to greater negative consequences from drug use among older adults. Alcohol abuse may not be identified because its effects on cognitive abilities may mimic changes associated with normal aging or degenerative brain disease. Also, depression may simply be attributed to more frequent losses rather than the depressant effects of alcohol, and the older adult may subsequently receive medical treatment for depression rather than alcoholism.

Injection Drug Users

In addition to the problem of addiction, **injection drug users (IDUs)** (those who self-administer intravenously or subcutaneously) are at risk for other health complications. Intravenous administration of drugs always carries a greater risk of overdose because the drug goes directly into the bloodstream. With illicit drugs, the danger is increased because the exact dosage is unknown. In addition, the drug may be contaminated with other chemicals, such as sugar, starch, or quinine, and these ingredients can cause negative consequences. Often IDUs make their own solution for intravenous administration, and any particles present can result in complications from emboli.

Addicts often share needles. Human immunodeficiency virus (HIV), hepatitis C, and other blood-borne diseases can be transmitted through contaminated needles. Infections and abscesses may develop secondary to dirty needles or poor administration techniques. IDUs represent the most rapidly growing source of new cases of acquired immunodeficiency syndrome (AIDS), and they are at the greatest risk for the spread of the virus in the heterosexual community. As of 2004, 20% of all new HIV infection cases occurred among IDUs, with a disproportionate effect on those in minority groups (Centers for Disease Control and Prevention, 2005a). Because of this trend, emphasis is being placed on reducing the transmission of this disease through contaminated needles. Abstinence is ideal but unrealistic for many addicts. Using the harm reduction model, the nurse should provide education on cleaning needles with bleach between uses and

on needle exchange programs to decrease the spread of the virus. Studies indicate that needle exchange programs have not increased injection drug abuse but have, in fact, increased the number of people entering treatment programs (Centers for Disease Control and Prevention, 2005b).

Drug Use during Pregnancy

Most drugs can negatively affect a fetus. Thus the use of any drug during pregnancy should be discouraged unless medically necessary. *Healthy People 2010* objectives address this issue. **Fetal alcohol syndrome (FAS)** has been identified as the leading preventable birth defect, causing mental and behavioral impairment (U.S. Department of Health and Human Services, 2005). One study found that women who are depressed during their pregnancy are more likely to binge drink. Thus depression screening and treatment as needed could be a useful adjunct to FAS/FAE intervention efforts (Homish et al, 2004). A Danish study of 24,768 women found an increasing risk of stillbirth with increasing moderate alcohol intake during pregnancy (Kesmodel et al, 2002). Another survey estimates that 12.4% of pregnant women drink alcohol. From 2003 to 2006 the percentage of pregnant women between the ages of 15 and 44 years who were engaged in binge drinking in the first trimester dropped from 10.6% to 4.6%. This may be due to the extensive information available about the effects of alcohol on the fetus (Substance Abuse and Mental Health Services Administration, 2007). Estimates of illicit drug use during pregnancy range from 1.3% of women ages 26 to 44 years to 12.9% of adolescent girls ages 15 to 17 years. Tobacco remains the most-used addictive substance during pregnancy, with about 18% of pregnant women smoking (Jones, 2006).

BRIEFLY NOTED

In some states, pregnant women who are using illicit drugs are reported to child protective services because of the potential harm to the fetus. Will this practice do more harm than good? What about women who drink alcohol or smoke cigarettes?

Despite the increased focus on drug abuse interventions, many pregnant women with drug problems do not receive the help they need. This may be a result of ignorance, poverty, lack of concern for the fetus, lack of available services, and fear of the consequences of revealing drug use. The fear of criminal prosecution may push addicted women further away from the health care system, cause them to conceal their drug use from medical providers, and cause them to avoid the critical treatment and medical care that they need (Brady and Ashley, 2005).

Use of Illicit Drugs

The strategy of "just say no" to drugs is both simplistic and misleading. Indiscriminant use of "good" drugs has caused more health problems from adverse reactions, drug interactions, dependence, addiction, and overdoses than use of "bad" drugs. However, the war on drugs focuses on illicit drugs and punishes illicit drug users. The black market associated with illicit drug use puts otherwise law-abiding citizens in close contact with criminals, prevents any quality control of the drugs, increases the risk of AIDS and hepatitis secondary to needle sharing, and hinders health care professionals' accessibility to the abuser or addict. Lack of quality control (unknown strength and purity) can cause unexpected overdoses or secondary effects of the impurities; for example, a synthetic analog of fentanyl (3-methylfentanyl) marketed as "heroin" is 6000 times as potent as morphine. Unsafe administration (contaminated needles) leads to local and systemic infections. The high cost of drugs on the black market leads to crime to support the addiction. In 2006, approximately 20.4 million (or 8.3%) Americans ages 12 years and older had used illicit drugs in the past month. Illicit drugs include marijuana/hashish, cocaine (including crack), heroin, hallucinogens, inhalants, or prescription-type psychotherapeutics that are used nonmedically. Marijuana was the most frequently used illicit drug (Substance Abuse and Mental Health Services Administration, 2007).

CODEPENDENCY AND FAMILY INVOLVEMENT

Drug addiction is often a family disease. One in four Americans experiences family problems related to alcohol abuse. One study found that 52.9% of Americans 18 years of age and older have a family history of alcoholism among first- or second-degree relatives (Dawson and Grant, 1998). People close to the addict often develop unhealthy coping mechanisms to continue the relationship. This behavior is known as **codependency**, a stress-induced preoccupation with the addicted person's life, leading to extreme dependence and excessive concern for the addict. Strict rules typically develop in a codependent family to maintain the relationships. The following are examples:

- Don't talk.
- Don't feel.
- Don't trust.
- Don't lose control.
- Don't seek help from outside the family.

Codependents try to meet the addict's needs at the expense of their own. Codependency may underlie medical complaints and emotional stress seen by health care providers such as ulcers, skin disorders, migraine headaches, chronic colds, and backaches. When the addicted person refuses to admit the problem, the family continues to adapt to emotionally survive the stress of the addict's irrational, inconsistent, and unpredictable behavior. Family members consequently develop roles that tend to be gross exaggerations of normal family roles, and they cling irrationally to these roles, even when they are no longer functional. One of the most significant roles a family member may assume is that of an enabler. **Enabling** is the act of shielding or preventing the addict from experiencing the consequences of the addiction. As a result, the addict does not always understand the cost of the addiction and thus is "enabled" to

continue to use. Although codependency and enabling are closely related, a person does not have to be codependent to enable. Anyone can be an enabler: a police officer, a boss or co-worker, and even a drug treatment counselor. Health care professionals who do not address the negative health consequences of drug use with the addicted person are enablers.

The nurse can help families recognize the problem of addiction and help them confront the addicted member in a caring manner. Whether or not the addicted family member is agreeable to treatment, the family members should be given some guidance about the resources and services available to help them cope more effectively. The nurse can help identify treatment options, counseling assistance, financial assistance, support services, and (if necessary) legal services for the family members. Children of ATOD abusers or addicts are themselves at a greater risk for developing an addiction and must be targeted for primary prevention.

TERTIARY PREVENTION AND THE ROLE OF THE NURSE

The nurse is in a key position to help the addict and the addict's family. The nurse's knowledge of community resources and how to mobilize them can significantly influence the quality of care clients receive.

DETOXIFICATION

Detoxification is the clearing of one or more drugs from the person's body and managing the withdrawal symptoms. Depending on the particular drug and the degree of dependence, the time required may range from a few days to several weeks. Because withdrawal symptoms vary (depending on the drug used) and range from uncomfortable to life-threatening, the setting for and management of withdrawal depends on the drug used. Stimulants or opiates may produce withdrawal symptoms that are very uncomfortable but not life-threatening. Detoxification from these drugs does not require direct medical supervision, but medical management of the withdrawal symptoms increases the comfort level. On the other hand, drugs such as alcohol, benzodiazepines, and barbiturates can produce life-threatening withdrawal symptoms. These clients should be under close medical supervision during detoxification and should receive medical management of the withdrawal symptoms to ensure a safe withdrawal. Of those who develop delirium tremens from alcohol withdrawal, 15% may not survive despite medical management; therefore, close medical management is initiated as the blood alcohol level begins to fall. A general rule in detoxification management is to wean the person off the drug by gradually reducing the dosage and frequency of administration. Thus a person with chronic alcoholism could be safely detoxified by a gradual reduction in alcohol consumption. In practice, however, the switch to another drug, usually a benzodiazepine, often offers a safer withdrawal from alcohol as well as an abrupt end to the intoxication from the drug of choice. For example, chlordiazepoxide (Librium) is commonly used for alcohol detoxification.

BRIEFLY NOTED

Outpatient or home detoxification for persons requiring medical detoxification for alcohol withdrawal can be a cost-effective treatment. Nurses can monitor and evaluate the client's health status in the home environment to reduce the risk of medical complications related to alcohol withdrawal, and to provide encouragement and support for the client to complete the detoxification.

ADDICTION TREATMENT

Addiction treatment differs from the management of negative health consequences of chronic drug abuse, overdose, and detoxification. **Addiction treatment** focuses on the addiction process. The goal is to help clients view addiction as a chronic disease and assist them to make lifestyle changes to halt the progression of the disease. According to the disease theory, addicts are not responsible for the symptoms of their disease; they arc, however, responsible for treating their disease. It is estimated that 18 million people who consume alcohol and almost 5 million who use illicit drugs need substance abuse treatment. However, less than 25% of those who need treatment get it, for various reasons. In 2006 4 million people ages 12 years or older (1.6% of the population) received some treatment for the use of alcohol or illicit drugs. More than half were treated at a self-help group. This contrasts to the estimated 23.6 million or 9.6% of the population ages 12 years and older who needed treatment (Substance Abuse and Mental Health Services Administration, 2007).

Most treatment facilities are multidisciplinary because the intervention strategies require a wide range of approaches. Their programs involve interactions between the addict, family, culture, and community. Strategies include medical management, education, counseling, vocational rehabilitation, stress management, and support services. The key to effective treatment is to match individual clients with the interventions most appropriate for them (National Institute on Drug Abuse, 2008).

For those addicted individuals unwilling or unable to completely abstain from psychoactive drugs, other medications can assist them in abstaining from their drug of choice. Methadone maintenance programs are used to treat heroin and other opioid addictions. Methadone, when administered in moderate or high daily doses, produces a **cross-tolerance** to other narcotics, thereby blocking their effects and decreasing the craving for heroin. The advantages of methadone are that it is long-acting and effective orally, does not produce a "high," is inexpensive, and has few known side effects. The oral use of methadone offers a solution to the danger of the spread of AIDS and other blood-borne infections that commonly occur among needle-sharing addicts. Although not recognized as a cure for heroin (or other opiate) addiction, methadone maintenance is effective in managing and is considered to be the gold standard of treatment for opioid addiction. Buprenorphine

(Suboxone ®) is a mixed agonist-antagonist given sublingually that has been introduced as a safer alternative to methadone. Protocols for this medication can be found at the U. S. website, www.buprenorphrine.samhsa.gov/. Total abstinence is the most frequently recommended treatment for ATOD addiction. People who are addicted to a particular drug (e.g., cocaine) are advised to abstain from the use of all psychoactive substances. The use of another drug may simply reinforce the craving for the original drug and cause relapse. More commonly, the addiction merely transfers to the replacement substance. Treatment may be on an inpatient or outpatient basis. In general, the more advanced the disease is, the greater the need for inpatient treatment. Inpatient treatment programs usually last 28 days, although the length of stay is often related to the amount of insurance coverage for this treatment. Once a person has completed detoxification (considered the first phase of the treatment process), the programs use counseling and group interaction to help the client stay "clean" long enough for the body chemistry to rebalance. This is often a difficult time for persons recovering from addictions because they may experience mood swings and difficulty sleeping and dealing with emotions.

The goal of the educational part of the programs is to provide information about the disease and how drugs affect a person physically and psychologically. Clients are informed of the various lifestyle changes that are recommended, and they learn about tools to assist them in making these changes. Discharge planning continues throughout treatment as clients build the support systems that they will need when they leave the controlled environment of a treatment center and face pressures and temptations (triggers) that may lead to relapse.

Long-term residential programs, also called *halfway houses,* can help to ease the person recovering from an addiction back into society. These facilities provide continued support and counseling in a structured environment for persons needing long-term assistance in adjusting to a drug-free lifestyle. The residents are expected to secure employment and take responsibility in managing their financial obligations.

Outpatient programs are similar in the education and counseling offered, but they allow the clients to live at home and continue to work while undergoing treatment. This method is effective for persons in the earlier stages of addiction who feel confident that they can abstain from drug use and who have established a strong support network.

Most programs include family counseling and education. In addition, specific programs address the needs of various populations such as adolescents, women during pregnancy, specific ethnic groups, gays and lesbians, as well as health care professionals. Recovery from addiction involves a lifetime commitment and may include periods of relapse. The addicted person must realize that modern medicine has not found a cure for addiction; therefore, returning to drug use may ultimately reactivate the disease process.

CASE STUDY

Ryan Swabbs is a masters degree-prepared nurse who works at a drug rehabilitation center in Mumfordsville. Mr. Swabbs provides individual and group counseling for clients in the process of controlling or stopping their drug addiction.

Tonya Lamburg is a teenage mother who has entered the drug rehabilitation center. She has a 2-year-old son who is staying with Ms. Lamburg's mother until Ms. Lamburg is able to return home. Ms. Lamburg is 16 years old and wants to end her problem with the use of alcohol and cocaine. Mr. Swabbs is assigned to her case.

At their first meeting, Mr. Swabbs assesses Ms. Lamburg's level of drug abuse and readiness for change. Ms. Lamburg has been at the center for 1 week and has not used any drugs since checking in. She shares that she has repeatedly tried to quit alcohol and cocaine "cold turkey" but started to feel "bad and shaky" and went back to using to stop the withdrawal symptoms. "I have no money. I cannot pay for food for my baby. Everything goes to pay for booze or to get high," said Ms. Lamburg. "I dropped out of school when I got pregnant. Everywhere I try to work I get fired. I decided to get help when I saw my baby get into my coke stash. I do not want my boy to die. I do not want to die."

SMOKING CESSATION PROGRAMS

Nearly 35 million Americans try to quit smoking each year. Fewer than 10% of those who try to quit on their own are able to stop for a year; those who use an intervention are more likely to be successful. Interventions that involve medications and behavioral treatments appear most promising (Anderson et al, 2002). For example, nicotine replacement therapy can be used to help smokers withdraw from nicotine while focusing their efforts on breaking the psychological craving or habit. Four types of nicotine replacement products are available: nicotine gum and skin patches are available over the counter, and nicotine nasal spray and inhalers are available by prescription. These products are about equally effective and can almost double the chances of successfully quitting. Other treatments include smoking cessation clinics, hypnosis, and acupuncture. The most effective way to get people to stop smoking and prevent relapse involves multiple interventions and continuous reinforcement, and most smokers require several attempts at cessation before they are successful. Farrelly et al (2008) evaluated whether state tobacco control programs were effective in decreasing the prevalence of adult smokers. They found that program expenditures more effectively influenced the habits of smokers 25 years of age and older versus those between ages 18 and 24. In the latter group the price of cigarettes had a greater effect on their smoking habits.

SUPPORT GROUPS

The founding of **Alcoholics Anonymous (AA)** in 1935 began a strong movement of peer support to treat a chronic illness. AA groups have developed around the world. Their success has led to the development of other support groups such as the following:

- Narcotics Anonymous (NA) for persons with narcotic addiction
- Pills Anonymous for persons with polydrug addictions
- Overeaters Anonymous
- Gamblers Anonymous

AA and NA help addicted people develop a daily program of recovery and reinforce the recovery process. The fellowship, support, and encouragement among AA members provide a vital social network for the person recovering from an addiction.

Al-Anon and Alateen are similar self-help programs for spouses, parents, children, or others involved in a painful relationship with an alcoholic (Nar-Anon for those in relationships with persons with narcotic addictions). Al-Anon family groups are available to anyone who has been affected by involvement with an alcoholic person. The purposes of Alateen include providing a forum for adolescents to discuss family stressors, learn coping skills from one another, and gain support and encouragement from knowledgeable peers. Adult Children of Alcoholics (ACOA) groups are also available in most areas to address the recovery of adults who grew up in alcoholic homes and are still carrying the scars and retaining dysfunctional behaviors.

For some persons, the AA program places too much emphasis on a higher power or focuses too much on the negative consequences of past drinking. Women for Sobriety focuses on rebuilding self-esteem, a core issue for many women with alcoholic problems. See www.womenforsobriety.org for additional information.

Rational Recovery has a cognitive orientation and is based on the assumption that ATOD addiction is caused by irrational beliefs that can be understood and overcome. See www.rational.org for additional information on this approach.

NURSE'S ROLE

Many people with alcoholism and drug addiction become lost in the health care system. If satisfactory care is not provided in one agency or the waiting list is months long, the person may give up rather than seek alternative sources of care. The nurse who knows the client's history, environment, and support systems and the local treatment programs can offer guidance to the most effective treatment modality (Center for Substance Abuse Treatment, 2006). **Brief interventions** by health care professionals who are not treatment experts can be effective in helping ATOD abusers and addicts change their risky behavior. Brief interventions may convince the ATOD abuser or addict to reduce substance consumption or follow through with a treatment referral (Whitlock et al, 2004). Box 24-1 describes six elements commonly included in brief interventions, using the acronym FRAMES. Strategies used with clients can vary depending on their readiness for change. Understanding the stages of change listed in Box 24-2 and recognizing which stage a client is in are important factors for determining which interventions and programs

Modified from Bien TH, Miller WR, Tonigan JS: Brief interventions for alcohol problems: a review, *Addictions* 88:315, 1993.

Box 24-1	**Brief Interventions Using the FRAMES Acronym**

- *Feedback.* Provide the client direct feedback about the potential or actual personal risk or impairment related to drug use.
- *Responsibility.* Emphasize personal responsibility for change.
- *Advice.* Provide clear advice to change risky behavior.
- *Menu.* Provide a menu of options or choices for changing behavior.
- *Empathy.* Provide a warm, reflective, empathetic, and understanding approach.
- *Self-efficacy.* Provide encouragement and belief in the client's ability to change.

Box 24-2	**Stages of Change**

Precontemplation

At this stage, the person does not intend to change in the foreseeable future. The person is often unaware of any problem. Resistance to recognizing or modifying a problem is the hallmark of precontemplation.

Contemplation

At this stage, the individual is aware that a problem exists and is seriously thinking about overcoming it but has not yet made a commitment to take action. The nurse can encourage the individual to weigh the pros and cons of the problem and the solution to the problem.

Preparation

Preparation was originally referred to as decision making. At this stage, the individual is prepared for action and may reduce the problem behavior but has not yet taken effective action (e.g., cuts down amount of smoking but does not abstain).

Action

At this stage, the individual modifies the behavior, experiences, or environment to overcome the problem. The action requires considerable time and energy. Modification of the target behavior to an acceptable criterion and significant overt efforts to change are the hallmarks of action.

Maintenance

In this stage, the individual works to prevent relapse and consolidate the gains attained during action. Stabilizing behavior change and avoiding relapse are the hallmarks of maintenance.

Modified from DiClemente CC, Schlundt D, Gemmell L: Readiness and stages of change in addiction treatment, *Am J Addictions* 13(2):103-120, 2004.

may be most helpful to the client (DiClemente et al, 2004). After the client has received treatment, the nurse can coordinate aftercare referrals and follow up on the client's progress. The nurse can provide additional support in the home as the client and family adjust to changing roles and the stress

involved with such changes. The nurse can support addicted persons who have relapsed by reminding them that relapses may well occur but that they and their families can continue to work toward recovery and an improved quality of life.

CLINICAL APPLICATION

Jane Doe, RN, is a home health case manager in a large, low-income housing area in her local community. She designs care plans and coordinates health care services for clients who need health care at home. She makes the initial visits to determine the level and frequency of care needed and then acts as supervisor of the volunteers and nurses aids who perform most of the day-to-day care. Single-parent families are the norm, and drug dealing is commonplace in this housing area.

Jane made a home visit to Anne, a 26-year-old mother of three. She takes care of her 62-year-old maternal grandfather, Mr. Jones, who is recovering from cardiac bypass surgery. Mr. Jones has a history of smoking two packs per day for almost 40 years. Since his surgery, he has decreased to one pack per day but he refuses to quit. He had a history of alcohol dependence, reportedly consuming up to a fifth of liquor a day, and a history of withdrawal seizures. Four years ago, Mr. Jones went through alcohol detoxification, but he refused to stay at the facility for continued treatment, stating he could stay sober on his own. Since that time he has had several binge episodes, but Anne says he has not been drinking since the surgery. A widower for 5 years, Mr. Jones now lives with his granddaughter and her children.

Anne is a widow and has two sons, ages 3 and 9 years, and a daughter, age 5 years. The oldest son's father is an alcoholic who is currently incarcerated for manslaughter while driving under the influence of alcohol, and the father of her two youngest children was killed by a stray bullet in a cocaine bust 3 years ago. She and her husband had smoked crack cocaine for several months but both stopped when she became pregnant with their youngest child and remained cocaine-free. Anne has been angry at the system and frightened of police officers ever since the drug raid in which her husband was killed. Other residents were also hurt, and less than $500 worth of cocaine was found three apartments away from hers.

Anne does not consume alcohol, but she smokes one to two packs of cigarettes per day. She quit smoking during her pregnancies but restarted soon after each birth.

A. *What type of interventions can Jane provide for Mr. Jones regarding his smoking?*
B. *How can Jane help Anne cope with the potential risk of Mr. Jones continuing to drink when he progresses to more independence?*
C. *How can Jane help Anne with her cigarette smoking?*
D. *Knowing that there is a genetic link to alcoholism and being aware of the high rate of drug problems in the housing area, how can Jane help prevent Anne and her children from developing substance abuse problems?*

> *E. What problems seem greater because of the drug laws, and what can Jane do to help make the environment safer and more nurturing?*
> *Answers are in the back of the book.*

REMEMBER THIS!

- Substance abuse is the number-one national health problem, linked to numerous forms of morbidity and mortality.
- Harm reduction is a new approach to ATOD problems; it deals with substance abuse primarily as a health problem rather than as a criminal problem.
- All persons have ideas, opinions, and attitudes about drugs that influence their actions.
- Social conditions such as a fast-paced life, excessive stress, and the availability of drugs influence the incidence of substance abuse.
- Important terms to understand when working with individuals, groups, or communities for whom substance abuse is prevalent are drug dependence, drug addiction, alcoholism, psychoactive drugs, depressants, stimulants, marijuana, hallucinogens, and inhalants.
- Primary prevention for substance abuse includes education about drugs and guidelines for use, as well as the promotion of healthy alternatives to drug use either for recreation or to relieve stress.
- Nurses can play a key role in developing community prevention programs.
- Secondary prevention depends heavily on careful assessment of the client's use of drugs. Such assessment should be part of all basic health assessments.
- High-risk groups include pregnant women, young people, older adults, intravenous drug users, and illicit drug users.
- Drug addiction is often a family problem, not merely an individual problem.
- Codependency describes a companion illness to the addiction of one person in which the codependent member is addicted to the addicted person.
- Brief interventions by a nurse can be as effective as treatment.
- Nurses are in ideal roles to assist with tertiary prevention for both the addicted person and the family.

WHAT WOULD YOU DO?

1. Read your local newspaper for 4 days and select stories that illustrate the effects of substance abuse on individuals, families, and the community. What interventions would you use? Who would you involve in your work? Are the interventions primary, secondary, or tertiary in nature? How would you evaluate your work?
2. For each of the stories in the newspaper related to substance abuse, describe preventive strategies that a nurse might have tried before the problem reached such a dire state.
3. Looking at your local community resources directory, the telephone book or the Internet, identify agencies that might serve as referral sources for individuals or families for whom substance abuse is a problem.
4. Attend an open AA or NA meeting and an Al-Anon meeting. Go alone if possible or with an alcoholic or a drug-addicted friend. As the members introduce themselves, give your first name and state, "I am a visitor." Plan to listen, and do not attempt to take notes. Respect the anonymity of the persons present. Discuss your experiences later in a group of your classmates.
   - Pay attention to your attitudes toward the attendees.
   - What are the themes of the meeting?
   - How could a nurse help the attendees?

■ REFERENCES

Abramson JL et al: Moderate alcohol consumption and risk of heart failure among older persons, *JAMA* 285(15):1971–1977, 2001.

Alcohol: *The Merck manual,* 2008, section 15, psychiatric disorders, chapter 198, drug use and dependence, Merck & Co., Inc. Retrieved Feb 05, 2009, from http://www.merck.com/mmpe/sec15/ch198/ch198g.html.

Amphetamines: *The Merck manual,* 2008, section 15, psychiatric disorders, chapter 198, drug use and dependence, Merck & Co., Inc. Retrieved Feb 5, 2009, from http://www.merck.com/mmpe/sec15/ch198/ch198k.html.

Anderson JE et al: Treating tobacco use and dependence: an evidence-based clinical practice guideline for tobacco cessation, *Chest* 121(3):932–941, 2002.

Barry M: *Health harms from secondhand smoke,* 2007, National Center for Tobacco-Free Kids, available at http://tobaccofreekids.org/research/factsheets/pdf/0103.pdf.

Bien TH, Miller WR, Tonigan JS: Brief interventions for alcohol problems: a review, *Addiction* 88:315, 1993.

Brady TM, Ashley OS, editors: *Women in substance abuse treatment: results from the Alcohol and Drug Services Study (ADSS).* (DHHS Publication No. SMA 04-3968, Analytic Series A-26). Rockville, Md, 2005, Substance Abuse and Mental Health Services Administration, Office of Applied Studies.

Centers for Disease Control and Prevention: Prevalence of cigarette use among 14 racial/ethnic populations—United States, 1999-2001, *MMWR Morb Mortal Wkly Rep* 53(3):49–52, 2004.

Centers for Disease Control and Prevention: *Access to sterile syringes,* fact sheet, 2005a. Retrieved Feb 29, 2008, from http://www.cdc.gov/idu/facts/AED_IDU_ACC.pdf.

Centers for Disease Control and Prevention: *Syringe exchange programs,* fact sheet, 2005b. Retrieved Feb 29, 2008, from http://www.cdc.gov/idu/facts/AED_IDU_SYR.pdf.

Centers for Disease Control and Prevention: *Tobacco information and prevention source (TIPS),* 2005c. Retrieved Feb 29, 2008, from http://www.cdc.gov/tobacco/research_data/health_consequences/mortali.htm.

Centers for Disease Control and Prevention: *Tobacco-related mortality,* fact sheet, 2006. Retrieved Feb 29, 2008, from http://www.cdc.gov/tobacco/data_statistics/Factsheets/tobacco_related_mortality.htm.

Center for Substance Abuse Treatment: *Substance abuse: clinical issues in intensive outpatient treatment.* Treatment Improvement Protocol (TIP) Series 47, DHHS Publication No. (SMA) 06–4182, Rockville, Md, 2006, Substance Abuse and Mental Health Services Administration.

Cocaine: *The Merck manual,* 2008, section 15, psychiatric disorders, chapter 198, drug use and dependence, Merck & Co., Inc. Retrieved Feb 05, 2009, from http://www.merck.com/mmpe/sec15/ch198/ch198j.html.

Courbasson CMA, de Sorkin AA, Dullerud B: Acupuncture treatment for women with substance use and anxiety/depression: an effective alternative therapy? *Fam Com Health* (30):112–120, 2007.

Dawson DA, Grant BF: Family history and gender: their combined effects on DSM-IV alcohol dependence and major depression, *J Stud Alcohol* 59(1):97–106, 1998.

DiClemente CC, Schlundt D, Gemmell L: Readiness and stages of change in addiction treatment, *Am J Addictions* 13(2):103–120, 2004.

Farrelly MC et al: The impact of tobacco control programs on adult smoking, *Am J Public Health* 98:304–309, 2008.

Gordon SM: *Heroin: challenge for the 21st century*, Wernersville, Pa, 2001, Caron Foundation.

Gordon SM: *Women and addiction: gender issues in abuse and treatment*, Wernersville, Pa, 2002, Caron Foundation.

Griffiths RD et al: Drink a little; take a few drugs: do nurses have knowledge to identify and manage in-patients at risk of drugs and alcohol? *Drug Alcohol Rev* (26):545–552, 2007.

Hallucinogens: *The Merck manual,* 2008, section 15, psychiatric disorders, chapter 198, drug use and dependence, Merck & Co., Inc. Retrieved Feb 27, 2008, from http://www.merck.com/mmpe/sec15/ch198/ch198l.html.

Homish G et al: Antenatal risk factors associated with postpartum comorbid alcohol use and depressive symptomatology, *Alcohol Clin Exp Res* 28(8):1242–1248, 2004.

Introduction: *The Merck manual,* 2008, section 15, psychiatric disorders, chapter 198, drug use and dependence, Merck & Co., Inc. Retrieved Feb 27, 2008, from http://www.merck.com/mmpe/sec15/ch198/ch198a.html.

Johnston LD, O'Malley PM, Bachman JG: Monitoring the future national survey results on drug use, *1975-2006, Col 1: Secondary school students.* NIH Publication No 07-6205. Bethesda, Md, 2007.

Jones HE: Drug addiction during pregnancy, *Cur Direct Psychol Sci* 15(3):126–130, 2006.

Juliano LM, Griffiths RR: A critical review of caffeine withdrawal: empirical validation of symptoms and signs, incidence, severity, and associated features, *Psychopharmacology* 176(1):1–29, 2004.

Kesmodel U et al: Moderate alcohol intake during pregnancy and the risk of stillbirth and death in the first year of life, *Am J Epidemiol* 155(4):305–312, 2002.

Marijuana. *The Merck manual,* 2008, section 15, psychiatric disorders, chapter 198, drug use and dependence, Merck & Co., Inc. Retrieved Feb 27. 2008, from http://www.merck.com/mmpe/sec15/ch198/ch198i.html.

Miller M: *Drug consumer safety rules,* Mosier, Ore, 2002, Mothers Against Misuse and Abuse, available at www.mamas.org.

National Institute on Alcohol Abuse and Alcoholism: Underage drinking: highlights from the Surgeon General's call to action to prevent and reduce underage drinking, *Alcohol Alert* (73):1–6, 2007.

National Institute on Drug Abuse: *NIDA Info Facts: Inhalants,* 2008. Retrieved March 21, 2009 at http://www.nida.nih.gov/infofacts/inhalants.html.

National Institute on Drug Abuse: *Principles of effective treatment,* 2008. Retrieved May 28, 2008, from http://www.drugabuse.gov/PODAT/PODAT1.html.

Opioids: *The Merck manual,* 2008, section 15, psychiatric disorders, chapter 198, drug use and dependence, Merck & Co., Inc. Retrieved Feb 05, 2009, from http://www.merck.com/mmpe/sec15/ch198/ch198f.html.

Physicians and Lawyers for National Drug Policy: *Policy priorities: summary.* Retrieved August 2008 from http://www.plndp.org.

Stott DG, Falconer A, Kerr GD, et al: Does low to moderate alcohol intake protect against cognitive decline in older people? *J Am Geriatric Soc* 56(12):2217–2224, 2008.

Substance Abuse and Mental Health Services Administration: *Results from the 2005 national survey on drug use and health: national findings,* Rockville, Md, 2006, SAMHSA.

Substance Abuse and Mental Health Services Administration: *Results from the 2006 national survey on drug use and health: national findings,* Rockville, Md, 2007, SAMHSA.

Substance Abuse and Mental Health Services Administration: *Chapter 6 – Family therapy. TIP 32: Treatment of adolescents with substance use disorders,* 2008, SAMHSA. Retrieved May 28, 2008, from http://www.ncbi.nlm.nih.gov/books/bv.fcgi?rid=hstat5.section.56538.

Substance Use in Children and Adolescents: *The Merck manual,* 2008, section 15, psychiatric disorders, chapter 198, drug use and dependence, Merck & Co., Inc. Retrieved Feb 05, 2009, from http://www.merck.com/mmpe/sec15/ch198/ch198qhtml.

U.S. Department of Health and Human Services: *Healthy People 2010: understanding and improving health,* ed 2 , Washington, DC, 2000, U.S. Government Printing Office.

U.S. Department of Health and Human Services: *U.S. Surgeon General releases advisory on alcohol use in pregnancy,* Washington, DC, 2005, HHS Press Office.

Weil A, Rosen W: *Chocolate to morphine: understanding mind-active drugs,* Boston, 1998, Houghton Mifflin.

West SL, O'Neal KK: Project D.A.R.E: outcome effectiveness revisited, *Am J Public Health* (94):1027–1029, 2004.

Whitlock EP et al: Screening and counseling to reduce alcohol misuse: Recommendations from the United States Preventive Services Task Force, *Am J Prev Med* 140(7):1–64, 2004.

evolve   http://evolve.elsevier.com/stanhope/foundations

Violence and Human Abuse

Kären M. Landenburger
Jacquelyn C. Campbell

ADDITIONAL RESOURCES

These related resources are found either in the appendix at the back of this book or on the book's website at http://evolve.elsevier.com/stanhope/foundations.

Evolve Website

• Community Assessment Applied

• Case Study, with questions and answers
• Quiz review questions
• WebLinks, including link to *Healthy People 2010* website

OBJECTIVES

After reading this chapter, the student should be able to:

1. Discuss the scope of the problem of violence in American communities, and describe at least three factors in most communities that encourage violence and human abuse.
2. Identify common predictors of potential child abuse and indicators of its presence.
3. Define the four general types of child abuse: neglect, physical, emotional, and sexual.

4. Discuss the dynamics and signs of female abuse by male partners.
5. Describe the growing community health problem of elder abuse.
6. Analyze the nursing role in working with survivors of violence.

CHAPTER OUTLINE

SOCIAL AND COMMUNITY FACTORS
INFLUENCING VIOLENCE
Work
Education
Media
Organized Religion
Population
Community Facilities
VIOLENCE AGAINST INDIVIDUALS OR ONESELF
Homicide

Assault
Sexual Violence Including Rape
Suicide
FAMILY VIOLENCE AND ABUSE
Development of Abusive Patterns
Types of Family Violence
Abuse of Older Adults
NURSING INTERVENTIONS

KEY TERMS

assault: a violent physical or verbal attack.

child abuse: active forms of maltreatment of children.

child neglect: physical or emotional neglect. Physical neglect refers to the failure to provide adequate food, clothing, shelter, hygiene, or necessary medical care; emotional neglect refers to the omission of basic nurturing, acceptance, and caring essential for healthy personal development.

emotional abuse: extreme debasement of a person's feelings so that he or she feels inept, uncared for, and worthless.

emotional neglect: the omission of the basic nurturing, acceptance, and caring essential for healthy personal development.

homicide: a killing of one human being by another.

incest: sexual abuse among family members, typically a parent and a child.

intimate partner violence (IPV): see spouse abuse.

neglect: the failure of a caregiver to provide services that are necessary for the physical and mental health of an individual.

older adult abuse: a form of family violence against older members. It may include neglect and failure to provide adequate food, clothing, shelter, and physical and safety needs; it can also include roughness in care and actual violent behavior toward the elderly.

physical abuse: one or more episodes of physical aggression often resulting in serious physical damage to the internal organs, bones, central nervous system, or sense organs.

physical neglect: failure to provide adequate food, proper clothing, shelter, hygiene, or necessary medical care.

rape: sexual intercourse forced on an unwilling person by threat of bodily injury or loss of life.

sexual abuse: coerced sexual acts ranging from fondling to rape or sexual degradation; it can happen to children or adults and be perpetrated by anyone inside or outside the family.

spouse abuse: physical, emotional, or sexual mistreatment of a partner or former partner.

suicide: the act or an instance of taking your own life voluntarily and intentionally.

violence: nonaccidental acts, interpersonal or intrapersonal, that result in physical or psychological injury to one or more of the people involved.

wife abuse: see spouse abuse.

The word *violence* comes from the Latin *violare,* meaning to violate, injure, or rape. Violence is a public health problem that has both emotional and physical effects. The United States, like many other countries, has a sizable problem with violence. Some societies are basically nonviolent, and for them violence is not a significant health problem. It remains unclear if violence stems from an innate aggressive drive or is a learned behavior. What is clear is that learned behavior and social norms can keep violence at low levels or even eliminate it. It is important to understand the conditions whereby aggression and violence are increased and, conversely, what keeps them in check and promotes nonviolent conflict resolution.

Violence is a concern for nurses. Significant mortality and morbidity result from violence. Nurses often care for the victims, the perpetrators, and those who witness physical and psychological violence. Nurses also can take an active role in the development of community responses to violence by contributing to the development of public policy and needed resources.

Violence is generally defined as those nonaccidental acts, interpersonal or intrapersonal, that result in physical or psychological injury to one or more persons. Violent behavior is predictable and thus preventable, especially with community action. Strategies have been developed in schools to prevent various forms of violence (Horton, 2001; Peterson, Larson, and Skiba, 2001). Poverty, including that resulting from unemployment, urban crowding, and racial inequality,

can influence violence. Knowledge of factors that contribute to violence serves as a starting point for social change and subsequently a change in the level of societal violence (Sampson, 2001). An increase in home-based services (Leventhal, 2001), the evaluation of current practices such as protection orders (Logan, Shannon, and Walker, 2005), and media campaigns (Gandy, 2001) are all examples of methods to prevent violence. Violence is a major cause of premature mortality and life-long disability, and violence-related morbidity is a significant factor in health care costs. An estimated 50,000 persons die annually in the United States from violence-related injuries. Homicide is the second leading cause of death for persons between the ages of 15 and 24, the third leading cause of death for those between the ages of 25 and 34, and the fourth leading cause of death for youth between the ages of 1 and 14. Suicide is the second leading cause of death for persons between the ages of 25 and 34 and the third leading cause of death for individuals between the ages of 10 and 24 (Centers for Disease Control and Prevention 2009). A section of the *Healthy People 2010* objectives is related to reducing violence (see the *"Healthy People 2010"* box).

This chapter examines violence as a public health problem and discusses how nurses can help individuals, families, groups, and communities prevent, cope with, and reduce violence and abuse. Nurses work with clients in many settings, including the home. Because they are in key positions to detect and intervene in community and family violence, nurses need to understand how community-level

National Objectives for Reducing Violence

15-32	Reduce homicides
15-33	Reduce maltreatment and maltreatment fatalities of children
15-34	Reduce the rate of physical assault by current or former intimate partners
15-35	Reduce the annual rate of rape or attempted rape
15-36	Reduce sexual assault other than rape
15-37	Reduce physical assault
15-38	Reduce physical fighting among adolescents
15-39	Reduce weapon carrying by adolescents on school property

From U.S. Department of Health and Human Services: *Healthy People 2010: national health promotion and disease prevention objectives,* ed 2, Washington, DC, 2000, U.S. Government Printing Office.

influences can affect all types of violence. Nurses are often considered the "first responders" when it comes to recognizing and dealing with violence (Trossman 2009).

SOCIAL AND COMMUNITY FACTORS INFLUENCING VIOLENCE

Many factors in a community can support or minimize violence. Changing social conditions, multiple demands on people, economic conditions, and social institutions influence the level of violence and human abuse. The following discussion of selected social conditions enumerates factors that influence violent behavior.

WORK

Productive and paid work is an expectation in mainstream American society. Work can be fulfilling and contribute to a sense of well-being; it can also be frustrating and unfulfilling, contributing to stress that may lead to aggression and violence. Some people are frustrated by jobs that are repetitive, boring, and lack stimulation. Others may report to supervisors whom they neither like nor respect. Workers may go home feeling physically and psychologically drained. They may have difficulty separating feelings generated at work from those at home. For example, a father arrives home feeling tired, angry, and generally inadequate because of a series of reprimands from his boss. Soon after he sits down, his 4-year-old son runs through the house pretending to fly a wooden airplane. After about three loud trips past his father, who keeps shouting for the child to be quiet and go outside, the airplane hits the father in the head. The father could hit the boy out of frustration and anger but that neither makes such violence acceptable nor completely explains it.

People hesitate to give up jobs even if they are frustrating, boring, or stressful. This is particularly true in times of economic downturns when jobs are scarce and competition for them is keen. Family needs may necessitate that

they keep the hated job. They feel trapped and may resent those who depend on them. This frustration and resentment may contribute to violent behavior. Unemployment is also associated with violence both within and outside the home. The inability to secure or keep a job may lead to feelings of inadequacy, guilt, boredom, dissatisfaction, and frustration. Young minority men have the highest rates of unemployment in the United States. This group also has the highest rate of violence. They may feel oppressed or discriminated against, and their lack of opportunities for jobs may encourage anger and violence. Most analyses conclude that the differential rates of violence between African-Americans and whites in the United States have more to do with economic realities, such as poverty, unemployment, and overcrowding, than with race (Sampson, Morenoff, and Raudenbusch, 2005; National Institute of Justice, 2004).

EDUCATION

In recent years, schools have assumed many responsibilities traditionally assigned to the family. Schools teach sexual development, discipline children, and often serve as a place to "dump" children who have no other place to go. Large classes often mean that teachers spend more time and energy monitoring and disciplining children than challenging and stimulating them to learn. In large classes, children who do not conform to expected behaviors are often isolated. The nonconforming child may be removed from the classroom, since there is little or no time to help the child learn alternative ways of behavior.

It is ironic that parents often punish children for hitting or biting other children by spanking them. Corporal punishment is still used in many U.S. schools. Such punishment only reinforces the child's tendency to strike out at others. Schools are often places in which the stressors and frustrations that can contribute to violence are abundant, and violence is learned rather than discouraged. However, school can be a powerful contributor to nonviolence. Youths can attend classes that teach peaceful conflict resolution and discuss the issues of date rape and potential sexual abuse. Parents need to know of the availability of such programs and encourage and support their children in participating (Knox and Roberts, 2005).

MEDIA

The media can influence the occurrence of violence. Television programs and print articles can inform and increase public awareness about family violence (Sampson et al, 2005). Abused women and rape victims benefit from media attention, which tends to decrease the stigma of such victimization and publicize available services. However, the media can indirectly lead people to choose violence. For example, television, movies, newspapers, and magazines show happy, fun-loving people. Television parades all the wonders money can provide; yet for many Americans, the hope of buying many of these nonessentials seems unrealistic. Such polarization between what is available and what is possible can foster the development of patterns of abuse. Frustration, unfilled dreams, and unmet wishes often result in hurting someone who cannot fight back.

The media cater to children by advertising products to buy and things to do. Parents may get angry when their children request the foods, toys, and clothes they see on television, in magazines or newspapers, or hear advertised on the radio. In addition, many toys and video games depict violence.

Often the media portray the world as a violent place. When the public is convinced that violence is rampant, there are two possible results. People may become blasé about violence and no longer feel outraged and galvanized to action when terrible things happen in their community. On the other hand, some become frightened of their neighbors, isolate themselves, and refuse to become involved when someone needs help. Neither response is useful in any community action program.

Hitting, kicking, stabbing, and shooting are seen daily as ways to handle anger and frustration. By the age of 18 years, the average child has seen 1800 murders and countless acts of nonfatal violence on television. Violence in schools, including colleges, has increased and become major news topics. This can either frighten people or inspire those with violent impulses. Frequent violence on television by children has been associated with aggressive behavior in longitudinal research (Wilson, Colvin, and Smith, 2002). On the other hand, the media can be a powerful force for increasing public awareness of various forms of violence and what can be done to address this issue (Sampson et al, 2005).

ORGANIZED RELIGION

Churches meet many human needs, including the need for stimulation, a sense of value, belonging, closeness, and worth, as well as the need for power. Religion generally teaches nonviolent conflict resolution. Churches, clergy, and members of church groups often provide positive role models and reinforce peaceful behavior. Historically, a seemingly contradictory relationship exists between abuse and religion. For example, many religious groups uphold the philosophy of "spare the rod, spoil the child." Also, some faiths support the victimization of women or spouses when they disapprove of divorce. Family members may stay together, although they are at emotional or physical war with one another, because of religious commitments (Fortune, 2001).

Although churches have been slow to recognize domestic violence, some changes are taking place. Male domination over women has become a major issue of discussion in some church groups, whereas in other groups women continue to be blamed for the abuse they sustain. Clergy need to be taught about the nature and dynamics of violence in the family, about religious messages and the potential for support, and about the need for collaboration between the church and advocates for the prevention of domestic violence.

POPULATION

A community's structure can influence the potential for violence. For example, when people are poor and live in crowded conditions the potential for tension and violence is greater. High-population-density communities can positively or negatively influence violence. Those with a sense of cohesiveness may have a lower crime rate than areas of similar size that lack social and cultural groups to support unity among members. Bonds formed among church groups, clubs, and professional organizations can promote harmony among members. In such groups, members can talk about stressors rather than responding with violence. For example, residents of public housing often form neighborhood associations to deal with situations common to many or all residents. Tension can be released in a productive way via projects carried out by the association.

Some residents of high-population areas feel powerless and helpless rather than cohesive. Lack of jobs and low-paying jobs can lead to feelings of inadequacy, despair, and social alienation. Social alienation and exclusion from opportunities can lead to decreased social cohesion and increased violence (Lee and Ousey, 2005; Lambert et al, 2004). Fear and apathy may cause community residents to withdraw from social contact. Withdrawal can foster crime because many residents assume someone else will report suspicious behavior, or they fear reprisals for such reports.

Youths may deal with feelings of powerlessness by forming gangs. Poverty and lack of education appear to be the overriding risk factors. A number of these young adults have attempted to deal with their feelings by turning to crime against people and property to release frustration. In many cities, these gangs have been highly destructive. Unfortunately, many programs have focused on family functioning, using secondary prevention through intervention with families, rather than focusing on primary prevention and the primary issues leading to gang membership (Polakow-Suransky, 2003).

Some high-population areas are characterized by a sense of confusion, resulting in disintegration and disorganization. These areas often have transient populations who have limited physical or emotional investment in the community. Lack of community concern allows crime and violence to go unchecked and may become a norm for the area. Also, as crime increases, residents who are able to move leave the area. This increases community disintegration because the residents who leave are often the most capable members of the population.

The potential for violence may increase among highly diverse populations. Differences in age, socioeconomic status, ethnicity, religion, citizenship, acculturation, or other cultural characteristics can disrupt community stability. Highly divergent groups may not communicate effectively and neither accept nor understand one another. These groups can become hostile and antagonistic toward other groups. Each may see the other as different and not belonging. The alienated group may become the focal point for the others' frustrations, anger, and fears. Racism, classism, and heterosexism are examples of major causes of community disintegration resulting in a vicious cycle of dishonesty, distrust, and hate.

COMMUNITY FACILITIES

Communities differ in the resources and facilities they provide to residents. Some are more desirable places to live, work, and raise families and have facilities that can reduce the potential for crime and violence. Recreational facilities such as playgrounds, parks, swimming pools, movie theaters, and tennis courts provide socially acceptable outlets for a variety of feelings, including aggression. These facilities are resources the residents can use for pleasure, personal enrichment, and group development. Spectator sports, such as football, baseball, basketball, soccer, or hockey, also allow community members to express feelings of anger and frustration. However, watching physically aggressive sports can encourage violence when people hit or shove one another. Familiarity with factors contributing to a community's violence or potential for violence enables nurses to recognize them and intervene accordingly.

VIOLENCE AGAINST INDIVIDUALS OR ONESELF

The potential for violence against individuals (e.g., murder, robbery, rape, assault) or oneself (e.g., suicide) is directly related to the level of violence in the community. Persons living in areas with high rates of crime and violence are more likely to become victims than those in more peaceful areas. The major categories of violence addressed in this chapter are described in terms of the scope of the problem in the United States and the underlying dynamics.

HOMICIDE

Homicide is the leading cause of death for young African-American women ages 15 to 34; it is the second leading cause of death for young Native American women ages 20 to 34; and it is the fourth, third, and fifth leading causes of death for white women ages 15 to 19, 20 to 24, and 25 to 34, respectively (Anderson and Smith, 2005). However, the African-American homicide rate has decreased significantly since 1970, whereas the white homicide rate has increased slightly (U.S. Department of Justice, 2004). Although the data are not adequate, it appears that Hispanic American men have a much higher rate of homicide than non-Hispanic American whites. Homicide is increasing the most among adolescents, but even among very young children in the United States homicide occurs at an alarming rate. The National Child Abuse and Neglect Data System (NCANDS) reported that in 2001 there were an estimated 1300 child fatalities, or 1.81 children per 100,000 in the general population. Children younger than 1 year of age accounted for 41% of the child fatalities, and those younger than 6 years of age accounted for 85% (U.S. Department of Health and Human Services, 2004). In recent years, 14% of all homicides were committed by a stranger. Homicides committed by spouses or family members equaled 15%. In two-thirds of homicides, victims were acquaintances of the offender or the relationship of the victim to the offender was unknown (U.S. Department of

Justice, 2007). When strangers are involved, many of these homicides are related to the illegal substance abuse network. Most homicides are committed by a friend, acquaintance, or family member during an argument. Prevention of homicide is an issue for both the public health system and the criminal justice system.

An alarming aspect of family homicide is that small children may witness the murder or find the body of a family member (Lewandowski et al, 2004). No automatic follow-up or counseling of these children occurs through the criminal justice or mental health system in most communities. These children are at great risk for emotional turmoil and for becoming involved in violence themselves.

The underlying dynamics of homicide within families vary greatly from those of other murders. Women are nine times more likely to be killed by an intimate partner than a stranger. The intimate partner may be a husband, boyfriend, same-sex partner, or ex-partner (Campbell et al, 2007). The top risk factor for intimate partner homicide (IPH) is previous domestic violence. Other risk factors are access to guns, estrangement, threats to kill and threats with a weapon, nonfatal strangulation, and a stepchild in the home if the victim is a female (Campbell et al, 2007). Thus prevention of family homicide involves working with abusive families. In a study of intimate partner homicide of women, 47% of the women who were killed had been seen in a health care setting during the year before they were killed by their husband, boyfriend, or ex-partner (Sharps Koziol-McLain et al, 2001). Nurses have a duty to warn family members of the possibility of homicide when severe abuse is present, just as they warn them of the hazards of smoking. Other nursing care issues are discussed further in the section on "Family Violence and Abuse."

ASSAULT

The death toll from violence is staggering, yet the physical injuries and emotional costs of **assault** are equally important issues in both the acute health care system and in the community. The ratio of nonfatal injuries to homicides was 94:1 in 2000. Although men were far more likely to be assaulted or killed than women, the ratio of nonfatal injuries to homicide was higher for females (144:1) than for males (78:1) (Centers for Disease Control and Prevention, 2002). The greatest risk factor for an individual's victimization through violence is age, and youths are at significantly higher risk. Whereas more males than females are victims of homicide and assault, women are more likely to be victimized by a relative, especially a male partner (U.S. Department of Justice, 2005). Sometimes the difference between a homicide and an assault is only the response time and the quality of emergency transport and treatment facilities. The same community measures used to address homicide can be used to combat assault. Also, nurses often see assaulted persons in home health care with long-term health problems such as head injuries, spinal cord injuries, and stomas from abdominal gunshot wounds. In addition to physical care, nurses must address the emotional trauma of a violent attack. They

Evidence-Based Practice

Although some research has demonstrated the problems associated with sexual assault in urban areas, rural areas have not been studied extensively. This literature review discusses 11 studies on sexual assault in rural areas and identifies several common concerns. The concerns include, but are not limited to, stranger versus acquaintance assault, hesitance to report assaults, blaming attitudes, and the need for additional, faster services.

Rural areas also present challenges that may not be as prevalent in other areas. These challenges are caused by the close proximity of the rural community, creating possible problems for the survivor when interacting with police, court officers, and hospital personnel who may be related to or acquainted with either the survivor or the perpetrator. This familiarity within the community may make it difficult for women to believe they can report assaults confidentially or seek proper care.

NURSE USE: Further research is needed in the area of rural sexual assault. Nurses can explore the physical and psychological impact of sexual assault in rural populations in order to better understand this underrepresented group. Such research can make clear the differences in sexual assault from the rural perspective so that appropriate interventions can be created and implemented.

From Annan SL: Sexual violence in rural areas: A review of the literature, *Family Commun Health* 29:164–168, 2006.

can help victims talk through their traumatic experience to try to make some sense of the violence and refer them for further counseling if anxiety, sleeping problems, or depression persists after the assault.

SEXUAL VIOLENCE INCLUDING RAPE

Sexual violence (SV) is sexual activity in which consent was not obtained or freely given (Centers for Disease Control and Prevention, 2007a). There are many kinds of SV including unwanted touching, **rape,** as well as sexual harassment, threats, intimidation, peeping, and taking nude photos. In the United Sates, 1 in 6 women and 1 in 33 men report an attempted or completed rape at some time in their lives (Centers for Disease Control and Prevention, 2007a). These numbers underestimate the extent of the problem since many cases are never reported. Victims may be ashamed, embarrassed, or afraid. They may think they will not be believed. Victim reporting of rape has improved. Hospital personnel, emergency personnel, and police have better protocols for victims of rape. Even though the collection of information leading to prosecution is emphasized, the protocols try to ensure respectful and supportive treatment for victims.

Sexual violence can affect health in many ways ranging from chronic pain, headaches, stomach problems, sexually transmitted diseases, unwanted pregnancies, generalized fear and anxiety, eating disorders, and depression. Victims may engage in negative health behaviors such as smoking, abusing alcohol, or drugs, or engaging in risky sexual behaviors.

It is necessary to be alert for signs of date and marital rape. Rape victims seldom offer sensitive information unless you specifically ask for it and make it clear that confidentiality will be upheld (Esposito, 2006). Rape results in about 32,000 pregnancies annually (Centers for Disease Control and Prevention, 2007a). Most of the violence against women is intimate partner violence. In the National Violence Against Women Survey (Tjaden and Thoennes, 2000), 64% of rapes, physical assaults, and stalkings were committed against women by either current or former intimate partners. Men, especially boys and young men, are also raped, but the statistics on the incidence of male rape are difficult to verify. It seems reasonable that the emotional trauma for a male rape victim is as serious as that for a woman, but there has been a lack of research in this area.

For reported rapes, cities constitute higher risk areas than do rural areas, and the hours between 8 pm and 2 am, the weekends, and the summer are the most critical times. In about 50% of rapes, the victim and the offender meet on the street, whereas in other cases the rapist either enters the victim's home or somehow entices or forces the victim to accompany him. The majority of rapists are known to the victim.

Prevention of rape, like that of other forms of human abuse, requires a broad-based community focus for educating both the community as a whole and key groups such as police, health providers, educators, and social workers. Rape rates and community-level variables such as community approval and legitimization of violence (e.g., violent network television viewing, permitting corporal punishment in schools) appear related and underscore the need for community-level intervention (Bachar and Koss, 2001).

A first step in intervening in the incidence and treatment of rape survivors is to change and clarify misconceptions about rape and victims of rape. Rape is a crime of violence, not a crime of passion. The underlying issues are hostility, power, and control rather than sexual desire. The defining issue is lack of consent of the victim. When a woman or man refuses any sexual activity, that refusal means "no." People have the right to change their mind, even when they seemed initially agreeable. Pressure from physical contact, threats, or deliberate inducement of drug or alcohol intoxication is a violation of the law. The myths that women say "no" to sex when they really mean "yes" and that the victims of rape are culpable because of the way they dress or act must end. On college campuses, negative attitudes toward acquaintance or date rape are slow to change. Women on college campuses underreport allegations of rape because of issues of confidentiality and fear of being discredited (Bachar and Koss, 2001).

During the act of rape, survivors are often hit, kicked, stabbed, and severely beaten. It is this violence as well as the violation of the sense of self that most traumatizes the person because of the fear for her life and her feelings of helplessness, lack of control, and vulnerability.

People react to rape differently, depending on their personality, past experiences, background, and support received after the trauma. Some cry, shout, or discuss the experience. Others withdraw and are afraid to discuss the attack. During the immediate as well as the follow-up stages, victims may blame themselves for what has happened. When working with rape victims help them identify the issues behind self-blame. Fault should not be placed on survivors; they should be taught to take control, learn assertiveness, and think they can take specific actions to prevent future rapes. Survivors need to talk about what happened and to express their feelings and fears in a nonjudgmental atmosphere. Nonjudgmental listening is important. In any psychological trauma, the right to privacy and confidentiality is crucial. Victims should be given privacy, respect, and assurance of confidentiality; told about health care procedures conducted immediately after the rape; given a complete physical examination by a trained nurse examiner (sexual assault or forensic nurse examiner); and linked with proper resources for ease of reporting.

Nurses often provide continuous care once the victim enters the health care system. Because many victims deny the event once the initial crisis is past, a single-session debriefing should be completed during the initial examination. The physical assessment, examination, and debriefing should be carried out by specially trained providers. In most states, nurses trained in sexual assault examination (sexual assault nurse examiner [SANE] nurses, a subspecialty of forensic nursing) perform the physical examination in the emergency department to gather evidence (e.g., hair samples, skin fragments beneath the victim's fingernails, evidence from pelvic examinations using colposcopy) for criminal prosecution of sexual assault. This crucial nursing intervention often takes time, and allows the nurse to begin communication with the victim. Nurses' evidence is credible and effective in court proceedings (Campbell R, 2004).

Rape is a situational crisis for which advance preparation is rarely possible. Therefore, nurses need to help victims cope with the stress and disruption of their lives caused by the attack. Counseling focuses on the crisis and the fears, feelings, and issues involved. Nurses can help survivors learn how to regroup personal forces. If posttraumatic stress disorder (PTSD) has developed, professional psychological or psychiatric treatment is indicated.

BRIEFLY NOTED

Forty to forty-five percent of physically abused women are also forced into sex. This has implications for the prevention of unintended and adolescent pregnancies, human immunodeficiency virus (HIV), acquired immunodeficiency syndrome (AIDS), and sexually transmitted diseases (STDs), as well as for women's healthy sexuality and self-esteem.

Many rape victims need follow-up mental health services to help them cope with the short-term and long-term effects of the crisis. The time after a rape is one of disequilibrium, psychological breakdown, and reorganization of attitudes about the safety of the world. Common, everyday tasks often tax a person's resources. Many individuals forget or fail to keep appointments. Nurses can make appropriate referrals and obtain permission from the victim to remain in contact through telephone conversations, which allows for ongoing

assessment of the victim's needs and opportunities to intervene when needed.

The best way to prevent sexual violence is to stop it before it begins. The Centers for Disease Control and Prevention advocates strategies such as (1) engaging high school students in mentoring programs or other skill-based activities that discuss health, sexuality, and dating behaviors; (2) helping parents and the media identify and address social and cultural influences that promote violent attitudes and actions; and (3) designing policies for school, work, and other public places that address sexual harassment (Centers for Disease Control and Prevention, 2007a). The CDC also uses a four-step approach to address public health problems such as sexual violence:
1. Define the problem
2. Identify risk and protective factors
3. Develop and test prevention strategies
4. Ensure widespread adoption (see www.cdc.gov/injury)

SUICIDE

In 2004, suicides were committed by 32,439 people in the United States (National Institute of Mental Health, 2004). This is equal to 89 suicides a day or one every 16 minutes (Centers for Disease Control and Prevention, 2007b). It is the eleventh leading cause of death in the United States; four times as many males as females commit **suicide** with firearms (Centers for Disease Control and Prevention, 2007b). The highest rate is for people 65 years and older. Women report attempting suicide about three times more often than men. Suicide rates are highest among men, American Indians/Alaska Natives, non-Hispanic whites, and persons ages 45 to 54. They most often occur in a house or apartment and involve a firearm (Centers for Disease Control and Prevention, 2009). Together, white males and white females accounted for more than 90% of all suicides (Centers for Disease Control and Prevention, 2004a).

Leading risk factors for suicide are depression and other mental disorders or substance-abuse disorders and intimate partner problems. Other risk factors include a prior suicide attempt, a family history of suicide, mental disorder, substance abuse or violence, firearms in the home, incarceration, and exposure to the suicidal behavior of others, i.e., family, peers or media figures (National Institute of Mental Health, 2004).

Nurses can aid in reducing suicide and in caring for victims, including the community, the family, and individuals. On a community level, nurses can be involved in a coordinated response for suicide prevention and the care of people who attempt suicide. Nurses can assist in developing policies and protocols for suicide prevention across the life span. Care may focus on family members and friends of suicide victims. Survivors often feel angry toward the dead person, yet may turn the anger inward. Likewise, survivors often question their own liability for the death. The impact of suicide can affect family, friends, co-workers, and the community. Survivors may find it hard to deal with their feelings toward the dead person. It may be difficult for them to concentrate, and they may limit their social activities because both their friends and family may be unable to talk about the suicide. Nurses can help survivors cope with the trauma of the loss and make referrals to a counselor or support groups.

FAMILY VIOLENCE AND ABUSE

Family violence, including sexual, emotional, and physical abuse, causes significant injury and death. These three forms tend to occur together as part of a system of coercive control. Generally, family violence is violence of the most powerful against the least powerful. Intimate partner violence is directed primarily toward wives (although they may physically fight back). According to the Bureau of Justice Statistics (U S. Department of Justice, 2005), 73% of victims of family violence were female and about 75% of their attackers were male.

Recognizing the battered child or spouse in the emergency department is relatively simple after the fact. It is unfortunate that by the time medical care is sought, serious physical and emotional damage may have already occurred. Nurses are in a key position to predict and deal with abusive tendencies. By understanding factors contributing to the development of abusive behaviors, nurses can identify abuse-prone families.

DEVELOPMENT OF ABUSIVE PATTERNS

To help abusive families, nurses need to understand that the factors that characterize people who become involved in family violence include upbringing, living conditions, and increased stress. Of these factors, the one most predictably present is previous exposure to some form of violence. As children, abusers were often beaten or saw siblings or parents beaten. They learned that violence is a way to manage conflict. Both men and women who witnessed abuse as children were more likely to abuse their children (Berman, Hardesty, and Humphreys, 2004). Childhood physical punishment teaches children to use violent conflict resolution as an adult. A child may learn to associate love with violence because a parent is usually the first person to hit a child. Children may think that those who love them also are those who hit them. The moral rightness of hitting other family members thus may be established when physical punishment is used to train children, especially when it is used more than occasionally. These experiences predispose children ultimately to use violence with their own children.

As well as having a history of child abuse themselves, people who become abusers tend to have hostile personality styles and be verbally aggressive. They often learn these behaviors from their own childhood experiences. Their parents may have set unrealistic goals, and when the children failed to perform accordingly, they were criticized, demeaned, punished, and denied affection. These children may have been told how to act, what to do, and how to feel, thereby discouraging the development of normal attachment, autonomy, problem-solving skills, and creativity (Dixon, Hamilton-Giachritsis, and Brown, 2005; Edwards et al, 2004). These children grow up feeling unloved and worthless. They may want a child of their own so that they will feel love.

To protect themselves from feelings of worthlessness and fear of rejection, abused children form a protective shell and may become hostile and distrustful of others. The behavior of potential abusers reflects a low tolerance for frustration, emotional instability, and the onset of aggressive feelings with minimal provocation. Because of their emotional insecurity, they often depend on a child or spouse to meet their needs of feeling valued and secure. When their needs are not met by others, they become overly critical. Critical, resentful behavior and unrealistic expectations of others lead to a vicious cycle. The more critical these people become, the more they are rejected and alienated from others. Abusive individuals often think the target of their hostility is "out to get" them. For example, a parent might think or say that an infant deliberately kept him or her awake all night. We know that infants do not intentionally keep parents awake. Rather, infants cry and fret for a reason of their own, not to annoy and inconvenience others.

A perceived or actual crisis may precede an abusive incident. Because a crisis reinforces feelings of inadequacy and low self-esteem, a number of events may occur in a short time to precipitate abusive patterns. Unemployment, marital strains, or an unplanned pregnancy can set off violence. The daily hassles of raising young children, especially in an economically strained household, intensify an already stressed atmosphere for which an unexpected and difficult event provokes violence. Stressful life events, poverty, and the number of small children in the home are often associated with family violence. Crowded living conditions can precipitate abuse. Several people living in a small space increases tensions and reduces privacy. Tempers flare due to the constant stimulation from others.

Social isolation reduces social support and can decrease a family's ability to cope with stress and lead to abuse. The problem may be intensified if a violent family member tries to keep the family isolated to escape detection. Therefore, if a family misses clinic or home visit appointments, nurses need to consider the possibility of abuse. Nurses can encourage involvement in community activities and can help neighbors reach out to one another to help prevent abuse.

Frequent moves disrupt social support systems, are associated with an increased stress level, and tend to isolate people, at least briefly. Mobility can have a serious negative effect on the abuse-prone family. These families do not readily initiate new relationships. They rely on the family for support. Resources may be unfamiliar or inaccessible to them. Because frequent moving may be both a risk factor for abuse and a sign of an abusive family trying to avoid detection, nurses should assess such families carefully for abuse.

TYPES OF FAMILY VIOLENCE

Family violence may not be limited to one family member; thus, nurses who detect child abuse should also suspect other forms of family violence. When older adult parents report that their (now adult) child was abused or has a history of violence toward others, the nurse should recognize the potential for elder abuse. **Physical abuse** of women may be accompanied by **sexual abuse**, both inside and outside the marital relationship. Severe wife abusers may commit other acts of violence, especially child abuse. Also, when one child is abused, others may be physically, sexually, or emotionally abused. Families who are verbally aggressive in conflict resolution (e.g., using name calling, belittling, screaming, and yelling) are more likely to be physically abusive. Although the various forms of family violence are discussed separately, they should not be thought of as totally separate phenomena. No member of the family is guaranteed immunity from abuse and **neglect.** Spouse abuse, child abuse, abuse of older adults, serious violence among siblings, and mutual abuse by members all occur. Although these examples are not inclusive, they demonstrate the scope of family violence. Remember abuse is about power and control. Emotional abuse and controlling behaviors often occur before physical abuse. Box 25-1 lists ways in which abusers can control and intimidate those whom they abuse. Remember that no one deserves to be treated this way.

Child Abuse

In 2005, U.S. state and local child protective services investigated 3.6 million cases in which it was reported that children were being neglected or abused. Of these, 899,000 were considered victims as follows: 63% neglect, 7% emotional abuse, 9% sexual abuse, and 17% physical abuse. These are probably conservative figures, because only the most severe cases are reported. Overall girls were slightly higher (51%) at risk than boys (47%) for all forms of maltreatment (Centers for Disease Control and Prevention, 2007c). Female children were four times more likely to be sexually abused than male children (U.S. Department of Health and Human Services, 2005). Child abuse tends to increase when there is increased family stress, especially during economic crunches. Babies are at risk for suffering brain injury when an adult, often feeling overwhelmed, violently shakes the baby whose muscles are too weak to hold his or her head steady thereby exposing the brain to injury (Goldberg 2009).

Many children witness domestic violence (Berman, Hardesty, and Humphreys, 2004). Children witnessing domestic violence may experience PTSD and exhibit aggressive behavior (Buka et al, 2001; Litrownik et al, 2003). Also children living in homes in which violence takes place between their parents are more likely to be abused themselves (Salzinger et al, 2002). Risk factors for children who are abused include parental factors such as limited family economic resources, lack of social support, parental domestic violence, and problems with substance abuse. Some of the risk factors are identified in Box 25-2. Children who witness parental domestic violence may react differently according to their age, level of development, and sex; their reactions are influenced by the severity and frequency of the abuse witnessed (Hurt et al, 2001).

The presence of child abuse signifies ineffective family functioning. Abusive parents who recognize their problem

---

Box 25-1   Abuse Is About Power and Control

All of these actions are unhealthy, and some are illegal.
Isolation: the abuser keeps the abused person:
- Away from seeing friends and family
- From going to work or school
- In an overly protective relationship and is jealous and possessive
- From using the car or otherwise traveling freely on his or her own

Threats: the abuser threatens to:
- Hurt or kill you or your family or friends
- Take your children away
- Report you to welfare or immigration authorities
- Hurt himself or herself

Intimidation: the abuser:
- Insults you, puts you down, calls you names or humiliates you in front of others
- Interrupts when you speak
- Stalks or harasses you, or tries to make you think you are crazy

Using children: the abuser:
- Calls you a bad parent, or tries to turn others against you
- Uses others, especially children, to deliver nasty messages to you
- Harasses with threats about custody, visitation, or family court orders

Being cruel: the abuser:
- Denies you food, sleep, or medical care
- Abuses or kills your pets
- Destroys your things such as clothes, photos, heirlooms, or other valued items

Withholds support: the abuser:
- Takes your money, fails to give you adequate money, or makes you account for everything you buy
- Denies access to bank accounts or credit cards

Sexual abuse: the abuser:
- Withholds sex or affection
- Prevents you from using birth control or condoms to protect against sexually transmitted diseases
- Forces you to engage in sexual acts

Modified from Health Bulletin: Domestic violence and abuse, *Health Ment Hygiene News* 2(10), 2003, New York City Department of Health and Mental Hygiene.

---

are often reluctant to seek assistance because of the stigma attached to being considered a child abuser. Children may be victims of abuse because they are small and relatively powerless. In many families, only one child is abused. Parents may identify with this particular child and be especially critical of the child's behavior. In some cases, the child may have certain qualities, such as looking like a relative, being handicapped, trying to resist the violence, or being particularly bright and capable or strong willed, that provoke the parent. However, in families in which child abuse occurs, there is an explicit or covert threat to children other than the one who is most severely abused. Thus, other children are affected by conflicting feelings such as guilt and relief. The targeted child is often coerced into silence by threats toward the sibling(s).

CASE STUDY

As nurse Marie Mason was preparing to visit a newborn and her mother, Vicki, she received word that two other children had been removed from Vicki's care in the past by Child Protective Services. During the initial visit and all other visits, Ms. Mason would unclothe the baby and assess her growth and development, as well as look for bruises or abrasions. Ms. Mason gained Vicki's trust during her weekly visits and for the first month thought all was progressing well. The father of the baby was often present, and he seemed caring of the child. Although the grandmother lived in the apartment at night, she spent her days at a treatment center for the mentally ill.

When the infant was 2 months old, the nurse noticed that Vicki did not support the infant's head despite her explanations that the baby needed that. Also, Vicki advanced the baby's diet to include pureed canned fruits and meats, well ahead of what had been advised. Vicki, who had diabetes mellitus type 1, also ate erratically and failed to test her own blood sugars. She was overweight but said she had been losing weight because she was only eating take-out Chinese food once a day. Ms. Mason set small goals with Vicki each week, such as adding an easy nutritious breakfast to her diet and testing her blood sugar at least once a day.

When the baby was 3 months old, Vicki told Ms. Mason that she had told the baby's father, Max, not to come back, since he had spoken harshly of her mother. Upon further questioning, Vicki revealed that she was afraid Max would hurt her and that he had slapped her on occasion. There was also a new man who seemed to be living in the house and was clearly fond of the mother and child.

Created by Deborah C. Conway, Assistant Professor,
School of Nursing, University of Virginia

Parents with low social support, a tendency toward depression, multiple stress factors, and a history of abuse are at risk for abusing their children (Ethier, Couture, and Lacharité, 2004). Abusive parents often have unrealistic expectations of a child's developmental abilities. They tend to have little involvement with and show minimal warmth toward their child (Gary, Campbell, and Humphreys, 2004). Parents who abuse their children use physical discipline more frequently, often in the form of physical punishment, and verbal abuse (Hines and Malley-Morrison, 2005; Straus, 2005). The nurse must teach normal parental behavior and also address the underlying emotional needs of the parents. They need to teach forms of parental control other than physical punishment. These parents often experience pain and poor emotional stability and need intervention as much as their children. The "How To" box lists some of the behavioral indicators of potentially abusive parents.

When child abuse is discovered, the child is often placed in a foster home. Unfortunately, not enough good foster care is available for all abused children. Also many foster care situations are abusive. Abused children generally want to

Box 25-2 Risk Factors for Child Abuse

Ask the following questions to determine if risk factors are present:
- What are the ages of the parents?
- Does the child come from a single-parent household or a family with a large number of children?
- Do the parents have the financial resources to care for a child?
- Are the parents communicative with each other and the nurse?
- Is there a support network that is willing to offer assistance?
- Does the mother of the child seem frightened of her partner?
- Does either of the parents have a history of child abuse?
- Do the parents have knowledge about child development?
- Does either parent or both have problems with substance abuse?
- Does the child suffer from recurrent injuries or unexplained illnesses?

Compiled from Barnett OW, Miller-Perrin CL, Perrin RD: *Family violence across the lifespan: an introduction,* Thousand Oaks, Calif, 1997, Sage; Pepler D et al.: Consider the children: research informing interventions for children exposed to domestic violence, *J Aggression Maltreatment Trauma* 3.1(5):37–57, 2000; Sedlak AJ, Broadhurst DD: *Executive summary of the Third National Incidence Study of Child Abuse and Neglect,* U.S. Department of Health and Human Services, Administration for Children and Families, Administration on Children, Youth and Families, National Center on Child Abuse and Neglect, Washington, DC, 1996, National Clearinghouse on Child Abuse and Neglect; Widom CS, Hiller-Sturmhöfel S: Alcohol abuse as a risk factor for and consequence of child abuse, *Alcohol Res Health* 25(1):52–57, 2001.

HOW TO Identify Potentially Abusive Parents

The following characteristics in couples expecting a child constitute warning signs of actual or potential abuse:
- Denial of the reality of the pregnancy, i.e., refusal to talk about the impending birth or to think of a name for the child
- An obvious concern or fear that the baby will not meet some predetermined standard: sex, hair color, temperament, or resemblance to family members
- Failure to follow through on the desire for an abortion
- An initial decision to place the child for adoption and a change of mind
- Rejection of the mother by the father of the baby
- Family experiencing stress and numerous crises so that the birth of a child may be the last straw
- Initial and unresolved negative feelings about having a child
- Lack of support for the new parents
- Isolation from friends, neighbors, or family
- Parental evidence of poor impulse control or fear of losing control
- Contradictory history
- Appearance of detachment
- Appearance of misusing drugs or alcohol
- Shopping for hospitals or health care providers
- Unrealistic expectations of the child
- Verbal, physical, or sexual abuse of the mother by the father, especially during pregnancy
- The child is not the biological offspring of the stepfather or the mother's current boyfriend
- Excessive talk of needing to "discipline" children and plans to use harsh physical punishment to enforce discipline

return to their parents, and most agencies try to keep natural families together as long as it is safe for the child. Nurses often monitor a family in which a formerly abused child is returned from foster care. Keen judgment and close collaboration with social services are essential. The nurse must ensure the safety of the child while working with the parents in an empathetic way. The nurse's goal is to enhance their parenting skills, not to be viewed as yet another watchdog. Remember also that abusive parents may try to replace a child who has been removed by the courts because of abuse. This is a normal response to the grief of losing a child. Rather than regarding another pregnancy as a sign of continued poor judgment or pathological behavior, the pregnancy can be perceived by the nurse as an opportunity for intensive intervention to prevent the abuse of the expected child. Generally, the parents are eager to avoid further problems if they are enlisted as partners in the project.

INDICATORS OF CHILD ABUSE. Nurses need to recognize the physical and behavioral indicators of abuse and neglect. **Child abuse** ranges from violent physical attacks to passive neglect. The children suffer physical injuries including cuts, bruises, burns, and broken bones; they may also be beaten, burned, kicked, or shook. Passive neglect may result in insidious malnutrition or other problems. Abuse is not limited to physical maltreatment but includes emotional abuse such as yelling at or continually demeaning, shaming, rejecting, withholding love from, threatening, and criticizing the child. Maltreatment can cause stress that can disrupt early brain development and, at extreme levels, can affect the development of the nervous and immune systems. Abused children are then at higher risk for adult health problems including alcoholism, depression, substance abuse, eating disorders, obesity, sexual proximity, smoking, suicide, and some chronic diseases (Centers for Disease Control and Prevention, 2006).

Children at risk for child maltreatment are those who (1) come from a family in which intimate partner violence is present; these children are at greater risk for physical and psychological abuse and child neglect (English, Marshall, and Stewart, 2003; Hines and Malley-Morrison, 2005); (2) are under age 4; these children are at the greatest risk for severe injury and death; (3) live in communities with a high level of violence and one that accepts child abuse; and (4) live in families with great stress, such as from substance abuse, poverty, and chronic illness, and who do not have nearby friends or relatives who can provide support and assistance (Centers for Disease Control and Prevention, 2006).

Emotional abuse involves extreme debasement of feelings and may result in the child feeling inadequate, inept, uncared for, and worthless. Victims of emotional abuse learn to hide their feelings to avoid incurring additional scorn. They may act out by performing poorly in school, becoming truant, and being hostile and aggressive. Children who are abused or who witness domestic violence can suffer developmentally; adolescents may run away from home as a direct result of domestic violence (Grella and Joshi, 2003).

HOW TO	**Recognize Actual or Potential Child Abuse**

Be alert to the following:
- An unexplained injury
- Skin: burns, old or recent scars, ecchymosis, soft tissue swelling, human bites
- Fractures: recent, or older ones that have healed
- Subdural hematomas
- Trauma to genitalia
- Whiplash (caused by shaking small children)
- Dehydration or malnourishment without obvious cause
- Provision of inappropriate food or drugs (alcohol, tobacco, medication prescribed for someone else, foods not appropriate for the child's age)
- Evidence of general poor care: poor hygiene, dirty clothes, unkempt hair, dirty nails
- Unusual fear of the nurse and others
- Considered to be a "bad" child
- Inappropriate dress for the season or weather conditions
- Reports or shows evidence of sexual abuse
- Injuries not mentioned in the history
- Seems to need to take care of the parent and speak for the parent
- Maternal depression
- Maladjustment of older siblings

Physical symptoms of stress from physical, sexual, or emotional abuse may include hyperactivity, withdrawal, overeating, dermatological problems, vague physical complaints, and exacerbation of stress-related physical problems such as asthma, stuttering, enuresis (bladder incontinence), and encopresis (bowel incontinence). Sadly, bedwetting is often a trigger for further abuse, which creates a particularly vicious cycle. When a child displays physical symptoms without clear physiological origin, ruling out the possibility of abuse should be part of the nurse's assessment process.

Child Neglect

Neglect is the failure to meet a child's basic needs including those for housing, food, clothing, education, and access to health care (Centers for Disease Control and Prevention, 2006). The two categories of **child neglect** are physical and emotional. **Physical neglect** is defined as failure to provide adequate food, proper clothing, shelter, hygiene, or necessary medical care. Physical neglect is most often associated with extreme poverty. In contrast, **emotional neglect** is the omission of basic nurturing, acceptance, and caring essential for healthy personal development. These children are largely ignored or in many cases treated as nonpersons. Such neglect usually affects the development of self-esteem. It is difficult for a neglected child to feel a great deal of self-worth because the parents have not demonstrated that they value the child. Neglect is more difficult to assess and evaluate than abuse because it is subtle and may go unnoticed. It is not directly related to poverty and occurs across the socioeconomic spectrum of families. Astute observations of children, their homes, and the way in which they relate to their caregivers can provide clues of neglect.

Sexual Abuse

Child abuse also includes sexual abuse. Approximately one in four female children and one in ten male children in the United States will experience some form of sexual abuse by the time they are 18 years of age. The exact prevalence is difficult to obtain because not all children have the cognitive ability to describe these experiences (Urbanic, 2004). This abuse ranges from unwanted sexual touching to intercourse. The majority of childhood sexual abuse is perpetrated by someone the child knows and trusts. Between one-third and one-half of all sexual abuse involves a family member (Hines and Malley-Morrison, 2005). Although sexual abuse is perpetrated by all categories of caregivers, a child's risk for abuse is higher with stepparents or nonrelated caregivers. Adults whom children and parents are inclined to trust, such as coaches, scout leaders, and even priests, have been reported sexual abusers. The long-term effects of sexual abuse include depression, sexual disturbances, and substance abuse (Hines and Malley-Morrison, 2005).

Research has shown that many of the characteristics of physically abusive and sexually abusive parents, such as unhappiness, loneliness, and rigidity, are shared by both groups. However, sexually abused children have more gastrointestinal symptoms and posttraumatic stress disorders than physically abused children (Ross, 2005).

Father–daughter **incest** is the type of intrafamilial sexual abuse most often reported. Although mother–son incest takes place, the incidence remains small. Many cases of parental incest go unreported because victims fear punishment, abandonment, rejection, or family disruption if they acknowledge the problem. Incest occurs in all races, religious groups, and socioeconomic classes. Although incest is receiving greater attention because of mandatory reporting laws, too often its incidence remains a family secret.

Because nurses are often involved in helping women deal with the aftermath of incest, it is crucial to understand the typical patterns and the long-term implications. A typical pattern is as follows. The daughter involved in paternal incest is usually about 9 years of age at the onset and is often the oldest or only daughter. The father or stepfather seldom uses physical force. He most likely relies on threats, bribes, intimidation, or misrepresentation of moral standards, or he exploits the daughter's need for human affection.

Nurses must be aware of the incidence, signs and symptoms, and psychological and physical trauma of incest. Symptoms include low self-esteem, depression, anxiety, and somatic symptoms of headaches, eating and sleeping disorders, menstrual problems, and gastrointestinal distress (Naar-King et al, 2002; Ross, 2005). Other symptoms include difficulties in social situations, especially in forming and maintaining close relationships with men, and behavioral symptoms such as substance abuse and sexual dysfunction. Children often try to avoid or escape the abusive behavior. Avoidance can take the form of either behavioral or mental

reactions, such as dressing to cover one's body or pretending that the abuse is not taking place. The child can escape either physically by running away or emotionally by withdrawing into other activities and thereby placing the sexual abuse in the background (Urbanic, 2004).

Adolescents may display inappropriate sexual activity or truancy or may run away from home. Running away is usually considered a sign of delinquency; however, an adolescent who runs away may be using a healthy response to a violent family situation. Therefore the assessment should include a thorough inquiry about sexual and physical abuse at home and an appropriate physical examination.

Intimate Partner Abuse

Most domestic violence is committed by men against women. However, men also abuse male partners and women abuse men. Men who abuse their partners are likely to abuse children (Health Bulletin, 2003). Of the approximately 3.5 million reports of family violence between 1998 and 2002, 73% of the victims were female, and most perpetrators were men (U.S. Department of Justice, 2005). Neither the term **wife abuse** nor the term **spouse abuse** takes into account violence in dating or cohabiting relationships or violence in same-sex relationships. **Intimate partner violence (IPV)** is defined as threatened, attempted, or completed physical, sexual, or emotional abuse by a current or former intimate partner. Within the realm of emotional or psychological abuse is financial abuse. The partner may be a spouse, ex-spouse, current or former boyfriend or girlfriend, or a dating partner (Centers for Disease Control and Prevention, 2008). Intimate partners can be of the same or opposite sex, and the incidence of violence in same-sex relationships is considered to be the same as in heterosexual relationships (Trossman, 2009; Centers for Disease Control and Prevention, 2004b). The abuse of female partners has the most serious community health ramifications because of the greater prevalence, the greater potential for homicide (Campbell et al, 2003), the effects on the children in the household, and the more serious long-term emotional and physical consequences.

Victims of child abuse and individuals who saw their mothers being battered are at risk of using violence toward an intimate partner, whether one is male or female (Centers for Disease Control and Prevention, 2004b). However, using evidence of a violent childhood to identify women at risk of abuse is less useful, because abuse cannot be predicted on the basis of characteristics of the individual woman. The violent background of an abusive male, combined with his tendencies to be possessive, controlling, and extremely jealous, is most predictive of abuse. Substance abuse is also associated with battering, although it cannot be said to cause the violence.

SIGNS OF ABUSE. Battered women often have bruises and lacerations of the face, head, and trunk of the body. Attacks are often carefully inflicted on parts of the body that can easily be disguised by clothing, such as breasts, abdomen, upper thighs, and back (Campbell and Sheridan, 2004). Ranging from physical restraint to murder, Schwartz (2007) lists these forms of physical abuse: hitting, kicking, punching, slapping, strangling, shaking, confining, burning, freezing, pushing, tripping, scratching, cutting, biting, pinching, throwing things, or hiding medications. Emotional, psychological, and verbal abuse includes coercion, manipulation, isolation, intimidation, mocking or criticizing, humiliating, lying, screaming, threatening, or using menacing forms of nonverbal behavior (Schwartz, 2007). Financial abuse is seen when a partner limits the other person's access to money as a method of control.

Once abused, women tend to exhibit low self-esteem and depression (Centers for Disease Control and Prevention, 2004b). Few are able to come right out and ask for help, which means that the nurse needs to communicate honestly, openly, and with sensitivity. Complete any screening in a quiet, private setting; do not ask anyone who accompanies them to translate or explain; it is best to have no one else present during the interview; and remember that any person accompanying the victim might be an abuser (Schwartz, 2007).

When a woman has a black eye or bruises about the mouth ask "Who hit you?" rather than "What happened to you?" The latter implies that the nurse is neither knowledgeable nor comfortable with violence, and this may prompt the woman to fabricate a more acceptable cause of her injury.

Abused women have more physical health problems than other women, specifically symptoms such as chronic pain (back, head, abdominal), neurological problems, problems sleeping, gynecological symptoms, urinary tract infections, and chronic gastrointestinal problems (Campbell, 2002). Ask "When did this happen?" and also ask "Where did this happen?" Write up what the person actually said using quotation marks and make note of grooming, posture, and mannerisms (Schwartz, 2007, p. 45).

ABUSE AS A PROCESS. According to Landenburger (1998) and Campbell et al (2004), women's emotional and behavioral reactions change over time as they respond to repeated battering. Initially they try to minimize the seriousness of the situation. The violence usually starts with a slight shove in the middle of a heated argument. All couples fight, and if there is any physical aggression, both the man and the woman tend to blame the incident on something external such as a particularly stressful day at work or drinking too much. The male partner usually apologizes for the incident, and as with any problem in a relationship, the couple tries to improve the situation. Although marital counseling may be useful at this early stage, it is generally contraindicated at all other stages because of the risk to the woman's safety. Unfortunately, abuse tends to escalate in frequency and severity over time, and the man's remorse tends to lessen. The risk is such that women who try to leave an abusive relationship are at significant risk for homicide (Campbell et al, 2004).

Because women often feel responsible for the success of a relationship, they may try to change their behavior to end the violence. They may even blame themselves for infuriating their spouse. Women who blame themselves for provoking the abuse are more likely to have low self-esteem and be depressed than those who do not blame themselves. Some women experience a moral conflict between their need to leave an abusive relationship and their sense that it is their responsibility to maintain relationships (Belknap, 1999). Women find that no matter what they do, the violence continues. During this period, the woman tries to hide the violence because of the stigma attached. She tries to placate her spouse and feels she is losing her sense of self (Landenburger, 1998). She is often concerned about her children whether she leaves or stays. Some women literally fear for their lives and those of their children. She fears that her partner will try to kill her, her children, or both if she attempts to leave. This fear may be justified. She may kill herself or her abuser to escape because she sees no other way out (Campbell et al., 2004). Because of the severity of the abuse, a woman may flee to a shelter to obtain physical safety for herself and her children (Bennett et al, 2004). As a woman tries to leave, the risk of homicide increases, creating a catch-22 situation. Often the woman thinks she will die if she stays or leaves the relationship. A nurse encountering a family in which there is severe abuse needs to consider the safety of the woman and her children as the priority. The woman will need an order of protection, a legal document specifically designed to keep the abuser away from her. She will also need help in getting to a safe place, such as a wife abuse shelter in an anonymous location. At the very least, the woman must design a carefully thought-out plan for escape and arrange for a neighbor or an adolescent child to call the police when another violent episode occurs.

Short-term help for women in abusive relationships can often be found. Many women, however, have identified a dearth of long-term and family-oriented services. Unfortunately, financial constraints sometimes factor into the decision-making process of whether to remain in abusive relationships. The high cost of attorney fees to obtain equitable divorces or child custody is a factor many women face when leaving these relationships (Lutenbacher, Cohen, and Mitzel, 2003).

An alternative to ending the relationship is the male partner's attendance at programs for batterers. These programs are most effective if they are court mandated and if the man's underlying values about women are addressed, as well as his violence (Tilley and Brackley, 2005). Abused women need affirmation, support, reassurances of the normalcy of their responses, accurate information about shelters and legal resources, and brainstorming about possible solutions. These needs can be met by other women in similar situations and by professionals such as nurses (Landenburger, Campbell, and Rodriguez, 2004). Women should not be pushed into actions that they are not ready to take.

After the abusive relationship has ended, a period of recovery ensues. This includes a normal grief response for the relationship that has ended and a search for meaning in the experience (Silva and Ludwig, 2002). Thus a formerly battered woman who is feeling depressed and lonely after the relationship has ended is exhibiting a normal response for which support is needed.

Nurses need to assess for intimate sexual abuse in which the battered woman is forced into sexual encounters. Serious physical and emotional damage can result from marital rape. Often women who have come to emergency departments because of abuse have not been screened for forced sex because the issue is considered too intrusive (Campbell and Soeken, 1999). Therefore, like intimate partner violence in the past, marital rape remains a private issue. There is also an alarming incidence of date rape, the dynamics of which may parallel marital rape. Adolescent boys are more likely to perpetrate sexual dating violence than are girls. Young women who have been victims of dating violence experience low self-esteem, depression, anger, and irritability (King and Ryan, 2004).

To assess for sexual assault, the question "Have you ever been forced into sex you did not wish to participate in?" should be used in all nursing assessments to see if marital rape, date rape, or rape of a male has occurred.

Health care providers should routinely inquire about family violence by asking clients directly about its occurrence within their family. Because many women have reported difficulty in disclosing abusive situations to health care providers, routine assessment will provide these women with opportunities to report their situations at their own pace. Routine screening can also serve to promote trust between client and provider and increase the likelihood of early identification of families at risk (Lutenbacher, Cohen, and Mitzel, 2003).

Battering during pregnancy has serious implications for the health of both women and their children. Approximately one in six pregnant women is physically battered during pregnancy, with a larger proportion (20%) of adolescents abused during pregnancy than adult women. Although abuse during pregnancy occurs across ethnic groups, white women experience a significantly higher severity of abuse than African-American or Hispanic women (Parker et al, 2004). These women are at risk for spontaneous abortion, premature delivery, low-birth weight infants, substance abuse during pregnancy, and depression (McFarlane and Parker, 2005). Abuse before pregnancy often precedes abuse during pregnancy. A man's control of contraception, a form of abusive controlling, may lead to unintended pregnancy and subsequent abuse. In addition, a man's refusal to use a condom places a woman at an increased risk of sexually transmitted diseases, including infection with HIV (Davila, 2002; Maman et al, 2002). Infants whose mothers were battered are often at high risk for child abuse. All pregnant women should be assessed for abuse at each prenatal care visit, and postpartum home visits should include assessment for child abuse and partner abuse.

ABUSE OF OLDER ADULTS

Older adult abuse is growing as a form of family violence. Between 1 million and 2 million Americans age 65 years or older have been injured, exploited, or otherwise mistreated

by someone on whom they depend for protection (Bonnie and Wallace, 2002). Like spouse abuse and child abuse, most cases of older adult abuse go unreported. As with other forms of human abuse, older adult maltreatment includes emotional, sexual, and physical neglect, as well as physical and sexual violence; financial abuse and violation of rights are particular issues for elders.

Older adults are neglected when the following occur:
- Others fail to provide adequate food, clothing, shelter, and physical care and to meet physiological, emotional, and safety needs.
- There is either lack of care or improper care; this can be considered criminal neglect.
- There is violation of their rights, medical abuse, and abandonment.
- There is financial abuse through fraud, coercion to relinquish property rights, and money mismanagement (Bonnie and Wallace, 2002).

Elders may also be abused by the following actions of caregivers:
- Rough handling that can lead to bruises and bleeding into body tissues because of the fragility of their skin and vascular systems. It is often difficult to determine if the injuries of older adults result from abuse, falls, or other natural causes. Careful assessment both through observation and discussion can help determine the cause of injuries.
- Imposing unrealistic toileting demands.
- Ignoring special needs and previous living patterns.
- Giving food that they cannot chew or swallow or that is contraindicated because of dietary restrictions or social or cultural preferences.
- Giving medication to induce confusion or drowsiness so that the elders will be less troublesome, will need less care, or will allow others to gain control of their financial and personal resources.

The most common form of psychological abuse is rejection or simply ignoring older adults, indicating that they are worthless and useless to others. Older adults may

HOW TO Identify Potential or Actual Older Adult Abuse

Be alert to the following:
- Financial mismanagement
- Withdrawal and passivity
- Depression
- Unexplained or repeated physical injuries
- Untreated health problems such as decubitus ulcers
- Poor nutrition
- Unexplained genital infections
- Physical neglect and unmet basic needs
- Social isolation
- Rejection of assistance by caregiver
- Lack of compliance to health regimens

From Butler RN: Warning signs of elder abuse, *Geriatrics* 54(3):3–4, 1999; Bonnie RJ, Wallace RB: *Elder mistreatment: abuse, neglect, and exploitation in aging America*, Washington, DC, 2002, National Academy Press.

HOW TO Assess for Intimate Partner Violence

Ask the following questions:
- Is somebody hurting you?
- You seem frightened of your partner. Has he hurt you?
- Did someone you know do this to you?

subsequently regress and become increasingly dependent on others, who tend to resent the imposition and demands on their time and lifestyles. The pattern becomes cyclical: as the person becomes more regressed, the level of dependence increases. Furthermore, the past accomplishments and present abilities of the older person may not be consistently acknowledged, causing them to feel even less capable. Indicators of actual or potential older adult abuse follow.

There are several precipitating factors for older adult abuse. The older person may be a physical, emotional, or financial burden on the caregiver, leading to frustration and resentment. Or the older adult may have previously been the abuser (Weeks et al, 2004). Children who have lived in abusive households learn that behavior. All older adults should be assessed for abuse. This is especially true for confused and frail elders. These illnesses place a high burden on the caregiver, with subsequent caregiver depression. Living with and providing care to a confused older adult is difficult. The round-the-clock tasks often exhaust family members. In addition, clients with Alzheimer's disease may become verbally and even physically aggressive as a result of their illness, which may trigger retaliatory violence. Family stress increases as members work harder to fulfill their other responsibilities in addition to meeting the needs of the older adults.

When families plan to care for an older family member at home, nurses must help them fully evaluate that decision and prepare for the stressors that will be involved. A plan for regular respite care is essential. Strategies for the primary and secondary prevention of abuse of older adults include victim support groups, senior advocacy volunteer programs, and training for providers working with older adults (Bonnie and Wallace, 2002).

Elderly people need to retain as much autonomy and decision-making ability as possible. Nurses have many ways to detect elder abuse, and they have the skills and responsibility for discovering it, giving treatment, and making referrals. Many families who care for older adult members exhaust their resources and coping ability. Nurses can help them find new sources of support and aid.

NURSING INTERVENTIONS

Primary prevention begins with a community approach that incorporates strategies from criminal justice, education, social services, community advocacy, and public health to prevent violence. Some communities have used the following:
- School-based curricula that teach children and youth how to cope with anger, stress, and frustration and that also teach communication and mediation skills.
- Family programs that teach parents how to deal with their children more effectively.
- Preschool programs to develop intellectual and social skills.
- Public education programs that can educate communities about different forms of violence and ways to get help and intervene (Meyer and Stein, 2004; Podnieks and Wilson, 2003).

- Nurse home visitation programs with families at risk may prevent child abuse and neglect.
- Lobbying for passage of legislation to outlaw physical punishment in schools and marital rape.

Strong community sanctions against violence in the home can reduce levels of abuse (Sullivan et al, 2005). Neighbors can watch what is happening and work together to address problems in other families; this is not an invasion of privacy but a sign of community cohesiveness. Nurses can work with advocate groups to make sure police deal with assault within marriage as swiftly, surely, and severely as assault between strangers. Nurses can encourage others to interfere when they see children beaten in a grocery store, notice that an older adult is not being properly cared for, see a neighborhood bully beat up his classmates, or hear a neighbor hitting his wife.

Second, people can take measures to reduce their vulnerability to violence by improving the physical security of their homes and learning personal defense measures. Nurses can encourage people to keep windows and doors locked, trim shrubs around their homes, and keep lights on during high-crime periods. Many neighborhoods organize crime watch programs and post signs to that effect. Other signs indicate that certain homes will assist children who need help; these homes are identified by the sign of a hand, usually posted in a window. Other neighbors informally agree to monitor one another's property and safety. Also, many law enforcement agencies evaluate homes for security and teach individual or neighborhood safety programs. Individuals install home security systems, participate in personal defense programs such as judo or karate, and purchase firearms for their protection.

Unfortunately, handguns are far more likely to kill family members than intruders (Hahn et al, 2005). Firearm accidents are a leading cause of death for young children, and handguns kept in the home are easy to use in moments of extreme anger with other family members or in extreme depression. The majority of homicides between family members and most suicides involve a handgun. Nursing assessments should include a question about guns kept in the home. The family should be made aware of the risk that a handgun holds for family members. If the family thinks that keeping a gun is necessary, safety measures should be taught, such as keeping the gun unloaded and in a locked compartment, keeping the ammunition separate from the gun and also locked away, and instructing children about the dangers of firearms. Lobbying for handgun-control laws is a primary prevention effort that can significantly decrease the rate of death and serious injury caused by handguns in the United States.

Identification of risk factors is an important part of primary prevention used by nurses who work with clients in a variety of settings. Although abuse cannot be predicted with certainty, several factors influence the onset and support the continuation of abusive patterns. Factors to include in an assessment for individual or family violence, or for potential family violence, are illustrated in Figure 25-1. Factors to be included when assessing a community for violence are shown in Box 25-3.

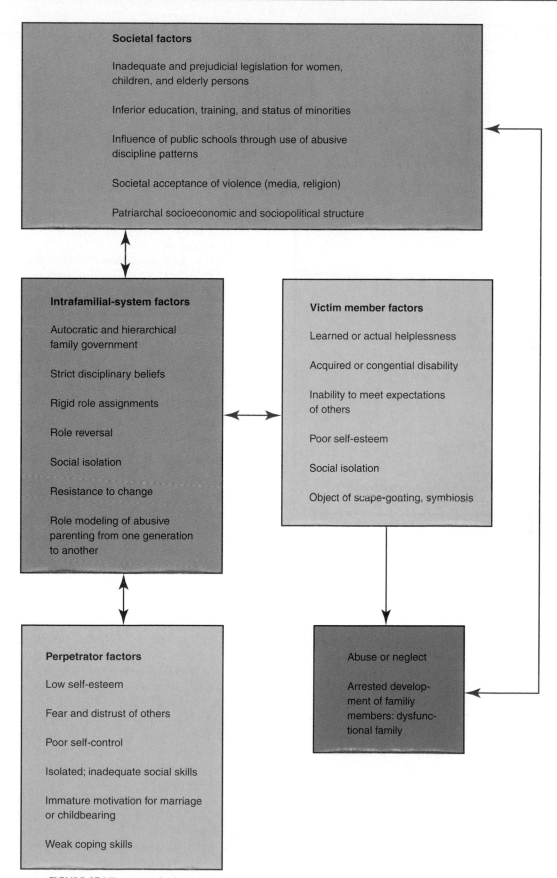

Societal factors

Inadequate and prejudicial legislation for women, children, and elderly persons

Inferior education, training, and status of minorities

Influence of public schools through use of abusive discipline patterns

Societal acceptance of violence (media, religion)

Patriarchal socioeconomic and sociopolitical structure

Intrafamilial-system factors

Autocratic and hierarchical family government

Strict disciplinary beliefs

Rigid role assignments

Role reversal

Social isolation

Resistance to change

Role modeling of abusive parenting from one generation to another

Victim member factors

Learned or actual helplessness

Acquired or congential disability

Inability to meet expectations of others

Poor self-esteem

Social isolation

Object of scape-goating, symbiosis

Perpetrator factors

Low self-esteem

Fear and distrust of others

Poor self-control

Isolated; inadequate social skills

Immature motivation for marriage or childbearing

Weak coping skills

Abuse or neglect

Arrested development of familiy members: dysfunctional family

FIGURE 25-1 Factors to include when assessing an individual's or family's potential for violence.

Box 25-3   **Assessing for Violence in a Community Context**

Individual Factors
- Signs of physical abuse (abrasions, contusions, burns)
- Physical symptoms related to emotional distress
- Developmental and behavioral difficulties
- Presence of physical disability
- Social isolation
- Decreased role performance within the family and in the job or school-related activities
- Mental health problems such as depression, low self-esteem, and anxiety
- Fear of intimate others
- Substance abuse

Familial Factors
- Economic stressors
- Presence of some form of family violence
- Poor communication
- Problems with childrearing
- Lack of family cohesion
- Recurrent familial conflict
- Lack of social support networks
- Poor social integration into the community
- Multiple changes of residence
- Access to guns
- Homelessness

Community Characteristics
- High crime rate
- High levels of unemployment
- Lack of neighborhood resources and support systems
- Lack of community cohesiveness

Box 25-4   **Prevention Strategies for Violence**

Individual and Family Levels
- Assess during routine examination (secondary)
- Assess for marital discord (secondary)
- Educate on developmental stages and the needs of children (primary)
- Counsel for at-risk parents (secondary)
- Teach parenting techniques (primary)
- Assist with controlling anger (secondary)
- Treat for substance abuse (tertiary)
- Teach stress-reduction techniques (primary)

Community Level
- Develop policy
- Conduct community resource mapping
- Collaborate with the community to develop systematic responses to violence
- Develop a media campaign
- Develop resources such as transition housing and shelters

Levels of Prevention   **Related to Violence**

PRIMARY PREVENTION

Strengthen the individual and family by teaching parenting skills.

SECONDARY PREVENTION

Reduce or end abuse by early screening; teach families how to deal with stress and how to have fun and enjoy recreation.

TERTIARY PREVENTION

When signs of abuse are evident, refer the client to appropriate community organizations.

As seen in the Levels of Prevention box and Box 25-4, primary prevention of violence can take place through community, family, and individual interventions. Nurses, in their work in schools, community groups, employee groups, daycare centers, and other community institutions, can foster healthy developmental patterns and identify signs of potential abuse. Nurses may participate in media campaigns that identify risk factors for abuse or in developing after-school programs and late-night programs to support youth in using their energies toward positive goals and in developing a constructive support network. Nurses can strengthen families by teaching parenting skills such as diapering, feeding, quieting, holding, rocking, and nonphysical disciplining. They can serve as role models during visits with the family and demonstrate by their actions positive behaviors toward the children.

When abuse occurs, nurses can initiate secondary prevention measures to reduce or terminate further abuse. Both developmental and situational crises present opportunities for abusive situations to develop. Nurses can help form groups to assist battered women. They can be primary leaders in the development of assessment practices in the health care arena. The development of training programs for health care providers can be an effective step toward identifying and respectfully treating victims of violence. Nurses can work closely with shelters in identifying the needs of individuals who seek sanctuary from abusive situations. On a family level, nurses can help family members discuss problems and seek ways to deal with the tension that led to the abusive situations. Injured persons must be temporarily or permanently placed in a safe location. Secondary preventive measures are most useful when potential abusers recognize their tendency to be abusive and seek help. For children, there is often a need for 24-hour child protection services or caregivers who can take care of the child until the acute family or individual crisis is resolved. Respite care is extremely important in families with frail older-adult family members. Telephone crisis lines can be used to provide immediate emergency assistance to families.

Effective communication with abusive families is important. Typically, these families do not want to discuss their problems and many are embarrassed to be involved in an abusive situation. Often feelings of guilt are present. Effective communication must be preceded by an attitude of acceptance. It is often difficult for nurses to value the worth of an individual who willfully abuses another. The behavior, not the person, must be condemned.

In addition, not all families know how to have fun. Nurses can assess how much recreation is integrated into the family's lifestyle. Through community assessment, nurses know what resources and facilities are available and how much they cost. Families may need counseling about the value of recreation and play in reducing tension and appropriately channeling aggressive impulses.

Although it may be difficult to form a trusting relationship with abusive families, nurses can engage in tertiary prevention by acting as a case manager and coordinating the other agencies and activities involved. Principles of giving care to families who are experiencing violence include the following:
- Intolerance for violence
- Respect and caring for all family members
- Safety as the first priority
- Absolute honesty
- Empowerment

Abusers often fear they will be condemned for their actions, so it is often difficult to make and maintain contact with abusive families. Although nurses convey an attitude of caring and concern for them, families may doubt the sincerity of this concern. They may avoid being home at the scheduled visit time because of fear of the consequences of the visit or an inability to believe that anyone really wants to help them. If the victim is a child, parents may fear that the nurse will try to remove the child. Nurses are mandatory reporters of child abuse, even when only suspected, in all states. They are also mandatory reporters of elder abuse and abuse of other physically and cognitively dependent adults, as well as of felony assaults of anyone in most states. The mandatory reporting laws also protect reporters from legal action on cases that are never substantiated. Even so, physicians and nurses are sometimes reluctant to report abuse. They may be more willing to report abuse in a poor family than in a middle-class one, or they may think that an older adult or child is better off at home than in a nursing home or foster home. Referral to protective service agencies is a way to get help, rather than an automatic step toward removal of the victim or criminal justice action. Families should be included in any reporting so they can have input. Absolute honesty about what will be reported to officials, what the family can expect, what the nurse is entering into records, and what the nurse is feeling is essential.

To further assist the family, the nurse needs to recognize and capitalize on the violent family's strengths, as well as to assess and deal with its problems. The nurse must use a nurse–family partnership rather than a paternalistic or authoritarian approach. Families can often generate many of their own solutions, which tend to be more culturally appropriate and individualized than those the nurse generates in isolation. Victims of direct attacks need information about their options and resources and reassurance that abuse is unfortunately rather common and that they are not alone in their dilemma. They also need reassurance that their responses are normal and that they do not deserve to be abused. Continued support

Box 25-5	**Common Community Services**

- Child protective services
- Child abuse prevention programs
- Adult protective services
- Parents Anonymous
- Wife abuse shelter
- Program for children of battered women
- Community support group
- 24-hour hotline
- Legal advocacy or information
- State coalition against domestic violence
- Batterer treatment
- Victim assistance programs
- Sexual assault programs

for their decisions must be coupled with nursing actions to ensure their safety.

Referral is an important component of tertiary prevention. Nurses should know about available community resources for abuse victims and perpetrators. Some of these resources are listed in Box 25-5. If attitudes and resources are inadequate, it is often helpful to work with local radio and television stations and newspapers to provide information about the nature and extent of human abuse as a community health problem. This also helps acquaint people with available services and resources. Frequently, people do not seek services early in an abusive situation because they simply do not know what is available to them. Ideally, a program or plan for abused people begins with a needs assessment to identify potential clients and to determine how to effectively serve this group. Nurses can help get programs started and provide public education.

CLINICAL APPLICATION

Mrs. Smith, a 75-year-old bedridden woman, consistently became rude and combative when her daughter, Mary, attempted to bathe her and change her clothes each morning. During a home visit, Mary told the nurse, Mrs. Jones, that she had gotten so frustrated with her mother on the previous morning that she had hit her. Mary felt terrible about her behavior. She stressed that her mother's incontinence made it essential that she be kept clean; her clothes had to be changed every day for her own safety and physical well-being.

A. *How should Mrs. Jones respond to this disclosure?*
B. *What specific nursing actions should be taken?*
C. *What ongoing services does the nurse need to provide?*
Answers are in the back of the book.

REMEMBER THIS!

- Violence and human abuse are not new phenomena, but they are growing community health concerns.
- People in communities across the United States are frustrated by increasing levels of violence.

- Nurses can evaluate and intervene in community and family violence.
- To intervene effectively, nurses must understand the dynamics of violence and human abuse.
- Factors influencing social and community violence include changing social conditions, economic conditions, population density, community facilities, and institutions within a community, such as organized religion, education, the mass communication media, and work.
- Violence and abuse of family members can happen to any family member: spouse, older adult, child, or physically or mentally compromised person.
- People who abuse family members were often abused themselves and react poorly to real or perceived crises. Other factors that characterize the abuser are the way the person was raised and the unique character of that person.
- Child abuse can be physical, emotional, or sexual. Incest is a common and particularly destructive form of child abuse.
- Spouse abuse is usually wife abuse. It involves physical, emotional, and, frequently, sexual abuse within a context of coercive control. It usually increases in severity and frequency and can escalate to homicide of either partner.
- Nurses can identify potential victims of family abuse because they see clients in a variety of settings, such as schools, businesses, homes, and clinics. Treatment of family abuse includes primary, secondary, and tertiary prevention and therapeutic intervention.

WHAT WOULD YOU DO?

1. For 1 week, keep a log or diary related to violence:
   a. Make a note of each time you feel as though you are losing your temper. Consider what it might take to cause you to react in a violent way.
   b. Think back. When was the last time you had a violent outburst? What precipitated it? What were your thoughts? What were your feelings? How might you have handled the situation or those feelings without reacting in a violent way?
   c. During this same week, make note of the episodes of violent behaviors you observe. For example, do parents hit children in the supermarket? What seems to precipitate such outbursts? What alternatives might exist for reacting in a less violent way?
2. If you learned, after a careful assessment of your community, that family violence is a significant community health problem, what plan of action could you take to intervene? Remember that the goal is to promote health. Outline a plan of action with objectives, timetables, implementation strategies, and evaluation plans for intervening in family violence in your community.
3. Complete a partial community assessment to determine the actual incidence and types of violence in your community.

4. What resources are available in your community for victims of violence?
   a. Interview a person who works in an agency that seeks to aid victims of violence.
   b. What is the role of the agency? Do its services seem adequate? Who is eligible? Is there a waiting list? What is the fee scale? Is the care culturally competent?

■ *REFERENCES*

Anderson RN, Smith BL: Deaths: Leading cause for 2002, *Natl Vital Stat Rep* 53:1–92, 2005.

Annan SL: Sexual violence in rural areas: a review of the literature, *Fam Commun Health* (29):164–168, 2006.

Bachar K, Koss MP: From prevalence to prevention: closing the gap between what we know about rape and what we do. In Renzetti CM, Edleson JL, Bergen RK, editors: *Sourcebook on violence against women*, Thousand Oaks, Calif, 2001, Sage, pp 117–142.

Belknap RA: Why did she do that? Issues of moral conflict in battered women's decision making, *Issues Ment Health Nurs* 20:387–404, 1999.

Bennett L, Riger S, Schewe P et al: Effectiveness of hotline, advocacy, counseling, and shelter services for victims of domestic violence: a statewide evaluation, *J Interpers Violence* 19: 815–829, 2004.

Berman H, Hardesty H, Humphreys J: Children of abused women. In Humphreys J, Campbell JC, editors: *Family violence and nursing practice*, Philadelphia, 2004, Lippincott Williams & Wilkins, pp 150–185.

Bonnie RJ, Wallace RB: *Elder mistreatment: abuse, neglect, and exploitation in aging America*, Washington, DC, 2002, National Academy Press.

Buka SL et al: Youth exposure to violence: prevalence, risks, and consequences, *Am J Orthopsychiatry* 71:298–310, 2001.

Butler RN: Warning signs of elder abuse, *Geriatrics* 54(3):3–4, 1999.

Campbell JC: Health consequences of intimate partner violence, *Lancet* 359(9314):1331–1336, 2002.

Campbell JC et al: Intimate partner homicide: review and implications of research and policy, *Trauma Violence Abuse* 8(3): 246-269, 2007.

Campbell JC, Sheridan DJ: Assessment of intimate partner violence and elder abuse. In Jarvis C, editor: *Physical assessment for clinical practice*, Philadelphia, 2004, Elsevier, pp 74–82.

Campbell JC, Soeken KL: Forced sex and intimate partner violence, *Violence Against Women* 5:1017–1035, 1999.

Campbell JC et al: Nursing care of survivors of intimate partner violence. In Humphreys J, Campbell JC, editors: *Family violence and nursing practice*, Philadelphia, 2004, Lippincott Williams & Wilkins, pp 307–360.

Campbell JC et al: Risk factors for femicide in abusive relationships, *Am J Public Health* 93(7):1089–1097, 2003.

Campbell R: *The effectiveness of sexual assault nurse examiner (SANE) programs*, 2004, Minnesota Center Against Violence and Abuse.

Centers for Disease Control and Prevention: Nonfatal physical assault-related injuries in hospital emergency departments, United States, 2000, *MMWR Morb Mortal Wkly Rep* 51(21): 460–463, 2002. Retrieved April 13, 2004, from http://www.cdc.gov/mmwr/preview/mmwrhtml/mm5121a3.htm.

Centers for Disease Control and Prevention: *Suicide fact sheet,* 2004a, available at http://www.cdc.org/ncip/factsheets/suifacts.htm.

Centers for Disease Control and Prevention: *Intimate partner violence fact sheet,* 2004b, available at http://www.cdc.org/ncipc/factsheets/ivpfacts.htm.

Centers for Disease Control and Prevention: *Understanding child maltreatment fact sheet,* 2006. Retrieved June 16, 2008, from http://www.cdc.gov/injury.

Centers for Disease Control and Prevention: *Sexual violence fact sheet,* 2007a. Retrieved June 16, 2008, from http://cdc.gov/injury.

Centers for Disease Control and Prevention: *Suicide facts at a glance,* 2007b. Retrieved June 16, 2008, from http://cdc.gov/injury.

Centers for Disease Control and Prevention: *Child Maltreatment facts at a glance,* 2007c. Retrieved June 16, 2008, from http://.cdc.gov/injury.

Centers for Disease Control and Prevention: Adverse health risk conditions and health risk behaviors associated with intimate partner violence: United States, 2005, *MMWR Morb Mortal Wkly Rep* 57(05):113–117, 2008. Retrieved Feb 7, 2008, from http://www.cdc.gov/mmwr/preview/mmwrhtml/mm5705a1.htm.

Centers for Disease Control and Prevention: Surveillance for violent deaths—national violent death reporting system 16 states, 2006, *MMWR Surveillance Summaries* 58(SSol):1–44, 2009.

Davila YR: Influence of abuse on condom negotiation among Mexican-American women involved in abusive relationships, *J Assoc Nurses AIDS Care* 13:46–56, 2002.

Dixon L, Hamilton-Giachritsis C, Brown K: Attributions and behaviours of parents abused as children: a meditational analysis of the intergenerational continuity of child maltreatment, *J Child Psychol Psychiatry* 46:59–68, 2005.

Edwards VJ et al: Adverse childhood experiences and health-related quality of life as an adult. In Tackett K, editor: *Health consequences of abuse in the family: a clinical guide for evidence-based practice. Application and practice in health psychology,* Washington, DC, 2004, American Psychological Association, pp 81–94.

English DJ, Marshall DB, Stewart AJ: Effects of family violence on child behavior and health during early childhood, *J Fam Violence* 18:43–57, 2003.

Esposito N: Women with a history of sexual assault, *Am J Nurs* 106:69–73, 2006.

Ethier LS, Couture G, Lacharité C: Risk factors associated with the chronicity of high potential of child abuse and neglect, *J Fam Violence* 19:13–24, 2004.

Fortune MM: Religious issues and violence against women. In Renzetti CM, Jeffery L, Bergen RK, editors: *Sourcebook on violence against women,* Thousand Oaks, Calif, 2001, Sage.

Gandy OH: Racial identity, media use, and the social construction of risk among African Americans, *J Black Studies* 31(5):600–618, 2001.

Gary FA, Campbell DW, Humphreys J: Theories of child abuse. In Humphreys J, Campbell JC, editors: *Family violence and nursing practice,* Philadelphia, 2004, Lippincott Williams & Wilkins, pp 252–287.

Goldberg C: Shaken baby cases on the increase: specialists link rise to economic stress, *Boston Globe,* March 19, 2009. Retrieved March 21, 2009, from www.boston.com.

Grella CE, Joshi V: Treatment processes and outcomes among adolescents with a history of abuse who are in drug treatment, *Child Maltreat* 8:7–18, 2003.

Hahn RA et al: Firearms laws and the reduction of violence: a systematic review, *Am J Prev Med* 28(suppl 1):40–71, 2005.

Health Bulletin: Domestic violence and abuse, *Health Ment Hygiene News* 2(10), 2003.

Hines DA, Malley-Morrison K: *Family violence in the United States,* Thousand Oaks, Calif, 2005, Sage.

Horton A: The prevention of school violence: new evidence to consider, *J Human Behav Soc Environ* 4(1):49–59, 2001.

Hurt H et al: Exposure to violence: psychological and academic correlates in child witnesses, *Arch Pediatr Adolesc Med* 155:1351–1356, 2001.

King MC, Ryan J: Nursing care and adolescent dating violence. In Humphreys J, Campbell JC, editors: *Family violence and nursing practice,* Philadelphia, 2004, Lippincott Williams & Wilkin, pp 288–306.

Knox KS, Roberts AR: Crisis intervention and crisis team models in schools, *Children Schools* 27:93–100, 2005.

Lambert SF et al: The relationship between perceptions of neighborhood characteristics and substance use among urban African American adolescents, *Am J Community Psychol* 34:205–218, 2004.

Landenburger K: *Exploration of women's identity: clinical approaches with abused women—empowering survivors of abuse: health care, battered women and their children,* Newbury Hills, Calif, 1998, Sage.

Landenburger K, Campbell DW, Rodriguez R: Nursing care of families using violence. In Humphreys J, Campbell JC, editors: *Family violence and nursing practice,* Philadelphia, 2004, Lippincott Williams & Wilkins, pp 220–251.

Lee MR, Ousey GC: Institutional access, residential segregation, and urban black homicide, *Sociol Inq* 75:31–54, 2005.

Leventhal JM: The prevention of child abuse and neglect: successfully out of the blocks, *Child Abuse Negl* 25(4):431–439, 2001.

Lewandowski L et al: "He killed my mommy!" Murder or attempted murder of a child's mother, *J Fam Violence* 19:211–220, 2004.

Litrownik AJ et al: Exposure to family violence in young at-risk children: a longitudinal look at the effects of victimization and witnessed physical and psychological aggression, *J Fam Violence* 18:59–73, 2003.

Logan TK, Shannon L, Walker R: Protection orders in urban and rural areas, *Violence Against Women* 11:876–911, 2005.

Lutenbacher M, Cohen A, Mitzel J: Do we really help? Perspectives of abused women, *Public Health Nurs* 20(1):56–64, 2003.

Maman S et al: HIV-positive women report more lifetime partner violence: findings from a voluntary counseling and testing clinic in Dar es Salaam, Tanzania, *Am J Public Health* 92:1331–1337, 2002.

McFarlane J, Parker B: *Abuse during pregnancy: a protocol for prevention and intervention,* White Plains, NY, 2005, March of Dimes Birth Defects Foundation.

Meyer H, Stein N: Relationship prevention education in schools: what's working, what's getting in the way, and what are some future directions, *Am J Health Ed* 35:198–204, 2004.

Naar-King S et al: Type and severity of abuse as predictors of psychiatric symptoms in adolescence, *J Fam Violence* 17:133–149, 2002.

National Institute of Justice: *When violence hits home: how economics and neighborhood play a role (NCJ 2050040),* 2004. Retrieved November 5, 2005, from http://www.ncjrs.gov/pdffiles1/nij/205004.pdf.

National Institute of Mental Health: *Suicide in the US: statistics and prevention (NIH 06-4594),* 2004. Retrieved February 8, 2008, from http://www.nimh.nih.gov/health/publications/suicide-in-the-us-statistics-and-prevention.shtml.

Parker B et al: Abuse during pregnancy. In Humphreys J, Campbell JC, editors: *Family violence and nursing practice,* Philadelphia, 2004, Lippincott Williams & Wilkins, pp 77–96.

Peterson RL, Larson J, Skiba R: School violence prevention: current status and policy recommendations, *Law Policy* 23(3):345–371, 2001.

Podnieks E, Wilson S: An exploratory study of responses to elder abuse in faith communities, *J Elder Abuse Neglect* 15:137–162, 2003.

Polakow-Suransky S: Boston's Ten Point Coalition: a faith-based approach to fighting crime in the inner city, *Responsive Community* 13:49–59, 2003.

Ross CA: Childhood sexual abuse and psychosomatic symptoms in irritable bowel syndrome, *J Child Sex Abus* 14:27–38, 2005.

Salzinger A et al: Effects of partner violence and physical child abuse on child behavior: a study of abused and comparison children, *J Fam Violence* 17:23–52, 2002.

Sampson RJ: Crime and public safety: insights from community-level perspectives on social capital. In Saegert S, Thompson JP, Warren MR, editors: *Social capital and poor communities,* New York, 2001, Russell Sage Foundation.

Sampson RJ, Morenoff JD, Raudenbusch S: Social anatomy of racial and ethnic disparities in violence, *Am J Public Health* 95(2):224–232, 2005.

Schwartz MR: When closeness breeds cruelty: helping victims of intimate partner violence, *Am Nurse Today* 2:42–46, 2007.

Sharps PW et al: Health care provider's missed opportunities for preventing femicide, *Prevent Med* 33:373–380, 2001.

Silva MC, Ludwig R: Domestic violence, nurses, and ethics: what are the links, *Online J Issues Nurs.* Retrieved May 12, 2002, from http://www.nursingworld.org/ojin/ethicol/ethics_8.htm.

Straus M: Children should never, ever be spanked no matter what the circumstances. In Loseke DR, Gelles R, Cavanaugh M, editors: *Current controversies on family violence,* Thousand Oaks, Calif, 2005, Sage, pp 137–157.

Sullivan M et al: Participatory action research in practice: a case study in addressing domestic violence in nine cultural communities, *J Interper Violence* 20:977–995, 2005.

Tilley DS, Brackley M: Men who batter intimate partners: a grounded theory study of the development of male violence in intimate partner relationships, *Issues Ment Health Nurs* 26:281–297, 2005.

Tjaden P, Thoennes N: *Full report of the prevalence, incidence, and consequences of violence against women: findings from the National Violence Against Women Survey, National Institute of Justice Centers for Disease Control and Prevention,* Washington, DC, 2000, U.S. Department of Justice.

Trossman S: Issues up close: ending the cycle, *Am Nurse Today* 4(1):26–28, 2009.

Urbanic JC: Sexual abuse in families. In Humphreys J, Campbell JC, editors: *Family violence and nursing practice,* Philadelphia, 2004, Lippincott Williams & Wilkins, pp 186–219.

U.S. Department of Health and Human Services: *Healthy People 2010: national health promotion and disease prevention objectives,* ed 2, Washington, DC, 2000, U.S. Government Printing Office.

U.S. Department of Health and Human Services: *Child maltreatment 2001: summary of key findings.* Retrieved April 13, 2004, from http://nccanch.acf.hhs.gov/pubs/factsheets/canstats.cfm.

U.S. Department of Health and Human Services, Administration on Children, Youth, and Families: *Child maltreatment 2003, 2005.* Retrieved Nov 8, 2005, from http://www.acf.hhs.gov/programs/cb/pubs/cm03/.

U.S. Department of Justice, Bureau of Justice Statistics: *Crime victimization 2003 (NCJ-205455), 2004.* Retrieved Nov 5, 2005, from http://www.ojp.usdoj.gov/bjs/abstract/cv03.htm.

U.S. Department of Justice, Bureau of Justice Statistics: *Family violence statistics: including statistics on strangers and acquaintances (NCJ-207846), 2005.* Retrieved Nov 6, 2005, from http://www.ojp.usdoj.gov/bjs/abstract/fvs.htm.

U.S. Department of Justice, Bureau of Justice Statistics: *Homicide trends in the United States, 2007.* Retrieved June 23, 2008, from http://www.ojp.usdoj.gov/bjs/homicide/homtrnd.htm#contents.

Weeks LE et al: A gendered analysis of the abuse of elder adults: evidence from professionals, *J Elder Abuse Neglect* 16:1–15, 2004.

Widom CS, Hiller-Sturmhöfel S: Alcohol abuse as a risk factor for and consequence of child abuse, *Alcohol Res Health* 25(1):52–57, 2001.

Wilson BJ, Colvin CM, Smith SL: Engaging in violence on American television: a comparison of child, teen, and adult perpetrators, *J Commun* 52:36–60, 2002.

Infectious Disease Prevention and Control

Francisco S. Sy
Susan C. Long-Marin

ADDITIONAL RESOURCES

These related resources are found either in the appendix at the back of this book or on the book's website at http://evolve.elsevier.com/stanhope/foundations.

Evolve Website

- Community Assessment Applied
- Case Study, with questions and answers
- Quiz review questions
- WebLinks, including link to *Healthy People 2010* website

Real World Community Health Nursing: An Interactive CD-ROM, second edition

If you are using this CD-ROM in your course, you will find the following activities related to this chapter:
- *Epidemiology: Report It* in **Epidemiology**
- *Investigation of an Outbreak* in **Epidemiology**

OBJECTIVES

After reading this chapter, the student should be able to:
1. Discuss the current effect and threats of infectious diseases on society.
2. Explain how the elements of the epidemiologic triangle interact to cause infectious diseases.
3. Provide examples of infectious disease control interventions at the three levels of public health prevention.
4. Explain the multisystem approach to the control of communicable diseases.
5. Define surveillance, and discuss the functions and elements of a surveillance system.
6. Discuss the factors contributing to newly emerging or reemerging infectious diseases.
7. Discuss the illnesses most likely to be associated with the intentional release of a biological agent.
8. Discuss issues related to obtaining and maintaining appropriate levels of immunization against vaccine-preventable diseases.
9. Describe issues and agents associated with foodborne illness and appropriate prevention measures.
10. Define the blood-borne pathogen reduction strategy, Universal Precautions.

CHAPTER OUTLINE

483

KEY TERMS

acquired immunity: the resistance acquired by a host as a result of previous natural exposure to an infectious agent; it may be induced by passive or active immunization.

active immunization: administration of all or part of a microorganism to stimulate an active response by the host's immunological system, resulting in complete protection against a specific disease.

agent: causative factor, such as a biological or chemical agent, invading a susceptible host through an environment favorable to produce disease.

anthrax: an acute disease caused by the spore-forming bacterium, *Bacillus anthracis.*

common vehicle: transportation of the infectious agent from an infected host to a susceptible host via water, food, milk, blood, serum, or plasma.

communicable diseases: diseases of human or animal origin caused by an infectious agent and resulting from transmission of that agent from an infected person, animal, or inanimate source to a susceptible host. Not all communicable diseases are communicated from host to host. For example, tetanus is transmitted from an inanimate source to a person but then cannot be passed from the infected person to another person.

communicable period: the time or times when an infectious agent may be transferred from an infected source directly or indirectly to a new host.

disease: an indication of a physiological dysfunction or a pathological reaction to an infection.

elimination: focuses on removing a disease from a large geographic area such as a country or region of the world.

emerging infectious diseases: diseases in which the incidence has increased in the past two decades or has the potential to increase in the near future.

endemic: the constant presence of an infectious disease within a specific geographic area.

environment: all of those factors internal and external to the client that constitute the context in which the client lives and that influence and are influenced by the host and agent–host interactions; the sum of all external conditions affecting the life, development, and survival of an organism.

epidemic: the occurrence of an infectious agent or disease within a specific geographic area in greater numbers than would normally be expected.

epidemiologic triangle: infectious agent, host, and environment.

eradication: the irreversible termination of all transmission of infection by extermination of the infectious agents worldwide.

herd immunity: immunity of a group or community.

horizontal transmission: person-to-person spread of infection through one or more of the following routes: direct or indirect contact, common vehicle, airborne, or vector-borne.

host: a living organism, human or animal, in which an infectious agent can exist under natural conditions.

incubation period: time interval beginning with the invasion by an infectious agent and continuing until the organism multiplies to sufficient numbers to produce a host reaction and clinical symptoms.

infection: the state produced by the invasion of a host by an infectious agent. Such infection may or may not produce clinical signs.

infectiousness: a measure of the potential ability of an infected host to transmit the infection to other hosts.

natural immunity: species-determined innate resistance to an infectious agent.

nosocomial infections: infections acquired during hospitalization or developed within a hospital setting. Nosocomial infections may involve clients, health care workers, visitors, or anyone who has contact with a hospital.

pandemic: a worldwide outbreak of an epidemic disease.

passive immunization: immunization by a transfer of a specific antibody from an immunized person to one who is not immunized.

resistance: the ability of the host to withstand infection.

severe acute respiratory syndrome (SARS): a previously unknown disease of undetermined etiology and no definitive treatment that was reported in early 2003 in places such as China and Hong Kong.

smallpox: an acute contagious febrile disease caused by a pox virus and characterized by skin eruption with pustules, sloughing, and scar formation.

surveillance: systematic and ongoing observation and collection of data concerning disease occurrence to describe phenomena and detect changes in frequency or distribution.

Universal Precautions: strategy to prevent exposure to pathogens transmitted through blood and other body fluids by requiring blood and body fluids from *all clients* to be handled as if they were infected with such pathogens.

vaccines: a preparation of killed microorganisms, living attenuated organisms, or living fully virulent organisms that is administered to produce or artificially increase immunity to a particular disease.

vectors: nonhuman organisms, often insects, that either mechanically or biologically play a role in the transmission of an infectious agent from source to host.

vertical transmission: passing the infection from parent to offspring via sperm, placenta, milk, or contact in the vaginal canal at birth.

There is worldwide concern about infectious diseases. This concern has increased with the growth of migration. As people move from one place to another they bring their diseases, levels of immunity and resistance to diseases, and the viruses or bacteria they may harbor that have not emerged as diseases in them. The topic is complex and includes the study of a wide range and variety of organisms and the pathology they may cause, as well as their diagnosis, treatment, prevention, and control. This chapter presents an overview of the communicable diseases with which nurses working in the community deal most often. Diseases are grouped according to descriptive category (by mode of transmission or means of prevention) rather than by individual organism (e.g., *Escherichia coli*) or taxonomic group (e.g., viral, parasitic). A detailed discussion of sexually transmitted diseases (STDs), human immunodeficiency virus (HIV), acquired immunodeficiency syndrome (AIDS), viral hepatitis, and tuberculosis (TB) is provided in Chapter 27. Although not all infectious diseases are directly communicable from person to person, the terms *infectious diseases* and *communicable diseases* are used interchangeably throughout this chapter.

BRIEFLY NOTED

Antibiotics are not effective against viral diseases, a fact found unacceptable to many clients looking for relief from the misery of a cold or flu. The inappropriate prescribing of antibiotics contributes to the growing problem of infectious agents that have developed resistance to once powerful antibiotics.

HISTORICAL AND CURRENT PERSPECTIVES

In 1900, communicable diseases were the leading causes of death in the United States. By 2000, improved nutrition and sanitation, vaccines, and antibiotics had put an end to the epidemics that once ravaged entire populations. In 1900, TB caused 11.3% of all deaths in the United States and was the second leading cause of death. In 2006, although TB was no longer on the list of leading causes of death, this formerly often fatal disease caused 646 deaths in the United States (Centers for Disease Control and Prevention, 2006a). As

people live longer, chronic diseases—heart disease, cancer, and stroke—have replaced infectious diseases as the leading causes of death. Infectious diseases, however, have not vanished. They are still the number one cause of death worldwide. In the United States, infectious diseases account for 25% of all physician visits each year (Directors of Health Promotion and Education, 2005). Organisms once susceptible to antibiotics are becoming increasingly drug resistant; this may result in vulnerability to diseases previously thought to no longer be a threat. And in the twenty-first century, infectious diseases have become a means of terrorism.

New killers are emerging, and old familiar diseases are taking on different, more virulent characteristics. Consider the following recent developments. The advent of the AIDS epidemic in the 1980s reminds us of plagues from the past and challenges our ability to contain and control infection like no other disease in this century. AIDS and injury are the leading killers of persons 25 to 44 years of age. Legionnaires' disease and toxic shock syndrome, unknown in the mid-twentieth century, have become part of our common vocabulary. The identification of infectious agents causing Lyme disease and ehrlichiosis has led to two new tick-borne diseases.

In the summer of 1993 in the southwestern United States, healthy young adults were stricken with a mysterious and unknown but often fatal respiratory disease that is now known as Hantavirus pulmonary syndrome. This syndrome was caused by a severe, invasive strain of *Streptococcus pyogenes* group A and was called by the press the "flesh-eating" bacteria. Consumption of improperly cooked hamburgers and unpasteurized apple juice contaminated with a highly toxic strain of *E. coli* (*Escherichia coli* O157:H7) caused illness and death in children across the country. In 1996, 10 states had outbreaks of diarrheal disease traced to imported fresh berries. The implicated organism in these outbreaks, *Cyclospora cayetanensis* (a coccidian parasite), was first diagnosed in humans in 1979 (Centers for Disease Control and Prevention, 2004a).

Also in 1996, the fear that "mad cow disease" (bovine spongiform encephalopathy, or BSE) could be transferred to humans through beef consumption led to the slaughter of thousands of British cattle and a ban on the international sale of British beef. Although not seen in the United States until 2003 when a BSE case was imported from Canada, BSE has been reported in many countries, including several in Europe, as well as in Japan, Canada, and Israel.

Vancomycin-resistant *Staphylococcus aureus* (VRSA) was reported in 1997; previously, vancomycin had been considered the only effective antibiotic against methicillin-resistant *Staphylococcus aureus* (MRSA). MRSA is increasingly a problem for people who acquire the bacteria in the hospital, and there is a growing incidence of community acquired MRSA. These latter outbreaks are associated with (but not limited to) places in which people share facilities such as locker rooms, prisons, and other close bathing areas.

Ebola hemorrhagic fever, a sporadic but highly fatal virus unknown to most people 30 years ago, is now the subject of movies and best-selling books. A 2002 outbreak in Gabon and the Republic of the Congo killed 79% of the affected individuals. And in 1999, the first Western Hemisphere activity of West Nile virus, a mosquito-transmitted illness that can affect livestock, birds, and humans, occurred in New York City. By 2002, West Nile virus, believed to be carried by infected birds and possibly mosquitoes in cargo containers, had spread across the United States as far west as California and was reported in Canada and Central America as well.

Also, in early 2003, severe acute respiratory syndrome (SARS), a previously unknown disease of undetermined etiology and no definitive treatment, emerged with major outbreaks in China, Hong Kong, Taiwan, Vietnam, Singapore, and Canada, with additional cases reported from 20 locations around the world. This syndrome ended as suddenly as it had begun with only a few cases being reported since 2003.

Worldwide, infectious diseases are the leading killer of children and young adults, accounting for more than 13 million deaths a year and for 50% of all deaths in developing countries. Of these infectious disease deaths, 90% result from six causes: pneumonia, diarrheal diseases, TB, malaria, measles, and HIV/AIDS (Institute of Medicine, 2001). The economic burden of infectious diseases is staggering. In the United States, treatment of non-AIDS STDs alone costs $5 billion annually. The annual costs of other infectious diseases are $30 billion for intestinal infections, $17 billion for influenza, $1 billion for salmonella, and $720 million for hepatitis B. Altogether, the cost of treatment and lost productivity associated with illness from infectious agents is about $120 billion per year (Directors of Health Promotion and Education, 2005). The societal costs of acute foodborne illness were estimated to be over $1.4 trillion in 2007 (Roberts, 2007).

Because of the morbidity, mortality, and associated cost of infectious diseases, the national health promotion and disease prevention goals outlined in *Healthy People 2010* list a number of objectives for reducing the incidence of these illnesses (see the "*Healthy People 2010*" box). Although infectious diseases may not be the leading cause of death in the United States at the beginning of the twenty-first century, they continue to present varied, multiple, and complex challenges to all health care providers. Nurses must know about these diseases to effectively participate in diagnosis, treatment, prevention, and control.

Healthy People 2010

Objectives Related to Communicable Diseases

14-1	Reduce or eliminate indigenous cases of vaccine-preventable disease
14-4	Reduce bacterial meningitis in young children
14-5	Reduce invasive pneumococcal infections
14-7	Reduce meningococcal disease
14-8	Reduce Lyme disease
14-11	Reduce tuberculosis
14-12	Increase the proportion of all tuberculosis patients who complete curative therapy within 12 months
14-13	Increase the proportion of contacts and other high-risk persons with latent tuberculosis infection who complete a course of treatment
14-14	Reduce the average time for a laboratory to confirm and report tuberculosis cases
14-15	Increase the proportion of international travelers who receive recommended preventive services when traveling in areas of risk for select diseases: hepatitis A, malaria, and typhoid
14-16	Reduce invasive early onset group B streptococcal disease
14-17	Reduce hospitalizations caused by peptic ulcer disease in the United States
14-18	Reduce the number of courses of antibiotics for ear infections for young children
14-19	Reduce the number of courses of antibiotics prescribed for the sole diagnosis of the common cold
14-22	Achieve and maintain effective vaccination coverage levels for universally recommended vaccines among young children
14-23	Maintain vaccination coverage levels for children in licensed day care facilities and children in kindergarten through the first grade
14-24	Increase the proportion of young children who receive all vaccines that have been recommended for universal administration for at least 5 years
14-26	Increase the proportion of children who participate in fully operational population-based immunization registries
14-27	Increase routine vaccination coverage levels of adolescents
14-29	Increase the proportion of adults who are vaccinated annually against influenza and ever vaccinated against pneumococcal disease
14-30	Reduce vaccine-associated adverse events

From U.S. Department of Health and Human Services: *Healthy People 2010: national health promotion and disease prevention objectives*, ed 2, Washington, DC, 2000, U.S. Government Printing Office.

TRANSMISSION OF COMMUNICABLE DISEASES

AGENT, HOST, AND ENVIRONMENT

The transmission of **communicable diseases** depends on the successful interaction of the infectious agent, the host, and the environment. These three factors make up the **epidemiologic triangle** (Figure 26-1) as discussed in Chapter 9. Changes in the characteristics of any of the factors may result in disease transmission. Consider the following examples. Not

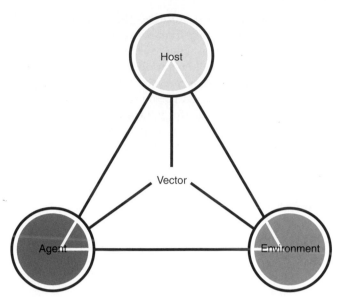

FIGURE 26-1 The epidemiologic triangle of a disease. (From Gordis L: *Epidemiology,* Philadelphia, 1996, Saunders.)

Box 26-1	Six Characteristics of an Infectious Agent

1. Infectivity: The ability to enter and multiply in the host.
2. Pathogenicity: The ability to produce a specific clinical reaction after infection occurs.
3. Virulence: The ability to produce a severe pathological reaction.
4. Toxicity: The ability to produce a poisonous reaction.
5. Invasiveness: The ability to penetrate and spread throughout a tissue.
6. Antigenicity: The ability to stimulate an immunological response.

only may antibiotic therapy eliminate a specific pathological agent but it may also alter the balance of normally occurring organisms in the body. As a result, one of these agents overruns another and disease, such as a yeast infection, occurs. HIV performs its deadly work not by directly poisoning the host but by destroying the host's immune reaction to other disease-producing agents. Individuals living in the temperate climate of the United States do not contract malaria at home, but they may become infected if they change their environment by traveling to a climate in which malaria-carrying mosquitoes thrive. As these examples illustrate, the balance among agent, host, and environment is often precarious and may be unintentionally disrupted. In the twenty-first century, the potential results of such disruption require attention as advances in science and technology, destruction of natural habitats, explosive population growth, political instability, and a worldwide transportation network combine to alter the balance among the environment, people, and the agents that produce disease.

Agent Factor

Four main categories of infectious agents can cause infection or disease: bacteria, fungi, parasites, and viruses. The individual **agent** may be described by its ability to cause disease and by the nature and the severity of the disease. *Infectivity, pathogenicity, virulence, toxicity, invasiveness,* and *antigenicity,* terms commonly used to characterize infectious agents, are defined in Box 26-1.

Host Factor

A human or animal **host** can harbor an infectious agent. The characteristics of the host that may influence the spread of disease are host resistance, immunity, herd immunity, and infectiousness of the host. **Resistance** is the ability of the host to withstand infection, and it may involve natural or acquired immunity.

Natural immunity refers to species-determined, innate resistance to an infectious agent. For example, opossums rarely contract rabies. **Acquired immunity** is the resistance acquired by a host as a result of previous natural exposure to an infectious agent. Having measles once protects against future infection. Acquired immunity may be induced by active or passive immunization. **Active immunization** refers to the immunization of an individual by administration of an antigen (infectious agent or vaccine) and is usually characterized by the presence of an antibody produced by the individual host. Vaccinating children against childhood diseases is an example of inducing active immunity. **Passive immunization** refers to immunization through the transfer of a specific antibody from an immunized individual to a nonimmunized individual, such as the transfer of antibody from mother to infant or by administration of an antibody-containing preparation (immune globulin or antiserum). Passive immunity from immune globulin is almost immediate but short-lived. It is often induced as a stopgap measure until active immunity has time to develop after vaccination. Examples of commonly used immune globulins include those for hepatitis A, rabies, and tetanus.

Herd immunity refers to the immunity of a group or community. It is the resistance of a group of people to invasion and spread of an infectious agent. Herd immunity is based on the resistance of a high proportion of individual members of a group to infection. It is the basis for increasing immunization coverage for vaccine-preventable diseases. Higher immunization coverage will lead to greater herd immunity, which in turn will block the further spread of the disease.

Infectiousness is a measure of the potential ability of an infected host to transmit the infection to other hosts. It reflects the relative ease with which the infectious agent is transmitted to others. Individuals with measles are extremely infectious; the virus spreads readily on airborne droplets. A person with Lyme disease cannot spread the disease to other people (although the infected tick can).

Environment Factor

The **environment** refers to all that is external to the human host, including physical, biological, social, and cultural factors. These environmental factors facilitate the transmission of an infectious agent from an infected host to other susceptible hosts. Reduction in communicable disease risk can be achieved by altering these environmental factors. Using mosquito nets and repellants to avoid bug bites, installing sewage systems to prevent fecal contamination of water supplies, and washing utensils after contact with raw meat to reduce bacterial contamination are all examples of altering the environment to prevent disease.

MODES OF TRANSMISSION

Infectious diseases can be transmitted horizontally or vertically. **Vertical transmission** is the passing of the infection from parent to offspring via sperm, placenta, milk, or contact in the vaginal canal at birth. Examples of vertical transmission are transplacental transmission of HIV and syphilis. **Horizontal transmission** is the person-to-person spread of infection through one or more of the following four routes: direct or indirect contact, common vehicle, airborne, or vector- borne. Most STDs are spread by direct sexual contact. Enterobiasis, or pinworm infection, can be acquired through direct contact or indirect contact with contaminated objects such as toys, clothing, and bedding. **Common vehicle** refers to transportation of the infectious agent from an infected host to a susceptible host via food, water, milk, blood, serum, saliva, or plasma. Hepatitis A can be transmitted through contaminated food and water; hepatitis B can be transmitted through contaminated blood. Legionellosis and TB are both spread via contaminated droplets in the air. **Vectors** can be arthropods such as ticks and mosquitoes or other invertebrates such as snails that can transmit the infectious agent by biting or depositing the infective material near the host.

DISEASE DEVELOPMENT

Exposure to an infectious agent does not always lead to an infection. Similarly, infection does not always lead to disease. Infection depends on the infective dose, the infectivity of the infectious agent, and the immunocompetence of the host. It is important to differentiate infection and disease, as clearly illustrated by the HIV/AIDS epidemic. **Infection** refers to the entry, development, and multiplication of the infectious agent in the susceptible host. **Disease** is one of the possible outcomes of infection, and it may indicate a physiological dysfunction or pathological reaction. An individual who tests positive for HIV is infected, but if that person shows no clinical signs, the individual is not diseased. Similarly, an individual who tests positive for HIV and also exhibits clinical signs of AIDS is both infected and diseased.

BRIEFLY NOTED

Discovered only in 1983, the infectious agent *Helicobacter pylori* is now recognized as the major factor in peptic ulcer disease.

Incubation period and communicable period are not synonymous. **Incubation period** is the time interval between invasion by an infectious agent and the first appearance of signs and symptoms of the disease. The incubation periods of infectious diseases vary from between 2 and 4 hours for staphylococcal food poisoning to between 10 and 15 years for AIDS. **Communicable period** is the interval during which an infectious agent may be transferred directly or indirectly from an infected person to another person. The period of communicability for influenza is 3 to 5 days after the clinical onset of symptoms. Hepatitis B-infected persons are infectious many weeks before the onset of the first symptoms and remain infective during the acute phase and chronic carrier state, which may persist for life.

DISEASE SPECTRUM

Persons with infectious diseases may exhibit a broad spectrum of disease that ranges from subclinical infection to severe and fatal disease. Those with subclinical or nonapparent infections are important from the public health point of view because they are a source of infection but may not be receiving the care that those with clinical disease are receiving. They should be targeted for early diagnosis and treatment. Those with clinical disease may exhibit localized or systemic symptoms and mild to severe illness. The final outcome of a disease may be recovery, death, or something in between, including a carrier state, complications requiring an extended hospital stay, or disability requiring rehabilitation.

At the community level, the disease may occur in endemic, epidemic, or pandemic proportion. **Endemic** refers to the constant presence of a disease within a geographic area or a population. Pertussis is endemic in the United States. **Epidemic** refers to the occurrence of a disease in a community or region in excess of normal expectancy. Although people tend to associate large numbers with epidemics, even one case can be termed *epidemic* if the disease is considered to have previously been eliminated from that area. For example, one case of polio, a disease that is considered to have been eliminated from the United States, would be considered epidemic. **Pandemic** refers to an epidemic that occurs worldwide and affects large populations. HIV/AIDS is both epidemic and pandemic, as the number of cases is growing rapidly across various regions of the world as well as in the United States. SARS is an emerging infectious disease and a recent example of a pandemic.

Severe Acute Respiratory Syndrome (SARS)

In February 2003, the world learned of a mysterious respiratory disease primarily infecting travelers and health care workers in Southeast Asia (Katz and Hirsch, 2003). Thought at first to be a form of influenza, the illness was soon recognized as an atypical and sometimes deadly pneumonia, transmitted easily through close contact and seemingly unresponsive to treatment with antibiotics and antivirals. Initially confined to mainland China, this disease of unknown etiology and no respect for national borders spread to Hong Kong and then quickly to Hanoi, Singapore, and Toronto, prompting the World Health Organization (WHO) to release a rare emergency travel advisory that heightened surveillance of clients with atypical pneumonia around the globe. Intense international investigation revealed that **severe acute respiratory syndrome (SARS),** as this illness came to be called, was associated with a new strain of coronavirus.

BRIEFLY NOTED

Between March 15 and April 15, 2003, 36 patients were diagnosed with SARS at the Queen Mary Hospital in Hong Kong. Reported common symptoms included cough, dyspnea, malaise, and fever (Tiwari et al, 2003).

SURVEILLANCE OF COMMUNICABLE DISEASES

During the first half of the twentieth century, the weekly publication of national morbidity statistics by the U.S. Surgeon General's Office was accompanied by the statement, "No health department, state or local, can effectively prevent or control disease without knowledge of when, where, and under what conditions cases are occurring" (Centers for Disease Control and Prevention, 1996**).** When conducting **surveillance** you gather the *who, when, where,* and *what;* these elements are then used to answer *why.* A good surveillance system systematically collects, organizes, and analyzes current, accurate, and complete data for a defined disease condition. The resulting information is promptly released to those who need it for effective planning, implementation, and evaluation of disease prevention and control programs.

Infectious disease surveillance incorporates and analyzes data from a variety of sources. Box 26-2 lists 10 commonly used data elements.

SURVEILLANCE FOR AGENTS OF BIOTERRORISM

Since September 11, 2001, greater emphasis has been placed on surveillance for any disease that might be associated with the intentional release of a biological agent. The concern is that because of the interval between exposure and disease, a covert release may go unrecognized and without response for some time if the resulting outbreak closely resembles a naturally occurring one. Health care providers are asked to be alert to (1) temporal or geographic clustering of illnesses (people who attended the same public gathering or visited

the same location), especially those with clinical signs that resemble an infectious disease outbreak—previously healthy people with unexplained fever accompanied by sepsis, pneumonia, respiratory failure, rash, or flaccid paralysis; (2) an unusual age distribution for a common disease (e.g., chickenpox-like disease in adults without a child source case); and (3) a large number of cases of acute flaccid paralysis such as that seen in *Clostridium botulinum* intoxication. Although more active infectious disease surveillance is being encouraged because of the potential for bioterrorism, the positive benefit is increased surveillance for other communicable diseases as well. Such heightened surveillance can just as easily warn of a community outbreak of salmonellosis or influenza (Lemon et al, 2007).

Nurses are frequently involved at different levels of the surveillance system. They collect data, make diagnoses, investigate and report cases, and provide information to the general public. Nursing activities include investigating sources and contacts in outbreaks of pertussis in school settings or shigellosis in day care; TB testing and contact tracing; collecting and reporting information pertaining to notifiable communicable diseases; and providing morbidity and mortality statistics to those who request them, including the media, the public, service planners, and grant writers.

LIST OF REPORTABLE DISEASES

Requirements for disease reporting in the United States are mandated by state rather than federal law. The list of reportable diseases varies by state. State health departments, on a voluntary basis, report cases of selected diseases to the Centers for Disease Control and Prevention (CDC) in Atlanta, Georgia. The disease conditions presently included in the National Notifiable Diseases Surveillance System (NNDSS) at the CDC are listed in Box 26-3 (Centers for Disease Control and Prevention, 2008c). The NNDSS data are collated and published weekly in the *Morbidity and Mortality Weekly Report* (*MMWR*). Final reports are published annually in the *Summary of Notifiable Diseases* (Centers for Disease Control and Prevention, 2008c).

EMERGING INFECTIOUS DISEASES

EMERGENCE FACTORS

Emerging infectious diseases are those in which the incidence has actually increased in the past two decades or has the potential to increase in the near future. These emerging diseases may include new or known infectious diseases. Consider the following examples. Hantavirus pulmonary syndrome was first detected in 1993 in the Four Corner area of Arizona and New Mexico, when a mysterious and deadly respiratory disease appeared to target young, healthy Native Americans. The disease was soon discovered to be a variant of, but to exhibit different pathology from, a rodent-borne virus previously known only in Europe and Asia. Transmission is thought to occur through aerosolization of rodent excrement. One explanation for the outbreak in the Southwest is that an unseasonably mild winter led to an unusual

---

Box 26-2	**Ten Basic Elements of Surveillance**

1. Mortality registration
2. Morbidity reporting
3. Epidemic reporting
4. Epidemic field investigation
5. Laboratory reporting
6. Individual case investigation
7. Surveys
8. Utilization of biological agents and drugs
9. Distribution of animal reservoirs and vectors
10. Demographic and environmental data

Box 26-3	Nationally Notifiable Infectious Diseases—United States 2008

1. Acquired Immunodeficiency Syndrome (AIDS)
2. Anthrax
3. Arboviral neuroinvasive and non-neuroinvasive diseases
   - California serogroup virus disease
   - Eastern equine encephalitis virus disease
   - Powassan virus disease
   - St. Louis encephalitis virus disease
   - West Nile virus disease
   - Western equine encephalitis virus disease
4. Botulism
   - Botulism, foodborne
   - Botulism, infant
   - Botulism, other (wound & unspecified)
5. Brucellosis
6. Chancroid
7. *Chlamydia trachomatis*, genital infections
8. Cholera
9. Coccidioidomycosis
10. Cryptosporidiosis
11. Cyclosporiasis
12. Diphtheria
13. Ehrlichiosis/Anaplasmosis
    - Ehrlichia chaffeensis
    - Ehrlichia ewingii
    - Anaplasma phagocytophilum
    - Undetermined
14. Giardiasis
15. Gonorrhea
16. *Haemophilus influenzae*, invasive disease
17. Hansen disease (leprosy)
18. Hantavirus pulmonary syndrome
19. Hemolytic uremic syndrome, post-diarrheal
20. Hepatitis, viral, acute
    - Hepatitis A, acute
    - Hepatitis B, acute
    - Hepatitis B virus, perinatal infection
    - Hepatitis C, acute
21. Hepatitis, viral, chronic
    - Chronic Hepatitis B
    - Hepatitis C Virus Infection (past or present)
22. HIV infection
    - HIV infection, adult ($\geq$13 years)
    - HIV infection, pediatric (<13 years)
23. Influenza-associated pediatric mortality
24. Legionellosis
25. Listeriosis
26. Lyme disease
27. Malaria
28. Measles
29. Meningococcal disease
30. Mumps
31. Novel influenza A virus infections
32. Pertussis
33. Plague
34. Poliomyelitis, paralytic
35. Poliovirus infection, nonparalytic
36. Psittacosis
37. Q Fever
38. Rabies
    - Rabies, animal
    - Rabies, human
39. Rocky Mountain spotted fever
40. Rubella
41. Rubella, congenital syndrome
42. Salmonellosis
43. Severe Acute Respiratory Syndrome-associated Coronavirus (SARS-CoV) disease
44. Shiga toxin-producing *Escherichia coli* (STEC)
45. Shigellosis
46. Smallpox
47. Streptococcal disease, invasive, Group A
48. Streptococcal toxic-shock syndrome
49. *Streptococcus pneumoniae*, drug resistant, invasive disease
50. *Streptococcus pneumoniae*, invasive disease non-drug resistant, in children less than 5 years of age
51. Syphilis
    - Syphilis, primary
    - Syphilis, secondary
    - Syphilis, latent
    - Syphilis, early latent
    - Syphilis, late latent
    - Syphilis, latent, unknown duration
    - Neurosyphilis
    - Syphilis, late, non-neurological
    - Syphilitic Stillbirth
52. Syphilis, congenital
53. Tetanus
54. Toxic-shock syndrome (other than Streptococcal)
55. Trichinellosis (Trichinosis)
56. Tuberculosis
57. Tularemia
58. Typhoid fever
59. Vancomycin - intermediate *Staphylococcus aureus* (VISA)
60. Vancomycin - resistant *Staphylococcus aureus* (VRSA)
61. Varicella (morbidity)
62. Varicella (deaths only)
63. Vibriosis
64. Yellow fever

From Centers for Disease Control and Prevention: *Nationally notifiable infectious diseases—United States 2008*, National Notifiable Diseases Surveillance System, Division of Public Health Surveillance and Informatics, available at http://www.cdc.gov/ncphi/disss/nndss/phs/infdis2008.htm; Centers for Disease Control and Prevention: *Nationally notifiable diseases surveillance system*, Division of Public Health Surveillance and Informatics, available at http://www.cdc.gov/ncphi/disss/nndss/nndsshis.htm.

increase in the rodent population; more people than usual were exposed to a virus that had until that point gone unrecognized in this country. Infection in Native Americans first brought attention to Hantavirus pulmonary syndrome because of a cluster of cases in a small geographic area, but no evidence suggests that any ethnic group is particularly

susceptible to this disease. Hantavirus pulmonary syndrome has now been diagnosed in sites across the United States. The best protection against this virus seems to be avoiding rodent-infested environments.

Not only is HIV/AIDS a relatively new disease but the resultant immunocompromise is largely responsible for the

Evidence-Based Practice

This article looks at an increasingly important topic: good hygiene in the home. With recent reminders that germs are readily transmitted via a variety of common surfaces such as door handles, telephone, television, and other devices that use remote controls, it is important to remind ourselves and our patients about good home health hygiene. The authors discuss the range of hygiene needs in the home, disease-causing microbes and their sources, how they spread, and how their transmission can be controlled by proper hygiene and household cleaning practices. They point out that in any given day, the home can provide the functions of a hotel, restaurant, day care center, medical center, and pet shop. Generally, the people in a home are healthy individuals but at times, some of them become acutely ill, have a chronic illness, or may be immunocompromised. When the latter three types of illnesses occur, the hygiene needs increase. Although nearly every sentence in this article has information valuable personally and to those working with individuals and families in the community, some of the key points are summarized here.

Kitchens, bathrooms, and the laundry are reservoirs for the growth of bacteria. The authors take a room by room look at the typical home and describe areas that pose unique hygiene risks. Areas that stay moist are prime sites for contamination. They also talk about cross-contamination such as what occurs when you cut a raw chicken and then use the same cutting board to cut vegetables. Ordinary household items such as sponges, dishcloths, and soiled laundry and activities such as grooming pets are havens for bacteria. They also describe what effect some common disinfecting agents have on germs. In general, some of the most effective are also some of the most economical: those containing alcohol, bleach, or phenolic. They then go on to talk about the various kinds of hand cleaners and also about sites other than the home in which microbes are readily transferred including day care centers for children and adults and schools.

NURSE USE: It is important that nurses be familiar with the content in this article about hand washing and organism transmission both in their own practices and in their health teaching to clients. Nurses who fail to practice what the article describes can easily carry microbes into patient areas at home, schools, and clinics.

From Aiello AE, Larson EL, Sedlak R: Personal health: bringing good hygiene home, *Am J Infect Control* 3(6):S152–165, 2008.

rising numbers of previously rare opportunistic infections such as cryptosporidiosis, toxoplasmosis, and *Pneumocystis* pneumonia. HIV may have existed in isolated parts of sub-Saharan Africa for years, and it emerged more recently into the rest of the world as the result of a combination of factors (e.g., new roads, increased commerce, prostitution). TB is a familiar face turned newly aggressive. After years of decline, it has resurged as a result of infection secondary to HIV/AIDS and the development of multidrug resistance.

West Nile virus (WNV) was first identified in Uganda in 1937. There are two lineages: one in Africa that seems to be enzootic (i.e., related to animals in a particular vicinity) and that does not result in severe human illness and a second associated with clinical human encephalitis that has been seen in Africa, Asia, India, Europe, and now North

America. How WNV first arrived in the United States may never be known, but the answer most likely involves infected birds or mosquitoes. Because the virus is new in this country and the outbreak of 2002 caused numerous deaths, WNV has garnered a great deal of media attention. However, for the majority of people, infection with WNV results in no clinical signs or only mild flu-like symptoms. In a small percentage of individuals—usually the young, the old, and the immunocompromised—a more severe, potentially fatal encephalitis may develop. After first appearing in New York City in 1999, the virus spent several years quietly spreading up and down the East Coast without remarkable morbidity or mortality. This situation changed abruptly in the summer of 2002, when WNV was reported across the country and was accompanied by significant avian, equine, and human mortality. By the fall of 2002, more than 3000 human cases with more than 180 deaths had been recorded. Especially hard hit were Illinois, Louisiana, Ohio, and Michigan. These periodic outbreaks appeared to result from a complex interaction of multiple factors, including weather—hot, dry summers followed by rain, which influenced mosquito breeding sites and population growth. Since the mid-1990s, outbreaks of WNV involving humans and horses appear to have increased in frequency in Europe, the Middle East, and the United States, with an apparent increase in severity of human disease and an accompanying high mortality rate in birds (Kramer, Styer, and Ebel, 2008). Because the ecology of WNV is not fully understood, the future pattern and nature of the virus in this country are uncertain; preventing human infection will continue to be a challenge for the foreseeable future. Currently, an equine vaccine exists and work is underway in developing vaccines for both birds and humans. The best way to prevent WNV is to avoid mosquito bites. Visit the CDC website on WNV (http://www.cdc.gov/ncidod/dvbid/westnile/) for more information.

CASE STUDY

Li Ming had emigrated to America from Tibet with her father and brother after her mother's death. During a trip to the emergency room with a fever, hemoptysis, and cough, she was diagnosed with drug-resistant tuberculosis and placed in directly observed therapy (DOT), which meant a nurse from the local health department had to witness her ingesting her medication daily. Ms. Ming found taking the medication a big problem; swallowing the pills caused her to gag. She was embarrassed to have to take them in front of a nurse and that made the whole situation even harder. Fortunately, all the rest of the family had negative purified protein derivative (PPD) skin tests and needed to be tested only periodically.

Ms. Ming was thin but not emaciated. She spoke English well enough to communicate with the nurse, Rachel Jones, who told her she could take her time swallowing the medication. They chatted each day about Ms. Ming's life in Tibet and her adjustment to America. Ms. Ming worked in a beauty salon washing hair. Although she was

25 years old, her father did not want her to date, and so she never had.

Ms. Jones worked to decrease Ms. Ming's anxiety. She taught Ms. Ming some relaxation exercises that Ms. Ming was able to use. During the first week of visits it took about an hour for the pills to be ingested. A month later the pill taking was down to 15 minutes and she no longer gagged.

Created by Deborah C. Conway

Several factors, operating singly or in combination, can influence the emergence of these diseases (Table 26-1) (Centers for Disease Control and Prevention, 1994). Except for microbial adaptation and changes made by the infectious agent, such as those likely in the emergence of *E. coli* O157:H7, most of the emergence factors are consequences of activities and behavior of the human hosts and of environmental changes such as deforestation, urbanization, and industrialization. The rise in households with two working parents has increased the number of children in day care, and with this shift has come an increase in diarrheal diseases such as shigellosis. Changing sexual behavior and illegal drug use influence the spread of HIV/AIDS, as well as other STDs. Before the use of large air-conditioning systems with cooling towers, legionellosis was virtually unknown. Modern transportation systems closely and quickly connect regions of the world that for centuries had little contact. Insects and animals as well as humans may carry disease between continents via ships and planes. Immigrants, legal and illegal, as well as travelers bring with them a variety of known and potentially unknown diseases. To prevent and control these emerging diseases, effective ways to educate people and change their behavior and to develop effective drugs and vaccines must be developed. Also, current surveillance systems must be strengthened and expanded to improve the detection and tracking of these diseases. Selected emerging infectious diseases, including a brief description of the diseases and symptoms they cause, their modes of transmission, and causes of emergence, are listed in Table 26-2.

PREVENTION AND CONTROL OF COMMUNICABLE DISEASES

Communicable disease can be prevented and controlled. The goal of prevention and control programs is to reduce the prevalence of a disease to a level at which it no longer poses a major public health problem. In some cases, diseases may even be eliminated or eradicated. The goal of **elimination** is to remove a disease from a large geographic area such as a country or region of the world. **Eradication** is the irreversible termination of all transmission of infection by extermination of the infectious agents worldwide. The World Health Assembly officially declared the global eradication of **smallpox** in 1980. After the successful eradication of smallpox, the eradication of other communicable diseases became a realistic challenge. The Americas were certified to be polio free in 1994 (an outbreak in Haiti and the Dominican Republic in 2000 was vaccine derived), the Western Pacific in 2000, and Europe in 2002 (World Health Organization, 2008).

PRIMARY, SECONDARY, AND TERTIARY PREVENTION

The three levels of prevention in public health are *primary, secondary,* and *tertiary.* In the prevention and control of infectious disease, primary prevention seeks to reduce the incidence of disease by preventing it before it happens, and in this, governments often provide assistance. Many interventions at the primary level, such as federally supplied vaccines and "no shots, no school" immunization laws, are population based because of public health mandate. Nurses deliver many of these childhood immunizations in public and community health settings, check immunization records in day care facilities, and monitor immunization records in schools.

The goal of secondary prevention is to prevent the spread of disease once it occurs. Activities center on rapid identification of potential contacts to a reported case. Contacts may be (1) identified as new cases and treated or (2) determined to be possibly exposed but not diseased and appropriately

---

Table 26-1	Factors That Can Influence the Emergence of New Infectious Diseases
Categories	**Specific Examples**
Societal events	Economic impoverishment, war or civil conflict, population growth and migration, urban decay
Health care	New medical devices, organ or tissue transplantation, drugs causing immunosuppression, widespread use of antibiotics
Food production	Globalization of food supplies, changes in food processing and packaging
Human behavior	Sexual behavior, drug use, travel, diet, outdoor recreation, use of child-care facilities
Environmental	Deforestation/reforestation, changes in water ecosystems, flood/drought, famine, global changes (e.g., warming)
Public health	Curtailment or reduction in prevention programs, inadequate communicable disease infrastructure surveillance, lack of trained personnel (epidemiologists, laboratory scientists, vector and rodent control specialists)
Microbial adaptation	Changes in virulence and toxin production, development of drug resistance, microbes as cofactors in chronic diseases

From Centers for Disease Control and Prevention: *Addressing emerging infectious disease threats: a prevention strategy for the U.S.,* Atlanta, 1994, CDC.

treated with prophylaxis. Public health disease control laws also assist in secondary prevention because they require investigation and prevention measures for individuals affected by a communicable disease report or outbreak. These laws can extend to the entire community if the exposure potential is deemed great enough, as could happen with an outbreak of smallpox or epidemic influenza. Much of the communicable disease surveillance and control work in this country is performed by nurses in community health. Whereas many infections are acute, with either recovery or death occurring

in the short term, some exhibit chronic courses (AIDS) or disabling sequelae (leprosy).

Tertiary prevention works to reduce complications and disabilities through treatment and rehabilitation.

ROLE OF NURSES IN PREVENTION

Prevention is at the center of public health and nurses often take the lead. Examples of such involvement include delivery of immunizations for vaccine-preventable diseases, especially childhood immunization, and the monitoring of immunization

Table 26-2 Examples of Emerging Infectious Diseases

Infectious Agent	Diseases/Symptoms	Mode of Transmission	Causes of Emergence
Borrelia burgdorferi	Lyme disease: rash, fever, arthritis, neurological and cardiac abnormalities	Bite of infective *Ixodes* tick	Increase in deer and human populations in wooded areas
Escherichia coli O157:H7	Hemorrhagic colitis, thrombocytopenia, hemolytic uremic syndrome	Ingestion of contaminated food, especially undercooked beef and raw milk	Likely to be caused by a new pathogen
Ebola-Marburg viruses	Fulminant, high mortality, hemorrhagic fever	Direct contact with infected blood, organs, secretions, semen	Unknown
Legionella pneumophila	Legionnaires' disease: malaise, myalgia, fever, headache, respiratory illness	Air-cooling systems, water supplies	Agent had caused illness in the past, but was only recognized/identified because a large group of people were infected, resulting in several deaths, and Centers for Disease Control and Prevention (CDC), on investigation, isolated the organism. Probably was the cause of many isolated incidences of respiratory infection in which an agent was never identified. Similar to Hantavirus in this country, which was first recognized because of a group outbreak in the Four Corners area of New Mexico.
Hantavirus	Hemorrhagic fever with renal syndrome, pulmonary syndrome	Inhalation of aerosolized rodent urine and feces	Human invasion of virus's ecological niche
Human immunodeficiency virus (HIV-1)	HIV infection, AIDS/HIV disease, severe immune dysfunction, opportunistic infections	Sexual contact with or exposure to blood or tissues of infected persons; perinatal	Urbanization, lifestyle changes, drug use, international travel, transfusions, transplant
Human papillomavirus	Skin and mucous membrane lesions (warts); strongly linked to cancer of the cervix and penis	Direct sexual contact, contact with contaminated surfaces	Newly recognized; changes in sexual lifestyle
Cryptosporidium	Cryptosporidiosis: infection of epithelial cells in gastrointestinal and respiratory tracts	Fecal–oral, person-to-person, waterborne	Development near watershed areas; immunosuppression
Pneumocystis carinii	Acute pneumonia	Unknown; possibly airborne or reactivation of latent infection	Immunosuppression
West Nile virus	No clinical signs to mild flu-like symptoms to fatal encephalitis	Bite of infected mosquitoes; infected birds serve as reservoirs	International travel and commerce

Data are from the Centers for Disease Control and Prevention: Addressing emerging infectious disease threats: a prevention strategy for the United States executive summary, *MMWR Morbid Mortal Wkly Rep* 43(RR-7):1, 1994; Ledeberg J, Shope RE, Oaks SC: *Emerging infections: microbial threats to health in the U.S.,* Washington, DC, 1992, National Academy Press; Peterson LR, Roehrig JT: West Nile virus: a re-emerging global pathogen, *Emerg Infect Dis* 7(4):612–614, 2001.

| Table 26-3 | A Multisystem Approach to Communicable Disease Control |

Goal	Example
Improve host resistance to infectious agents and other environmental hazards	Improved hygiene, nutrition, and physical fitness; increased immunization coverage; provision of chemoprophylaxis and chemotherapy; stress control and improved mental health
Improve the safety of the environment	Improved sanitation, provision of safe water and clean air; proper cooking and storage of food; control of vectors and animal reservoir hosts
Improve public health systems	Increased access to health care; adequate health education; improved surveillance systems
Facilitate social and political changes to ensure better health for all people	Individual, organizational, and community action; legislation

Modified from Wenzel RP: Control of communicable diseases: overview. In Wallace RB, editor: *Public health and preventive medicine,* ed 14, Stamford, Conn, 1998, Appleton & Lange.

Levels of Prevention ▶ Related to Infectious Disease Interventions

PRIMARY PREVENTION

Goal: To prevent the occurrence of disease:
- Responsible sexual behavior
- Malaria chemoprophylaxis
- Tetanus boosters, flu shots
- Rabies preexposure immunization
- Safe food-handling practices in the home
- Repellants for preventing vector-borne disease
- Following childhood immunizations recommendations and "no shots, no school" laws
- Regulated and inspected municipal water supplies
- Blood-borne pathogen regulations
- Restaurant inspections
- Federal regulations protecting American cattle from exposure to bovine spongiform encephalopathy (BSE)

SECONDARY PREVENTION

Goal: To prevent the spread of disease:
- Immunoglobulin after hepatitis A exposure
- Immunization and chemoprophylaxis as appropriate in meningococcal outbreak
- Rabies postexposure immunization
- Tuberculosis screening for health care workers
- Sexually transmitted disease (STD) partner notification
- Human immunodeficiency virus (HIV) testing and treatment
- Quarantine

TERTIARY PREVENTION

Goal: To reduce complications and disabilities through treatment and rehabilitation:
- *Pneumocystis carinii* pneumonia (PCP) chemoprophylaxis for people with AIDS
- Regular inspection of hands and feet as well as protective footwear and gloves to avoid trauma and infection for leprosy clients who have lost sensation in those areas

status in clinic, day care, school, and home settings. Nurses work in communicable disease surveillance and control, teach and monitor blood-borne pathogen control, and advise on prevention of vector-borne disease. They teach methods for responsible sexual behavior, screen for STDs, and provide HIV counseling and testing. They screen for TB, iden-

tify TB contacts, and deliver directly observed TB treatment in the community (see "Levels of Prevention" box).

MULTISYSTEM APPROACH TO CONTROL

Communicable diseases represent an imbalance in the harmonious relationship between the human host and the environment. This state of imbalance provides the infectious agent with an opportunity to cause illness and death in the human population. Given the many factors that can disrupt the agent–host–environment relationship, a multisystem approach to control of communicable diseases (Table 26-3) must be developed (Wenzel, 1998).

BRIEFLY NOTED

When dealing with a communicable disease that has outbreak potential, include family members and close contacts as well as the sick person when developing a treatment and prevention plan.

AGENTS OF BIOTERRORISM

Both the attacks of September 11, 2001 and the subsequent anthrax attacks demonstrated the possibilities for the intentional release of a biological agent, or bioterrorism. The CDC suggests that the biological agents most likely to be employed in a bioterrorist attack are those that both have the potential for high mortality and can be easily disseminated, with the results of major public panic and social disruption. The following six infectious agents are of the highest concern: anthrax *(Bacillus anthracis)*, plague *(Yersinia pestis)*, smallpox (variola major), botulism *(Clostridium botulinum)*, tularemia *(Francisella tularensis)*, and selected hemorrhagic viruses (Filoviridae and Arenaviridae). Visit the CDC Emergency Preparedness and Response website (http://www.bt.cdc.gov/) for more information.

ANTHRAX

Until the fall of 2001, **anthrax** was more commonly a concern of veterinarians and military strategists than the general public. After September 11, the news of deaths caused by letters deliberately contaminated with anthrax and sent through the postal service profoundly changed our view of this infectious disease. Anthrax is an acute disease caused by the spore-forming bacterium *Bacillus anthracis*. Anthrax may have caused the biblical fifth and sixth plagues of Exodus as well as the Black Bane of Europe in the 1600s. In 1881 anthrax became the first bacterial disease for which immunization was available. More commonly seen in cattle, sheep, and goats, anthrax in modern times has rarely and sporadically affected humans (Centers for Disease Control and Prevention, 2006b).

Anthrax is an organism that perpetuates itself by forming spores. When animals dying from anthrax suffer terminal hemorrhage and infected blood comes into contact with the air, the bacillus organism sporulates. These spores are highly resistant to disinfection and environmental destruction and may remain in contaminated soil for many years. In the United States, anthrax zones are said to follow the cattle drive trails of the 1800s. Sometimes referred to as *wool-handler's disease,* anthrax has commonly posed the greatest risk to people who work directly with dying animals, such as veterinarians, or those who handle infected animal products such as hair, wool, and bone or bone meal, or products made from these materials such as rugs and drums. Products made from infected materials may result in the transmission of this disease around the world. Person-to-person transmission is rare (Heymann, 2004).

Anthrax disease may manifest in one of three syndromes: cutaneous, gastrointestinal, and respiratory or inhalational. Cutaneous anthrax, the form most commonly seen, occurs when spores come in contact with abraded skin surfaces. Itching is followed in 2 to 6 days by the development of a characteristic black eschar, usually surrounded by some degree of edema and possibly secondary infection. The lesion itself is usually not painful. If untreated, infection may spread to the regional lymph nodes and bloodstream, resulting in septicemia and death. The fatality rate for untreated cutaneous anthrax is between 5% and 20%, but if it is appropriately treated, death seldom occurs. Before 2001, the last cutaneous case in the United States was reported in 1992. Gastrointestinal anthrax is considered very rare and occurs from eating undercooked contaminated meat. The initial symptoms are nausea, loss of appetite, vomiting, and fever. These are typically followed by abdominal pain, vomiting of blood, and severe diarrhea (Centers for Disease Control and Prevention, 2005c).

Inhalational anthrax is also rare; it is usually seen in occupational exposure such as hide tanning or bone processing. Before 2001, the last case reported in the United States was in 1976. Initially, symptoms are mild and nonspecific and may include fever, malaise, mild cough, or chest pain. These symptoms are followed 3 to 5 days later, often after an apparent improvement, by fever and shock, rapid deterioration, and death. Untreated cases of inhalational anthrax are fatal; treated cases may show as high as a 95% fatality rate if treatment is initiated more than 48 hours after the onset of symptoms.

HOW TO **Distinguish Chickenpox from Smallpox**

Despite the availability of a vaccine, chickenpox is still a common disease of childhood and may be seen in susceptible adults as well. Although many health care providers are familiar with chickenpox, most have never seen a case of smallpox. Because of the potential for smallpox to be used as a bioweapon, the Centers for Disease Control and Prevention (CDC) suggests that nurses and other practitioners familiarize themselves with the differences in presentation between the two diseases. The rash pattern for each disease is distinctive, but it has been observed that in the first 2 to 3 days of development, the two may be indistinguishable. Infectious disease texts and posters provide a pictorial description. If a smallpox infection is suspected, the local health department should be notified immediately.

Chickenpox (varicella)	Smallpox (historical variola major)
Sudden onset with slight fever and mild constitutional symptoms (both may be more severe in adults). Rash is present at onset.	Sudden onset of fever, prostration, severe body aches, and occasional abdominal pain and vomiting, as in influenza. Clear-cut prodromal illness, rash follows 2–4 days after fever begins decreasing.
Rash progression is maculopapular for a few hours, vesicular for 3–4 days, followed by granular scabs.	Progression is macular, papular, vesicular, and pustular, followed by crusted scabs that fall off after 3–4 weeks if the patient survives.
Rash is "centripetal" with lesions most abundant on the trunk or areas of the body usually covered by clothing.	Rash is "centrifugal" with lesions most abundant on the face and extremities.
Lesions appear in "crops" and can be at various stages in the same area of the body.	Lesions are all at the same stage in all areas.
Vesicles are superficial and collapse on puncture; mild scarring may occur.	Vesicles are deep-seated and do not collapse on puncture; pitting and scarring are common.

From Heymann, DL editor: *Control of communicable diseases manual,* ed 18, Washington, DC, 2004, American Public Health Association; Henderson DA: Smallpox: clinical and epidemiologic features, *Emerg Infect Dis* 5(4):537–539, 1999.

Because of factors such as the ability to become an aerosol, the resistance to environmental degradation, and a high fatality rate, inhalational anthrax is considered to have an extremely high potential for being the single greatest biological warfare threat (Fauci et al, 2008).

Any threat of anthrax should be reported to the Federal Bureau of Investigation and to local and state health departments. Anthrax is sensitive to a variety of antibiotics including the penicillins, chloramphenicol, doxycycline, and the fluoroquinolones. In cases of possible bioterrorism activity, individuals with a credible threat of exposure, a confirmed exposure, or who are at high risk of exposure are immediately started on antibiotic prophylaxis, preferably fluoroquinolones. Immunization is recommended as well. People who have been exposed are not contagious, so quarantine is not appropriate (Heymann, 2004).

SMALLPOX

Formerly a disease found worldwide, smallpox has been considered eradicated since 1979. The last known natural death from smallpox occurred in Somalia in 1977. The United States stopped routinely immunizing for smallpox in 1982. The only documented existing virus sources are located in freezers at the CDC in Atlanta and a research institute in Novosibirsk, Russia. Controversy exists over the destruction of these viral stocks, and despite an earlier call by WHO for destruction in 2002, this date has been postponed to allow for additional research needed should clandestine supplies fall into terrorist hands.

Smallpox could be a leading candidate as an agent for bioterrorism. Susceptibility is 100% in the unvaccinated (those vaccinated before 1982 are not considered protected, although they may possess some immunity), and the fatality rate is estimated at 30% or higher (Centers for Disease Control and Prevention, 2008d). Vaccinia vaccine, the immunizing agent for smallpox, is available through the CDC and is effective even after exposure. A second generation vaccinia vaccine, the immunizing agent for smallpox that was licensed by the FDA in 2007, is available through the CDC and can be effective even several days after exposure (U.S. Food & Drug Administration, 2007). Because of the potential for bioterrorism and the fact that many health care providers have never seen this disease, it is important to become familiar with the clinical and epidemiologic features of smallpox and how it is differentiated from chickenpox (see the "How To" box).

VACCINE-PREVENTABLE DISEASES

Vaccines are one of the most effective methods of preventing and controlling communicable diseases. The smallpox vaccine, which left distinctive scars on so many shoulders, is no longer in general use because the smallpox virus has been declared totally eradicated from the world's population. Despite threats of bioterrorism, there are no plans to reintroduce universal smallpox immunization with existing vaccine because of potential side effects. Diseases such as polio, diphtheria, pertussis, and measles, which previously occurred in epidemic proportions, are now controlled by routine childhood immunization. They have not, however, been eradicated, so children need to be immunized against these diseases. In the United States, "no shots, no school" legislation has resulted in the immunization of most children by the time they enter school. However, many infants and toddlers, the group most vulnerable to these potentially severe diseases, do not receive scheduled immunizations on time despite the availability of free vaccines. Surveys show that inner-city children from minority and ethnic groups are particularly at risk for incomplete immunization. *Healthy People 2010* contains several objectives about obtaining and maintaining appropriate levels of immunization in all age groups (U.S. Department of Health and Human Services, 2000).

Because many children receive their immunizations at public health departments, nurses play a major role in increasing immunization coverage of infants and toddlers. Nurses track children known to be at risk for underimmunization and call or send reminders to their parents. They help avoid missed immunization opportunities by checking the immunization status of every young child encountered, whether the clinic or home visit is related to immunization or not. In addition, they organize immunization outreach activities in the community that deliver immunization services; provide answers to parents' questions and concerns about immunization; and educate parents about why immunizations are needed, about inappropriate contraindications to immunization, and about the importance of completing the immunization schedule on time.

ROUTINE CHILDHOOD IMMUNIZATION SCHEDULE

Routine immunization against the following 15 diseases is recommended for children 0-6 years in the United States: hepatitis A and B, diphtheria, tetanus, pertussis, measles, mumps, rubella, polio, *Haemophilus influenzae* type B, meningitis, varicella (chickenpox), *Streptococcus pneumoniae*-related illnesses, rotavirus, and influenza (Centers for Disease Control and Prevention, 2009b). The recommended vaccine schedule is a rather complex and frequently changing document that makes continuing adjustments for the latest research and recommendations. The newest addition is the pneumococcal conjugate vaccine (PCV), licensed in 2000 to prevent diseases caused by *S. pneumoniae,* including pneumonia, sinusitis, meningitis, and acute otitis media (Centers for Disease Control and Prevention, 2007a). To the undoubted relief of parents who feared days of work lost to caring for children miserable with chickenpox, the varicella vaccine was licensed for general use in 1995. In 1996, acellular pertussis transformed the former diphtheria, pertussis, and tetanus combination from DTP to DTaP, and in 1999, orally delivered live polio vaccine (OPV) was totally replaced in the schedule by inactivated polio vaccine (IPV). Measles, mumps, and rubella (MMR) remain in combination but are now given as early as 12 months. Because most of these vaccines require three to four doses, they ideally should begin when an infant is 2 months old to achieve recommended immunization levels by 2 years of age. Additional doses may be required before a child enters school and at adolescence or on entering college. Booster doses of tetanus should be given every 10 years. The Advisory Committee on Immunization Practices, the American Academy of Pediatrics, and the American Academy of Family Physicians regularly update recommended immunization schedules. Examples of other vaccines available for use in special circumstances include those against meningococcal meningitis, plague, rabies, yellow fever, and human papilloma virus (HPV).

MEASLES

Measles is an acute, highly contagious disease that although considered a childhood illness, is often seen in the United States in adolescents and young adults. Symptoms include fever, sneezing and coughing, conjunctivitis, small white spots on the inside of the cheek (Koplik spots), and a red, blotchy rash beginning several days after the respiratory signs. Measles is caused by the rubeola virus and is transmitted by inhalation of infected aerosol droplets or by direct contact with infected nasal or throat secretions or with articles freshly contaminated with the same nasal or throat secretions. Its very contagious nature, combined with the fact that people are most contagious before they know they are infected, makes measles a disease that can spread rapidly through the population. Infection with measles confers lifelong immunity (Heymann, 2004).

Measles and malnutrition form a deadly combination for many children in the developing world. Much of this mortality is preventable by immunizing all infants. Immunization has dramatically decreased the number of measles cases in the United States. Measles are currently not considered endemic in the United States.

With first-dose vaccine coverage of preschool children at more than 90% and schools in 49 states requiring two doses of vaccine, the pattern of infection has shifted from underimmunization of infants and school-aged children to disease acquired from other countries. Of the 131 cases of measles reported during the first 7 months of 2008, 89% were imported from or associated with importations from other countries, particularly counties in Europe where several outbreaks are ongoing. These recent outbreaks in the United States highlight the risk of measles importations from other countries by people who travel (Centers for Disease Control and Prevention, 2008a). Groups who remain at greatest risk for infection are those who do not routinely accept immunization, such as people with religious or philosophical objections, students in schools that do not require two doses of vaccine, and infants in areas in which immunization coverage is low (Centers for Disease Control and Prevention, 2002).

Healthy People 2010 calls for the sustained elimination of indigenous cases of vaccine-preventable disease. Efforts to meet this goal will require (1) rapid detection of cases and implementation of appropriate outbreak control measures, (2) achievement and maintenance of high levels of vaccination coverage among preschool-aged children in all geographic regions, (3) continued implementation and enforcement of the two-dose schedule among young adults, (4) the determination of the source of all outbreaks and sporadic infections, and (5) cooperation among countries in measles control efforts. Nurses receive reports of cases, investigate them, initiate control measures for outbreaks, and use every opportunity to immunize adolescents and young adults who lack documentation of two doses of measles vaccine. Nurses who work in regions in which undocumented residents are common, where groups obtain exemption from immunization on religious grounds, where preschool coverage is low, and/or where international visitors are frequent need to be especially alert for cases of measles and the need for prompt outbreak control among particularly susceptible populations.

RUBELLA

The rubella (German measles) virus causes a mild febrile disease characterized by enlarged lymph nodes and a fine, pink rash that is often difficult to distinguish from measles or scarlet fever. In contrast to measles, rubella is only moderately contagious. Transmission is through inhalation of or direct contact with infected droplets from the respiratory secretions of infected persons. Children may show few or no symptoms, while adults usually experience several days of low-grade fever, headache, malaise, runny nose, and conjunctivitis before the rash appears. Many infections occur without a rash (Heymann, 2004).

Since the introduction of a vaccine in 1969, cases of rubella in the United States have dropped greatly. This decrease has changed the epidemiology of the disease. Although still considered a childhood illness, rubella increasingly occurs in adolescents and young adults. When children are well immunized, infections in older populations become more important. Until recently, outbreaks in adolescents and adults were often seen in institutions, universities, and the military, but now they are appearing in the workplace and the community. Immigration may play a large role in this shift in age group, ethnicity, and outbreak location, as rubella is increasingly seen in young male Hispanics, ages 15 to 44 years, who come from countries without or with newly introduced rubella control programs. Unimmunized immigrants do not necessarily import disease, but their unimmunized status leaves them vulnerable to infection once they arrive.

For many years, because it caused only a mild illness, rubella was considered to be of minor importance. Then, in 1941, the link between maternal rubella and certain congenital defects was recognized, and the disease suddenly assumed major public health significance. Congenital rubella syndrome (CRS) occurs in up to 90% of infants born to women who are infected with rubella during the first trimester of pregnancy (Heymann, 2004). Rubella infection, in addition to causing intrauterine death and spontaneous abortion, may result in anomalies that can affect single or multiple organ systems. Defects include cataracts, congenital glaucoma, deafness, microcephaly, mental retardation, cardiac abnormalities, and diabetes mellitus.

Eliminating rubella and CRS will require many of the same efforts discussed for measles, including achievement and maintenance of high rates of immunization among preschoolers, emphasizing early detection and outbreak control, taking advantage of opportunities such as high school and college entrance to immunize susceptible adolescents, and extending immunization opportunities to religious groups that traditionally do not seek health care. Because of the large percentage of cases reported in Hispanic communities, outreach to adolescents and young adults, especially women of childbearing age, from countries that may have only recently begun to vaccinate routinely against rubella is of critical importance.

PERTUSSIS

Pertussis (whooping cough) begins as a mild upper respiratory infection that progresses to an irritating cough and in 1 to 2 weeks may become paroxysmal (a series of repeated violent coughs). The repeated coughs occur without intervening breaths and can be followed by a characteristic inspiratory "whoop." Pertussis is caused by the bacterium *Bordetella pertussis* and is transmitted via an airborne route through contact with infected droplets (Goldrick, 2004a, b). It is highly contagious and is considered endemic in the United States. Vaccination against pertussis, delivered in combination with diphtheria and tetanus, is a part of the routine childhood immunization schedule. Treatment of infected individuals with antibiotics such as erythromycin may shorten the period of communicability but does not relieve symptoms unless given early in the course of the infection. A 2-week treatment with antibiotics is recommended for family members and close contacts of infected individuals, regardless of immunization status (Heymann, 2004).

Before the development of a whole-cell vaccine in the 1940s, pertussis led to hundreds of thousands of cases and thousands of deaths per year, the majority in children younger than 5 years. After vaccine licensure and the introduction of universal vaccination, reported cases in the United States steadily declined, hitting a record low of just more than 1000 in 1976. However, beginning in the early 1980s, pertussis cases began to show cyclical increases every 3 to 4 years until 2004, in which more than 25,000 cases were reported. This was the highest number of reported cases since 1959. Currently, pertussis causes substantial morbidity in the United States and is the only childhood vaccine preventable disease showing an upward trend in reported cases (Centers for Disease Control and Prevention, 2005d).

Although the largest increase in pertussis cases has been among adolescents and adults, the annual reported incidence remains highest among infants under 1 year of age. Pertussis in very young children, especially those younger than 6 months, is attributed to being underimmunized or nonimmunized because of age. Cases in older children result largely from underimmunization, and in adolescents and adults with histories of complete immunization, cases are thought to be the result of waning immunity. Some of the rise in cases in adolescents and adults may be attributed to increased awareness and improved reporting. However, the decrease in cases to fully immunized 1 to 4 year olds and the stability of cases in 5 to 9 year olds suggest the increase of incompletely or nonimmunized infant cases represents an actual rise in pertussis circulation (Centers for Disease Control and Prevention, 2005d). The increase in adolescent and adult pertussis is alarming not because of increased morbidity—their cases are often mild or inapparent—but because they serve as a reservoir of infection for infants, especially those younger than 6 months, who are the most vulnerable to pertussis and the most likely to suffer complications resulting in hospitalization and death.

Although natural infection with pertussis results in permanent immunity, immunization through vaccination does not. Before 2005, pertussis vaccines were not labeled for use in individuals older than 6 years of age, making catching up children with missing doses and boostering for waning immunity not an option. The introduction of Tdap, a combination booster for tetanus, pertussis, and diphtheria, has produced a new tool for combating waning immunity. Preteens should get Tdap at the age of 11 to 12 years, and adults who never received Tdap can take one dose as a substitute for their next Td tetanus booster. Prevention efforts should be directed at maintaining high rates of immunization, publicizing Tdap, increasing awareness of pertussis in adolescents and adults among providers, and promptly implementing treatment and control in the face of outbreaks (Centers for Disease Control and Prevention, 2009c).

Nurses may expect periodic outbreaks of pertussis because of its cyclical nature. Working with the community to maintain the highest possible levels of immunization coverage can minimize these occurrences. Because of the contagious nature of pertussis, nurses play a major role in limiting transmission during outbreaks by ensuring appropriate treatment of family members, classmates, and other close contacts.

INFLUENZA

Influenza (flu) is a viral respiratory infection often indistinguishable from the common cold or other respiratory diseases. Transmission is airborne and through direct contact with infected droplets. Unlike many viruses that do not survive long in the environment, the flu virus may survive for many hours in dried mucus. Outbreaks are common in the winter and early spring in areas in which people gather indoors, such as in schools and nursing homes. Gastrointestinal and respiratory symptoms are common. Because symptoms do not always follow a characteristic pattern, many viral diseases that are not influenza are often called *flu*. The most important factors to note about influenza are its epidemic nature and the mortality that may result from pulmonary complications, especially in older adults.

There are three types of influenza viruses: A, B, and C. Type A is usually responsible for large epidemics, whereas outbreaks from type B are more regionalized; type C epidemics are less common and usually result in only mild illness. Influenza viruses often change in the nature of their surface appearance or their antigenic makeup. Types B and C are fairly stable viruses, but type A changes constantly. Minor antigenic changes are referred to as *antigenic drift,* and they result in yearly epidemics and regional outbreaks. Major changes such as the emergence of new subtypes are called *antigenic shift;* these occur only with type A viruses. Antigenic shift and drift lead to epidemic outbreaks every few years and pandemic outbreaks every 10 to 40 years. Mortality rates associated with epidemics may be higher than those in nonepidemic situations (Heymann, 2004).

In 1997 in Hong Kong, the first known cases of human illness associated with an avian influenza virus, A (H5N1), were reported. Referred to in the press as *Hong Kong bird flu,* this virus appears to have been transmitted to people through contact with infected poultry. As a result of this association, Hong Kong officials ordered the slaughter of all chickens in and around Hong Kong, which appears to have stopped the spread of this disease. No cases were reported outside Hong Kong, and despite recurring outbreaks of avian flu, no further outbreaks of A (H5N1) have been reported.

The preparation of influenza vaccine each year is based on the best possible prediction of what type and variant of virus will be most prevalent that year. Because of the changing nature of the virus, yearly immunization is necessary and in the United States is given in early fall before the flu season begins. Immunization is highly recommended for children ages 6 months to 19 years, pregnant women, people 50 years of age and older, individuals of any age with certain chronic medical conditions, individuals who live in long-term care facilities, and those who live with or care for persons at risk for complications from the flu. Although immunization is recommended for the previously mentioned groups, any individual may benefit from this protection. Flu shots do not always prevent infection, but they do result in milder disease symptoms. Because of small quantities of egg protein found in the vaccine, individuals with egg sensitivity should consult their physician to determine if immunization should be administered.

The use of influenza antiviral drugs should be considered in nonimmunized persons or in groups at high risk for complications such as older persons in institutions or nursing homes. The neuraminidase inhibitors (oseltamivir, zanamivir) have activity against influenza A and B viruses, whereas the adamantanes (amantadine, rimantadine) have activity only against influenza A viruses. Since January 2006, the neuraminidase inhibitors have been the only recommended influenza antiviral drugs because of widespread resistance to the adamantanes among influenza A (H3N2) virus strain. In 2007 to 2008, a significant increase in the prevalence of oseltamivir resistance was reported among influenza A (H1N1) viruses worldwide. Also during the 2007 to 2008 influenza season, 10.9% of H1N1 viruses tested in the United States were resistant to oseltamivir. Current guidelines indicate that antiviral treatment should be guided by surveillance data on circulating viruses and confirmatory testing of viral subgroups (Centers for Disease Control and Prevention, 2008e).

Novel influence A (H1N1) is a new flu virus that was first detected in Mexico and the United States in March and April 2009. While it has a swine origin, it quickly began spreading from person-to-person. It is spread in the same way that regular seasonal influenza viruses spread which is primarily through the coughs and sneezes of people who have the virus or by touching objects soiled with the virus and then touching their nose or mouth. Because this is a new virus most people have little or no immunity to it, and there is no vaccine to prevent this virus at present. The symptoms for this virus are similar to those for human seasonal influenza and include fever, lethargy, body aches, headache, chills, loss of appetite and coughing. Some infected people may have a runny nose, sore throat, nausea, vomiting and diarrhea.

Antiviral agents can reduce the severity and duration of illness, and these drugs must be taken under a physician's prescription. Prevention of this virus requires the same precautionary measures as those of many other communicable diseases including:

- Wash hands properly or use alcohol-based handrub, and this is especially necessary after you cough or sneeze.
- Avoiding touching your mouth, nose or eyes.
- Cover your mouth when you cough or sneeze and do not spit.
- Do not go to work or school if you develop influenza symptoms
- If you develop flulike symptoms stay home for 7 days after the symptoms begin or until you have been symptom-free for 24 hours (Centers for Disease Control and Prevention 2009d).

On June 11, 2009, the World Health Organization (WHO) raised the worldwide pandemic alert level to phase 6. This designation indicates that the flu has spread to many countries and that a global pandemic is underway. The designation does not address the severity of the flu but rather the extent of the spread of the virus (Centers for Disease Control and Prevention, 2009d).

Healthy People 2010 suggests increasing the proportion of the population vaccinated annually against influenza and ever vaccinated against pneumococcal disease. Nurses often spearhead influenza immunization campaigns that target older adults. Examples include conducting flu clinics at polling places during elections or at community centers and churches during "senior vaccination Sundays." Inhabitants of residences and nursing homes for older adults are at risk, because influenza can spread rapidly with severe consequences through such living arrangements. As with children, nurses should check immunization history and encourage immunization for every adult encountered in a clinic or home visit.

FOODBORNE AND WATERBORNE DISEASES

Foodborne illness, sometimes referred to as "food poisoning," can be categorized as either a food infection or food intoxication. Food infection results from bacterial, viral, or parasitic infection of food and includes salmonellosis, hepatitis A, and trichinosis. Food intoxication results from toxins produced by bacterial growth, chemical contaminants (heavy metals), and a variety of disease-producing substances found naturally in certain foods such as mushrooms and some seafood. Examples of food intoxications are botulism, mercury poisoning, and paralytic shellfish poisoning. Table 26-4 presents some of the most common

Table 26-4	Commonly Encountered Food Intoxications			
Casual Agent	**Incubation Period**	**Duration**	**Clinical Presentation**	**Associated Food**
Staphylococcus aureus	30 min to 7 hr	1–2 days	Sudden onset of nausea, cramps, vomiting, and prostration, often accompanied by diarrhea; rarely fatal	All foods, especially those likely to come into contact with food-handlers' hands that may be contaminated from infections of the eyes and skin
Clostridium perfringens (strain A)	6–24 hr	1 day or less	Sudden onset of colic and diarrhea, maybe nausea; vomiting and fever unusual; rarely fatal	Inadequately heated meats or stews; food contaminated by soil or feces becomes infective when improper storage or reheating allows multiplication of organism
Vibrio parahaemolyticus	4–96 hr	1–7 days	Watery diarrhea and abdominal cramps; sometimes nausea, vomiting, fever, and headache; rarely fatal	Raw or inadequately cooked seafood; period of time at room temperature usually required for multiplication of organisms
Clostridium botulinum	12–36 hr, sometimes days	Slow recovery, could be months	Central nervous system signs; blurred vision, difficulty in swallowing and dry mouth, followed by descending symmetrical flaccid paralysis of an alert person; "floppy baby" in infant; fatality <15% with antitoxin and respiratory support	Home-canned fruits and vegetables that have not been preserved with adequate heating; infants have become infected from ingesting honey

Data from Heymann DL, editor: *Control of communicable diseases manual,* ed 18, Washington, DC, 2004, American Public Health Association.

agents of food intoxication, their incubation period, source, symptoms, and pathology. Although it is not a hard-and-fast rule, food infections are associated with incubation periods of 12 hours to several days after ingestion of the infected food, whereas food intoxications become obvious within minutes to hours after ingestion. Some botulism is a clear exception to this rule, with an incubation period of a week or more in adults. The expression *ptomaine poisoning,* often used when discussing foodborne illness, does not refer to a specific causal organism.

Salmonella and *Campylobacter* are most likely to cause illness, and *Salmonella, Listeria,* and *Toxoplasma* are most frequently involved with deaths. FoodNet is a CDC sentinel surveillance system targeting seven states and collecting information on seven bacterial and two parasitic agents. Confirmed foodborne outbreaks are reported by states to the CDC through the Foodborne Disease Outbreak Surveillance System; on average, 1300 outbreaks have been reported every year since 1998. In June 2001, the CDC launched an Electronic Foodborne Outbreak Reporting System (EFORS).

In recent years, publicity has surrounded foodborne outbreaks affecting people nationwide. Examples include the illness and, in some cases, deaths of individuals after eating fresh spinach contaminated with a virulent strain of *E. coli;* peanut butter infected with salmonella; cans of corned beef, chili, and beef stew pulled from grocery shelves because of possible botulism; and a warning not to eat fresh tomatoes for fear of contracting an unusual strain of salmonella, although the actual culprit turned out to be chili peppers. Although the young, the old, and the debilitated are most susceptible, anyone can acquire a foodborne illness. However, a new, particularly susceptible population is emerging as the adult population ages and chronic diseases (e.g., AIDS) and advanced medical treatment (e.g., chemotherapy, organ transplants) result in growing numbers of immunosuppressed individuals. At the same time, centralized food processing draws from multiple producers and suppliers outside the country as well as within, and markets through widespread distribution networks increase the potential for any contamination to result in a large-scale foodborne outbreak, compounding the difficulty in attempting to trace the source. Public health officials think the reported cases of foodborne illness vastly underestimates the true number of cases and that this number is likely to increase.

TEN GOLDEN RULES FOR SAFE FOOD PREPARATION

It is complex, costly, and time consuming to protect a nation's food supply from contamination by all virulent microbes. However, much foodborne illness, regardless of causal organism, can be prevented by simple changes in food preparation, handling, and storage to destroy or denature contaminants and prevent their further spread. Because these measures are so important in preventing foodborne disease, *Healthy People 2010* has included an objective directed toward them, and the WHO has developed the "Ten Golden Rules for Safe Food Preparation" presented in Box 26-4 (Heymann, 2004).

Box 26-4	Ten Golden Rules for Safe Food Preparation

1. Choose food processed for safety.
2. Cook food thoroughly.
3. Eat cooked food immediately.
4. Store cooked food carefully.
5. Reheat cooked foods thoroughly.
6. Avoid contact between raw foods and cooked foods.
7. Wash hands repeatedly.
8. Keep all kitchen surfaces meticulously clean.
9. Protect foods from insects, rodents, and other animals.
10. Use pure water.

From Heymann DL, editor: *Control of communicable diseases manual,* ed 18, Washington, DC, 2004, American Public Health Association.

BRIEFLY NOTED

Irradiation of meat and poultry is one option being used to prevent outbreaks of foodborne disease.

SALMONELLOSIS

Salmonellosis is a bacterial disease characterized by a sudden onset of headache, abdominal pain, diarrhea, nausea, sometimes vomiting, and almost always fever. Onset is typically within 48 hours of ingestion, but the clinical signs are impossible to distinguish from other causes of gastrointestinal distress. Diarrhea and lack of appetite may last several days, and dehydration may be severe. Although morbidity can be significant, death is uncommon except among infants, older adults, and the debilitated. The rate of infection is highest among infants and small children. It is estimated that only a small proportion of cases is recognized clinically and that only 1% of clinical cases are reported. The number of salmonella infections yearly may actually number in the millions (Heymann, 2004).

Outbreaks occur commonly in restaurants, hospitals, nursing homes, and institutions for children. The transmission route is eating food derived from an infected animal or food contaminated by feces of an infected animal or person. Meat, poultry, and eggs are the foods most often associated with salmonella outbreaks. However, recently regional and national outbreaks have resulted from vegetables (e.g., lettuce, green onions, tomatoes, chili peppers) and peanut butter. Animals are the common reservoir for the various *Salmonella* serotypes, although infected humans may also fill this role. Animals are more likely to be chronic carriers. *Salmonella* carriers include reptiles such as iguanas, pet turtles, poultry, cattle, swine, rodents, dogs, and cats. Person-to-person transmission is an important consideration in day care and institutional settings.

ESCHERICHIA COLI O157:H7

Escherichia coli O157:H7 belongs to the enterohemorrhagic category of *E. coli* serotypes that produce a strong cytotoxin that can cause a potentially fatal hemorrhagic colitis. This pathogen was first described in humans in 1992 after two outbreaks of illness were associated with eating hamburgers from a fast-food restaurant chain. Undercooked hamburger has been implicated in several outbreaks, as have roast beef, alfalfa sprouts, unpasteurized milk and apple cider, municipal water, jalapenos, spinach, and person-to-person transmission in day care centers. Infection with *E. coli* O157:H7 causes bloody diarrhea, abdominal cramps, and, infrequently, fever. Children and older adults are at highest risk for clinical disease and complications. Hemolytic uremic syndrome is seen in 5% to 10% of cases and may result in acute renal failure. The case fatality rate is 3% to 5% (Heymann, 2004).

Hamburger is often involved in outbreaks since the grinding process exposes pathogens on the surface of the whole meat to the interior of the ground meat, effectively mixing the once-exterior bacteria thoroughly throughout the hamburger so that searing the surface no longer suffices to kill all bacteria. Tracking the contamination is complicated by the fact that hamburger is often made of meat ground from several sources. The best protection against this pathogen, as with most foodborne agents, is to thoroughly cook food before eating it (see "Evidence-Based Practice" box on p. 491).

WATERBORNE DISEASE OUTBREAKS AND PATHOGENS

Waterborne pathogens usually enter water supplies through animal or human fecal contamination and often cause enteric disease. They include viruses, bacteria, and protozoans. Hepatitis A virus is probably the best known waterborne viral agent, although other viruses may also be transmitted by this route (enteroviruses, rotaviruses, and paramyxoviruses). The most important waterborne bacterial diseases are cholera, typhoid fever, and bacillary dysentery. However, other *Salmonella* types, *Shigella, Vibrio,* and various coliform bacteria including *E. coli* O157:H7 may be transmitted in the same manner. In the past, the most important waterborne protozoans have been *Entamoeba histolytica* (amebic dysentery) and *Giardia lamblia,* but outbreaks of cryptosporidiosis in municipal water have called attention to the importance of protecting sources of water. Protozoans do not respond to traditional chlorine treatment as do enteric and coliform bacteria, and their small size requires special filtration.

The CDC defines an outbreak of waterborne disease as an incident in which two or more persons experience similar illness after consuming water that epidemiologic evidence implicates as the source of that illness. Only a single incident is required in cases of chemical contamination. The CDC and the Environmental Protection Agency (EPA) maintain a collaborative surveillance program for collection and periodic reporting of data on the occurrence and causes of waterborne disease outbreaks.

VECTOR-BORNE DISEASES

Vector-borne diseases refer to illnesses for which the infectious agent is transmitted by a carrier, or vector, usually an arthropod (mosquito, tick, fly), either biologically

cycles; infected humans have simply somehow managed to get in their way. Means of transmission include animal bites, inhalation, ingestion, direct contact, and arthropod intermediates. This last transmission route means that some vector-borne diseases may also be zoonoses. Other than vector-borne diseases, some of the more common zoonoses in the United States include toxoplasmosis *(Toxoplasma gondii)*, cat-scratch disease *(Bartonella henselae)*, brucellosis *(Brucella* species), listeriosis *(Listeria monocytogenes)*, salmonellosis *(Salmonella* serotypes), and rabies (family Rhabdoviridae, genus *Lyssavirus).*

RABIES (HYDROPHOBIA)

One of the most feared of human diseases, rabies has the highest case fatality rate of any known human infection—essentially 100%. In the 1970s, three cases of presumed rabies recovery were reported. All had received preexposure or postexposure prophylaxis. During 2004, one rabies patient in the United States recovered and remains the only rabies patient to have survived without the administration of rabies vaccination. A significant public health problem worldwide with as many as 50,000 deaths a year, mostly in developing countries, rabies in humans in the United States is a rare event because of the widespread vaccination of dogs begun in the 1950s. Today, the major carriers of rabies in the United States are not dogs but wild animals—raccoons, skunks, foxes, coyotes, and bats. Small rodents, rabbits and hares, and opossums rarely carry rabies. Epidemiologic information should be consulted concerning the potential carriers for a given geographic region. When the virus spreads from wild to domestic animals, cats are often involved. During 2007, 49 states and Puerto Rico reported 7258 cases of rabies in animals and one in a human to the Centers for Disease Control and Prevention (Blanton et al, 2008).

Rabies is transmitted to humans by introducing virus-carrying saliva into the body, usually via an animal bite or scratch. Transmission may also occur if infected saliva comes into contact with a fresh cut or intact mucous membranes. Rabies is found in neural tissue and is not transmitted via blood, urine, or feces. Airborne transmission has been documented in caves with infected bat colonies. Transmission from human to human is theoretically possible but has only been documented in the case of organ transplants harvested from individuals who died of undiagnosed rabies. Guidelines for organ donation exist to minimize this possibility (Centers for Disease Control and Prevention, 2004d). The best protection against rabies remains vaccinating domestic animals—dogs, cats, cattle, and horses. If a person is bitten, clean the bite wound thoroughly with soap and water and immediately consult a physician. Suspicion of rabies should exist if the bite is from a wild animal or an unprovoked attack from a domestic animal. Even when there is no suspicion of rabies, a physician should be contacted because tetanus or antibiotic prophylaxis may be indicated.

No successful treatment exists for rabies once symptoms appear, but if given promptly and as directed, postexposure prophylaxis with human rabies immune globulin and rabies vaccine can prevent the development of the disease. Three products are licensed for use as rabies vaccine in the United States: human diploid cell vaccine (HDCV), rabies vaccine adsorbed (RVA), and purified chick embryo cell (PCEC) culture (RabAvert) (Centers for Disease Control and Prevention, 2008b). The vaccine is administered in a series of five 1-ml doses injected into the deltoid muscle. Reactions to the vaccine are fewer and less serious than with previously used vaccines. Individuals who deal frequently with animals, such as zookeepers, laboratory workers, and veterinarians, may choose to receive the vaccine as preexposure prophylaxis. The decision to administer the vaccine to a bite victim depends on the circumstances of the bite and is made on an individual basis.

Recommendations for providing postexposure prophylaxis treatment are provided by the Advisory Committee for Recommendations on Immunization Practices and are available through local public health officials or the CDC. In general, cats and dogs that have bitten someone and have verified rabies vaccinations are confined for 10 days for observation. Treatment is initiated only if signs of rabies are observed during this period. If the animal is known or suspected to be rabid, treatment begins immediately. If the animal is unknown to the victim and escapes, public health officials should be consulted for help in deciding whether treatment is indicated. With wild animal bites, treatment is begun immediately. With bites from livestock, rodents, and rabbits, treatment is considered on an individual basis. Decisions to treat become more complicated for possible nonbite exposure to saliva from known infected animals, and again public health officials are helpful in making these treatment decisions (Centers for Disease Control and Prevention, 2008b).

PARASITIC DISEASES

Parasitic diseases are more prevalent in developing countries than in the United States because of tropical climate and inadequate prevention and control measures. A lack of cheap and effective drugs, poor sanitation, and a scarcity of funding lead to high reinfection rates even when control programs are attempted. Parasites are classified into four groups: nematodes (roundworms), cestodes (tapeworms), trematodes (flukes), and protozoa (single-celled animals). Nematodes, cestodes, and trematodes are all referred to as *helminths.* Table 26-5 presents examples of diseases caused by parasites from these groups. Nurses and other health professionals should be aware of the growing numbers of reported parasitic infections in the United States.

INTESTINAL PARASITIC INFECTIONS

Enterobiasis (pinworm) is the most common helminthic infection in the United States, with an estimated 42 million cases a year. Pinworm infection is seen most often among children and is most prevalent in crowded and institutional settings. Pinworms resemble small pieces of white thread and can be seen with the naked eye. Diagnosis is usually accomplished by pressing cellophane tape to the perianal

Table 26-5	Selected Parasite Categories
Category	**Parasite and Disease**
Intestinal nematodes	*Ascaris lumbricoides* (roundworm)
	Trichuris trichiura (whipworm)
	Ancylostoma, Necator (hookworm)
	Enterobius vermicularis (pinworm)
Blood and tissue nematodes	*Wuchereria bancrofti* (filariasis)
	Onchocerca volvulus (river blindness)
Cestodes	*Taenia solium* (pork tapeworm)
	Taenia saginata (beef tapeworm)
Trematodes	*Schistosoma* species (schistosomiasis)
Protozoans	*Giardia lamblia* (giardiasis)
	Entamoeba histolytica (amebiasis)
	Plasmodium species (malaria)
	Leishmania species (leishmaniasis)
	Trypanosoma species (African sleeping sickness, Chagas' disease)
	Toxoplasma gondii (toxoplasmosis)

Data from Brown H, Neva FA: *Basic clinical parasitology,* ed 6, Norwalk, Conn, 1994, Appleton & Lange; and Centers for Disease Control and Prevention, 2005, available at cdc.gov/ncidod/dpd/parasiticpathways/default.htm.

region early in the morning. Treatment with oral vermicides results in a cure rate of 90% to 100%. According to the CDC, the most common parasitic infections are caused by the following parasites: *Trichomonas, Giardia lamblia, Cryptosporidium,* and *Toxoplasma* (Centers for Disease Control and Prevention, 2008c). The opportunities for widespread indigenous transmission of these intestinal parasites are reduced because of improved sanitary conditions in this country. Effective drug treatment is available for these intestinal parasitic infections.

PARASITIC OPPORTUNISTIC INFECTIONS

Some of the common parasitic opportunistic infections in clients with AIDS and others who are immunocompromised include *Pneumocystis carinii* pneumonia (PCP), cryptosporidiosis, microsporidiosis, isosporiasis, and toxoplasmosis. All of these infections cause diarrheal disease and are transmitted by fecal–oral contact. However, since the introduction of routine prophylactic treatment and highly active antiretroviral therapy (HAART), the incidence of opportunistic infections in AIDS patients has declined significantly. Toxoplasmosis, PCP, cryptosporidiosis, and microsporidiosis have declined in AIDS patients but have not disappeared. Isosporiasis is rare for these patients (Katlama, 2004). Toxoplasmosis and PCP are more likely to occur in people who either lack access to health care or do not know that they have AIDS.

CONTROL AND PREVENTION OF PARASITIC INFECTIONS

Correct diagnosis by nurses and other health care workers allows the provision of appropriate treatment and client education for preventing and controlling parasitic infections. The diagnosis of parasitic diseases is based on history of travel,

characteristic clinical signs and symptoms, and the use of appropriate laboratory tests to confirm the clinical diagnosis. Knowing what specimens to collect, how and when to collect them, and what laboratory techniques to use are all important in establishing a correct diagnosis. Effective drug treatment is available for most parasitic diseases. The high cost of the drugs, drug resistance, and toxicity are some of the common therapeutic problems. Measures for prevention and control of parasitic diseases include early diagnosis and treatment, improved personal hygiene, safer sex practices, community health education, vector control, and improvements in sanitary control of food, water, and waste disposal.

NOSOCOMIAL INFECTIONS

Nosocomial infections are infections acquired during hospitalization or developed within a hospital setting. They may involve clients, health care workers, visitors, or anyone who has contact with a hospital. Invasive diagnostic and surgical procedures, broad-spectrum antibiotics, and immunosuppressive drugs, along with the original underlying illness, leave hospitalized clients particularly vulnerable to exposure to virulent infectious agents from other clients and indigenous hospital flora from health care staff. In this setting, the simple act of performing hand hygiene before approaching every client becomes critical. Each year, hospital-acquired infections may affect as many as 2 million people, result in 88,000 deaths, and add $5 billion to health costs (Centers for Disease Control and Prevention, 2000). Also, nosocomial infections may involve and contribute to antibiotic resistance. The CDC maintains the National Nosocomial Infection Surveillance (NNIS) system, the only source of national data on the epidemiology of nosocomial infections in the United States.

Infection control practitioners play a key role in hospital infection surveillance and control programs. Without a qualified and well-trained person in this position, the infection control program is ineffective. More than 95% of infection control practitioners are nurses. Their common job titles are *infection control nurse, infection control coordinator,* and *nurse epidemiologist.*

UNIVERSAL PRECAUTIONS

In 1985, in response to concerns about the transmission of HIV infection during health care procedures, the CDC recommended a **Universal Precautions** policy for all health care settings. This strategy requires that blood and body fluids from *all clients* be handled as if infected with HIV or other blood-borne pathogens. When in a situation in which potential contact with blood or other body fluids exists, health care workers must always perform hand hygiene and wear gloves, masks, protective clothing, and other indicated personal protective barriers. Needles and sharp instruments must be used and disposed of properly. The CDC also made recommendations for preventing transmission of HIV and hepatitis B during medical, surgical, and dental procedures (Centers for Disease Control and Prevention, 1997).

CLINICAL APPLICATION

The rising numbers of foreign-born residents in communities that did not previously have large immigrant populations provide a challenge to those involved with communicable disease control, especially in outbreak situations. Language barriers, specific cultural practices, and undocumented status all contribute to opportunities for infection and present obstacles to prevention and control. It is common for diseases such as TB, brucellosis, measles, hepatitis B, and parasitic infections to originate in other countries and be diagnosed only after arrival of the person in the United States. People coming from countries without, with newly established, or with poorly enforced vaccination programs may be unimmunized. These people are particularly susceptible to infection in outbreak situations. For example, many people coming from Latin America have not been immunized against rubella. Differences in cultural practices can lead to outbreaks of foodborne illness. Listeriosis outbreaks have been traced to the use of unpasteurized milk in cottage industry cheese production.

In the face of a single infectious disease report or an outbreak situation, when working with communities whose members speak little English, it is vital (1) to have a means of communication, (2) to be able to provide a culturally appropriate message, and (3) to have an established level of trust. Ideally, these requirements are addressed before an outbreak occurs, allowing a prompt and efficient response when immediate action is needed.

A. *What would be a useful first step in building trust with a largely non-English-speaking immigrant community?*
   1. *Hold a health fair in the community.*
   2. *Provide incentives to use health department services.*
   3. *Identify trusted community leaders such as religious leaders and ask their help in developing a plan.*
   4. *Distribute a brochure in the target community language.*
B. *What might best encourage undocumented residents to respond to a request to be immunized during an outbreak situation?*
   1. *Use an already established public health program to provide interpreter services, making it clear that proof of immigration status is not required for services.*
   2. *Place a request in the newspaper in the language of the targeted individuals.*
   3. *Involve trusted community leaders in making the request.*
   4. *Emphasize to the individuals the severity of the consequences if immunization does not occur.*
C. *What means of communication would work best when targeting largely non-English-speaking communities of recent immigrants?*
   1. *Publish newspaper articles in the target language.*
   2. *Request radio announcements in the target language.*
   3. *Post fliers in the target language in the community.*
   4. *Enlist trusted community leaders to make announcements.*

D. *How would public health officials best go about developing information to effectively reach a largely non-English-speaking community of recent immigrants?*
   1. *Use the services of the local university communications department.*
   2. *Ask community leaders to work with translators and prevention specialists to develop messages using their own words.*
   3. *Hire a professional to translate an existing well-developed English-language brochure.*
   4. *Use brochures provided by the state health department.*

Answers are in the back of the book.

REMEMBER THIS!

- The burden of infectious diseases is high in both human and economic terms. Preventing these diseases must be given high priority in our present health care system.
- The successful interaction of the infectious agent, host, and environment is necessary for disease transmission. Knowledge of the characteristics of each of these three factors is important in understanding the transmission, prevention, and control of these diseases.
- Effective intervention measures at the individual and community levels must be aimed at breaking the chain linking the agent, host, and environment. An integrated approach focused on all three factors simultaneously is an ideal goal to strive for but may not be feasible for all diseases.
- Health care professionals must constantly be aware of vulnerability to threats posed by emerging infectious diseases. Most of the factors causing the emergence of these diseases are influenced by human activities and behavior.
- Communicable diseases are preventable. Preventing infection through primary prevention activities is the most cost-effective public health strategy.
- Health care professionals must always apply infection control principles and procedures in the work environment. They should strictly practice the universal blood and body fluid precautions strategy to prevent transmission of HIV and other blood-borne pathogens.
- Effective control of communicable diseases requires the use of a multisystem approach focusing on improving host resistance, improving safety of the environment, improving public health systems, and facilitating social and political changes to ensure health for all people.
- Communicable disease prevention and control programs must move beyond providing drug treatment and vaccines. Health promotion and education aimed at changing individual and community behavior must be emphasized.
- Nurses play a key role in all aspects of prevention and control of communicable diseases. Close cooperation with other members of the interdisciplinary health care team must be maintained. Mobilizing community participation is essential to successful implementation of programs.

- The successful global eradication of smallpox proved the feasibility of the eradication of communicable diseases. As professionals and concerned citizens of the global village, health care workers must support the current global eradication campaigns against poliomyelitis and dracunculiasis.

WHAT WOULD YOU DO?

1. Ride with a nurse who makes home visits. Discuss living situations and other risk factors that may contribute to the development of infectious diseases, as well as possible points at which the nurse may intervene to help prevent these diseases, such as checking the immunization status of all individuals in the household. What are realistic interventions, and how much responsibility should a nurse take in attempting to affect the living situation?
2. To become familiar with the reportable diseases that are a problem in your community, look at how many cases have been reported during the past month, 6 months, and year. Contrast these numbers with national and state statistics. How is your county or city different from or similar to these larger jurisdictions? If different, what environmental, political, or demographic features may contribute to this difference?
3. Spend time with the persons who are responsible for reporting and investigating communicable disease in your community. Discuss types of surveillance conducted and outbreak procedures that may accompany the reporting of some of these diseases. If possible, go on an outbreak investigation. Would the existing surveillance systems and outbreak control policies be sufficient in the case of a bioterrorism event?
4. Review the demographic profile of your community including trends from the past 10 years and projections for the next decade. Pay special attention to growth patterns of particular populations such as racial and ethnic groups or specific age groups (e.g., children younger than 18 years, adults ages 65 years and older). How do changes in these populations affect the delivery of interventions for infectious disease control such as immunization?
5. Visit a clinic that serves a refugee, immigrant, or migrant labor population to observe the infectious diseases commonly seen in these groups. Compare and contrast this visit with a visit to a clinic that serves an inner-city population and a visit to a clinic that serves a rural population. How are the infectious disease control issues different and/or similar for these varied populations?
6. Sit in a clinic waiting room for immunization services and talk with parents about their concerns and the barriers they may perceive in obtaining immunizations for their children. How can this information be used to better facilitate immunization services?
7. Spend time with a school nurse to see what infectious diseases are routinely encountered in the educational setting. Discuss risk factors for disease in school-aged youths and the strategies employed to prevent infectious diseases in this age group. Do school policies support the strategies needed for the prevention of infectious diseases in students?
8. Visit a day care center. Observe potential situations for the communication of infectious diseases, and discuss with the director the steps taken to prevent and control infection, including immunization requirements and procedures for hand hygiene and food preparation. Does the center have specific infection control policies and procedures, and do the staff members appear to be following them?

■ REFERENCES

Blanton JD et al: Rabies surveillance in the United States during 2007, *J Am Vet Med Assoc* 233(6):884-897, 2008.
Brown H, Neva FA: *Basic clinical parasitology*, ed 6, Norwalk, Conn, 1994, Appleton & Lange.
Centers for Disease Control and Prevention: *Addressing emerging infectious disease threats: a prevention strategy for the U.S.*, Atlanta, 1994, CDC.
Centers for Disease Control and Prevention: Notifiable disease surveillance and notifiable disease statistics—United States, June 1946 and June 1996, *MMWR Morb Mortal Wkly Rep* 45(530), 1996.
Centers for Disease Control and Prevention: Immunization of health-care workers: recommendations of the advisory committee on immunization practices (ACIP) and the hospital infection control practices advisory committee (HICPAC), *MMWR Morb Mortal Wkly Rep* 46(RR-18):1–42, 1997.
Centers for Disease Control and Prevention: *Hospital infections cost U.S. billions of dollars annually*, Atlanta, 2000, CDC, Media Relations. Retrieved April 25, 2007, from http://www.cdc.gov/od/media/ressrel/r2k0306b.htm.
Centers for Disease Control and Prevention: Notice to readers: recommended childhood immunization schedule, *MMWR Morb Mort Wkly Rep* 49(RR05):1–2, 2002.
Centers for Disease Control and Prevention: *Cyclospora infection, cyclosporiasis*, 2004a, available at http://www.cdc.gov/ncidod/dpd/parasites/cyclospora/2004-cyclospora-fs.pdf.
Centers for Disease Control and Prevention: Lyme disease—United States, 2001-2002, *MMWR Morb Mortal Wkly Rep* 53:365–369, 2004b.
Centers for Disease Control and Prevention: *Nationally notifiable infectious diseases*, CDC, Division of Public Health Surveillance and Informatics, 2004c, available at cdc.gov/epo/dphsi/phs/infdis2004.htm.
Centers for Disease Control and Prevention: Recovery of a patient from clinical rabies-Wisconsin, 2004, *MMWR Morb Mort Wkly Rep* 53(50):1171–1173, 2004d.
Centers for Disease Control and Prevention: Summary of notifiable diseases—United States 2003, *MMWR Morb Mortal Wkly Rep* 52:1–85, 2005a.
Centers for Disease Control and Prevention: Recommended childhood and adolescent immunization schedule, United States, 2005, *MMWR Morb Mortal Wkly Rep* 53:Q1–Q3, 2005b.
Centers for Disease Control and Prevention: *Questions and answers about anthrax*, March 2005c, available at www.bt.cdc.gov/agent/anthrax/faq/index.asp.
Centers for Disease Control and Prevention: Recommended antimicrobial agents for the treatment and postexposure prophylaxis of pertussis, 2005, CDC guidelines, *MMWR Morb Mortal Wkly Rep* 54(RR14):1–2, 2005d.
Centers for Disease Control and Prevention: Inhalation anthrax associated with dried animal hides–Pennsylvania and NYC, 2006, *MMWR Morb Mortal Wkly Rep* 55(10): 280–283, 2006a.

Centers for Disease Control and Prevention: *Reported tuberculosis in the U.S. executive summary,* 2006b. Retrieved June 22, 2008, from cdc.gov/tb/surv/surv2006/pdf.

Centers for Disease Control and Prevention: *Pneumococcal disease in children—Q & A,* 2007a. Retrieved April 2007 from cdc.gov/vaccines/vpd-vac/pneumo/dis-faqs.htm.

Centers for Disease Control and Prevention: *Malaria facts,* 2007b, available at cdc.gov/malaria/facts/htm.

Centers for Disease Control and Prevention: *Update: Measles--United States, January-July 2008, MMWR Morb Mortal Wkly Rep* 57(33):893–896, 2008a.

Centers for Disease Control and Prevention: Human rabies prevention—United States, 2008, *MMWR Morb Mortal Wkly Rep* 57(RR03): 1–26, 28, 2008b.

Centers for Disease Control and Prevention: *About parasites,* 2008c, available at cdc.gov/ncidod/dpd/aboutparasites.htm.

Centers for Disease Control and Prevention: *Smallpox: what everyone should know,* 2008d. Retrieved Sept 17, 2008, from http://www.cdc.gov.smallpox.

Centers for Disease Control and Prevention: *Nationally notifiable infectious diseases,—United States, 2008,* National Notifiable Diseases Surveillance System, Division of Public Health Surveillance and Informatics, 2008e. Retrieved Jan 20, 2009, from http://www.cdc.gov/ncphi/disss/nndss/phs/infdis2008.htm.

Centers for Disease Control and Prevention, CDC Health Advisory: *CDC issues interim recommendations for the use of influenza antiviral medications in the setting of oseltamivir resistance among circulating Influenza A (H1N1) viruses, 2008-2009 Influenza season,* 2008f. Retrieved Jan 20, 2009, from http://www2a.cdc.gov/HAN/ArchiveSys/ViewMsgV.asp?AlertNum=00279.

Centers for Disease Control and Prevention: *Nationally notifiable diseases surveillance system,* Division of Public Health Surveillance and Informatics, 2009a. Retrieved Jan 20, 2009, from http://www.cdc.gov.ncphi/disss/nsdss/nndsshis.htm.

Centers for Disease Control and Prevention: *Recommended immunization schedule for persons 0 through 6 years—United States,* 2009b. Retrieved Jan 20, 2009, from http://www.cdc.gov/vaccines/recs/schedules/downloands/child/2009/09 0-6 yrs_ chart_ only.jpg.

Centers for Disease Control and Prevention: *Vaccines and preventable diseases, pertussis (whooing cough)—what you need to know,* 2009c. Retrieved Jan 20, 2009, from http://www.cdc.gov/vaccines/vpd-vac/pertussis/default.htm.

Centers for Disease Control and Prevention: *Novel H1N1 flu situation update,* June 12, 2009d available at http://www.cdc.gov/h1n1flu/update.htm.

Directors of Health Promotion and Education: *Addressing infectious disease threats,* 2005, available at http://www.dhpe.org/infectintro.asp.

Fauci AS et al: *Harrison's principles of international medicine,* ed 17, Columbus, Ohio, 2008, McGraw-Hill.

Goldrick BA: 21st-Century emerging and reemerging infections, *Am J Nurs* 104(1):67–70, 2004a.

Goldrick BA: Vaccine-preventable infections in children, *Am J Nurs* 104(2):34–38, 2004b.

Henderson DA: Smallpox: clinical and epidemiologic features, *Emerg Infect Dis* 5(4):537–539, 1999.

Heymann DL editor: *Control of communicable diseases manual,* ed 18, Washington, DC, 2004, American Public Health Association.

Institute of Medicine: *Emerging infectious diseases from the global to the local perspective—workshop report,* Washington, DC, 2001, National Academy Press.

Katlama C: HIV and AIDS-parasitic diseases. In Cohen J, Powderly WG, editors: *Infectious diseases,* ed 2, 2004. Retrieved April 2007 from www.mdconsult.com.

Katz JR, Hirsh AM: When global health is local health, *Am J Nurs* 103(12):75–79, 2003.

Kramer LD, Styer LM, Ebel GD: A global perspective of the epidemiology of West Nile virus, *Annu Rev Entomol* 153:61–81, 2008.

Ledeberg J, Shope RE, Oaks SC: *Emerging infections: microbial threats to health in the U.S.,* Washington, DC, 1992, National Academy Press.

Lemon SM et al: *Global infectious disease surveillance and detection: assessing the challenges, finding solutions,* Washington, DC, 2007, National Academies Press.

Peterson LR, Roehrig JT: West Nile virus: a re-emerging global pathogen, *Emerg Infect Dis* 7(4):612-614, 2001.

Roberts T: WTP estimates of the societal costs of US food-borne illness, *Am J Agricultural Economics* 89(5):1183-1188, 2007.

Tiwari A et al: Severe acute respiratory syndrome (SARS) in Hong Kong: patients' experiences, *Nurs Outlook* 51(5):212–219, 2003.

U.S. Department of Health and Human Services: *Healthy People 2010: national health promotion and disease prevention objectives,* Washington, DC, 2000, U.S. Government Printing Office.

U.S. Food and Drug Administration: *FDA approves second-generation smallpox vaccine,* September 1, 2007. Retrieved Jan 20, 2009, from http://www.fda.gov/bbs/topics/NEWS/2007/NEW01693.html.

Wenzel RP: Control of communicable diseases: overview. In Wallace RB, editor: *Public health and preventive medicine,* ed 14, Stamford, Conn, 1998, Appleton & Lange.

World Health Organization: *Poliomyelitis,* 2008. Retrieved June 24, 2008, from www.who.int/mediacentre/factsheets/smallpox/en/index/html.

HIV, Hepatitis, Tuberculosis, and Sexually Transmitted Diseases

Patty J. Hale

ADDITIONAL RESOURCES

These related resources are found either in the appendix at the back of this book or on the book's website at http://evolve.elsevier.com/stanhope/foundations.

Appendix

- Appendix C.1: Summary Description of Hepatitis A–E and G
- Appendix C.2: Recommendations for Prophylaxis of Hepatitis A
- Appendix C.3: Recommended Postexposure Prophylaxis for Percutaneous or Permucosal Exposure to Hepatitis B Virus
- Appendix D.5: Summary of Recommendations for Adult Immunizations

Evolve Website

- Community Assessment Applied
- Case Study, with questions and answers
- Quiz review questions
- WebLinks, including link to *Healthy People 2010* website

Real World Community Health Nursing: An Interactive CD-ROM, second edition

If you are using this CD-ROM in your course, you will find the following activities related to this chapter:
- *IIIV/AIDS Epidemiology: Evaluate the Trends* in **Epidemiology**
- *What's My Line?* in **Community/Public Health Nursing History**

OBJECTIVES

After reading this chapter, the student should be able to:
1. Describe the natural history of human immunodeficiency virus (HIV) infection and plan appropriate client education at each stage.
2. Discuss the clinical signs of HIV, hepatitis, and sexually transmitted diseases (STDs).
3. Describe the scope of the problem with HIV, STDs, hepatitis, and tuberculosis (TB) and identify groups that are at greatest risk.
4. Analyze behaviors that place people at risk of contracting selected communicable diseases.
5. Describe nursing actions to prevent these diseases and care for people who experience these diseases.

CHAPTER OUTLINE

HUMAN IMMUNODEFICIENCY VIRUS INFECTION
Natural History of HIV
Transmission
Epidemiology and Surveillance of HIV/AIDS
HIV Testing
Caring for Clients with AIDS in the Community

SEXUALLY TRANSMITTED DISEASES
Gonorrhea
Syphilis
Chlamydia
Herpes Simplex Virus 2 (Genital Herpes)
Human Papillomavirus Infection

HEPATITIS
Hepatitis A Virus
Hepatitis B Virus
Hepatitis C Virus
TUBERCULOSIS

NURSE'S ROLE IN PROVIDING PREVENTIVE CARE
FOR COMMUNICABLE DISEASES
Primary Prevention
Secondary Prevention
Tertiary Prevention

KEY TERMS

acquired immunodeficiency syndrome (AIDS): AIDS can affect the immune and central nervous systems and cause infections or cancers. It is caused by the human immunodeficiency virus (HIV).

chlamydia: a sexually transmitted disease caused by the organism *Chlamydia trachomatis,* which causes infection of the urethra and cervix. Infections may be asymptomatic and if untreated result in severe morbidity.

directly observed therapy (DOT): a system of providing medications for persons with tuberculosis infection in which the client is monitored to ensure that the medication is taken and to maximize adherence to the treatment.

genital herpes: a virus that attacks the genitals and sacral nerve. Infection is characterized by painful lesions that present as vesicles and progress to ulcerations on the male and female genitals, buttocks, or upper thighs.

genital warts: cauliflower-type growths that are caused by human papillomavirus.

gonorrhea: a sexually transmitted disease caused by a bacterium, *Neisseria gonorrhoeae,* that results in inflammation of the urethra and cervix and dysuria, or may result in no symptoms.

hepatitis A virus (HAV): a virus that is transmitted by the fecal–oral route. The clinical course of hepatitis A ranges from mild to severe and often requires prolonged convalescence. The onset is usually characterized by acute fever, nausea, lack of appetite, malaise, and abdominal discomfort, followed after several days by jaundice.

hepatitis B virus (HBV): a virus that is transmitted through exposure to body fluids. Infection results in a clinical picture that ranges from a self-limited acute infection to fulminant hepatitis or hepatic carcinoma, possibly leading to death.

hepatitis C virus (HCV): a virus that is transmitted through exposure to blood and body fluids. Hepatitis C virus infection may present with such mild symptoms that it goes unrecognized. It is the most common chronic blood-borne infection in the United States.

HIV antibody test: a laboratory procedure that detects antibodies to HIV. Enzyme-linked immunosorbent assay (ELISA) is the test commonly used in screening blood for the antibody to HIV; the Western blot is used as a confirmatory test.

human immunodeficiency virus (HIV): the virus that causes acquired immunodeficiency syndrome (AIDS) and HIV infection.

human papillomavirus (HPV): a sexually transmitted disease that results in genital warts (condyloma acuminata) that grow in the vulva, vagina, cervix, urinary meatus, scrotum, or perianal area. A link exists between HPV infections and cancer.

incidence: in epidemiology, the number of new cases of infection or disease that occur in a defined population in a specified period of time.

incubation period: the time interval beginning with invasion by an infectious agent and continuing until the organism multiplies to sufficient numbers to produce a host reaction and clinical symptoms.

injection drug use: includes intravenous and subcutaneous drug injection; the latter is usually over the abdominal area.

nongonococcal urethritis (NGU): inflammation of the urethra from microorganisms other than *Neisseria gonorrhoeae; Chlamydia trachomatis* has been implicated as the cause of 50% of cases.

partner notification: identifying and locating contacts of persons who have been diagnosed with a transmissible disease to notify them of their exposure and to encourage them to seek medical treatment.

pelvic inflammatory disease (PID): infection of the female reproductive organs, specifically the fallopian tubes and endometrium, resulting in infertility and/or ectopic pregnancy. Acute symptoms and signs include lower abdominal pain, increased vaginal discharge, urinary frequency, vomiting, and fever. PID results from untreated gonorrhea and chlamydia.

sexually transmitted diseases (STDs): communicable diseases such as gonorrhea, chlamydia, and HIV infection that can be transmitted by sexual activity.

syphilis: an infectious STD caused by a bacterium, *Treponema pallidum;* it is characterized by the appearance of lesions or chancres that may involve any tissue. Relapses are frequent, and after the initial chancre and secondary symptoms, syphilis may exist without symptoms for years.

tuberculosis (TB): an infectious disease caused by a bacterium, *Mycobacterium tuberculosis.* It is transmitted by airborne droplets, resulting in pulmonary symptoms and wasting. Infection can be latent and asymptomatic, later progressing to active infection.

Healthy People 2010

Objectives Related to HIV, Hepatitis, and Sexually Transmitted Diseases

13-1   Reduce AIDS among adolescents and adults

13-2   Reduce the number of new AIDS cases among adolescent and adult men who have sex with men

13-3   Reduce the number of new AIDS cases among females and males who inject drugs

13-4   Reduce the number of new AIDS cases among adolescent and adult men who have sex with men and inject drugs

13-5   Reduce the number of cases of HIV infection among adolescents and adults

13-6   Increase the proportion of sexually active persons who use condoms

13-11   Increase the proportion of adults with tuberculosis (TB) who have been tested for HIV

13-12   Increase the proportion of adults in publicly funded HIV counseling and testing sites who are screened for common bacterial sexually transmitted diseases (STDs) (chlamydia, gonorrhea, and syphilis) and are immunized against hepatitis B virus

13-13   Increase the proportion of HIV-infected adolescents and adults who receive testing, treatment, and prophylaxis, consistent with current Public Health Service treatment guidelines

13-14   Reduce deaths from HIV infection

13-15   Extend the interval of time between an initial diagnosis of HIV infection and AIDS diagnosis in order to increase years of life of an individual infected with HIV

13-16   Increase the years of life of an HIV-infected person by extending the interval of time between an AIDS diagnosis and death

13-17   Reduce new cases of perinatally acquired HIV infection

14-2   Reduce chronic hepatitis B virus infections in infants and young children (perinatal infections)

14-3   Reduce hepatitis B

14-6   Reduce hepatitis A

14-9   Reduce hepatitis C

14-10   Increase the proportion of persons with chronic hepatitis C infection identified by state and local health departments

14-11   Reduce tuberculosis

14-12   Increase the proportion of all tuberculosis patients who complete curative therapy within 12 months

14-28   Increase hepatitis B vaccine coverage among high-risk groups

25-1   Reduce the proportion of adolescents and young adults with *Chlamydia trachomatis* infections

25-2   Reduce gonorrhea

25-3   Eliminate sustained domestic transmission of primary and secondary syphilis

25-4   Reduce the proportion of adults with genital herpes infection

25-5   Reduce the proportion of persons with human papillomavirus (HPV) infection

25-6   Reduce the proportion of females who have ever required treatment for pelvic inflammatory disease (PID)

25-7   Reduce the proportion of childless females with fertility problems who have had an STD or who have required treatment for PID

25-8.1 Reduce HIV infections in adolescent and young adult females aged 13 to 24 years that are associated with heterosexual contact

25-19   Increase the proportion of all sexually transmitted disease clinic patients who are being treated for bacterial STDs (chlamydia, gonorrhea, and syphilis) and who are offered provider referral services for their sex partners

25-10   Reduce neonatal consequences from maternal STDs, including chlamydial pneumonia, gonococcal and chlamydial ophthalmia neonatorum, laryngeal papillomatosis (from human papillomavirus infection), neonatal herpes, and preterm birth and low birth weight associated with bacterial vaginosis

27-1   Increase the proportion of adolescents who abstain from sexual intercourse or use condoms if currently sexually active

27-2   Increase the proportion of sexually active females aged 25 years and under who are screened annually for genital chlamydia infections

27-3   Increase the proportion of pregnant females screened for STDs (including HIV infection and bacterial vaginosis) during prenatal health care visits, according to recognized standards

From U.S. Department of Health and Human Services: *Healthy People 2010: understanding and improving health,* ed 2, Washington, DC, 2000, U.S. Government Printing Office.

A considerable amount of information is available about the risk of communicable diseases. Concern about infectious diseases prompted the development of standards for **sexually transmitted diseases (STDs), human immunodeficiency virus (HIV)** and **acquired immunodeficiency syndrome (AIDS)**, hepatitis, and tuberculosis (TB) in the *Healthy People 2010* report. The *Healthy People 2010* box lists some objectives used to evaluate progress toward decreasing communicable diseases by the year 2010. Since these diseases are often acquired through behaviors that can be avoided or changed, nursing actions focus considerably on disease prevention. Prevention can take the form of vaccine administration (as for hepatitis A and hepatitis B), early

detection (for TB), or teaching clients about abstinence or safer sex. Individuals who live with these chronic infections can transmit them to others. This chapter describes selected communicable diseases and their nursing management including primary, secondary, and tertiary prevention.

HUMAN IMMUNODEFICIENCY VIRUS INFECTION

In 2006, over 1 million persons in the United States were living with HIV/AIDS, and there were 56,300 new HIV infections that year. This is a relatively newly diagnosed disease that has grown enormously. On June 5, 1981, the *Morbidity and Mortality Weekly Report (MMWR)* published by the Centers for Disease Control and Prevention reported on five cases of *Pneumocystis carinii* pneumonia in healthy young men in Los Angeles, California. These cases became the first recognized reports of AIDS in the United States. Since then HIV/AIDS has become one of the world's greatest public health challenges (Centers for Disease Control and Prevention, 2006b; Centers for Disease Control and Prevention, 2008j).

Although there have been several successes in the prevention of and treatment for this disease, challenges remain. First, between 252,000 and 312,000 people are unaware that they are HIV infected. This places them at high risk because they do not take advantage of available treatments. It also poses risks for those with whom they have sexual contact. Also, some populations remain at higher risk, including men who have sex with men, especially those who are young or are from racial and ethnic minority groups. Gay and bisexual men accounted for a significantly higher proportion of estimated new infection in 2006 than any other risk group (Centers for Disease Control and Prevention, 2008j). In 2006, women accounted for 25% of all new HIV/AIDS diagnoses, and black women were at especially high risk. The economic costs of HIV/AIDS result from premature disability and treatment. Because 88% of afflicted persons are between the ages of 20 and 49 years, many families become disrupted and lose creative and economic productivity. The health care costs for this group are supported primarily by Medicaid and Medicare. Many people with HIV qualify for Medicaid or Medicare because they are indigent or fall into poverty when paying for health care over the course of the illness.

BRIEFLY NOTED

In 2006 there were more than 1 million persons known to be living with HIV/AIDS in the United States (Centers for Disease Control and Prevention, 2006b).

The Ryan White Comprehensive AIDS Resource Emergency (CARE) Act was passed in 1990 to provide services for persons with HIV infection (U.S. Department of Health and Human Services, 2008). This program provides funds for health care in the geographic areas with the largest number of AIDS cases. Covered health services include emergency services, services for early intervention and care (sometimes including coverage of health insurance), and drug reimbursement programs for HIV-infected individuals. The AIDS Drug Assistance Programs (ADAPs) are awards that pay for medications on the basis of the estimated number of persons living with AIDS in the individual state (Health Resources and Services Administration, 2008).

NATURAL HISTORY OF HIV

The natural history of HIV includes three stages (Gandhi, 2006):
1. The primary infection (within about 1 month of contracting the virus)

2. Clinical latency, a period with no obvious symptoms
3. A final stage of symptomatic disease

When HIV enters the body, it can cause a flu-like syndrome referred to as a *primary infection* or *acute retroviral syndrome.* This may go unrecognized. Initially the body's CD4 white blood cell count drops for a brief time when the virus is most plentiful in the body. The immune system increases antibody production in response to this initial infection, which is a self-limiting illness. The symptoms are lymphadenopathy, myalgias, sore throat, lethargy, rash, and fever (Gandhi, 2006). An antibody test at this stage is usually negative, so it is often not recognized as HIV.

After about 6 weeks to 3 months, HIV antibodies appear in the blood. Although most antibodies serve a protective role, HIV antibodies do not. Their presence does help in the detection of HIV infection because tests show their presence in the bloodstream.

During this prolonged **incubation period**, clients experience a gradual deterioration of the immune system and can transmit the virus to others. The use of highly active antiretroviral therapy (ART) has greatly increased the survival time of persons with HIV/AIDS.

AIDS is the last stage on the long continuum of HIV infection and may result from damage caused by HIV, secondary cancers, or opportunistic organisms. AIDS is defined as a disabling or life-threatening illness caused by HIV; it is diagnosed in a person with a $CD4^+$ T-lymphocyte count of less than 200/ml with or without documented HIV infection (Gandhi, 2006).

Many of the AIDS-related opportunistic infections are caused by microorganisms that are commonly present in healthy individuals but do not cause disease in persons with an intact immune system. These microorganisms increase in persons with HIV/AIDS due to a weakened immune system. Opportunistic infections may be caused by bacteria fungi, viruses, or protozoa. The most common opportunistic diseases are *Pneumocystis carinii* pneumonia and oral candidiasis. TB, an infection that is becoming more prevalent because of HIV infection, can spread rapidly among immunosuppressed individuals. Thus HIV-infected persons who live near one another, such as in long-term care facilities, correctional facilities, drug treatment facilities, or other settings, must be carefully screened and deemed noninfectious before admission to such settings.

TRANSMISSION

HIV is transmitted through exposure to blood, semen, vaginal secretions, and breast milk (Heymann, 2004). It is not transmitted through casual contact such as touching or hugging someone who has HIV infection. It is not transmitted by insects, coughing, sneezing, office equipment, or sitting next to or eating with someone who has HIV infection. The modes of transmission are listed in Box 27-1. The exposure categories of AIDS are shown in Figure 27-1. Rare transmission methods include accidental needle stick injury, organ transplants, and artificial insemination with donated semen (Gandhi, 2006).

| Box 27-1 | **Modes of Transmission of Human Immunodeficiency Virus (HIV)** |

HIV can be transmitted in the following ways:

- Sexual contact, involving the exchange of body fluids, with an infected person
- Sharing or reusing needles, syringes, or other equipment used to prepare injectable drugs
- Perinatal transmission from an infected mother to her fetus during pregnancy or delivery or to an infant when breastfeeding
- Transfusions or other exposure to HIV-contaminated blood or blood products, organs, or semen

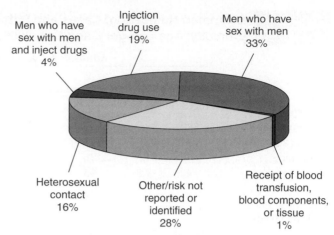

FIGURE 27-I Adult AIDS cases by exposure category from June 2000 through June 2001, United States. NOTE: The category "*other/risk not reported*" includes three children who were exposed to HIV-infected blood; one child was infected after intentional inoculation with HIV-infected blood, and two children were exposed to HIV-infected blood in a household setting. The category "*receipt of blood transfusion, components, or tissue*" includes 41 adults and adolescents and 2 children who developed AIDS after receiving blood screened negative for HIV antibody. Thirteen additional adults developed AIDS after receiving tissue organs or artificial insemination from HIV-infected donors. Four of the 13 received tissue, organs, or artificial insemination from a donor who was negative for HIV antibody at the time of donation. (Data from Centers for Disease Control and Prevention: *HIV/AIDS surveillance report* 13[1]:12, 2001.)

Potential blood and tissue donors are interviewed to screen for a history of high-risk activities, and they are screened with the HIV antibody test. Blood or tissue is not used from individuals who have a history of high-risk behavior or who are HIV infected. In addition to being screened, coagulation factors used to treat hemophilia and other blood disorders are made safe through heat treatments to inactivate the virus. Screening has significantly reduced the risk of transmission of HIV by blood products and organ donations. The presence of an STD infection such as chlamydia or gonorrhea increases the risk of HIV infection, and HIV may also increase the risk for other STDs. This may result from any of the following: open lesions providing a portal of entry for pathogens; STDs decreasing the host's immune status, resulting in a rapid progression of HIV infection; and HIV changing the natural history of STDs or the effectiveness of medications used in treating STDs (Heymann, 2004).

Nurses can educate people about the modes of transmission and can be role models for how to behave toward and provide supportive care for those with HIV infection. An understanding of how transmission does and does not occur will help family and community members feel more comfortable in relating to and caring for persons with HIV.

EPIDEMIOLOGY AND SURVEILLANCE OF HIV/AIDS

Nurses must identify the trends of HIV infection in the populations they serve so that they can screen clients who may be at risk and can adequately plan prevention programs and illness care resources. For example, knowing that AIDS disproportionately affects minorities assists the nurse to set priorities and plan services for these groups. Factors such as geographic location, age, and ethnic distribution are tracked to more effectively target programs. Since the first cases of AIDS were identified in 1981, approximately 1,147,697 HIV or AIDS cases have been diagnosed and reported to the CDC (Centers for Disease Control and Prevention, 2006b). The majority occur in men and disproportionally in those in racial and ethnic groups. From 1981 to 2004, 522,723 deaths of persons with AIDS were reported to the CDC. Survival after diagnosis has increased significantly since 1996. The 2-year survival rate was 44% for those diagnosed between 1981 and 1992 and 85% for those diagnosed from

1996 to 2000 (Centers for Disease Control and Prevention, 2006b) (see "Evidence-Based Practice" box on p. 515).

Initially, the groups with the highest **incidence** of HIV infection were homosexual and bisexual men, injection drug users and their sexual partners, and hemophiliacs. Although men who have sex with men (MSM) still make up the largest group with AIDS in the United States, the number of persons contracting HIV through heterosexual transmission is increasing at a faster rate. Heterosexual transmission has surpassed **injection drug use** as the primary mode of HIV transmission in women. A high proportion of infected females are associated with sexual contact with older males (Centers for Disease Control and Prevention, 2004). African-American women are at particular risk. In 2006 more infections occurred among young people under the age of 30 years than any other age group. Also, although persons over age 50 continue to represent a relatively small proportion of new infection, those who have unprotected sex, consume alcohol, or inject drugs are at higher risk for contracting HIV/AIDS than younger people with the same lifestyle characteristics. Aging brings a decline in the immune response and decreased organ reserves, which slows the person's ability to deal with risk factors for HIV/AIDS (Stark, 2007; Centers for Disease Control and Prevention, 2008j). Also, the geographic distribution of HIV infections is more concentrated in urban areas.

The distribution of pediatric AIDS reflects the infection rate in women. The number of perinatally acquired AIDS

Table 27-1   **Estimated Numbers of Cases and Rates (per 100,000 Population) of AIDS, by Race/Ethnicity, Age Category, and Sex, 2006: 50 States and the District of Columbia**

| | Adults or Adolescents | | | | | | Children (less than 13 years) | | Total* | |
| | Males | | Females | | Total* | | | | | |
Race/ethnicity	No.	Rate	No.	Rate	No.	Rate	No.	Rate	No.	Rate
White, not Hispanic	9,267	11.2	1,659	1.9	10,926	6.4	4	0.0	10,929	5.4
Black, not Hispanic	11,540	82.9	6,391	40.4	17,930	60.3	30	0.4	17,960	47.6
Hispanic	5,388	31.3	1,516	9.5	6,903	20.8	3	0.0	6,907	15.6
Asian/Pacific Islander	423	7.5	95	1.6	518	4.4	1	0.0	519	3.7
American Indian/ Alaska Native	118	12.2	37	3.6	155	7.8	0	0.0	155	6.2
Total†	**26,989**	**22.4**	**9,801**	**7.8**	**36,790**	**14.9**	**38**	**0.1**	**36,828‡**	**12.3**

From Centers for Disease Control and Prevention: *HIV/AIDS surveillance report,* 2006, Vol. 18, Atlanta, 2008, U.S. Department of Health and Human Services, Centers for Disease Control and Prevention.
NOTE: These numbers do not represent reported case counts. Rather, they are point estimates, which result from adjustments of reported case counts. The reported case counts have been adjusted for reporting delays, but not for incomplete reporting.
Data exclude cases for which the state or area of residence of the person is unknown, as well as cases from U.S.-dependent areas, for which census information about race and age categories is lacking.
*Because row totals were calculated independently of the values for the subpopulations, the values in each row may not sum to the row total.
† Includes person of unknown race or multiple races. Because column totals were calculated independently of the values for the subpopulations, the values in each column may not sum to the column total.
‡ Includes 358 persons of unknown race or multiple races.

cases has decreased dramatically because of prenatal care that includes HIV testing, zidovudine drug therapy for the mother, and cesarean delivery. If left untreated, the clinical picture of pediatric HIV infection involves a shorter incubation period than in adults and symptoms may occur within the first year of life. The physical signs and symptoms in children are also different from those in adults. These include failure to thrive, diarrhea, developmental delays, and bacterial infections such as otitis media and pneumonia. Detection of HIV infection in infants of infected mothers is through tests different from those used in children older than 18 months. The enzyme-linked immunosorbent assay (EIA) test is not valid because it tests for antibodies, which in the infant reflect passively acquired maternal antibodies. Thus a diagnosis of HIV infection in early infancy requires the use of other tests, such as HIV culture or polymerase chain reaction (PCR) results (Centers for Disease Control and Prevention, 2001b). Despite having an infected mother, many children do not acquire AIDS. However, one or both parents may die as a result of HIV infection. The families of many children with AIDS are impoverished, with limited financial, emotional, social, and health care resources. The added strain of this illness makes many individuals and families unable to provide for the emotional, physical, and developmental needs of affected children.

Between 1996 and 2000, adult cases of AIDS decreased in all ethnic categories. As depicted in Table 27-1, AIDS has disproportionately affected minority groups. In a study that included 29 states, non-Hispanic black and Hispanic populations constituted 21% of the population yet these

groups accounted for 84% of heterosexually acquired HIV from 1999 to 2002. The disproportionate incidence in these groups is attributed to "lack of knowledge about HIV, decreased perception of risk, use of drugs or alcohol, and different interpretations of so-called 'safe sex'" (Centers for Disease Control and Prevention, 2004, p. 128).

Although AIDS is a reportable condition, reporting varies among states. Studies of diagnosed cases of AIDS do not reveal current HIV infection patterns because of the long interval between infection with HIV and the onset of clinical disease. Since antiretroviral drugs are more likely to be effective if given early in the HIV infection before symptoms occur, the CDC encourages mandatory reporting. Since 2000, 35 areas including Guam and the U.S. Virgin Islands had laws or regulations that required confidential name-based HIV infection reporting (Centers for Disease Control and Prevention, 2006b). Opponents to the reporting express concerns about the government's ability to maintain confidential registries and about potential invasions into personal lives, particularly as related to discrimination in housing, employment, and insurance.

HIV TESTING

The **HIV antibody test** is the most commonly used screening test for determining infection. It may be conducted with oral fluids or blood samples. The rapid test, also called the same-day test, can provide test results within the hour. These tests indicate if the antibody to HIV is present. They do not reveal if a person has AIDS, nor do they isolate the virus. The most commonly used form of this test is the EIA, which effectively screens blood and other donor products. Cases

Evidence-Based Practice

The need to develop effective interventions preventing the infection of sexually transmitted HIV among Latino adolescents is growing as this population continues to be affected by the disease. In 2001, the incidence of AIDS for adult and adolescent Latinos was 5.3 times higher than for their non-Hispanic white peers. One cause for this increase is low condom use by Latino adolescents in heterosexual contact, which is the major mode of transmission.

Despite the fact that adolescents and young adults made up 40.5% of the overall Latino population in 2000, sexually transmitted HIV prevention research and education for this population remain scarce. Villarruel, Jemmott, and Jemmott attempted to address this issue in their 2005 study by examining the influence of cultural and contextual variables and the role of the community in order to create an effective curriculum to address the issue of HIV. Their study built on successful intervention models and used focus groups to determine the best way to approach Latino adolescents about reducing their risk of sexually transmitted HIV. The curriculum that emerged, called *¡Cuídate!*, sought to influence attitudes and beliefs about HIV risk-reduction behaviors such as abstinence and condom use while discussing the detection and prevention of HIV and other sexually transmitted diseases.

The *¡Cuídate!* curriculum was evaluated and feedback was gathered from facilitators and participants after the program concluded. Comments were positive overall, particularly from the participants, who said that they learned a great deal from the program and that it was fun to participate in it. By using Latino music and video in the program, *¡Cuídate!* was able to reach adolescents on their level in order to deliver a life-saving message of great importance to their community.

NURSE USE: The *¡Cuídate!* curriculum was created in order to address concerns about the spread of HIV in the adolescent Latino population. Culturally based interventions such as this are increasingly important in a multicultural world because of the varying approaches to healthcare in diverse populations. Because sexually transmitted HIV research in the Latino population was lacking, the research team used a myriad of methods to address the issue and build their curriculum. By outlining the strategies used to create such an intervention, other culturally based programs can be created while a body of research is accumulated. This partnering of research and practice is critical as culturally focused health care becomes a part of daily life for researchers and practitioners alike.

From Villaruel AM, Jemmott LS, Jemmott JB: Designing a culturally based intervention to reduce HIV sexual risk for Latino adolescents, *J Assoc Nurses AIDS Care* 16(12):23–31, 2005.

of positive results with the EIA are confirmed to be false by testing with the Western blot. False-negative results may also occur after infection and before antibodies are produced. Sometimes referred to as the *window period,* this can last from 6 weeks to 3 months. Testing for HIV infection is offered at many locations including health department STD clinics and family planning clinics, primary care offices, and freestanding HIV-counseling and HIV-testing sites. Voluntary screening programs for HIV may be either confidential or anonymous; the process for each is unique. Confidential testing involves reporting the person's name and address;

this information is considered privileged. With anonymous testing, the client is given an identification code number that is attached to all records of the test results. Demographic data such as the person's sex, age, and race may be collected, but there is no record of the client's name and address. An advantage of anonymous testing may be that it increases the number of people who are willing to be tested, because many of those at risk are engaged in illegal activities. The anonymity eliminates their concern about the possibility of arrest or discrimination.

CARING FOR CLIENTS WITH AIDS IN THE COMMUNITY

Because AIDS is a chronic disease, affected individuals continue to live and work in the community. They have bouts of illness interspersed with periods of wellness in which they are able to return to school or work. When they are ill, much of their care is provided in the home. The nurse teaches families and significant others about personal care and hygiene, medication administration, Standard Precautions to ensure infection control, and healthy lifestyle behaviors such as adequate rest, balanced nutrition, and exercise. The Americans with Disabilities Act of 1990 and other laws protect persons with HIV/AIDS against discrimination in housing, at work, and in other public situations. In 1998, the Supreme Court ruled that antidiscrimination protection also covered HIV-infected persons who were asymptomatic (Centers for Disease Control and Prevention, 2001a). Policies regarding school and worksite attendance have been developed by most states and localities on the basis of these laws.

Nurses can rely on these policies to provide direction for the community's response when an individual develops HIV infection. Nursing actions include the following:

- Identifying resources such as social and financial support services
- Interpreting school and work policies
- Assisting employers by educating managers about how to deal with ill or infected workers to reduce the risk of breaching confidentiality or wrongful actions such as termination

HIV-infected children should attend school, because the benefits of attendance far outweigh the risks of transmitting or acquiring infections. None of the cases of HIV infection in the United States has been transmitted in a school setting. An interdisciplinary team made up of the child's physician, public health personnel, the child's parent or guardian, and the nurse should make decisions about educational and care needs. Individual decisions about risk to the infected child or others should be based on the behavior, neurological development, and physical condition of the child. Attendance may be inadvisable if cases of childhood infections, such as chickenpox or measles, are in the school, since the immunosuppressed child is at greater risk of suffering complications. Alternative arrangements, such as homebound instruction, might be instituted if a child is unable to control body secretions or displays biting behavior.

BRIEFLY NOTED

Because of impaired immunity, children with HIV infection are more likely to get childhood diseases and suffer serious sequelae. Therefore DPT (diphtheria, pertussis, tetanus), IPV (inactivated polio virus), and MMR (measles, mumps, rubella) vaccines should be given at regularly scheduled times for children infected with HIV. HiB (*Haemophilus influenzae* type B), hepatitis B, pneumococcus, and influenza vaccines may be recommended after medical evaluation.

A growing number of services are available for persons with HIV/AIDS. Voluntary and faith-based groups, such as community organizations or AIDS support organizations, are available in some localities to address their many needs. Services include counseling, support groups, legal aid, personal care services, housing programs, and community education programs. Nurses collaborate with workers from community organizations in the client's home and may advise these groups in their supportive work. The federal government and many organizations have established toll-free numbers and websites to provide information. Box 27-2 presents contact numbers for several of these organizations.

Eliminating HIV/AIDS is complex and beyond the scope of one group or agency. Public health partnerships that bring together public and private persons and groups will be essential, as well as greater access to mandatory HIV testing. Prevention messages should be culturally appropriate and should talk about the role alcohol and drug abuse play in HIV risk. An additional strategy focuses on improved monitoring of HIV infections in order to refine the targeting and delivery of efforts at prevention (Centers for Disease Control and Prevention, 2006b).

Considerable work has been done and progress is being made in finding effective treatment for HIV. In 2008, the U.S. Food and Drug Administration approved raltegravir (Isentress) tablets, which can be used in combination with other antiretroviral drugs for adults who have developed a drug resistance. Patients need to be taught about the warning signs of adverse effects, especially those related to creatine kinase elevations.

Box 27-2	**Sexually Transmitted Diseases Resources**

- American Social Health Association's STI Resource Center Hotline (800-227-8922)
- National AIDS Hotline (800-342-2437) or online at http://www.ashastd.org/nah
- CDC Hepatitis Hotline (888-443-7232) or online at http://www.cdc.gov/ncidod/diseases/hepatitis/index.htm
- CDC National Prevention Information Network (800-458-5231)
- AIDS Info (800-HIV-0440) or online at http://www.aidsinfo.nih.gov/
- Hemophilia and AIDS/HIV Network for Dissemination of Information (HANDI) (800-42-HANDI) or online at http://www.hemophilia.org/
- AIDS Treatment News (800-873-2812) or online at http://www.aidsnews.org/

SEXUALLY TRANSMITTED DISEASES

Sexually transmitted diseases are a major public health challenge in the United States. There are an estimated 19 million new infections annually, and almost half of them are in people between the ages of 15 and 24 years. Chlamydia and gonorrhea are the two most common infectious diseases in the United States. Although 1.5 million cases of these diseases were reported in 2007, it is thought that the majority go undetected. If chlamydia and gonorrhea are not treated, both can lead to infertility (Centers for Disease Control and Prevention, 2009a). The rates for the two most infectious types of syphilis, primary and secondary, decreased during the 1990s and reached an all time low in the year 2000. However, the rate began increasing in 2000 with the rate increasing in men by 17.9% in 2007 (Centers for Disease Control and Prevention, 2009a). This rate increase is being driven by gay and bisexual men. The common STDs listed in Table 27-2 are grouped according to their having either a bacterial or viral cause. The bacterial infections include gonorrhea, syphilis, and chlamydia. Most of these infections are cured with antibiotics. The exceptions are the newly emerging antibiotic-resistant strains of gonorrhea. In contrast, STDs caused by viruses cannot be cured. These are chronic diseases leading to a lifetime of symptom management and infection control. The viral infections include herpes simplex virus and human papillomavirus (HPV), also referred to as *genital warts*. The hepatitis A and hepatitis B viruses, which may also be transmitted via sexual activity, are discussed in the "Hepatitis" section of this chapter on pp. 520-523.

GONORRHEA

Neisseria gonorrhoeae is a gram-negative intracellular diplococcal bacterium that infects the mucous membranes of the genitourinary tract, rectum, and pharynx. It is transmitted through genital–genital contact, oral–genital contact, and anal–genital contact. **Gonorrhea** is identified as either uncomplicated or complicated. Uncomplicated gonorrhea refers to limited cervical or urethral infection. Complicated gonorrhea includes salpingitis, epididymitis, systemic gonococcal infection, and gonococcal meningitis. The signs and symptoms of infection in males are purulent and copious urethral discharge and dysuria. An estimated 10% to 20% of males are asymptomatic.

When gonococcal infection is asymptomatic, treatment may not be sought, and it continues to be spread to others through sexual activity. Some individuals, even when symptomatic, continue to be sexually active and infect others (National Institute of Allergy and Infectious Diseases, 2007). Because up to 40% of those infected with gonorrhea are coinfected with *Chlamydia trachomatis,* treatment effective against both organisms, such as doxycycline or

Table 27-2	Summary of Sexually Transmitted Diseases				
Disease/Pathogen	Incubation	Signs and Symptoms	Diagnosis	Treatment	Nursing Implications
Bacterial					
Chlamydia: *Chlamydia*	3–21 days	*Male:* Nongonococcal urethritis (NGU); painful urination and urethral discharge; epididymitis *Female:* None or mucopurulent cervicitis (MPC), vaginal discharge; if untreated, progresses to symptoms of PID: diffuse abdominal pain, fever, chills	Tissue culture; Gram stain of endocervical or urethral discharge: presence of PMNs without gram-negative intracellular diplococci suggests NGU	One of the following treatments: • Doxycycline 100 mg PO twice a day × 7 days • Azithromycin 1 g PO × 1 • Erythromycin 500 mg four times a day × 7 days • Ofloxacin 300 mg PO twice a day × 7 days • Doxycycline—effective and cheap • Azithromycin—good because a single dose is sufficient	Refer partners of past 60 days; counsel client to use condoms and to avoid sex until therapy is complete and symptoms are gone in both client and partners; medication teaching Annual screening recommended for all sexually active women under 25 years, and women over 25 years if new or multiple sexual partners
Gonorrhea: *Neisseria gonorrhoeae*	3–21 days	*Male:* Urethritis, purulent discharge, painful urination, urinary frequency; epididymitis *Female:* None, or symptoms of PID	Culture of discharge; Gram stain of urethral discharge, endocervical or rectal smear	One of the following treatments: • Ceftriaxone 125 mg IM × 1 If chlamydial infection is not ruled out, give azithromycin 1 g PO × 1	Refer partners of past 60 days; return for evaluation if symptoms persist; counsel client to use therapy until complete and symptoms are gone in both client and partners; medication teaching
Syphilis: *Treponema pallidum*	10–90 days	Primary: Usually single, painless chancre; if untreated, heals in a few weeks	Visualization of pathogen on darkfield microscopic examination; single painless ulcer (chancre), FTA-ABS or MHA-TP, VDRL (reactive 14 days after appearance of chancre)	Penicillin G 2.4 million units, IM once. If penicillin allergy: • Doxycycline 100 mg PO twice a day × 2 weeks • Tetracycline 500 mg four times a day × 14 days	Counsel to be tested for HIV; screen all partners of the past 3 months; reexamine the client at 3 and 6 months
	6 weeks to 6 months	Secondary: Low-grade fever, malaise, sore throat, headache, adenopathy, and rash	Clinical signs of secondary syphilis	Tetracycline hydrochloride should not be administered to pregnant women or those with neurosyphilis or congenital syphilis	
	Within 1 year of infection	Early latency: Asymptomatic, infectious lesions may recur	VDRL: FTA-ABS or MHA-TP	Early latent: Benzathine penicillin G 2.4 million units IM once	
	After 1 year from date of infection	Late latency: Asymptomatic; noninfectious except to fetus of pregnant women	Lumbar puncture, CSF cell count, protein level determination, and VDRL	Late latent: Benzathine penicillin G 7.2 million units total in three doses of 2.4 million units each	
	Late active: 2–40 years 20–30 years 10–30 years	Gummas of skin, bone, mucous membranes, heart, liver CNS involvement: Paresis, optic atrophy Cardiovascular involvement: Aortic aneurysm, aortic valve insufficiency		In general, penicillins are prescribed in varying doses depending on diagnosis	

Continued

Table 27-2 **Summary of Sexually Transmitted Diseases—cont'd**

Disease/Pathogen	Incubation	Signs and Symptoms	Diagnosis	Treatment	Nursing Implications
Viral					
Human immunodeficiency virus (HIV)	4–6 weeks Seroconversion: 6 weeks to 3 months AIDS: month to years (average, 11 years)	Possible: Acute mononucleosis-like illness (lymphadenopathy, fever, rash, joint and muscle pain, sore throat) Appearance of HIV antibody Opportunistic diseases: most commonly *Pneumocystis carinii* pneumonia, oral candidiasis, Kaposi's sarcoma	HIV antibody test: EIA or the OraSure Western blot test; SmithKline Beecham)—an oral HIV-1 antibody testing system—test results in about 3 days CD4+ T-lymphocyte count of less than 200/mcl with documented HIV infection, or diagnosis with clinical manifestations of AIDS as defined by the CDC	Prophylactic administration of zidovudine (ZDV) immediately after exposure may prevent seroconversion Asymptomatic infection with HIV-1 and CD4+ counts ≤500/mm³. Treat with ZDV 500–600 mg/day; treatment can be held in those with asymptomatic infection and CD4+ counts between 500 and 200/mm³ until symptoms appear or CD4+ counts rise Symptomatic infection: Start ZDV 20 mg every 8 hours; alternatives to ZDV: didanosine (ddI), stavudine (d4t), zalcitabine (ddC), and a combination of ZDV and ddI; additional treatments are necessary for opportunistic infections	HIV education and counseling; partner referral for evaluation; medication education; assessment and referral Men who have sex with men should be tested annually for HIV, chlamydia, syphilis, and gonorrhea
Genital warts: human papillomavirus (HPV)	4–6 weeks most common; up to 9 months	Often subclinical infection; painless lesions near vaginal openings, anus, shaft of penis, vagina, cervix; lesions are textured, cauliflower appearance; may remain unchanged over time	Visual inspection for lesions; Pap smear; hybrid capture 2 HPV DNA test; colposcopy	No cure; one-third of lesions will disappear without topical treatment *Patient-applied:* Topical podofilox 0.5% or imiquimod 5% cream *Provider administered:* Podophyllum resin 10–25%, or tricloroacetic acid 80–90%—repeat weekly if needed; cryotherapy with liquid nitrogen, laser, or surgical removal	Warts and surrounding tissues contain HPV, so removal of warts does not completely eradicate the virus; examination of partners is not necessary, as treatment is only symptomatic; condom use may reduce transmission; medication application
Genital herpes: herpes simplex virus 2 (HSV-2)	2–20 days; average, 6 days	Vesicles, painful ulceration of penis, vagina, labia, perineum, or anus; lesions last 5–6 weeks and recurrence is common; may be asymptomatic	Presence of vesicles; viral culture (obtained only when lesions present and before they have scabbed over)	No cure; treatment may be episodic or suppressive for frequent recurrence Episodic treatment: acyclovir 800 mg PO twice a day × 5 days, or acyclovir 200 mg five times a day × 5 days, or valacyclovir 1 g PO daily × 5 days	Refer partners for evaluation; teach clients about the likelihood of recurrent episodes and the ability to transmit to others even if asymptomatic; condom use; annual Pap smear

From Centers for Disease Control and Prevention: Sexually transmitted diseases treatment guidelines 2006, *MMWR Morb Mortal Wkly Rep* 55:(RR-11), 2006; Centers for Disease Control and Prevention: Update to CDC's sexually transmitted diseases treatment guidelines, 2006: Fluoroquinolones no longer recommended for treatment of gonococcal infections–United States, 2007, *MMWR Morb Mortal Wkly Rep* 56(14): 332-336, 2007.
AIDS, Acquired immunodeficiency syndrome; *CDC,* Centers for Disease Control and Prevention; *CNS,* central nervous system; *CSF,* cerebrospinal fluid; *DNA,* deoxyribonucleic acid; *EIA,* enzyme-linked immunosorbent assay; *FTA-ABS,* fluorescent treponemal antibody absorption test; *MHA-TP,* microhemagglutination—*Treponema pallidum; Pap,* Papanicolaou; *PID,* pelvic inflammatory disease; *PMN,* polymorphonuclear neutrophil; *VDRL,* Venereal Disease Research Laboratory test for syphilis.

azithromycin, is recommended (AIDS Education and Training Centers National Resource Center, 2008).

Although the rates have been fairly stable for the past decade, there were 355,991 cases of gonorrhea reported in 2007 (Centers for Disease Control and Prevention, 2009a). Declines before 1998 were the result of testing of asymptomatic women and follow-up with their partners to prevent reinfection. Health care providers may underreport gonorrhea, leading to a difference between the actual cases and reported cases. Also, asymptomatic clients may not seek treatment and are therefore not identified. Groups with the highest incidence of gonorrhea are African-Americans, persons living in the southern United States, and persons 15 to 24 years of age (Division of STD Prevention, 2007).

The number of antibiotic-resistant cases of gonorrhea in the United States has risen at an alarming rate. Penicillin-resistant gonorrhea was first identified in 1976 when 15 cases were reported (Phillips, 1976). The increase in antibiotic-resistant infections is partly attributed to the increased and often illicit use of antibiotics as a prophylactic measure by those who have multiple sexual partners. To ensure proper treatment and cure, those diagnosed with gonorrheal infection should return for health care if symptoms persist, have their partner evaluated for infection, and remain sexually abstinent until antibiotic therapy is completed (Centers for Disease Control and Prevention, 2008b).

The development of **pelvic inflammatory disease (PID)** is a risk for asymptomatic women who do not seek treatment. PID, which is a serious infection involving the fallopian tubes (salpingitis) and is the most common complication of gonorrhea, may also result from chlamydia infection. Its symptoms include fever, abnormal menses, and lower abdominal pain, but PID may not be recognized because the symptoms vary among women. PID can result in ectopic pregnancy and infertility related to fallopian-tube scarring and occlusion (Centers for Disease Control and Prevention, 2008d).

SYPHILIS

Syphilis, caused by *Treponema pallidum*, infects moist mucosal or cutaneous membranes and is spread through direct contact, usually by sexual contact or from mother to fetus. In sexual transmission, microscopic breaks in the skin and mucous membranes during sexual contact create a point of entry for the bacteria (Chin, 2000). Transmission via blood transfusion can occur if the donor is in the early stages of the disease (Heymann, 2004). The clinical signs of syphilis are divided into primary, secondary, and tertiary infections. Latency, a period during which an individual is free of symptoms, may occur during the early and late stages. As defined by the United States Public Health Service, the early stage is the first full year after infection and includes the primary, secondary, and early latent stages. The late stage is the time after this first year and includes late latency and tertiary syphilis. During latency, no clinical signs of infection are present but the person has historical or serological evidence of infection. The possibility of relapse exists.

The first stage is called *primary syphilis*. When the disease is acquired sexually, the bacteria produce infection in the form of a chancre at the site of entry. The lesion begins as a macula, progresses to a papule, and later ulcerates. If left untreated, this chancre persists for 3 to 6 weeks and then heals spontaneously (Heymann, 2004). *Secondary syphilis* occurs when the organism enters the lymph system and spreads throughout the body. Signs include rash, lymphadenopathy, and mucosal ulceration. Symptoms of secondary syphilis include sore throat, malaise, headaches, weight loss, variable fever, and muscle and joint pain. *Tertiary syphilis* can lead to blindness, congenital damage, cardiovascular damage, or syphilitic psychoses, as well as the development of lesions of the bones, skin, and mucous membranes, known as *gummas*. Tertiary syphilis usually occurs several years after initial infection and is rare in the United States because the disease is usually cured in its early stages with antibiotics. Tertiary syphilis does, however, remain a major problem in developing countries. Congenital syphilis rates have declined dramatically, but the effects are devastating. Syphilis is transmitted transplacentally and if untreated can cause premature stillbirth, blindness, deafness, facial abnormalities, crippling, or death. Signs include jaundice, skin rash, hepatosplenomegaly, or pseudoparalysis of an extremity. Treatment consists of penicillin given intravenously or intramuscularly (Centers for Disease Control and Prevention, 2008f).

CHLAMYDIA

Chlamydia infection, from the bacterium *Chlamydia trachomatis,* infects the genitourinary tract and rectum of adults and causes conjunctivitis and pneumonia in neonates. Transmission occurs when mucopurulent discharge from infected sites, such as the cervix or urethra, comes into contact with the mucous membranes of a noninfected person. Like gonorrhea, the infection is often asymptomatic in women and, if left untreated, can result in PID. When chlamydia infection is present, symptoms in women include dysuria, urinary frequency, and purulent vaginal discharge. In men the urethra is the most common site of infection, resulting in **nongonococcal urethritis (NGU)**. The symptoms of NGU are dysuria and urethral discharge. Epididymitis is a possible complication.

Chlamydia is the most common reportable infectious disease in the United States. Because it causes PID, ectopic pregnancy, infertility, and neonatal complications, it is a major focus of preventive efforts (Centers for Disease Control and Prevention, 2008a). Rates of chlamydia have increased in recent years, partly because of improved diagnosis and reporting. Risk factors that positively correlate with chlamydial infection are age less than 25 years, multiple sexual partners, and a history of infection with other STDs (Centers for Disease Control and Prevention, 2008a). The high frequency of chlamydial infections in individuals infected with gonorrhea requires that effective treatment for both organisms be given when a gonorrheal infection is identified (Centers for Disease Control and Prevention, 2008b).

HERPES SIMPLEX VIRUS 2 (GENITAL HERPES)

Herpes viruses infect genital and nongenital sites. Herpes simplex virus 1 (HSV-1) primarily causes nongenital lesions such as cold sores that may appear on the lip or mouth. Herpes simplex virus 2 (HSV-2) is the primary cause of **genital herpes**. Like other viral STDs, there is no cure for HSV-2 infection, and it is considered a chronic disease. The virus is transmitted through direct exposure and infects the genitalia and surrounding skin. After the initial infection, the virus remains latent in the sacral nerve of the central nervous system and may reactivate periodically with or without visible vesicles.

Signs and symptoms of HSV-2 infection include the presence of painful lesions that begin as vesicles and ulcerate and crust within 1 to 4 days. The first episode is typically longer and is usually characterized by more lesions than seen in subsequent infections. Lesions may occur on the vulva, vagina, upper thighs, buttocks, and penis and have an average duration of 11 days. The vesicles can cause itching and pain and may be accompanied by dysuria or rectal pain. Although the ability to pass the infection to others is higher with active lesions, some individuals can spread the virus even when they are asymptomatic. Approximately 50% of people experience a prodromal phase. This may include a mild, tingling sensation up to 48 hours before eruption or shooting pains in the buttocks, legs, or hips (American Social Health Association, 2008; National Institute of Allergy and Infectious Diseases, 2008).

Nationwide, at least 45 million people ages 12 years and older, or one out of five adolescents and adults, have had genital HSV infection. Between the late 1970s and early 1990s, the number of Americans with genital herpes infection increased by 30% (Centers for Disease Control and Prevention, 2005a). Since a large number of people have no symptoms and HSV-2 is difficult to identify, the prevalence may be underrated.

The consequences of HSV-2 are of particular concern for women and their children. HSV-2 infection is linked with the development of cervical cancer. There is also an increased risk of spontaneous abortion and risk of transmission to the newborn during vaginal delivery (Centers for Disease Control and Prevention, 2005a). The clinical infection in infants may cause skin or mouth sores, eye infections, or brain or internal organ infections (March of Dimes, 2005). A pregnant woman who has active lesions at the time of giving birth should have a cesarean delivery before the rupture of amniotic membranes to avoid fetal contact with the herpetic lesions, whereas those who have no clinical evidence of herpes lesions should be delivered vaginally. A small number of infants are infected *in utero* (Corey and Wald, 1999).

HUMAN PAPILLOMAVIRUS INFECTION

Human papillomavirus (HPV), also called **genital warts,** can infect the genitals, anus, and mouth. Transmission of HPV occurs through direct contact with warts that result from HPV. However, HPV has been detected in semen, and exposure to the virus through body fluids is also possible. Genital warts are most commonly found on the penis and scrotum in men and the vulva, labia, vagina, and cervix in women. They appear as textured surface lesions, with what is sometimes described as a *cauliflower* appearance. The warts are usually multiple and vary between 1 and 5 mm in diameter. They may be difficult to visualize, so careful examination is required. HPV is common in young sexually active women (Division of STD Prevention, 2007). As with genital herpes, it is hard to know the actual prevalence since this is not a reported disease and many infections are subclinical.

Complications of HPV infection are especially serious for women. The link between HPV infection and cervical cancer has been established and is associated with specific types of the virus. Pap smears are important since they allow for microscopic examination of cells to detect HPV and tumors. The tumors can often be surgically removed if found early (Heymann, 2004). HPV infection is exacerbated in both pregnancy and immune-related disorders, which are believed to result from a decrease in cell-mediated immune functioning. HPV may infect the fetus during pregnancy and can result in a laryngeal papilloma that can obstruct the infant's airway. Genital warts may enlarge and become friable during pregnancy, and therefore surgical removal may be recommended.

A vaccine to protect against specific types of HPV that cause cervical cancer is available (Centers for Disease Control and Prevention, 2009d). The vaccine, Gardasil, stimulates the immune system to block HPV infection before it occurs. Once HPV infection occurs, the goal is to eliminate the lesions (warts). Genital warts spontaneously disappear over time, as do skin warts. However, because the condition is worrisome for the client and HPV may lead to the development of cervical neoplasia, treatment of the lesions through surgical removal, cytotoxic agents, or immunotherapies is often used. There is also some controversy about the vaccine. A good source is the Centers for Disease Control and Prevention for current updates on this topic.

BRIEFLY NOTED

The challenge of HPV prevention is that condoms do not necessarily prevent infection. Warts may grow where barriers, such as condoms, do not cover, and skin-to-skin contact may occur.

HEPATITIS

Viral hepatitis refers to a group of infections that primarily affect the liver. These infections have similar clinical presentations but different causes and characteristics. Brief profiles of the types of hepatitis are presented in Table 27-3.

Table 27-3 Viral Hepatitis Profiles

	Hepatitis A	Hepatitis B	Hepatitis C	Hepatitis D	Hepatitis E	Hepatitis G
Incubation period	Average, 30 days; range, 15–50 days	Average, 75 days; range, 40–120 days	Average, 45 days; range, 17–175 days	Average, 28 days; range, 14–43 days	Average, 40 days; range, 15–60 days	Unknown
Mode of transmission	Fecal–oral, waterborne, sexual	Blood-borne, sexual, perinatal	Primarily blood-borne; also sexual and perinatal	Superinfection or coinfection of hepatitis B case	Fecal–oral	Blood-borne; may facilitate other strains of viral hepatitis to progress more rapidly
Incidence	125,000–200,000 cases/year in the United States	140,000–320,000 cases/year in the United States	28,000–180,000 cases/year in the United States	7500 cases/year in the United States	Low in the United States, epidemic outbreaks worldwide	0.3% of all acute viral hepatitis
Chronic carrier state?	No	Yes, 0.1–15% of cases	Yes, 85% or more of cases	Yes, 70–80% of cases	No	Yes, 90–100% of cases
Diagnosis	Serological test (anti-HAV), viral isolation	Serological test (HBsAg), viral isolation	Serological test (anti-HCV)	Serological test (anti-HDV), liver biopsy	Serological test (anti-HEV)	None currently
Sequelae	No chronic infection	Chronic liver disease; liver cancer	Chronic liver disease; liver cancer	Chronic liver disease; liver cancer	No chronic infection	Rare or may not occur
Vaccine availability	Yes, vaccination of preschool children recommended; travelers to endemic regions; men who have sex with men	Yes, vaccination of infants recommended; individual with exposure risks; men who have sex with men	No	No	No	No
Control and prevention	Personal hygiene; proper sanitation	Preexposure vaccination; reduce exposure risk behaviors	Screening of blood/organ donors; reduce exposure risk behaviors	Preexposure or postexposure prophylaxis for HBV	Protection of water systems from fecal contamination	Unknown

HAV, Hepatitis A virus; *HBsAg,* hepatitis B surface antigen; *HBV,* hepatitis B virus; *HCV,* hepatitis C virus; *HDV,* hepatitis D virus; *HEV,* hepatitis E virus.

HEPATITIS A VIRUS

Hepatitis A virus (HAV) is most often transmitted through the fecal–oral route. Sources may be water, food, or sexual contact. The virus level in the feces appears to peak 1 to 2 weeks before symptoms appear, making individuals highly contagious before they realize they are ill (Heymann, 2004). Although there has been a vaccine for this disease since 1995, hepatitis A infection remains one of the most frequently reported vaccine-preventable diseases. Persons most at risk for HAV infection are travelers to countries with high rates of infection, children living in areas with high rates of infection, injection drug users, men who have sex with men, and persons with clotting disorders or chronic liver disease.

Hepatitis A is found worldwide. In developing countries where sanitation is inadequate, epidemics are not common because most adults are immune from childhood infection. In countries with improved sanitation, outbreaks are common in day care centers whose staff must change diapers, among household and sexual contacts of infected individuals, and among travelers to countries where hepatitis A is endemic. In the United States, cases are most common among schoolchildren between the ages of 5 and 14 years. In many outbreaks, one individual is the source of an infection that may become communitywide. In other cases, hepatitis A is spread through food contaminated by an infected food-handler, contaminated produce, or contaminated water. The source of infection may never be identified in as many as 25% of outbreaks. Children are often infected but show no symptoms, so they play an extremely important role in HAV transmission and are a source of infection for others. Since 1996 when routine childhood vaccination was recommended, the overall rate of hepatitis A has declined, with the greatest accomplishments seen in children (Centers for Disease Control and Prevention, 2007a).

The clinical course of hepatitis A ranges from mild to severe and may entail a prolonged convalescence. Onset is usually acute, with fever, nausea, lack of appetite, malaise, and abdominal discomfort, followed after several days by jaundice. Good sanitation and personal hygiene are the best means of preventing infection. People who travel often or for long periods in countries in which the disease is endemic should have the HAV vaccine. Until 2007, an injection of immune globulin (IG) was the only recommended way to protect people who had been exposed to hepatitis A. In June 2007, U.S. guidelines were revised to allow the use of the hepatitis A vaccine after exposure to prevent infection in healthy person between 1 and 40 years of age. Candidates for IG administration and vaccine after exposure to HAV are listed in Box 27-3 (Centers for Disease Control and Prevention, 2008i; Centers for Disease Control and Prevention, 2007b; Heymann, 2004).

HEPATITIS B VIRUS

The number of new cases of **hepatitis B virus (HBV)** in the United States has been decreasing as a result of the use of HBV vaccine. The groups with the highest prevalence are

---

Box 27-3	People who Require Protection by Administration of Immune Globulin (IG) for Hepatitis A Virus or Hepatitis A Vaccine

Those with close personal contact:
- All household and sexual contacts of persons with hepatitis A virus (HAV)
- Persons who have shared illicit drugs with someone with hepatitis A
- Regular babysitter or staff of day care centers if a case of HAV occurs among children or staff
- Household members whose diapered children attend a day care center where three or more families are infected
- Staff and residents of prisons or institutions for developmentally disabled persons, if they have close contact with persons with HAV
- Hospital employees if exposed to feces of infected clients
- Food-handlers who have a co-worker infected with HAV; patrons only in limited situations

---

injection drug users, persons with STDs, men who have sex with men, people who were born in geographic regions with a hepatitis B surface antigen (HBsAg) prevalence of 2% or greater, health care workers, hemodialysis clients, and inmates of long-term correctional institutions.

The HBV is spread through blood and body fluids and, like HIV, is referred to as a *blood-borne pathogen*. It has the same transmission properties as HIV, and thus individuals should take the same precautions to prevent the spread of both HIV and HBV. A major difference is that HBV remains alive outside the body for a longer time than does HIV and thus has greater infectivity. The virus can survive for at least 1 week dried at room temperature on environmental surfaces, and therefore infection control measures are paramount in preventing transmission from client to client (Centers for Disease Control and Prevention, 2005b).

Infection with HBV results in either acute or chronic HBV infection. The acute infection is self-limited, and individuals develop an antibody to the virus and successfully eliminate the virus from the body. They subsequently have lifelong immunity against the virus. Symptoms range from mild, flu-like symptoms to a more severe response that includes jaundice, extreme lethargy, nausea, fever, and joint pain. Any of these more severe symptoms may result in hospitalization. A second possible outcome from infection is chronic HBV infection, which occurs in 2% to 6% of infected adults (Centers for Disease Control and Prevention, 2005b). These individuals cannot rid their bodies of the virus and remain lifelong carriers of the hepatitis B surface antigen (HBsAg). As carriers, they can transmit the HBV to others. They may develop hepatic carcinoma or chronic active hepatitis. The signs and symptoms of chronic hepatitis B include anorexia, fatigue, abdominal discomfort, hepatomegaly, and jaundice.

HBV infection can be prevented by immunization, prevention of nosocomial occupational exposure, and prevention of sexual and injection drug-use exposure. Vaccination is recommended for persons with occupational risk, such as health care workers, and for children. Protection from HBV consists of a series of three intramuscular injections, with the second and third doses administered 1 and 6 months after the first (Centers for Disease Control and Prevention, 2005b). Testing continues to be recommended for pregnant women, infants born to HBsAg-positive mothers, household contacts and sexual partners of HBV-infected persons, individuals who may be exposed to blood or body builds that are contaminated (e.g., a needle-stick injury in a health care worker), or persons infected with HIV (Centers for Disease Control and Prevention, 2008k). The CDC published new testing guidelines in 2008 that recommend testing for HBsAg for persons born in geographic regions with HBsAg prevalence of 2% or greater, U.S. born persons who were not vaccinated as infants and whose parents came from geographic regions with HBsAg prevalence of 2% or greater, injection-drug users, men who have sex with men, persons with elevated *alanine aminotransferase* and *aspartate aminotransferase*(ALT/AST) of unknown origin, and persons with selected medial conditions who need immunosuppressive therapy (Centers for Disease Control and Prevention, 2008l). All pregnant women should be tested for HBsAg, and if the mother is positive, newborns require hepatitis B immune globulin in addition to the hepatitis B vaccine at birth, and then at 1 and 6 months thereafter (Centers for Disease Control and Prevention, 2008e). Hepatitis B immune globulin is given after exposure to provide passive immunity and thus prevent infection.

In 1992, the Occupational Safety and Health Administration (OSHA) released *Occupational Exposure to Bloodborne Pathogens* (Occupational Safety and Health Administration, 1992), the standard that mandates specific activities to protect workers from HBV and other blood-borne pathogens. Potential exposures for health care workers are needlestick injuries and mucous membrane splashes. The OSHA standard requires employers to identify the risk of blood exposure to various employees. If employees perform work that involves a potential exposure to the body fluids of other people, employers are mandated to offer the HBV vaccine to the employee at the employer's expense and to offer annual educational programs on preventing HBV and HIV exposure in the workplace. Employees have the right to refuse the vaccine.

HEPATITIS C VIRUS

Hepatitis C virus (HCV) infection is the most common chronic blood-borne infection in the United States (Wise et al, 2008). The hepatitis C virus is transmitted when blood or body fluids of an infected person enter an uninfected person. This infection has been called "the silent stalker" since it is now the leading cause of chronic liver disease, end-stage liver disease, liver cancer, and liver transplants in the United States (Harkness, 2003). High-risk groups include health care workers and emergency personnel who are accidentally exposed, infants who are born to infected mothers, and injection drug users who share needles or other drug-use equipment. Others at risk include people who have sex with multiple partners, people on hemodialysis (from dialysis

equipment shared with infected persons), and recipients of donor organs and blood products before 1992 (Centers for Disease Control and Prevention, 2007, 2008g).

During the 1980s, HCV spread rapidly. It is estimated that 3.2 million people are infected in the United States, and they are the source of HCV transmission to others (Centers for Disease Control and Prevention, 2007). In 2005, chronic liver disease from hepatitis C was the leading cause for liver transplantation in the United States (Wise et al, 2008).

The clinical signs of hepatitis C may be so mild that an infected individual does not seek medical attention. The incubation period ranges from 2 weeks to 6 months with an average of 7 to 8 weeks. Clients may experience fatigue and other nonspecific symptoms such as anorexia, malaise, weight loss, right-sided pain, and occasionally jaundice and signs of possible chronic illness (Harkness, 2003). Clients infected with HCV often have an elevated level of the liver enzyme *alanine aminotransferase* (ALT), which may rise and fall during HCV infection. About 15% of infected persons will have spontaneous resolution of the infection, but most develop chronic liver disease. HCV infection may lead to cirrhosis or hepatocellular carcinoma (Centers for Disease Control and Prevention, 2007, 2008h).

Primary prevention of HCV infection includes screening of blood products and donor organs and tissue; risk reduction counseling and services, including obtaining the sexual and injection drug use (IDU) history; and infection control practices. Secondary prevention strategies include testing of high-risk individuals, including those who seek HIV testing and counseling, and appropriate medical follow-up of infected clients. HCV testing should be offered to persons who received blood or an organ transplant before 1992, health care workers after exposure to blood or body fluids, children born to HCV-positive women, and persons who have ever injected drugs or been on dialysis. Routine testing for HCV is not recommended for health care workers, pregnant women, household contacts of HCV-positive persons, or the general population, though anyone who wants to get tested should talk to a health care professional (Centers for Disease Control and Prevention, 2008g).

TUBERCULOSIS

Tuberculosis (TB) is a mycobacterial disease caused by *Mycobacterium tuberculosis*. Transmission is usually by exposure to the tubercle bacilli in airborne droplets from persons with pulmonary TB during talking, coughing, or sneezing. The disease is not an easy one to catch and typically requires breathing the same air as an infected person for hours with close contact (Ruppert, 2007). Common symptoms are cough, fever, hemoptysis, chest pains, fatigue, and weight loss. The incubation period is 4 to 12 weeks. The most critical period for the development of clinical disease is the first 6 to 12 months after infection. About 5% of those initially infected may develop pulmonary TB or extrapulmonary involvement. The infection in about 95% of those initially infected becomes latent and may be reactivated later in life. Reactivation of latent infections is common in older adults; immunocompromised persons; substance abusers; underweight and undernourished persons; and those with diabetes, silicosis, or gastrectomy (Heymann, 2004).

In terms of the epidemiology of TB, the World Health Organization estimates that one-third of the world's population is infected with TB, and it is a leading cause of death worldwide among infectious diseases (World Health Organization, 2007). The incidence of TB in the United States showed a steady decline during the 1970s and early 1980s but increased between 1985 and 1992. The national TB rate fell in 2008 to an all time low of 4.2 cases per 100,000 people. However, this disease continues to affect the foreign born and persons representing a racial or ethnic minority at higher rates. Specifically, foreign-born persons are affected 10 times more than U.S. born persons. Hispanics are seven times more likely to contract TB than whites. Also in 2008, more TB cases were reported among Hispanics than among any other racial/ethnic group, followed by Asians and blacks (Centers for Disease Control and Prevention, 2009b). This increase is believed to have been the result of the deterioration of community services for TB, the HIV epidemic, immigration from countries in which TB is endemic, and the onset of multidrug-resistant TB.

BRIEFLY NOTED

Tuberculosis, hepatitis B, and congenital syphilis have been identified by experts as diseases for which a strategy for elimination from the United States has been identified. To accomplish this objective for TB, recommendations include the expansion of directly observed therapy (DOT) and the development of a safe and effective vaccine to prevent the development of TB in individuals who have been exposed to TB (World Health Organization, 2007).

TB screening tests include skin testing with purified protein derivative (PPD), followed by chest radiography for persons with a positive skin reaction and pulmonary symptoms. Persons who are immunosuppressed by drugs or who have diseases such as advanced TB, AIDS, or measles may be unable to mount an immune response to the PPD, so the result may be a false-negative skin test reaction because of anergy (nonreaction). Confirmatory tests include stained sputum smears and other body fluids with the presence of the acid-fast bacilli (for presumptive diagnosis) and culture of the tubercle bacilli for definitive diagnosis. Although doing a culture test remains the gold standard in TB diagnosis, the Centers for Disease Control and Prevention (2009c) recommend that nucleic acid amplification (NAA) be performed on at least one respiratory specimen from each person with signs and symptoms of pulmonary TB when a diagnosis is considered but has not been confirmed. How to read a PPD test is described in the "How To" box.

| **HOW TO** | **Perform a Purified Protein Derivative (PPD) Test** |

Apply and Read the PPD Test
- For the Mantoux test, inject 0.1 ml containing 5 tuberculin units of PPD tuberculin.
- Read the reaction 48 to 72 hours after injection.
- Measure only induration.
- Record results in millimeters.

Interpret the PPD Test
Test is positive if the induration is greater than or equal to 5 mm in the following:
- Persons known to have human immunodeficiency virus (HIV) infection
- Persons whose chest radiograph is suggestive of previous tuberculosis (TB)
- Close contacts of a person with infectious TB

Test is positive if the induration is greater than or equal to 10 mm in the following:
- Persons with certain medical conditions, such as diabetes, alcoholism, or drug abuse
- Persons who inject drugs (if HIV negative)
- Foreign-born persons from areas in which TB is common
- Medically underserved, low-income populations
- Residents and staff of long-term care facilities, jails, and prisons
- Children younger than 4 years of age

Test is positive if the induration is greater than or equal to 15 mm in the following:
- All persons over 4 years of age with no risk factors for TB

From Chin J: *Control of communicable diseases manual,* Washington, DC, 2000, American Public Health Association.

CASE STUDY

Jill Miles is the nurse epidemiologist for the Warren County Health Department. Part of Ms. Miles' role at the health department is to administer tuberculosis (TB) screening to at-risk populations and to track TB cases seen in the county. Ms. Miles has identified the homeless population in Warren County as a high-risk population for TB.

Ms. Miles has already implemented a TB education program at the homeless shelter. Every other month, she goes to the shelter and teaches a class about TB: what it is, who is at risk, and why to get a TB screening test. Furthermore, every person who wishes to stay at the shelter must receive a TB screening test.

Yesterday, the homeless shelter contacted Ms. Miles and reported that one of the men staying at the shelter tested positive for active TB but they now cannot find him. The shelter director suspects the man has left to work at one of the rural farms that offer temporary work, but he does not know which farm.

Ms. Miles talks to the men at the shelter who spoke with the client. She learns that the client, Jose, is in his 30s and speaks only Spanish. The friends give Ms. Miles some leads of possible farms to which Jose may have gone. Ms. Miles calls the farms and speaks to the farm managers. Luckily, Ms. Miles discovers one of the farm managers had recently been at the shelter to recruit workers. She visits the farm and, through interviewing the newly hired men, finds Jose, the missing person with active TB. Because of Jose's transient lifestyle, Ms. Miles decides to enroll him in directly observed therapy (DOT) for TB treatment. DOT will provide a hotel room and meals for him while he receives TB treatment.

Clients with TB should be treated promptly with the appropriate combination of multiple antimicrobial drugs. Effective drug regimens used in the United States include isoniazid (INH), rifampin, and pyrazinamide. Treatment regimens for persons with active symptomatic infection may be different from the regimens used for persons with latent TB infection or with HIV (U.S. Department of Health & Human Services, 2008). Multidrug-resistant TB (MDR TB) refers to a type of TB that does not respond to the best drugs: IHN and rifampin. Resistance can develop when there is poor adherence by clients in taking the medication or when the wrong drug is prescribed (World Health Organization, 2007; Ruppert, 2007). Nurses administer tuberculin skin tests and provide education on the importance of compliance to long-term therapy. They may also be involved in directly observed therapy (DOT) and contact investigations of cases in the community.

NURSE'S ROLE IN PROVIDING PREVENTIVE CARE FOR COMMUNICABLE DISEASES

From prevention to treatment, the nurse functions as a counselor, educator, advocate, case manager, and primary care provider. Appropriate interventions for primary, secondary, and tertiary prevention are reviewed. In primary prevention, the nursing process is used to care for clients with communicable diseases. Nurses are in an ideal position to affect the outcomes of communicable diseases, and their influence begins with primary prevention.

PRIMARY PREVENTION

Primary prevention aims to keep people healthy and avoid the onset of disease. First, assess for risk behavior and provide relevant intervention through education on how to avoid infection, mostly through healthy behaviors. To assess the risk of acquiring an infection, take a history that focuses on potential exposure, which varies with the specific organism being studied and its mode of transmission. The questions to be asked can be especially challenging with STD clients. The nurse should obtain a sexual and injection drug use history for clients and their partners. The sexual history provides information that leads to the need for specific diagnostic tests, treatment approaches, and partner notification. It also facilitates evaluation of risk factors and is necessary for the nurse to be able to provide relevant education for the client's lifestyle.

A thorough sexual history requires obtaining personal and sensitive information. Ask about the types of relationships, the number of sexual partners and encounters, and the types of sexual behaviors practiced. The confidential nature

---

Levels of Prevention | Related to Nursing Interventions

PRIMARY PREVENTION

- Provide community education about prevention of communicable diseases to well populations.
- Vaccinate for hepatitis A virus (HAV) or hepatitis B virus (HBV).
- Provide community outreach for education and needle exchange.

SECONDARY PREVENTION

- Administer purified protein derivative (PPD).
- Test and counsel for human immunodeficiency virus (HIV).
- Notify partners and trace contacts.

TERTIARY PREVENTION

- Educate caregivers of persons with HIV about Standard Precautions.
- Initiate directly observed therapy (DOT) for tuberculosis treatment.
- Identify community resources for providing supportive care (e.g., funds for purchasing medications).
- Set up support groups for persons with herpes simplex virus 2.

---

of the information and how it will be used should be shared with the client to establish open communication and goal-directed interaction. Most clients feel uneasy disclosing such personal information. The nurse can ease this discomfort by remaining supportive and open during the interview to facilitate honesty about intimate activities. The nurse serves as a model for discussing sensitive information in a candid manner. When discussing precautions, use direct and simple language to describe specific behaviors. This encourages the client to openly discuss sexuality during this interaction and with future partners.

Nurses who are uncomfortable discussing topics such as sexual behavior or sexual orientation are likely to avoid assessing risk behaviors with the client and therefore may compromise data collection. Nurses can gain confidence in conducting sexual risk assessments by understanding their own values and feelings about sexuality and realizing that the purpose of the interaction is to improve the client's health. The nurse's comfort in discussing sexual behavior can be improved by using role-playing to practice assessments of sexual and IDU behavior and by contracting with clients to make behavior changes.

Identifying the number of sexual and injection-drug-using partners and the number of contacts with these partners provides information about the client's risk. The chance of exposure decreases as the number of partners decreases, so people in mutually monogamous relationships are at low risk for acquiring STDs. You can obtain this information by asking, "How many sex (or drug) partners have you had over the past 6 months?" It is important to avoid basing assumptions about the sexual partner or partners on the client's sex, age, ethnicity, or any other factor. Stereotypes and assumptions about who people are and what they do are common problems that keep interviewers from asking the questions that lead to obtaining useful information. For example, it should not be taken for granted that if a man is homosexual, he always has more than one partner. Be aware also that the long incubation of HIV and the subclinical phase of many STDs lead some monogamous individuals to assume erroneously that they are not at risk.

It is important to determine whether the person has sexual contact with men, women, or both. This information can be obtained simply by asking. This lets the client know that the nurse is open to hearing about these behaviors, and thus the nurse is more likely to obtain information that is relevant to sexual practices and risk. Women who are exclusively lesbian are at low risk for acquiring STDs, but bisexual women may transmit STDs between male and female partners. In addition, it is possible for men to have sexual contact with other men and not label themselves as homosexual. Therefore education to reduce risk that is aimed at homosexual men will not be heeded by men who do not see themselves as homosexual. In such situations the nurse can ask, "When was the last time you had sex with another man?"

Certain sexual practices are more likely to result in exposure to and transmission of STDs. Dangerous sexual activities include unprotected anal or vaginal intercourse, oral–anal contact, and insertion of finger or fist into the rectum. These practices introduce a high risk of transmission of enteric organisms or result in physical trauma during sexual encounters. The nurse can obtain information about sexual encounters by asking, "Can you tell me the kinds of sexual practices in which you engage? This will help determine what risks you may have and the type of tests we should do." Clients who engage in genital–anal, oral–anal, or oral–genital contact will need throat and rectal cultures for some STDs, as well as cervical and urethral cultures.

Drug use is linked to STD transmission in several ways. Drugs such as alcohol put people at risk because these drugs can lower inhibitions and impair judgment about engaging in risky behaviors. Addictions to drugs may cause individuals to acquire the drug or money to purchase the drug through sexual favors. This increases both the frequency of sexual contacts and the chances of contracting STDs. Thus the nurse should obtain information on the type and frequency of drug use and the presence of risk behaviors. The administration of vaccines to prevent infection such as for hepatitis A and hepatitis C is an example of primary prevention.

Interventions to prevent infection are aimed at preventing specific infections. These interventions can take several forms and include, for example, education on how to prevent infection or the availability of vaccines. For example, on the basis of the information obtained in the sexual history and risk assessment just described, the nurse can identify specific education and counseling needs of the client. The nursing interventions focus on contracting with clients to change behavior and reduce their risk in regard to sexual practice.

Safer Sex

Sexual abstinence is the best way to prevent STDs. However, for many people sexual abstinence is not realistic, and teaching how to make sexual behavior safer is critical. Safer sexual behavior includes masturbation, dry kissing, touching, fantasy, and vaginal and oral sex with a condom.

If used correctly and consistently, condoms can prevent both pregnancy and STDs because they prevent the exchange of body fluids during sexual activity. Although the failure rate of condoms has been estimated to be less than 2%, this is believed to be related to incorrect use rather than condom failure (Centers for Disease Control and Prevention, 2005c). Thus information about proper use of condoms and how to communicate with a partner is also necessary. The nurse has many opportunities to convey this information during counseling. Condom use may be viewed as inconvenient, as messy, or as decreasing sensation. Consuming alcohol may accompany sexual activity and decrease condom use. Nurses can use role playing to assist clients gain skill in discussing safer sex by role modeling and by practicing communication skills.

Female condoms can also be a barrier to body fluid contact and therefore protect against pregnancy and STDs. The main advantage of the female condom is that its use is controlled by the woman. Because it is made of polyurethane, it is also useful if a latex sensitivity develops to regular male condoms. Symptoms of latex allergy include penile, vaginal, or rectal itching or swelling after use of a male condom or diaphragm. The female condom consists of a sheath over two rings, with one closed end that fits over the cervix. The cost is about $3 per condom.

Clients should understand that it is important to know the risk behavior of their sexual partners, including a history of injection drug use and STDs, bisexuality, and any current symptoms. This is because each sexual partner is potentially exposed to all the STDs of all the persons with whom the other partner has been sexually active.

Drug Use

Injection drug use is risky because the potential for injecting blood-borne pathogens, such as HIV and HBV, exists when needles and syringes are shared. During IDU, small quantities of drugs are repeatedly injected. Blood is withdrawn into the syringe and is then injected back into the user's vein. Individuals should be advised against using injectable drugs and sharing needles, syringes, or other drug paraphernalia. If equipment is shared, it should be in contact with full-strength bleach for 30 seconds and then rinsed with water several times to prevent injecting bleach. People who inject drugs are difficult to reach for health care services. Effective outreach programs include using community peers, increasing accessibility of drug treatment programs combined with HIV testing and counseling, and long-term repeat contacts after completion of the program.

BRIEFLY NOTED

When obtaining a client's sexual history do the following:
- Remain supportive and open to facilitate honesty.
- Use terms the client will understand (be prepared to suggest multiple terms).
- Speak candidly so the client will feel comfortable talking.

Community Outreach, Education, and Evaluation

Because of the illegal nature of injectable drugs and the poverty associated with HIV, many people at risk have neither the inclination nor the resources to seek health care. Nurses may work to establish programs within communities because the opportunities for counseling on the prevention of HIV and other STDs are increased by bringing services into the neighborhoods of those at risk. Workers go into communities to disseminate information on safer sex, drug treatment programs, and discontinuation of drug use or safer drug-use practices (e.g., using new needles and syringes with each injection). Some programs provide sterile needles and syringes, condoms, and literature about anonymous test sites.

Using primary prevention, nurses can educate healthy groups about prevention of communicable diseases. Information about modes of transmission, testing, availability of vaccines, and early symptoms can be provided to groups in the community and can help prevent the spread of STDs and HIV. Effective and convenient places to hold these educational sessions include schools, businesses, and churches. When talking with groups about HIV infection, be sure to discuss the following:
- The number of people who are diagnosed with AIDS
- The number infected with HIV
- Modes of transmission of the virus
- How to prevent infection
- Common symptoms of illness
- The need for a compassionate response to those afflicted
- Available community resources
- Content about other STDs, since the mode of transmission (sexual contact) is the same
- Information on these diseases, including the distribution, incidence, and consequences of the infection for individuals and society

Evaluation is based on whether risky behavior has changed to safe behavior and, ultimately, whether illness is prevented. Condom use is evaluated for consistency of use if the client is sexually active. Other behaviors, such as abstinence or monogamy, can be evaluated for their implementation. At the community level, behavioral surveys can be done to measure reported condom use and condom sales, and measures of disease incidence and prevalence can be calculated to evaluate the effectiveness of intervention.

SECONDARY PREVENTION

Secondary prevention includes screening for diseases to ensure their early identification and treatment, and follow-up with contacts to prevent further spread. In general, client teaching and counseling should include education about preventing self-reinfection, managing symptoms, and preventing the infection of others. HIV screening is recommended for all patients in health care settings unless the patient declines testing. Persons at high risk should be tested annually. This includes people with one or more of the following:
- A history of STDs
- Multiple sex partners
- Injection drug use
- Who have had intercourse without using a condom; who have had intercourse with someone who has another partner; and who have had sex with a prostitute
- Men with a history of homosexual or bisexual activity
- Who have been a sexual partner to anyone in one of these groups
- Who have had a blood transfusion between January 1978 and March 1985 (Centers for Disease Control and Prevention, 2001c).

If HIV infection is discovered before the onset of symptoms, the disease process and CD4 lymphocyte counts or viral loads can be monitored early. In addition, prophylactic therapy with antibiotics or antiretroviral therapy may be started and may delay the onset of symptomatic illness. Thus testing enables clients to benefit from early detection and treatment, as well as risk-reduction education.

HIV Test Counseling

An important part of care is counseling about the HIV antibody test. First, clients must know that the antibody test is not diagnostic for AIDS but is indicative of HIV infection. During initial counseling the nurse should do the following:
- Assess risk
- Discuss risk behaviors and how to avoid engaging in them
- Develop with the client a risk-reduction plan
- Set a follow-up appointment to receive test results and posttest counseling

   PRETEST COUNSELING. During pretest counseling do the following:
- Conduct the actual risk assessment
- Provide relevant teaching as described in the "Primary Prevention" section, beginning on p. 525.
- Tell the client who will have access to the test results; although AIDS is reported nationally, the reporting of HIV infection varies among states

In the case of rapid tests, inform the client that a second test is needed if the rapid test is positive.

Because there is no cure or vaccine available, preventing the transmission of HIV requires a risk assessment of the client's behavior and counseling on how to reduce identified risks. Sexually active individuals who have multiple partners must be encouraged to abstain, to enter a mutually monogamous relationship, or to use condoms. Injection drug users should be advised to enter a treatment program or discontinue drug use. If they continue to use drugs, they should be warned not to share needles, syringes, or any other drug paraphernalia.

POSTTEST COUNSELING. Persons who have a negative test result should be counseled about risk-reduction activities to prevent any future transmission. They need to understand that the test may not be truly negative, because it does not identify infections that may have been acquired within 3 months before the test. As noted earlier, the appearance of HIV antibody can take up to 12 weeks. The client must be aware of the means of viral transmission and how to avoid infection. The HIV-infected person needs to do the following:

* Have regular medical evaluations and follow-up care
* Avoid donating blood, plasma, body organs, other tissue, and sperm
* Take precautions against exchanging body fluids during sexual activity
* Inform sexual or injection-drug-using partners of potential exposure to HIV, or arrange to have the health department notify them
* Inform health care providers of the HIV infection
* Consider the risk of perinatal transmission and use contraceptives

Be sure to counsel anyone who is antibody positive about the need to reduce risks and notify partners. If the client is unwilling or hesitant to notify past partners, partner notification (or contact tracing, as described in the section that follows) can be done by the nurse. Psychosocial counseling is indicated when positive HIV test results precipitate acute anxiety, depression, or suicidal ideation. Inform the client about available counseling services and support systems. Caution the person to consider carefully who should be informed of the test results. Many individuals have told others about their HIV-positive test, only to experience isolation and discrimination. Help the client explore plans for the future, and advise them to avoid stress, drugs, and infections to maintain optimal health.

Partner Notification/Contact Tracing

Partner notification, also known as *contact tracing,* is an example of a population-level intervention aimed at controlling communicable diseases. Partner notification programs usually occur in conjunction with reportable disease requirements and are carried out by most health departments. It is done by confidentially identifying and notifying exposed individuals of those found to have reportable diseases. This could result in, for example, family members and close contacts of individuals with TB being given a PPD test, which may be administered in the home.

Individuals diagnosed with a reportable STD are asked to provide the names and locations of their partners so that they can be informed of their exposure and obtain the necessary treatment. Clients may be encouraged to notify their partners and to encourage them to seek treatment. If the client agrees to do so, suggestions on how to tell partners and how to deal with possible reactions may be explored. In some instances, clients may feel more comfortable if the nurse notifies those who are exposed. If clients contact their partners about possible infection, the nurse contacts health care providers or clinics to verify the examination of exposed partners.

If the client prefers not to participate in notifying partners, the nurse contacts them—often by a home visit—and counsels them to seek evaluation and treatment. The client is offered literature describing treatment, risk reduction, and the clinic's location and hours of operation. The identity of the infected client who provides the names of sexual and IDU partners cannot be revealed. Maintaining confidentiality is critical with all persons with STDs, but particularly with those who are HIV positive, because discrimination may still occur.

BRIEFLY NOTED

Assessing a client's risk of acquiring an STD should be done with all sexually active individuals. Such risk assessments should be included as baseline assessment data for those attending all clinics and those who receive school health, occupational health, public health, and home nursing services.

TERTIARY PREVENTION

Tertiary prevention can apply to many of the chronic viral STDs and TB. For viral STDs, focus your efforts on managing symptoms and providing psychosocial support regarding future interpersonal relations. Many clients report feeling contaminated, and support groups may be available to help clients cope with chronic STDs.

Observed Therapy

In **directly observed therapy (DOT)** programs for TB medication the nurse observes and documents individual clients taking their TB drugs. When clients prematurely stop taking TB medications, there is a risk of the TB becoming resistant to the medications. This can affect an entire community of people who are susceptible to this airborne disease. Health professionals share in the responsibility of adhering to treatment, and DOT ensures that TB-infected clients have adequate medication. Thus DOT programs are aimed at the population level to prevent antibiotic resistance in the community and to ensure effective treatment at the individual level. Many health departments have DOT home health programs to ensure adequate treatment. Directly observed treatment, short course (DOTS), is a variation applied in specific countries of the world to combat multidrug-resistant TB (World Health Organization, 2007).

The management of AIDS in the home may include monitoring physical status and referring the family to additional care services for maintaining the client in the home. Case management is important in all phases of HIV infection. It is especially important at this stage to ensure that clients have adequate services to meet their needs. This may include ensuring that medication can be obtained by identifying funding resources, maintaining infection control standards, reducing risk behaviors, identifying sources of respite care for caretakers, or referring clients for home or hospice care. Nursing interventions include teaching families about managing symptomatic illness by preventing deteriorating conditions such as diarrhea, skin breakdown, and inadequate nutrition.

Standard Precautions

The importance of teaching caregivers about infection control in home care is vital. Concerns about the transmission of HIV may be expressed by clients, families, friends, and other groups. Whereas fear may be expressed by some, others who are caring for loved ones with HIV may not take adequate precautions such as wearing gloves because of concern about appearing as though they do not want to touch a loved one. Others may believe myths that suggest they cannot be infected by someone they love. Standard Precautions must be taught to caregivers in the home setting. All blood and articles soiled with body fluids must be handled as if they were infectious or contaminated by blood-borne pathogens. Gloves should be worn whenever hands will be expected to touch nonintact skin, mucous membranes, blood, or other fluids. A mask, goggles, and gown should also be worn if there is any potential for splashing or spraying of infectious material during any care. All protective equipment should be worn only once and then disposed of. If the skin or mucous membranes of the caregiver come in contact with body fluids, the skin should be washed with soap and water and the mucous membranes should be flushed with water as soon as possible after the exposure. Thorough hand washing with soap and water—a major infection control measure—should be conducted whenever hands become contaminated and whenever gloves or other protective equipment (mask, gown) are removed. Soiled clothing or linen should be washed in a washing machine filled with hot water using bleach as an additive and should be dried on a hot-air cycle of a dryer.

CLINICAL APPLICATION

Yvonne Jackson is a 20-year-old woman who visits the Hopetown City Health Department's maternity clinic. Examination reveals she is at 14 weeks of gestation. She is single but has been in a steady relationship for the past 6 months with Phil. She states that she has no other children. The HIV test is routinely performed during the initial prenatal visit. The results are positive.

Yvonne is shocked and emotionally distraught about the positive test results. Understanding that Yvonne will not be able to concentrate on all of the questions and information that need to be covered, the nurse sets priorities regarding essential information to obtain and provide during this visit.

A. *List the relevant factors to consider on the basis of this information.*
B. *What questions do you need to ask with regard to controlling the spread of HIV to others?*
C. *What information is most important to give to Yvonne at this time?*
D. *What follow-up does the nurse need to arrange for Yvonne?*

Answers are in the back of the book.

- Nearly all communicable diseases discussed in this chapter are preventable because they are transmitted through specific, known behaviors.
- STDs are among the most serious public health problems in the United States. Not only is there an increased incidence of drug-resistant gonococcal infection, but other STDs, such as HPV (genital warts), HIV, and HSV (genital herpes), are associated with cancer.
- STDs affect certain groups in greater numbers. Factors associated with risk include being younger than 25 years, being a member of a minority group, residing in an urban setting, being impoverished, and using crack cocaine.
- It is important for nurses to educate clients about ways to prevent communicable diseases.
- Many STDs do not produce symptoms in clients.
- Aside from death, the most serious complications caused by STDs are pelvic inflammatory disease, infertility, ectopic pregnancy, neonatal morbidity and mortality, and neoplasia.
- Hepatitis A is often silent in children, and children are a significant source of infection to others.
- The emergence of multidrug-resistant TB has prompted the use of directly observed therapy (DOT) in the United States and other countries to ensure adherence with drug treatment regimens.
- Early detection of communicable diseases is important because it results in early treatment and prevention of additional transmission to others. Treatment includes effective medications, stress reduction, and proper nutrition.
- Partner notification, or contact tracing, is done by identifying, contacting, and ensuring evaluation and treatment of persons exposed to sexual and injectable drug-using partners. Contact tracing is also conducted with TB and HAV.
- Most of the care (both home and outpatient) that is provided for HIV is done within the community setting, which reduces direct health care costs but increases the need for financial support of home and community health services.

WHAT WOULD YOU DO?

1. Identify the number of reported cases of AIDS and the number of reported cases of HIV infection in your community and state (if this is reportable in your state). How are the cases distributed by age, sex, geographic location, and race? How does this rate compare with the national average?
2. Identify the location or locations of HIV testing services in your community. Are the test results anonymous or confidential? Describe how and to whom the results are reported. Do you agree with how this reporting is handled, or would you do it differently if you were in charge? If so, how?
3. Identify counseling and home care services that are available in your community to people with HIV. Are they adequate? What do they cost? Can you see improvements or changes that you would recommend?

4. Form small groups and role-play a nurse–client interaction involving risk assessment and counseling regarding safer sex and injection drug use practices.

■ *REFERENCES*_____

AIDS Education & Training Centers National Resource Center: *Gonorrhea and chlamydia,* 2008, available at http://www.aidsetc.org/aidsetc?page=cm-526_gonorrhea.

American Social Health Association: *Learn about herpes,* 2008. Retrieved May 20, 2008, from ashastd.org/herpes/herpes_learn_symptoms.cfm.

Centers for Disease Control and Prevention: *HIV/AIDS surveillance report* 13(1):12, 2001a.

Centers for Disease Control and Prevention: Revised recommendations for HIV screening of pregnant women, *MMWR Morb Mortal Wkly Rep* 50(RR-10):59–86, 2001b.

Centers for Disease Control and Prevention: Revised guidelines for HIV counseling, testing, and referral, *MMWR Morb Mortal Wkly Rep* 50(RR-19), 2001c.

Centers for Disease Control and Prevention: Heterosexual transmission of HIV—29 states, 1999-2002, *MMWR Morb Mortal Wkly Rep* 53(6), 2004.

Centers for Disease Control and Prevention: *Genital herpes fact sheet,* 2005a, available at http://www.cdc.gov/std/herpes/std-fact_herpes.htm.

Centers for Disease Control and Prevention: *Hepatitis B prevention,* 2005b, available at www.cdc.gov/ncidod/diseases/hepatitis/msw/hbv_wsw_fact.htm.

Centers for Disease Control and Prevention: *Basic facts about condoms and their use in preventing HIV infection and other STDs,* 2005c, available at www.thebody.com/cdc/factcond.html.

Centers for Disease Control and Prevention: Sexually transmitted diseases treatment guidelines 2006, *MMWR Morb Mortal Wkly Rep* 55:(RR-11), 2006a.

Centers for Disease Control and Prevention: Twenty-five years of HIV/AIDS—United States, 1981–2006, *MMWR Morb Mortal Wkly Rep* 55(21)189–193, 2006b.

Centers for Disease Control and Prevention: Surveillance for acute viral hepatitis—United States, 2005, *MMWR Morb Mortal Wkly Rep* 56(SS03)1–24, 2007a.

Centers for Disease Control and Prevention: Update: prevention of hepatitis A after exposure to hepatitis A virus and international travelers. Updated recommendations of the advisory committee on immunizations practices-United States, 2007, *MMWR Morb Mortal Wkly Rep* 41:1080–1084, 2007b.

Centers for Disease Control and Prevention: *Chlamydia—CDC fact sheet,* 2008a, available at http://www.cdc.gov/std/chlamydia/STDFact-Chlamydia.htm.

Centers for Disease Control and Prevention: *Gonorrhea—CDC fact sheet,* 2008b, available at http://www.cdc.gov/std/Gonorrhea/STDFact-gonorrhea.htm.

Centers for Disease Control and Prevention: *HIV/AIDS surveillance report, 2006,* vol 18, Atlanta, 2008c, U.S. Department of Health and Human Services, Centers for Disease Control and Prevention.

Centers for Disease Control and Prevention: *Pelvic inflammatory disease—CDC fact sheet,* 2008d, available at http://www.cdc.gov/std/PID/STDFact-PID.htm.

Centers for Disease Control and Prevention: *Pregnancy and hepatitis B: frequently asked questions,* 2008e, available at http://www.cdc.gov/ncidod/diseases/hepatitis/b/faqb-pregnancy.htm.

Centers for Disease Control and Prevention: *Syphilis: fact sheet,* 2008f, available at http://www.cdc.gov/std/syphilis/STDFact-Syphilis.htm#cure.

Centers for Disease Control and Prevention: *Viral hepatitis C: fact sheet,* 2008g, available at http://www.cdc.gov/ncidod/diseases/hepatitis/c/fact.htm.

Centers for Disease Control and Prevention: *Viral hepatitis C: frequently asked questions about hepatitis C,* 2008h, available at http://www.cdc.gov/ncidod/diseases/hepatitis/c/faq.htm#1a.

Centers for Disease Control and Prevention: *MMWR Morb Mortal Wkly Rep,* Synopsis for March 20, 2008. World TB Day. Press release, 2008i.

Centers for Disease Control and Prevention: *Estimate of new HIV infections in the United States-CDC HIV/AIDS facts,* 2008j. Retrieved March 25, 2009, from http://www.cdc.gov/hiv/topics/surveillance/resources/factsheets/pdf/incidence.pdf.

Centers for Disease Control and Prevention: *Viral hepatitis A: frequently asked questions about hepatitis A,* 2008k. Retrieved January 15, 2009, from http://www.cdc.gov/hepatitis/HAV/HAVfaq.htm#protection.

Centers for Disease Control and Prevention: *Viral hepatitis-testing and public health management of persons with chronic hepatitis B virus infection,* 2008l. Retrieved January 15, 2009, from http://www.cdc.gov/hepatitis/HBV/TestingChronic.htm.

Centers for Disease Control and Prevention: *Trends in reportable sexually transmitted diseases in the United States, 2007. National surveillance data for Chlamydia, gonorrhea, and syphilis,* 2009a. Retrieved January 15, 2009, from http://www.cdc.gov/STD/stats07/trends.htm.

Centers for Disease Control and Prevention: *Trends in tuberculosis—United States,* 2008, *MMWR Morb Mortal Wkly* 58(10): 249-253, 2009b.

Centers for Disease Control and Prevention: Updated guidelines for the use of nucleic acid amplification tests in the diagnosis of tuberculosis-United States, 2009, *MMWR Morb Mortal Wkly Rep* 58(01):7–10, 2009c.

Centers for Disease Control and Prevention: *Reports of health concerns following HPV vaccination,* 2009d. Retrieved March 25, 2009, from http://www.cdc.gov.vaccines.

Chin J: *Control of communicable diseases manual,* Washington, DC, 2000, American Public Health Association.

Corey L, Wald A: Genital herpes. In Holmes KK, et al, editors: *Sexually transmitted diseases,* New York, 1999, McGraw-Hill.

Division of STD Prevention: *Sexually transmitted disease surveillance—2006 ,* Atlanta, 2007, CDC.

Gandhi M: *Medical encyclopedia: AIDS,* Washington, DC, 2006, U.S. National Library of Medicine and the National Institutes of Health.

Harkness GA: Hepatitis C: the "silent stalker," *Am J Nurs* 103(9): 24–25, 2003.

Health Resources and Services Administration: *AIDS drug assistance program (ADAP),* 2008, available at http://hab.hrsa.gov/treatmentmodernization/partb.htm#ADAP.

Heymann D: *Control of communicable diseases manual,* Washington, DC, 2004, American Public Health Association.

March of Dimes: *Genital herpes and pregnancy,* 2005, available at http://www.marchofdimes.com/professionals/14332_1201.asp.

National Institute of Allergy and Infectious Diseases: *Sexually transmitted infections,* 2007, available at http://www3.niaid.nih.gov/healthscience/healthtopics/sti/default.htm.

National Institute of Allergy and Infectious Diseases: *Herpevac trial for women: about herpes.* Retrieved June 17, 2008, from http://www.niaid.nih.gov/dmid/stds/herpevac/about_herpes.htm.

Occupational Safety and Health Administration: *Occupational exposure to bloodborne pathogens,* Richmond, Va, 1992, Department of Labor and Industry.

Phillips I: Beta-lactamase producing, penicillin-resistant gonococcus, *Lancet* 2:656, 1976.

Ruppert R: Tuberculosis today: fighting an ancient adversary, *Am Nurse Today* 2(11):32–36, 2007.

Stark SW: The aging face of HIV/AIDS, *Am Nurse Today* 2(6): 30–34, 2007.

U.S. Department of Health and Human Services: *Healthy People 2010: understanding and improving health,* ed 2, Washington, DC, 2000, U.S. Government Printing Office.

U.S. Department of Health and Human Services: *The Ryan White HIV/AIDS program: a living history, toward passage – 1990.* Retrieved May 20, 2008, from http://hab.hrsa.gov/livinghistory/timeline/1986-1990/1990.html.

U.S. Department of Health and Human Services: *Tuberculosis.* Retrieved June 18, 2008, from http://www.hhs.gov/tb/.

Villaruel AM, Jemmott LS, Jemmott JB: Designing a culturally based intervention to reduce HIV sexual risk for Latino adolescents, *J Assoc Nurses AIDS Care* 16(12):23–31, 2005.

Wise M et al: Changing trends in hepatitis-C related mortality in the United States, 1995–2004, *Hepatology* 47(4):1128–1135, 2008.

World Health Organization: *Tuberculosis: fact sheet,* 2007, available at http://www.who.int/mediacentre/factsheets/fs104/en/index.html.

PART VII

Nursing Practice in the Community: Roles and Functions

Chapter 28

Nursing Practice at the Local, State, and National Levels in Public Health

Diane B. Downing

ADDITIONAL RESOURCES

These related resources are found either in the appendix at the back of this book or on the book's website at http://evolve.elsevier.com/stanhope/foundations.

Appendix
- Appendix E.3: The Health Insurance Portability and Accountability Act (HIPAA): What Does It Mean for Public Health Nurses?

Evolve Website
- Community Assessment Applied
- Case Study, with questions and answers
- Quiz review questions
- WebLinks, including link to *Healthy People 2010* website

OBJECTIVES

After reading this chapter, the student should be able to:

1. Define public health, public health nursing, and local, state, and national roles.
2. Identify trends in public health nursing.
3. Describe examples of public health nursing roles.
4. Discuss emerging public health issues that affect public health nursing practice.
5. Describe collaborative partnerships for nursing.
6. Identify educational preparation of public health nurses and competencies necessary to practice.
7. Demonstrate understanding of team concepts in public health settings.

CHAPTER OUTLINE

ROLES OF LOCAL, STATE, AND FEDERAL PUBLIC HEALTH AGENCIES

HISTORY AND TRENDS OF PUBLIC HEALTH

SCOPE, STANDARDS, AND ROLES OF NURSING IN PUBLIC HEALTH

ISSUES AND TRENDS IN PUBLIC HEALTH

EDUCATION AND KNOWLEDGE REQUIREMENTS FOR PUBLIC HEALTH NURSES

CERTIFICATION FOR NURSES IN PUBLIC AND COMMUNITY HEALTH

NATIONAL HEALTH OBJECTIVES

FUNCTIONS OF PUBLIC HEALTH NURSES

The authors wish to thank Mary Eure Fisher for her foundational work on this chapter.

KEY TERMS

advocate: one who works to protect the rights of the client while supporting the client's responsibility for self-determination.

assessor: a health professional who uses data in a systematic way to help identify needs, questions to be addressed, abilities, and available resources.

case manager: a nurse who works to enhance continuity and provide appropriate care for clients whose health problems are actually or potentially chronic and complex.

community health: meeting collective needs by identifying problems and managing behaviors within the community and between the community and the larger society.

disaster responders: people who work as members of a team in a disaster to feed back information to relief workers to facilitate rapid rescue and recovery.

educator: a nurse who provides information to clients or staff for the purpose of facilitating learning.

federal public health agencies: federal level government agencies that develop regulations that implement policies formulated by Congress and provide a significant amount of funding to state and territorial health agencies for public health activities.

local public health agencies: the agencies responsible for implementing and enforcing local, state, and federal public health codes and ordinances and providing essential public health programs to a community.

outreach workers: health workers who make a special, focused effort to find people with specific health problems for the purpose of increasing their access to health services.

primary caregivers: health care professionals who are primarily responsible for providing for the health care needs of clients.

public health: organized efforts designed to fulfill society's interest in ensuring conditions in which people can be healthy.

public health nursing: "the practice of promoting and protecting the health of populations using knowledge from nursing, social, and public health sciences" (APHA Public Health Nursing Section, 1996, p. 1).

public health programs: programs designed with the goal of improving a population's health status.

referral resource: an agency or source in the community with whom nurses communicate and to which clients are sent for assistance.

role model: a person who is an example of professional or personal behavior for others.

state public health agency: each of the U.S. states and territories has a single identified official state public health agency, managed by a state health commissioner.

All public health involves partnerships. **Public health programs** are designed with the goal of improving a population's health status. They go beyond the administration of health care to include the following:
- Community health assessment
- Analysis of health statistics
- Public education
- Outreach
- Record keeping
- Professional education for providers
- Surveillance
- Compliance to regulations for some institutions and/or agencies and school systems
- Follow-up of population health problems
  The following are examples requiring follow-up care:
- Persons with active, untreated tuberculosis
- Pregnant women who have not kept prenatal visits
- Underimmunized children

Public health programs are frequently implemented by the development of partnerships or coalitions with other providers, agencies, and groups in the location being served. Nurses are involved in these activities in various ways depending on the public health agency (local, state, or federal) and the identified needs.

Public health is not a branch of medicine; it is an organized community approach designed to prevent disease, promote health, and protect populations. It works across many disciplines and is based on the scientific core of epidemiology (Institute of Medicine, 1988; Centers for Disease Control and Prevention, 2005). Nurses in public health work with multidisciplinary teams of people both within the public health areas and in other human services agencies. A critical partnership that shapes public health in the United States is the interaction of local, state, and federal agencies.

ROLES OF LOCAL, STATE, AND FEDERAL PUBLIC HEALTH AGENCIES

In the United States, the local–state–federal partnership includes federal agencies, the state and territorial public health agencies, and the 3200 local public health agencies. The interaction of these agencies is critical to effectively use precious resources, financial and personnel, and to address the health of populations. Nurses working in all of these agencies work together to identify, develop, and implement interventions that will improve and maintain the nation's health.

Federal public health agencies develop regulations that implement policies formulated by Congress and provide a significant amount of funding to state and territorial health agencies to do the following (Institute of Medicine, 1988, 2003):
- Provide public health activities
- Survey the nation's health status and health needs

Box 28-1	**Public Health Agency Functions**

Generally, local public health agencies perform the following functions:
- Provide and disseminate health information
- Provide leadership in health planning
- Provide essential public health and environmental services
- Analyze statistics on births to monitor community health status
- File a certificate for every birth or death in that area

- Set practices and standards
- Provide expertise that facilitates evidence-based practice
- Coordinate public health activities that cross state lines
- Support health services research

The U.S. Department of Health and Human Services (US-DHHS) and the Environmental Protection Agency (EPA) are the federal agencies that most influence public health activities at the state and local levels. The USDHHS includes the Centers for Disease Control and Prevention (CDC), the Health Resources and Services Administration (HRSA), the Agency for Healthcare, Research and Quality (AHRQ), and the Food and Drug Administration (FDA). The USDHHS is the agency that facilitates development of the nation's *Healthy People* objectives (U.S. Department of Health and Human Services, 2000).

Each of the states and territories has a single identified official **state public health agency** that is managed by a state health commissioner. The structure of state public health agencies varies. Some states require that the state health commissioner be a physician. A growing number of states do not limit the position to physicians but, rather, require specific public health experience. California, Maryland, Iowa, Washington, and Michigan are examples of states that focus on public health experience as a requirement for the state health commissioner position. This allows for the appointments of nurses and other professionals to this position. State public health agencies are responsible for monitoring health status and enforcing laws and regulations that protect and improve the public's health. These agencies receive funding from federal agencies for the implementation of public health interventions. The following are examples:
- Communicable disease programs
- Maternal and child health programs
- Chronic disease prevention programs
- Injury prevention programs

The agencies distribute federal and state funds to the local public health agencies to implement programs at the community level, and they provide oversight and consultation for local public health agencies. State health agencies also delegate some public health powers, such as the power to quarantine, to local health officers.

Local public health agencies have responsibilities that vary depending on the locality, but they are the agencies that are responsible for implementing and enforcing local, state, and federal public health codes and ordinances and providing essential public health programs to a community. The goal of the local public health department is to safeguard the public's health and to improve the community's health status. The health department's authority is delegated by the state for specific functions (Box 28-1). As with state health departments, some states require that local health directors be physicians, whereas others focus on public health experience. For example, public health nurses in Maryland, Washington, Wisconsin, and California hold local health director positions. The duties of local health departments vary depending on the state and local public health codes and ordinances and the responsibilities assigned by the state and local governments. Usually, the local public health department provides for the administration, regulatory oversight, public health, and environmental services for a geographic area.

The majority of local, state, and federal public health agencies will be involved in the following:
- Collecting and analyzing vital statistics
- Providing health education and information to the population served
- Receiving reports about and investigating and controlling communicable diseases
- Protecting the environment to reduce the risk to health
- Providing some health services to particular populations at risk or with limited access to care (local public health agencies, guided by state and federal policies and goals and community needs)
- Planning for and responding to natural and man-made disasters and emergencies
- Identifying public health problems for at-risk and high-risk populations
- Conducting community assessments to identify community assets and gaps
- Partnering with other organizations to develop and implement responses to identified public health concerns

Nurses in public health work for local, state, and federal agencies. They work in partnership with each other, other public health staff, other governmental agencies, and the community to fulfill the functions of providing some health services to individuals, families, and groups who may have limited access to health care. They also engage in case finding to identify persons at risk for disease and/or being lost to the health care system.

Other public health agency staffs include the following:
- Physicians
- Nutritionists
- Environmental health professionals
- Health educators
- Various laboratory workers
- Epidemiologists
- Health planners
- Paraprofessional home visitors
- **Outreach workers**

Examples of community-based organizations include the following:
- The United Way
- The American Red Cross
- Free clinics

- Head Start programs
- Day care centers
- Community health centers
- Hospitals
- Senior centers
- Advocacy groups
- Churches
- Academic institutions
- Businesses

Other government agencies include the fire and emergency services department, law enforcement agencies, schools, parks and recreation departments, and elected officials. Changes in local, state, and federal governments affect public health services, and nursing has to develop strategies for dealing with these changes. To meet the changing needs of a community, nurses must identify public health concerns and work in programs to provide needed services.

HISTORY AND TRENDS OF PUBLIC HEALTH

A person born today can expect to live 30 years longer than a person born in 1900. Medical care accounts for 5 years of that increase, but public health is responsible for the additional 25 years through prevention efforts brought about by changes in social policies, community actions, and individual and group changes in behavior (U.S. Department of Health and Human Services, 2000). Historically, nurses working in public health were valued by and important to society and functioned in an autonomous setting. They worked with populations and in settings that were not of interest to other health care disciplines or groups. Much public health service was delivered to the poor and to women and children, who did not have political power or voice. During the course of the twentieth century, public health responsibilities expanded beyond communicable disease prevention, occupational health, and environmental health programs to include reproductive health, chronic disease prevention, and injury prevention activities.

As a result of Medicaid managed care, many public health agencies were no longer providing personal health care services. Public health agencies began to shift emphasis from a focus on primary health care services to a focus on core public health activities such as the investigation and control of diseases and injuries, community health assessment, community health planning, and involvement in environmental health activities. As the twentieth century came to a close, genetics, newly emerging communicable diseases, preventing bioterrorism and violence, and handling and disposing of hazardous waste were emerging as additional public health issues (Centers for Disease Control and Prevention, 2002).

The Institute of Medicine (IOM, 2003) identified the following seven priorities for public health in the twenty-first century:

- Understand and emphasize the broad determinants of health
- Develop a policy focus on population health

- Strengthen the public health infrastructure
- Build partnerships
- Develop systems of accountability
- Emphasize evidence-based practice
- Enhance communication (Institute of Medicine, 2003)

BRIEFLY NOTED

Changes are occurring and will continue to occur in public health nursing. Public health nurses have to learn to function in an environment that must deal with many changes, as changes occur continually because of the many internal and external factors from people, programs, politics, and the unknown, as well as known local, state, and federal actions. Which skills help the public health nurse adapt to changes?

Public health activities at the beginning of the twenty-first century were shaped by the September 11, 2001, airplane attacks of the World Trade Center, the Pentagon, and a field in Pennsylvania, in which thousands were murdered. However, public health activities at the federal, state, and local levels were even more dramatically affected by a series of anthrax exposures that occurred shortly after the airplane attacks. In addition to anthrax exposures in Florida and New York, a month after the plane attacks, thousands of workers at the Brentwood Post Office and the Senate Building in Washington, D.C., were exposed to an especially virulent strain of anthrax from a contaminated letter. The anthrax exposures alerted policymakers to the weakening public health infrastructure required to respond to bioterrorism events.

By the end of the twentieth century, resources for communicable disease services had decreased as surveillance and containment activities and protection of water and food supplies produced decreasing rates of communicable disease. Nurses in public health are facing issues such as unprecedented influenza, tetanus, and childhood vaccine shortages and emerging infections that compete with bioterrorism activities for resources. As an example, in 2008 a pertussis epidemic occurred in the United States.

During the twentieth century, public health nurses were a major force in the nation, achieving immunization rates that accounted for the dramatic decrease in measles. In 1996, nearly 900,000 fewer cases of measles were reported than in 1941 (Turnock, 2004). However, the general public was not informed about how this immunization activity was accomplished or about its effect on improving health and lowering health care cost. For public health services to receive adequate funding, it is necessary for the public and the government to be aware of the benefits provided to a community by nurses. A prime example of emerging infectious diseases is the severe acute respiratory syndrome (SARS), caused by a virus, that brought illness and death to many in 2003. The disease spread quickly from China to other countries, being transported by airline passengers traveling internationally.

BRIEFLY NOTED

Many of the epidemics of the future will be defined by social problems such as substance abuse, teen pregnancy, lack of jobs, lack of affordable housing, as well as newly identified communicable diseases such as SARS and avian flu.

SCOPE, STANDARDS, AND ROLES OF NURSING IN PUBLIC HEALTH

In 1920, C.E.A. Winslow defined **public health** as "the science and art of preventing disease, prolonging life and promoting health and efficiency through organized community effort" (Turnock, 2004, p. 9). This definition is still used in public health textbooks because it focuses on the relationship between social conditions and health across all levels of society. Nursing practice in public health focuses on the individuals, families, and groups in areas in which nurses live, work, and play. Nurses educated as public health nurses work with communities and populations.

Additional knowledge, skills, and aptitudes are necessary for a nurse to go beyond focusing on the health needs of the individual to focusing on the health needs of populations (see Chapter 1). This additional knowledge distinguishes the public health nurse from the nurses in community health and others who are practicing in the community setting. Nursing practice in **community health** is the synthesis of nursing theory and public health theory applied to promoting, preserving, and maintaining the health of populations through the delivery of personal health care services to individuals, families, and groups. The focus of practice is the health of individuals, families, and groups. Care is provided within the context of preventing disease and disability and promoting and protecting the health of the community as a whole.

A variety of settings and a diversity of perspectives are available to nurses interested in developing a career in public health. Nurses working at the federal, state, and local levels integrate community involvement and knowledge about the entire population with clinical understandings of the health and illness experiences of individuals and families in the population. They translate and articulate the health and illness experiences of diverse, often vulnerable individuals and families in the population to health planners and policymakers, and they help members of the community voice their problems and aspirations. Nurses are knowledgeable about multiple strategies for intervention, focusing primarily on those for the family and the individual. They translate knowledge from the health and social sciences to individuals and population groups through targeted interventions, programs, and advocacy. Nurses are directly engaged in the interdisciplinary activities of the core public health functions of assessment, assurance, and policy development. In any setting, the role of the nurse focuses on the prevention of illness, injury, or disability and on the promotion and maintenance of the health of populations (Public Health Nursing Section, 2001).

Nurses in public health deliver services within the framework of ever-constricting resources coupled with emerging and complex public health issues. This requires the efficient, equitable, and evidence-based use of resources. The National Public Health Performance Standards Program (Centers for Disease Control and Prevention, 2004), a federal, state, and local partnership, has developed evaluation instruments that can be used to collect and analyze data on the programs provided through state and local public health systems. The instruments link with the 10 essential services of public health that define the core functions of public health (see Chapter 1).

Nurses make a significant difference in improving the health of a community by monitoring and assessing critical health status indicators such as the following:
• Immunization levels
• Infant mortality rates
• Communicable diseases

On the basis of their assessment and in partnership with the community, nurses advocate for evidence-based interventions to respond to negative health status indicators. Nurses provide the link for people who need personal health services and ensure health care when it is needed and not available elsewhere (U.S. Department of Health and Human Services, 2000).

A shift in the focus of public health from being the primary care provider of last resort to developing partnerships to meet the health promotion and disease prevention needs of populations in a community has raised concerns about available health care for the uninsured and underinsured. The nurses' role in this ongoing shift in health care delivery is still being developed for many agencies. Nurses retain responsibility for ensuring that all populations have access to affordable, quality health care services. They accomplish this by:
• Providing clinical preventive services to certain high-risk populations.
• Establishing programs and services to meet special needs.
• Recommending clinical care and other services to clients and their families in clinics, homes, and the community.
• Providing referrals through community links to needed care.
• Participating in community provider coalitions and meetings to educate others and to identify service centers for community populations.
• Providing clinical surveillance and identification of communicable disease.

Case management at the community level is a renewed effort in nursing. Through case management activities, nurses link persons with needed health care providers (see Chapter 13).

Uninsured individuals seek services on a sliding payment scale from sources such as university clinics, public hospital clinics, neighborhood health centers, or one of the variety of free clinics. Nurses serve as a bridge between these populations and the resource needs for this at-risk group by approaching health care providers on behalf of individuals

Levels of Prevention	Related to Nurses in Public Health

PRIMARY PREVENTION

- Partner with the community to conduct a community health assessment to identify community assets and gaps.
- Partner with the community to develop programs in response to identified gaps.
- Provide information about safe-sex practices.
- Educate day care centers and families about the dangers of lead-based paint.
- Educate day care centers, schools, and the general community about the importance of hand hygiene to prevent transmission of communicable diseases.
- Inspect day care centers, nursing homes, and hospitals to ensure client safety and quality of care.
- Advocate for issues such as mandatory seatbelt legislation, smoke-free environments, and universal access to health care.
- Provide no-charge infant car seats accompanied by classes in the use of safety seats.
- Identify environmental hazards such as housing quality, playground safety, pedestrian safety, and product safety hazards, and work with the community and policymakers to mitigate the identified hazards.
- Conduct ongoing disease surveillance for communicable diseases.

SECONDARY PREVENTION

- Identify and treat clients in a sexually transmitted disease clinic.
- Identify and treat clients in a tuberculosis clinic.
- Provide directly observed therapy (DOT) for clients with active tuberculosis.
- Conduct contacting and tracing for individuals exposed to a client with an active case of tuberculosis or a sexually transmitted disease.
- Conduct lead-screening activities for children.
- Implement screening programs for genetic disorders and metabolic deficiencies in newborns; breast, cervical, and testicular cancer; diabetes; hypertension; and sensory impairments in children, and ensure follow-up services for clients with positive results.
- Implement control measures when an outbreak is identified.

TERTIARY PREVENTION

- Provide case management services that link clients with chronic illnesses to health care and community support services.
- Provide case management services that link clients with serious mental illnesses to mental health and community support services.

seeking medical and/or health services and keeping the needs of this population on the political agenda. Frequently, low-income populations or populations with multiple chronic illnesses lack the knowledge and skills to negotiate the complex health care system. This population needs the following:

- Education and training in identifying their problems
- Approaches to self-care
- Illness prevention strategies
- Lifestyle choices that will have an effect on their health

The nurse understands the barriers these populations confront, such as transportation and difficulty understanding and following health care provider instructions.

Although vulnerable populations have always benefited from nursing services, the populations that are most acutely in need of public health services have changed dramatically over the past two decades. Of particular concern are the number of young women and their partners who are substance abusers and have risky behaviors that put their pregnancy or children at high risk of injury or abuse. Nurses at the federal, state, and local levels have developed innovative, collaborative approaches to prepare staff to work effectively with this population.

ISSUES AND TRENDS IN PUBLIC HEALTH

The discovery and development of antibiotics in the 1940s, coupled with immunization programs and improvements in sanitation, contributed to the decrease in infectious disease-related morbidity and mortality during the twentieth century (Centers for Disease Control and Prevention, 2002). Twenty-first century issues facing nurses in public health include the following:

- Increasing rates of drug resistance to community-acquired pathogens
- Social issues such as welfare reform
- Racial and ethnic disparities in health outcomes
- Behaviorally influenced issues (e.g., chronic diseases, violence in society, substance abuse)
- Emergency preparedness activities
- Unequal access to health care

Nurses must keep abreast of the issues that affect all of society. Assessments need to be changed to include the factors that affect the populations they serve.

For example, a major twenty-first century public health challenge is emerging infections resulting from drug-resistant organisms. The widespread, often inappropriate, use of antimicrobial drugs has resulted in a loss of effectiveness for some community-acquired infections such as gonorrhea, pneumococcal infections, and tuberculosis (TB) and increasing rates of drug resistance in community-acquired pathogens such as *Streptococcus pneumonia, Escherichia coli,* and *Salmonella* spp. (Rubin, 2001). The nurse can influence this trend by objecting to inappropriate use of antibiotics by providers and educating individuals, families, health care providers, and the community about the dangers of misuse and overuse of antibiotics.

Social issues such as welfare reform will influence a population's ability to obtain preventive health services either because they lose government-sponsored health care coverage or because the low-wage jobs they take do not allow time off for health care.

When childcare is an issue for the welfare mother returning to work, effects on the individual, family, community, and population must be considered. Nurses assess the problem and determine what is wrong with a system that forces parents to go to work so they can be removed from welfare rolls but that does not provide for childcare. The question to be answered by a nurse is "What will it take to change the system?"

Partnerships and collaboration among groups are much more powerful in making change than the individual client and nurse working alone. As another example, the depressed, nonfunctional mother in need of counseling is a significant public health concern because the needs of the mother, children, and family are not being met. Frequently, the problem may not be obvious to the health professional who sees this woman for the first time. Nurses have special preparation to help them both identify the individual's problem and look at its effects on the broader community. In this example, consider the following:

• The children may grow to be adults with mental health problems.
• The mental health services of the community services will need to be able to handle the increase in this population.
• Children may become violent adults, resulting in a need for more correction facilities.
• Mothers may need additional mental health services.
• Children may be absent from school often and may not be able to contribute to society.
• Adults may be nonproductive in the workplace because absence from school leads to lack of skills.

Often, one problem of the single individual places great burdens on the community.

Healthy People 2010 includes objectives to address racial and ethnic disparities in health outcomes (U.S. Department of Health and Human Services, 2000). The Institute of Medicine (2002) reports that disparities in health care treatment account for some of the gaps in health outcomes between racial and ethnic groups. This report found that minority groups receive lower-quality health care than white people do, regardless of insurance status, income, and severity of the condition. Nurses work as case managers and at the policy level to promote equal access to health care, including health literature and spoken services that reflect the community in which the services are being delivered. The nurse working directly as a case manager or in a clinic setting can promote culturally and linguistically appropriate services by partnering with other community agencies such as interpreter services. Equal access to health care can be facilitated by identifying and alerting the community to gaps in services available in the community. For example, some communities may appear to have an adequate number of pediatricians to meet the community's needs. However, a community assessment may reveal that the community is home to a high number of children who rely on Medicaid as payment for services or to families whose primary language is not English. Matching this information with the pediatrician population may reveal that none of the pediatricians accepts Medicaid as payment for services or that they all deliver services in English only.

EDUCATION AND KNOWLEDGE REQUIREMENTS FOR PUBLIC HEALTH NURSES

The Association of Community Health Nursing Educators states that the educational preparation of community health nurses should be at least a baccalaureate degree. Those who have associate degrees are encouraged to seek further degrees because of the increasing complexity of better care delivery in public health.

The Council on Linkages Between Academia and Public Health Practice (2001) examined a decade of work to identify a list of core public health competencies that represent a set of skills, knowledge, and attitudes necessary for the broad practice of public health. They capture the crosscutting competencies necessary for all disciplines that work in public health, including nurses, physicians, environmental health specialists, health educators, and epidemiologists. The competencies are applied (at the three skill levels of *aware, knowledgeable,* and *proficient*) to three job categories of frontline staff, senior-level staff, and supervisory and management staff. A detailed list of core competencies by job category and skill level is available at http://www.TrainingFinder.org/competencies (see Appendix H.3). In addition to having the core public health competencies, public health nurses have specialized competencies as described in the *Scope and Standards of Public Health Nursing Practice* (American Nurses Association, 2007). The core public health competencies are divided into the following eight domains:

1. Analytic assessment skills
2. Basic public health sciences skills
3. Cultural competency skills
4. Communication skills
5. Community dimensions of practice skills
6. Financial planning and management skills
7. Leadership and systems thinking skills
8. Policy development and program planning skills

Many of these core public health competencies are provided by nurses who have learned these skills in the workplace while gaining knowledge through years of practice. Rapid changes in public health are providing a challenge to nurses in that neither the time nor the staff is available to provide as much on-the-job training as is needed to learn and upgrade skills and knowledge of staff. Nurses with baccalaureate or master's preparation are needed to provide a strong public health system (see Chapter 1).

CERTIFICATION FOR NURSES IN PUBLIC AND COMMUNITY HEALTH

One level of certification is available for nurses working in community health. The examination is offered through the American Nurses' Credentialing Center. Although certification is voluntary, being recognized as competent in a specialty area indicates to clients and employers that the nurse has the knowledge and skills essential to **public health**

nursing practice. The nurse who is certified focuses on a holistic approach to care of the total population, including the promotion and maintenance of health, health education, case management, coordination, and the provision of continuity of care. Individuals eligible to take the certification examination must be a registered nurse and licensed in the United States or its territories, have a baccalaureate degree in nursing with a masters or higher degree in public health, and have a minimum of 500 hours of faculty-supervised practice in public health nursing. The preferred credentials for certification are a registered nurse license, a masters, postmasters, or doctorate degree in nursing, and 500 hours of faculty-supervised clinical practice in the specialty. Nurses are examined on topics such as foundations of public health, human development, epidemiology, biostatistics, evaluation and research, assessment, health promotion and disease prevention, population and community education, health systems, and leadership. Nurses are recognized as advanced practice public health nurses (American Nurses Credentialing Center, 2008).

CASE STUDY

Four-year-old David had a near-sudden infant death episode when he was 4 months old. His father was able to revive David with cardiopulmonary resuscitation (CPR) but not before his brain had become anoxic. David was left a blind quadriplegic with little or no ability to communicate even after having spent many months in a hospital.

When nurse Margaret Moore first started visiting David, he was receiving tube feedings and personal care from his mother. (His father had left the home, saying he could not stand seeing his son in this debilitated state.) David's mother, Brandy Johnson, received emotional support from her mother and sister, who stopped by when they could. David was enrolled three mornings a week in a special education program for children with cerebral palsy and other severe disabilities. Those mornings Ms. Johnson worked at a minimum wage job bagging groceries. Some days she made extra money caring for a niece after school in her home. The rest of the time she cared for David; her only outlet was to write mournful poetry when he slept.

Ms. Moore's visits involved checking David's physical status and determining what care and support the two needed. One week she realized that David was getting too big for his car seat since he had grown to 45 pounds, yet regular car seats assumed that a child that size could sit by himself. She had to find a source and some funding for the specially adapted $250 car seat he needed.

Ms. Moore worried about Ms. Johnson's mental health given that she was a young woman alone, with no car, and unable to have the normal experiences of a young woman. The nurse found a community support group for parents of disabled children, located on the bus line, in which parents could share their experiences with one another. She also found a group that met once a month that was interested in poetry writing. Ms. Johnson had trouble getting her calls returned from the program in which she needed to enroll David to get some help caring for her son. Ms. Moore also got no response to her calls to that agency, so she made a visit in person; she was able to get David enrolled quickly.

Created by Deborah C. Conway

NATIONAL HEALTH OBJECTIVES

Since 1979, the U.S. surgeon general has worked with local, state, and federal agencies, the private sector, and the U.S. population to develop health objectives for the nation. These objectives are revisited every 10 years. In 2000, the USDHHS released *Healthy People 2010: Understanding and Improving Health.* These objectives will guide the work of public health nurses over the next decade.

State health departments play a key role in implementing the *Healthy People* objectives. Examples of state *Healthy People 2010* goals can be located on the Public Health Foundation website at www.phf.org. State health departments help set local goals using the *Healthy People 2010* objectives as a framework. Knowing that public health departments do not have the resources to accomplish these goals independently, collaboration is essential to quality nursing practice and is encouraged at the local level with existing groups. New partnerships are developed related to specific goals. Communities develop coalitions to address selected objectives, based on community needs, to include all of the local community stakeholders such as social services, mental health, education, recreation, government, and businesses. Membership varies from community to community depending on that community's formal and informal structure. The groups join the coalition for a variety of reasons. For example, businesses see the value of developing a productive workforce that will be of importance to them and the community in the future.

The *Healthy People 2010* objectives are developed to achieve the two major goals of increasing quality and years of healthy life and eliminating health disparities (U.S. Department of Health and Human Services, 2000). Nurses help clients identify unhealthy behaviors and then help them develop strategies to improve their health. Some of the behaviors addressed by nurses are tobacco use, physical activity, and nutritional habits that lead to obesity, all of which affect quality and years of healthy life. Nurses also organize the community to conduct community health assessments to identify where health disparities exist and to target interventions to address those disparities. For example, community health assessments may disclose that certain populations are at higher risk for the following:

- Asthma
- Diabetes
- Low immunization rates
- High cigarette smoking behavior
- Exposure to environmental hazards

●Healthy People 2010

Objectives to Improve Pregnancy Outcomes

9-1 Increase the proportion of pregnancies that are intended

9-2 Reduce the proportion of births occurring within 24 months of a previous birth

9-3 Increase the proportion of females at risk of unintended pregnancy (and their partners) who use contraception

9-4 Reduce the proportion of females experiencing pregnancy despite use of a reversible contraceptive method

9-5 Increase the proportion of health care providers who provide emergency contraception

9-6 Increase male involvement in pregnancy prevention and family planning efforts

9-7 Reduce pregnancies among adolescent females

9-8 Increase the proportion of adolescents who have never engaged in sexual intercourse before age 15 years

9-9 Increase the proportion of adolescents who have never engaged in sexual intercourse

9-10 Increase the proportion of sexually active, unmarried adolescents aged 15 to 17 years who use contraception that both effectively prevents pregnancy and provides barrier protection against disease

9-11 Increase the proportion of young adults who have received formal instruction before turning age 18 years on reproductive health issues, including all of the following topics: birth control methods, safer sex to prevent HIV, prevention of sexually transmitted diseases, and abstinence

9-12 Reduce the proportion of married couples whose ability to conceive or maintain a pregnancy is impaired

9-13 Increase the proportion of health insurance policies that cover contraceptive supplies and services

From U.S. Department of Health and Human Services: *Healthy People 2010: understanding and improving health,* ed 2, Washington, DC, 2000, U.S. Government Printing Office.

The following are some *Healthy People 2010* communicable disease areas of focus:
- Vaccine-preventable infectious diseases
- Emerging antimicrobial resistance
- Human immunodeficiency virus (HIV)
- Acquired immunodeficiency syndrome (AIDS)
- Sexually transmitted diseases (STDs)

To help clients reduce their risk of acquiring a communicable disease, nurses provide clients with instructions on the use of barrier methods of contraception and information on the hazards of multiple sexual partners and street drug use. Getting a complete sexual history on all clients coming to the health department for services takes special skills but is essential to determine the behaviors that have brought the client to the local health department. Abstinence as a birth control method can be addressed with all populations. Education of young persons before they become sexually active has helped reduce the incidence of some sexually transmitted diseases in this population.

FUNCTIONS OF PUBLIC HEALTH NURSES

Nurses in public health have many functions, depending on the needs and resources of an area. **Advocate** is one of the many roles of the nurse. As an advocate, the nurse collects, monitors, and analyzes data and discusses with the client which services are needed and whether the client is an individual, a family, or a group. The nurse and the client then develop the most effective plan and approach to take, and the nurse helps the client implement the plan so that the client can become more independent in making decisions and obtaining the services needed.

Case manager is a major role for nurses. Nurses use the nursing process of assessing, planning, implementing, and evaluating outcomes to meet clients' needs. Clear and complex communications are frequently an important component of case management. Other health and social agency participants may not be familiar with the home and community living conditions that are known to the nurse. It is the nurse who has been there and seen the living conditions and who can tell the story for the client or assist the individual or family with the telling of their story. Case managers assist clients in identifying and obtaining the services they need the most at the least cost. For example, a nurse may go into the home to visit a new mother and baby. Upon assessment she may find that the mother needs help in finding a new job, childcare, and a pediatrician and assistance in finding health insurance. The nurse helps the mother in the following ways:
- Assists with prioritizing the problems
- Helps make a plan for resolving the problems
- Contacts other agencies on behalf of the mother when needed
- Follows up with the mother to see that the problems are being resolved
- Follows up with the agencies, such as social services, to make certain the mother's request to enroll her children in the State Children's Health Insurance Program has been honored

Nurses are a major **referral resource**. They maintain current information about health and social services available within the community. They know what resources will be acceptable to the client within the social and cultural norms for that group. The nurse educates clients to enable them to use the resources and to learn self-care. Nurses refer to other services in the area, and other services refer to the nurse for care or follow-up. For example, the mother and new baby may be referred to the nurse for postnatal care with postpartum home visit follow-up.

Assessor of literacy is a large part of nursing in public health. Many individuals are limited in their ability to read, write, and communicate clearly. The nurse has to be culturally sensitive and aware of the specific areas of unique problems of clients, such as financial limitations that may in turn limit educational opportunities. Frequently, when persons go to a physician's office, clinic, or hospital, they are clean and neatly dressed. The assumption is made that

Evidence-Based Practice

The purpose of this project was to identify and better understand the health risk behaviors of a group of urban adolescents in the seventh grade. The study described (1) the types of health risk behaviors being undertaken, (2) the frequency of participation in the health risk behaviors, and (3) the age at which the health risk behavior first occurred. A sample of 54 urban seventh graders was found to have many health needs after participating in a Youth Risk Behaviors Surveillance System (YRBSS) Questionnaire. Students were found to smoke regularly and to use alcohol. The rating of their health was good or excellent, but they rarely met the daily requirements for intake of fruits and vegetables. Although they rated their weight as being acceptable, most were trying to lose weight. Differences between the boys and girls were noted in weight perception, with girls more likely than boys to use smoking as a primary method of weight control.

NURSE USE: Nurses can provide effective health care interventions and community health outreach to this adolescent population to reduce their participation in risky behaviors such as smoking, drinking, and inadequate nutrition. Instruments such as the YRBSS questionnaire provide a good assessment of the health needs of clients and can be used to plan health education individually or in groups.

From Dowdell EB, Santucci ME: Health risk behavior assessment: nutrition, weight, and tobacco use in urban seventh-grade class, *Public Health Nurs* 21(2):128–136, 2004.

when they nod at the health care provider it means that they understand what has been said. This is frequently not the case, but the client is embarrassed to admit that he or she does not understand what has been said. Being illiterate does not mean a person is mentally slow. It is important for the nurse to follow up on the many contacts the individual or family has with medical, social, and legal services to clarify what is understood and to find an answer to the questions that have not been asked by the client or answered by the services.

The nurse is an **educator**, teaching to the level of the client so that information received is information that can be used. Patience and repetitions over time are necessary to develop the trust and to enable the client to use the relationship with the nurse for more information. As educator, the public health nurse identifies community needs (e.g., playground safety, hand hygiene, pedestrian safety, safe-sex practices) and develops and implements educational activities aimed at changing behaviors over time (see "Evidence-Based Practice" box).

Nurses in public health are direct **primary caregivers** in many situations both in the clinic and in the community. Where the nurse provides primary care is determined by community assessment and is usually in response to an identified gap to which the private sector is unable to respond, coupled with an assessment of the effect of the gap in services on the health of the population. Examples include the following:

- Prenatal services for uninsured women
- Free or low-cost immunization services for targeted populations

- Directly observed therapy for clients with active TB
- Treatment for STDs

Nurses ensure that direct care services are available in the community for at-risk populations by working with the community to develop programs that will meet the needs of those populations. Currently, no system of outreach service in the medical models of care addresses the multiple needs of high-risk populations. High-risk populations frequently do not understand the medical, social, educational, or judicial system and the professional languages, codes of behavior, or expected outcomes of these services. Clients need a case manager, a health educator, an advocate, and a **role model** to enable them to benefit from these services and to teach them how to avoid complex and expensive problems in the future. The local nurse in public health fills these roles and many more for this population. These are examples of the difficult clinical issues that nurses face in making ethical and professional decisions.

The nurse's role in public health is unique and essential in many situations. Access to homes gives the nurse information that usually cannot be gathered in the hospital or clinic setting. The nurse learns to ask intimate questions creatively and to seek information that will facilitate case management and provide the clinical and social care needed, including other community resources. Careful attention must be paid to privacy and confidentiality in delivering these nursing services. The credibility of the nurse and the agency depends on the professional handling of the public health information of each staff member.

When an emergency or a disaster occurs, nurses at the local, state, and federal levels have multiple roles in assessment, planning, implementing, and evaluating needs and resources for the different populations being served. Whether the disaster is local or national, small or large, natural or caused by humans, nurses are skilled professionals essential to the team. As a health care facility, the local public health department has an emergency operations plan, as well as a role in the local, regional, and state disaster plans. Nurses' roles include the following:

- Providing education that will prepare communities to cope with disasters
- Establishing mass dispensing clinics
- Conducting enhanced communicable disease surveillance
- Working with environmental health specialists to ensure safe food and water for disaster victims and emergency workers
- Serving on the local emergency planning committee

Their presence may be required in other regions of the state or country to provide official nursing duties in a time of crisis, such as a hurricane, that requires a lengthy period of recovery. Each governmental jurisdiction has an emergency plan. The public health agency is expected to provide planning and staffing during a disaster. These local emergency preparedness plans may be multigovernmental, which requires coordination among communities.

Essential and unique roles for nurses in public health exist in the area of communicable disease control. Nursing

skills are necessary for education, prevention, surveillance, and outbreak investigation. Nurses can do the following:
- Find infected individuals
- Notify contacts
- Refer to other health providers or agencies for care
- Administer treatments
- Educate the individual, family, community, professionals, and populations
- Act as advocates
- Be state-of-the-art resources to reduce the rate of communicable disease in the community

The communicable disease role is one of the most important roles for nursing during disasters. During the September 11, 2001 airplane attacks, nurses at the federal, state, and local levels immediately implemented active enhanced surveillance activities. Information about communicable diseases seen at the local level was passed on to the state public health agency and finally to the CDC. At each step, the data were analyzed for evidence of unusual disease trends.

BRIEFLY NOTED

It is important for nurses in public health to practice confidentiality when they have knowledge about an individual, family, communicable disease outbreak, community-level problem, or any special knowledge obtained in the public health work setting.

When October 2001 alerts from the CDC began presenting information about a photo editor in Florida who had been hospitalized with inhalation of anthrax, nurses in public health and hospital infection control practitioners throughout the nation increased activity. Public health response to disasters requires that resources be redirected temporarily from other programs while maintaining programs that will prevent additional outbreaks. Therefore nurses not normally involved in communicable disease activities can be shifted to this function. The exposures resulting from the anthrax-tainted letters presented unprecedented public health challenges. The Washington, D.C. anthrax exposures resulted in thousands of possible work-related exposures, five cases of inhalation anthrax in the region, and two deaths over a period of months. Public health at the federal, state, and local levels was looked to for coordinated leadership and answers to a` situation in which experience was limited and answers were uncertain. Although communicable disease control is a core public health service, the role of public health as incident commander in a widespread public health emergency is a new role. The following were issues to be addressed:
- How to conduct mass treatment in response to a bioterrorism event
- Which jurisdiction is in charge
- How to communicate uncertain information to the public
- Who should take antibiotics and for how long had to be rapidly resolved across jurisdictional and agency lines

The anthrax exposures are typical of the nature of public health emergencies. They unfold as the communicable disease moves through communities.

Nurses in public health are essential partners in disaster drills. In Virginia, an electrical company has a nuclear plant that requires annual multijurisdictional disaster drills. These disaster planning and practice sessions are an opportunity for local nurses to get to know other agencies' representatives and to let them know what nursing can offer. Because nurses are out in the communities and have assessment skills, they are essential in evaluating how the disaster was handled and in making suggestions about how future events might be managed. To be most effective as **disaster responders**, nurses have to be a part of the team *before* an emergency. Knowing what type of disaster is likely to occur in a community is essential for planning. Types of disasters vary from place to place, but there is a history of past events and how they were handled, as well as resources and training from regional, state, and federal agencies. Nurses can help educate the public about the individual responsibilities and preparations that can be in place both for the person and for the community. Nurses at the local, state, and federal levels work in partnership to accomplish each function (see "Levels of Prevention" box on p. 538).

CLINICAL APPLICATION

A retirement community in a small town reported to the local health department 24 cases of severe gastrointestinal illness that had occurred among residents and staff of the facility during the past 24 to 36 hours. It was determined that the ill clients became sick within a short, well-defined period and that most recovered within 24 hours without treatment. The communicable disease outbreak team, composed of nurses, public health physicians, and an environmental health specialist, was called to respond to this possible epidemic.

How should they respond to this situation?
A. *Call the Centers for Disease Control and Prevention and ask for help with surveillance.*
B. *Send all the ill persons in the retirement community to the hospital.*
C. *Evaluate the agent, host, and environment relationships to determine the cause of the problem.*
D. *Close the dining room and find another source to provide food to the residents.*
Answer is in the back of the book.

REMEMBER THIS!

- Local public health departments are responsible for implementing and enforcing local, state, and federal public health codes and ordinances while providing essential public health services.
- The goal of the local health department is to safeguard the public's health and improve the community's health status.

- Nursing in community health is the practice of promoting and protecting the health of populations using knowledge from nursing and social and public health sciences.
- Public health is based on the scientific core of epidemiology.
- Marketing of nursing in public health is essential to inform both professionals and the public about the opportunities and challenges of populations in public health care.
- A driving force behind nursing changes is the economy and the increase in managed care.
- Nurses need ongoing education and training as public health changes.
- Some of the roles in which nurses function are advocate, case manager, referral source, counselor, primary care provider, educator, outreach worker, and disaster responder.
- Nurses have an important role in helping with local disasters, including planning, staffing, and evaluating events.

WHAT WOULD YOU DO?

1. What are some of the roles of the nurse in the local, state, and federal public health systems? Explain why they may be different from one another.
2. How can nurses prepare themselves for change? Illustrate what you mean.
3. What can nurses learn from the past practice of public health nurses?
4. Describe collaborative partnerships that nurses have developed. How do partnerships help solve public health problems?
5. What are some external factors that have an effect on nursing in public health?
6. If you were a nurse in public health for a day, what would you like to accomplish?
7. How would you determine the most pressing public health issue in your community?

■ REFERENCES

American Nurses Association: *Public health nursing: scope and standards of practice*, Silver Spring, Md, 2007, ANA.

American Nurses Credentialing Center: *Certification*, Silver Spring, Md, 2008, ANA.

American Public Health Association: *Definition of public health nursing*, Washington, DC, 1996, Public Health Nursing Section, American Public Health Association.

Centers for Disease Control and Prevention: Achievements in public health, 1900–1999: control of infectious diseases, *MMWR Morb Mortal Wkly Rep* 48:621–629, 2002.

Centers for Disease Control and Prevention: *National Public Health Performance Standards Program, state public health system performance assessment instrument, version: state tool*, Atlanta, Ga, May 2004, CDC, available at http://www.phppo.cdc.gov/nphpsp/Partners.asp.

Centers for Disease Control and Prevention: *The national public health performance standards, an overview, slide 9, 2005.* Retrieved Aug 27, 2005, from http://www.cdc.gov/od/ocphp/nphpsp/Presentationlinks.htm.

Council on Linkages between Academia and Public Health Practice: *Core competencies for public health professionals*, Washington, DC, 2001, Public Health Foundation.

Dowdell EB, Santucci ME: Health risk behavior assessment: nutrition, weight, and tobacco use in urban seventh-grade class, *Public Health Nurs* 21(2):128–136, 2004.

Institute of Medicine: *The future of public health*, Washington, DC, 1988, National Academy Press.

Institute of Medicine: *Unequal treatment: confronting racial and ethnic disparities in health care*, Washington, DC, 2002, National Academy Press.

Institute of Medicine: *The future of public health in the 21st century*, Washington, DC, 2003, National Academies Press.

Public Health Nursing Section, Minnesota Department of Health: *Public health interventions—applications for public health nursing practice,* St. Paul, Minn, 2001, Department of Health, American Public Health Association.

Rubin S: Antibiotic resistance in outpatient populations, *Clin Updates Infect Dis* 5:108, 2001.

Turnock BJ: *Public health: what it is and how it works*, Gaithersburg, Md, 2004, Aspen.

U.S. Department of Health and Human Services: *Healthy People 2010: understanding and improving health*, ed 2, Washington, DC, 2000, U.S. Government Printing Office.

The Faith Community Nurse

Cynthia Z. Gustafson

ADDITIONAL RESOURCES

These related resources are found either in the appendix at the back of this book or on the book's website at http://evolve.elsevier.com/stanhope/foundations.

Evolve Website

• Community Assessment Applied
• Case Study, with questions and answers

• Quiz review questions
• WebLinks, including link to *Healthy People 2010* website

OBJECTIVES

After reading this chapter, the student should be able to:

1. Describe the heritage of health and healing in faith communities.
2. Describe models of the parish nurse.
3. Demonstrate an awareness of the nurse's role as parish nurse in faith communities for health promotion and disease prevention.
4. Recognize the role of holistic health care for wellness in faith communities.

5. Help communities of faith include *Healthy People 2010* guidelines in program planning.
6. Collaborate with key partners to implement health ministries relevant for the faith community.
7. Discuss the legal, ethical, and financial issues related to parish nursing.

CHAPTER OUTLINE

KEY TERMS

congregants: people who gather as part of a faith community of the congregation of a church.

congregational model: parish nurse arrangement in an individual community of faith in which the nurse is accountable to the congregation and its governing body.

faith communities: distinct groups of people acknowledging specific faith traditions and gathering in churches, cathedrals, synagogues, or mosques.

healing: strengthening the inner spiritual connectedness and choosing healthy lifestyles.

health ministries: activities and programs in faith communities directed at improving the health and well-being of individuals, families, and communities across the life span.

holistic care: understanding the body, mind, and spirit relationship of persons in an environment that is always changing.

holistic health centers: comprehensive health teams that include family and clergy and encourage personal responsibility for health and preventive health practices.

institutional model: parish nurse arrangement in a larger partnership under contract with hospitals, medical centers, long-term care facilities, or educational institutions.

neighborhood nurse: also known as block nurse, the nurse responds to a defined community or "locality."

parish nurse coordinator: a parish nurse who has completed a certificate program designed to develop the nurse as a coordinator of a parish nursing service.

parish nurses: nurses who respond to health and wellness needs within the faith context of populations of faith communities and are partners with the church in fulfilling the mission of the health ministry.

parish nursing: a community-based and population-focused professional nursing practice with faith communities to promote whole person health to its parishioners, usually focused on primary prevention.

partnerships: relationships between individuals, groups, or organizations in which the parties are working together to achieve a joint goal; it is often used synonymously with coalitions and alliances, although partnerships usually have focused goals, such as jointly providing a specific program. Partnerships generally involve shared power.

pastoral care staff: faith community leaders including clergy, nurses, and educational and youth ministry staff.

polity: the policy, governances, expectations, and mission of a specific faith community.

wellness committee: a health cabinet supporting healthy, spiritually fulfilling lives; it is made up of a nurse and members of the congregation.

Parish nursing has long established roots in the healing and health professions (Patterson, 2003). Historical accounts of nursing document the importance of caring for members of communities. The earliest accounts of concern for others stem from communities of faith. Wholeness in health and being in relationships with the Creator have sustained individuals and groups during times of illness, brokenness, stress, and incurable conditions (Hale and Koenig, 2003; Solari-Twadell and McDermott, 2006). Today parish nurses work in close relationships with individuals, families, and faith communities to establish programs and services that significantly affect health, healing, and wholeness (Chase-Ziolek, 2005; Nist, 2003; O'Brien, 2003; Patterson, 2003; Shelly, 2002; Solari-Twadell and McDermott, 2006; Tuck, Pullen, and Wallace, 2001). Parish nurses balance knowledge and skill in the role and facilitate the faith community to become a caring place—a place that is a source of health and healing.

Parish nurses address universal health problems of individuals, families, and groups of all ages. The members of congregations experience the following:
- Birth
- Death
- Acute and chronic illness
- Stress
- Dependency concerns

- Challenges of life transitions
- Growth and development
- Decisions regarding healthy lifestyle choices

Faith members live in communities that make decisions regarding policies for financing and managing health care and for keeping environments safe and communities healthy for present and future generations. Parish nurses encourage partnering with other community health resources to arrive at creative responses to health issues and concerns.

Parish nursing is gaining prominence as nurses reclaim their traditions of healing, acknowledge gaps in service delivery, and, along with the rise of nursing centers, affirm the independent functions of nursing (Nist, 2003; Solari-Twadell, 2006). In 1998 the American Nurses Association (ANA) accepted parish nursing as the most recognized term for the practice of nurses working with congregations or faith communities. With the Health Ministries Association (HMA), the ANA published the *Scope and Standards of Parish Nursing* (Health Ministries Association and American Nurses Association, 1998). In the 2005 revision of the *ANA Scope and Standards of Practice,* the term *faith community nurse* was adopted to be inclusive of the titles of parish nurse, congregational nurse, health ministry nurse, crescent nurse, or health and wellness nurse (American Nurses Association and Health Ministries Association, 2005).

Although most parish nurses are in Protestant congregations, they may be found in most faith communities, including communities that serve diverse cultures (Minden, 2005; Schweitzer, 2004; Simpson, 2004). Parish nurses are also serving faith communities in South Korea, Canada, Australia, New Zealand, Swaziland, Russia, and the United Kingdom (Berry et al, 2000; Gustafson, 2003; Lukits, 2000; Roberts, 2003; Van Loon, 2004; Woodworth, 2005).

DEFINITIONS IN FAITH COMMUNITY NURSING

Faith communities are groups of people that gather in churches, cathedrals, synagogues, or mosques and acknowledge common faith traditions. **Parish nursing** is the most commonly used term that denotes the professional nursing practice in this context. **Parish nurses** respond to health and wellness needs of populations of faith communities and are partners with the church in fulfilling the mission of the health ministry. The inclusive term of *faith community nursing,* as adopted by the ANA and the HMA, defines nursing practice with an intentional focus on *spiritual care* as central to promoting "wholistic" health and prevention of illness (American Nurses Association and Health Ministries Association, 2005, p. 1).

The faith community includes persons throughout the life span: active and less active members, those confined to homes, or those in nursing homes. Often the faith community's mission also includes individuals and groups in the geographic or common cultural community who are not designated members. The services may be extended to those beyond the congregation. The parish nurse emphasizes the nursing discipline's spiritual dimension while incorporating physical, emotional, and social aspects of nursing with individuals, families, and faith communities (see "Evidence-Based Practice" box).

Health ministries are those activities and programs in faith communities organized around health and healing to promote wholeness in health across the life span (Chase-Ziolek, 2005). The services may be specifically planned or may be more informal. A professional or a lay person may provide them. These services include the following:
• Visiting the homebound
• Providing meals for families in crisis or when returning home after hospitalization
• Participating in prayer circles
• Volunteering in community acquired immunodeficiency syndrome (AIDS) care groups
• Serving "healthy heart" church suppers
• Holding regular grief support groups (Hale and Koenig, 2003).

Popular parish nurse models include the **congregational model** and the **institutional model** (Box 29-1).

The development of a parish nurse and health ministry program arises from the individual community of faith. The nurse is accountable to the congregation and its governing body. The institutional model includes greater collaboration and partnership; the nurse may be in a contractual relationship with hospitals, medical centers, long-term care establishments, or educational institutions. In either model, nurses work closely with professional health care members, faith community **pastoral care staff**, and lay volunteers who represent various aspects of the life of the congregational community (Vandecreek and Mooney, 2002). To promote **healing**, the nurse builds on strengths to encourage integrating inner spiritual knowledge and healthy lifestyle choices for optimal wellness. The intentional and compassionate presence of a spiritually mature professional nurse in individual or group situations is vital. In this role, providing such holistic care with congregation populations is important. **Holistic care** is concerned with the relationship of body, mind, and spirit in a constantly changing environment (Dossey, Keegan, and Guzzetta, 2005). The nurse and

---

Box 29-1 Parish Nurse Models

• *Congregation-based model,* in which the nurse is usually autonomous. The development of a parish nurse/health ministry program arises from the individual community of faith. The nurse is accountable to the congregation and its governing body.
• *Institution-based model,* which includes greater collaboration and partnerships. The nurse may be in a contractual relationship with hospitals, medical centers, long-term care establishments, or educational institutions.

Evidence-Based Practice

The relationship between prayer and health outcomes was studied in a mail survey of a randomly selected population of members of a mainstream denomination in the United States. The study's purpose was to examine the relationship of prayer to eight categories of physical and mental health. Health status was measured by the Medical Outcomes Study Short-Form 36 Health Survey. The mail survey provided self-reports of health and resulted in an overall high level of functioning. Those persons who prayed more frequently scored lower in physical functioning and in the ability to carry out role activities, and they scored higher in pain. However, these same persons also had significantly higher mental health scores than did those who prayed less. These persons of advanced age and poor physical health were praying more than younger healthy members. The study also reinforced other research that showed that persons pray more often as failing health accompanies aging. One explanation for the increased prayer was that as the individual perceived that increased vulnerability would accompany the disabilities, increased efforts toward gaining strength and comfort were made. The study affirms the protective results of prayer on the persons' mental health.

NURSE USE: Parish nurses can be encouraged to continue to support members of faith communities in prayer; help them find the space and moments to pray during times of stress, illness, and grief; and encourage support groups to assist persons to enhance prayer and meditation practices.

From Meisenhelder JB, Chandler EN: Prayer and health outcomes in church members, *Altern Ther Health Med* 6(4):56–60, 2000.

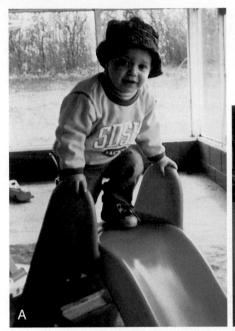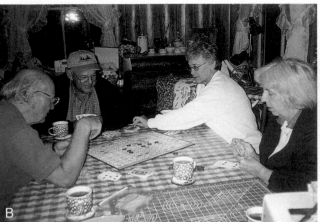

FIGURE 29-I Promoting healthy activities across the life span in church and community activities.

Box 29-2	**Resources for Parish Nursing**

International Parish Nurse Resource Center
Eden Theological Seminary
475 East Lockwood Avenue
St. Louis, MO 63119
314-918-2559
ann.solari-twadell@advocatehealth.com
(Publication: *Parish Nurse Perspectives*)

Health Ministries Association
P.O. Box 529
Queen Creek, AZ 85242
1-800-280-9919
hmasso@mindspring.com
(Publication: *Connections*)

Interfaith Health Program of the Carter Center
1256 Briarcliff Road
Atlanta, GA 30306
(Publication: *Faith & Health*)

See the WebLinks on this book's website at http://evolve.elsevier.
com/stanhope/foundations for further information about resources.

members of the congregation assess, plan, implement, and evaluate programs. The process of providing holistic care is enhanced by an active **wellness committee** or health cabinet (Chase-Ziolek, 2005).

These committees are most effective when members represent the broad spectrum of the life of the church (Figure 29-1). The parish nurse uses all the knowledge and skills of this specialty to provide effective services. The outcome is a truly caring congregation that supports healthy, spiritually fulfilling lives. Box 29-2 lists resources for parish nursing.

BRIEFLY NOTED

Parish nurses are employed by senior living complexes and nursing homes to offer a spiritual focus to the nursing practice within various levels of living arrangements for elders, in addition to serving one or more congregations in the community.

HERITAGE AND HORIZONS

FAITH COMMUNITIES

In the roots of many faith communities are concerns for justice, mercy, and the need for spiritual and physical healing. The appeal for caring, the healing of diseases, and acknowledging periods of illness and wellness are universal. Throughout a major portion of the twentieth century religion played an important role in the lives of many in this country. An important aspect of living one's spirituality and religion is being a part of a community of faith from birth to death, throughout wellness and illness. Participating as individuals or as families, all benefit from the associations with the supportive faith community or congregation (Carson and Koenig, 2002).

Support from members of groups that are meaningful to a person's total well-being aids in recovery and healing (Buijs and Olson, 2001; Hurley and Mohnkern, 2004). Asking for help and using strengths from earliest faith, traditions, family support, and teachings assist individuals, groups, and communities in interpreting brokenness, disasters, joys, births, deaths, illness, and recovery. Throughout history, health existed at the center of the human interaction with the Creator.

The integration of faith and health within the caring community results in beneficial outcomes. Persons who are assaulted with physical and emotional illness and brokenness and who are able to call upon their faith beliefs and religious traditions are able to increase coping skills and realize spiritual growth. These coping skills and spiritual strengths extend beyond the current situation and help with future life challenges and total well-being (Taylor, 2003).

Some of the major Christian faith communities in the late nineteenth and early twentieth centuries used missionaries to develop multipurpose activities in communities, which included education and health activities along with religious messages. Hospitals were built in the United States and abroad, and underserved populations were targeted. As political and economic forces have changed through the years, so health ministries of the faith communities have altered their approaches. Some groups have identified with community development efforts in helping people empower themselves to meet their needs for food, education, clean environments, social support, and primary health care.

Some groups have also recognized and increased their emphasis on the following:
- Individual responsibility
- The escalating cost of health care
- The need for cost containment
- The increasing numbers of uninsured and underserved
- The ever-increasing dilemma of interpreting the many changes in the health care delivery system
- Issues of domestic violence
- Issues of substance abuse
- Issues with human immunodeficiency virus (HIV)/AIDS

These efforts have been translated into a variety of positions endorsed by the governing bodies of the faith communities.

The **holistic health centers** of the 1970s emphasized a comprehensive team approach to total health care. The teams in those centers included family and clergy, who emphasized personal responsibility for health and encouraged preventive health practices. The formation of parish nursing in the early 1980s built on the strengths of the holistic health centers and focused on the team of nurses and clergy, working with individuals and with their families. Nurses used their abilities to listen to the spoken and unspoken concerns of individuals and made assessments and judgments based on their knowledge of the health sciences and humanities. As with the early history of the development of public health nursing in this country, parish nurses found that health promotion services were needed in underserved and rural areas (Baldwin et al, 2001; Wallace et al, 2002). Nurses identified the following:
- Gaps in the delivery of service
- Acknowledged strength within persons to increase healing
- The vital role of families in healthy outcomes
- The community support needed for individuals and families

BRIEFLY NOTED

The International Parish Nurse Resource Center (IPNRC)/ Advocate Health Care resources are the outgrowth of the early visions of the Rev. Granger Westberg. As a Lutheran clergyman who was involved with the W.K. Kellogg Wholistic Health Centers, Westberg recognized that nurses were central to the endeavors and that they enhanced minister and doctor communication to promote a "whole person" approach. In the mid-1980s Westberg suggested placing nurses on the staff of churches and proposed the church as another "health agency" in the community (Solari-Twadell et al, 1994).

FAITH NURSE COMMUNITY

The beginnings of the parish nurse movement coincided with the following (Baldwin et al., 2001; Wallace et al, 2002):
- Recognition of more independent functions of the nurse
- Articulation and proliferation of advanced practice nursing roles
- The growth of nursing centers
- Technological advances
- Diagnosis-related groups (DRGs), which resulted in hospitals discharging clients earlier and clients returning to their homes sicker with few, if any, caregivers available
- Caregivers faced with multiple tasks of coordinating employment and finances, learning new caregiving tasks, and maintaining former and ongoing family responsibilities
- Increased consumer demand for involvement in health care decisions
- Society's emphasis on individual responsibility for health because many diseases were indeed preventable and health care costs had to be cut
- Recognition that fragmented care and inadequate caregiver training and availability were problems for the disenfranchised, underserved, uninsured, economically well situated, and better-educated persons
- Challenges faced by suburban and rural families to seek ways to best meet the multiple demands of young children, teens, and aging parents

These numerous interacting and overlapping forces were burdens for the population. Parish nurse services were one way to coordinate care and foster continuity of care. The parish nurse services emphasized health promotion and disease prevention and provided the benefits of holistic care through the supportive faith community.

The mission of the International Parish Nurse Resource Center (IPNRC) is the promotion and development of quality parish nurse programs through research, education, and consultation (International Parish Nurse Resource Center, 1998). Information about accessing the Center appears in Box 29-2. The Center has also endorsed curricula for the parish nurse and **parish nurse coordinator** (Patterson, 2003; Solari-Twadell and McDermott, 2006). Throughout the years, the IPNRC has been vigilant in addressing emerging issues such as documentation accountability, certification for parish nurses, and accreditation concerns (related to the Joint Commission on Accreditation of Healthcare Organizations [The Joint Commission]) for parish nurses connected with institutional hospital systems.

Nurses functioning as parish nurses need to have the following:
- Leadership skills
- Astute, articulate nonverbal and verbal communication
- Negotiation and collaboration skills

As with other population groups, the parish nurse attempts to include those persons who are less vocal or visible in the community of faith. If the vision of the congregation extends beyond its immediate membership, those outside of the immediate faith community who would benefit from the services are also potential recipients. This may be accomplished by including the block nurse or **neighborhood nurse** in the area surrounding the faith community.

HEALTH CARE DELIVERY

The health care delivery system is challenged to work within parameters of tighter financial constraints while also welcoming advanced technology and addressing new health concerns. Consumer demand for involvement in health care decisions continues to increase, and society emphasizes individual responsibility for health. Simultaneously, consumers have increased interest in their own well-being and have expressed needs for more current health information to be available in a wider variety of formats (Loeb, O'Neill, and Gueldner, 2001; Swinney et al, 2001). These numerous interacting and overlapping forces are both a challenge and a burden for the population.

In addition to consumer interest and a heightened awareness of responsibility for our own health, health care providers and managed care systems have found it financially advantageous for their participants to be healthy and remain out of the system. Thus with rising costs of care, scarce resources for populations, and the complex system demands on individuals and families to seek health care, the challenge for the consumer now is how to cope with these forces. Consumers and health care providers are still muddling through the complexity and fragmentation of the delivery system as it affects the young, old, and very old; the poor, middle-income, and affluent; persons of diverse ethnic origins; and those affected by disparities within society (Baldwin et al, 2001). Advanced practice nurses are addressing these consumer needs for primary care by practicing in the faith community setting (Bitner and Woodward, 2004).

A primary focus of the nurse in the past few decades has been to coordinate care and to link health care providers, groups, and community resources as the client tries to understand diverse health plans. Negotiating with individuals, agencies, and community partnerships within the complex maze of the broader health care environment demands a knowledgeable and seasoned professional. Nurses are aware of the necessity of collaborative practices and the formation of **partnerships** to care for groups and individuals

throughout the age span. These nurses recognize the need for health promotion and disease prevention at all levels; they regularly assess the need to interpret care plans given to clients by health care providers. They advocate for healthy lifestyle choices in exercise, nutrition, substance use, and stress management. They realize that information and guidance must be available via media and in schools, workplaces, faith communities, and residential neighborhoods. Parish nurses share these and other important nursing functions as they serve populations through faith communities (Anderson, 2004; Chase-Ziolek and Iris, 2002).

FAITH COMMUNITY NURSING PRACTICE

CHARACTERISTICS OF THE PRACTICE

The goal of parish nursing is to develop and sustain health ministries within faith communities. Health ministries promote wholeness in health, emphasize health promotion and disease prevention, and do this within the context of linking healing with the person's faith belief and level of spiritual maturity. Parish nurse Ruth Berry, the previous author of this chapter, participated in a 1994 invitational conference that included 26 professionals consisting of nurse educators, practicing parish nurses, and the staff of the IPNRC; their purpose was to discuss and design a document outlining educational guidelines for the rapidly growing new nursing specialty. The final product included the following five characteristics identified as central to the philosophy of parish nursing (Solari-Twadell, 2006):

1. The spiritual dimension is central to the practice of parish nursing. Nursing embodies the physical, psychological, social, and spiritual dimensions of clients into professional practice. Although parish nursing includes all four, it focuses on intentional and compassionate care, which stems from the spiritual dimension of all humankind.

2. The roots of the role balance both knowledge and skills of nursing, using nursing sciences, the humanities, and theology. The nurse combines nursing functions with pastoral care functions. Visits in the office, home, hospital, or nursing home often involve prayer and may include a reference to scripture, symbols, sacraments, and liturgy of the faith community represented by the nurse. The values and beliefs of the faith community are integral to the supportive care given. Nurses also assist with worship services as appropriate within the faith community.

3. The focus of the specialty is the faith community and its ministry. The faith community is the source of health and healing partnerships, which result in creative responses to health and health-related concerns. Partnerships may be among individuals, groups, and health care professionals within the congregation. They may also be among various congregations or community agencies, institutions, or individuals. Partnerships also evolve as the congregation visualizes its health-related mission beyond the walls, stones, and steeples of its own place of worship.

4. Parish nurse services emphasize the strengths of individuals, families, and communities. Parish nurses endorse this fourth characteristic in their practice. As congregations realize the need for care and care for one another, their individual and corporate relationship with their Creator is often enhanced. This provides additional coping strength for future crisis situations within the family and community.

5. Health, spiritual health, and healing are considered an ongoing, dynamic process. Because spiritual health is central to well-being, influences are evident in the total individual and noted in a healthy congregation. Well-being and illness may occur simultaneously; spiritual healing or well-being can exist in the absence of cure.

The Third Invitational Parish Nurse Educational Colloquium sponsored by the IPNRC affirmed assumptions of the practice of parish nursing (Solari-Twadell, McDermott, and Matheus, 2000; Solari-Twadell, 2006). Those gathered affirmed that the term *client* in parish nursing embraces individuals, families, congregations, and communities across the life span. The practice includes the full cultural and geographic community regardless of ethnicity, lifestyle, sex, sexual orientation, or creed. The nurse in the practice incorporates faith and health and employs the nursing process in providing services to the faith community, as well as to the community served by that faith community. Facilitating collaborative health ministries in the faith communities is an important component of the practice. In addition, the group affirmed that although the curricula stem from a Judeo-Christian theological framework, parish nursing respects diverse traditions of faith communities and encourages adaptation of the programs to these faith traditions.

BRIEFLY NOTED

The Wisconsin Women's Health Foundation has joined forces with parish nurses to establish the GrapeVine Project. This highly successful program provides health information and resources to rural women using parish nurses as the primary message bearers. As parish nurses inform women about the importance of general health and disease prevention, they connect them and their communities, like a cluster of grapes, to other women and communities along a continuous grapevine. Parish nurses are viewed as a trusted resource for rural women all over the state since they are based out of faith communities and are prepared to address both the spiritual and the physical needs of clients.

SCOPE AND STANDARDS OF FAITH COMMUNITY NURSING PRACTICE

Nursing: Scope and Standards of Practice (American Nurses Association, 2004) describes what nursing is, what nurses do, and the responsibilities for which they are accountable. This document serves as the template for the specialties within the profession, and therefore is the foundation for

Levels of Prevention — Related to Overweight, Obesity, and Physical Activity

PRIMARY PREVENTION

- Hold classes on healthy eating and explain the food pyramid appropriate for various age levels (elementary school, adolescents, new parents).
- Promote and encourage age-appropriate activities that include physical exercise in youth group meetings, retreats, trips, vacation church school, and nursery programs.
- Encourage a variety of activities and discourage extended inactivity.
- Encourage healthy snacks and meals for youth outings and at educational hour and parenting sessions.
- Write house-of-worship newsletter articles informing parents of the need for adequate exercise and proper nutrition for healthy lifestyles in growing and adult years.
- Encourage parents to be proactive in school parenting councils and in neighborhood recreation leagues to ensure exercise programs and activities so that children and youths expend energy to promote proper weight maintenance and prevent accumulation of fat.
- Encourage faith community leaders to sponsor a safe indoor/outdoor activity area for neighborhood or at-risk children.

SECONDARY PREVENTION

- Provide health assessment and counseling during home visits for health promotion initiated for other family members—for example, at visits after a hospitalization or a birth.
- Be available for health counseling for teens before and after youth activities.
- In schools associated with faith communities, assist with height and weight screening to identify young persons needing attention.

TERTIARY PREVENTION

- Collaborate closely with faith education teachers and youth ministers and counselors about sessions that deal with nutrition behavior change, exercise behavior modification, injury prevention guidelines, health problems of overweight young persons, and the advantages of reduced weight, support, stress management, and improved quality of life.
- Follow up and monitor the health care provider's plan of care for young persons who have been identified as overweight; support and encourage them to withstand peer ridicule during changes in behavior.
- Assist in making choices for behavior change (suggest avoiding calorie-rich or nutritionally lacking foods during school meal and snack times; suggest possible paths for walking and bicycling; identify courts and gyms available for more strenuous exercise).
- In youth groups and parenting groups discuss the need for loving, caring friends and the support needed for long-term behavior modification programs that are life-long efforts.

Faith Community Nursing: Scope and Standards of Practice (American Nurses Association and Health Ministries Association, 2005). This revised scope and standards describes the who, what, where, when, why, and how of the practice of faith community nursing. Nurses well versed in the parish nursing practice field compiled this revision of the 1998 *Scope and Standards of Parish Nursing Practice*

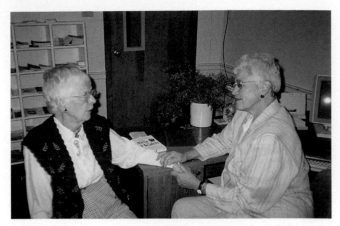

FIGURE 29-2 A parish nurse provides support for spiritual and emotional needs as well as physical needs.

Intervene in Maternal and Infant Health

- Visit a family immediately after the birth of a new infant to further assess parenting skills and parent and infant bonding, reinforce a holistic reflection of life transitions, and plan for faith community support as indicated in those areas not addressed by family or other community agencies.
- Augment community prenatal classes or facilitate classes in the faith community stressing growth and development in the prenatal and postnatal period, family transitions, and adequate health monitoring needed by parents, children, and new family members.
- Facilitate an expectant parent support group to reinforce positive health during pregnancy, interpret plans negotiated with the health care provider, promote spiritual reflection of family life transitions, and encourage a connection with the Creator and the beliefs of the faith community; provide emotional, social, and community support to the family.

by a thorough review of the practice, public comments, and dialogue of practicing parish nurses. Specialty areas within professional nursing achieve a major milestone when the standards and scope common to that practice are recognized.

The specialized practice of faith community nursing focuses on intentional *spiritual care* as an integral part of the process of promoting wholistic health and preventing or minimizing illness in the faith community (American Nurses Association and Health Ministries Association, 2005) (see the "How To" box).

The *Scope and Standards* delineate examples of the parish nurse's independent functions. These functions are in compliance with and reflect current nursing practice, client health promotion needs, professional standards, and the legal scope of professional nursing practice. Nurses function within the nurse practice act of their jurisdiction (state). If dependent functions are practiced, parish nurses must be in compliance with the legal criteria of the jurisdiction's nurse practice act (American Nurses Association and Health Ministries Association, 2005). For example, when influenza vaccine or immunization clinics are offered, appropriate arrangements are made to use nurses from the cooperating agency (health department), or the parish nurse must have a contractual policy agreement with the cooperating agency to provide the immunizations. In addition to a narrative description and glossary of terms, the 1998 document outlines standards of care and standards of professional performance. In keeping with the wise use of persons and materials, standards of professional performance elaborate on the coordination of care and consultation. Faith community nurses are "vital partners in advancing the nation's health initiatives such as *Healthy People 2010* to increase the quality of years of healthy life and eliminate health disparities" (American Nurses Association and Health Ministries Association, 2005, p. 9) (Figure 29-2).

BRIEFLY NOTED

The parish nurse benefits from several years of practical experience after the basic undergraduate preparation, because the nature of the position demands a seasoned professional.

EDUCATIONAL PREPARATION FOR THE FAITH COMMUNITY NURSE

Current educational preparation for the parish nurse includes the successful completion of extensive continuing education contact hours or designated coursework in parish nurse preparation at the baccalaureate or graduate level, as well as a thorough grasp of the *Scope and Standards* of the practice (American Nurses Association and Health Ministries Association, 2005). Such preparation is held in colleges, universities, health care institutions, and parish nurse networks across the United States and other countries as well as online and distance delivery (Gustafson, 2006). Many of these programs are in partnership with the IPNRC for ongoing support and revision (Patterson, 2003). These basic programs provide an orientation to the role and functions of the parish nurse as well as worship experiences for the process of ministry (McDermott and Solari-Twadell, 2006). Parish nurses are then able to adapt this knowledge, combined with an in-depth understanding of the beliefs of their faith tradition, to meet the holistic health needs of their local community of faith. According to *Faith Community Nursing: Scope and Standards of Practice* (American Nurses Association and Health Ministries Association, 2005), the preferred minimum preparation for the specialty includes educational preparation at the baccalaureate or higher level with content in community nursing, experience as a registered nurse, knowledge of the health care assets of a community, specialized knowledge of the spiritual practices of a given faith community, and specialized skills and knowledge to implement the *Scope and Standards*. Both the annual Westberg Symposium offered by the IPNRC and the annual meeting of the HMA offer comprehensive sessions and a forum for nurses to network, gain new knowledge, and stay abreast of current resources, trends, and issues in the practice.

Advanced practice opportunities also enrich a specialty practice. Master's-prepared nurses (with a specialization in public health nursing, holistic nursing, or mental health nursing) and nurse practitioners have found niches in parish nursing. Major universities have had creative arrangements for faculty and student clinical options at the undergraduate and graduate levels (Kotecki, 2002; Rouse, 2000; Swinney et al, 2001; Trofino, Hughes, and Hay, 2000). A 1500-member congregation in Florida employed a full-time master's-prepared nurse certified in holistic nursing by the American Holistic Nurses Association (AHNA). Faculty practice arrangements at the University of Kentucky (with a 1000-member congregation), collaborations between the Divinity School and nursing programs to form the Health and Nursing Ministries Program at Duke University, University of Colorado faculty arrangements offering opportunities for doctoral and master's-level students, and the pioneering Parish Health Nurse program at Georgetown University are notable.

Many parish nurses function in a part-time capacity. Some nurses are responsible for service with several congregations, whereas others engage in parish nursing as part of a full-time commitment in other capacities. Working in several arenas adds distinctive perspectives to a parish nurse service. Depending on the practice model, the nurse has a narrowly defined or a wider realm of responsibility. Parish nurse practices may be integrated into a health care facility or into practices that collaborate with related professional practice areas such as health departments or colleges of nursing. Practices in which several parish nurses are supervised by a coordinator have built-in opportunities for sharing, partnering, and mentoring. Parish nurses may also have regional responsibilities that correspond to intermediate governing areas of the faith community. These regions may be clusters of churches or areas such as districts, synods, presbyteries, or jurisdictions.

Parish nurses accept responsibility for ongoing professional education within nursing and pastoral care arenas. Preparation and continuing education must continue to include the basics and enrichment courses and updates in the following (Louis and Alpert, 2000):

- Nursing
- Theological/pastoral care field
- Public health
- Medicine
- Sociology
- Cultural diversity
- Human growth and development throughout the life span
- Improving collaboration, negotiation, and coordination skills
- Consultation
- Leadership
- Management
- Research skills

The challenge for the practice is to document trends, maintain and enhance the quality of the preparation and services offered, engage in evidence-based practice, use increased numbers of advanced practice nurses, network within professional organizations, and become involved

in outcomes-oriented research. To remain at the cutting edge of the profession and recognize competency among practitioners, the specialty must pursue professional certification.

ISSUES IN FAITH COMMUNITY NURSING PRACTICE

Every new discipline or care area must be alert to issues of accountability to populations served and to those who entrust the nurse with the responsibility to serve a designated population. This facilitates positive outcomes and avoids conflicts with individual and group rights and state regulations.

- Discussions of health promotion plans must include the individual, the family, and the faith community.
- Negotiations with the pastoral staff, congregations, institutions, and the wider community may be involved in job description preparation or program planning.
- Issues such as privacy, confidentiality, group concerns, access, and record management must be discussed with the pastoral staff or the contracting agency at the outset of any parish nurse agreement.

PROFESSIONAL ISSUES

Annual and periodic evaluations are required of parish nurse practices and services needed. These evaluations may be self, peer, congregational, and/or institutional. Personnel committees provide guidance and contribute to the evaluation. They also advocate for parish nurse services and raise awareness with the congregational staff members and programs. Professional appraisal is standard in nursing practice. The appraisals guide professional development and program development and planning. Because the scope of parish nursing practice is broad and focuses on the independent practice of the discipline, the nurse must consider a wide variety of issues:

- Position descriptions
- Professional liability
- Professional education
- Experiential preparation
- Collaborative agreements
- Working with lay volunteers as well as retired professionals

Abiding by the professional nursing code is understood; however, the nurse must also know the **polity**, expectations, and mission of the particular faith community. The nurse also continually interprets the profession for the faith community.

The nurse is required to be the following:

- Knowledgeable about lines of authority and channels of communication in the congregation and in the collaborative institutions
- Well acquainted with the personnel committees of the congregation
- An advocate for well-being to highlight justice issues in local and national legislation

- A contributor of information to policymakers about the implications for health and well-being for the parish and the local and global communities
- An active participant in political activities that contribute to spiritual growth and healthy functioning

BRIEFLY NOTED

Developing a keen sense of the value of the faith community within the geopolitical community and appreciating its associations within the local and wider community are beneficial.

ETHICAL ISSUES

Issues evolve from client, faith community, and professional arenas. The nurse's interventions are guided by professional responsibilities that include the following:
- Code for Nurses (American Nurses Association, 2005)
- Individual and group rights
- Statements of faith
- Polity of the faith community served

Professional and therapeutic relationships are maintained at all times; consulting and counseling with minors and individual members of the opposite sex are conducted using professional ethical principles. Policies about these issues are established at the outset of the practice with the pastoral team, the wellness committee, the parish nurse, and the local congregation's governing body.

As in other community health situations, the parish nurse, along with the client, does the following:
- Identifies parameters of ethical concerns
- Plans ahead with clients to consider healthy options in making ethical decisions
- Supports clients in their journey to choose alternatives that will strengthen coping skills
- Allows the client to grow stronger in faith and health
- Considers the "virtue ethics, such as caring, forgiveness, and compassion, in their decision making" (American Nurses Association and Health Ministries Association, 2005, p. 19)

Communities of faith strive to be caring communities and value the fellowship among its members. However, confidentiality is of utmost importance in parish nursing practice. The parish nurse values client confidentiality while delicately assisting the client and the client's family to "share" concerns with the pastoral staff and fellow **congregants**. This sharing gains valuable support to promote optimal healing. The nurse is often the staff member who helps the family to the stage of acceptance of a health concern. How much to share and when to share a concern is indeed a private affair and a part of the important journey of healing. A joyous event for one family may be a devastating event or even a depressing reminder of a past event for another family. The celebrations and joys of a healthy new infant one week may raise guilt and ambivalence for congregational members when, within a brief time, another family's long-awaited child dies at birth.

BRIEFLY NOTED

A young couple who has contributed their time, enthusiasm, and skills assisting as church youth group leaders are expecting their first child. What a valuable learning experience for the teens, the parish nurse contends. Having a couple experience healthy life events is indeed beneficial for youth. Upon birth, the infant is diagnosed with Down syndrome. Now the typical celebrations and visions for the future have changed. Instead of parties, what information is to be shared, and with whom and when? How much privacy is granted? The manner in which the family, other youth leaders, and the nurse work with the team, use the strengths of the congregation, and reflect on the spiritual needs of all concerned is important for healthy outcomes. The learning opportunities are valuable growth experiences for the young teens and for the new parents. Having opportunities to describe your feelings and dealing with them in supportive groups benefit the healing process.

LEGAL ISSUES

As an advocate of client and group rights, the nurse does the following:
- Identifies and reports neglect, abuse, and illegal behaviors to the appropriate legal sources
- Appropriately refers members to pastoral or community resources if the scope of the problem is beyond the realm of the professional nurse
- Refers to another health care professional if conflict between the nurse and client is such that no further progress is possible

The parish nurse who has a positive relationship that values open dialogue with the pastoral team will be supported in efforts to select the most appropriate community resources for clients.

The nurse must personally and professionally abide by the parameters of the nurse practice act of the jurisdiction and maintain an active license of that state. The following are additional legal concerns:
- Institutional contractual agreements
- Records management
- Release of information
- Volunteer liability

Resources would include the faith community's legal consultant, the faith community's national position statements, and those of the HMA and IPNRC (Solari-Twadell and McDermott, 2006).

FINANCIAL ISSUES

Innovative arrangements for variations of the basic models mentioned previously call for sustained financial support. The nurse is called on to partner in finding funds and networking with potential supporters. The nurse is accountable for money spent and for fundraising, whether the position is salaried or volunteer. Educational and promotional materials, equipment, travel time, continuing education, and malpractice insurance are selected areas that need to be included in the budget of the parish nurse. If these materials are not budget items, services may be limited, and this needs to be interpreted to the faith community. Money, time, and people are never sufficient to meet the needs of a parish nurse ministry, but it is up to the nurse to use a resource assessment in advance of a project to be able to come to a clear understanding of what is possible given the specific faith community resources (Solari-Twadell and McDermott, 2006).

NATIONAL HEALTH OBJECTIVES AND FAITH COMMUNITIES

The *Healthy People 2010* leading health indicators encourage communities to cooperatively lend support to individuals and families to attain an improved health status that can be passed on to future generations. One of the oldest and strongest partnerships is that established between communities and religious or faith communities. The Carter Center in Atlanta and the Park Ridge Center in Chicago collaborated with health care professionals and leaders of faith traditions to identify roles of faith communities to address national health objectives and approaches to improving overall public health.

Examples of congregational models addressing the specific objectives encouraging *Healthy People 2000* guidelines are increasingly being documented (Baldwin et al, 2001; Buijs and Olson, 2001; Hale and Bennett, 2000; Kolb et al, 2003; Swinney et al, 2001; Weis et al, 2002). In addition, the National Heart, Lung and Blood Institute urges partnerships with faith communities and offers suggestions for program planning.

Specific national objectives dealing with nutrition; physical activity; use of tobacco, alcohol, and other drugs; immunization status; environmental health; and injury and violence are within the realm of the health education role of the parish nurse. Activities include age-appropriate discussions of preventive activities with various groups; classes on the use and misuse of alcohol, tobacco, and other drugs; and discussions regarding responsible sexual behavior in the context of faith values. Parish nurses can also aid the local public health nurse in activities for screening and prevention of communicable disease such as tuberculosis (Toth et al, 2004).

Another national level effort to strengthen the potential partnerships between faith communities and health care professionals is the Caucus on Public Health and the Faith Community of the American Public Health Association (APHA). The first gathering of the caucus at the 1995 APHA annual meeting was addressed by then-APHA President Dr. Caswell Evans. Health care professionals of many faiths welcomed the opportunity to voice their interest in holistically supporting their communities and clients.

Wellness committees and parish nurses with the faith community's input may regularly review the various health status objectives, make comparisons between national and specific state objectives, and then assess the extent to which the specific congregation or groups of congregations are in need of reducing their risk. Health promotion activities such as regular blood pressure screening and monitoring activities focus on heart disease and stroke prevention and disability.

- Age-appropriate discussion of preventive activities can be held with various groups.
- Signs and symptoms of heart attack and stroke can be noted and described in newsletters and posted in strategic areas.
- The nurse can coordinate healthy low-fat church suppers.
- The nurse can encourage "moms and tots" groups to choose healthy fruit and vegetables as snacks after their faith discussion meetings.
- The nurse can coordinate a series of classes for families of adolescents on stress management and sessions on the use and misuse of alcohol, tobacco, and other drugs.
- The nurse can encourage regular exercise for individuals as a part of ongoing church activities.

Examples of interventions related to selected portions of *Healthy People 2010* objectives that could be addressed by parish nurses are listed in the "*Healthy People 2010*" box.

The congregation's health and wellness committee can similarly address other objectives to identify activities in which to engage individuals, groups, or the congregation as a whole. To promote healthy families, faith communities can address objectives with a maternal and infant health focus. Most advantageous for the faith community would be to engage in partnership activities with other community efforts such as health fairs. Health fairs are effective strategies for health promotion efforts guided by the *Healthy People 2010* framework. These and similar activities promote the increased health of the entire community and include persons of all ages, encourage enthusiastic fellowship and leisure, and reduce duplication of effort.

● Healthy People 2010

Overweight and Obesity

Nutrition and overweight priority: promote good nutrition and healthier weights

19-3	Reduce the proportion of children and adolescents who are overweight and obese
19-3.a	Reduce childhood obesity rates from 11% to 5%

Physical Activity

Priority: promote daily physical activity

22-7	Increase the proportion of adolescents who engage in vigorous physical activity that promotes cardiorespiratory fitness 3 or more days per week for 20 or more minutes per occasion

From U.S. Department of Health and Human Services: *Healthy People 2010: national health promotion and disease prevention objectives*, Washington, DC, 2000, U.S. Department of Health and Human Services.

Healthy People 2010 categories will incorporate leading health indicators. The 2010 authors hope that use of "leading health indicators" will result in a more precise and accurate way to reflect the intent of *Healthy People 2010*. Communities of faith are among the new health-related partners, which include members such as managed care organizations and business partners.

Parish nurses working with groups are pivotal as supportive links to implementing healthy behaviors. The recognition that persons are at greater risk of human immunodeficiency virus (HIV) infection when other sexually transmitted diseases (STDs) are present is another cue for faith communities to encourage community-based programs to prevent STDs, especially among adolescents and minorities. As young persons develop values and make lifestyle choices, their growth in character in a faith community can provide direction, support, and coping skills to select healthy options.

CASE STUDY

Jeremy Black is the community nursing professor at a school of nursing. Looking for new clinical experiences, Mr. Black was advised to examine parish nursing experiences for his students. He contracted with a Baptist church to bring health services to the church through himself and his students.

With Mr. Black's prompting, volunteers from the church joined together to form the church's Wellness Committee. The goal of the Wellness Committee was to identify the needs of the church members and to provide direction for Mr. Black and his students. Through interviews and surveys, the Wellness Committee and Mr. Black identified "increase knowledge of health promotion activities" as one of the needs the nursing students could address.

Mr. Black decided the nursing students would plan and organize a health fair for the church. Pairs of students were assigned to develop booths. Students were expected to research their topic, develop educational materials, and then teach at the fair. The five booths were as follows: blood pressure screening and information, osteoporosis screening and information, body mass index screening and information, self-screening information for certain cancers (e.g., skin, breast), and vision and hearing screenings and information. Mr. Black would provide the necessary equipment for the various screenings.

The health fair was given on a Sunday morning after worship services. Church members walked through and visited booths in which they were interested. Church members commented to the students how nice the booths looked and how glad they were to obtain the information.

FUNCTIONS OF THE FAITH COMMUNITY NURSE

Examples of parish nursing interventions have been cited throughout this chapter. This section summarizes and expands some of the usual functions and describes activities.

A primary independent function is that of *personal health counseling*. Parish nurses discuss the following:
- Health risk appraisals
- Spiritual assessments
- Plans for healthier lifestyles
- Support and guidance related to numerous acute and chronic actual and potential health problems

Parish nurses carry out their practice in groups or individually. They make visits to homes, hospitals, and nursing homes. They see persons in the faith community's house of worship. Some nurses have designated offices, whereas others use space that is most conducive to the particular activity or client need.

A second function is that of *health education*. Parish nurses participate in health education as follows:
- Publish information in congregation news bulletins
- Distribute information
- Have available a variety of resources for the physical, mental, and spiritual health of the congregation
- Hold classes to address identified needs
- Provide individual teaching as needed
- Hold discussions for targeted groups or meetings
- Strive to promote wholeness in health
- Create a fuller understanding of total physical, mental, and spiritual well-being

As a *liaison* between resources in the faith community and the local community, the parish nurse's responsibilities again are as follows:
- Help clients know what resources are available to solve their problems
- Help individuals and families match the appropriate resource to their problem
- Link clients with the appropriate services

The parish nurse is also a *facilitator*. The nurse does the following:
- Links congregational needs to the establishment of and referral to support groups
- Facilitates changes in the congregation to increase disability access or to extend meals and services to those who are homebound
- May also work with the volunteer coordinator to train volunteers or ensure that interested persons acquire training to function as lay caregivers to meet congregational needs

Box 29-3 is an example of how the parish nurse works with other providers and community resources to meet the health needs of a client.

Underlying all of the previously mentioned functions is *pastoral care,* which the nurse fulfills as follows:
- Stresses the spiritual dimension of nursing
- Lends support during times of joy and sorrow
- Guides the person through health and illness throughout life
- Helps identify the spiritual strengths that assist in coping with particular events

The nurse may use hymns, favorite scripture verses, psalms, pictures, church windows, stories, or other images that are important for the individual or group to hold to the connectedness between faith, health, and well-being.

Box 29-3	Parish Nursing as Healing Ministry: An Adult Daughter's Reflection

What a pleasure to be able to commend [parish nurse's] personal friendship and professional help! Without her support it would have been difficult, if not impossible, for my father to live at home during his last 6 years. But she had, along with his doctor, the sure feeling that it was the right thing for him and that it could be done. When the time came that he needed caregivers around the clock, she skillfully conveyed suggestions in such a way that the caregivers' cultural differences were not a barrier. She helped them grow as caregivers, appreciating their accomplishments, even to having a blackberry-picking "outing" at her home.

My father in his earlier years had been a deacon and had loved visiting shut-ins. It brought him so much happiness that he in turn received his church's caring, healing ministry through his parish nurse. He attended church on Sundays beyond what one would expect of one in his 90s, and almost his last Sunday was the day he celebrated turning 96.

Thank you, [parish nurse], for our "Mission Accomplished"!

With permission, A.F.H.

Numerous healthy activities should be encouraged in congregations, and the nurse often works with the congregation to expand its immediate borders to augment services in the community that promote health and wellness. Congregations are keenly aware that more than half of the members of mainstream churches are part of the growing aging population of our country. Increased numbers of persons who are either uninsured or underinsured are in their communities. Thus services offered may include the following:

- Food pantries
- Day care for seniors
- Congregate meals
- Preschool and latch-key arrangements
- Tutoring
- Meals on Wheels
- Visits to less-mobile members
- Outreach for vulnerable populations

Box 29-4 lists several selected activities of parish nurses (Berry, 2004). However, the creative implementing of the parish nurse concept by each individual nurse within a unique faith community will result in a wealth of possibilities.

CLINICAL APPLICATION

The nursing process is a method that can be used to begin program planning and evaluation with faith communities. Such an approach can involve congregational members and parish nurses in a dynamic endeavor to jointly learn about the members' individual health status as well as that of the faith community and the local and broader geographic community. Parish nurse programs are derived in various ways. Initially, the impetus for parish nursing may stem from an unmet health need within the congregation, from visions of a lay or health professions member concerned

Box 29-4	A Sampling of Parish Nurse Interventions and Activities

- Sharing the joys of a new member in the family; sharing the sorrows of losses
- Anticipating changes in health status or in growth and development
- Being present for questions that seem difficult or unacceptable to ask the health care provider
- Explaining and assisting in considering choices when new living and care arrangements must be made
- Listening to the concerns of a youngster anticipating diagnostic procedures
- Praying with the spouse of a dying parishioner
- Helping individuals and families make decisions regarding advance directives in light of faith beliefs
- Helping teens consider options when overwhelmed with serious life issues
- Providing information, support, and prayer regarding advance directives
- Seeking community resources and opportunities for fitness and nutrition classes
- Working with the wellness committee to ensure that fellowship meals meet the nutritional and spiritual needs of the elderly
- Offering educational opportunities about changes in health care legislation and its influence on the congregation and community
- Accompanying a faith community member to a 12-step meeting
- Participating in worship leadership with the pastoral staff

From Berry R: A parish nurse. In *Office of Resourcing Committees on Preparation for Ministry: a day in the life of.... a kaleidoscope of specialized ministries,* Louisville, Ky, 2004, Presbyterian Church (USA), Distribution Management Service.

about caring within the congregation, or from discussions of a committee dealing with health and wellness issues. *Which of the following activities is most likely to increase the interest and involvement of the congregation's members?*

A. *Writing a contract for parish nursing services.*
B. *Surveying the faith communities' environment.*
C. *Gathering information on leaders and valued activities in the congregation through focus groups of pastoral staff.*
D. *Assessing the needs of the congregational members through a survey.*
E. *Holding a health fair.*
Answer is in the back of the book.

REMEMBER THIS!

- Parish nurse services respond to health, healing, and wholeness within the context of the church. Although the emphasis is on health promotion and disease prevention throughout the life span, the spiritual dimension of nursing is central to the practice.
- The parish nurse partners with the wellness committee and volunteers to plan programs and consider health-related concerns within faith communities.

- To promote a caring faith community, the usual functions of the parish nurse include personal health counseling, health teaching, facilitating linkages and referrals to congregation and community resources, advocating and encouraging support resources, and providing pastoral care.
- Parish nurses collaborate to plan, implement, and evaluate health promotion activities considering the faith community's beliefs, rituals, and polity. *Healthy People 2010* guidelines are basic to the partnering for programs.
- Nurses in congregational or institutional models enhance the health ministry programs of the faith communities if carefully chosen partnerships are formed within the congregation, with other congregations, and also with local health and social community agencies.
- Nurses working in the parish nursing specialty must seek to attain adequate educational and skill preparation and to be accountable to those served and to those who have entrusted the nurse to serve.
- Nurses are encouraged to consider innovative approaches to creating caring communities. These may be in congregations as parish nurses, among several faith communities in a single locale, or regionally; or in partnership with other community agencies.
- To be sustained as a parish nurse healer, the nurse needs to heal and nurture herself or himself while supporting individuals, families, and congregation communities in their healing process.

WHAT WOULD YOU DO?

1. Contact the local council of churches to see if there is a parish nurse in your community. If so, arrange to spend a day with the nurse.
   a. Interview the nurse regarding the role functions of the parish nurse.
   b. Ask how the standards of practice of the parish nurse are integrated into the practice.
2. Discuss with classmates the similarities and differences between parish nursing and other nurses in community health. Review the content in this chapter, and compare your answers.
3. Choose a *Healthy People 2010* objective to implement in a parish nursing setting. Discuss plans for implementing the objective and evaluating the outcomes. What data did you use to develop a plan for implementing? How did you choose your population?

■ REFERENCES

American Nurses Association: *Code for nurses with interpretive statements*, Washington, DC, 2005, ANA.

American Nurses Association: *Nursing: scope and standards of practice*, Silver Spring, Md, 2004, ANA, available at nursebooks.org.

American Nurses Association and Health Ministries Association: *Faith community nursing: scope and standards of practice*, Silver Spring, Md, 2005, ANA, available at nursebooks.org.

Anderson C: The delivery of health care in faith-based organizations: parish nurses as promoters of health, *Health Commun* 16:117-128, 2004.

Baldwin KA et al: Perceived needs of urban African American church congregants, *Public Health Nurs* 18:295-303, 2001.

Berry R: A parish nurse. In *Office of Resourcing Committees on Preparation for Ministry: a day in the life of...: a kaleidoscope of specialized ministries*, Louisville, Ky, 2004, Presbyterian Church (USA), Distribution Management Service.

Berry R et al: Weaving international parish nurse experiences: sharing the story of Korea. In Solari-Twadell A, coordinator: *Weaving parish nursing into the new millennium*, proceedings of the 14th Annual Westberg Symposium, Itasca, Ill, 2000.

Bitner KL, Woodward M: Advanced practice parish nursing: a clinical narrative, *Clin Excell Nurse Pract* 8:159-165, 2004.

Buijs R, Olson J: Parish nurses influencing determinants of health, *J Community Health Nurs* 18:13-23, 2001.

Carson VB, Koenig HG: *Parish nursing: stories of services and health care*, Philadelphia, 2002, Templeton Foundation Press.

Chase-Ziolek M: *Health, healing and wholeness*, Cleveland, 2005, Pilgrim.

Chase-Ziolek M, Iris M: Nurses' perspectives of the distinctive aspects of providing nursing care in a congregational setting, *J Community Health Nurs* 19:173-186, 2002.

Dossey BM, Keegan L, Guzzetta CE: *Holistic nursing: a handbook for practice*, ed 4, Sudbury, Mass, 2005, Jones and Bartlett.

Gustafson CZ: From Montana to Swaziland: nurses reaching out in hope, *Parish Nurse Perspect* 2:13, 2003.

Gustafson CZ: Distance delivery of parish nurse education. In Solari-Twadell PA, McDermott MA, editors: *Parish nursing: development, education, and administration*, St. Louis, 2006, Elsevier.

Hale WD, Bennett RG: *Building healthy communities through medical-religious partnerships*, Baltimore, Md, 2000, Johns Hopkins University.

Hale WD, Koenig HG: *Healing bodies and souls: a practical guide for congregations*, Minneapolis, 2003, Fortress.

Health Ministries' Association and American Nurses Association: *Scope and standards of parish nursing practice*, Washington, DC, 1998, ANA.

Hurley JE, Mohnkern S: Mobilize support groups to meet congregational needs, *J Christian Nurs* 21:34-39, 2004.

International Parish Nurse Resource Center: *Role of parish nurse, mission and resource* (brochure), Park Ridge, Ill, 1998, International Parish Nurse Resource Center.

Kolb SE et al: Ministerio de Salud: development of a mission driven partnership, *J Multicult Nurs Health* 9:6-12, 2003.

Kotecki CN: Community-based strategies. Incorporating faith-based partnerships into the curriculum, *Nurse Educ* 27:13-15, 2002.

Loeb SJ, O'Neill J, Gueldner SH: Health motivation: a determinant of older adults' attendance at health promotion programs, *J Community Health Nurs* 18:151-165, 2001.

Louis M, Alpert P: Spirituality for nurses and their practice, *Nurs Leadersh Forum* 5:43-51, 2000.

Lukits A: Parish nurses fill gap in health care system, *Reg Nurse J* 12:10-12, 2000.

McDermott MA, Solari-Twadell PA: Parish nurse curricula, In Solari-Twadell PA, McDermott MA, editors: *Parish nursing: development, education, and administration*, St. Louis, 2006, Elsevier, pp 121-131.

Meisenhelder JB, Chandler EN: Prayer and health outcomes in church members, *Altern Ther Health Med* 6(4):56-60, 2000.

Minden P: Parish nursing: inclusive or exclusive? *Holis Nurs Practice* 19:49, 2005.

Nist JA: Parish nursing programs: through them, faith communities are reclaiming a role in healing, *Health Prog* 84:50–54, 2003.

O'Brien ME: *Parish nursing: health care ministry within the church*, Sudbury, Mass, 2003, Jones and Bartlett.

Patterson DL: *The essential parish nurse*, Cleveland, 2003, Pilgrim.

Roberts F: Faith community nurses fill gap in primary care, *Kai Tiaki Nurs New Zealand* 9:11, 2003.

Rouse DP: Parish nursing as community-based pediatric clinical experience, *Nurse Educ* 25:8–11, 2000.

Schweitzer R: Shleimut: a multidisciplinary approach to Jewish healing, healing and wholeness, *Parish Nurse Perspect* 3:7–8, 2004.

Shelly JA: *Nursing in the church*, Madison, Wis, 2002, NCF Press.

Simpson J: Featured parish nurse: "Crescent Nurse," *Parish Nurse Perspect* 3:2, 2004.

Solari-Twadell PA: Uncovering the intricacies of the ministry of parish nursing practice through research. In Solari-Twadell PA, McDermott MA, editors: *Parish nursing: development, education, and administration*, St. Louis, 2006, Elsevier, pp 17–34.

Solari-Twadell PA, McDermott MA, editors: *Parish nursing: development, education, and administration*, St. Louis, 2006, Elsevier.

Solari-Twadell PA, McDermott MA, Matheus R, editors: *Parish nursing education: preparation for parish nurse managers/coordinators: promoting congregational health, healing and wholeness for the twenty-first century*, Park Ridge, Ill, 2000, IPNRC, Advocate Health Care.

Solari-Twadell PA et al: *Assuring viability for the future: guideline development for parish nurse education programs*, Park Ridge, Ill, 1994, Lutheran General Health System.

Swinney J et al: Community assessment: a church community and the parish nurse, *Public Health Nurs* 18:40–44, 2001.

Taylor EJ: Prayer's clinical issues and implications, *Holistic Nurs Pract* 17:179–188, 2003.

Toth A et al: Tuberculosis prevention and treatment: all nursing roles are key, *Can Nurse* 100:27–30, 2004.

Trofino J, Hughes CB, Hay KM: Primary care parish nursing: academic, service and parish partnerships, *Nurs Admin Q* 24:59–74, 2000.

Tuck I, Pullen L, Wallace D: Comparative study of the spiritual perspectives and interventions of mental health and parish nurses, *Issues Ment Health Nurs* 22:593–606, 2001.

U.S. Department of Health and Human Services: *Healthy People 2010* [CD-ROM], Rockville, Md, 2000, U.S. Government Printing Office, available at http://www.health.gov/healthypeople.

Vandecreek L, Mooney S: *Parish nurses, health care chaplains, and community clergy*, New York, 2002, Haworth Press.

Van Loon A: Faith community nursing, *ACCNS J Community Nurs* 9:7, 2004.

Wallace DC et al: Client perceptions of parish nursing, *Public Health Nurs* 19:128–135, 2002.

Weis et al: Parish nurse practice with client aggregates, *J Community Health Nurs* 19:105–113, 2002.

Woodworth H: News from "across the pond," *Parish Nurse Perspect* 4:8, 2005.

The Nurse in Home Health and Hospice

Juliann G. Sebastian
Karen S. Martin

ADDITIONAL RESOURCES

These related resources are found either in the appendix at the back of this book or on the book's website at http://evolve.elsevier.com/stanhope/foundations.

Appendix

- Appendix A.2: Schedule of Clinical Preventive Services
- Appendix B.1: OASIS: Start of Care Assessment
- Appendix E.1: Infection Control Guidelines for Home Care
- Appendix E.3: Health Insurance Portability and Accountability Act (HIPAA): What Does It Mean for Public Health Nurses?
- Appendix E.4: Living Will Directive
- Appendix G.4: Omaha System Problem Classification Scheme with Case Study Application
- Appendix H.2: American Nurses Association Standards of Care of Public Health Nursing Practice.

⊖Evolve Website

- Community Assessment Applied
- Quiz review questions
- WebLinks, including link to *Healthy People 2010* website

Real World Community Health Nursing: An Interactive CD-ROM, second edition

If you are using this CD-ROM in your course, you will find the following activities related to this chapter:

- *Prioritize Your Day* in **A Day in the Life of a Community Health Nurse**

OBJECTIVES

After reading this chapter, the student should be able to do the following:

1. Describe the history of nursing in home care.
2. Compare different types of home care, including home-based nursing programs, home health, and hospice.
3. Explain the professional standards and educational requirements for nursing in home care.
4. Explain how nurses in home care work with interprofessional teams.

5. Analyze reimbursement mechanisms, issues, and trends related to home care.
6. Recognize how nurses in home care use quality improvement strategies and promote client safety.
7. Assess trends in home care as related to promoting the achievement of national health objectives.
8. Describe key components of the Omaha System.

CHAPTER OUTLINE

HISTORY OF HOME CARE
TYPES OF HOME CARE NURSING
Population-Focused Home Care
Transitional Care in the Home

Home-Based Primary Care
Home Health
Hospice
Home Care of the Dying Child

KEY TERMS

accreditation: a credentialing process used to recognize health care agencies or educational programs for provision of quality services and programs.

benchmarking: comparing national standards and guidelines with other agencies.

care coordination: linking clients with services.

certification: a mechanism, usually by means of written examination, that provides an indication of professional competence in a specialized area of practice.

client outcomes: changes in client health status as a result of care or program implementation.

family caregiving: assisting the client to meet his or her basic needs and providing direct care such as personal hygiene, meal preparation, medication administration, and treatments.

hospice: palliative system of health care for terminally ill people; it takes place in the home with family involvement under the direction and supervision of health professionals, especially the visiting nurse. Hospice care takes place in the hospital when severe complications of terminal illness occur or when the family becomes exhausted or does not fulfill commitments.

interprofessional collaboration: a working agreement in which each home health care provider carefully

analyzes his or her role in determining the best plan for the client's care.

Outcomes and Assessment Information Set (OASIS): an instrument to collect client data for doing outcome assessments in home health.

palliative care: alleviating symptoms of, meeting the special needs of, and providing comfort for the dying clients and their families by the nurse.

prospective payment system: a mechanism whereby Medicare will pay home health agencies a set amount of money to care for a client who meets the criteria of 1 of 80 home health resource groups (the diagnosis is based on severity, functional status, and number of services needed).

regulations: specific statements of law that relate to and clarify individual pieces of legislation.

reimbursement system: the process by which home health care agencies receive payment, either by the client or three major funding sources: Medicare, Medicaid, and third-party funding.

skilled care: care provided to a client that requires the knowledge and skill of a registered nurse.

telehealth: health information sent from one site to another by electronic communication.

This chapter explains the development and current status of nursing in home care. Home care refers to care provided by a formal caregiver such as a nurse, speech or physical therapist, or physician within a client's home. Home care by formal caregivers is complemented by self-care provided by the client and caregiving by family members and friends. Home care differs from other areas of health care in that health care providers practice in the client's home environment. The home is where nurses have provided care for more than a century in the United States. Home care enables clients and families to receive health care in their usual home environment where they may feel more comfortable and where it may be easier to learn how to make health-related lifestyle changes. For clients who are homebound, home care may be a necessity.

Home care includes disease prevention, health promotion, and episodic illness-related services provided to people in their places of residence. Home may be a house, an apartment, a trailer, a boarding and care home, a shelter, a car, or any other place in which someone lives.

Home care does not refer only to home health; it is much broader than that. It is an approach to care that is provided in people's homes because theory or research suggests this is the optimum location for certain health and nursing services. Home care includes home health services, in-home hospice services, home visiting by public health nurses, and a variety of home-based health care programs focused on specific populations such as new mothers, frail elders, and people with certain chronic health problems. Home health nursing in particular "refers to the practice of nursing applied to a client

Levels of Prevention   Applied to Home Care

PRIMARY PREVENTION

Prepartum and postpartum home visiting models can help vulnerable mothers learn how to cope successfully with stressful life events (Izzo et al, 2005).

SECONDARY PREVENTION

The nurse assesses clients in their homes for early signs of new health problems, contacts the physician, and initiates prompt treatment to prevent the condition from worsening. An example is assessing clients for the development of side effects from medications.

TERTIARY PREVENTION

The nurse provides counseling on dietary modifications and insulin injections to the newly diagnosed diabetic client. The purpose of these interventions is to prevent the development of complications from diabetes. The diabetic client and his or her family implement the therapeutic plan with the goal of maintaining health at the highest possible level.

---

with a health condition in the client's place of residence... Home health nursing is a specialized area of nursing practice with its roots firmly placed in nursing in the community" (American Nurses Association [ANA], 2007, p. 3).

BRIEFLY NOTED

Despite the current nursing shortage, increased client load, complex technological needs of clients in the home, and reimbursement regulations that focus on secondary and tertiary care, it remains an ethical responsibility of the home care nurse to promote health and prevent illness in the home and community.

It is essential to work with the family in the provision of care to an individual client. Family is defined by the individual and includes any caregiver or significant person who assists a client in need of care at home. **Family caregiving** includes assisting clients to meet their basic needs and providing direct care such as personal hygiene, meal preparation, medication administration, and treatments. Today, caregivers provide care in the home that in the past was provided in a hospital. Caregivers and clients themselves also provide health maintenance care between the visits of the professional provider. Levels of prevention in home care, including health maintenance care, are discussed in the "Levels of Prevention" box.

Client goals include health promotion, maintenance, and restoration. By maximizing the level of independence and self-care abilities, nurses help their clients function at the highest possible level. In addition, nurses contribute to the prevention of complications in chronically ill persons and help minimize the effects of disability and illness.

In any form of home care, nurses continually assess the client's response to interventions, report their findings to the client's physician or other health care provider as appropriate, and collaborate to modify the treatment plan or interventions as needed. Interventions are modified based on the client's responses. Services are coordinated through an agency obligated to maintain quality care and to provide continuity whether that agency is a home health agency, hospice, community nursing program, clinic, or hospital. Thus the range of services provided in home care is extensive.

Nurses practice autonomously with little structure in the home setting; therefore, competence and creativity are essential (Snow, 2000). The home environment lacks many resources typically found in institutions, so it is essential that nurses have good organizational skills, be able to adapt to different settings, and demonstrate interpersonal ability to work with the diverse needs of people in their homes.

When working in a client's home, the nurse is a guest and, to be effective, must earn the trust of the family and establish a partnership with the client and family. Client safety is of utmost concern in home care just as in other health care settings.

HISTORY OF HOME CARE

Home care provided by formal caregivers can be traced back to the nineteenth century (Buhler-Wilkerson, 2002). At that time, ladies' charitable organizations provided care to the sick in their own homes by hiring nurses. By the late nineteenth and early twentieth centuries, Lillian Wald had established the Henry Street Settlement House in New York City and expanded home care to include community health needs. In Wald's Henry Street Settlement House, nurses and social workers visited people in their homes and provided instruction on basic hygiene, assessed health status, educated people about good nutrition, and provided support and immunizations. Although much home care was provided by voluntary organizations such as visiting nurse associations in the early twentieth century, it was coordinated with governmental agencies such as health departments (Barkauskas and Stocker, 2000).

Home care began changing from its charitable and public health-oriented beginnings when payers added it to their benefit plans (Buhler-Wilkerson, 2002). Wald persuaded the Metropolitan Life Insurance Company to include home care as a benefit in the early 1900s. Later home care was included as a benefit for Medicare enrollees following passage of Medicare legislation in 1965.

Inclusion of home care in the benefit packages of the Metropolitan Life Insurance Company and later in Medicare began to change the nature of the services (Buhler-Wilkerson, 2002). Services focused on clients with specific functional and health problems who could not be cared for elsewhere. Nurses provided more technical care as time progressed. Home health as an industry expanded following the shift to prospective payment for hospital care with the federal Tax Equity and Financial Responsibility Act in 1982 (Tieman, 2003). This occurred because clients were discharged more quickly from hospitals and needed more high-acuity nursing care in the home. The 1997 federal Balanced Budget Act (Zhu, 2004) required moving reimbursement for home health services to a prospective payment system, which again meant pressure to care for clients with acute illnesses that were likely to improve. Attention continues to be paid to efficiency and cost-effectiveness of care. This often means that care is targeted toward very specific client populations and is highly organized and closely documented.

Historically, nurses who worked in people's homes were social reformers, living in immigrant communities and providing nursing clinics, health education, and care for the sick. They provided for the nutritional needs of their communities as well as clothing, hygiene, and adequate shelter. They were responsible for developing needed programs and providing necessary services in communities, including prenatal care, postpartum visits to new mothers and babies, hot-lunch school programs, preschool clinics, transportation services, summer camp programs, tuberculosis screening, blood typing, immunization for polio, and "sick room" equipment programs.

This combination of preventive services and illness care shifted following the introduction of Medicare in 1966. The Medicare program emphasized care for more acutely ill people rather than illness prevention and health promotion.

Hospice care, or care of the dying client and his or her significant others, was introduced in the United States in the 1970s by Dr. Florence Wald, Dean of the Yale University School of Nursing, with the input of Dr. Cicely Saunders, a British physician who had developed the modern hospice concept in England in the 1960s (Von Gunter and Ryndes, 2005). Elisabeth Kübler-Ross's book *On Death and Dying* (1964) highlighted the need to provide more humane and sensitive care at the end of life. The concept of hospice grew out of a commitment to provide compassionate and dignified end-of-life care to people in the comfort of their homes (Hoffmann, 2005). Later hospice models included **palliative care**, which is symptom management, with a focus on **care coordination** and comprehensive support (Higginson and Koffman, 2005) often in specialized inpatient hospice units. Both home-based and inpatient hospice care models share a focus on comfort, pain relief, and mitigation of other distressing symptoms.

TYPES OF HOME CARE NURSING

Several different types of home care nursing will be described in this chapter. They are population-focused home care, transitional care in the home, home-based primary care, home health, and hospice (Turk et al, 2000). These new models do not always rely on short-term, curative skilled nursing approaches. Instead they often incorporate aspects of traditional public health nursing in which nurses visited people in their homes to provide comprehensive assessments, nursing care, and linkages with community agencies.

POPULATION-FOCUSED HOME CARE

Research has demonstrated that home-based approaches to care delivery produce better outcomes for certain populations. Population-focused home care is directed toward the needs of specific groups of people, including those with high-risk health needs such as mental health problems, cardiovascular disease, or diabetes; families with infants or young children; or older adults (Inglis et al, 2004). These models commonly include structured approaches to regular visits with assessment protocols, focused health education, counseling, and health-related support and coaching. In one example, an interdisciplinary home care program included psychiatric nurses who made home visits to elders who lived in public housing and had psychiatric symptoms (Rabins et al, 2000). The nurses conducted comprehensive psychiatric assessments of older adults who had been referred to them by building personnel. They provided counseling, coaching, medication monitoring, referrals, and coordinated care with social workers and physicians. The program was effective in reducing psychiatric symptoms. Interdisciplinary collaboration is a required process in home health care.

The Program of All-Inclusive Care for the Elderly (PACE) is a managed care model of integrated health and personal care services (Nadash, 2004; Turk et al, 2000). Interprofessional care is provided in adult day care centers with home-based assessments and supportive services also provided. Because of the model's success, it is now included in Medicare and Medicaid capitation plans.

These are examples of population-focused home care. This approach to home care uses care delivery models developed using research evidence to improve health and cost outcomes for high-risk populations (see "Evidence-Based Practice" box on p. 567).

TRANSITIONAL CARE IN THE HOME

Transitional care programs in the home are designed for populations who have complex or high-risk health problems and are making a transition from one level of care to another (Brooten et al, 2002; Naylor, 2006). Examples of high-risk groups for whom transitional care programs have been tested include adults with cognitive impairments (Naylor et al, 2005), women with high-risk pregnancies (Brooten et al, 2002), and older adults with heart failure (Naylor et al, 2006). These programs facilitate a smooth and coordinated health care experience for clients receiving health services across sites of care. An example would be an adult with diabetes who visits an ambulatory care clinic, is hospitalized, and is then discharged home. A transitional care program would involve assessment, planning, teaching, making referrals, and following up on the referrals by nurses at each stage of care to foster independence and self-care. Nursing care might include intensive teaching about self-care and telephone calls to ensure that the client and caregiver understood and were able to implement the instructions (Naylor et al, 2005).

BRIEFLY NOTED

Home care nurses can facilitate smooth transitions from one level of care to another by working closely with hospital discharge planners (Brooten et al, 2002). Because clients and caregivers may find it difficult to learn while the client is hospitalized, home care nurses should communicate clearly with discharge planners about the therapeutic plan, medication regimens, what clients have been taught about self-care, and symptoms that should be reported to the physician.

HOME-BASED PRIMARY CARE

Home-based primary care is another form of home care delivery. The emphasis in these programs is delivering primary care in the homes of people for whom it is difficult to come into a primary care clinic, community center, or physician's office due to functional or other health problems (Turk et al, 2000). One example is the Veterans Affairs Administration Hospital-Based Home Care Program (Turk et al, 2000). These programs are interprofessional and emphasize self-care and help clients feel that the care experience is well coordinated across sites of care. Nurses provide health education to clients and caregivers in addition to primary care services such as health assessment, medication management, referrals, case management, and screening for new health problems. Comprehensive home care services are part of the Veterans Health Administration's goals to create more client-centered care arrangements that promote coordination of the care experience across sites of care (Perlin, Kolodner, and Roswell, 2004).

House call programs represent another example of primary care in the home. Nurse practitioners or physicians may provide primary care to clients who would find it difficult to visit a primary care office because of their health problems, or interprofessional teams that include nurses, physicians, or other health professionals may provide primary care (Muramatsu, Mensah, and Cornwell, 2004).

HOME HEALTH

Home health agencies are divided into the following five general types based on administrative and organizational structures (Figure 30-1):
- Official
- Private and voluntary
- Combination
- Hospital based
- Proprietary

These types differ in organization and administration but are similar in terms of the standards they must meet for licensure, certification, and accreditation.

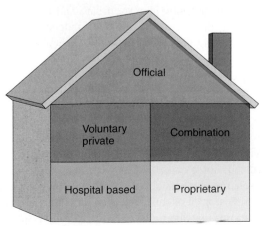

FIGURE 30 I Types of home health agencies.

Official or public agencies include those agencies operated by the state, county, city, or other local government units, such as health departments. Nurses employed in these settings may also provide well-child clinics, immunizations, health education programs, and home visits for preventive health care. Official agencies are funded primarily by tax funds and are nonprofit. Home care services are reimbursed through Medicare, Medicaid, and private insurance companies.

Voluntary and private agencies are grouped together as nonprofit home health agencies. Voluntary agencies are supported by charities such as United Way; by Medicare, Medicaid, and other third-party payers; and by client payments. Traditionally, visiting nurse associations (VNAs) were the principal type of voluntary home health agency. With the initiation of Medicare in 1966, private nonprofit agencies emerged as alternatives to publicly supported programs.

Boards of directors that represent the communities they serve govern voluntary and private nonprofit agencies. These agencies are nongovernmental organizations and are exempt from federal income tax. Historically, voluntary agencies were responsible for the development of nursing in the home that was based on the client's need for service rather than the ability to pay. In some communities, official and voluntary home health agencies have merged into combination agencies to provide home health care and decrease cost and prevent duplication of services. The services remain the same, and either the board members come from the two existing agencies or a new board is formed. The nurse may serve in several population-focused nursing roles, as does the nurse in the official type of agency.

In the 1970s, hospital-based agencies emerged in response to the recognized need for continuity of care from the acute care setting and also because of the high cost of institutionalization.

In 1983 implementation of the **prospective payment system** for acute hospital care by the federal government caused a fundamental change in home care. Costs of care dictated earlier patient discharge to control expenses. Home health agencies including hospital-based agencies increased in number and developed services to improve quality along with controlling costs (Tieman, 2003).

Agencies that are not eligible for income tax exemption are called proprietary (profit-making) agencies. Proprietary agencies can be licensed and certified for Medicare by the state licensing agency. The owner of the agency is responsible for governing. Reimbursement is primarily from third-party payers and individual clients if agencies do not accept Medicare.

The changing environment in home health care has several implications for the nurse providing care in the home. Because clients are discharged from acute care at earlier stages of treatment, a highly skilled level of care at home is needed. For example, many home health agencies provide infusion therapies in the home, such as administration of antibiotics, blood products, chemotherapy, and parenteral nutrition therapies (e.g., see Dobson, 2001). To survive in the competitive arena, agencies must continue to provide quality care and be cost-effective without compromising accountability.

HOSPICE

Historically, the word *hospice* referred to a place of refuge for travelers. The contemporary meaning refers to palliative care of the very ill and dying, reducing distress from physical, emotional, and spiritual symptoms (Hanley, 2004). Originating in nineteenth-century England, the earliest hospices first provided palliative care to terminally ill clients in hospitals and later extended the services into homes. In 1970 the hospice movement in the United States gained momentum in response to awakened public interest generated by Dr. Elisabeth Kübler-Ross's work on death and dying (Kübler-Ross, 1969). Public-sponsored hospices, successful in meeting the special needs of the dying client, attracted the attention of Congress. Medicare reimbursement for hospice services became available in 1982; services not covered by Medicare may be covered by other insurance plans or charitable organizations (Hoffmann, 2005).

A variety of hospice care models in the United States use institutional services, home care, or both. In addition to prescribed home care services, core services offered through hospice include volunteers, chaplain support, respite care, financial help with medicines and equipment, and bereavement support for the family after the client's death.

One criterion for hospice is that the disease process or condition has progressed to the extent that further treatment cannot cure. It is the goal of hospice to increase the quality of remaining life. The hospice team is usually medically directed and nurse coordinated. Pain management, symptom control, and emotional support are key interventions.

Hospice provides on-call nursing 24 hours a day to monitor changes in the client's condition and attend to the needs of the client and family. After the death of the client, hospice provides bereavement counseling and services for up to 1 year.

Hospice programs may be integrated with a home health, hospital, or skilled nursing agency, or they may be freestanding (Hospice Association of America, 2001). The philosophy of care requires that the interprofessional team have the knowledge, skill, compassion, and experience to work with the unique needs of this population. The primary goal is to help maintain the client's dignity and comfort (McClement et al, 2004). Alleviating pain; encouraging the client, family, and friends to communicate with each other about essential sensitive issues related to death and dying; and coordinating care to ensure a comfortable, peaceful death contribute to palliative care. Although providing comfort transcends cultures, nurses should incorporate an understanding of unique cultural values, expectations, and preferences into hospice and palliative care (Doorenbos and Schim, 2004; Jensen, 2003; Lorenz et al, 2004).

Health care providers who work with the dying often experience unique stress. Staff stress must be identified and appropriately addressed to help in the delivery of quality care and to maintain the care provider's well-being. Nurses should be aware of signs of physical or emotional fatigue and design their own self-care strategies to prevent these problems (Sherman, 2004). The hospice nurse needs a firm foundation in home care skills, knowledge of community resources, the ability to function constructively as a team member, comfort with death and dying, and the mature ability to meet personal emotional needs as well as the emotional needs of the hospice client and family.

End-of-life care is of great concern to nursing, and many issues are debated by the public (e.g., client choice, available hospice services, reimbursement status, admission criteria, and assisted suicide). *The Code of Ethics for Nurses With Interpretive Statements* (American Nurses Association, 2005) and involvement in a formal interdisciplinary ethics committee can assist nurses in resolving these dilemmas (see the "How To" box).

HOW TO ▸ Use a Hospice Approach to Care in Any Setting

The hospice philosophy of care means providing comfort measures to an individual before death. The circumstances of death vary. The individual may be any age, from infancy to the older adult. A nurse may be faced with the death of a single individual or of many people during a limited time. Death may occur in the individual's home, in a hospital setting, or in an uncontrolled setting such as the community. How can nursing care be adapted to any situation? What basic skills of professional caregivers can be applied in any situation or setting? How do caregivers adapt to a hospice home death, inpatient death, or a sudden, unexpected death where, for example, many people have died as a result of a natural disaster or a terrorist act?

- Be prepared now. Consider your own philosophy of death so that you can assist others without distraction when that time comes.
- Cultures vary in their beliefs about and responses to death. Know the differences in cultural responses so that you can effectively help people in their time of need.
- Death events cannot be totally controlled—even in a hospice environment in which family and friends and the dying individual have been prepared for the death. Expect the unexpected and take cues from the client and the loved ones regarding their needs.
- Shock, disbelief, and crisis reactions occur even with prepared hospice deaths. Ask family and caregivers what they need; provide them with the basics such as food or blankets; provide comfort; if it is not contraindicated, provide the family and friends with personal effects or mementos of the individual; give sensitive, caring support. Sit with them and listen.
- In a disaster, when many people are affected, the philosophy of care is to provide the greatest good to the greatest number of people. In a triage situation, the needs of those with less severe injuries have priority over the needs of those who are closer to death (Mistovich et al, 2000). Responsibilities of caregivers and health professionals will be stretched to the maximum. How do we care for the needs of the dying? How do we attend to the responses of the public to their loved ones? Someone needs to be present to support them. A specified leader to a group of clients must delegate responsibility to a caregiver who can assist the dying and their loved ones.

From Mistovich J, Hafen B, Karren K: *Prehospital emergency care,* ed 6, Upper Saddle River, NJ, 2000, Prentice-Hall.

HOME CARE OF THE DYING CHILD

In most situations, the terminally ill child desires to be home with his or her parents in familiar surroundings. That secure place is where families can provide the greatest comfort. The needs of the dying child and family are unique partly because society does not expect death to occur to the young or to have the child die before the parent.

Knowledge of the child's physical, cognitive, psychosocial, and spiritual development will enable the nurse to provide appropriate pain management, assist the child and family to communicate with each other, advocate for their needs in the community, and refer to key players who can offer them assistance such as volunteers, counselors, or clergy.

Bereavement telephone calls or visits by hospice staff may continue for the family up to 1 year after the death of the child, at anniversaries of the child's death, and on holidays and the child's birthday. The family (including parents, grandparents, and siblings) can participate in community memorial services and support groups that are offered by the hospice program or other bereavement organizations. More research is needed on the most effective nursing interventions for dying children and their families (Hinds et al, 2005).

SCOPE OF PRACTICE

As with other types of nursing practice, health promotion and disease prevention activities are a fundamental component of practice. Because some home care may be intermittent, primary objectives for the nurse are to facilitate self-care, prevent further illness, and promote the client's well-being. The nurse facilitates the development of positive health behaviors for the individual who has had an episode of illness.

A client may be recuperating at home after suffering a cerebrovascular accident (CVA, or stroke) and may be unable to perform activities of daily living without assistance. Such clients can be instructed to perform these activities in a modified form. In this way they have some control over their lives and self-care activities, and they can be taught to prevent possible losses in other self-care areas. Although self-care is considered the ideal outcome of home health interventions, in reality many clients require assistance. The concept of self-management is used to help chronically ill clients promote health and prevent illness (Lorig et al, 2005; Wagner et al, 2001).

Nursing in home care involves both direct and indirect activities.

DIRECT AND INDIRECT CARE

Direct care refers to the actual physical aspects of nursing care—anything requiring physical contact and face-to-face interactions. In home care, direct care activities include performing a physical assessment on the client, changing a dressing on a wound, giving medication by injection, inserting an indwelling catheter, or providing intravenous

HOW TO | Maintain Infection Control Standards for Home Care

The practice of universal precautions means that all blood and body fluids are treated as potentially infectious. Universal precautions are implemented to prevent exposure and infection of caregivers. It is an important practice because many infections are subclinical.
- Use extreme care to prevent injuries when handling needles, scalpels, and razors. Do not recap, bend, break, or remove the needle from a syringe before disposal. Discard needles and syringes in puncture-resistant containers made of plastic or metal and dispose of them in a local landfill or as directed by your agency.
- Barrier precautions, such as gloves, masks, eye covering, and gowns, should be worn when contact with blood and body fluids is expected.
- Soiled dressings or other materials contaminated with body fluids should be double bagged in polyethylene garbage bags.
- Kitchen counters, dishes, and laundry should be cleaned in warm water and detergent after use. Bathrooms may be cleaned with a household disinfectant.
- Hand hygiene is the most important practice in preventing infections. Hand hygiene should be performed before and after providing client care and before and after preparing food, eating, feeding, or using the bathroom.

therapy. Direct care also involves teaching clients and family caregivers how to perform a certain procedure or task. By serving as a preeminent model, the nurse helps the client and family develop positive health behaviors. When in the home, nurses need to be aware of infection control guidelines for self-protection and to protect the client (see the "How To" box on infection control).

Nursing care in home health is covered by Medicare and other third-party payers as long as the care being delivered is **skilled care**. To determine whether a service performed by the nurse is skilled nursing care, several factors are evaluated and must be adequately documented. Examples of skilled nursing services include the following:
- Evaluating a client's health status and condition
- Administering treatments, rehabilitative exercises, and medications; inserting catheters; irrigating colostomies; and providing wound care
- Teaching the client and family to implement the therapeutic plan such as treatments, therapeutic diets, and taking medications
- Reporting changes in the client's condition to the physician and arranging for medical follow-up as indicated

Indirect care activities are those that a nurse does on behalf of clients to improve or coordinate care. These activities include consulting with other nurses and health providers in a multidisciplinary approach to care, organizing and participating in client care team conferences, advocating for clients with the health care system and insurers, supervising home health aides, obtaining results of diagnostic tests, and documenting care. The example below illustrates direct and indirect care activities in a home health agency.

Mr. Jones, 70 years old, was discharged from the hospital yesterday after heart surgery for coronary artery disease. Today he is admitted to home health services for skilled nursing, for an assessment of his cardiovascular status. Direct care involves teaching Mr. and Mrs. Jones about medications, exercise, nutrition, and the signs and symptoms of possible postoperative cardiac problems. In addition, the nurse will assess Mr. Jones' cardiovascular status and the healing of his incisions, and help him return to an optimal state of functioning. The family's psychosocial adaptation and needs will also be addressed, and Mr. Jones' adjustment to his postsurgical status and his level of self-care will be assessed. The nurse also teaches Mr. Jones how he can prevent an exacerbation of his condition by maintaining medical follow-up and adapting his lifestyle to increase his adherence to the programs established for him Primary prevention assessment strategies and counseling include environmental issues such as safety in the home and neighborhood, immunizations (e.g., influenza, pneumococcus), and reduction of stress factors. One of the nurse's indirect care activities might be consulting with the pharmacist about optimal strategies for monitoring and preventing medication side effects. Another would be contacting a social service agency to facilitate Mr. Jones' access to financial assistance for his medications.

NURSING ROLES IN HOME CARE

Nurses fulfill roles such as the following:
- Clinician
- Case manager
- Client advocate
- Educator
- Mentor
- Researcher
- Administrator
- Consultant

Home care nurses in staff positions are clinicians who provide direct nursing care to clients and families. They are also educators because they teach clients and families the "how to" and "why" of self-care.

Nurses function as case managers, coordinating care with and for clients over time and across settings. They function according to client needs, either providing the care to meet those needs or making referrals and coordinating care (Zink, 2005). In some cases, home care nurses provide disease management services, in which the emphasis is on the use of research evidence, guidelines, and protocols for managing populations with chronic illnesses (Huffman, 2005). Nurse care coordination has been found to improve outcomes for older adults with chronic health problems (Marek et al, 2006).

Nurses also act as mentors, participating in the ongoing education of their colleagues, both formally, providing inservice education, and informally as team members. Additionally, they may teach classes to community groups regarding health education topics. The researcher role in home care is increasingly important, as the efficacy, or quality, and cost-effectiveness of care become mandated by Medicare and other payers. Home care nurses often provide the data required for clinical or administrative changes to occur within their agency of employment. Home care nurses have a variety of opportunities to participate in research. All nurses should

Evidence-Based Practice

Finding ways to help clinicians adopt and consistently use evidence-based clinical practices is an example of translating research into practice. Murtaugh and colleagues (Murtaugh et al, 2005) tested two interventions designed to help home health nurses use evidence-based practices for clients with heart failure. The study participants were nurses in a large nonprofit home health agency in an urban area. A total of 354 nurses employed by the agency were randomly assigned to the control group or one of two intervention groups. The control group received the usual care. One intervention group of nurses received basic e-mail reminders to follow the agreed-upon evidence-based practices for clients with heart failure. These reminders were sent when the nurse admitted a client with heart failure to care. The other intervention group received the e-mail reminders, patient education materials for use with their clients, and information regarding outreach and consultation with a clinical nurse specialist. Data were collected via chart reviews of participating nurses' clients. Although both intervention groups significantly increased their adherence to heart failure evidence-based practice guidelines, the group that also received patient education materials and clinical nurse specialist consultation had the best results.

NURSE USE: This study shows how important it is to plan ways to facilitate evidence-based practice and that simple reminder and support strategies can be effective.

From Murtaugh CM et al: Just-in-time evidence-based email "reminders" in home health care: impact on nurse practices, *Health Serv Res* 40:849–864, 2005.

use appropriate and current research to improve practice. Staff nurses can participate in research by suggesting clinical problems in need of research and participating in clinical research teams. Research must be a priority in the future if quality and cost-effectiveness are to be maintained. A home care administrator can be a nurse who has had advanced education with public health experience; requirements are stipulated by both federal and state rules and regulations. Finally, consultants may provide advice and counsel to staff and clients.

The *Code of Ethics for Nurses With Interpretive Statements* (American Nurses Association, 2005) is a guide for nurses facing ethical dilemmas. It is the "profession's nonnegotiable ethical standard" (p. 5). The home care nurse acts as a client advocate, maintaining client confidentiality, promoting informed consent, and making and following up on contacts to see that community resources are available to clients. Ethical conflicts and dilemmas are identified and resolved through formal agency mechanisms designed to address such issues. The nurse is responsible for building a trusting relationship with the family, determining whether the home is a safe and appropriate place to provide care for the particular client, and staying abreast of current research and ethical issues related to home care. The nurse acts in the area of professional obligations through political and social reform that affects client- and population-based care. The client privacy guidelines from the Health Insurance Portability and Accountability Act of 1996 (HIPAA) require ethical conduct by the nurse in the protection of all forms of personal health information (Wilson, 2004). This is becoming an even greater concern as health data are stored and transmitted electronically with electronic health records and electronic billing.

The nurse uses appropriate agency and community resources, including delegating tasks to other caregivers, to provide good benefits at reasonable cost to the client. The nurse helps the client become an informed consumer to assist in empowerment and self-advocacy. A study of home health clients before and after implementation of Medicare prospective payment for home health (Anderson et al, 2005) showed that those who were readmitted to the hospital following implementation of prospective payment were older and sicker, and experienced less continuity of care. This suggests that some health clients have more complicated health needs than in the past and that it is especially important for nurses to work with clients and other home care professionals to plan clinical interventions carefully to obtain the best possible outcomes.

STANDARDS OF HOME NURSING PRACTICE

Home health nurses practice in accordance with the *Scope and Standards of Home Health Nursing Practice* developed by the ANA (American Nurses Association, 2007). Nurses providing hospice care in the home use the *Scope and Standards of Hospice and Palliative Nursing Practice* (Hospice and Palliative Nurses Association and American Nurses Association, 2007). Periodically, the profession revises the scope of practice and standards of specialty practice to reflect the ongoing changes in the health care system and their effects on nursing care. These ANA standards contain two parts: Standards of Care, which follow the six steps of the nursing process, and eight Standards of Professional Performance. The Standards of Care are assessment, diagnosis, outcome identification, planning, implementation, and evaluation. The Standards of Professional Performance include quality of care, performance appraisal, education, collegiality, ethics, collaboration, research, and resource use. Other clinical standards of practice either from the American Nurses Association or from specialty professional organizations guide population-focused home care, transitional care in the home, and home-based primary care.

BRIEFLY NOTED

Home care nurses should establish both short- and long-term goals with clients and families. The goals provide for continuity of care and state the criteria for evaluating the client's condition and progress toward an optimum level of self-care.

EDUCATIONAL REQUIREMENTS FOR HOME NURSING PRACTICE

Nurses come to home care from a variety of educational and practice backgrounds. Differences in both experience and educational preparation influence the contributions that nurses make to home care. Home care nurses should be educated to function at a high level of competency so that they can be relied on not only by their professional colleagues but also by the community. A baccalaureate degree in nursing should be the minimum requirement for entry into professional practice in any community health setting.

In home care, the nurse with a baccalaureate degree functions in the role of a generalist, providing skilled nursing and coordinating care for a variety of home health clients. The nurse with a master's degree is prepared for the advanced practice role as clinical specialist, nurse practitioner, researcher, administrator, or educator. As home care continues to play a larger role in community nursing practice, the need for specialized nurse clinicians will increase to meet the highly technological and complex care that has been moved from the hospital into the home setting. In managed care, more clinical specialists will be needed to provide case management and to develop programs to meet the needs of the population served by the managed care network. Nurse practitioners can provide primary care to frail older adults and other homebound clients. Educational programs are increasing to prepare nurses for advanced practice roles in home health.

CERTIFICATION

Home health nurses can seek **certification** as a generalist home health nurse, home health clinical nurse specialist, nursing case manager, or an advanced practice public health nurse through the American Nurses Credentialing Center. The National Hospice Organization will certify hospice nurses. A baccalaureate degree in nursing is required for the generalist examination and a master's degree for the advance practice examinations. Nurses must also demonstrate current practice. In the highly competitive health care environment, certification is expected to become more necessary to ensure the competence and quality of care for the public.

INTERPROFESSIONAL CARE

The responsibilities and functions of other health professions in home care are dictated by Medicare regulations, professional organizations, and state licensing boards. Other specialized services can be provided in home care such as the following:

- Enterostomal therapy
- Podiatry
- Pharmaceutical therapy
- Nutrition counseling
- Intravenous therapy
- Respiratory therapy
- Psychiatric or mental health nursing

Many of these services can be provided on a consulting basis, either in the form of staff education or through direct

Box 30-1	Factors for Successful Interprofessional Functioning

Knowledge

1. Understand how the group process can be used to achieve group goals.
2. Understand problem solving.
3. Understand role theory.
4. Understand what other professionals do and how they view their roles.
5. Understand the differences between client levels of acuity across levels of care, including acute care, home care, ambulatory care, and long-term care.

Skill

1. Use principles of group process effectively.
2. Communicate clearly and accurately.
3. Communicate without using the profession's jargon.
4. Express yourself clearly and concisely in writing.

Attitude

1. Feel confident in your role as a professional.
2. Trust and respect other professionals.
3. Share tasks with other professionals.
4. Work effectively toward conflict resolution.
5. Be flexible.
6. Adopt an attitude of inquiry.
7. Be timely.

care. The interprofessional team may be composed of any or all of the following providers:

- Physician
- Physical therapist
- Occupational therapist
- Social worker
- Homemaker
- Home health aide
- Speech pathologist

Each client in Medicare-funded home care programs must be under the current care of a doctor of medicine, podiatry, or osteopathy to certify that the client has a medical problem. The physician must certify a plan of treatment before care is provided to the client.

Successful **interprofessional collaboration** and functioning depend on numerous factors, including the knowledge, skills, and attitudes of each team member. Factors necessary for successful interdisciplinary team functioning are shown in Box 30-1. The plan of care should be implemented and reinforced by all involved disciplines. For example, nurses must reinforce the teaching by the physical therapist of the exercise regimen and gait training.

ACCOUNTABILITY AND QUALITY MANAGEMENT

QUALITY IMPROVEMENT AND CLIENT SAFETY

Quality improvement activities are a crucial part of nursing care delivery. Nurses participate in the following:

- Monitoring care

- Seeing and analyzing opportunities for improving care
- Developing guidelines to improve care
- Collecting data
- Making recommendations
- Implementing activities to enhance quality of care

Results of these activities are used to make changes in health care delivery. According to the National Association of Home Care (NAHC) (2001), outcomes to determine quality indexes in Medicare are taken from the OASIS-B1 database and integrated into Outcome Based Quality Improvement (OBQI). The OBQI is a quality improvement system for home health care (Shaughnessy et al, 2002).

Quality management activities include peer review and other forms of performance appraisal. Professional development and lifelong learning are increasing in importance as home care changes rapidly to meet society's health care needs. Both the nurse and the employing agency are encouraged to endorse nursing participation in ongoing professional development, which includes continuing education and competence in home care nursing. The nurse likewise exhibits collegiality by sharing expertise with others as appropriate and participating in the education and evaluation of students and other colleagues.

Since the beginning of Medicare, home health agencies have monitored the quality of care to their clients as a mandatory requirement for certification as a home health agency. All agencies, whether home health, hospice, or a clinic, hospital, or program providing home care, are accountable to their clients, to their reimbursement sources, to themselves as health care providers, and to professional standards.

Clinical data are of great importance in assessing the quality of care. The care and services the client receives and any communication between the physicians and other home care providers must be documented. Increasingly this documentation occurs in electronic health records, often by entering data into a laptop computer while in the home. It is in the clinical record that nurses demonstrate that they are delivering quality care and are also identifying means to improve the quality of care. It is the legal method by which the quality of care can be assessed. This documentation also demonstrates the client's ongoing need for services and shows how the multiple disciplines arrange for continuity and comprehensive care.

As an example, during the initial home visit, the nurse assesses the status of the client and family. This information becomes a permanent part of the clinical record. Subsequent integration of health services must be noted. In addition to clinical notes of all home visits, progress notes must be sent to the client's physician, including the assessment of the client to verify the implementation of the plan of care.

The **Outcomes and Assessment Information Set (OASIS)** measures outcomes for quality improvement and client satisfaction with care. Funded by the Centers for Medicare and Medicaid Services (CMS) and the Robert Wood Johnson Foundation, OASIS underwent extensive testing and is required for use by Medicare-certified home health agencies (Hittle et al, 2003).

The OASIS was revised and renamed in 1998 and is now OASIS-B1. OASIS data are measured and reported to the

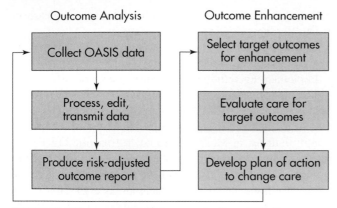

FIGURE 30-2 Two-stage QBQI framework. (From U.S. Department of Health and Human Services and Centers for Medicare and Medicaid Services: *Outcome-based quality improvement (OBQI) implementation manual,* Washington, DC, 2002b, U.S. Department of Health and Human Services, pp 2.4, 2.10.)

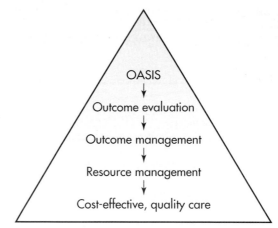

FIGURE 30-3 The outcome paradigm. (From U.S. Department of Health and Human Services and Centers for Medicare and Medicaid Services: *Outcome-based quality improvement (OBQI) implementation manual,* Washington, DC, 2002b, U.S. Department of Health and Human Services, pp 2.4, 2.10.)

CMS on the client's admission to home health care, after an episode of hospitalization, at the time of recertification, and on discharge from care. Data are submitted by each agency to a national databank, and agencies receive both results and comparisons with similar agencies to determine areas needing improvement. See Appendix B.1 for one part of this assessment.

Using the OASIS-B1 data, outcome analysis and improvement strategies can be accomplished through the Outcome Based Quality Improvement (OBQI) framework (Shaughnessy et al, 2002). The OBQI is a two-stage framework that includes "outcome analysis" and "outcome enhancement" (Figure 30-2). The first stage, data analysis, enables an agency to compare its performance to a national sample, identify factors that may affect outcomes, and identify final outcomes that show improvement in or stabilization of a client's condition. The second stage, known as outcome enhancement, involves the selection of specific **client outcomes** and then determining strategies to improve care (U.S. Department of Health and Human Services, 2002b; Centers for Medicare and Medicaid, 2002). Figure 30-3 shows the OBQI outcome paradigm. The goals of the OASIS and OBQI are the provision of cost-effective, quality care.

Accrediting organizations also mandate reporting outcomes as a performance standard. Performance improvement programs are based on measurable data, including **benchmarking**, which means comparing yourself with national standards and guidelines and with other agencies. Clinical guidelines, pathways, and clinical maps are other methods that agencies are using to standardize care and control costs.

ACCREDITATION

Accreditation is a voluntary process; an agency chooses to participate. The accreditation decision is based on the data in a self-study, the report of a site visit team, and other relevant information. In the future, accreditation may become a requirement for licensure of all home health agencies. Today, home health agencies may be accredited through The Joint Commission (TJC) or the Community Health Accreditation Program of the National League for Nursing (CHAP). Both

organizations look at the organizational structure through which care is delivered, the process of care through home visits, and the outcomes of client care, focusing on improved health status. Performance improvement must be ongoing in the agency.

Ensuring client safety is of primary concern in home care. Although client safety problems in home care may differ somewhat from those in acute care, they are still serious issues and must be prevented. With the emphasis on self-care by clients and families, safety problems may relate to clients having good understanding of their health behaviors. Home care clients may experience the following:

* Care errors as a result of inaccurate communications around referrals
* Cognitive deficits from health problems
* Socioeconomic problems such as lack of money for food or medications

The Joint Commission has National Patient Safety Goals (Friedman, 2003) that apply to home care and hospices accredited by them.

FINANCIAL ASPECTS OF HOME CARE

REIMBURSEMENT MECHANISMS

The **reimbursement system** for home health care is complicated and standardized. Medicare and Medicaid are the principal funding sources for home health care, with third-party health insurance providing another major source. Budgeted funds for public health from taxes cover preventive home care visits to the clients of public health agencies. Other home care services such as health education, risk reduction, case management, or primary care may be reimbursed from a variety of sources. These include program funds, grants, contracts, or third-party billing.

If a client has both Medicare and Medicaid or a private insurance plan, Medicare is used as the primary payment source provided the services being delivered to the client meet the definition of *skilled.* After Medicare pays, then private insurance is used. When the client is no longer eligible

Table 30-1	Comparison of the Two Major Federally Supported Programs for Home Health Care

Medicare (Title XVIII)	Medicaid (Title XIX)
Federal insurance program administered by the Social Security Administration	Federal and state assistance program administered by the state
Age 65 years and over or disabled	Income-based eligibility
Conditions of participation	Conditions of participation
Homebound status	Not necessarily homebound status
Intermittent service	Intermittent service
Skilled service	Not necessarily skilled service
Restorative program	Custodial and maintenance program
Physician certification	Physician certification
Therapist, medical, or social service	State option—therapist, medical, or social service
Pays for rental and purchase	Pays for purchase of equipment
Reimbursement by prospective payment	Reimbursement—maximum allowed at the state level
Based on national rates	Based on a negotiated rate between the federal government and state

for home care under Medicare, the Medicaid benefits can be used. Table 30-1 illustrates the differences between Medicare and Medicaid programs.

COST-EFFECTIVENESS

Because of the increased number of home health agencies and increasing costs, the federal government instituted a prospective payment system on October 1, 2000. This system prevents the abuse or fraudulent use of Medicare funding. Evaluation results show that the prospective payment system has increased efficiencies and reduced certain costs and that it has generally not been associated with declines in quality (Schlenker et al, 2005).

Nurses in many settings are not directly exposed to the financial aspects of health care. In home health, nurses must be "cost-conscious" so that they can explain to clients what Medicare will or will not cover. It is often difficult for older clients to understand why Medicare will not pay for the nurse to make home visits to take their blood pressure if their condition remains stable. Medicare pays for services only if the client's condition is unstable, the client is homebound, and the client requires skilled, intermittent, and part-time care.

LEGAL AND ETHICAL ISSUES

In any health care system there is the potential for illegal and unethical activity. Much publicity has been given to Medicare fraud and abuse. Examples of such practices include inappropriate use of home health services, inaccurate billing

for services, excessive administrative staff, "kickbacks" for referrals, and billing for noncovered medical supplies.

Home care nurses are confronted with multiple issues in everyday practice. Third-party payers have interpreted the definition of skilled care inconsistently over the years. The home care nurse must abide by established federal **regulations** when delivering care to clients, even when the needs are greater than what is reimbursed. Frequency of visits poses another issue. Only intermittent visits are reimbursed. If the frequency increases, then full-time skilled services may be required. Continual reassessment of client and family needs is imperative to avoid inappropriate use and overuse of services. Home care nurses must be knowledgeable about which medical supplies are covered. This information is readily available and nurses must work within regulatory guidelines and educate the community as to what should be covered and what is actually covered. Evidence-based nursing practice is essential.

Home care nurses are at risk for malpractice claims related to the complexity of care needed and actual or alleged negligence from rushed visits or failure to adhere to standards of practice (Dailey and Newfield, 2005). Performance improvement programs, use of evidence-based practice guidelines, and appropriate use of information technology for communication and telehealth are strategies that can help reduce these risks (Dailey and Newfield, 2005).

TRENDS IN HOME CARE

NATIONAL HEALTH OBJECTIVES

Because nurses are working with clients and families in the home and community, they are in a position to promote the achievement of some of the key *Healthy People 2010* objectives. The nurse can assess the client's status related to key objectives, identify available resources and gaps to meet client needs, and coordinate care with other providers and community agencies.

The "*Healthy People 2010*" box highlights the objectives home care nurses can assist the nation in meeting through their nursing care and case management activities. Many of these objectives relate to lifestyle issues. With appropriate health education and referral to community resources for assistance, morbidity and mortality can be reduced and chronic disabilities decreased. In this way the nurse can contribute to meeting the national health objectives on a one-to-one client-provider level.

FAMILY RESPONSIBILITY, ROLES, AND FUNCTIONS

The family plays an important role in the delivery of home care. The term family, as discussed previously, refers to a caregiver responsible for the client's well-being. Women have traditionally been the caregivers for children and older adults in the United States. Now, however, women are less available to provide this care without assistance, because they are often working outside the home. Similarly, other family members may be employed or have multiple obligations, creating new challenges for family caregiving and for nurses designing care delivery strategies in home care.

Examples of National Health Objectives for the Year 2010

2-4	Increase the proportion of adults aged 18 years and older with arthritis who seek help in coping if they experience personal and emotional problems
3-1	Reduce the overall death rate from cancer
3-11	Increase the proportion of women who receive a Pap test
3-12	Increase the proportion of adults who receive a colorectal cancer screening examination
3-13	Increase the proportion of women ages 40 years and older who have received a mammogram within the preceding 2 years
4-2	Reduce deaths from cardiovascular disease in persons with chronic kidney failure
4-7	Reduce kidney failure due to diabetes
5-1	Increase the proportion of persons with diabetes who receive formal diabetes education
5-2	Prevent diabetes
5-5	Reduce the death rate from diabetes
5-7	Reduce deaths from cardiovascular disease in persons with diabetes
5-9	Reduce the frequency of foot ulcers in persons with diabetes
5-17	Increase the proportion of persons with diabetes who perform self blood glucose monitoring at least once daily
6-3	Reduce the proportion of adults with disabilities who report feelings such as sadness, unhappiness, or depression that prevent them from being active
6-11	Reduce the proportion of people with disabilities who report not having the assistive devices and technology needed
12-6	Reduce hospitalizations of older adults with heart failure as the principal diagnosis
12-7	Reduce deaths from stroke
12-8	Increase the proportion of adults who are aware of the early warning symptoms and signs of a stroke
12-10	Increase the proportion of adults with high blood pressure whose blood pressure is under control
14-5	Reduce invasive pneumococcal infections
15-13	Reduce deaths caused by unintentional injuries
15-14	Reduce the number of nonfatal unintentional injuries
15-25	Reduce residential fire deaths
15-27	Reduce deaths from falls
15-28	Reduce hip fractures among older adults
24-10	Reduce deaths from chronic obstructive pulmonary disease (COPD) among adults
26-2	Reduce deaths from cirrhosis

From U.S. Department of Health and Human Services: *Healthy People 2010: national health promotion and disease prevention objectives,* Washington, DC, 2001, U.S. Department of Health and Human Services.

BRIEFLY NOTED

Convene a family care conference to discuss issues with a client and family, develop a consistent team approach, and clarify roles and responsibilities.

Home care programs and reimbursement systems may be set up to provide family services or may reserve those services for families in crisis (Hokenstad et al, 2005). Nurses must find creative ways to include family caregivers as partners in the client's care, and provide the teaching, coaching, and support needed. Nurses in home care should advocate for policy changes when necessary to foster effective evidence-based family care strategies.

Assistance from social support systems helps families cope with the stress of caring for an ill family member. The goal is to maintain the client at home for as long as possible and to provide high-quality care. To do this, resources must be used appropriately and effectively. However, developing a public consensus to resolve these issues has been challenging.

TECHNOLOGY AND TELEHEALTH

The incentives and pressures for cost control and improved health outcomes have increased the development and use of telehealth technology in the home care setting (West and Milio, 2004). At the same time, some technologies have been simplified and their reliability increased, facilitating their safe use in the home. Telehealth, parenteral nutrition, chemotherapy, intravenous therapy for hydration and antibiotics, intrathecal pain management, ventilators, apnea monitors, chest tubes, and skeletal traction are examples of current home care technologies. The home care nurse must be prepared to evaluate the cost and safety of technology for the home. Clients must be screened and meet specific admission criteria for use of particular technologies.

Telehealth has emerged as a viable and acceptable way to provide health care. **Telehealth** is defined as sharing health information between the client and clinicians using either synchronous or asynchronous electronic communications via telephone, videophone, or a biometric monitoring unit (West and Milio, 2004). Examples of the uses of telehealth include telephone triage and advice, and biometric telemonitoring equipment to measure vital signs, cardiac function, and point-of-care diagnostics. The WebTV and ViaTV phones are two examples of telecommunication devices that can be used to communicate between client and health care provider through the Internet to transmit data, write e-mails, obtain medical information, and monitor or assess changes in condition (Finkelstein and Friedman, 2000). Telehealth has been used successfully to improve health outcomes for clients with diabetes (Chumbler et al, 2005), heart failure (Jerant et al, 2003), and chronic wounds (Kobza and Scheurich, 2000).

BRIEFLY NOTED

Telemonitoring is increasingly being used to supplement care provided for chronically ill clients in their homes. It also is being used for infants and women with high-risk pregnancies. New technologies are being developed such as nanotechnology, handheld biosensors, and virtual reality that will expand the capabilities of telemonitoring and strengthen the abilities of clients to provide self-care with professional support (Meystre, 2005).

HEALTH INSURANCE PORTABILITY AND ACCOUNTABILITY ACT OF 1996

In 1996 Congress passed the Health Insurance Portability and Accountability Act (HIPAA), which was initially related specifically to the portability of health insurance. The full scope of the legislation had a far-reaching impact on protecting the privacy and security of personal health information. All health care organizations were required to meet HIPAA federal privacy standards by April 14, 2003. This legislation protects the client's private information through the electronic transfer of health records, allows individuals full access to their personal medical records, provides clear information (informed consent) specifying the medical use of the client's personal health information and records to allow the client to have control over that information, and ensures legal protection, with significant criminal and civic penalties to those individuals or agencies that do not comply with the privacy requirements (U.S. Department of Health and Human Services, 2002a).

More recent federal efforts have stimulated the use of electronic health records (Brailer, 2004), and it seems likely that more health care agencies will invest in comprehensive electronic information systems and that systems will be compatible across agencies. This has the potential to make seamless care delivery and client safety more likely, although safeguards need to be included to protect the privacy and confidentiality of personal health information.

OMAHA SYSTEM

Nurses, other practitioners, managers, and administrators in community settings face urgent practice, documentation, and information management challenges (Martin, 2005; Monsen and Martin, 2002a, b). Because of the magnitude and speed of changes in the health care system and developments in information technology, those in community settings face critical needs for the following:

1. Timely, valid, and reliable data that describe clients' demographic characteristics, the severity and acuity of their needs, the type and location of services, and reimbursement methods
2. Timely, valid, and reliable data that quantify the clients receiving care, the services they receive, and the costs and outcomes of that care
3. Verbal and automated methods for nurses to communicate with other nurses and health care practitioners

The American Nurses Association (2006) has addressed these challenges; their website summarizes the Omaha System and other recognized terminologies that can describe clinical data, improve and standardize practice, and increase interoperability—the ability to exchange coded data.

DESCRIPTION OF THE OMAHA SYSTEM

As early as 1970, the staff and administrators of the Visiting Nurse Association (VNA) of Omaha, Nebraska, began addressing nursing practice, documentation, and information management concerns. At that time, no systematic

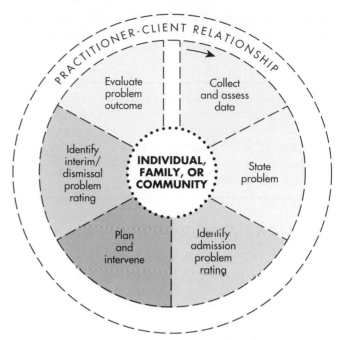

FIGURE 30-4 Omaha System model of the problem-solving process. (From Martin K: *The Omaha System: a key to practice, documentation, and information management*, St. Louis, 2005, Elsevier.)

nomenclature or classification of client problems existed that could be used with a problem-oriented record systems, and practitioners were not using computers. These realities provided the incentive for initiating research.

During the next 20 years, the VNA of Omaha staff conducted four extensive, federally funded Omaha System development, reliability, validity, and usability research projects. The result of the research was the Problem Classification Scheme, the Intervention Scheme, and the Problem Rating Scale for Outcomes (Martin, 2005). As shown in Figure 30-4, the theoretical framework of the Omaha System is based on the dynamic, interactive nature of the nursing or problem-solving process, the practitioner–client relationship, and concepts of diagnostic reasoning, clinical judgment, and quality improvement. The client as an individual, a family, or a community appears at the center of the model; this location shows the many ways the Omaha System can be used and the essential partnership between clients and practitioners.

The Omaha System is the only ANA-recognized terminology developed inductively (initially) by and for practicing nurses in the community. The goals of the Omaha System research were:

1. To develop a structured and comprehensive system that could be both understood and used by members of various disciplines
2. To foster collaborative practice

Therefore the Omaha System was designed to guide practice decisions, sort and document pertinent client data uniformly, and provide a framework for an agency-wide, multidisciplinary clinical information management system capable of meeting the needs of practitioners, managers, and administrators (Martin, 2005; Monsen and Martin, 2002b).

See the tools in Appendix G.4 for the Omaha System Problem Classification Scheme with Case Study for Application.

BRIEFLY NOTED

More provider agencies are using computers and clinical information software so nurses can document their care and client outcomes wherever they are in the community. In Minnesota, 85% of all counties now have one or more public health or home care agencies or schools and colleges of nursing using Omaha System software.

CLINICAL APPLICATION

The home visit is the hallmark of nursing in home care. When a nurse enters a client's home, she or he is a guest and must recognize that the services offered can be accepted or rejected. The first visit sets the stage for success or failure. The initial assessment of the client, the support system, and the environment is critical.

A. *What strategies would the nurse consider to develop a trusting relationship during the first visit?*

B. *What would be the most important elements to assess in the home environment?*

C. *What should the nurse do to establish a partnership with the client?*

D. *What should the nurse include in the client contract?*

E. *How can the nurse assess the preferred learning style?*

Answers are in the back of the book.

REMEMBER THIS!

- Home care differs from other areas of health care because health care providers practice in the client's environment. This unique characteristic affects several components of nursing practice in the home care setting including establishing trust, developing care partnerships, selecting interventions, collecting outcomes and data, ensuring client safety, and promoting quality.
- Family members, including any caregiver or significant person who takes the responsibility to assist the client in need of care at home, are an integral part of home health care.
- Home nursing care has its roots in public health nursing, with an emphasis on health promotion, illness prevention, and caring for people in the contexts of their communities.
- Home care reached a turning point with the arrival of Medicare, which provided regulations for certain forms of home care practice and reimbursement mechanisms.
- Although many think of home health when thinking of home care, there are many other approaches to home care. Five types of home care are described in this chapter: population-focused home care, transitional care in the home, home-based primary care, home health, and hospice. Home care nurses should learn about current and new models of home care and use those that are most effective for the situation.

- Home health agencies are divided into the following five general types on the basis of administrative and organizational structures: official, private and voluntary, combination, hospital based, and proprietary.
- Standards of home nursing practice originate from ANA and specialty organizations.
- Demonstration of professional competency is essential for home health care nurses.
- The home health care nurse practices in accordance with the *Scope and Standards of Home Health Nursing Practice* developed by the American Nurses Association, Council of Community Health Nurses (1999). Hospice nurses use the *Scope and Standards of Hospice and Palliative Nursing Practice* jointly developed by the Hospice and Palliative Care Nurses Association and the ANA (2002).
- Interdisciplinary collaboration is a required process in home health care. It is inherent in the definition of home care.
- In home care, as in other care settings, professionals experience stress associated with changing roles and overlapping responsibilities. In collaborating, home health care providers should carefully analyze one another's roles to determine whether overlapping occurs and adjust the plan of care as needed.
- Since the advent of Medicare, home health agencies have monitored the quality of care to their clients as a mandatory requirement for certification as a home health agency. All agencies are accountable to clients and families, to their reimbursement sources, to themselves as a health care provider, and to professional standards.
- Nurses in any home care setting should work to establish and use quality improvement processes and design care systems to ensure client safety.
- The home care nurse today faces many challenges. Ethical issues (reimbursement criteria and access to care), role development (high-technology nursing and hospice nursing), and opportunities for research (quality of care, cost-effectiveness, and client safety) affect nursing practice in the home.
- Home care agencies may be accredited through The Joint Commission or the Community Health Accreditation Program.
- The Omaha System was developed and refined through a process of research. Reliability and validity were established for the entire system.
- The Omaha System is unique in that it is the only comprehensive vocabulary developed initially by and for practicing population-focused nurses.
- The Omaha System was designed to follow specific principles. The system consists of a Problem Classification Scheme, an Intervention Scheme, and a Problem Rating Scale for Outcomes.
- The Omaha System offers benefits in three principal areas: practice, documentation, and information management. These areas are of concern to community health educators and students as well as community health practitioners and administrators.

WHAT WOULD YOU DO?

1. Make a home visit with an experienced home care nurse and do the following:
   A. Describe the process of the visit.
   B. Observe and discuss whether that nurse uses a client problem/nursing diagnosis, intervention, or outcome measurement system or framework. Is it important to use a system or framework approach? Explain.
2. Make a joint home visit with another health care professional and assess as in the preceding activity. Also, attend a client/family care conference meeting and write a summary of the process of the group. How has your attitude concerning an issue changed or not changed according to those expressed by various family members?
3. Review a client record. What client outcomes were met through home health care? What specific outcomes showed an improvement or a stabilizing condition?
4. Review your state's laws governing advance directives. Consider the legal and ethical advantages and disadvantages of having such directives. How would you write an advance directive for yourself?

■ REFERENCES

American Nurses Association: *Public health nursing: scope and standards practice*, Washington, DC, 2007, ANA.

American Nurses Association: *Code of ethics for nurses with interpretive statements*, Kansas City, Mo, 2005, ANA.

American Nurses Association: *ANA recognized terminologies and data element sets*. Retrieved June 2006 from http://www. nursingworld.org/npii/terminologies.htm.

Anderson MA et al: Hospital readmission from home health care before and after prospective payment, *J Nurs Schol* 37:73–79, 2005.

Barkauskas VH, Stocker J: Public health and home care: historical roots and current partnerships, *Caring* 19(11):6–10, 2000.

Brailer DJ: EHRs: the Fed's big push. Interview by Ken Terry, *Med Econ* 81:26, 28–29, 2004.

Brooten D et al: Lessons learned from testing the Quality Cost Model of Advanced Practice Nursing (APN) Transitional Care, *J Nurs Schol* 34:369–375, 2002.

Buhler-Wilkerson K: No place like home: a history of nursing and home care in the U.S., *Home Health Nurse* 20:641–647, 2002.

Centers for Medicare and Medicaid: *2002 data compendium*, available at http://www.cms.gov/researchers/pubs/datacompendium/.

Chumbler NR et al: Evaluation of a care coordination home-telehealth program for veterans with diabetes, *Eval Health Prof* 28:464–478, 2005.

Dailey M, Newfield J: Legal issues in homecare: current trends, risk-reduction strategies, and opportunities for improvement, *Home Care Manag Pract* 17:93–100, 2005.

Dobson PM: A model for home infusion therapy and maintenance, *J Infus Nurs* 24:385–394, 2001.

Doorenbos AZ, Schim SM: Cultural competence in hospice, *Am J Hosp Palliat Care* 21:28–32, 2004.

Finkelstein J, Friedman R: Potential role of telecommunication technologies in the management of chronic health conditions, *Dis Manag Health Outcomes* 8:57–63, 2000.

Friedman MM: The Joint Commission's National Patient Safety Goals: implications for home care and hospice organizations, *Home Health Nurse* 21:481–488, 2003.

Hanley E: The role of home care in palliative care services, *Care Manag J* 5:151–157, 2004.

Higginson IJ, Koffman J: Public health and palliative care, *Clin Geriatr Med* 21:45–55, 2005.

Hinds PS et al: Key factors affecting dying children and their families, *J Palliat Med* 8(suppl 1):570–578, 2005.

Hittle DF et al: A study of reliability and burden of home health assessment using OASIS, *Home Health Care Serv Q* 22:43–63, 2003.

Hoffmann RL: The evolution of hospice in America: nursing's role in the movement, *J Gerontol Nurs* 31:(26–34), 53–54, 2005.

Hokenstad A et al: Closing the home care case: clinicians' perspectives on family caregiving, *Home Health Care Manag Pract* 17:388–397, 2005.

Hospice Association of America: *Hospice facts and statistics*, Washington, DC, 2001, HAOA.

Hospice and Palliative Nurses Association and American Nurses Association: *Scope and standards of hospice and palliative nursing practice*, Silver Spring, Md, 2007, ANA.

Huffman M: A case study in home health disease management, *Home Health Nurse* 23:636–638, 2005.

Inglis S et al: A new solution for an old problem? Effects of a nurse-led, multidisciplinary, home-based intervention on readmission and mortality in clients with chronic atrial fibrillation, *J Cardiovasc Nurs* 19:118–127, 2004.

Izzo CV et al: Reducing the impact of uncontrollable stressful life events through a program of nurse home visitation for new parents, *Prev Sci* 6:269-274, 2005.

Jensen R: Cross-cultural perspectives in palliative care, *J Pain Palliat Care Pharmacother* 17:223–229, 2003.

Jerant AF et al: A randomized trial of telenursing to reduce hospitalization for heart failure: patient-centered outcomes and nursing indicators, *Home Health Care Serv Q* 22:1–20, 2003.

Kobza L, Scheurich A: The impact of telemedicine on outcomes of chronic wounds in the home care setting, *Ostomy Wound Manag* 46:48–53, 2000.

Kübler-Ross E: *On death and dying*, New York, 1969, McMillan.

Lorenz KA et al: Accommodating ethnic diversity: a study of California hospice programs, *Med Care* 42:871–874, 2004.

Lorig KR et al: A national dissemination of an evidence-based self-management program: a process evaluation study, *Patient Educ Couns* 59:69–79, 2004, Epub 2004.

Marek KD et al: Nurse care coordination in community-based long-term care, *J Nurs Schol* 38:80–86, 2006.

Martin KS: *The Omaha System: a key to practice, documentation, and information management*, St. Louis, 2005, Elsevier.

McClement SE et al: Dignity-conserving care: application of research findings to practice, *Int J Palliat Nurs* 10:173–179, 2004.

Meystre S: The current state of telemonitoring: a comment on the literature, *Telemed J E Health* 211:63–69, 2005.

Mistovich J, Hafen B, Karren K: *Prehospital emergency care*, ed 6, Upper Saddle River, NJ, 2000, Prentice Hall.

Monsen KA, Martin KS: Developing an outcomes management program in a public health department, *Outcomes Manag* 6:62–66, 2002a.

Monsen KA, Martin KS: Using an outcomes management program in a public health department, *Outcomes Manag* 6:120–124, 2002b.

Muramatsu N, Mensah E, Cornwell T: A physician house call program for the homebound, *Jt Comm J Qual Saf* 30:266–276, 2004.

Murtaugh CM et al: Just-in-time evidence-based email "reminders" in home health care: impact on nurse practices, *Health Serv Res* 40:849–864, 2005.

Nadash P: Two models of managed long-term care: comparing PACE with a Medicaid-only plan, *Gerontologist* 44:644–654, 2004.

National Association of Home Care: *Basic statistics about home care*, Washington, DC, 2001, NAHC.

Naylor MD: Transitional care: a critical dimension of the home healthcare quality agenda, *J Health Qual* 28:48–54, 2006.

Naylor MD et al: Cognitively impaired older adults: from hospital to home, an exploratory study of these clients and their caregivers, *AJN* 105:52–61, 2005.

Perlin JB, Kolodner RM, Roswell RH: The Veterans' Health Administration: quality, value, accountability, and information as transforming strategies for client-centered care, *J Health Manag* 50:828–836, 2004.

Rabins PV et al: Effectiveness of a nurse-based outreach program for identifying and treating psychiatric illness in the elderly, *JAMA* 283:2802–2809, 2000.

Schlenker RE et al: Initial home health outcomes under prospective payment, *Health Serv Res* 40:177–193, 2005.

Shaughnessy PW et al: Improving patient outcomes of home health care: findings from two demonstration trials of outcome-based quality improvement, *J Am Geriatr Soc* 50:1354–1364, 2002.

Sherman DW: Nurses' stress and burnout: how to care for yourself when caring for patients and their families with life-threatening illness, *AJN* 104:48–56, 2004.

Snow M: Competency: assuring competent RN infusion therapy in the home care setting, *Chart* 97:8, 2000.

Tieman J: It was 20 years ago today… some say it's complex and vulnerable to political whims, but Medicare's PPS has helped impose order on hospital finances, *Mod Health* 33:(6–7), 25–28, 2003.

Turk L et al: A new era in home care, *Semin Nurse Manag* 8:143–150, 2000.

U.S. Department of Health and Human Services: *Healthy People 2010: national health promotion and disease prevention objectives*, Washington, DC, 2001, U.S. Department of Health and Human Services.

U.S. Department of Health and Human Services: *HHS fact sheet: administrative simplification under HIPAA: national standards for transactions, security and privacy*, Washington, DC, Jan 22, 2002a, USDHHS, Public Health Service, available at http://www.hhs.gov/news.

U.S. Department of Health and Human Services and Centers for Medicare and Medicaid Services: *Outcome-based quality improvement (OBQI) implementation manual*, Washington, DC, 2002b, U.S. Department of Health and Human Services, pp 2.4, 2.10.

Von Gunter CF, Ryndes T: The academic hospice, *Ann Intern Med* 143:655–658, 2005.

Wagner EH et al: Improving chronic illness care: translating evidence into action, *Health Affairs* 20:64–78, 2001.

West VL, Milio N: Organizational and environmental factors affecting the utilization of telemedicine in rural home healthcare, *Home Health Care Serv Q* 23:49–67, 2004.

Wilson HP: HIPAA: The big picture for hospice and home care, *Home Health Care Manag Pract* 16:127–137, 2004.

Zhu CW: Effects of the balanced budget act on Medicare home health utilization, *J Am Geriatr Soc* 52:989–994, 2004.

Zink MR: Episodic case management in home care, *Home Health Nurse* 23:655–662, 2005.

The Nurse in the Schools

Janet T. Ihlenfeld

ADDITIONAL RESOURCES

These related resources are found either in the appendix at the back of this book or on the book's website at http://evolve.elsevier.com/stanhope/foundations.

Evolve Website

- Community Assessment Applied
- Case Study, with questions and answers
- Quiz review questions
- WebLinks, including link to *Healthy People 2010* website

Real World Community Health Nursing: An Interactive CD-ROM, second edition

If you are using this CD-ROM in your course, you will find the following activities related to this chapter:
- *Describe Your Roles* in **A Day in the Life of a Community Health Nurse**

OBJECTIVES

After reading this chapter, the student should be able to:
1. Discuss professional standards expected of school nurses.
2. Differentiate between the many roles and functions of school nurses.
3. Describe the different variations of school health services and coordinated school health programs.
4. Assess the nursing care given in schools in terms of the primary, secondary, and tertiary levels of prevention.
5. Identify future trends in school nursing.

CHAPTER OUTLINE

KEY TERMS

American Academy of Pediatrics (AAP): a professional organization for pediatricians that sets policy statements for child health.

Americans With Disabilities Act (ADA): an act passed in 1990 that mandated that individuals with mental and physical disabilities be brought into the mainstream of American life.

case manager: a school nurse who performs a number of general activities concerning health problems of the children.
Centers for Disease Control and Prevention (CDC): a branch of the U.S. Public Health Service whose primary responsibility is to propose, coordinate, and evaluate changes in the surveillance of disease in the United States.
community outreach: a role of a nurse who gives care outside one defined setting.
consultant: someone who provides professional advice, services, or information.
counselor: a role of a nurse when mental health support is provided.
crisis teams: school staff designated to deal with crises at school.
direct caregiver: a role of a nurse giving health care to the ill or injured.
do-not-resuscitate (DNR) orders: physician's orders to not medically intervene when death is about to occur.
emergency plan: procedures to effectively give care in a crisis situation.
full-service school-based health centers (FSSBHCs): a federal program providing comprehensive health care at a site within a school to all including social services, day care, and job training.
health educator: a role of a nurse in providing instruction on health topics.
individualized education plans (IEPs): plans to decide educational accommodations for disabled children.
individualized health plans (IHPs): plans to decide the health needs of disabled children in school.

National Association of School Nurses (NASN): a professional organization for school nurses that sets standards and guidelines for them.
PL 93-112 Section 504 of the Rehabilitation Act of 1973: federal law requiring services for persons with handicaps.
PL 94-142 Education for All Handicapped Children Act: federal law requiring education for all children with handicaps.
PL 105-17 Individuals With Disabilities Education Act (IDEA): educational services that must be provided for disabled children from birth through age 22 years.
primary prevention: health promotion and education.
researcher: a role of a nurse to investigate phenomena related to health.
Safe Kids Campaign: a federal program to provide education to children about safety.
school-based health centers (SBHCs): a federal program providing health care, dental care, and mental health care to children and families in schools.
School Health Policies and Programs Study 2000 (SHPPS 2000): a federal study of CDC-funded school health programs.
school-linked program: a school health program run by a community health agency.
secondary prevention: screening and providing health care.
Standard Precautions: procedures to prevent exposure to blood-borne diseases.
tertiary prevention: continued long-term health care.

According to the U.S. Department of Health and Human Services (USDHHS), in 2004 more than 53 million children attended one of 120,000 schools every day (Centers for Disease Control and Prevention, 2004). These children need health care during their school day, and this is the job of the school nurse. Approximately 47,600 school nurses are in the public schools (Pfizer Pharmaceuticals, 2001).

It is commonly thought that school nurses do nothing but put bandages on cuts and soothe children with stomachaches. However, that is not their major role. School nurses give comprehensive nursing care to the children and the staff at the school. At the same time, they coordinate the health education program of the school and consult with school officials to help identify and care for other persons in the community.

The school nurse gives care to the children not only in the school building itself but in other settings in which there are children—for example, in juvenile detention centers, in preschools and day care centers, during field trips, at sporting events, and in the children's homes (National Association of School Nurses, 2001).

The school nurse, therefore, must be flexible in providing nursing care, education, and help to those who need it. This chapter discusses the history of nursing in the schools and the functions of school nurses today. In addition, the standards

of practice for school nurses are discussed, as the nurse takes on a variety of roles. Different types of school health services are reviewed, including government-financed programs.

The primary, secondary, and tertiary levels of nursing care that nurses give to children in the schools are presented. The most common health problems that the school nurse encounters are also discussed under their appropriate prevention levels. The chapter ends with a discussion of the ethical dilemmas that may arise for school nurses. The future of nursing in the schools is predicted for ever-changing communities.

HISTORY OF SCHOOL NURSING

The history of school nursing began with the earliest efforts of nurses to care for people in the community.
- In the late 1800s in England, the Metropolitan Association of Nursing provided medical examinations for children in the schools of London.
- By 1892, nurses in London were responsible for checking the nutrition of the children in the schools (Ross, 1999).
- In 1897, nurses in New York City schools began to identify ill children. They then excluded these children from classes so that other children would not be infected (Hawkins, Hayes, and Corliss, 1994).

- Many states had laws in the late 1800s mandating that within the schools nurses teach about the abuse of alcohol and narcotics (Veselak, 2001).

In the early 1900s in the United States, the main health problem in the community was the spread of infectious diseases. On October 2, 1902, in New York City, Lillian Wald's Henry Street Settlement nurses began going into homes and schools to assess children. At first these public health nurses were in only four schools caring for about 10,000 children. They made plans to identify children with lice and other infestations and children with infected wounds, tuberculosis (TB), and other infectious diseases (Hawkins, Hayes, and Corliss, 1994; Kalisch and Kalisch, 2004).

The need for school nurses was immediately recognized by the health care community.

- By 1910, Teachers College in New York City added a course on school nursing to their curriculum for nurses.
- In 1916 a school superintendent requested that a public health nurse be sent to the schools to care for children of immigrants (Kalisch and Kalisch, 2004).
- By the 1920s, school nurse teachers were employed by most municipal health departments.
- In the 1940s, the nurses were employed mostly by the school districts directly.
- The nurses also provided home nursing and health education for the children and their parents (Hawkins, Hayes, and Corliss, 1994).

After World War II and into the 1950s, as a result of the increased use of immunizations and antibiotics, the number of children with communicable disease in the schools decreased.

- School nurses then turned their attention to screening children for common health problems and for vision and hearing.
- School nurses were less likely to teach health concepts in the children's classrooms and more likely to consult with teachers about health education (Hawkin, Hayes, and Corliss, 1994).
- There was an increased emphasis on employee health, and school nurses began screening teachers and other school staff for health problems (Veselak, 2001).
- In the 1960s there was an upsurge in the call for higher levels of education for school nurses.

- A position paper delivered at the 1960 American Nurses Association (ANA) convention called for a Bachelor of Science degree in nursing as the minimum educational preparation for school nurses.

FEDERAL LEGISLATION IN THE 1970S, 1980S, 1990S, AND 2000S

Community involvement in health in schools was a major thrust in the 1970s and 1980s.

- Counseling and mental health services were added to the responsibilities of school nurses, who began to directly teach children concepts of health.
- Children were no longer just being screened for illnesses (Hawkins, Hayes, and Corliss, 1994).
- Because of federal laws that required schools to make accommodations for handicapped children, medically fragile children were attending schools, often for the first time.

One of these laws, **Public Law (PL) 93-112 Section 504 of the Rehabilitation Act of 1973,** was an important step in helping all children enjoy a normal educational experience (Betz, 2001; Moses, Gilchrest, and Schwab, 2005). This law was followed by **PL 94-142 Education for All Handicapped Children Act**, which required that children with disabilities have services provided for them in the schools.

After the passing of the **Americans With Disabilities Act (ADA)** in 1992, **PL 105-17 Individuals With Disabilities Education Act (IDEA)** passed in 1997. Both of these laws required that more children be allowed to attend schools. Schools had to make allowances for their special needs, which included ensuring that their school experience was in balance with their health care needs by developing **individualized education plans (IEPs)** and **individualized health plans (IHPs).** That meant that more children with human immunodeficiency virus (HIV), acquired immunodeficiency syndrome (AIDS), chronic illnesses, or mental health problems were in the classrooms and needed more attention from the school nurse (Betz, 2001; Moses et al, 2005). The No Child Left Behind Act of 2001 requires a healthy environment in the schools, which also affects children who have health problems (Whalen et al, 2004). Table 31-1 summarizes the effects of these laws on school nurses and schoolchildren.

Table 31-1 Federal Legislation Affecting School Nursing

Law	Effect on School Nurses and Children
1973: PL 93-112, Section 504 of the Rehabilitation Act	Children cannot be excluded from schools due to a handicap. The school must provide health services that each child needs.
1975: PL 94-142, Education for All Handicapped Children Act	All children should attend school in the least restrictive environment. Requires school district's committee on the handicapped to develop individualized education plans (IEPs) for children.
1992: Americans With Disabilities Act	Persons with disabilities cannot be excluded from activities.
1997: PL 105-17, Individuals With Disabilities Education Act (IDEA)	Educational services must be offered by the schools for all disabled children from birth through age 22 years.

Compiled from Betz CL: Use of 504 plans for children and youth with disabilities: nursing application, *Pediatr Nurs* 27(4): 347–352, 2001.

Table 31-2 **High Points in School Nursing History**

Decade	Major Events in School Nursing
1890s	English and American nurses are used in schools to examine children for infectious diseases and to teach about alcohol abuse.
1900s	Henry Street Settlement in New York City sends nurses into schools and homes to investigate the children's overall health.
1910s	School nursing course added to Teachers College nursing program.
1920s and 1930s	School nurses are employed by community health departments.
1940s	School districts employ school nurses.
1950s	Children are screened in schools for common health problems.
1960s	Educational preparation for school nurses is debated.
1970s	School nurse practitioner programs are begun. Increased emphasis is put on mental health counseling in schools.
1980s	Children with long-term illness or disabilities attend schools.
1990s	School-based and school-linked clinics are started. Total family and community health care is offered.
2000s	School nurses provide comprehensive primary, secondary, and tertiary levels of nursing care.

Also during the 1990s, the responsibilities of the school nurse were extended to include the development of complete clinics and health care agency centers within or attached to the schools (Hawkins, Hayes, and Corliss, 1994). These school-based clinics are discussed later in this chapter. By 2002, some school nurses were responsible for several schools, and they gave care under a variety of nursing roles. Table 31-2 highlights the history of school nursing over the past century.

STANDARDS OF PRACTICE FOR SCHOOL NURSES

The professional body for school nurses is the **National Association of School Nurses (NASN)**, headquartered in Washington, D.C. This association provides general guidelines and support for all school nurses. Along with the American Nurses Association, the NASN revised the standards of professional practice for school nurses in 2005. These standards include assessment, diagnosis, outcomes identification, planning, implementation, and evaluation.

In addition, the professional performance standards include quality of practice, education, professional practice evaluation, collegiality, collaboration, ethics, research, resource utilization, leadership, and program management (National Association of School Nurses/American Nurses Association, 2005). In general, the NASN standards (Box 31-1) compare very well with those developed by the **American Academy of Pediatrics (AAP)** regarding the provision of health care to students in the schools. The AAP (2001c) developed its own ideas about how nurses function in schools based on their assessment of schoolchildren's health needs. These guidelines are very similar to those written by the NASN. The AAP stated that school nurses should ensure the following:

- That children get the health care they need, including emergency care in the school
- That the nurse keeps track of the state-required vaccinations that children have received

Box 31-1 **Summary of Major Concepts of NASN Standards**

- Give and evaluate appropriate up-to-date nursing care.
- Collaborate well with other health providers and school staff.
- Maintain school health office policies including privacy and safety of health records.
- Teach health promotion and maintenance to children, families, and communities.

Modified from National Association of School Nurses: *Scope and standards of professional school nursing practice,* Washington, DC, 2005, National Association of School Nurses.

- That the nurse carries out the required screening of the children based on state law
- That children with health problems are able to learn in the classroom

The AAP recommends that the nurse be the head of a health team that includes a physician (preferably a pediatrician), school counselors, the school psychologist, members of the school staff including the administrator, and teachers. The goal is for children to obtain complete health care in the schools.

EDUCATIONAL CREDENTIALS OF SCHOOL NURSES

The NASN recommends that school nurses be registered nurses who also have bachelor's degrees in nursing and a special certification in school nursing (National Association of School Nurses, 2005). The AAP has the same recommendations (American Academy of Pediatrics, 2001c). However, not all nurses have been educated this way. There are no general laws regarding the educational background of school nurses. School nurses in some states are required to be registered nurses, but licensed practical nurses are also seen in some schools. Only about 50% of all U.S. states require some form of additional study for school nurse specialty certification (Kolbe, Kann, and Brener, 2001).

School nurses do not start their nursing careers in the schools. All have prior experience in nursing—most from working either in hospitals or communities. In addition, most have spent years working with children, so they are aware of their special health needs.

ROLES AND FUNCTIONS OF SCHOOL NURSES

School nurses give care to children as direct caregivers, educators, counselors, consultants, and case managers. They must coordinate the health care of many students in their schools with the health care that the children receive from their own health care providers.

In *Healthy People 2010*, objective 7-4 states that there should be one nurse for every 750 children in each school (U.S. Department of Health and Human Services, 2000). Most schools have not achieved this objective. In 1994, approximately 28% of the nation's schools met that standard. The new objective is that 50% of the country's elementary, middle, junior high, and senior high schools have this many nurses by 2010. Having fewer nurses in the schools means that the nurses are expected to perform many different functions. It is therefore possible that they are unable to provide the amount of comprehensive care that the students need (Broussard et al, 2004).

In 2003 the National Association of School Nurses adopted a resolution recommending that there be a school nurse at all times in every school. The recommendation was based on requirements of the IDEA Act and CDC health recommendations (National Association of School Nurses, 2003).

BRIEFLY NOTED

Many schools do not have a nurse in the building every day.

SCHOOL NURSE ROLES

Direct Caregiver

The school nurse is expected to give immediate nursing care to the ill or injured child or school staff member. **Direct caregiver** is the traditional role of the school nurse.

Although most school nurses are in public or private schools and give care only during school hours, the nurse in a boarding school gives nursing care to children 24 hours a day and 7 days a week. In boarding schools, the children live at school and go home only for vacations. The nurse also lives at the school and may be on call all the time. The nurse in the boarding school is very important to the children because this nurse is the gatekeeper to their complete health care (Thackaberry, 2001). The nurse makes all of the health care decisions for the child and has a referral system to contact other health care providers, such as physicians and psychological counselors, if needed.

Healthy People 2010

Objectives Related to School Health and School Nursing

6-9	Increase the proportion of children and youth with disabilities who spend at least 80% of their time in regular education programs
7-2	Increase the proportion of middle, junior high, and senior high schools that provide comprehensive school health education to prevent health problems in the following areas: unintentional injury; violence; suicide; tobacco use and addiction; alcohol or other drug use; unintended pregnancy, HIV/AIDS, and STD infection; unhealthy dietary patterns; inadequate physical activity; and environmental health
7-4	Increase the proportion of the nation's elementary, middle, junior high, and senior high schools that have a nurse-to-student ratio of at least 1:750
9-11	Increase the proportion of young adults who have received formal instruction before turning age 18 years on reproductive health issues, including all of the following topics: birth control methods, safer sex to prevent HIV, prevention of sexually transmitted diseases, and abstinence
14-23	Maintain vaccination coverage levels for children in licensed day care facilities and children in kindergarten through the first grade
14-24	Increase the proportion of young children who receive all vaccines that have been recommended for universal administration for at least 5 years
14-27	Increase routine vaccination coverage levels of adolescents
15-31	Increase the proportion of public and private schools that require the use of appropriate head, face, eye, and mouth protection for students participating in school-sponsored sports
15-39	Reduce weapon carrying by adolescents on school property
16-23	Increase the proportion of territories and states that have service systems for children with special health care needs
21-13	Increase the proportion of school-based health centers with an oral health component
22-8	Increase the proportion of the nation's public and private schools that require daily physical education for all students
24-5	Reduce the number of school or work days missed by persons due to asthma
26-9	Increase the age and proportion of adolescents who remain alcohol and drug free
27-11	Increase smoke-free and tobacco-free environments in schools, including all school facilities, property, vehicles, and events
28-2	Increase the proportion of preschool children aged 5 years and under who receive vision screening
28-4	Reduce blindness and visual impairment in children and adolescents aged 17 years and under

From U.S. Department of Health and Human Services: *Healthy People 2010: understanding and improving health,* ed 2, Washington, DC, 2000, U.S. Government Printing Office.

2001a). The SBHCs can range in size from small to large. There are school clinics open to the community only during the school year and also health centers that are open 24 hours a day all year. An example of the more limited clinic is the SBHC in Gulfport, Mississippi, in which 12 clinics are run in the schools by the local hospital during the school-year months of August through May (Hospitals' Outreach, 2000).

Another example of a clinic is the **school-linked program**, which is coordinated by the school but has community ties (American Academy of Pediatrics, 2001a). An example of this is the *Collaborative Model for School Health* in Pitts County, North Carolina. The nurses employed by the local hospital in that area provide health care for children in kindergarten through fifth grade. The county health department, the local university's nursing school, and other private health care providers collaborate to provide primary, secondary, and tertiary nursing care. An evaluation of the program has shown that the children's school attendance and learning have increased as a result of the presence of more complete school health services (Farrior et al, 2000).

At a center in Texas, an urban SBHC is located in a school district in which many of the children lack health insurance. The school nurses there are assisted by three part-time nurse practitioners and one nurse in community health. The school nurse is responsible for keeping records on the children's immunizations, does the screening, provides first aid to injured children, and refers children who need additional health care to the SBHC in the school. Parents like the program because they trust the school nurse. They also like its location inside the school because everyone can receive health care without having to travel far to get to a clinic (Carpenter and Mueller, 2001).

FULL-SERVICE SCHOOL-BASED HEALTH CENTERS

Because the SBHCs have been so successful, in some areas they have grown into **full-service school-based health centers (FSSBHCs)** (U.S. Department of Health and Human Services, 2001b). These centers give care not only to students in a comprehensive health care setting but also to other persons in the community. They may provide social services, day care, job training, and educational counseling in addition to the medical and nursing care, mental health counseling, and dental care seen in smaller school-based centers (U.S. Department of Health and Human Services, 2001b).

For example, there are three different sites of federally funded FSSBHCs in Modesto, California, run by the Golden Valley Health Center. Each of these clinics is open 40 hours a week to provide health care for the children and families of migrant and seasonal farmworkers in the area. This program is successful because it provides health care in the school for entire families in an area in which some families may not have access to health care. Because the building has separate entrances, the center can be open after the school day has ended, so it is used often (U.S. Department of Health and Human Services, 2001b).

SCHOOL NURSES AND *HEALTHY PEOPLE 2010*

Many *Healthy People 2010* objectives are directed toward the health of children. In addition, several point directly at the care that nurses give to children in the schools. The "*Healthy People 2010*" box lists the objectives that involve school-age children. These objectives are concerned with children with disabilities in the schools, the number of children with major health problems, and the ratio of nurses to children in the schools. Nurses can accomplish these goals using the three levels of prevention, as discussed next.

THE LEVELS OF PREVENTION IN THE SCHOOLS

The three levels of prevention (primary, secondary, and tertiary) have always been a part of health care in the schools (Wold and Dagg, 2001). **Primary prevention** provides health promotion and education to prevent health problems in children. **Secondary prevention** includes the screening of children for various illnesses, monitoring their growth and development, and caring for them when they are ill or injured. **Tertiary prevention** in the schools is the continued care of children who need long-term health care services, along with education within the community (Figure 31-2).

PRIMARY PREVENTION IN THE SCHOOLS

Children need continued health services in the schools. The school nurse sees them on an almost daily basis and is usually the person who is given the role of teaching them about and promoting their health.

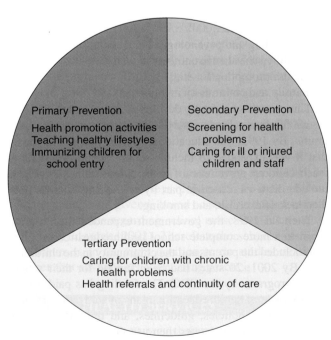

FIGURE 31-2 Levels of prevention in schools.

CASE STUDY

Samantha Smith is the registered nurse for Green Hills Elementary School and Rising Stars Elementary School. Ms. Smith spends 2½ days at each school providing health care in the nursing clinics and helping the science teachers incorporate health into their curriculum. This week Ms. Smith is performing vision screenings for grades kindergarten, 1, 3, and 5 at both schools.

At the beginning of the school year, Ms. Smith asked parents to volunteer to help with vision and hearing screenings. Shortly before the day of the vision screening, Ms. Smith met with and trained the five parents who had volunteered to help.

The day before the screening, Ms. Smith spoke to the students in each classroom that would receive screening. She talked to the students about their five senses and how to keep them healthy. Ms. Smith explained the vision screening process so that the students would know what to expect the next day. On the day of the screening, Ms. Smith sets up the screening charts and calls each grade level separately for screening. Students who fail the screening are rescreened by Ms. Smith and then referred to their ophthalmologist for vision correction.

The school nurse may have the opportunity to go into the classroom to teach health promotion concepts—for example, hand-washing or tooth-brushing skills. They may spend time with the teachers, providing the latest information on healthy lifestyles for children or how to spot a child who may be ill or in need of counseling.

School nurses use the nursing process while they care for children in the schools. In their primary prevention efforts, they do the following:
- Assess children and families to determine their level of knowledge about health issues
- Find out whether children are at risk for preventable problems
- Analyze the assessment findings
- Make plans to develop teaching plans or health promotion activities
- Implement these activities
- Evaluate and revise the plan
    The school nurse focuses on the following areas of primary prevention:
- Preventing childhood injuries
- Preventing substance abuse behaviors
- Reducing the risk of the development of chronic diseases
- Monitoring the immunization status of children

Prevention of Childhood Injuries

Injuries are the leading cause of death in children and teenagers (Deal et al, 2000). The school nurse educates children, teachers, and parents about preventing injuries. Working with the national **Safe Kids Campaign**, the school nurse can provide educational programs reminding children to use

- Keep the lesson to no more than 10 minutes in length.
- Use a lot of examples, pictures, and stuffed animals in the talk.
- Always remember the developmental stage of the children when teaching them.

---

their seatbelts or bicycle helmets to prevent injuries. Other classes can focus on crossing the street, water safety, and fire safety. The school nurse, as the trusted person at school, is able to quickly provide information on injury prevention, since most injuries are preventable (Rubsam, 2001).

School nurses also provide information on how to prevent playground injuries. They assess school playgrounds for equipment safety on the basis of the U.S. Consumer Product Safety Commission guidelines (Bernardo, Gardner, and Seibel, 2001) and promote skateboard and scooter safety by providing health educational workshops to children and their families (American Academy of Pediatrics, 2002).

These programs can be implemented by the nurse on a community-wide scale. Research has shown that once behaviors of children related to safety are taught, their effects spread quickly throughout the community. This makes the entire community safer (Klassen et al, 2000).

Substance Abuse Prevention Education

Primary prevention interventions by the school nurse include educating children and adolescents about the effects of alcohol and other drugs on their bodies. Preventing use of and "saying no" to drugs have been part of the school health program for many years. Teenagers are taught by the school nurse to stay away from drugs: marijuana, cocaine, crack, heroin, and alcohol.

There has been an increase in the use of "club drugs" such as lysergic acid diethylamide (LSD), ketamine, gamma-hydroxybutyrate (GHB), Rohypnol, and 3,4-methylene-dioxymethamphetamine (MDMA [Ecstasy]). The school nurse can inform students about the serious side effects of Ecstasy, in particular, that it causes a very high body temperature that can lead to death. Teaching the teenagers about the dangers of all drugs is the responsibility of the school nurse. In addition, the school nurse can teach parents and other members of the community about the latest drug fads, increasing everyone's awareness of these dangerous trends (Wood and Synovitz, 2001).

Disease Prevention Education

The nurse has the opportunity to teach children healthy lifestyles to reduce their risk of disease later in life. For example, children can be taught ways to reduce their risk of getting heart disease. In one school program in North Carolina, teachers taught third-graders and fourth-graders about eating healthy foods, getting exercise, and not smoking (Harrell et al, 2001). The school nurse can then reinforce the teachers' educational plans or develop the program further for other age-groups to teach them how to take care of their heart.

Getting health promotion information to the parents of the children is often a challenge for the school nurse. In the West Seneca school district near Buffalo, New York, one of the district's school nurses has a column in the *District Newsletter* that is sent to all residents of the town. Each newsletter focuses on a different area of health promotion, which in March/April 2002 was on sun exposure and use of tanning booths (Krystofik, 2002a). In this way, the school nurse was able to promote the health of not only the schoolchildren but the community as well.

Required Vaccinations for Schoolchildren

All states have laws that require that children receive immunizations, or vaccinations, against communicable diseases before they attend school (Boyer-Chuanroong and Deaver, 2000). School nurses must be up to date on the latest laws on immunizations for children in their own state.

For children entering kindergarten, these vaccinations include diphtheria, pertussis, and tetanus (the DPT series); measles, mumps, and rubella (the MMR series); polio; and others.

The school nurse must keep a complete file of all of the children's vaccination records to meet the state's laws. These files should contain the following:
- Student's name
- Date of birth
- Address
- Telephone number
- Parents'/guardians' names
- Contact information
- Primary health care provider's name, telephone number, and address
- All the vaccinations with the dates the child received booster shots

This makes it easy for the school nurse to find out which children still need immunizations or boosters.

Because children are prevented from attending school if they have not had the required shots, the school nurse must make every effort to find missing data in the immunization record.
- The nurse must contact the parents to get the immunization history for the child.
- Written notes should be sent to each child's home at least 1 year before each new immunization is needed so that the parents have time to get the child to their health care provider for the shots.
- If the parents or guardians do not speak English, these notes should be translated into the family's language (Boyer-Chuanroong and Deaver, 2000).
- If the parents have lost the information that gives the child's immunization history, the nurse should encourage them to contact their physician or nurse practitioner to get it.

Many problems with children not being immunized or having incomplete vaccination records may occur in families who have moved many times or who may not have a

regular physician. The parents may have no idea whether the child has even received the shots. Families may not have health care insurance to pay for the immunizations, or they may have insurance that does not pay for preventive care. In these cases, the parents have to pay for the immunizations, which can be expensive. Certain low-income families without health care insurance may qualify for federal programs that provide free immunizations to children. Each state has its own program, so school nurses should become familiar with what their state provides.

SECONDARY PREVENTION IN THE SCHOOLS

Because secondary prevention involves caring for children when they need health care, this is the largest responsibility for the school nurse. This includes caring for ill or injured students and school employees. It also involves screening and assessing children and referral to appropriate health agencies or providers. The school nurse uses the nursing process during secondary prevention activities. When an ill or injured child comes to the school's health office, the nurse must immediately assess the child for the degree of illness or injury.

Children seek out the school nurse for a variety of different needs:
- Headaches
- Stomachaches
- Diarrhea
- Anxiety over being separated from the parents
- Cuts, bruises, or other injuries

In addition, children may seek reassurance from the school nurse or even appear to hide in the nurse's office. This may be caused by harassment or bullying from other children in the school (Sweeney and Sweeney, 2000).

Once the assessment data are gathered, the nurse determines the course of action and follows it through the implementation and evaluation phases. This occurs for direct child health care as well as for screening children for other health problems. If assessment data identify a child as having a health problem, the school nurse continues to follow the nursing process to further care for that child.

BRIEFLY NOTED

The health records of children in schools are to be kept private, just as they are in hospitals and other health agencies.

Nursing Care for Emergencies in the School

The school nurse cares for children who are injured or become ill in the school. The school nurse should therefore have an **emergency plan** in place so that a routine can be followed when emergencies occur. This plan should include the following:
- Making an assessment of the emergency and surveying the scene
- Treating the injured or ill children or teachers
- Calling for backup help from the community's emergency medical units if needed

The AAP and the American Health Association (AHA) have recommended that plans be developed in the schools in case of an emergency when a child or staff member needs immediate care. The school nurse should develop this plan so that a staff member in the school, for example the principal or an athletic coach, can follow it in case the nurse is not in the building at the time of the emergency. The following recommendations are based on the AAP/AHA guidelines (American Academy of Pediatrics, 2001b; Hazinski et al, 2004).

The plan should include the following:
- When to call 911 for local emergency personnel
- How to make arrangements to transfer a child to the hospital via ambulance in case more care is needed
- If the nurse is not in the school at all times, at least two different staff members identified as responsible for determining if emergency care is needed

These persons should be educated by the school nurse on proper first-aid techniques so that correct care is given until further help arrives.

All staff in the schools should be taught **Standard Precautions**. These policies should be written into the emergency plan.
- Members of the athletic staff such as coaches and physical education teachers should also be up to date on emergency health procedures.
- If they are not, the school nurse should teach them about the policies and provide a means to review first-aid procedures with them on a regular basis.

Individualized emergency plans should be made for all students who may have a health problem that could result in an emergency situation in the school. This plan could be for the following:
- Children with food allergies (e.g., to peanuts)
- Children who have a sensitivity to insect bites that could result in anaphylactic shock
- Children with chronic illnesses such as asthma, diabetes, or hemophilia

The children in the schools should be taught basic first-aid procedures by the nurse, including Standard Precautions related to blood exposure. This lesson, depending on the age and grade level of the children, would allow the children to help in a playground accident while the adults are being summoned to the scene.

All emergency procedures should be written and easily accessible to anyone in the school. Research has shown that the nurse may not always be at the school and the emergency may have to be handled by a teacher, administrator, secretary, custodian, or coach (Sapien and Allen, 2001). Along with the procedures and an emergency manual written or obtained by the school nurse, the following are required:
- An injury or illness log should be maintained by personnel so that the emergency is accurately recorded.
- Procedures should be available for notifying the parents or legal guardians about the emergency, what was done for the child, and where the child was sent if transfer to a hospital or other medical agency was required.

Because nursing care may have to be given to a child or adult in respiratory or cardiac arrest, the nurse should have current certification in cardiopulmonary resuscitation (CPR) and the use of the automated external defibrillator (AED) (Hazinski et al, 2004). Other education in the area of emergency nursing would also be helpful to the school nurse, including pediatric advanced life support (PALS) or emergency nursing for pediatrics certification (ENPC) (Sapien and Allen, 2001).

Emergency Equipment in the School Nurses' Office

The school nurse needs much equipment to deal with emergencies in the school. These needs are based on the guidelines of the AAP (American Academy of Pediatrics, 2001b). The health office should have basic items on hand. Necessary equipment includes the following:
- Full oxygen tanks with oxygen masks of different kinds (bag-valve masks, resuscitation masks), splints for sprained or broken limbs
- Cervical spine collars to keep a child's head in proper alignment
- Sterile dressings

Various sizes of these items are needed because children of different ages are in the school. Another recommended item for the nurse's office is an epinephrine autoinjector kit in case a child goes into anaphylactic shock after exposure to an allergen (American Academy of Pediatrics, 2001b; Sapien and Allen, 2001). This should be locked in a medication cabinet because there is a needle in the kit. Of course, gloves should also be available to meet Standard Precautions guidelines. A telephone should be available for calling emergency personnel and parents. Next to the telephone should be paper and pen so that instructions from the emergency personnel can be written down.

Giving Medication in School

The school nurse, as part of secondary prevention, may be responsible for giving medications to children during the school day (McCarthy, Kelly, and Reed, 2000). These may include the following:
- Prescribed medications
- Medications that the parents have asked the school's nurse to give (e.g., cold remedies)
- Vitamins

In all instances, the nurse should develop a series of guidelines to help with the legal administration of medications in the school. Parents should be sure to tell the school nurse if the child is on any medications (American Academy of Pediatrics, 2001d).
- The prescribed drug should have the original prescription label on it and be in the original container so that there are no errors.
- The AAP (2004) recommended that the physician inform the school nurse about possible side effects of the medication that may occur during the school day.
- If the physician does not contact the nurse first, the nurse should call the physician and ask.

- A current, signed parental consent form for giving the medication should also be in the student's file.
- A current medication (drug) book should be in the nurse's office so that it can be consulted for information.

The school nurse should also have a means of contacting a pharmacist to ask questions regarding the medication if needed.

Assessing and Screening Children at School

The AAP Committee on School Health (American Academy of Pediatrics, 2004) has developed guidelines for the school nurse to use when screening children in the schools. The plans are for the state-required screening of children as well as for more complete health examinations for children in the school.

- Children should receive screening for vision, hearing, height and weight, oral health, TB, and scoliosis in the schools (Centers for Disease Control and Prevention, 2004).
- For each of these areas, the school nurse should keep a confidential record of all of the screening results for the children in the school, according to Health Insurance and Portability and Accountability Act (HIPPA) rules.
- Each state has different laws regarding the screenings, and the nurse should be aware of these laws. The nurse needs to know the requirements for each of the states.

In addition, some children may not have a regular physician or other primary health care provider such as a nurse practitioner to provide health care. For these children, the AAP (2000a) has recommended the following:

- Children have a physical and developmental examination in the school setting
- Children provide information on their language skills and their motor abilities
- Children be tested on their social abilities and their height and weight
- Children have an assessment of their level of physical growth as well as their sexual maturation
- Children have dental assessments

Physical examinations to play in a school sport are also given in the school. The school nurse would arrange for the sports physicals and would help monitor the examinations being done by the school's physician or nurse practitioner.

Screening for TB in schoolchildren is also done in several states. This can be a problem because children must have the Mantoux test (tuberculin skin test [TST]) given to them first. Then they have to return to have the test site read by the nurse. If the site is positive, the child has been exposed to TB and needs further health screening. One study showed that it was more efficient to have the children screened for TB at the clinic and then have the school nurse read the test and send that information to the health clinic for follow-up (DeLago et al, 2001).

The school nurse can also screen children and adolescents for hypertension (high blood pressure). One study in a city's middle high schools found that some teenagers had high blood pressure (Meninger et al, 2001). These teens can be taught techniques to reduce their blood pressure and so reduce their risk of cardiovascular disease as they get older.

Screening Children for Lice

School nurses also must screen children for lice infestation. According to one study, between 6 and 12 million cases of lice occur every year in the United States and most are in school-aged children. Lice are found most often in white middle-class children and are more often seen in clean hair as well. Therefore the suggestion that lice are associated with unclean homes in poverty areas is incorrect (Kirchofer, Price, and Telljohann, 2001). The school nurse needs to check children for lice because in many areas, children with lice are excluded from school. Check on the local school district policies. During the "lice check," the nurse must check the children's hair for both lice and nits (Ten Steps, 2000).

The following are responsibilities of the school nurse (Kirchofer, Price, and Telljohann, 2001):

- Teach children, parents, and teachers how to prevent lice and treat cases of infestation
- Teach children not to share combs and hats
- Teach parents how to completely treat the child with the antilice medications
- Teach parents to remove all nits from the head with a fine-toothed comb
- Teach parents to wash all bed linens and clothing

Identification of Child Abuse or Neglect

The school nurse is mandated by state laws to report suspected cases of child abuse or neglect. These laws differ from state to state, and the nurse should be aware of the particular requirements for reporting in each state.

A nurse who identifies a child who may be abused or receives information from a teacher or other staff member that leads to the belief that a child has been abused must contact the appropriate legal authorities as well as the school's principal. A confidential file should be made about the incident. However, the nurse should let the government authorities, usually the state or county child protection department, look into the suspected case. In all cases, the child should be protected from harm, and those who have no right to know that child abuse or neglect is suspected should not be given any information.

Communicating with Health Care Providers

The school nurse often makes an assessment of a child that requires referral to the child's family physician or other health care provider. The findings from these assessments must be communicated accurately to the child's parent and the provider. The nurse must be able to get the information quickly and accurately to the child's parents. Be aware of the HIPAA privacy rules (Bergren, 2004).

One way to do this is to write a detailed report about the findings. This information can be given to the child to give to his or her parents. However, the child may lose the report before it gets to them. The information can be mailed to the parents, but this takes more time. Perhaps the best way is to telephone the parents, telling them that the child needs to see the physician or nurse practitioner and that the child will be bringing the information home that day. In this way, the parents can ask the child for the report and the child is aware that the parents expect it.

One state, Nebraska, developed a plan in which the school nurse writes the health care problem information on a referral card for the parents to give to the child's physician. Then the physician can follow up on the problem and write information that the school nurse needs to know regarding the child's diagnosis, the plan of care, and special needs in the school for the child's care.

This *School Nurse Referral Care Program* is one way to help the nurse know what was found in the health care appointment that the nurse recommended (Nebraska school nurses improve communication, 2000).

Suicide and Other Mental Health Problems

Suicide is the third leading cause of death in teenagers. Recommendations have been made about reducing the incidence of suicide in teenagers. A suicide prevention program developed in one school district, discussed below, contains ideas for the school nurse to use. Suicide prevention must be addressed by school nurses, who can do the following:
- Lead educational programs within the schools to emphasize coping strategies and stress management techniques for children and adolescents who have problems and to teach about the risk factors
- Teach faculty members to look for the risk factors
- Help organize a peer assistance program to help teenagers cope with school stresses (King, 2001)

If a student threatens suicide at school, the school nurse should intervene by ensuring the safety of the student and by removing him or her from the school situation immediately. While parents are being notified, the nurse should assess the child's suicide risk and refer the child or teenager to crisis intervention or mental health services.

In the unfortunate instance in which a teenager who attended the school has committed suicide, the school nurse is called upon to help the school population, both students and teachers, cope with the death. Grief counseling should be set up and coordinated by the school nurse. In addition, further assessments should be made regarding the suicide potential among the deceased teenager's friends, because suicide clusters have been seen to occur. Adolescents may have early signs of mental or emotional problems such as behavior problems in class or severe class or test anxiety. Families may be in crisis, and this translates into problems for the children (Leighton, Worraker, and Nolan, 2003; Leighton et al, 2003).

Children who are homeless have special problems. Children who do not have a stable address have probably moved from school to school very frequently (Nabors and Weist, 2002). Children whose parents are addicted to drugs or alcohol can also benefit from support from the school nurse (Gance-Cleveland, 2004). This lack of a stable environment may make it more likely that they may develop mental or emotional problems. The school nurse can be an advocate for these children and their families.

Violence at School

In the past several years, school shootings by students have occurred involving other students and teachers. This has happened in at least eight states and two foreign countries. In each of these cases, a student or students brought firearms to school and used them, resulting in injuries and deaths of students and teachers (Freed, 2005; Steger, 2000; Williams and Kalkenberg, 2002).

The school nurse may be able to help identify students who will act in this way. Furthermore, the nurse can provide health education classes to help children learn positive ways of dealing with conflict.

The mother of a murdered girl in Paducah, Kentucky, herself a registered nurse, stated that six characteristics may help point out a student who may be thinking about such drastic violence (Steger, 2000):
1. *Venting:* having mood swings
2. *Vocalizing:* threatening others
3. *Vandalizing:* damaging property
4. *Victimizing:* seeing himself or herself as a victim
5. *Vying:* belonging to gangs
6. *Viewing:* witnessing the abuse of others

By helping to identify the student who might be considering school violence or by teaching students and teachers about these warning signs in students, the school nurse may be able to help prevent violent actions through education and follow-up of children who need help.

School Crisis Teams: Responding to Disasters

Events that occur in or near schools may cause a crisis for children, teachers, and staff. Possible crises include the following (Chemtob, Nakashima, and Hamada, 2002):
- The death of a student or teacher as a result of accident, injury, homicide, or suicide
- An accident or fire in the school or community
- A disaster in the community that affects many children's families, such as a tornado, hurricane, or earthquake

Schools should have crisis plans in place to help the children, teachers, parents, and community cope with the sudden event. **Crisis teams** should be in place to help everyone respond quickly to the crisis, to ensure the safety of the school, and to follow up on the effects of the crisis on the members of the school.

The crisis plan should include the following:
- An administrative policy made either for the entire school district or, if the schools are large, for each individual school
- The names of the persons on the crisis team: the superintendent of the school district, the school nurse, the guidance counselor, the school psychologist or social worker, teachers, police or school security, clergy from the community, and parents

The school nurse is involved with triaging injured people, working with the emergency medical personnel as they care for the injured or ill, and assessing the degree of shock, stress, or grieving in the children, teachers, parents, and others in or near the school. The school nurse is also there to be a counselor to help everyone cope with the emotional parts of this serious event (Starr, 2002) (Box 31-2).

The nurse can help the crisis team make a checklist for everyone to follow that tells what to do in every possible crisis situation. Then, at the end of the crisis, the crisis team should take time to counsel all of the people who helped in the crisis including the teachers, emergency personnel, and parents, as well as the children. In that way, everyone can talk about the crisis. The crisis plan should be reviewed every year to see what parts of the plan need updating (National School Boards Association, 2003).

TERTIARY PREVENTION IN THE SCHOOLS

Using the nursing process, the school nurse gives nursing care related to tertiary prevention when working with children who have long-term or chronic illnesses or children with special needs. The nurse participates in developing an individual education plan (IEP) for students with long-term health needs. The nurse's responsibilities include the following:

- The nurse must have information about the child's medications to be given during school hours.
- The nurse must know if the child needs any therapy during the school day, such as physical or occupational therapy.
- The nurse must know if the child has a hearing or vision problem.
- The nurse must ask the teacher to seat the child in the best place in the classroom so the child can better see or hear the teacher and other children.

If a child is in a wheelchair or uses crutches, the school building itself may need to be altered so that the child can get around the school and use the restrooms. It is the responsibility of the nurse to tell the school's administrators about any needs such as these (American Academy of Pediatrics, 2004a).

BRIEFLY NOTED

Children with disabilities who live in residential care facilities because of their long-term health needs go to school every day.

Children with Asthma

Asthma is the leading cause of absenteeism among children with a chronic illness (Swartz et al, 2005). Children may be hospitalized with an asthma attack, or they may have just returned home from the hospital. Asthma can also be caused by allergic triggers that affect children in the school. The following are possible culprits:

- Chalk dust from the blackboards
- Molds or mildew in the school
- Dander from pets that live in some classrooms

There may also be concerns about the quality of the air in the school building because many doors are shut. Industrial arts classes and other sources of air pollution are in the

Box 31-2	Dealing with a Disaster: Responsibilities of the School Nurse

- Provide triage.
- Communicate with emergency medical personnel.
- Assess the school community for the presence of shock and stress.
- Recommend reduced television viewing of the disaster.
- Provide grief counseling.
- Communicate with the children, parents, and school personnel.
- Follow up with assessment of children for anxiety, depression, regression, and posttraumatic stress disorder.

Modified from Calarco C: Preparing for a crisis: crisis team development, *J Sch Nurs* 15(1):46–48, 1999; Starr NB: Helping children and families deal with the psychological aspects of disaster, *J Pediatr Health Care* 16(1):36–39, 2002.

school (Pike-Parris, 2004; U.S. Environmental Protection Agency, 2003). The school nurse can keep track of the indoor air quality of the school so that school administrators have data about what can affect the children. Figure 31-3 contains the questions developed by the U.S. Environmental Protection Agency that the school nurse should answer regarding the air quality of the school.

The nurse uses tertiary prevention when helping children who have asthma. This includes the following (Sander, 2002):

- Administering or helping children use their inhalers or other asthma rescue medications
- Teaching the teachers, children, and parents about asthma and ways that can reduce the factors to which the child may be allergic in the classroom

Many schools have management programs in place to help children with asthma (Taras et al, 2004).

Children with Diabetes Mellitus

The school nurse must establish a plan of care for children with diabetes. This includes plans to monitor blood glucose and give insulin or other medications during the school day. Special nutritional needs also must be discussed (Meyers, 2005; National Association of School Nurses, 2005).

Children Who Are Autistic

Because all children are expected to attend some school regardless of their illness, children with autism go to regular schools in most cases. Because a child with autism has severe communication problems, the school nurse helps the child, the teachers, and the parents so that the child's school day is pleasant, as follows (Cade and Tidwell, 2001):

- The nurse can give the child prescribed medications for mood or prevention of seizures.
- The nurse is responsible for preparing the teachers about the communication problems that the child may have.
- The nurse may recommend the use of sign language, picture boards, or other types of communication devices that are used by the child.
- The nurse can teach the parents about autism.

Health Officer/School Nurse

This checklist discusses three major topic areas:
Student Health Records Maintenance
Public Health and Personal Hygiene Education
Health Officer's Office

Instructions:
1. Read the IAQ *Backgrounder.*
2. Read each item on this Checklist.
3. Check the diamond(s) as appropriate or check the circle if you need additional help with an activity.
4. Return this checklist to the IAQ Coordinator and keep a copy for future reference.

Name: _____

Room or Area: _____

School: _____

Date Completed: _____

Signature: _____

MAINTAIN STUDENT HEALTH RECORDS

There is evidence to suggest that children, pregnant women, and senior citizens are more likely to develop health problems from poor air quality than most adults. Indoor Air Quality (IAQ) problems are most likely to affect those with preexisting health conditions and those who are exposed to tobacco smoke. Student health records should include information about known allergies and other medically documented conditions, such as asthma, as well as any reported sensitivity to chemicals. Privacy considerations may limit the student health information that can be disclosed, but to the extent possible, information about students' potential sensitivity to IAQ problems should be provided to teachers. This is especially true for classes involving potential irritants (e.g., gaseous or particle emissions from art, science, industrial/vocational education sources). Health records and records of health-related complaints by students and staff are useful for evaluating potential IAQ-related complaints.

Include information about sensitivities to IAQ problems in student health records
• Allergies, including reports of chemical sensitivities.
• Asthma.
◇ Completed health records exist for each student.
◇ Health records are being updated.
○ Need help obtaining information about student allergies and other health factors.

Track health-related complaints by students and staff
• Keep a log of health complaints that notes the symptoms, location and time of symptom onset, and exposure to pollutant sources.
• Watch for trends in health complaints, especially in timing or location of complaints.
◇ Have a comprehensive health complaint logging system.
◇ Developing a comprehensive health complaint logging system.
○ Need help developing a comprehensive health complaint logging system.

Recognize indicators that health problems may be IAQ
• Complaints are associated with particular times of the day or week.
• Other occupants in the same area experience similar problems.

• The problem abates or ceases, either immediately or gradually, when an occupant leaves the building and recurs when the occupant returns.
• The school has recently been renovated or refurnished.
• The occupant has recently started working with new or different materials or equipment.
• New cleaning or pesticide products or practices have been introduced into the school.
• Smoking is allowed in the school.
• A new warm-blooded animal has been introduced into the classroom.
◇ Understand indicators of IAQ-related problems.
○ Need help understanding indicators of IAQ-related problems.

HEALTH AND HYGIENE EDUCATION

Schools are unique buildings from a public health perspective because they accommodate more people within a smaller area than most buildings. This proximity increases the potential for airborne contaminants (germs, odors, and constituents of personal products) to pass between students. Raising awareness about the effects of personal habits on the well-being of others can help reduce IAQ-related problems.

Obtain *Indoor Air Quality: An Introduction for Health Professionals*
• Contact IAQ INFO, 800-438-4318.
◇ Already have this EPA guidance document.
◇ Guide is on order.
○ Cannot obtain this guide.

Inform students and staff about the importance of good hygiene in preventing the spread of airborne contagious diseases
• Provide written materials to students (local public health agencies may have information suitable for older students).
• Provide individual instruction/counseling where necessary.
◇ Written materials and counseling available.
◇ Compiling information for counseling and distribution.
○ Need help compiling information or implementing counseling program.

FIGURE 31-3 Indoor air quality checklist. (From U.S. Environmental Protection Agency: Indoor air quality [IAQ] tools for schools: health officer/school nurse checklist, 2003, available at http://www.epa.gov/iaq/schools/tfs/healthof.html.)

Continued

Provide information about IAQ and health
- Help teachers develop activities that reduce exposure to indoor air pollutants for students with IAQ sensitivities, such as those with asthma or allergies (contact the American Lung Association [ALA], the National Association of School Nurses [NASN], or the Asthma and Allergy Foundation of America [AAFA]). Contact information is also available in the IAQ Coordinator's Guide.
- Collaborate with parent-teacher groups to offer family IAQ education programs.
- Conduct a workshop for teachers on health issues that covers IAQ.
◇ Have provided information to parents and staff.
◇ Developing information and education programs for parents and staff.
○ Need help developing information and education program for parents and staff.

Establish an information and counseling program regarding smoking
- Provide free literature on smoking and secondhand smoke.
- Sponsor a quit-smoking program and similar counseling programs in collaboration with the ALA.
◇ "No Smoking" information and programs in place.
◇ "No Smoking" information and programs in planning.
○ Need help with a "No Smoking" program.

HEALTH OFFICER'S OFFICE

Since the health office may be frequented by sick students and staff, it is important to take steps that can help prevent transmission of airborne diseases to uninfected students and staff (see your IAQ Coordinator for help with the following activities).

Ensure that the ventilation system is properly operating
- Ventilation system is operated when the area(s) is occupied.
- Provide an adequate amount of outdoor air to the area(s). There should be at least 15 cubic feet of outdoor air supplied per occupant.
- Air filters are clean and properly installed.
- Air removed from the area(s) does not circulate through the ventilation system into other occupied areas.
◇ Ventilation system operating adequately.
○ Need help with ventilation-related activities.

☐ **No Problems to Report.** I have completed all the activities on this checklist, and I do not need help in any areas.

FIGURE 31-3, cont'd

The nurse can help parents work with others in the health care system so that the child can have a positive learning experience at school.

Children with Special Needs in the Schools

Also attending school are children who need the following:
- Urinary catheterization
- Dressing changes
- Peripheral or central line intravenous catheter maintenance
- Tracheotomy suctioning
- Gastrostomy or other tube feedings
- Intravenous medication

The following are included in the nurse's responsibilities:
- To supervise a health aide who is assigned to the child to care for complex nursing needs
- To provide tertiary care to maintain the child's health
- To maintain the skills needed to assess the child's well-being
- To teach another person in the school how to care for the child in case the nurse is not in the building when the child needs help

It is the responsibility of the school nurse to keep up with the latest health care information through in-service programs (Krystofik, 2002b).

Children with HIV or AIDS may also attend school. Because of privacy and confidentiality laws, the school nurse may not even know that a child with HIV/AIDS attends the school. In these cases, the nurse may be aware of the child's HIV status either by direct notification from the parents or physician or just by knowing that certain drugs the child is taking during the school day are anti-HIV

medications. In all cases, the nurse cannot release that information to anyone.
- As part of regular health education in the school, the school nurse can provide education to the children, school employees, and community about HIV/AIDS prevention and risks (American Academy of Pediatrics, 2004).
- The school nurse should also be part of the school health advisory committee to develop an HIV/AIDS health curriculum that teaches not only about HIV/AIDS prevention but also about the disease itself, so that children and families are not afraid to go to school with children who have the disease.
- Continuing education programs can be useful to teach the teachers and parents about the disease (American Academy of Pediatrics, 2004).

Children with DNR Orders and the School Nurse

As part of tertiary prevention, the school nurse also maintains the health of children with terminal diseases who go to school. These children have been largely mainstreamed into the regular school population. The PL 92-142 Education for All Handicapped Children Act stated in 1975 that all children should go to school in the "least restrictive environment" (American Academy of Pediatrics, 2004b). Therefore there may be children who have **do-not-resuscitate (DNR) orders** at school, and some may die at school. DNR orders are signed by the parents and the physician according to the state's law. Under law, the school nurse is bound to obey the DNR order; however, it is not clear how the schools view them.

When a child dies in school, the nurse is responsible for helping the children who witnessed the death. The nurse becomes a grief counselor and helps the children and teachers cope with the death. Further education about death and dying given by the school nurse would also help the school community cope with death in the schools.

Homebound Children

Even though the laws regarding disabled persons state that all children should go to school, some children cannot do so. Instead, they may be taught in the home or in another institutional setting such as the hospital. In these situations, the school nurse functions as follows (American Academy of Pediatrics, 2004c):

- Should be a liaison between the child's teacher, physician, school administrators, and parents regarding the child's needs
- Helps these individuals make up the child's IEP so that it is appropriate for the child and does not remove necessary learning from the plan
- Allows the child to go to school when he or she is able
- Coordinates the child's health care needs and classes

Pregnant Teenagers and Teenage Mothers at School

Many teenage girls who are pregnant attend school. Therefore the school nurse may provide ongoing care to the mother. Although this may appear to be primary prevention, it is tertiary prevention because adolescent pregnancies are considered to be at high risk.

CONTROVERSIES IN SCHOOL NURSING

School nursing has evolved into a complex health care role, and some areas of the field still cause controversy—for example, birth control education and giving birth control to students in the schools. Because opinions differ relating to sex education and reproductive services in the schools, the school nurse should make an effort to communicate with the community, school board, teachers, parents, and students about what they think about different types of services in the school (Wang et al, 2002).

ETHICS IN SCHOOL NURSING

The school nurse may be faced with ethical issues in the schools, such as the following:

- A child may have a DNR order that the parents wish to be used if the child dies at school (see earlier), but following the DNR order may be against the nurse's personal beliefs.
- Perhaps a girl asks the nurse where she can get an abortion and wishes to talk to the school nurse about how she feels, but the nurse is against abortions.
- A teenager asks for emergency contraception, which the nurse does not wish to give (Roye and Johnsen, 2002).

In these cases the following action should be taken:

- The nurse must give nursing care to the student client and keep personal beliefs out of the discussion.

Table 31-3 Online Resources for School Nurses

Organization	Internet Address
The American Academy of Child and Adolescent Psychiatry	http://www.aacap.org
American Academy of Pediatrics	http://www.aap.org
National Association of School Nurses	http://www.nasn.org
Center for Health and Health Care in the Schools	http://www.healthinschools.org
National Youth Violence Prevention Resource Center	http://www.safeyouth.org
U.S. Department of Education Emergency Preparedness	http://www.ed.gov/ emergencyplan
Healthy Schools Network	http://www.healthyschools.org

- If the nurse feels so strongly that he or she cannot work with the situation, another school nurse should be called for help.
- The student should be referred to other health providers who can give the care the student needs.

FUTURE TRENDS IN SCHOOL NURSING

The future of school nursing is strong. The amount of health care being given in the schools is increasing. In the future, school nursing will use telehealth and telecounseling to teach health education (National Association of School Nurses, 2002). School nurses will use the Internet to work with children and parents. Online resources are listed in Table 31-3. The school nurse is responsible for keeping up with the latest changes in health care and health practice so that the health of children in the schools can be enhanced by new trends in health care.

CLINICAL APPLICATION

Erin and Sandy, student nurses in their last semester of nursing school, were invited by their former high school to give a talk on nursing as a career at the school's career day. During their presentation, which included a multimedia PowerPoint video presentation on nursing, a student asked, "Why would I want to be a school nurse? Ours just sits in the office handing out bandages."

How should Erin and Sandy respond?

A. *Talk about the many things that school nurses are responsible for.*
B. *Ask how other high school students in the room feel about this comment.*
C. *Use the classroom's intercom to ask the school nurse to come to the classroom.*
D. *Discuss the ways the school nurse prevents injuries from becoming infected.*

Answer is in the back of the book.

REMEMBER THIS!

- School nurses provide health care for children and families.
- In the early 1900s, school nurses screened children for infectious diseases.
- By 2002, school nurses provided direct care, health education, counseling, case management, and community outreach.
- The National Association of School Nurses (NASN) is the professional organization for school nurses.
- School nurses have varying educational levels depending on state laws.
- The U.S. government supports school-based health centers, school-linked programs, and full-service school-based health centers.
- *Healthy People 2010* has objectives to enhance the health of children in the schools.
- Primary prevention provides health promotion and education to prevent childhood injuries and substance abuse.
- The school nurse monitors the children for all of their state-mandated immunizations for school entry.
- Secondary prevention involves screening children for illnesses and providing direct nursing care.
- School nurses develop plans for emergency care in the schools.
- Giving medications to children in the school must be monitored carefully to prevent errors.
- School health nurses are mandated to tell the authorities about suspected cases of child abuse and/or neglect.
- Tertiary prevention includes caring for children with long-term health needs, including asthma and disabling conditions.
- School nurses carry out catheterizations, suctioning, gastrostomy feedings, and other skills in the schools.
- Some ethical dilemmas in the schools are related to women's health care.
- Some nurses use the Internet to help communicate with children and their families.

WHAT WOULD YOU DO?

1. For the state in which you live, make a list of the immunizations required for children attending schools. Then contrast this to the immunizations you received when in school. How has this changed over the years?
2. Arrange to visit an elementary school health office during screening activities. Observe the interaction between the nurse and the children. Describe how the nurse is using the nursing process during the screening process.
3. On the Internet, focus on your state's health department. What trends do you see relating to health in the schools?

■ REFERENCES

Allers-Korostynski M: Adult learning center: a unique adventure for a school nurse, *J Sch Nurs* 16:50–51, 2000.

American Academy of Pediatrics, Committee on Pediatric AIDS: Human immunodeficiency virus/acquired immunodeficiency syndrome education in schools, 1998 (reaffirmed 2001), *Pediatric clinical practice guidelines & policies: a compendium of evidence-based research for pediatric practice*, ed 4, 2004, AAP, p 936.

American Academy of Pediatrics, Committee on School Health: School health centers and other integrated school health services, *Pediatrics* 107:198–201, 2001a, available at http://www.aap.org/policy/re0030.html.

American Academy of Pediatrics, Committee on School Health: Guidelines for emergency medical care in school, *Pediatrics* 107:435–436, 2001b, available at http://www.aap.org/policy/re9954.html.

American Academy of Pediatrics, Committee on School Health: The role of the school nurse in providing school health services, *Pediatrics* 108:1231–1232, 2001c.

American Academy of Pediatrics, Committee on School Health: Guidelines for the administration of medication in school, *Pediatrics* 92(3):499–500, 1993 (reaffirmed 2001d), available at http://www.aap.org/policy/04524.html.

American Academy of Pediatrics, Committee on School Health: School health assessments, 2000a (reaffirmed 2003), *Pediatric clinical practice guidelines & policies: a compendium of evidence-based research for pediatric practice*, ed 4, 2004a, AAP, p 958.

American Academy of Pediatrics, Committee on School Health and Committee on Bioethics: Do not resuscitate orders in schools, 2000b (reaffirmed 2003), *Pediatric clinical practice guidelines & policies: a compendium of evidence-based research for pediatric practice*, ed 4, 2004b, AAP, p 928.

American Academy of Pediatrics, Committee on School Health: Home, hospital, and other non-school-based instruction for children and adolescents who are medically unable to attend school, 2000c (reaffirmed 2003), *Pediatric clinical practice guidelines & policies: a compendium of evidence-based research for pediatric practice*, ed 4, 2004c, p 935, AAP.

American Academy of Pediatrics, Committee on Injury and Poison Prevention: Skateboard and scooter injuries, *Pediatrics* 109:542–543, 2002.

American Academy of Pediatrics, Committee on School Health: Guidelines for the administration of medication in school, 2003, *Pediatric clinical practice guidelines & policies: a compendium of evidence-based research for pediatric practice*, ed 4, 2004, AAP, p 932.

Bergren MD: Privacy questions from practicing school nurses, *J Sch Nurs* 20:296–301, 2004.

Bernardo LM, Gardner MJ, Seibel K: Playground injuries in children: a review and Pennsylvania trauma center experience, *J Soc Pediatr Nurs* 6:11–20, 2001.

Betz CL: Use of 504 plans for children and youth with disabilities: nursing application, *Pediatr Nurs* 27:347–352, 2001.

Boyer-Chuanroong L, Deaver P: Meeting the preteen vaccine law: a pilot program in urban middle schools, *J Sch Health* 70:39–44, 2000.

Broussard L: School nursing: not just band-aids any more? *J Soc Pediatr Nurs* 9:77–83, 2004.

Cade M, Tidwell S: Autism and the school nurse, *J Sch Health* 71:96–100, 2001.

Calarco C: Preparing for a crisis: crisis team development, *J Sch Nurs* 15:46–48, 1999.

Carpenter LM, Mueller CS: Evaluating health care seeking behaviors of parents using a school-based health clinic, *J Sch Health* 71:497–499, 2001.

Centers for Disease Control and Prevention: *Adolescent and school health,* Washington, DC, 2004, CDC, available at www.cdc.gov/programs/health01.pdf.

Centers for Disease Control and Prevention: *Healthy youth! Coordinated school health program,* Washington, DC, 2005, CDC, available at http://www.cdc.gov/HealthyYouth/CSHP/index.htm.

Chemtob CM, Nakashima JP, Hamada RS: Psychosocial intervention for postdisaster trauma symptoms in elementary school children: a controlled community field study, *Arch Pediatr Adolesc Med* 156:211–216, 2002.

Croghan E: Do not underestimate the school nurse, *Nurs Times* 95(20):47, 1999.

Croghan E, Johnson C: Occupational health and school health: a natural alliance? *J Adv Nurs* 45:155–161, 2004.

Deal LW et al: Unintentional injuries in childhood: analysis and recommendations, *Future Child* 10:4–22, 2000.

DeLago CW et al: Collaboration with school nurses: improving the effectiveness of tuberculosis screening, *Arch Pediatr Adolesc Med* 155:1369–1373, 2001.

Duncan C: Health hangout for east enders, *Nurs Times* 96(30):33, 2000.

Edwards LH: Research priorities in school nursing: a Delphi process, *J Sch Health* 72:173–177, 2002.

Farrior KC et al: A community pediatric prevention partnership: linking schools, providers, and tertiary care services, *J Sch Health* 70:79–83, 2000.

Freed J: Shooting rampage by student leaves 10 dead in Minnesota, *Buffalo News* pp A-1–A-2, March 22, 2005.

Gance-Cleveland B: Qualitative evaluation of a school-based support group for adolescents with an addicted parent, *Nurs Res* 53:379–386, 2004.

Guajardo AD, Middleman AB, Sansaricq KM: School nurses identify barriers and solutions to implementing a school-based hepatitis B immunization program, *J Sch Health* 72:128–130, 2002.

Hawkins JW Hayes ER, Corliss CP: School nursing in America—1902–1994: a return to public health nursing, *Public Health Nurs* 11:416–425, 1994.

Hazinski et al: Response to cardiac arrest and selected life-threatening medical emergencies: the medical emergency response plan for schools—a statement for healthcare providers, policymakers, school administrators, and community leaders, *Circulation* 109:278–291, 2004.

Harrell JS et al: School-based interventions to improve the health of children with multiple cardiovascular risk factors. In Funk SG, editors: *Key aspects of preventing and managing chronic illness,* New York, 2001, Springer.

Hospitals' Outreach: Hospitals' outreach program offers more than a "school nurse," *AHA News* 36(10):6, 2000.

Kalisch PA, Kalisch BJ: *American nursing: a history,* ed 4, Philadelphia, 2004, Lippincott Williams & Wilkins.

King KA: Developing a comprehensive school suicide prevention program, *J Sch Health* 71:132–137, 2001.

Kirchofer GM, Price JH, Telljohann SK: Primary grade teacher's knowledge and perceptions of head lice, *J Sch Health* 71:448–452, 2001.

Klassen TP et al: Community-based injury prevention interventions, *Future Child* 10:83–110, 2000.

Kolbe LJ, Kann L, Brener ND: Overview and summary of findings: School Health Policies and Programs Study 2000, *J Sch Health* 71:253–259, 2001.

Krystofik DA: Nurse's corner: too much sun is not a good thing, *Our Schools: West Seneca Central Schools Newsletter,* p 7, March/April 2002a.

Krystofik DA: Nurse's corner: staff development day provides day of professional growth for school nurses, *Our Schools: West Seneca Central Schools Newsletter,* p 7, March/April 2002b.

Leighton S, Worraker A, Nolan P: School nurses and mental health part 1, *Ment Health Pract* 7:14–16, 2003.

Leighton S et al: School nurses and mental health part 2, *Ment Health Pract* 7:17–20, 2003.

McCarthy AM, Kelly MW, Reed D: Medication administration practices of school nurses, *J Sch Health* 70:371–376, 2000.

Meninger JC et al: Identification of high-risk adolescents for interventions to lower blood pressure. In Funk SG, et al: *Key aspects of preventing and managing chronic illness,* New York, 2001, Springer.

Meyers L: Safe at school. Treating diabetes in the classroom, *Diabetes Forecast* 44–48, May 2005.

Moses M, Gilchrest C, Schwab NC: Section 504 of the Rehabilitation Act: determining eligibility and implications for school districts, *J Sch Nurs* 21:48–58, 2005.

Nabors LA, Woist MD: School mental health services for homeless children, *J Sch Health* 72:269, 2002.

National Association of School Nurses/American Nurses Association: *Scope and standards of professional school nursing practice,* Washington, DC, 2005, American Nurses Association.

National Association of School Nurses, National Association of School-Based Health Care, American School Health Association: *Joint statement on the school nurse/school-based health center partnership,* 2001, available at http://www.nasn.org/statements/schoolbasedjoint.htm.

National Association of School Nurses: *NASN resolution: access to a school nurse,* 2003, available at http://www.nasn.org/statements/resolutionaccess.htm.

National Association of School Nurses: NASN resolution: telehealth technology, Silver Spring, Md, 2002, National Association of School Nurses.

National School Boards Association and Division of Adolescent and School Health, Centers for Disease Control and Prevention: *Schools and terrorism: a supplement to the National Advisory Committee on Children and Terrorism. Recommendations to the Secretary,* Washington, DC, 2003, CDC.

Nebraska school nurses improve communication: Providers, parents and nurses interact on students' health, *Nation's Health* 30:7, 2000.

Pfizer Pharmaceuticals: *Opportunities to care: the Pfizer guide to careers in nursing,* New York, 2001, Pfizer Pharmaceuticals Group.

Pike-Paris A: Indoor air quality: Part I—what it is, *Pediatr Nurs* 30:430–433, 2004.

Ross SK: The clinical nurse specialist's role in school health, *Clin Nurs Spec* 13:28–33, 1999.

Roye CF, Johnsen JRM: Adolescents and emergency contraception, *J Pediatr Health Care* 19:3-9, 2002.

Rubsam JM: Identification of risk factors and effective intervention strategies corresponding to the major causes of childhood death from injury, *J NY State Nurses Assoc* 32:4-8, 2001.

Sander N: Making the grade with asthma, allergies, and anaphylaxis, *Pediatr Nurs* 28:593–595, 598, 2002.

Sapien RE, Allen A: Emergency preparation in schools: a snapshot of a rural state, *Pediatr Emerg Care* 17:329–333, 2001.

Starr NB: Helping children and families deal with the psychological aspects of disaster, *J Pediatr Health Care* 16:36–39, 2002.

Steger S: Killed at school, *RN* 63:36–38, 2000.

Swartz MK, Banasiak NC, Meadows-Oliver M: Barriers to effective pediatric asthma care, *J Pediatr Health Care* 19:71–79, 2005.

Sweeney JF, Sweeney DD: Frequent visitors to the school nurse at two middle schools, *J Sch Health* 70:387–389, 2000.

Taras H et al: Impact of school nurse case management on students with asthma, *J Sch Health* 74:213–219, 2004.

Ten steps to keep schools louse-free: *Dermatol Times* 21:42, 2000.

Thackaberry J: Who cares for the health of your school? *Independent School* 60:94–97, 2001.

U.S. Department of Health and Human Services: *Healthy People 2010: understanding and improving health*, ed 2, Washington, DC, 2000, U.S. Government Printing Office.

U.S. Department of Health and Human Services, Bureau of Primary Health Care, Health Resources and Services Administration: *Healthy schools, healthy communities program,* 2001a, available at http://bphc.hrsa.gov/hshc.

U.S. Department of Health and Human Services, Center for School-Based Health, Bureau of Primary Health Care, Health Resources and Services Administration: *Beyond access to care for students, full service school-based health centers,* 2001b, available at http://www.bphc.hrsa.org.

U.S. Environmental Protection Agency: *Indoor air quality (IAQ) tools for schools: health officer/school nurse checklist,* 2003, available at http://www.epa.gov/iaq/schools/tfs/healthof.html.

Veselak KE: Historical steps in the development of the modern school health program, *J Sch Health* 71:369–372, 2001. (Reprinted from *J Sch Health* 9:262–269, 1959.)

Wang LY, Burstein GR, Cohen DA: An economic evaluation of a school-based sexually transmitted disease screening program, *Sex Transm Dis* 29:737–745, 2002.

Whalen LG et al: *Profiles 2002. School health profiles. Surveillance for characteristics of health programs among secondary schools,* Washington, DC, 2004, Centers for Disease Control and Prevention, U.S. Department of Health and Human Services.

Williams CJ, Kalkenberg P: Germany in shock after school bloodbath, *Buffalo News* pp A-1, A-6, April 27, 2002.

Wold SJ, Dagg NV: School nursing: a framework for practice, *J Sch Health* 71:401–404, 2001. (Reprinted from *J Sch Health* 48:111–114, 1978.)

Wolfe LC Selekman J: School nurses: what it was and what it is, *Pediatr Nurs* 28:403–407, 2002.

Wood R, Synovitz LB: Addressing the threats of MDMA (Ecstasy): implications for school health professionals, parents and community members, *J Sch Health* 71:38–41, 2001.

Chapter 32

The Nurse in Occupational Health

evolve http://evolve.elsevier.com/stanhope/foundations

Bonnie Rogers

ADDITIONAL RESOURCES

These related resources are found either in the appendix at the back of this book or on the book's website at http://evolve.elsevier.com/stanhope/foundations.

Appendix

- Appendix G.3: Comprehensive Occupational and Environmental Health History

Evolve Website

- Community Assessment Applied
- Case Study, with questions and answers
- Quiz review questions
- WebLinks, including link to *Healthy People 2010* website

Real World Community Health Nursing: An Interactive CD-ROM, second edition

If you are using this CD-ROM in your course, you will find the following activities related to this chapter:
- *Visit OSHA: Investigate Worksite Injuries* in **A Day in the Life of a Community Health Nurse**
- *Find Your Professional Organization* in **A Day in the Life of a Community Health Nurse**
- *Compare NIOSH and OSHA* in **A Day in the Life of a Community Health Nurse**

OBJECTIVES

After reading this chapter, the student should be able to:
1. Describe the nursing role in occupational health.
2. Describe current trends in the American workforce.
3. Describe examples of work-related illness and injuries.
4. Use the epidemiologic model to explain work–health interactions.
5. Cite at least three host factors associated with increased risk from an adverse response to hazardous workplace exposure.

6. Explain one example each of biological, chemical, environmental/mechanical, physical, and psychosocial workplace hazards.
7. Complete an occupational health history.
8. Describe the functions of OSHA and NIOSH.
9. Describe an effective disaster plan.

CHAPTER OUTLINE

DEFINITION AND SCOPE OF OCCUPATIONAL HEALTH NURSING
HISTORY AND EVOLUTION OF OCCUPATIONAL HEALTH NURSING
ROLES AND PROFESSIONALISM IN OCCUPATIONAL HEALTH NURSING
WORKERS AS A POPULATION AGGREGATE
Characteristics of the Workforce

Characteristics of Work
Work–Health Interactions
APPLICATION OF THE EPIDEMIOLOGIC MODEL
Host
Agent
Environment
ORGANIZATIONAL AND PUBLIC EFFORTS TO PROMOTE WORKER HEALTH AND SAFETY
On-Site Occupational Health and Safety Programs

NURSING CARE OF WORKING POPULATIONS
Worker Assessment
Workplace Assessment
HEALTHY PEOPLE 2010 RELATED
TO OCCUPATIONAL HEALTH

LEGISLATION RELATED TO OCCUPATIONAL HEALTH

DISASTER PLANNING AND MANAGEMENT

KEY TERMS

agents: causative factors invading a host through an environment favorable to produce disease, such as a biological or chemical agent.

environment: all those factors internal and external to the client that influence and are influenced by the host and agent–host interactions.

Hazard Communication Standard: the "right-to-know" standard that requires all manufacturing firms to inventory toxic agents, label them, develop information sheets, and educate employees about these agents.

host: a human or animal that provides adequate living conditions for any given infectious agent.

National Institute for Occupational Safety and Health (NIOSH): the branch of the U.S. Public Health Service that is responsible for investigating workplace illnesses, accidents, and hazards.

occupational health hazards: dangerous processes, conditions, or materials within a work environment that can result in harm to an employee.

occupational health history: questions added to a health assessment that provide data necessary to rule out or confirm job-induced symptoms or illnesses.

Occupational Safety and Health Administration (OSHA): the federal agency charged with improving worker health and safety by establishing standards and regulations and by educating workers.

work–health interactions: the influence of work on health shown by statistics on illnesses, injuries, and deaths associated with employment.

Workers' Compensation: compensation given to an employee for an injury that occurred while the employee was working.

worksite walk-through: an assessment of the workplace conducted by the nurse.

In America, work is viewed as important to our life experiences, with most adults spending about one-third of their time at work (Rogers, 2003). Work—when fulfilling, fairly compensated, healthy, and safe—can help build long and contented lives and strengthen families and communities. Although some workers may never face more than minor adverse health effects from exposures at work, such as occasional eye strain resulting from poor office lighting, every industry grapples with serious hazard. No work is completely risk free, and all health care professionals should have some basic knowledge about workforce populations, work and related hazards, and methods to control hazards and improve health.

Many substantial changes have occurred in the following:
- The nature of work
- Workplace risks
- The work environment
- Workforce composition and demographics
- Health care delivery mechanisms

An analysis of these trends suggests that work–health interactions will continue to grow in importance, affecting the following:
- How work is done
- How hazards are controlled or minimized
- How health care is managed and integrated into workplace health delivery strategies

As a result, significant developments are occurring in occupational health and safety programs designed to prevent and control work-related illness and injury and to create environments that foster and support health-promoting activities. Occupational health nurses have performed critical roles in planning and delivering worksite health and safety services. In addition, the continuing increase of health care costs and the concern about health care quality have prompted the inclusion of primary care and management of non-work-related health problems in the health services programs. In some settings, family services are also provided. This chapter describes the role of the nurse in relation to the working population.

DEFINITION AND SCOPE OF OCCUPATIONAL HEALTH NURSING

Adapted from the American Association of Occupational Health Nurses (American Association of Occupational Health Nurses, 1999), *occupational health nursing* is defined as follows:

> *The specialty practice that focuses on the promotion, prevention, and restoration of health within the context of a safe and healthy environment. It involves the prevention of adverse health effects from occupational and environmental hazards. It provides for and delivers occupational and environmental health and safety services to workers, worker populations, and community groups. It is an autonomous specialty, and nurses make independent nursing judgments in providing health care.*

Occupational health nurses work in traditional manufacturing, industry, service, health care facilities, construction sites, and government settings. Their scope of practice is broad and includes the following:

- Worker and workplace assessment and surveillance
- Primary care
- Case management
- Consulting
- Counseling
- Health promotion and protection
- Administration and management
- Research
- Legal–ethical monitoring
- Community orientation

The knowledge in occupational health and safety is applied to the workforce aggregate.

HISTORY AND EVOLUTION OF OCCUPATIONAL HEALTH NURSING

Ada Mayo Stewart, hired in 1885 by the Vermont Marble Company in Rutland, Vermont, is often considered the first industrial nurse. Riding a bicycle, Miss Stewart visited sick employees in their homes, provided emergency care, taught mothers how to care for their children, and taught healthy living habits (Felton, 1985). In the early days of occupational health nursing, the nurse's work was family centered and holistic. Nursing care for workers in industry began in 1888 and was called *industrial nursing*. A group of coal miners hired Betty Moulder, a graduate of the Blockley Hospital School of Nursing in Philadelphia (later called the Philadelphia General Hospital), to take care of their ailing co-workers and families (American Association of Occupational Health Nurses, 1976).

Employee health services grew rapidly during the early 1900s as companies recognized that the provision of worksite health services led to a more productive workforce. At that time, workplace accidents were seen as an inevitable part of having a job. However, the public did not support this attitude, and a system for **Workers' Compensation** arose that remains in place today (McGrath, 1995).

Industrial nursing grew rapidly during the first half of the twentieth century. Educational courses and professional societies were established. By World War II there were approximately 4000 industrial nurses (Brown, 1981). The American Association of Industrial Nursing (AAIN), now called the *American Association of Occupational Health Nurses,* was established as the first national nursing organization in 1942. The aim of the AAIN was to improve industrial nursing education and practice and to promote interdisciplinary collaborative efforts (Rogers, 1994).

The passing of several laws in the 1960s and 1970s to protect workers' safety and health led to an increased need for occupational health nurses. In particular, the passing of the landmark *Occupational Safety and Health Act* in 1970, which created the *Occupational Safety and Health Administration* (OSHA) and the *National Institute for Occupational Safety and Health* (NIOSH), discussed later in this chapter, created a large need for nurses at the worksite to meet the demands of the many standards being implemented. The Act focused primarily on education and research. In 1988, the first occupational health nurse was hired by OSHA to provide technical assistance in standards development, field consultation, and occupational health nursing expertise. In 1993, the Office of Occupational Health Nursing was established within the agency.

ROLES AND PROFESSIONALISM IN OCCUPATIONAL HEALTH NURSING

As American industry has shifted from agrarian (agriculture) to industrial to highly technological processes, the role of the occupational health nurse has continued to change. The focus on work-related health problems now includes the spectrum of human responses to multiple, complex interactions of biopsychosocial factors that occur in community, home, and work environments. The customary role of the occupational health nurse has extended beyond emergency treatment and prevention of illness and injury. The interdisciplinary nature of occupational health nursing has become more critical as occupational health and safety problems require more complex solutions. The occupational health nurse frequently collaborates closely with multiple disciplines, industry management, and representatives of labor.

Occupational health nurses constitute the largest group of occupational health professionals (U.S. Department of Health and Human Services, 2001). Their role is unique in that the nurse adapts to an agency's needs as well as to the needs of specific groups of workers.

The professional organization for occupational health nurses is the American Association of Occupational Health Nurses (AAOHN). The AAOHN's mission is comprehensive. It supports the work of the occupational health nurse and advances the specialty. The AAOHN also does the following:

- Promotes the health and safety of workers
- Defines the scope of practice and sets the standards of occupational health nursing practice
- Develops the Code of Ethics for occupational health nurses with interpretive statements
- Promotes and provides continuing education in the specialty
- Advances the profession through supporting research
- Responds to and influences public policy issues related to occupational health and safety

See "Evidence-Based Practice" box on p. 605.

The AAOHN describes 10 job roles for occupational health nurses: clinician, case manager, coordinator, manager, nurse practitioner, corporate director, health promotion specialist, educator, consultant, and researcher (American Association of Occupational Health Nurses, 1999). The majority of occupational health nurses work as solo clinicians, but increasingly, additional roles are being included in the specialty practice. In many companies, the occupational health nurse has assumed expanded responsibilities in job analysis, safety, and benefits management. Many occupational health nurses also work as independent contractors or have their own businesses providing occupational health and safety services to industry, as well as consultation. With the current changes in health care delivery and the movement toward managed care, occupational health nurses will need increased skills in primary care, health promotion, and disease prevention. Occupational health nurses devote much attention to keeping workers and, in some cases, their families healthy and free from illness and worksite injuries. Specializing in the field is often a requirement.

Academic education in occupational health and safety is generally at the graduate level; however, many nurses with an associate degree in nursing (ADN) or a bachelor's degree in nursing (BSN) work in occupational health. Certification in occupational health nursing is provided by the American Board for Occupational Health Nurses (ABOHN). Requirements include experience, continuing education, professional activities, and examination.

WORKERS AS A POPULATION AGGREGATE

The population of the United States was expected to increase from approximately 272 million people in 1999 to an estimated 297 million people by the year 2010. However, by 2008, the population had grown to almost 304 million people, far exceeding the estimates (Central Intelligence Agency, 2008). By 2010 the U.S. population will be older. The greatest growth will be among people older than 65 years, with a reduction in the number of those younger than 25 years. This will be reflected in the workforce, with a decrease in the number of young job seekers. It is estimated that by the year 2010, 67% of the workforce will be between the ages of 25 and 54 years and 17% will be older than 55 years (Institute of Medicine, 2000). The number of adults ages 65 years and older will more than double between now and the year 2050. By that year, one in five Americans will be an older adult.

In 2008 there were more than 154 million civilian wage and salary workers in the United States, employed in about 63,000 different worksites (Bureau of Labor Statistics, 2009). Neither of these statistics indicates the full number of individuals who have potentially been exposed to work-related health hazards. Although some individuals may currently be unemployed or retired, they continue to bear the health risks of past occupational exposures. The number of affected individuals may be even larger as work-related illnesses are found among spouses, children, and neighbors of exposed workers.

Americans are employed in diverse industries that range in size from one to tens of thousands of employees. Types of industries include the following:
- Traditional manufacturing (e.g., automotive, appliances)
- Service industries (e.g., banking, health care, restaurants)
- Agriculture
- Construction
- Newer high-technology firms, such as computer chip manufacturers

Approximately 95% of business organizations are considered small, employing fewer than 500 people (Bureau of Labor Statistics, 2003a). Although some industries are noted for the high degree of hazards associated with their work (e.g., manufacturing, mines, construction, agriculture), no worksite is free of occupational health and safety hazards. The larger the company, the more likely it is to sponsor health and safety programs for employees. Smaller companies are more apt to rely on the external community to meet their needs for health and safety services.

CHARACTERISTICS OF THE WORKFORCE

The U.S. workplace and workforce are rapidly changing (Bureau of Labor Statistics [BLS], 2003a):
- Jobs in the economy continue to shift from manufacturing to service.
- Longer hours, compressed work weeks, shift work, reduced job security, and part-time and temporary work are realities of the modern workplace (Institute of Medicine, 2000).
- New chemicals, materials, processes, and equipment are developed and marketed at an ever-increasing pace.
- As the U.S. workforce grows to approximately 155 million by the year 2010, it will become older and more racially diverse (Institute of Medicine, 2000).
- By the year 2005, minorities represented 16% of the workforce and women represented approximately 47% of the workforce.

These changes will present new challenges to protecting worker safety and health.

In an era in which it was expected that the demand for workers would outstrip the available supply, businesses were concerned about strategies to increase health status, employment longevity, and satisfaction of workers. However, the 2008 downturn in the economy changed the picture with record high unemployment rates (Bureau of Labor Statistics, 2009). By the year 2010, minorities are projected to constitute 32% of the workforce and women approximately 48% of the workforce. These changes will present new challenges to protecting worker safety and health (U.S. Department of Health and Human Services, National Institute for Safety and Health, 2004a). In 2005, Hispanics made up 16% and women 47% of the workforce.

The demographic trends in the U.S. workforce indicate a changing population aggregate that has implications for the prevention services targeted to that group. Major changes in the working population are reflected in the increasing numbers of women, older individuals, and those with chronic illnesses who are part of the workforce. Because of changes in the economy, extension of life span, legislation, and society's acceptance of working women, the proportion of the employed population that these three groups represent will probably continue to grow.

CHARACTERISTICS OF WORK

Over time, there has been a dramatic shift in the types of jobs held by workers. Following the evolution from an agrarian (agriculture) economy to a manufacturing society and then

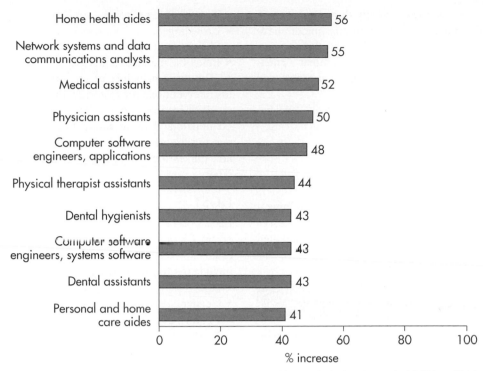

Occupation	% increase
Home health aides	56
Network systems and data communications analysts	55
Medical assistants	52
Physician assistants	50
Computer software engineers, applications	48
Physical therapist assistants	44
Dental hygienists	43
Computer software engineers, systems software	43
Dental assistants	43
Personal and home care aides	41

% increase

FIGURE 32-1 Occupations projected to have the most rapid growth during the period 2004 to 2014. (From the Bureau of Labor Statistics: *Employment and wages,* Washington, DC, 2005, U.S. Department of Labor.)

to a highly technological workplace, the greatest proportion of paid employment was in the following occupations:
- Service (e.g., health care, information processing, banking, insurance)
- Professional technical positions (e.g., managers, computer specialists)
- Clerical work (e.g., word processors, secretaries)

During the period from 1996 to 2000, service-providing industries accounted for most of the job growth. Health services, business services, social services, and engineering, management, and related services are expected to account for almost one in every two worker jobs (Institute of Medicine, 2000).

This change in the nature of work was accompanied by many new occupational hazards such as the following:
- Complex chemicals
- Nanotechnology
- Nonergonomic workstation design (the adaptation of the workplace or work equipment to meet the employee's health and safety needs)
- Job stress
- Burnout
- Exhaustion

In addition, the emergence of the global economy with free trade and multinational corporations presented new challenges for health and safety programs that were culturally relevant.

WORK–HEALTH INTERACTIONS

The influence of work on health, or **work–health interactions**, is shown by statistics on illnesses, injuries, and deaths associated with employment. In 2005, 4.2 million workers reported work-related illnesses and injuries, of which 2.2 million resulted in lost time from work. Of these, approximately 5% were severe enough to result in temporary or permanent disabilities that prevented the workers from returning to their usual jobs (Bureau of Labor Statistics, 2006a). Ten occupations, which accounted for nearly one-third of the 2.2 million injuries and illnesses involving days away from work, are shown in Figure 32-1. Truck drivers, nonconstruction laborers, and nursing aides and orderlies were the top three occupations representing days away from work, with registered nurses being the occupation with the tenth highest number of lost days from work.

Employers reported 4.6 work injuries and occupational illnesses per 100 workers in 2005. That same year, occupational injuries alone cost billions of dollars in lost wages and lost productivity, administrative expenses, health care, and other costs (Bureau of Labor Statistics, 2006b). This figure does not include the cost of occupational diseases.

These figures are often described as the "tip of the iceberg" because many work-related health problems go unreported. But even the recorded statistics are significant in describing the amount of human suffering, financial loss, and decreased productivity associated with workplace hazards.

The high number of work injuries and illnesses can be drastically reduced. In fact, significant progress has been made in improving worker protection since Congress passed the 1970 Occupational Safety and Health Act. For example, vinyl chloride-induced liver cancers and brown lung disease (byssinosis) from cotton dust exposure have been almost eliminated. Reproductive disorders associated with certain glycol ethers have been recognized and controlled. Fatal work injuries have declined substantially through the years. Notably, since 1970, fatal injury rates in coal miners have been reduced by more than 75%, and there has been a general downward trend in the prevalence of coal miner's pneumoconiosis (National Institute for Occupational Safety and Health, 2000).

The U.S. workplace has been rapidly changing and becoming more diverse. Major changes have been occurring:

- In the way work is organized
- With increased shiftwork
- With reduced job security
- In part-time and temporary work
- As new chemicals, materials, processes, and equipment (e.g., latex gloves in health care; fermentation processes in biotechnology) continue to be developed and marketed at an ever-accelerating pace

APPLICATION OF THE EPIDEMIOLOGIC MODEL

The epidemiologic triad can be used to understand the relationship between work and health (Figure 32-2).

With a focus on the health and safety of the employed population, the *host* is described as any susceptible human being. Because of the nature of work-related hazards, nurses must assume that all employed individuals and groups are at risk of being exposed to occupational hazards. The agents, factors associated with illness and injury, are occupational exposures that are classified as *biological, chemical, ergonomic, physical,* or *psychosocial* (Box 32-1).

The third element, the **environment**, includes all external conditions that influence the interaction of the host and agents. These may be workplace conditions such as the following:

- Temperature extremes
- Crowding
- Shiftwork
- Inflexible management styles

The basic principle of epidemiology is that health status interventions for restoring and promoting health are the result of complex interactions among these three elements. To understand these interactions and to design effective nursing strategies for dealing with them in a proactive manner, nurses must look at how each element influences the others.

HOST

Each worker represents a **host** within the worker population group. Certain host factors are associated with increased risk of adverse response to the hazards of the workplace. These include the following (Rogers, 2003):

- Age
- Gender
- Health status
- Work practices
- Ethnicity
- Lifestyle factors

For example, the population group at greatest risk for experiencing work-related accidents with subsequent injuries is new workers with less than 1 year of experience on the current job (Bureau of Labor Statistics, 2003b). The host factors of age, gender, and work experience combine to increase this group's risk of injury because of characteristics such as risk taking, lack of knowledge, and lack of familiarity with the new job.

Older workers may be at increased risk in the workplace because of diminished sensory abilities, the effects of chronic illnesses, and delayed reaction times.

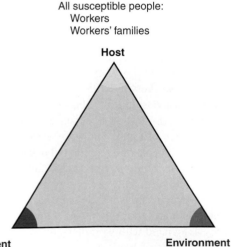

All susceptible people:
Workers
Workers' families

Host

Agent

Workplace hazards:
Biological
Chemical
Ergonomic
Physical
Psychosocial

Environment

All other external
factors that influence
host-agent interactions:
Physical
Social

FIGURE 32-2 The epidemiologic triad.

Box 32-1	**Categories of Work-Related Hazards**

- *Biological and infectious hazards.* Infectious and biological agents, such as bacteria, viruses, fungi, or parasites, that may be transmitted via contact with infected patients or contaminated body secretions and fluids to other individuals
- *Chemical hazards.* Various forms of chemicals, including medications, solutions, gases, vapors, aerosols, and particulate matter, that are potentially toxic or irritating to the body system
- *Enviromechanical hazards.* Factors encountered in the work environment that cause or potentiate accidents, injuries, strain, or discomfort (e.g., unsafe and/or inadequate equipment or lifting devices, slippery floors, workstation deficiencies)
- *Physical hazards.* Agents within the work environment, such as radiation, electricity, extreme temperatures, and noise, that can cause tissue trauma
- *Psychosocial hazards.* Factors and situations encountered or associated with a job or work environment that create or potentiate stress, emotional strain, or interpersonal problems

From Rogers B: *Occupational health nursing: concepts and practice,* ed 2, St. Louis, 2003, Elsevier.

A third population group that may be very susceptible to workplace exposure is women in their child-bearing years because of the following:

- The hormonal changes during these years
- The increased stress of new roles and additional responsibilities
- Transplacental exposures

These are host factors that may influence this group's response to potential toxins. In addition to these host factors, there may be other, less-understood individual differences in responses to occupational hazard exposures. Even if employers maintain exposure levels below the level recommended by occupational health and safety standards, 15% to 20% of the population may have health reactions to the "safe" low-level exposures (Levy and Wegman, 2006). This group has been termed *hypersusceptible*. The following are host factors that appear to be associated with this hypersusceptibility:

- Light skin
- Malnutrition
- Compromised immune system
- Glucose 6-phosphate dehydrogenase deficiency
- Serum alpha 1-antitrypsin deficiency
- Chronic obstructive pulmonary disease
- Sickle cell trait
- Hypertension

Individuals who have known hypersusceptibility to chemicals that are respiratory irritants, hemolytic chemicals, organic isocyanates, and carbon disulfide may also be hypersusceptible to other agents in the work environment (Levy and Wegman, 2006). Although this has prompted some industries to consider preplacement screening for such risk factors, the associations between these individual health markers and hypersusceptible response are unclear.

AGENT

Work-related hazards, or **agents** (see Box 32-1), present potential and actual risks to the health and safety of workers in the millions of business establishments in the United States. Any worksite commonly presents multiple and interacting exposures from all five categories of agents. Table 32-1 lists some of the more common workplace exposures, their known health effects, and the types of jobs associated with these hazards.

Biological Agents

Biological agents are living organisms whose excretions or parts are capable of causing human disease, usually by an infectious process. Biological hazards are common in workplaces such as health care facilities and clinical laboratories in which employees are potentially exposed to a variety of

Table 32-1 Selected Job Categories, Exposures, and Associated Work-Related Diseases and Conditions

Job Categories	Exposures	Work-Related Diseases and Conditions
All workers	Workplace stress	Hypertension, mood disorders, cardiovascular disease
Agricultural workers	Pesticides, infectious agents, gases, sunlight	Pesticide poisoning, "farmer's lung," skin cancer
Anesthetists	Anesthetic gases	Reproductive effects, cancer
Automobile workers	Asbestos, plastics, lead, solvents	Asbestosis, dermatitis
Butchers	Vinyl plastic fumes	Meat wrapper's asthma
Caisson workers	Pressurized work environments	"Caisson disease," "the bends"
Carpenters	Wood dust, wood preservatives, adhesives	Nasopharyngeal cancer, dermatitis
Cement workers	Cement dust, metals	Dermatitis, bronchitis
Ceramic workers	Talc, clays	Pneumoconiosis
Demolition workers	Asbestos, wood dust	Asbestosis
Drug manufacturers	Hormones, nitroglycerin, etc.	Reproductive effects
Dry cleaners	Solvents	Liver disease, dermatitis
Dye workers	Dyestuffs, metals, solvents	Bladder cancer, dermatitis
Embalmers	Formaldehyde, infectious agents	Dermatitis
Felt makers	Mercury, polycyclic hydrocarbons	Mercury poisoning
Foundry workers	Silica, molten metals	Silicosis
Glass workers	Heat, solvents, metal powders	Cataracts
Hospital workers	Infectious agents, cleansers, radiation	Infections, latex allergies, unintentional injuries
Insulators	Asbestos, fibrous glass	Asbestosis, lung cancer, mesothelioma
Jackhammer operators	Vibration	Raynaud's phenomenon
Lathe operators	Metal dusts, cutting oils	Lung disease, cancer
Office computer workers	Repetitive wrist motion on computers and eye strain	Tendonitis, carpal tunnel syndrome, tenosynovitis

infectious agents, including viruses, fungi, and bacteria. Of particular concern in occupational health are infectious diseases transmitted by humans (e.g., from client to worker or from worker to worker) in a variety of work settings. Blood-borne and airborne pathogens represent a significant class of exposures for the U.S. health care worker. Occupational transmission of blood-borne pathogens (including the hepatitis B and C viruses and the human immunodeficiency virus [HIV]) occurs primarily by means of needlestick injuries but also through exposures to the eyes or mucous membranes (Panililio et al, 2005).

Transmission of tuberculosis (TB) within health care settings (especially multidrug-resistant TB) has reemerged as a major public health problem. Since 1989, outbreaks of this type of TB have been reported in hospitals, and some workers have developed active drug-resistant TB. In addition, among workers in health care, social service, and corrections facilities who work with populations at increased risk of TB, hundreds have experienced tuberculin skin test conversions. Reliable data are lacking on the extent of possible work-related TB transmission among other groups of workers at risk for exposure.

Many workers in these settings are employed as maintenance workers, security guards, aides, or cleaning people, who tend not to be well protected from inadvertent exposures, which include contaminated bed linen in the laundry, soiled equipment, and trash containing contaminated dressings or specimens (Jensen et al, 2005).

Chemical Agents

More than 300 billion pounds of *chemical agents* are produced annually in the United States. Of the approximately 2 million known chemicals in existence, less than 0.1% have been adequately studied for their effects on humans. Of those chemicals that have been linked to carcinogens, approximately half test positive as animal carcinogens. Most chemicals have not been studied epidemiologically to determine the effects of exposure on humans (Levy and Wegman, 2006). As a consequence of general environmental contamination with chemicals from work, home, and community activities, a variety of chemicals are found in the body tissues of the general population (U.S. Department of Health and Human Services, 2000).

In many workplaces, significant exposure to a daily, low-level dose of chemicals may be below the exposure standards but may still involve a potentially chronic and perhaps cumulative assault on workers' health. Predicting human responses to such exposures is further complicated because several chemicals are often combined to create a new chemical agent. Human effects may be associated with the interaction of these agents rather than with a single chemical. Another concern about occupational exposure to chemicals is effects on reproductive health. Workplace reproductive hazards have become important legal and scientific issues. Toxicity to male and female reproductive systems has been demonstrated from exposure to common agents such as lead, mercury, cadmium, nickel, and zinc, as well as to

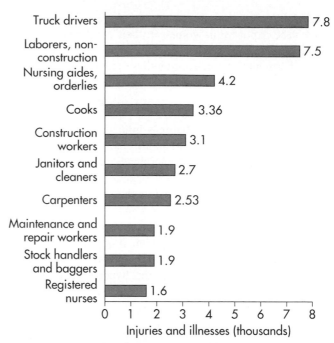

FIGURE 32-3 Ten occupations with the most injuries and illnesses involving days away from work, 2005. The total number of injuries and illnesses involving days away from work was 2.2 million. (From Bureau of Labor Statistics: Lost work time injuries and illnesses: characteristics and resulting time away from work, Washington, DC, 2006, U.S. Department of Labor.)

antineoplastic drugs. Because data for predicting human responses to many chemical agents are inadequate, workers should be assessed for all potential exposures and cautioned to work preventively with these agents. High-risk or vulnerable workers should be carefully screened and monitored for optimal health protection, such as those workers with latex allergy, which is a widely recognized health hazard (Petsonk and Levy, 2005; Weissman and Lewis, 2002).

Environmental and Mechanical Agents

Environmental and *mechanical agents* are those agents that can potentially cause injury or illness, that are related to the work process, or that can cause musculoskeletal or other strains that can produce negative health effects when certain tasks are performed repeatedly. Examples are repetitive motions, poor workstation–worker fit, and lifting heavy loads. Carpal tunnel syndrome, tendonitis, and tenosynovitis are the most frequently seen occupational diseases observed in workers who are chronically exposed to repetitive motion. The most frequently reported upper-extremity musculoskeletal disorders affect the hand and wrist region.

In 2005, sprains and strains were by far the most frequent disabling conditions, accounting for 40.7% of days away from work. Bruises accounted for 9.0%, and cuts and lacerations accounted for another 7.4% (Figure 32-3). The back and shoulders were the body parts most often affected by disabling work incidents. Repeated trauma disorders accounted for 35% of the nonfatal cases of occupational illness recorded in 2001. Included in this category are carpal tunnel syndrome (CTS) and tendonitis (Bureau of Labor Statistics, 2003b).

Physical Agents

Physical agents are those agents that produce adverse health effects through the transfer of physical energy. Commonly encountered physical agents in the workplace include the following:

- Temperature extremes
- Vibration
- Noise
- Radiation
- Laser
- Lighting

For example, vibration, which accompanies the use of power tools and vehicles such as trucks, affects internal organs, supportive ligaments, the upper torso, and the shoulder-girdle structure.

Localized effects are seen with handheld power tools; the most common is Raynaud's phenomenon. The control of worker exposure to these agents is usually accomplished through engineering strategies such as eliminating or containing the offending agent. In addition, workers must use preventive actions, such as practicing safe work habits and wearing personal protective equipment when needed. Examples of safe work habits include taking appropriate breaks from environments with temperature extremes and not eating or smoking in radiation-contaminated areas. Personal protective equipment includes the following:

- Hearing protection
- Eye guards
- Protective clothing
- Devices for monitoring exposures to agents such as radiation

This class of agents is considered one of the most easily controlled.

Psychosocial Agents

Psychosocial agents involve conditions that create a threat to the psychological and/or social well-being of individuals and groups (Rogers, 2003). A psychosocial response to the work environment occurs as an employee acts selectively toward the environment in an attempt to achieve a harmonious relationship. When such a human attempt at adaptation to the environment fails, an adverse psychosocial response may occur. Work-related stress or burn-out is fast becoming a significant problem for many individuals (Rogers, 2003). Responses to negative interpersonal relationships, particularly those with authority figures in the workplace, are often the cause of vague health symptoms and increased absenteeism. Epidemiologic work in mental health has pointed to environmental variables such as these in the incidence of mental illness and emotional disorder.

The psychosocial environment includes characteristics of the work itself, as well as the interpersonal relationships required in the work setting and shiftwork. An estimated 10% of Americans do some form of shiftwork, which has the potential to lead to a variety of psychological and physical problems, including exhaustion, depression, anxiety, and gastrointestinal disturbance.

Evidence-Based Practice

The authors collected data on 200 firefighters during physical examinations to determine the presence of risk factors for developing cardiovascular disease. Evidence-based guidelines and the Framingham risk scoring process were used to predict future cardiovascular disease among the firefighters. Firefighters ranged in age from 22 to 64 years (mean = 41 years) and were assessed for body mass index, elevated total cholesterol, elevated blood pressure, high-density lipoprotein (HDL) and low-density lipoprotein (LDL), and glucose levels. These firefighters were found to have obesity, elevated total cholesterol, and elevated blood pressure that exceeded the *Healthy People 2010* target levels. They also exceeded the general population prevalence rates for obesity, high LDLs, and low HDLs.

NURSE USE: The occupational health nurse can use this approach to examine firefighters and other workers for cardiovascular risk factors and develop worksite health policies and fitness programs to prevent the development of coronary heart disease. The nurse can assess the work environment for factors that may contribute to the development of risk factors, such as nutritional choices and stressors in the workplace.

From Byczek L et al: Cardiovascular risks in firefighters: implications for occupational health nurse practice, *AAOHN J* 52(2):66–76, 2004.

Strategies to minimize the adverse effects of shiftwork such as rotating shifts clockwise are beneficial. Job characteristics associated with an increased risk of heart disease among clerical and blue-collar workers are low autonomy, poor job satisfaction, and limited control over the pace of work.

Interpersonal relationships among employees and co-workers or bosses and managers are often sources of conflict and stress. Another aspect is *organizational culture*. This refers to the norms and patterns of behavior that are sanctioned within a particular organization. Such norms and patterns set guidelines for the types of work behaviors that will enable employees to succeed within a particular firm. The following are examples:

- Following organizational norms for working overtime
- Expressing constructive dissatisfaction with management
- Making work a top priority (U.S. Department of Health and Human Services, National Institute for Occupational Safety and Health, 2002a)

These factors and the employee's response to them must be assessed if strategies for influencing the health and safety of workers are to be effective.

Nonfatal violence in the health care worker's workplace is a serious problem that seems to be underreported. Much of the study of health care worker violence has been in psychiatric settings; however, reports in other areas such as the emergency department have occurred. Risk factors associated with this type of violence must be identified and strategies implemented to reduce the risk (U.S. Department of Health and Human Services, National Institute for Occupational Safety and Health, 2004b).

predispose the client to increased health risks of certain jobs. The **occupational health history** is an indispensable component of the health assessment of individuals (Rogers, 2003) (see Appendix G.3). Because work is a part of life for most people, including an occupational health history in all routine nursing assessments is essential. Many workers in the United States do not have access to health care services in their workplaces. Yet it is not unusual to find health care providers in the community who have little or no knowledge about workplaces or expertise in occupationally related illnesses and injuries. Because of the large number of small businesses that do not have the resources to maintain on-site health care, injured and ill workers are first seen in the public and private health care sector (e.g., in clinics, emergency rooms, physicians' offices, hospitals, health maintenance organizations [HMOs], ambulatory care centers). Nurses are often the first-line assessors of these individuals and perhaps the only contact for education about self-protection from workplace hazards.

Identifying workplace exposures as sources of health problems may influence the client's course of illness and rehabilitation and also prevent similar illnesses among others with potential for exposure (Levy and Wegman, 2006). Including occupational health data in client assessments begins with recognizing the possible relationship between health and occupational factors. The next step is to integrate into the history-taking procedure some routine assessment questions that will provide the data necessary to confirm or rule out occupationally induced symptoms. Symptoms of hazardous workplace exposures may be indicated by vague complaints involving any body system. These complaints are often similar to common medical problems. The occupational health histories should include the following points:

- A list of current and past jobs the client has held, including specific job titles, or history of exposure
- Questions about current and past exposures to specific agents and relationships between the symptoms and activities at work
- Other factors that may enhance the client's susceptibility to occupational agents (e.g., life history such as smoking, underlying illness, previous injury, disability)

Questions about the employee's occupational history can be included in existing assessment tools. The more complete the data collected, the more likely the nurse is to notice the influence of work-health interactions. All employees should be questioned about their employment history. To describe only a current status of "retired" or "housewife" may lead to the omission of needed data. The nurse should be aware that not all workers are well-informed about the materials with which they work or about potential hazards. For this reason the nurse must develop basic knowledge about the types of jobs held by clients and the possible hazards associated with them. Because there is an increased likelihood that multiple exposures from other environments such as home and yard may interact with workplace exposures, the nurse should extend the questioning to include this information.

Identifying work-related health problems does not require an extensive knowledge of occupational agents and their effects. A systematic approach for evaluating the potential for workplace exposures is the most effective intervention for detecting and preventing occupational health risks. Figure 32-4 shows one short assessment tool that can be incorporated into routine history taking. Similar questions can be included in the assessment of workers' spouses and dependents, who may have indirect exposure to occupational hazards.

During these health assessments, the nurse has the opportunity to provide instruction about workplace hazards and preventive measures the worker can use. At the same time, the nurse is obtaining information that will be valuable in optimizing work-job fit. Such assessments may be done as follows:

- As preplacement examinations before the client begins a job
- On a periodic basis during employment
- With the onset of a work-related health problem or exposure
- When an employee is being transferred to another job with different requirements and exposures
- At termination
- At retirement

The goal of these assessments is to identify agent and host factors that could place the employee at risk and to determine prevention steps that can be taken to eliminate or minimize the exposure and potential health problem. When the health data from such assessments are considered collectively, the nurse may determine some patterns in risk factors associated with the occurrence of work-related injuries and illnesses in a total population of workers. For example, a nurse practitioner in a clinic noted a dramatic increase in the number of dermatitis cases among her clients. When she looked at factors in common among these individuals, she determined that they all worked at a company with solvent exposure commonly associated with dermal irritations. She worked with the union and the company to assess the environment/agent exposure to the employees. This nursing intervention led to a safer work environment and a decrease in dermatitis in this population group. Such an approach can be

I.   Present Job

   A.   What is your job title? _____

   B.   What do you do for a living? _____

   C.   How long have you had this job? _____

   D.   Describe the specific tasks of this job: _____
       _____

   E.   What product or service is produced by the company where you work? _____ _____
       _____

   F.   Are you exposed to any of the following on your present job?
       Metals   Radiation   Stress
       Vapors, gases   Vibration   Others: _____
       Dusts   Loud noise
       Solvents   Extreme heat or cold

   G.   Do you feel you have any health problems that may be associated with your work?
       If yes, describe: _____
       _____

   H.   How would you describe your satisfaction with your job? _____
       _____

   I.   Have any of your co-workers complained of illness or injuries that they associate with their jobs?
       If yes, describe: _____
       _____

II. All Past Work

   Starting with your first job, please provide the following information:

Job title	Years held	Description of work	Exposures	Injuries/Illnesses	Personal protection equipment used

III. Other Exposures

   A.   Do you have any hobbies which involve exposure to chemicals, metals, or any of the other agents mentioned
       before? If yes, describe: _____

   B.   Are any other members of your household exposed to any of the substances listed above? If yes, describe:
       _____

   C.   Do you live near any factories, dump sites, or other sources of pollution? If yes, describe: _____
       _____

FIGURE 32-4 Occupational health history form.

Name of company: _____   Date: _____
Address: _____
Telephone: _____
Parent company (if any): _____
Location of corporate offices: _____
SIC code: _____

The Work:

Major products: _____
Major processes and operations, raw materials, by-products: _____
_____
Type of jobs: _____
_____
Potential exposures: _____
_____

Work Environment
General conditions: _____
Safety signs: _____
Physical environment: _____

Worker Population
Employees
Total number: _____   Number in production: _____   Others: _____
% Full-time: _____   % Men: _____   % Women: _____
% First shift: _____   % Second shift: _____   % Third shift: _____
Age distribution: _____
% Unionized: _____   Names of unions: _____

Human Resources Management
Corporate commitment to health
Personnel
Policies/procedures
Input/surveys/committees
Record keeping

Health Data
Work-related illnesses, injuries, deaths per annum: _____
OSHA recordable: _____   Workers' compensation: _____
Other: _____   Most frequent complaints: _____
Average number of monthly calls to the health unit: _____
Absenteeism rate: _____

Occupation Health and Safety Services
Examinations
Employee assistance
Treatment of illness/injury
Health education
Physical fitness, health promotion activities
Mandatory programs
Safety audits
Environmental monitoring
Health risk appraisal
Screenings
Health promotion

Control Strategies
Engineering
Work practice
Administrative
Personal protective equipment

FIGURE 32-5 Worksite assessment guide.

used at the company, industry, and community levels. The initial collection of data and the questioning about workplace exposures are vital steps for any intervention.

BRIEFLY NOTED

There is an acceptable level of risk in any job.

WORKPLACE ASSESSMENT

The nurse may conduct a similar assessment of the workplace itself. The purpose of this assessment, known as a **worksite walk-through** or survey, is to learn the following (Rogers, 2003):

- About the work processes and the materials
- The requirements of various jobs
- The presence of actual or potential hazards
- The work practices of employees

Figure 32-5 shows a brief outline that can be used to guide a worksite assessment.

More complex surveys are performed by industrial hygienists and safety professionals when the purpose of the walk-through is environmental monitoring or a safety audit. However, most occupational health nurses have developed expertise in these areas and include such tasks as part of their functions. For any health care provider who assesses workers, this information makes up an important database. For the on-site health care provider, worksite walk-throughs assist the professional in developing rapport and establishing credibility with the employees.

A worksite survey begins with an understanding of the type of work that occurs in the workplace. All business organizations are classified within the North American Industry Classification System (NAICS) with a numerical code. This code, usually a two-digit to four-digit number, indicates a company's product and, therefore, the possible types of **occupational health hazards** that may be associated with the processes and materials used by its employees. NAICS codes are used to collect and report data on businesses. For example, the illness and injury rates of one company are compared with the rates of other companies of similar size with the same NAICS code to determine whether the company is experiencing an excess of illness or injury.

By knowing the NAICS code of a company, a health care professional can access reference books that describe the usual processes, materials, and by-products of that kind of company.

The nurse should review the work processes and work areas by jobs or locations in the workplace. These preliminary data provide clues about what hazards may be present and an understanding of the types of jobs and health requirements that may be involved in a particular industry. A description of the work environment is next and provides an overall picture of the general appearance, physical layout, and safety of the environment. Are safety signs posted and readable where needed? Is clutter or dampness on the floor that could cause slips or falls?

| HOW TO | **Assess a Worker and the Workplace** |

Assessing the worker for a work-related problem is a critical practice element. The nurse should do the following:
- Take a complete general and occupational health history with emphasis on workplace exposure assessment, job hazard analysis, and list of previous jobs.
- Conduct a health assessment to identify agent and host factors that interact to place workers at risk.
- Identify patterns of risk associated with illness and injury.

Assessing the work environment is necessary to determine workplace exposures that create worker health risk. The nurse should do the following:
- Understand the work being done.
- Evaluate the work-related hazards.
- Understand the work process.
- Gather data about the incidence and prevalence of work-related illness and injuries and related hazards.
- Examine the control strategies in place for eliminating exposures.

A description of the employee group is vital to understanding the demographics and the work distribution in the company. Knowing about shiftwork and productivity can be helpful in pinpointing potential stressors. Human resources management and corporate commitment to health and safety are necessary to develop a support culture for effective and efficient programming. Assessing the status of policies and procedures and assessing opportunities for input into improving service are important to establish the organization's strength in occupational health and safety management. Gathering data about the incidence and prevalence of work-related illnesses and injuries and the cost patterns for these conditions provides useful epidemiologic trends. It also targets high-cost areas. It is important to know the types of occupational safety and health services and programs. This will indicate whether required programs are being offered and whether they include health-promotion and disease-prevention strategies.

Finally, examining control strategies that are effective in eliminating or reducing exposure is important in determining risk reduction. Engineering controls can reduce worker exposure by modifying the exposure source, such as putting needles in a puncture-proof container (see the "How To" box).

CASE STUDY

Brenda Dowell is an occupational health nurse. Ms. Dowell works in the employee health clinic of a teaching hospital. This morning, Cindy True visits Ms. Dowell after accidentally sticking herself with a needle she just used to draw blood from one of her patients.

Ms. True tells Ms. Dowell that she graduated last year from nursing school and has been working on the cancer unit for the past 8 months. Ms. True usually works the night shift, but she was called to fill in for an evening shift nurse who was out sick. Ms. True was not accustomed to the evening shift routine and felt disoriented. One of Ms. True's patients was admitted to the floor 1 hour before her shift started and needed several laboratory tests. The day-shift nurse did not have time to draw blood for the laboratory studies and passed the task on to Ms. True. This was her second time drawing blood for laboratory tests, and she was having difficulty finding the vein. Ms. True was relieved when the blood was finally drawn, but as she was cleaning up her supplies she felt a sharp tinge of pain on her hand. She looked down and saw the used needle in her finger. The nurse-manager for her unit sent Ms. True to employee health.

Ms. Dowell counsels Ms. True about the risks from needle-stick injuries and about the seriousness of Ms. True's exposure and explains the testing for blood-borne pathogens Ms. True will have to undergo.

Work practice controls include good hygiene, waste disposal, and housekeeping. Administrative controls reduce exposure through job rotation, workplace monitoring, and employee training and education. Personal protective control is the last resort and requires the worker to actively engage in strategies for protection, such as use of gloves, masks, and gowns to prevent exposure to blood and body fluid (Rogers, 2003).

BRIEFLY NOTED

Both corporate culture and cost-effective programs are key factors in influencing the development of occupational health services.

The more information that can be collected before the walk-through, the more efficient will be the process of the survey. After the survey is conducted, the nurse can use the information with the aggregate health data to evaluate the effectiveness of the occupational health and safety program and to plan future programs.

HEALTHY PEOPLE 2010 RELATED TO OCCUPATIONAL HEALTH

In an attempt to meet the goal of increasing the quality and years of healthy life for Americans, health education and health protection strategies are proposed to address the needs of large population groups such as the American workforce.

Healthy People 2010 identifies the national health objectives aimed at reducing the risk of occupational illnesses and promoting safety.

LEGISLATION RELATED TO OCCUPATIONAL HEALTH

The occupational health and safety services provided by an employer are influenced by specific legislation at federal and state levels. Although the relationship between work and health has been known since the second century (Ramazzini,

● Healthy People 2010

Objectives Focusing on Occupational Health

20-1	Reduce deaths from work-related injuries
20-2	Reduce work-related injuries resulting in medical treatment, lost time from work, or restricted work activity
20-3	Reduce the rate of injury and illness cases involving days away from work due to overexertion or repetitive motion
20-4	Reduce deaths due to pneumoconiosis
20-5	Reduce deaths from work-related homicides
20-6	Reduce work-related assault
20-7	Reduce the number of persons who have elevated blood lead concentrations due to work exposures
20-8	Reduce occupational skin diseases or disorders among full-time workers
20-9	Increase the proportion of worksites employing 50 or more persons that provide programs to prevent or reduce employee stress
20-10	Reduce occupational needlestick injuries among health care workers
20-11	Reduce new cases of work-related noise-induced hearing loss

From U.S. Department of Health and Human Services: *Healthy People 2010*: *national health promotion and disease prevention objectives*, Washington, DC, 2000, U.S. Government Printing Office.

1713), public policy that effectively controlled occupational hazards was not enacted until the 1960s. The Mine Safety and Health Act of 1968 was the first legislation that specifically required certain prevention programs for workers. This was followed by the Occupational Safety and Health Act of 1970, which established two agencies to carry out the Act's purpose of ensuring "safe and healthful working conditions for working men and women" (Public Law 91-596, 1970).

Within the context of the Occupational Health and Safety Act, the **Occupational Safety and Health Administration (OSHA)**, a federal agency within the U.S. Department of Labor, was created to develop and enforce workplace safety and health regulations. OSHA sets the standards that regulate workers' exposure to potentially toxic substances, enforcing these at the federal, regional, and state levels. Specific standards and information about compliance can be obtained from federal, regional, and state OSHA offices (www.osha.org).

The **National Institute for Occupational Safety and Health (NIOSH)** was established by the Occupational Safety and Health Act of 1970 and is part of the Centers for Disease Control and Prevention (CDC). The NIOSH agency identifies, monitors, and educates about the incidence, prevalence, and prevention of work-related illnesses and injuries and examines potential hazards of new work technologies and practices (U.S. Department of Health and Human Services, National Institute for Occupational Safety and Health, 2002b). Although NIOSH and OSHA were both created by the same act of Congress, they have discrete functions (Box 32-3).

Box 32-3	Functions of Federal Agencies Involved in Occupational Health and Safety

Occupational Safety and Health Administration (OSHA)

- Determine and set standards for hazardous exposures in the workplace.
- Enforce the occupational health standards (including the right of entry for inspection).
- Educate employers about occupational health and safety.
- Develop and maintain a database of work-related injuries, illnesses, and deaths.
- Monitor compliance with occupational health and safety standards.

National Institute for Occupational Safety and Health (NIOSH)

- Conduct research and review research findings to recommend permissible exposure levels for occupational hazards to OSHA.
- Identify and research occupational health and safety hazards.
- Educate occupational health and safety professionals.
- Distribute research findings relevant to occupational health and safety.

From U.S. Department of Health and Human Services—National Institute for Occupational Safety and Health: *National occupational research agenda,* Pub No 99-108, Washington, DC, 2003, U.S. Government Printing Office.

BRIEFLY NOTED

NIOSH publications, many of which are free, are online at http://www.cdc.gov/niosh/homepage.html.

Many standards have been established by OSHA and promulgated to protect worker health. One example is the **Hazard Communication Standard**. This standard is based on the premise that while working to reduce and eliminate potentially toxic agents in the work environment, an important line of defense is to provide the work community with information about hazardous chemicals so as to minimize exposures. The Hazard Communication Standard, which was first established in 1983, requires that all worksites with hazardous substances inventory their toxic agents, label them, and provide information sheets, called *material safety data sheets (MSDSs),* for each agent. In addition, the employer must have in place a hazard communication program that provides workers with education about these agents. This education must include agent identification, toxic effects, and protective measures. Numerous standards have been established by OSHA for specific chemicals and programs. A standard familiar to all health care professionals is the *Bloodborne Pathogens Standard.*

Workers' Compensation acts are important state laws that govern financial compensation of employees who suffer work-related health problems. These acts vary by state; each state sets rules for the reimbursement of employees with occupational health problems for medical expenses and lost work time associated with the illness or injury. Workers' Compensation claims and the experience-based insurance premiums paid by industry have been important motivators for increasing the health and safety of the workplace.

DISASTER PLANNING AND MANAGEMENT

Although disaster planning and management have been functions of occupational health and safety programs, this is an area of new legislation that affects businesses and health professionals. The legislation of the *Superfund Amendment and Reauthorization Act* (SARA) requires that written disaster plans of industries be shared with key resources in the community, such as fire departments and emergency departments. Concern about disasters, such as the terrorist attacks on the World Trade Center and Pentagon on September 11, 2001, the methyl isocyanate leak in Bhopal, India, the community exposure to chemicals at Times Beach, Missouri, and the effects of hurricanes such as Katrina, has mandated more attention to disaster planning.

The goals of a disaster plan are to prevent or minimize injuries and deaths of workers and residents, minimize property damage, provide effective triage, and facilitate necessary business activities. A disaster plan requires the cooperation of different personnel within the company and community. The nurse is often a key person on the disaster planning team, along with safety professionals, physicians, industrial hygienists, the fire chief, and company management. The potential for disaster (e.g., explosions, fires, leaks) must be identified; this is best achieved by completing an exhaustive chemical and hazard inventory of the workplace. The MSDSs and plant blueprints are critical for correctly identifying substances and work areas that may be hazardous. Worksite surveys are the first step to completing this inventory.

Effective disaster plans are designed by those with knowledge of the work processes and materials, the workers and workplace, and the resources in the community. Specific steps must be detailed for actions to be put in place by specific individuals in the event of a disaster, as follows:

- The written plan must be shared with all who will be involved.
- Employees should be prepared in first aid, cardiopulmonary resuscitation (CPR), and fire brigade procedures.
- Plans must be clear, specific, and comprehensive (i.e., covering all shifts and all work areas) and must include activities to be conducted within the worksite and those that require community resources.
- Transportation plans, fire response, and emergency response services should be coordinated with the agencies that would be involved in an actual disaster.
- The disaster plan, emergency and safety equipment, and the first response team's abilities should be tested at least annually with a drill.
- Practice results should be carefully evaluated, with changes made as needed.

- Hospitals and other emergency services, such as fire departments, should be involved in developing the disaster plan and should receive a copy of the plan and a current hazard inventory.
- The occupational health nurse or another company representative should provide emergency health care providers with updated clinical information on exposures and appropriate treatment.
- It should never be assumed that local services will have current information on substances used in industry.
- Representatives of these agencies should visit the worksite and accompany the nurse on a worksite walk-through so that they are familiar with the operations.

In disaster planning, the nurse often assumes or is assigned to the following:

- Coordinating the planning and implementing efforts
- Working with appropriate key people within the company and in the community to develop a workable, comprehensive plan
- Providing ongoing communication to keep the plan current
- Planning the drills
- Educating the employees, management, and community providers
- Assessing the equipment and services that may be used in a disaster

In the event of a disaster, the nurse should play a key role in coordinating the response. Principles of triage may be used as the response team determines the extent of the disaster and the ability of the company and community to respond. Postdisaster nursing interventions are also critical. Examples include identifying ongoing disaster-related health needs of workers and community residents, collecting epidemiologic data, and assessing the cause of and the necessary steps to prevent a recurrence.

CLINICAL APPLICATION

When an insurance company renovated its claims processing office area, all typewriters were replaced with video display terminals (VDTs) and associated hardware for handling all future work by computer. The company's occupational health nurse noticed an increase in visits to the health unit for complaints of headaches, stiff neck muscles, and visual disturbances. These health problems have been associated with VDT operation.

To conduct a complete investigation of this problem, the nurse assessed the workers, the new agent (the VDTs), previously existing potential agents, and the work environment. Interventions focused on designing a program to resolve the health hazard by changing the work process, if possible. In the present example, the first level of intervention was the design of the workstation, the component used by the VDT operations in doing the work. Minimizing the possible hazards of the agent involved recommendations for desks, chairs, and lighting designs that would accommodate the individual worker and allow shielding of the VDT. The nursing interventions included strengthening

the resistance of the host by prescribing appropriate rest breaks, eye exercises, and relaxation strategies. Recognizing that previous cervical neck injury or impaired vision may increase the risk of adverse effects from VDT work, the nurse would include assessment for these factors in employees' preplacement and periodic health examinations.

For the environmental concerns, the nurse educated the manager about the health risks of paced, externally controlled work expectations and recommended alternatives. *This case is an example of which of the following?*
A. *The application of the occupational health history*
B. *A worksite assessment or walk-through*
C. *A work–health interaction*
D. *The use of the epidemiologic triad in exploring occupational health problems*
Answer is in the back of the book.

REMEMBER THIS!

- Occupational health nursing is an autonomous practice specialty.
- The scope of occupational health nursing practice is broad, including worker and workplace assessment and surveillance, case management, health promotion, primary care, management and administration, business and finance skills, and research.
- The workforce and workplace are changing dramatically, requiring new knowledge and new occupational health services.
- The type of work has shifted from primarily manufacturing to service and technological jobs.
- Workplace hazards include exposure to biological, chemical, environmental and mechanical, physical, and psychosocial agents.
- The Occupational Safety and Health Act of 1970 states that workers must have a safe and healthful work environment.
- The interdisciplinary occupational health team usually consists of the occupational health nurse, occupational medicine physician, industrial hygienist, and safety specialist.
- Work-related health problems must be investigated and control strategies implemented to reduce exposure.
- Control strategies include engineering, work practice, administration, and personal protective equipment.
- The Occupational Safety and Health Administration enforces workplace safety and health standards.
- The National Institute for Occupational Safety and Health is the research agency that provides grants to investigate the causes of workplace illness and injuries.
- Workers' Compensation Acts are important laws that govern financial compensation of employees who suffer work-related health problems.
- The occupational health nurse should play a key role in disaster planning and coordination.
- Academic education in occupational health nursing is generally at the graduate level; however, many nurses with associate degrees in nursing (ADNs) and bachelor's degrees in nursing (BSNs) work in occupational health.

WHAT WOULD YOU DO?

1. Arrange to visit a local industry to observe work processes and discuss working conditions. See if you can identify the work-related hazards and make recommendations for eliminating them.
2. Interview the occupational health nurse in an industry setting and ask questions about scope of practice, job functions, and contributions to the business.
3. Contact the American Association of Occupational Health Nurses and ask what the most pressing trends are in the specialty.
4. Obtain a proposed standard for the Occupational Safety and Health Administration, critique it, and submit your comments.
5. Attend a Worker's Compensation hearing, analyze the problem, and critique the outcome.

■ REFERENCES

American Association of Occupational Health Nurses: *The nurse in industry*, New York, 1976, American Association of Occupational Health Nurses.

American Association of Occupational Health Nurses: *Code of ethics*, Atlanta, Ga, 2003, AAOHN.

American Association of Occupational Health Nurses: *Standards for occupational health nursing practice*, Atlanta, 1999, American Association of Occupational Health Nurses.

Brown M: Occupational health nursing, New York, 1981, Mac Millian.

Bureau of Labor Statistics: *Handbook of labor statistics,* Washington, DC, 2003a, U.S. Department of Labor.

Bureau of Labor Statistics: *Survey of occupational injuries and illnesses. Nonfatal (OSHA recordable) injuries and illnesses. Industry incidence rates and counts,* Washington, DC, 2003b, U.S. Department of Labor.

Bureau of Labor Statistics: *Employment and wages*, Washington, DC, 2005, U.S. Department of Labor.

Bureau of Labor Statistics: *Handbook of labor statistics,* Washington, DC, 2006a, U.S. Department of Labor.

Bureau of Labor Statistics: *Survey of occupational injuries and illnesses. Nonfatal (OSHA recordable) injuries and illnesses. Industry incidence rates and counts,* Washington, DC, 2006b, U.S. Department of Labor.

Bureau of Labor Statistics: *Employment and wages*, Washington, DC, 2009, U.S. Department of Labor.

Byczek L et al: Cardiovascular risks in firefighters: implications for occupational health nurse practice, *AAOHN J* 52(2):66–76, 2004.

Central Intelligence Agency: *World fact book*, Washington, DC, 2008, CIA.

Felton J: The genesis of American occupational health nursing, part 1, *Occup Health Nurs* 33:615, 1985.

Institute of Medicine: *Safe work in the 21st century*, Washington, DC, 2000, National Academy Press.

Jensen PA et al: Guidelines for preventing the transmission of Mycobacterium tuberculosis in health care settings, *MMWR Morb Mortal Wkly Rep* 54(RR17), 2005.

Levy BS, Wegman DH: *Occupational health: recognizing and preventing occupational disease*, Philadelphia, 2006, Lippincott Williams & Wilkins.

McGrath B: Fifty years of industrial nursing, *Public Health Nurs* 37:119, 1995.

National Institute for Occupational Safety and Health: *Workplace injury/illness rates*, Washington, DC, 2000, U.S. Government Printing Office.

O'Donnell M: *Health promotion in the workplace*, New York, 2002, Delmar.

Panililio A et al: Updated U.S. Public Health Service guidelines for the management of occupational exposures to HIV and recommandations for post exposure prophylaxis, *MMWR Morb Mortal Wkly Rep* 54(RR9), 2005.

Petsonk L, Levy B: Latex allergy. *In Preventing occupational disease and injury*, Washington, DC, 2005, American Public Health Association, pp 298–301.

Public Law 91-596: *Occupational Health and Safety Act, U.S. Congress*, Washington, DC, 1970, U.S. Government Printing Office.

Ramazzini B: *De Morbis Artificum [Diseases of Workers], 1713* (Wright WC, translator), Chicago, 1940, University of Chicago.

Rogers B: *Occupational health nursing: concepts and practice*, ed 2, Philadelphia, 1994, Saunders.

Rogers B: *Occupational health nursing: concepts and practice*, St. Louis, 2003, Elsevier.

Sofie JK: Creating a successful occupational safety and health program, *AAOHN J* 48:125–130, 2000.

U.S. Department of Health and Human Services: *Healthy People 2010: understanding and improving health*, ed 2, Washington, DC, 2000, U.S. Government Printing Office.

U.S. Department of Health and Human Services: *Data from the national sample survey of registered nurses*, Rockville, Md, 2001, Bureau of Health Professions.

U.S. Department of Health and Human Services, National Institute for Occupational Safety and Health: *The changing organization of work and the safety and health of working people*, Pub No 2002-116, Cincinnati, 2002a, U.S. Department of Health and Human Services.

U.S. Department of Health and Human Services, National Institute for Occupational Safety and Health: *National occupational research agenda*, Washington, DC, 2002b, U.S. Government Printing Office.

U.S. Department of Health and Human Services, National Institute for Occupational Safety and Health: *National occupational research agenda*, Washington, DC, 2003, U.S. Government Printing Office.

U.S. Department of Health and Human Services, National Institute for Occupational Safety and Health: *Workers health chartbook, 2004*, Pub No. 2004-16, Washington, DC, 2004a, U.S. Government Printing Office.

U.S. Department of Health and Human Services, National Institute for Occupational Safety and Health: *National occupational research agenda*, Pub No 2004-100D, Washington, DC, 2004b, U.S. Government Printing Office.

Weissman DN, Lewis DH: Allergic and latex specific sensations: route, frequency, and amount of exposure that are required to initiate IgE production, *J Allergy Clin Immunol* 110:557–563, 2002.

Whelton PK, Gordis L: Epidemiology of clinical medicine, *Epidemiol Rev* 22(1):140–144, 2000.

Appendixes

APPENDIX H   Essential Elements of Public Health Nursing

Appendixes

International and National Agendas for Health Care Delivery

A.1 NATIONAL HEALTH OBJECTIVES 2010

1. ACCESS TO QUALITY HEALTH SERVICES
Goal: Improve access to comprehensive high-quality health care services.

2. ARTHRITIS, OSTEOPOROSIS, AND CHRONIC BACK CONDITIONS
Goal: Prevent illness and disability related to arthritis and other rheumatic conditions, osteoporosis, and chronic back conditions.

3. CANCER
Goal: Reduce the number of new cancer cases as well as the illness, disability, and death caused by cancer.

4. CHRONIC KIDNEY DISEASE
Goal: Reduce new cases of chronic kidney disease and its complications, disability, death, and economic costs.

5. DIABETES
Goal: Through prevention programs, reduce the disease and economic burden of diabetes, and improve the quality of life for all persons who have or are at risk for diabetes.

6. DISABILITY AND SECONDARY CONDITIONS
Goal: Promote the health of people with disabilities, prevent secondary conditions, and eliminate disparities between people with and without disabilities in the U.S. population.

7. EDUCATIONAL AND COMMUNITY-BASED PROGRAMS
Goal: Increase the quality, availability, and effectiveness of educational and community-based programs designed to prevent disease and improve health and the quality of life.

8. ENVIRONMENTAL HEALTH
Goal: Promote health for all through a healthy environment.

9. FAMILY PLANNING
Goal: Improve pregnancy planning and spacing and prevent unintended pregnancy.

10. FOOD SAFETY
Goal: Reduce foodborne illnesses.

11. HEALTH COMMUNICATION
Goal: Use communication strategically to improve health.

12. HEART DISEASE AND STROKE
Goal: Improve cardiovascular health and quality of life through the prevention, detection, and treatment of risk factors; early identification and treatment of heart attacks and strokes; and prevention of recurrent cardiovascular events.

13. HIV
Goal: Prevent HIV infection and its related illness and death.

14. IMMUNIZATION AND INFECTIOUS DISEASES
Goal: Prevent disease, disability, and death from infectious diseases, including vaccine-preventable diseases.

15. INJURY AND VIOLENCE PREVENTION
Goal: Reduce injuries, disabilities, and deaths due to unintentional injuries and violence.

16. MATERNAL, INFANT, AND CHILD HEALTH
Goal: Improve the health and well-being of women, infants, children, and families.

17. MEDICAL PRODUCT SAFETY
Goal: Ensure the safe and effective use of medical products.

18. MENTAL HEALTH AND MENTAL ILLNESS
Goal: Improve mental health and ensure access to appropriate, quality mental health services.

19. NUTRITION AND OVERWEIGHT
Goal: Promote health and reduce chronic disease associated with diet and weight.

20. OCCUPATIONAL SAFETY AND HEALTH
Goal: Promote the health and safety of people at work through prevention and early intervention.

21. ORAL HEALTH
Goal: Prevent and control oral and craniofacial diseases, conditions, and injuries and improve access to related services.

22. PHYSICAL FITNESS AND ACTIVITY
Goal: Improve health, fitness, and quality of life through daily physical activity.

23. PUBLIC HEALTH INFRASTRUCTURE
Goal: Ensure that Federal, Tribal, State, and local health agencies have the infrastructure to provide essential public health services effectively.

24. RESPIRATORY DISEASES
Goal: Promote respiratory health through better prevention, detection, treatment, and education efforts.

25. SEXUALLY TRANSMITTED DISEASES
Goal: Promote responsible sexual behaviors, strengthen community capacity, and increase access to quality services to prevent sexually transmitted diseases (STDs) and their complications.

26. SUBSTANCE ABUSE
Goal: Reduce substance abuse to protect the health, safety, and quality of life for all, especially children.

27. TOBACCO USE
Goal: Reduce illness, disability, and death related to tobacco use and exposure to secondhand smoke.

28. VISION AND HEARING
Goal: Improve the visual and hearing health of the Nation through prevention, early detection, treatment, and rehabilitation.

From U.S. Department of Health and Human Services: *Healthy People 2010: understanding and improving health,* Washington, DC, 2000, U.S. Department of Health and Human Services, available at http:///www.health.gov/healthypeople/document/html/uih/uih_6.htm.

A.2 SCHEDULE OF CLINICAL PREVENTIVE SERVICES

1. BIRTH TO 10 YEARS
Interventions considered and recommended for the periodic health examination

Leading Causes of Death
Conditions originating in the perinatal period
Congenital anomalies
Sudden infant death syndrome (SIDS)
Unintentional injuries (non–motor vehicle)
Motor vehicle injuries

INTERVENTIONS FOR THE GENERAL POPULATION

Screening
Height and weight
Blood pressure
Vision screen
Hemoglobinopathy screen (birth)[1]
Phenylalanine level (birth)[2]
Thyroxine (T_4) and/or thyroid-stimulating hormone (TSH) (birth)[3]

Counseling
Injury prevention
Child safety car seats (age <5 yr)
Lap-shoulder belts (age ≥5 yr)
Bicycle helmet; avoid bicycling near traffic
Smoke detector, flame retardant sleepwear
Hot water heater temperature <120 °F to 130 °F
Window/stair guards, pool fence
Safe storage of drugs, toxic substances, firearms, and matches
Syrup of ipecac, poison control phone number
Cardiopulmonary resuscitation (CPR) training for parents/ caretakers
Diet and exercise
Breastfeeding, iron-enriched formula and foods (infants and toddlers)
Limit fat and cholesterol; maintain caloric balance; emphasize grains, fruits, vegetables (age ≥2 yr)
Regular physical activity*
Substance use
Effects of passive smoking*
Antitobacco message*
Dental health
Regular visits to the dental care provider*
Floss, brush with fluoride toothpaste daily*
Advice about baby bottle tooth decay*

Immunizations
Diphtheria–tetanus–pertussis (DTP)[4]
Oral poliovirus (OPV)[5]
Measles–mumps–rubella (MMR)[6]

---

[1]Whether screening should be universal or targeted to high-risk groups will depend on the proportion of high-risk individuals in the screening area and other considerations.
[2]If done during first 24 hr of life, repeat by age 2 wk.
[3]Optimally between days 2 and 6, but in all cases, before newborn nursery discharge.

[4]2, 4, 6, and 12 to 18 mo; once between ages 4 and 6 yr (DtaP [diphtheria, tetanus, and pertussis] may be used at 15 mo and older).
[5]2, 4, and 6 to 18 mo; once between ages 4 and 6 yr.
[6]12 to 15 mo and ages 4 to 6 yr.

Haemophilus influenzae type b (Hib) conjugate[7]
Hepatitis B[8]
Varicella[9]

Chemoprophylaxis
Ocular prophylaxis (birth)

---

[7]2, 4, 6, and 12 to 15 mo; no dose needed at 6 mo if PRP-OMP (*Haemophilus* b conjugate) vaccine is used for first two doses.
[8]Birth, 1, 6 mo; or 0 to 2 mo, 1 to 2 mo later, and 6 to 18 mo. If not done in infancy: current visit, and 1 and 6 mo later.
[9]12 to 18 mo; or any child without hx of chickenpox or previous immunization. Include information on risk in adulthood, duration of immunity, and potential need for booster doses.

Interventions for High-Risk Populations

Population	Potential Interventions
Preterm or low birth weight	Hemoglobin/hematocrit (HR1)
Infants of mothers at risk for HIV	HIV testing (HR2)
Low income; immigrants	Hemoglobin/hematocrit (HR1); PPD (HR3)
TB contacts	PPD (HR3)
Native American/Alaskan Native	Hemoglobin/hematocrit (HR1); PPD (HR3); hepatitis A vaccine (HR4); pneumococcal vaccine (HR5)
Travelers to developing countries	Hepatitis A vaccine (HR4)
Residents of long-term care facilities	PPD (HR3); hepatitis A vaccine (HR4); influenza vaccine (HR6)
Certain chronic medical conditions	PPD (HR3); pneumococcal vaccine (HR5); influenza vaccine (HR6)
Increased individual or community lead exposure	Blood lead level (HR7)
Inadequate water fluoridation	Daily fluoride supplement (HR8)
Family history of skin cancer; nevi; fair skin, eyes, hair	Avoid excess/midday sun, use protective clothing* (HR9)

*The ability of clinician counseling to influence this behavior is unproven.
HIV, Human immunodeficiency virus; *HR,* high-risk definition; *PPD,* purified protein derivative; *TB,* tuberculosis.

High-Risk Definitions
HR1 = Infants ages 6 to 12 months who are living in poverty, black, Native American or Alaskan Native, immigrants from developing countries, preterm and low-birth-weight infants, or infants whose principal dietary intake is unfortified cow's milk
HR2 = Infants born to high-risk mothers whose HIV (human immunodeficiency virus) status is unknown. Women at high risk include past or present injection drug users; persons who exchange sex for money or drugs, and their sex partners; injection drug users, bisexual, or HIV-positive sex partners currently or in the past; persons seeking treatment for sexually transmitted diseases (STDs); or blood transfusion during 1978 to 1985
HR3 = Persons infected with HIV, close contacts of persons with known or suspected tuberculosis (TB), persons with medical risk factors associated with TB, immigrants from countries with a high TB prevalence, medically underserved low-income populations (including the homeless), and residents of long-term care facilities
HR4 = Persons ≥2 years living in or traveling to areas in which the disease is endemic and in which periodic outbreaks occur (e.g., countries with high or intermediate endemicity; certain Alaskan Native, Pacific Islander, Native American, and religious communities). Consider for institutionalized children ages ≥2 years. Clinicians should also consider local epidemiology.

HR5 = Immunocompetent persons ≥2 years with certain medical conditions, including chronic cardiac or pulmonary disease, diabetes mellitus, and anatomic asplenia. Immunocompetent persons ≥2 years living in high-risk environments or social settings (e.g., certain Native American and Alaskan Native populations)
HR6 = Annual vaccination of children >6 months who are residents of chronic care facilities or who have chronic cardiopulmonary disorders, metabolic diseases (including diabetes mellitus), hemoglobinopathies, immunosuppression, or renal dysfunction
HR7 = Children about age 12 months who (1) live in communities in which the prevalence of lead levels requiring individual intervention, including residential lead hazard control or chelation, is high or undefined; (2) live in or frequently visit a home built before 1950 with dilapidated paint or with recent or ongoing renovation or remodeling; (3) have close contact with a person who has an elevated lead level; (4) live near a lead industry or heavy traffic; (5) live with someone whose job or hobby involves lead exposure; (6) use lead-based pottery; or (7) take traditional ethnic remedies that contain lead
HR8 = Children living in areas with inadequate water fluoridation (<0.6 ppm)
HR9 = Persons with a family history of skin cancer, a large number of moles, atypical moles, poor tanning ability, or light skin, hair, and eye color

2. AGES 11 TO 24 YEARS
Interventions considered and recommended for the periodic health examination

Leading Causes of Death
Motor vehicle/other unintentional injuries
Homicide
Suicide
Malignant neoplasms
Heart diseases

INTERVENTIONS FOR THE GENERAL POPULATION

Screening
Height and weight
Blood pressure[1]
Papanicolaou (Pap) test[2] (females)
Chlamydia screen[3] (females <20 yr)
Rubella serology or vaccination hx[4] (females >12 yr)
Assess for problem drinking

Counseling
Injury prevention
Lap/shoulder belts
Bicycle/motorcycle/all-terrain vehicle (ATV) helmets*
Smoke detector*
Safe storage/removal of firearms*

Substance use
Avoid tobacco use
Avoid underage drinking and illicit drug use*
Avoid alcohol/drugs use while driving, swimming, boating, etc.*
Sexual behavior
STD prevention: abstinence; avoid high-risk behavior*; use condoms/female barrier with spermicide*
Unintended pregnancy: contraception
Diet and exercise
Limit fat and cholesterol; maintain caloric balance; emphasize grains, fruits, vegetables
Adequate calcium intake (females)
Regular physical activity*
Dental health
Regular visits to dental care provider*
Floss, brush with fluoride toothpaste daily*

Immunizations
Tetanus–diphtheria (Td) boosters (11 to 16 yr)
Hepatitis B[5]
MMR (11 to 12 yr)[6]
Varicella (11 to 12 yr)
Rubella[4] (females >12 yr)

Chemoprophylaxis
Multivitamin with folic acid (females planning/capable of pregnancy)

---

[1]Periodic blood pressure (BP) measurement for persons ages ≥21 yr.
[2]If sexually active at present or in the past: ≤3 yr. If sexual history is unreliable, begin Pap tests at age 18 yr.
[3]If sexually active.
[4]Serologic testing documenting vaccination history and routine vaccination against rubella (preferably with MMR [measles, mumps, rubella]) are equally acceptable alternatives.

[5]If not previously immunized: current visit, 1 and 6 mo later.
[6]If susceptible to chickenpox.
*The ability of clinician counseling to influence this behavior is unproven.

Interventions for High-Risk Populations

Population	Potential Interventions
High-risk sexual behavior	RPR/VDRL (HR1); screen for gonorrhea (female) (HR2), HIV (HR3), chlamydia (female) (HR4); hepatitis A vaccine (HR5)
Injection or street drug use	RPR/VDRL (HR1); HIV screen (HR3); hepatitis A vaccine (HR5); PPD (HR6); advice to reduce infection risk (HR7)
TB contacts; immigrants; low-income	PPD (HR6)
Native Americans/Alaskan Natives	Hepatitis A vaccine (HR5); PPD (HR6); pneumococcal vaccine (HR8)
Travelers to developing countries	Hepatitis A vaccine (HR5)
Certain chronic medical conditions	PPD (HR6); pneumococcal vaccine (HR8); influenza vaccine (HR9)
Settings where adolescents and young adults congregate	Second MMR (HR10)
Susceptible to varicella, measles, mumps	Varicella vaccine (HR11); MMR (HR12)
Blood transfusion between 1975 and 1985	HIV screen (HR3)
Institutionalized persons; health care/laboratory vaccine workers	Hepatitis A vaccine (HR5); PPD (HR6); influenza (HR9)
Family history of skin cancer; nevi; fair skin, eyes, hair	Avoid excess/midday sun, use protective clothing* (HR13)
Prior pregnancy with neural tube defect	Folic acid 4.0 mg (HR14)
Inadequate water fluoridation	Daily fluoride supplement (HR15)

---

*The ability of clinician counseling to influence this behavior is unproven.
VDRL, Venereal Disease Research Laboratory.

High-Risk Definitions

HR1 = Persons who exchange sex for money or drugs, and their sex partners; persons with other STDs (including HIV); and sexual contacts of persons with active syphilis. Clinicians should also consider local epidemiology.

HR2 = Females who have had two or more sex partners in the last year; a sex partner with multiple sexual contacts; exchanged sex for money or drugs; or a history of repeated episodes of gonorrhea. Clinicians should also consider local epidemiology.

HR3 = Males who had sex with males after 1975; past or present injection drug use; persons who exchange sex for money or drugs, and their sex partners; injection drug-using, bisexual, or HIV-positive sex partner currently or in the past; blood transfusion from 1978 to 1985; persons seeking treatment for STDs. Clinicians should also consider local epidemiology.

HR4 = Sexually active females with multiple risk factors, including a history of prior STD; new or multiple sex partners; ages younger than 25 years; nonuse or inconsistent use of barrier contraceptives; cervical ectopy. Clinicians should consider local epidemiology of the disease in identifying other high-risk groups.

HR5 = Persons living in, traveling to, or working in areas in which the disease is endemic and in which periodic outbreaks occur (e.g., countries with high or intermediate endemicity; certain Alaskan Native, Pacific Islander, Native American, and religious communities); men who have sex with men; injection or street drug users. Vaccine may be considered for institutionalized persons and workers in these institutions, military personnel, and day care, hospital, and laboratory workers. Clinicians should also consider local epidemiology.

HR6 = HIV positive, close contacts of persons with known or suspected TB, health care workers, persons with medical risk factors associated with TB, immigrants from countries with high TB prevalence, medically underserved low-income populations (including homeless), alcoholics, injection drug users, and residents of long-term facilities

HR7 = Persons who continue to inject drugs

HR8 = Immunocompetent persons with certain medical conditions, including chronic cardiac or pulmonary disease, diabetes mellitus, and anatomic asplenia. Immunocompetent persons who live in high-risk environments or social settings (e.g., certain Native American and Alaskan Native populations).

HR9 = Annual vaccination of residents of chronic care facilities; persons with chronic cardiopulmonary disorders, metabolic diseases (including diabetes mellitus), hemoglobinopathies, immunosuppression, or renal dysfunction; and health care providers for high-risk patients

HR10 = Adolescents and young adults in settings in which such individuals congregate (e.g., high schools and colleges), if they have not previously received a second dose

HR11 = Healthy persons ages ≥13 years without a history of chickenpox or previous immunization. Consider serologic testing for presumed susceptible persons ages ≥13 years.

HR12 = Persons born after 1956 who lack evidence of immunity to measles or mumps (e.g., documented receipt of live vaccine on or after the first birthday, laboratory evidence of immunity, a history of physician-diagnosed measles or mumps)

HR13 = Persons with a family or personal history of skin cancer, a large number of moles, atypical moles, poor tanning ability, or light skin, hair, and eye color

HR14 = Women with a prior pregnancy affected by neural tube defect who are planning pregnancy

HR15 = Persons ages <17 years living in areas with inadequate water fluoridation (<0.6 ppm)

3. AGES 25 TO 64 YEARS
Interventions considered and recommended for the periodic health examination

Leading Causes of Death

Malignant neoplasms

Heart diseases

Motor vehicle and other unintentional injuries

Human immunodeficiency virus (HIV) infection

Suicide and homicide

INTERVENTIONS FOR THE GENERAL POPULATION

Screening

Blood pressure

Height and weight

Total blood cholesterol (men ages 35 to 64 yr, women ages 45 to 64 yr)

Papanicolaou (Pap) test (women)[1]

Fecal occult blood test[2] and/or sigmoidoscopy (≥50 yr)

Mammogram, clinical breast examination[3] (women ages 50 to 69 yr)

Assess for problem drinking

Rubella serology or vaccination hx[4] (women of childbearing age)

Counseling

Substance use

Tobacco cessation

Avoid alcohol/drug use while driving, swimming, boating, etc.*

Diet and exercise

Limit fat and cholesterol; maintain caloric balance; emphasize grains, fruits, vegetables

Adequate calcium intake (women)

Regular physical activity*

Injury prevention

Lap/shoulder belts

Motorcycle/bicycle/ATV helmets*

Smoke detector

Safe storage/removal of firearms*

Sexual behavior

STD prevention: avoid high-risk behavior,* use condoms/female barrier with spermicide

Unintended pregnancy: contraception

Dental health

Regular visits to dental care provider*

Floss, brush with fluoride toothpaste daily*

---

[1]Women who are or have been sexually active and who have a cervix: every 3 yr or less.

[2]Annually.

[3]Mammogram every 1–2 yr, or mammogram every 1–2 yr with annual clinical breast examination.

*The ability of clinician counseling to influence this behavior is unproven.

Immunizations
Tetanus–diphtheria (Td) boosters
Rubella[4] (women of childbearing age)

---

[4]Serologic testing, documented vaccination history, and routine vaccination (preferably with MMR) are equally acceptable.

Chemoprophylaxis
Multivitamin with folic acid (women planning or capable of pregnancy)
Discuss hormone prophylaxis (perimenopausal and postmenopausal women)

Interventions for High-Risk Populations

Population	Potential Interventions
High-risk sexual behavior	RPR/VDRL (HR1); screen for gonorrhea (female) (HR2), HIV (HR3), chlamydia (female) (HR4); hepatitis B vaccine (HR5); hepatitis A vaccine (HR6)
Injection or street drug use	RPR/VDRL (HR1); HIV screen (HR3); hepatitis B vaccine (HR5); hepatitis A vaccine (HR6); PPD (HR7); advice to reduce infection risk (HR8)
Low income; TB contacts; immigrants, alcoholics	PPD (HR7)
Native Americans/Alaskan Natives	Hepatitis A vaccine (HR6); PPD (HR7); pneumococcal vaccine (HR9)
Travelers to developing countries	Hepatitis B vaccine (HR5); hepatitis A vaccine (HR6)
Certain chronic medical conditions	PPD (HR7); pneumococcal vaccine (HR9); influenza vaccine (HR10)
Blood product recipients	HIV screen (HR3); hepatitis B vaccine (HR5)
Susceptible to measles, mumps, or varicella	MMR (HR11); varicella vaccine (HR12)
Institutionalized persons	Hepatitis A vaccine (HR6); PPD (HR7); pneumococcal vaccine (HR9); influenza vaccine (HR10)
Health care/lab workers	Hepatitis B vaccine (HR5); hepatitis A vaccine (HR6); PPD (HR7); influenza vaccine (HR10)
Family history of skin cancer: fair skin, eyes, hair	Avoid excess/midday sun, use protective clothing* (HR13)
Previous pregnancy with neural tube defect	Folic acid 4.0 mg (HR14)

*The ability of clinician counseling to influence this behavior is unproven.

High-Risk Definitions

HR1 = Persons who exchange sex for money or drugs, and their sex partners; persons with other STDs (including HIV); and sexual contacts of persons with active syphilis. Clinicians should also consider local epidemiology.

HR2 = Women who exchange sex for money or drugs, or who have had repeated episodes of gonorrhea. Clinicians should also consider local epidemiology.

HR3 = Men who had sex with men after 1975; past or present injection drug use; persons who exchange sex for money or drugs, and their sex partners; injection drug-using, bisexual, or HIV-positive sex partner currently or in the past; blood transfusion from 1978 to 1985; persons seeking treatment for STDs. Clinicians should also consider local epidemiology.

HR4 = Sexually active women with multiple risk factors, including a history of STD; new or multiple sex partners; nonuse or inconsistent use of barrier contraceptives; cervical ectopy. Clinicians should also consider local epidemiology.

HR5 = Blood product recipients (including hemodialysis patients), persons with frequent occupational exposure to blood or blood products, men who have sex with men, injection drug users and their sex partners, persons with multiple recent sex partners, persons with other STDs (including HIV), travelers to countries with endemic hepatitis B

HR6 = Persons living in, traveling to, or working in areas in which the disease is endemic and in which periodic outbreaks occur (e.g., countries with high or intermediate endemicity; certain Alaskan Native, Pacific Islander, Native American, and religious communities); men who have sex with men; injection or street drug users. Consider for institutionalized persons and workers in these institutions, military personnel, and day care, hospital, and laboratory workers. Clinicians should also consider local epidemiology.

HR7 = HIV positive, close contacts of persons with known or suspected TB, health care workers, persons with medical risk factors associated with TB, immigrants from countries with high TB prevalence, medically underserved low-income populations (including homeless), alcoholics, injection drug users, and residents of long-term care facilities

HR8 = Persons who continue to inject drugs

HR9 = Immunocompetent institutionalized persons ages ≥50 years and immunocompetent persons with certain medical conditions, including chronic cardiac or pulmonary disease, diabetes mellitus, and anatomic asplenia. Immunocompetent persons who live in high-risk environments or social settings (e.g., certain Native American and Alaskan Native populations)

HR10 = Annual vaccination of residents of chronic care facilities; persons with chronic cardiopulmonary disorders, metabolic diseases (including diabetes mellitus), hemoglobinopathies, immunosuppression or renal dysfunction; and health care providers for high-risk patients

HR11 = Persons born after 1956 who lack evidence of immunity to measles or mumps (e.g., documented receipts of live vaccine on or after the first birthday, laboratory evidence of immunity, a history of physician-diagnosed measles or mumps)

HR12 = Healthy adults without a history of chickenpox or previous immunization. Consider serologic testing for presumed susceptible adults.

HR13 = Persons with a family or personal history of skin cancer, a large number of moles, atypical moles, poor tanning ability, or light skin, hair, and eye color

HR14 = Women with a previous pregnancy affected by neural tube defect who are planning pregnancy

4. AGES 65 YEARS AND OLDER
Interventions considered and recommended for the periodic health examination

Leading Causes of Death
Heart diseases
Malignant neoplasms (lung, colorectal, breast)
Cerebrovascular disease
Chronic obstructive pulmonary disease
Pneumonia and influenza

INTERVENTIONS FOR THE GENERAL POPULATION

Screening
Blood pressure
Height and weight
Fecal occult blood test[1] and/or sigmoidoscopy
Mammogram and/or clinical breast examination[2] (women <69 yr)
Papanicolaou (Pap) test (women)[3]
Vision screening
Assess for hearing impairment
Assess for problem drinking

---

[1]Annually.
[2]Mammogram every 1–2 yr or mammogram every 1–2 yr with annual clinical breast examination.
[3]All women who are or have been sexually active and who have a cervix: every 3 yr or less. Consider discontinuation of testing after age 65 yr if previous regular screening has consistently normal results.

Counseling
Substance use
Tobacco cessation
Avoid alcohol/drug use while driving swimming, boating, etc.*
Diet and exercise
Limit fat and cholesterol; maintain caloric balance; emphasize grains, fruits, vegetables
Adequate calcium intake (women)
Regular physical activity*
Injury prevention
Lap/shoulder belts
Motorcycle and bicycle helmets*
Fall prevention*
Safe storage/removal of firearms*
Smoke detector*
Set hot water heater to 120 °F to 130 °F.
Cardiopulmonary resuscitation (CPR) training for household members
Dental health
Regular visits to dental care provider*
Floss, brush with fluoride toothpaste daily*
Sexual behavior
STD prevention: avoid high-risk sexual behavior*; use condoms

Immunizations
Pneumococcal vaccine
Influenza[1]
Tetanus–diphtheria (Td) boosters
Chemoprophylaxis
Discuss hormone prophylaxis (perimenopausal and postmenopausal women)

---

*The ability of clinician counseling to influence this behavior is unproven.

Interventions for High-Risk Populations

Population	Potential Interventions
Institutionalized persons	PPD (HR1); hepatitis A vaccine (HR2); amantadine/rimantadine (HR4)
Chronic medical conditions; TB contacts; low income; immigrants; alcoholics	PPD (HR1)
Persons ≥75 years; or ≥70 years with risk factors for falls	Fall prevention intervention (HR5)
Cardiovascular disease risk factors	Consider cholesterol screening (HR6)
Family history of skin cancer; nevi; fair skin, eyes, hair	Avoid excess/midday sun, use protective clothing* (HR7)
Native Americans/Alaskan Natives	PPD (HR1); hepatitis A vaccine (HR2)
Travelers to developing countries	Hepatitis A vaccine (HR2); hepatitis B vaccine (HR8)
Blood product recipients	HIV screen (HR3); hepatitis B vaccine (HR8)
High-risk sexual behavior	Hepatitis A vaccine (HR2); HIV screen (HR3); hepatitis B vaccine (HR8); RPR/VDRL (HR9)
Injection or street drug use	PPD (HR1); hepatitis A vaccine (HR2); HIV screen (HR3); hepatitis B vaccine (HR8); RPR/VDRL (HR9); advice or reduce infection risk (HR10)
Health care/lab workers	PPD (HR1); hepatitis A vaccine (HR2); amantadine/rimantadine (HR4); hepatitis B vaccine (HR8)
Persons susceptible to varicella	Varicella vaccine (HR11)

*The ability of clinician counseling to influence this behavior is unproven.

High-Risk Definitions

HR1 = HIV positive, close contacts of persons with known or suspected TB, health care workers, persons with medical risk factors associated with TB, immigrants from countries with high TB prevalence, medically underserved low-income populations (including homeless), alcoholics, injection drug users, and residents of long-term care facilities

HR2 = Persons living in, traveling to, or working in areas in which the disease is endemic and in which periodic outbreaks occur (e.g., countries with high or intermediate endemicity; certain Alaskan Native, Pacific Islander, Native American, and religious communities); men who have sex with men; injection or street drug users. Consider for institutionalized persons and workers in these institutions, and day care, hospital, and laboratory workers. Clinicians should also consider local epidemiology.

HR3 = Men who had sex with men after 1975; past or present injection drug use; persons who exchange sex for money or drugs, and their sex partners; injection drug-using, bisexual, or HIV-positive sex partner currently or in the past; blood transfusion from 1978 to 1985; persons seeking treatment for STDs. Clinicians should also consider local epidemiology.

HR4 = Consider for persons who have not received influenza vaccine or are vaccinated late; when the vaccine may be ineffective due to major antigenic changes in the virus; for unvaccinated persons who provide home care for high-risk persons; to supplement protection provided by vaccine in persons who are expected to have a poor antibody response; and for high-risk persons in whom the vaccine is contraindicated

HR5 = Persons ages 75 years and older; or ages 70 to 74 years with one or more additional risk factors, including the use of certain psychoactive and cardiac medications (e.g., benzodiazepines, antihypertensives); use of four or more prescription medications; impaired cognition, strength, balance, or gait. Intensive individualized home-based multifactorial fall prevention intervention is recommended in settings in which adequate resources are available to deliver such services.

HR6 = Although evidence is insufficient to recommend routine screening in elderly persons, clinicians should consider cholesterol screening on a case-by-case basis for persons ages 65 to 75 years with additional risk factors (e.g., smoking, diabetes, hypertension).

HR7 = Persons with a family or personal history of skin cancer, a large number of moles, atypical moles, poor tanning ability, or light skin, hair, and eye color

HR8 = Blood product recipients (including hemodialysis patients), persons with frequent occupational exposure to blood or blood products, men who have sex with men, injection drug users and their sex partners, persons with multiple recent sex partners, persons with other STDs (including HIV), travelers to countries with endemic hepatitis B

HR9 = Persons who exchange sex for money or drugs, and their sex partners; persons with other STDs (including HIV); and sexual contacts of persons with active syphilis. Clinicians should also consider local epidemiology.

HR10 = Persons who continue to inject drugs

HR11 = Healthy adults without a history of chickenpox or previous immunization. Consider serologic testing for presumed susceptible adults.

5. PREGNANT WOMEN*

Interventions considered and recommended for the periodic health examination

INTERVENTIONS FOR THE GENERAL POPULATION

Screening

First visit

Blood pressure

Hemoglobin/hematocrit

Hepatitis B surface antigen (HbsAg)

Rapid plasma reagin (RPR)/VDRL

Chlamydia screen (<25 yr)

Rubella serology or vaccination history

D(Rh) typing, antibody screen

Offer chorionic villus sampling (CVS) (<13 wk)[1] or amniocentesis (15 to 18 wk)[1] (ages ≥35 yr)

Offer hemoglobinopathy screening

Assess for problem or risk drinking

Offer HIV screening[2]

Follow-up visits

Blood pressure

Urine culture (12 to 16 wk)

Offer amniocentesis (15 to 18 wk)[1] (age ≥35 yr)

Offer multiple marker testing[1] (15 to 18 wk)

Offer serum α-fetoprotein[1] (16 to 18 wk)

Counseling

Tobacco cessation; effects of passive smoking

Alcohol/other drug use

Nutrition, including adequate calcium intake

Encourage breastfeeding

Lap/shoulder belts

Infant safety car seats

STD prevention: avoid high-risk sexual behavior; use condoms

Chemoprophylaxis

Multivitamin with folic acid

High-Risk Definitions

HR1 = Women with history of STD or new or multiple sex partners. Clinicians should also consider local epidemiology. Chlamydia screen should be repeated in third trimester if at continued risk.

HR2 = Women younger than age 25 years with two or more sex partners in the last year, or whose sex partner has multiple sexual contacts; women who exchange sex for money or drugs; and women with a history of repeated episodes of gonorrhea. Clinicians should also consider local epidemiology. Gonorrhea screen should be repeated in the third trimester if at continued risk.

HR3 = In areas in which universal screening is not performed because of the low prevalence of HIV infection, pregnant women with the following individual risk factors should be screened: past or present injection drug use; women who exchange sex for money or drugs; injection drug-using, bisexual, or HIV-positive sex partner currently or in the past; blood transfusion from 1978 to 1985; persons seeking treatment for STDs

---

[1]Women with access to counseling and follow-up services, reliable standardized laboratories, skilled high-resolution ultrasound, and, for those receiving serum marker testing, amniocentesis capabilities.

[2]Universal screening is recommended for areas (states, counties, or cities) with an increased prevalence of HIV infection among pregnant women. In low-prevalence areas, the choice between universal and targeted screening may depend on other considerations.

*See Appendixes A.2-2 and A.2-3 for other preventive services recommended for women of this age group.

HR4 = Women who are initially HbsAg negative who are at high risk because of injection drug use, suspected exposure to hepatitis B during pregnancy, multiple sex partners

HR5 = Women who exchange sex for money or drugs, women with other STDs (including HIV), and sexual contacts of persons with active syphilis. Clinicians should also consider local epidemiology.

HR6 = Women who continue to inject drugs

HR7 = Unsensitized D-negative women

HR8 = Prior pregnancy affected by Down syndrome, advanced maternal age (≥35 yr), known carriage of chromosome rearrangement

HR9 = Women with a previous pregnancy affected by neural tube defect

Interventions for High-Risk Populations

Population	Potential Interventions
High-risk sexual behavior	Screen for chlamydia (1st visit) (HR1), gonorrhea (1st visit) (HR2), HIV (1st visit) (HR3) HbsAg (third trimester) (HR4); RPR/VDRL (third trimester) (HR5)
Blood transfusion 1978 to 1985	HIV screen (First visit) (HR3)
Injection drug use	HIV screen (HR3); HbsAg (third trimester) (HR4); advice to reduce infection risk (HR6)
Unsensitized D-negative women	D(Rh) antibody testing (24–28 wk) (HR7)
Risk factors for Down syndrome	Offer CVS[1] (first trimester), amniocentesis[1] (15–18 wk) (HR8)
Prior pregnancy with neural tube defect	Offer amniocentesis* (15–18 wk), folic acid 4.0 mg[3] (HR9)

*Women with access to counseling and follow-up services, reliable standardized laboratories, skilled high-resolution ultrasound, and, for those receiving serum marker testing, amniocentesis capabilities.

6. CONDITIONS FOR WHICH CLINICIANS SHOULD REMAIN ALERT

Condition	Population
Symptoms of peripheral arterial disease	Older persons, smokers, diabetic persons
Skin lesions with malignant features	General population, particularly those with established risk factors
Symptoms and signs of oral cancer and premalignancy	Persons who use tobacco, older persons who drink alcohol regularly
Subtle or nonspecific symptoms and signs of thyroid dysfunction	Older persons, postpartum women, persons with Down syndrome
Signs of ocular misalignment	Infants and children
Symptoms and signs of hearing impairment	Infants and young children (<3 yr)
Large spinal curvatures	Adolescents
Changes in functional performance	Older persons
Depressive symptoms	Adolescents, young adults, persons at increased risk for depression
Evidence of suicidal ideation	Persons with established risk factors for suicide
Various presentations of family violence	General population
Symptoms and signs of drug abuse	General population
Obvious signs of untreated tooth decay or mottling, inflamed or cyanotic gingival, loose teeth, and severe halitosis	General population
Evidence of early childhood caries	Children
Mismatching of upper and lower dental arches, dental crowding or malalignment, premature loss of primary posterior teeth (baby molars), and obvious mouth breathing	

From *The guide to clinical preventive services 2006—recommendations of the U.S. Preventive Services Task Force: pocket guide*, Rockville, Md, Agency for Healthcare Research and Quality, June 2006. AHRQ Publication No. 06-0588, available at http://www.ahrq.gov/clinic/pocketgd06/.

A.3 Declaration of Alma-Ata

The International Conference on Primary Health Care, meeting in Alma-Ata this twelfth day of September in the year nineteen hundred and seventy-eight, expressing the need for urgent action of all governments, all health and development workers, and the world community to protect and promote the health of all the people of the world, hereby makes the following Declaration:

I

The Conference strongly reaffirms that health, which is a state of complete physical, mental, and social well-being, and not merely the absence of disease or infirmity, is a fundamental human right and that the attainment of the highest possible level of health is a most important worldwide social goal, whose realization requires the action of many other social and economic sectors in addition to the health sector.

II

The existing gross inequality in the health status of the people, particularly between developed and developing countries and within countries, is politically, socially, and economically unacceptable and is therefore of common concern to all countries.

III

Economic and social development, based on a new international economic order, is of basic importance to the fullest attainment of health for all and to the reduction of the gap between the health status of developing and developed countries. The promotion and protection of the health of the people are essential to sustained economic and social development and contribute to a better quality of life and to world peace.

IV

The people have the right and duty to participate individually and collectively in the planning and implementation of their health care.

V

Governments have a responsibility for the health of their people, which can be fulfilled only by the provision of adequate health and social measures. In the coming decades a main social target of governments, international organizations, and the whole world community should be the attainment by all peoples of the world by the year 2000 of a level of health that will permit them to lead a socially and economically productive life. Primary health care is the key to attaining this target as part of development in the spirit of social justice.

VI

Primary health care is essential health care based on practical, scientifically sound, and socially acceptable methods and technology made universally accessible to individuals and families in the community through their full participation and at a cost that the community and country can afford to maintain at every stage of their development in the spirit of self-reliance and self-determination. It forms an integral part both of the country's health system, of which primary health care is the central function and main focus, and of the overall social and economic development of the community. It is the first level of contact for individuals, the family, and the community with the national health system bringing health care as close as possible to where people live and work, and it constitutes the first element of a continuing health care process.

VII

Primary health care

1. Reflects and evolves from the economic conditions and sociocultural and political characteristics of the country and its communities and is based on the application of the relevant results of social, biomedical, and health services research and public health experience;
2. Addresses the main health problems in the community, providing promotive, preventive, curative, and rehabilitative services accordingly;
3. Includes at least education concerning prevailing health problems and the methods of preventing and controlling them; promotion of food supply and proper nutrition; an adequate supply of safe water and basic sanitation; maternal and child health care, including family planning; immunization against the major infectious diseases; prevention and control of locally endemic diseases; appropriate treatment of common diseases and injuries; and provision of essential drugs;
4. Involves, in addition to health sector, all related sectors and aspects of national and community development, in particular agriculture, animal husbandry, food industry, education, housing, public works, communication, and other sectors; and demands the coordinated efforts of all those sections;
5. Requires and promotes maximum community and individual self-reliance and participation in the planning, organization, operation, and control of primary health care making fullest use of local, national, and other available resources; and to this end, develops through appropriate education the ability of communities to participate;
6. Should be sustained by integrated, functional, and mutually supportive referral levels, leading to the progressive improvement of comprehensive health care for all, and giving priority to those most in need;
7. Relies, at local and referral levels, on health workers, including physicians, nurses, midwives, auxiliaries, and community workers, as applicable, as well as on traditional practitioners as needed, suitably trained socially and technically to work as a health team and to respond to the expressed health needs of the community.

VIII

All governments should formulate national policies, strategies, and plans of action to launch and sustain primary health care as part of a comprehensive national health system and in coordination with other sectors. To this end, it will be necessary to exercise political will, to mobilize the country's resources, and to use available external resources rationally.

IX

All countries should cooperate in a spirit of partnership and service to ensure primary health care for all people because the attainment of health by people in any one country directly concerns and benefits every other country. In this context the joint WHO-UNICEF report* on primary health care constitutes a solid basis for the further development and operation of Primary Health Care throughout the world.

---

*World Health Organization: *Primary health care: report of the International Conference on Primary Health Care,* Alma-Ata, USSR, September 6–12, 1978, Geneva, 1978, WHO.

X

An acceptable level of health for all the people of the world by the year 2000 can be attained through a fuller and better use of the world's resources, a considerable part of which is now spent on armaments and military conflicts. A genuine policy of independence, peace, détente, and disarmament could and should release additional resources that could well be devoted to peaceful aims and in particular to the acceleration of social and economic development of which primary health care, as an essential part, should be allotted its proper share.

Individual Assessment Tools

B.1 OASIS: START OF CARE ASSESSMENT

Outcome and Assessment Information Set (OASIS-B1)

START OF CARE VERSION
(also used for Resumption of Care Following Inpatient Stay)

Items to be Used at this Time Point--M0080-M0825

CLINICAL RECORD ITEMS

(M0080)   Discipline of Person Completing Assessment:
☐ 1-RN   ☐ 2-PT   ☐ 3-SLP/ST   ☐ 4-OT

(M0090)   Date Assessment Completed: _ _/_ _/_ _ _ _
month day   year

(M0100)   This Assessment Is Currently Being Completed for the Following Reason:

Start/Resumption of Care
☐   1 -   Start of care—further visits planned
☐   3 -   Resumption of care (after inpatient stay)

DEMOGRAPHICS AND PATIENT HISTORY

(M0175)   From which of the following Inpatient Facilities was the patient discharged during the past 14 days?
(Mark all that apply.)

☐   1 -   Hospital
☐   2 -   Rehabilitation facility
☐   3 -   Skilled nursing facility
☐   4 -   Other nursing home
☐   5 -   Other (specify) _____
☐ NA -   Patient was not discharged from an inpatient facility [**If NA, go to *M0200***]

(M0180)   Inpatient Discharge Date (most recent):
_ _/_ _/_ _ _ _
month   day   year

☐ UK -   Unknown

629

(M0190)   Inpatient Diagnoses and ICD-9-CM code categories (three digits required; five digits optional) <u>for only those conditions treated during an inpatient facility stay within the last 14 days</u> (no surgical or V-codes):

<u>Inpatient Facility Diagnosis</u>   <u>ICD-9-CM</u>

a. _____   (__ __ __.__ __)

b. _____   (__ __ __.__ __)

Effective 10/1/2003

List each Inpatient Diagnosis and ICD-9-CM code at the level of highest specificity for only those conditions treated during an inpatient stay within the last 14 days (no surgical, E-codes, or V-codes):

<u>Inpatient Facility Diagnosis</u>   <u>ICD-9-CM</u>

a. _____   (__ __ __.__ __)

b. _____   (__ __ __.__ __)

(M0200)   Medical or Treatment Regimen Change Within Past 14 Days: Has this patient experienced a change in medical or treatment regimen (e.g., medication, treatment, or service change due to new or additional diagnosis, etc.) within the past 14 days?

☐   0 - No   **[If No, go to *M0220*]**

☐   1 - Yes

(M0210)   List the patients Medical Diagnoses and ICD-9-CM code categories (three digits required; five digits optional) <u>for those conditions requiring changed medical or treatment regimen</u> (no surgical or V-codes):

<u>Changed Medical Regimen Diagnosis</u>   <u>ICD-9-CM</u>

a. _____   (__ __ __.__ __)

b. _____   (__ __ __.__ __)

c. _____   (__ __ __.__ __)

d. _____   (__ __ __.__ __)

Effective 10/1/2003

List the patient's Medical Diagnoses and ICD-9-CM codes at the level of highest specificity for those conditions requiring changed medical or treatment regimen (no surgical, E-codes, or V-codes):

<u>Changed Medical Regimen Diagnosis</u>   <u>ICD-9-CM</u>

a. _____   (__ __ __.__ __)

b. _____   (__ __ __.__ __)

c. _____   (__ __ __.__ __)

d. _____   (__ __ __.__ __)

(M0220)   Conditions Prior to Medical or Treatment Regimen Change or Inpatient Stay Within Past 14 Days: If this patient experienced an inpatient facility discharge or change in medical or treatment regimen within the past 14 days, indicate any conditions which existed <u>prior to</u> the inpatient stay or change in medical or treatment regimen. **(Mark all that apply.)**

☐   1   -   Urinary incontinence

☐   2   -   Indwelling/suprapubic catheter

☐   3   -   Intractable pain

☐   4   -   Impaired decision-making

☐   5   -   Disruptive or socially inappropriate behavior

☐   6   -   Memory loss to the extent that supervision required

☐   7   -   None of the above

☐ NA   -   No inpatient facility discharge <u>and</u> no change in medical or treatment regimen in past 14 days

☐ UK   -   Unknown

(M0230/M0240)   Diagnoses and Severity Index: List each medical diagnosis or problem for which the patient is receiving home care and ICD-9-CM code category (three digits required; five digits optional—no surgical or V-codes) and rate them using the following severity index. (Choose one value that represents the most severe rating appropriate for each diagnosis). ICD-9-CM sequencing requirements must be followed if multiple coding is indicated for any diagnoses.

Effective 10/1/2003

List each diagnosis and ICD-9-CM code at the level of highest specificity (no surgical codes) for which the patient is receiving home care. Rate each condition using the following severity index. (Choose one value that represents the most severe rating appropriate for each diagnosis.) E-codes (for M0240 only) or V-codes (for M0230 or M0240) may be used. ICD-9-CM sequencing requirements must be followed if multiple coding is indicated for any diagnoses. If a V-code is reported in place of a case mix diagnosis, then M0245 Payment Diagnosis should be completed. Case mix diagnosis is primary or first secondary diagnosis that determines the Medicare PPS case mix group.

Severity Rating

0 - Asymptomatic, no treatment needed at this time
1 - Symptoms well controlled with current therapy
2 - Symptoms controlled with difficulty, affecting daily functioning; patient needs ongoing monitoring
3 - Symptoms poorly controlled, patient needs frequent adjustment in treatment and dose monitoring
4 - Symptoms poorly controlled, history of rehospitalizations

	(M0230) Primary Diagnosis	ICD-9-CM	Severity Rating
a.	_____	(__ __ __.__ __)	☐0 ☐1 ☐2 ☐3 ☐4

	(M0240) Other Diagnoses	ICD-9-CM	Severity Rating
b.	_____	(■__ __ __.__ __)	☐0 ☐1 ☐2 ☐3 ☐4
c.	_____	(■__ __ __.__ __)	☐0 ☐1 ☐2 ☐3 ☐4
d.	_____	(■__ __ __.__ __)	☐0 ☐1 ☐2 ☐3 ☐4
e.	_____	(■__ __ __.__ __)	☐0 ☐1 ☐2 ☐3 ☐4
f.	_____	(■__ __ __.__ __)	☐0 ☐1 ☐2 ☐3 ☐4

Effective 10/1/2003

(M0245)   Payment Diagnosis (optional): If a V-code was reported in M0230 in place of a case mix diagnosis, list the primary diagnosis and ICD-9-CM code, determined in accordance with OASIS requirements in effect before October 1, 2003–no V-codes, E-codes, or surgical codes allowed. ICD-9-CM sequencing requirements must be followed. Complete both lines (a) and (b) if the case mix diagnosis is a manifestation code or in other situations where multiple coding is indicated for the primary diagnosis; otherwise, complete line (a) only.

	(M0245) Primary Diagnosis	ICD-9-CM
a.	_____	(__ __ __.__ __)
	(M0245) First Secondary Diagnosis	ICD-9-CM
b.	_____	(__ __ __.__ __)

(M0250)   Therapies the patient receives <u>at home</u>: **(Mark all that apply.)**

☐   1 - Intravenous or infusion therapy (excludes TPN)
☐   2 - Parenteral nutrition (TPN or lipids)
☐   3 - Enteral nutrition (nasogastric, gastrostomy, jejunostomy, or any other artificial entry into the alimentary canal)
☐   4 - None of the above

(M0260)   Overall Prognosis: BEST description of patient's overall prognosis for <u>recovery from this episode of illness</u>.

☐   0   - Poor: little or no recovery is expected and/or further decline is imminent
☐   1   - Good/Fair: partial to full recovery is expected
☐ UK - Unknown

(M0270)   Rehabilitative Prognosis: BEST description of patient's prognosis for <u>functional status</u>.

☐   0   - Guarded: minimal improvement in functional status is expected; decline is possible
☐   1   - Good: marked improvement in functional status is expected
☐ UK - Unknown

(M0280)   Life Expectancy: (Physician documentation is not required.)

☐   0   - Life expectancy is greater than 6 months
☐   1   - Life expectancy is 6 months or fewer

(M0290)   High-Risk Factors characterizing this patient: **(Mark all that apply.)**

☐   1   - Heavy smoking
☐   2   - Obesity
☐   3   - Alcohol dependency
☐   4   - Drug dependency
☐   5   - None of the above
☐ UK - Unknown

LIVING ARRANGEMENTS

(M0300)   Current Residence:

☐   1   - Patient's owned or rented residence (house, apartment, or mobile home owned or rented by patient/couple/significant other)
☐   2   - Family member's residence
☐   3   - Boarding home or rented room
☐   4   - Board and care or assisted living facility
☐   5 - Other (specify) _____

(M0340)   **Patient Lives With: (Mark all that apply.)**

- ☐   1 -   Lives alone
- ☐   2 -   With spouse or significant other
- ☐   3 -   With other family member
- ☐   4 -   With a friend
- ☐   5 -   With paid help (other than home care agency staff)
- ☐   6 -   With other than above

SUPPORTIVE ASSISTANCE

(M0350)   **Assisting Persons(s) Other than Home Care Agency Staff: (Mark all that apply.)**

- ☐   1 -   Relatives, friends, or neighbors living outside the home
- ☐   2 -   Person residing in the home (EXCLUDING paid help)
- ☐   3 -   Paid help
- ☐   4 -   None of the above **[If None of the above, go to *M0390*]**
- ☐ UK -   Unknown **[If Unknown, go to *M0390*]**

(M0360)   **Primary Caregiver** taking <u>lead</u> responsibility for providing or managing the patient's care, providing the most frequent assistance, etc. (other than home care agency staff):

- ☐   0 -   No one person **[If No one person, go to *M0390*]**
- ☐   1 -   Spouse or significant other
- ☐   2 -   Daughter or son
- ☐   3 -   Other family member
- ☐   4 -   Friend or neighbor or community or church member
- ☐   5 -   Paid help
- ☐ UK -   Unknown **[If Unknown, go to *M0390*]**

(M0370)   **How Often** does the patient receive assistance from the primary caregiver?

- ☐   1 -   Several times during day and night
- ☐   2 -   Several times during day
- ☐   3 -   Once daily
- ☐   4 -   Three or more times per week
- ☐   5 -   One to two times per week
- ☐   6 -   Less often than weekly
- ☐ UK -   Unknown

(M0380)   **Type of Primary Caregiver Assistance: (Mark all that apply.)**

- ☐   1 -   ADL assistance (e.g., bathing, dressing, toileting, bowel/bladder, eating/feeding)
- ☐   2 -   IADL assistance (e.g., meds, meals, housekeeping, laundry, telephone, shopping, finances)
- ☐   3 -   Environmental support (housing, home maintenance)
- ☐   4 -   Psychosocial support (socialization, companionship, recreation)
- ☐   5 -   Advocates or facilitates patient's participation in appropriate medical care
- ☐   6 -   Financial agent, power of attorney, or conservator of finance
- ☐   7 -   Health care agent, conservator of person, or medical power of attorney
- ☐ UK -   Unknown

SENSORY STATUS

(M0390)   **Vision** with corrective lenses if the patient usually wears them:

- ☐   0 -   Normal vision: sees adequately in most situations; can see medication labels, newsprint.
- ☐   1 -   Partially impaired: cannot see medication labels or newsprint, but <u>can</u> see obstacles in path, and the surrounding layout; can count fingers at arm's length.
- ☐   2 -   Severely impaired: cannot locate objects without hearing or touching them <u>or</u> patient nonresponsive.

(M0400)   **Hearing and Ability to Understand Spoken Language** in patient's own language (with hearing aids if the patient usually uses them):

- ☐   0 -   No observable impairment. Able to hear and understand complex or detailed instructions and extended or abstract conversation.
- ☐   1 -   With minimal difficulty, able to hear and understand most multistep instructions and ordinary conversation. May need occasional repetition, extra time, or louder voice.
- ☐   2 -   Has moderate difficulty hearing and understanding simple, one-step instructions and brief conversation; needs frequent prompting or assistance.
- ☐   3 -   Has severe difficulty hearing and understanding simple greetings and short comments. Requires multiple repetitions, restatements, demonstrations, additional time.
- ☐   4 -   <u>Unable</u> to hear and understand familiar words or common expressions consistently, <u>or</u> patient nonresponsive.

(M0410)   Speech and Oral (Verbal) Expression of Language (in patient's own language):

- ☐ 0 - Expresses complex ideas, feelings, and needs clearly, completely, and easily in all situations with no observable impairment.
- ☐ 1 - Minimal difficulty in expressing ideas and needs (may take extra time; makes occasional errors in word choice, grammar or speech intelligibility; needs minimal prompting or assistance).
- ☐ 2 - Expresses simple ideas or needs with moderate difficulty (needs prompting or assistance, errors in word choice, organization or speech intelligibility). Speaks in phrases or short sentences.
- ☐ 3 - Has severe difficulty expressing basic ideas or needs and requires maximal assistance or guessing by listener. Speech limited to single words or short phrases.
- ☐ 4 - <u>Unable</u> to express basic needs even with maximal prompting or assistance but is not comatose or unresponsive (e.g., speech is nonsensical or unintelligible).
- ☐ 5 - Patient nonresponsive or unable to speak.

(M0420)   Frequency of Pain interfering with patient's activity or movement:

- ☐ 0 - Patient has no pain or pain does not interfere with activity or movement
- ☐ 1 - Less often than daily
- ☐ 2 - Daily, but not constantly
- ☐ 3 - All of the time

(M0430)   Intractable Pain: Is the patient experiencing pain that is <u>not easily relieved</u>, occurs at least daily, and affects the patient's sleep, appetite, physical or emotional energy, concentration, personal relationships, emotions, or ability or desire to perform physical activity?

- ☐ 0 - No
- ☐ 1 - Yes

INTEGUMENTARY STATUS

(M0440)   Does this patient have a **Skin Lesion** or an **Open Wound**? This excludes "OSTOMIES."

- ☐ 0 - No **[If No, go to *M0490*]**
- ☐ 1 - Yes

(M0445)   Does this patient have a **Pressure Ulcer**?

- ☐ 0 - No **[If No, go to *M0468*]**
- ☐ 1 - Yes

(M0450)   Current Number of Pressure Ulcers at Each Stage: (Circle one response for each stage.)

Pressure Ulcer Stages	Number of Pressure Ulcers				
a) Stage 1: Nonblanchable erythema of intact skin; the heralding of skin ulceration. In darker-pigmented skin, warmth, edema, hardness, or discolored skin may be indicators.	0	1	2	3	4 or more
b) Stage 2: Partial thickness skin loss involving epidermis and/or dermis. The ulcer is superficial and presents clinically as an abrasion, blister, or shallow crater.	0	1	2	3	4 or more
c) Stage 3: Full-thickness skin loss involving damage or necrosis of subcutaneous tissue which may extend down more to, but not through, underlying fascia. The ulcer presents clinically as a deep crater with or without undermining of adjacent tissue.	0	1	2	3	4 or more
d) Stage 4: Full-thickness skin loss with extensive destruction, tissue necrosis, or damage to muscle, bone, or supporting more structures (e.g., tendon, joint capsule, etc.)	0	1	2	3	4 or more
e) In addition to the above, is there at least one pressure ulcer that cannot be observed due to the presence of eschar or a nonremovable dressing, including casts? ☐ 0 - No ☐ 1 - Yes					

(M0460)   **Stage of Most Problematic (Observable) Pressure Ulcer:**

     ☐   1 - Stage 1
     ☐   2 - Stage 2
     ☐   3 - Stage 3
     ☐   4 - Stage 4
     ☐   NA - No observable pressure ulcer

(M0464)   **Status of Most Problematic (Observable) Pressure Ulcer:**

     ☐   1 - Fully granulating
     ☐   2 - Early/partial granulation
     ☐   3 - Not healing
     ☐   NA - No observable pressure ulcer

(M0468)   Does this patient have a **Stasis Ulcer?**

   ☐   0 - No **[If No, go to *M0482*]**
   ☐   1 - Yes

(M0470)   **Current Number of Observable Stasis Ulcer(s):**

     ☐   0 - Zero
     ☐   1 - One
     ☐   2 - Two
     ☐   3 - Three
     ☐   4 - Four or more

(M0474)   Does this patient have at least one **Stasis Ulcer that Cannot be Observed** due to the presence of a nonremovable dressing?

     ☐   0 - No
     ☐   1 - Yes

(M0476)   **Status of Most Problematic (Observable) Stasis Ulcer:**

     ☐   1 - Fully granulating
     ☐   2 - Early/partial granulation
     ☐   3 - Not healing
     ☐   NA - No observable stasis ulcer

(M0482)   Does this patient have a **Surgical Wound?**

   ☐   0 - No **[If No, go to *M0490*]**
   ☐   1 - Yes

(M0484)   **Current Number of (Observable) Surgical Wounds:** (If a wound is partially closed but has <u>more</u> than one opening, consider each opening as a separate wound.)

     ☐   0 - Zero
     ☐   1 - One
     ☐   2 - Two
     ☐   3 - Three
     ☐   4 - Four or more

(M0486)   Does this patient have at least one **Surgical Wound that Cannot be Observed** due to the presence of a nonremovable dressing?

     ☐   0 - No
     ☐   1 - Yes

(M0488)   **Status of Most Problematic (Observable) Surgical Wound:**

     ☐   1 - Fully granulating
     ☐   2 - Early/partial granulation
     ☐   3 - Not healing
     ☐   NA - No observable surgical wound

RESPIRATORY STATUS

(M0490)   When is the patient dyspneic or noticeably **Short of Breath?**

   ☐   0 - Never, patient is not short of breath
   ☐   1 - When walking more than 20 feet, climbing stairs
   ☐   2 - With moderate exertion (e.g., while dressing, using commode or bedpan, walking distances less than 20 feet)
   ☐   3 - With minimal exertion (e.g., while eating, talking, or performing other ADLs) or with agitation
   ☐   4 - At rest (during day or night)

(M0500)   **Respiratory Treatments** utilized at home: **(Mark all that apply.)**

   ☐   1 - Oxygen (intermittent or continuous)
   ☐   2 - Ventilator (continually or at night)
   ☐   3 - Continuous positive airway pressure
   ☐   4 - None of the above

ELIMINATION STATUS

(M0510)   Has this patient been treated for a **Urinary Tract Infection** in the past 14 days?

- ☐   0 - No
- ☐   1 - Yes
- ☐ NA - Patient on prophylactic treatment
- ☐ UK - Unknown

(M0520)   Urinary Incontinence or Urinary Catheter Presence:

- ☐   0 - No incontinence or catheter (includes anuria or ostomy for urinary drainage) **[If No, go to *M0540*]**
- ☐   1 - Patient is incontinent
- ☐   2 - Patient requires a urinary catheter (i.e., external, indwelling, intermittent, suprapubic) **[Go to *M0540*]**

(M0530)   When does Urinary Incontinence occur?

- ☐   0 - Timed-voiding defers incontinence
- ☐   1 - During the night only
- ☐   2 - During the day and night

(M0540)   Bowel Incontinence Frequency:

- ☐   0 - Very rarely or never has bowel incontinence
- ☐   1 - Less than once weekly
- ☐   2 - One to three times weekly
- ☐   3 - Four to six times weekly
- ☐   4 - On a daily basis
- ☐   5 - More often than once daily
- ☐ NA - Patient has ostomy for bowel elimination
- ☐ UK - Unknown

(M0550)   Ostomy for Bowel Elimination: Does this patient have an ostomy for bowel elimination that (within the last 14 days): a) was related to an inpatient facility stay, <u>or</u> b) necessitated a change in medical or treatment regimen?

- ☐   0 - Patient does <u>not</u> have an ostomy for bowel elimination.
- ☐   1 - Patient's ostomy was <u>not</u> related to an inpatient stay and did <u>not</u> necessitate change in medical or treatment regimen.
- ☐   2 - The ostomy <u>was</u> related to an inpatient stay or <u>did</u> necessitate change in medical or treatment regimen.

NEURO/EMOTIONAL/BEHAVIORAL STATUS

(M0560)   Cognitive Functioning: (Patient's current level of alertness, orientation, comprehension, concentration, and immediate memory for simple commands.)

- ☐   0 - Alert/oriented, able to focus and shift attention, comprehends and recalls task directions independently.
- ☐   1 - Requires prompting (cuing, repetition, reminders) only under stressful or unfamiliar conditions.
- ☐   2 - Requires assistance and some direction in specific situations (e.g., on all tasks involving shifting of attention), or consistently requires low stimulus environment due to distractibility.
- ☐   3 - Requires considerable assistance in routine situations. Is not alert and oriented or is unable to shift attention and recall directions more than half the time.
- ☐   4 - Totally dependent due to disturbances such as constant disorientation, coma, persistent vegetative state, or delirium.

(M0570)   When Confused (Reported or Observed):

- ☐   0 - Never
- ☐   1 - In new or complex situations only
- ☐   2 - On awakening or at night only
- ☐   3 - During the day and evening, but not constantly
- ☐   4 - Constantly
- ☐ NA - Patient nonresponsive

(M0580)   When Anxious (Reported or Observed):

- ☐   0 - None of the time
- ☐   1 - Less often than daily
- ☐   2 - Daily, but not constantly
- ☐   3 - All of the time
- ☐ NA - Patient nonresponsive

(M0590) Depressive Feelings Reported or Observed in Patient: (Mark all that apply.)

- ☐   1 - Depressed mood (e.g., feeling sad, tearful)
- ☐   2 - Sense of failure or self-reproach
- ☐   3 - Hopelessness
- ☐   4 - Recurrent thoughts of death
- ☐   5 - Thoughts of suicide
- ☐   6 - None of the above feelings observed or reported

(M0610)   **Behaviors Demonstrated <u>at Least Once a Week</u> (Reported or Observed): (Mark all that apply.)**

☐   1 -   Memory deficit: failure to recognize familiar persons/places, inability to recall events of past 24 hours, significant memory loss so that supervision is required

☐   2 -   Impaired decision-making: failure to perform usual ADLs or IADLs, inability to appropriately stop activities, jeopardizes safety through actions

☐   3 -   Verbal disruption: yelling, threatening, excessive profanity, sexual references, etc.

☐   4 -   Physical aggression: aggressive or combative to self and others (e.g., hits self, throws objects, punches, dangerous maneuvers with wheelchair or other objects)

☐   5 -   Disruptive, infantile, or socially inappropriate behavior (**excludes** verbal actions)

☐   6 -   Delusional, hallucinatory, or paranoid behavior

☐   7 -   None of the above behaviors demonstrated

(M0620)   **Frequency of Behavior Problems (Reported or Observed)** (e.g., wandering episodes, self-abuse, verbal disruption, physical aggression, etc.):

☐   0 -   Never

☐   1 -   Less than once a month

☐   2 -   Once a month

☐   3 -   Several times each month

☐   4 -   Several times a week

☐   5 -   At least daily

(M0630)   Is this patient receiving **Psychiatric Nursing Services** at home provided by a qualified psychiatric nurse?

☐   0 -   No

☐   1 -   Yes

ADL/IADLS

> **For M0640–M0800, complete the "Current" column for all patients. For these same items, complete the "Prior" column only at start of care and at resumption of care; mark the level that corresponds to the patient's condition 14 days prior to start of care date (M0030) or resumption of care date (M0032). In all cases record what the patient is *able to do*.**

(M0640)   **Grooming:** Ability to tend to personal hygiene needs (i.e., washing face and hands, hair care, shaving or make up, teeth or denture care, fingernail care).

Prior   Current

☐   ☐   0 -   Able to groom self unaided, with or without the use of assistive devices or adapted methods.

☐   ☐   1 -   Grooming utensils must be placed within reach before able to complete grooming activities.

☐   ☐   2 -   Someone must assist the patient to groom self.

☐   ☐   3 -   Patient depends entirely upon someone else for grooming needs.

☐   UK -   Unknown

(M0650)   **Ability to Dress <u>Upper</u> Body** (with or without dressing aids) including undergarments, pullovers, front-opening shirts and blouses, managing zippers, buttons, and snaps:

Prior   Current

☐   ☐   0 -   Able to get clothes out of closets and drawers, put them on and remove them from the upper body without assistance.

☐   ☐   1 -   Able to dress upper body without assistance if clothing is laid out or handed to the patient.

☐   ☐   2 -   Someone must help the patient put on upper body clothing.

☐   ☐   3 -   Patient depends entirely upon another person to dress the upper body.

☐   UK -   Unknown

(M0660)   **Ability to Dress <u>Lower</u> Body** (with or without dressing aids) including undergarments, slacks, socks or nylons, shoes:

Prior   Current

☐   ☐   0 -   Able to obtain, put on, and remove clothing and shoes without assistance.

☐   ☐   1 -   Able to dress lower body without assistance if clothing and shoes are laid out or handed to the patient.

☐   ☐   2 -   Someone must help the patient put on undergarments, slacks, socks or nylons, and shoes.

☐   ☐   3 -   Patient depends entirely upon another person to dress lower body.

☐   UK -   Unknown

(M0670)   **Bathing:** Ability to wash entire body. **Excludes** grooming (washing face and hands only).

Prior   Current

☐   ☐   0 -   Able to bathe self in <u>shower or tub</u> independently.

☐   ☐   1 -   With the use of devices, is able to bathe self in shower or tub independently.

☐   ☐   2 -   Able to bathe in shower or tub with the assistance of another person:

         (a)   for intermittent supervision or encouragement or reminders, <u>OR</u>

         (b)   to get in and out of the shower or tub, <u>OR</u>

         (c)   for washing difficult to reach areas.

☐   ☐   3 -   Participates in bathing self in shower or tub, <u>but</u> requires presence of another person throughout the bath for assistance or supervision.

☐   ☐   4 -   <u>Unable</u> to use the shower or tub and is bathed in <u>bed or bedside chair.</u>

☐   ☐   5 -   Unable to effectively participate in bathing and is totally bathed by another person.

☐   UK -   Unknown

(M0680)   Toileting: Ability to get to and from the toilet or bedside commode.

Prior	Current			
☐	☐	0	-	Able to get to and from the toilet independently with or without a device.
☐	☐	1	-	When reminded, assisted, or supervised by another person, able to get to and from the toilet.
☐	☐	2	-	<u>Unable</u> to get to and from the toilet but is able to use a bedside commode (with or without assistance).
☐	☐	3	-	<u>Unable</u> to get to and from the toilet or bedside commode but is able to use a bedpan/urinal independently.
☐	☐	4	-	Is totally dependent in toileting.
☐		UK	-	Unknown

(M0690)   Transferring: Ability to move from bed to chair, on and off toilet or commode, into and out of tub or shower, and ability to turn and position self in bed if patient is bedfast.

Prior	Current			
☐	☐	0	-	Able to independently transfer.
☐	☐	1	-	Transfers with minimal human assistance or with use of an assistive device.
☐	☐	2	-	<u>Unable</u> to transfer self but is able to bear weight and pivot during the transfer process.
☐	☐	3	-	<u>Unable</u> to transfer self and is <u>unable</u> to bear weight or pivot when transferred by another person.
☐	☐	4	-	Bedfast, unable to transfer but is able to turn and position self in bed.
☐	☐	5	-	Bedfast, unable to transfer and is <u>unable</u> to turn and position self.
☐		UK	-	Unknown

(M0700)   Ambulation/Locomotion: Ability to <u>SAFELY</u> walk, once in a standing position, <u>or</u> use a wheelchair, once in a seated position, on a variety of surfaces.

Prior	Current			
☐	☐	0	-	Able to independently walk on even and uneven surfaces and climb stairs with or without railings (i.e., needs no human assistance or assistive device).
☐	☐	1	-	Requires use of a device (e.g., cane, walker) to walk alone <u>or</u> requires human supervision or assistance to negotiate stairs or steps or uneven surfaces.
☐	☐	2	-	Able to walk only with the supervision or assistance of another person at all times.
☐	☐	3	-	Chairfast, <u>unable</u> to ambulate but is able to wheel self independently.
☐	☐	4	-	Chairfast, unable to ambulate and is <u>unable</u> to wheel self.
☐	☐	5	-	Bedfast, unable to ambulate or be up in a chair.
☐		UK	-	Unknown

(M0710)   Feeding or Eating: Ability to feed self meals and snacks. **Note: This refers only to the process of <u>eating</u>, <u>chewing</u>, and <u>swallowing</u>, <u>not</u> preparing the food to be eaten.**

Prior	Current			
☐	☐	0	-	Able to independently feed self.
☐	☐	1	-	Able to feed self independently but requires:
				(a) meal set-up; <u>OR</u>
				(b) intermittent assistance or supervision from another person; <u>OR</u>
				(c) a liquid, pureed or ground meat diet.
☐	☐	2	-	<u>Unable</u> to feed self and must be assisted or supervised throughout the meal/snack.
☐	☐	3	-	Able to taken in nutrients orally <u>and</u> receives supplemental nutrients through a nasogastric tube or gastrostomy.
☐	☐	4	-	<u>Unable</u> to take in nutrients orally and is fed nutrients through a nasogastric tube or gastrostomy.
☐	☐	5	-	Unable to take in nutrients orally or by tube feeding.
☐		UK	-	Unknown

(M0720)   Planning and Preparing Light Meals (e.g., cereal, sandwich) or reheat delivered meals:

Prior	Current			
☐	☐	0	-	(a) Able to independently plan and prepare all light meals for self or reheat delivered meals; <u>OR</u>
				(b) Is physically, cognitively, and mentally able to prepare light meals on a regular basis but has not routinely performed light meal preparation in the past (i.e., prior to this home care admission).
☐	☐	1	-	<u>Unable</u> to prepare light meals on a regular basis due to physical, cognitive, or mental limitations.
☐	☐	2	-	Unable to prepare any light meals or reheat any delivered meals.
☐		UK	-	Unknown

(M0730)   Transportation: Physical and mental ability to <u>safely</u> use a car, taxi, or public transportation (bus, train, subway).

Prior	Current			
☐	☐	0	-	Able to independently drive a regular or adapted car; <u>OR</u> uses a regular or handicap-accessible public bus.
☐	☐	1	-	Able to ride in a car only when driven by another person; <u>OR</u> able to use a bus or handicap van only when assisted or accompanied by another person.
☐	☐	2	-	<u>Unable</u> to ride in a car, taxi, bus, or van, and requires transportation by ambulance.
☐		UK	-	Unknown

Appendixes

(M0740) **Laundry:** Ability to do own laundry—to carry laundry to and from washing machine, to use washer and dryer, to wash small items by hand.

Prior Current

☐ ☐ 0 - (a) Able to independently take care of all laundry tasks; OR
         (b) Physically, cognitively, and mentally able to do laundry and access facilities, but has not routinely performed laundry tasks in the past (i.e., prior to this home care admission).

☐ ☐ 1 - Able to do only light laundry, such as minor hand wash or light washer loads. Due to physical, cognitive, or mental limitations, needs assistance with heavy laundry such as carrying large loads of laundry.

☐ ☐ 2 - Unable to do any laundry due to physical limitation or needs continual supervision and assistance due to cognitive or mental limitation.

☐   UK - Unknown

(M0750) **Housekeeping:** Ability to safely and effectively perform light housekeeping and heavier cleaning tasks.

Prior Current

☐ ☐ 0 - (a) Able to independently perform all housekeeping tasks; OR
         (b) Physically, cognitively, and mentally able to perform all housekeeping tasks but has not routinely participated in housekeeping tasks in the past (i.e., prior to this home care admission).

☐ ☐ 1 - Able to perform only light housekeeping (e.g., dusting, wiping kitchen counters) tasks independently.

☐ ☐ 2 - Able to perform housekeeping tasks with intermittent assistance or supervision from another person.

☐ ☐ 3 - Unable to consistently perform any housekeeping tasks unless assisted by another person throughout the process.

☐ ☐ 4 - Unable to effectively participate in any housekeeping tasks.

☐   UK - Unknown

(M0760) **Shopping:** Ability to plan for, select, and purchase items in a store and to carry them home or arrange delivery.

Prior Current

☐ ☐ 0 - (a) Able to plan for shopping needs and independently perform shopping tasks, including carrying packages; OR
         (b) Physically, cognitively, and mentally able to take care of shopping, but has not done shopping in the past (i.e., prior to this home care admission).

☐ ☐ 1 - Able to go shopping, but needs some assistance:
         (a) By self is able to do only light shopping and carry small packages, but needs someone to do occasional major shopping; OR
         (b) Unable to go shopping alone, but can go with someone to assist.

☐ ☐ 2 - Unable to go shopping, but is able to identify items needed, place orders, and arrange home delivery.

☐ ☐ 3 - Needs someone to do all shopping and errands.

☐   UK - Unknown

(M0770) **Ability to Use Telephone:** Ability to answer the phone, dial numbers, and effectively use the telephone to communicate.

Prior Current

☐ ☐ 0 - Able to dial numbers and answer calls appropriately and as desired.

☐ ☐ 1 - Able to use a specially adapted telephone (i.e., large numbers on the dial, teletype phone for the deaf) and call essential numbers.

☐ ☐ 2 - Able to answer the telephone and carry on a normal conversation but has difficulty with placing calls.

☐ ☐ 3 - Able to answer the telephone only some of the time or is able to carry on only a limited conversation.

☐ ☐ 4 - Unable to answer the telephone at all but can listen if assisted with equipment.

☐ ☐ 5 - Totally unable to use the telephone.

☐ ☐ NA - Patient does not have a telephone.

☐   UK - Unknown

MEDICATIONS

(M0780) **Management of Oral Medications:** Patient's ability to prepare and take all prescribed oral medications reliably and safely, including administration of the correct dosage at the appropriate times/intervals. **Excludes injectable and IV medications. (NOTE: This refers to ability, not compliance or willingness.)**

Prior Current

☐ ☐ 0 - Able to independently take the correct oral medication(s) and proper dosage(s) at the correct times.

☐ ☐ 1 - Able to take medication(s) at the correct times if:
         (a) individual dosages are prepared in advance by another person; OR
         (b) given daily reminders; OR
         (c) someone develops a drug diary or chart.

☐ ☐ 2 - Unable to take medication unless administered by someone else.

☐ ☐ NA - No oral medications prescribed.

☐   UK - Unknown

(M0790) **Management of Inhalant/Mist Medications:** Patient's ability to prepare and take all prescribed inhalant/mist medications (nebulizers, metered dose devices) reliably and safely, including administration of the correct dosage at the appropriate times/intervals. **Excludes all other forms of medication (oral tablets, injectable and IV medications).**

Prior Current

☐ ☐ 0 - Able to independently take the correct medication and proper dosage at the correct times.

☐ ☐ 1 - Able to take medication at the correct times if:
         (a) individual dosages are prepared in advance by another person, OR
         (b) given daily reminders.

☐ ☐ 2 - Unable to take medication unless administered by someone else.

☐ ☐ NA - No inhalant/mist medications prescribed

☐   UK - Unknown

(M0800)   Management of Injectable Medications: <u>Patient's ability</u> to prepare and take <u>all</u> prescribed injectable medications reliably and safely, including administration of correct dosage at the appropriate times/intervals. <u>**Excludes**</u> **IV medications.**

Prior	Current			
☐	☐	0	-	Able to independently take the correct medication and proper dosage at the correct times.
☐	☐	1	-	Able to take injectable medication at correct times if:
				(a) individual syringes are prepared in advance by another person, <u>OR</u>
				(b) given daily reminders.
☐	☐	2	-	<u>Unable</u> to take injectable medications unless administered by someone else.
☐	☐	NA	-	No injectable medications prescribed.
☐		UK	-	Unknown

EQUIPMENT MANAGEMENT

(M0810)   Patient Management of Equipment (includes <u>ONLY</u> oxygen, IV/infusion therapy, enteral/parenteral nutrition equipment or supplies): <u>Patient's ability</u> to set up, monitor and change equipment reliably and safely, add appropriate fluids or medication, clean/store/dispose of equipment or supplies using proper technique. **(NOTE: This refers to ability, not compliance or willingness.)**

- ☐   0 - Patient manages all tasks related to equipment completely independently.
- ☐   1 - If someone else sets up equipment (i.e., fills portable oxygen tank, provides patient with prepared solutions), patient is able to manage all other aspects of equipment.
- ☐   2 - Patient requires considerable assistance from another person to manage equipment, but independently completes portions of the task.
- ☐   3 - Patient is only able to monitor equipment (e.g., liter flow, fluid in bag) and must call someone else to manage the equipment.
- ☐   4 - Patient is completely dependent on someone else to manage all equipment.
- ☐   NA - No equipment of this type used in care **[If NA, go to** *M0825***]**

(M0820)   Caregiver Management of Equipment (includes <u>ONLY</u> oxygen, IV/infusion equipment, enteral/parenteral nutrition, ventilator therapy equipment or supplies): <u>Caregiver's ability</u> to set up, monitor, and change equipment reliably and safely, add appropriate fluids or medication, clean/store/dispose of equipment or supplies using proper technique. **(NOTE: This refers to ability, not compliance or willingness.)**

- ☐   0 - Caregiver manages all tasks related to equipment completely independently.
- ☐   1 - If someone else sets up equipment, caregiver is able to manage all other aspects.
- ☐   2 - Caregiver requires considerable assistance from another person to manage equipment, but independently completes significant portions of task.
- ☐   3 - Caregiver is only able to complete small portions of task (e.g., administer nebulizer treatment, clean/store/dispose of equipment or supplies).
- ☐   4 - Caregiver is completely dependent on someone else to manage all equipment.
- ☐   NA - No caregiver
- ☐   UK   Unknown

THERAPY NEED

(M0825)   Therapy Need: Does the care plan of the Medicare payment period for which this assessment will define a case mix group indicate a need for therapy (physical, occupational, or speech therapy) that meets the threshold for a Medicare high-therapy case mix group?

- ☐   0 - No
- ☐   1 - Yes
- ☐   NA - Not applicable

Appendixes

B.2 CULTURAL ASSESSMENT GUIDE

There must be an awareness of your own ethnocultural heritage, both as a person and as a nurse. In addition, an awareness and sensitivity must be developed to the health beliefs and practices of a client's heritage. This awareness and sensitivity can be developed through careful assessment of a client's heritage and cultural beliefs. The factors that must be explored during a multicultural nursing assessment are as follows:

CULTURAL IDENTITY/ANCESTRY/HERITAGE
- Place of birth of patient and his or her parents/ancestors
- Reason for immigration

Ethnohistory
- Length of time in the United States
- Age of immigration
- Degree of acculturation

Social Organization
- Living arrangements
- Family composition, definition and degree of contact with family members
- Position in the family hierarchy and decision making
- Social support
- Family roles, expectations of each other, gender-appropriate roles
- Extent of family participation in the care desired

Socioeconomic Status
- Occupation before and after immigration
- Educational attainment
- Type of residence
- Medical insurance
- Primary care provider, other care providers and specialists used

BIOCULTURAL ECOLOGY AND HEALTH RISKS
- Purpose of visit/consultation/hospitalization
- Perceived cause of the problem
- Terms used to describe problem, feelings

- Preponderance of the problem within the family and community
- Folk treatment
- Effect of the problem on self and family
- Expectations of care to be provided
- Presence of health risks

LANGUAGE AND COMMUNICATION
- Languages spoken and written
- Preferred language when speaking and reading
- Need and preference for an interpreter (gender, age, etc.)
- Literacy level and English proficiency

RELIGION/SPIRITUALITY
- Religion, spiritual leader, contact for religious/spiritual leader
- Religious/spiritual needs
- Religious rituals observed
- Dietary practices observed

CARING BELIEFS AND PRACTICES
- Measures to promote health
- Caring practices when sick
- Practices relevant to activities of daily living
- Folk and professional healers sought
- Healing modalities used for problem
- Expectations about care to be given
- Hygiene, dietary, and mobility concerns
- Age and gender considerations
- Beliefs and practices with regard to life transitions

EXPERIENCE WITH PROFESSIONAL HEALTH CARE
- Evaluations of previous experiences
- Attributes of valued caregivers

From Potter PA, Perry AG: *Basic nursing: essentials for practice*, ed 6, St. Louis, 2007, Mosby.

Hepatitis Information

C.1 SUMMARY DESCRIPTION OF HEPATITIS A–E AND G

Type	Definition	Risk	Symptoms	Precautions	Prevention of Spread
A	Liver disease caused by picornavirus; commonly called "infectious hepatitis"	Live in house with infected person Inject drugs Travel internationally to areas with a high prevalence of hepatitis A Eat infected shellfish Consume contaminated food and water	Skin, eye yellowing Loss of appetite Nausea Vomiting Fever Fatigue Diarrhea Stomach/joint pain Unable to work for extended periods	Stricter handwashing by foodhandler Improved sanitary conditions Improved personal hygiene	Immune gamma globulin injections Hepatitis A vaccine
B	A major cause of acute and chronic liver disease that can lead to cirrhosis and hepatocellular cancer; "serum hepatitis"	Exposure to human blood Live with someone who is a carrier Inject drugs Have a sex partner infected with hepatitis B Have sex with more than one partner A child born in Asia, Africa, Amazon, South America, Pacific Islands, or the Middle East	Skin, eye yellowing Loss of appetite Nausea Vomiting Diarrhea Stomach/joint pain No symptoms (carrier) Itching Skin eruptions	Vaccinate: • Babies at birth • Adolescents and others who have sex or inject drugs • Persons whose job places them at risk	Hepatitis B vaccine
C	Virus causing chronic liver disease, found in blood, caused by non-A and non-B hepatitis virus. May develop cirrhosis and liver failure	Drug injection Exposure to human blood Hemodialysis patients Receipt of blood transfusion Multiple sex partners Live with person with hepatitis C	Same as hepatitis B	Do not take blood, organs, tissue, or sperm from person with hepatitis C Do not share toothbrushes, razors, or other items possibly contaminated with blood (including needles) Cover open sores or other skin breaks	Practice safe sex Have only one sex partner Routine screening of blood/other donors

continued

Type	Definition	Risk	Symptoms	Precautions	Prevention of Spread
D	An incomplete virus requiring hepatitis B to be present to cause infection. This results in a more severe acute liver disease, leading to chronic liver disease with cirrhosis	Injection drug users Hemophilia clients Developmentally disabled persons who are hospitalized	Same as hepatitis B	Avoid sexual contact with injection drug users Do not use needle used by others Proper sterilization technique in institutions	Individual screening for hepatitis B Blood screening for hepatitis B and hepatitis D Early vaccination for hepatitis B
E	Enterically transmitted non-A and non-B hepatitis virus. Usually acute and does not usually cause chronic disease	Ingestion of fecally contaminated water Pregnant women International travelers Persons in Asia and Indian countries	Same as hepatitis B	Avoid contaminated waters	None at this time
G	Non-A–E hepatitis virus described as a flavivirus. Present in 1%–2% of blood donors in the United States. Causes acute liver disease	Any intravenous (IV) therapy Injected drugs End-stage renal disease Pregnancy Hemophilia	Same as hepatitis B Liver inflammation Liver failure	Avoid multiple transfusions Avoid IV drug use Check new babies for perinatal transmission Avoid all unnecessary IVs Monitor persons on hemodialysis	Individual screening for hepatitis G virus (HGV) See precautions

Data from Centers for Disease Control and Prevention, Atlanta, 2007, 2008; *Science News* 149(15):238, 1996; National Institutes of Health: HCV International Symposium, June 1999.

C.2   RECOMMENDATIONS FOR PROPHYLAXIS OF HEPATITIS A

General information: Persons who have been exposed to hepatitis A (HAP) recently and who have not been vaccinated should be given a single dose of single-antigen hepatitis A vaccine or immune globulin (IG) (0.02 mL/kg) as soon as possible and within 2 weeks of the exposure. Note: the guidelines vary by age and health status, so consult the Centers for Disease Control and Prevention website under Hepatitis A for specific information. Read below for who requires protection with either IG or hepatitis A vaccine after exposure.

1. *Close personal contacts:* This includes close personal contacts of persons who have been confirmed by a blood test to have hepatitis A and persons in the household including babysitters or caretakers, as well as those with whom the person has sexual contacts or shares illicit drugs.

2. *Day-care centers.* Day care facilities with children in diapers can be important settings for hepatitis A virus (HAV) transmission. IG or hepatitis A vaccine should be administered to all staff and attendees of day care centers or homes if (1) one or more hepatitis A cases are recognized among children or employees, or (2) cases are recognized in two or more households of center attendees. When an outbreak (hepatitis cases in three or more families) occurs, IG or hepatitis A vaccine should also be considered for members of households whose diapered children attend. In centers not enrolling children in diapers, IG need be given only to classroom contacts of an index case.

3. *Schools.* Contact at elementary and secondary schools is usually not an important means of transmitting hepatitis A. Routine administration of IG or hepatitis A vaccine is not indicated for pupils and teachers in contact with a patient. However, when epidemiologic study clearly shows the existence of a school- or classroom-centered outbreak, IG or hepatitis A vaccine may be given to those who have close personal contact with patients.

4. *Institutions for custodial care.* Living conditions in some institutions, such as prisons and facilities for the developmentally disabled, favor transmission of hepatitis A. When outbreaks occur, giving IG or hepatitis A vaccine to residents and staff who have close contact with patients with hepatitis A may reduce the spread of the disease. Depending on the epidemiologic circumstances, prophylaxis can be limited or can involve the entire institution.

5. *Hospitals.* Routine hepatitis A postexposure prophylaxis is not routinely indicated when a single case occurs. Rather, sound hygienic practices should be emphasized. Staff education should point out the risk of exposure to hepatitis A and emphasize precautions regarding direct contact with potentially infective materials. Outbreaks of hepatitis A among hospital staff occur occasionally, usually in association with an unsuspected index patient who is fecally incontinent. Large outbreaks have occurred among staff and family contacts of infected infants in neonatal intensive care units. In outbreaks, prophylaxis of persons exposed to feces of infected patients may be indicated.

6. *Offices and factories.* Routine hepatitis A postexposure prophylaxis is not indicated under the usual office or factory conditions for persons exposed to a fellow worker with hepatitis A. Experience shows that casual contact in the work setting does not result in virus transmission.
7. *Common-source exposure.* IG or hepatitis A vaccine might be effective in preventing foodborne or waterborne hepatitis A if exposure is recognized in time. However, postexposure prophylaxis is not recommended for persons exposed to a common source of hepatitis infection after cases have begun to occur in those exposed, because the 2-week period during which prophylaxis is effective will have been exceeded.

If a food-handler is diagnosed as having hepatitis A, common-source transmission is possible but uncommon. Prophylaxis should be administered to other food-handlers but is usually not recommended for patrons. However, IG or hepatitis A vaccine administration of patrons may be considered if (1) the infected person is directly involved in handling, without gloves, foods that will not be cooked before they are eaten; (2) the hygienic practices of the food-handler are deficient; and (3) patrons can be identified and treated within 2 weeks of exposure. Situations in which repeated exposures may have occurred, such as in institutional cafeterias, may warrant stronger consideration of IG or hepatitis A vaccine use.

C.3   RECOMMENDED POSTEXPOSURE PROPHYLAXIS FOR PERCUTANEOUS OR PERMUCOSAL EXPOSURE TO HEPATITIS B VIRUS

Vaccination and Antibody Response Status of Exposed Person	HBsAg-Positive Source	HBsAg-Negative Source	Source Not Tested or Status Unknown
Unvaccinated	HBIG × 1; initiate hepatitis B vaccine series	Initiate hepatitis B vaccine series	Initiate hepatitis B vaccine series
Previously vaccinated			
Known responder*	No treatment	No treatment	No treatment
Known nonresponder	HBIG × 2 or HBIG × 1 and initiate revaccination	No treatment	If known high-risk source, treat as if source were HBsAg positive
Antibody response unknown	Test exposed person for anti-HBs 1. If adequate,* no treatment 2. If inadequate,* HBIG × 1 and vaccine booster	No treatment	Test exposed person for anti-HBs 1. If adequate,* no treatment 2. If inadequate,* initiate revaccination

Centers for Disease Control and Prevention: Update: prevention of hepatitis A after exposure to hepatitis A virus and in international travelers. Updated recommendations of the advisory committee on immunization practices (ACIP), *MMWR Morb Mortal Wkly Rev* 56(41):1080–1084, 2007.
*Responder is defined as a person with adequate levels of serum antibody to hepatitis B surface antigen (e.g., anti-HBs >10 mIU/ml); inadequate response to vaccination defined as serum anti-HBs <10 mIU/ml.
HBsAg, Hepatitis B surface antigen; *HBIG,* hepatitis B immune globulin; dose 0.06 ml/kg intramuscularly; *anti-HBs,* antibody to hepatitis B surface.

Immunization Information

D.1 RECOMMENDED IMMUNIZATION SCHEDULE FOR PERSONS AGED 0 THROUGH 6 YEARS—UNITED STATES • 2009

For those who fall behind or start late, see the catch-up schedule

Vaccine ▼ Age ▶	Birth	1 month	2 months	4 months	6 months	12 months	15 months	18 months	19–23 months	2–3 years	4–6 years
Hepatitis B[1]	HepB	HepB		*see footnote 1*		HepB					
Rotavirus[2]			RV	RV	*RV*[2]						
Diphtheria, Tetanus, Pertussis[3]			DTaP	DTaP	DTaP	*see footnote 3*	DTaP				DTaP
Haemophilus influenzae type b[4]			Hib	Hib	*Hib*[4]	Hib					
Pneumococcal[5]			PCV	PCV	PCV	PCV				PPSV	
Inactivated Poliovirus			IPV	IPV		IPV					IPV
Influenza[6]						Influenza (Yearly)					
Measles, Mumps, Rubella[7]						MMR		*see footnote 7*			MMR
Varicella[8]						Varicella		*see footnote 8*			Varicella
Hepatitis A[9]						HepA (2 doses)				HepA Series	
Meningococcal[10]										MCV	

Range of recommended ages

Certain high-risk groups

This schedule indicates the recommended ages for routine administration of currently licensed vaccines, as of December 1, 2008, for children aged 0 through 6 years. Any dose not administered at the recommended age should be administered at a subsequent visit, when indicated and feasible. Licensed combination vaccines may be used whenever any component of the combination is indicated and other components are not contraindicated and if approved by the Food and Drug Administration for that dose of the series. Providers should consult the relevant Advisory Committee on Immunization Practices statement for detailed recommendations, including high-risk conditions: http://www.cdc.gov/vaccines/pubs/acip-list.htm. Clinically significant adverse events that follow immunization should be reported to the Vaccine Adverse Event Reporting System (VAERS). Guidance about how to obtain and complete a VAERS form is available at http://www.vaers.hhs.gov or by telephone, 800-822-7967.

1. Hepatitis B vaccine (HepB). *(Minimum age: birth)*
 At birth:
 • Administer monovalent HepB to all newborns before hospital discharge.
 • If mother is hepatitis B surface antigen (HBsAg)-positive, administer HepB and 0.5 mL of hepatitis B immune globulin (HBIG) within 12 hours of birth.
 • If mother's HBsAg status is unknown, administer HepB within 12 hours of birth. Determine mother's HBsAg status as soon as possible and, if HBsAg-positive, administer HBIG (no later than age 1 week).
 After the birth dose:
 • The HepB series should be completed with either monovalent HepB or a combination vaccine containing HepB. The second dose should be administered at age 1 or 2 months. The final dose should be administered no earlier than age 24 weeks.
 • Infants born to HBsAg-positive mothers should be tested for HBsAg and antibody to HBsAg (anti-HBs) after completion of at least 3 doses of the HepB series, at age 9 through 18 months (generally at the next well-child visit).
 4-month dose:
 • Administration of 4 doses of HepB to infants is permissible when combination vaccines containing HepB are administered after the birth dose.

2. Rotavirus vaccine (RV). *(Minimum age: 6 weeks)*
 • Administer the first dose at age 6 through 14 weeks (maximum age: 14 weeks 6 days). Vaccination should not be initiated for infants aged 15 weeks or older (i.e., 15 weeks 0 days or older).
 • Administer the final dose in the series by age 8 months 0 days.
 • If Rotarix® is administered at ages 2 and 4 months, a dose at 6 months is not indicated.

3. Diphtheria and tetanus toxoids and acellular pertussis vaccine (DTaP). *(Minimum age: 6 weeks)*
 • The fourth dose may be administered as early as age 12 months, provided at least 6 months have elapsed since the third dose.
 • Administer the final dose in the series at age 4 through 6 years.

4. *Haemophilus influenzae* type b conjugate vaccine (Hib). *(Minimum age: 6 weeks)*
 • If PRP-OMP (PedvaxHIB® or Comvax® [HepB-Hib]) is administered at ages 2 and 4 months, a dose at age 6 months is not indicated.
 • TriHiBit® (DTaP/Hib) should not be used for doses at ages 2, 4, or 6 months but can be used as the final dose in children aged 12 months or older.

5. Pneumococcal vaccine. *(Minimum age: 6 weeks for pneumococcal conjugate vaccine [PCV]; 2 years for pneumococcal polysaccharide vaccine [PPSV])*
 • PCV is recommended for all children aged younger than 5 years. Administer 1 dose of PCV to all healthy children aged 24 through 59 months who are not completely vaccinated for their age.

 • Administer PPSV to children aged 2 years or older with certain underlying medical conditions (see *MMWR* 2000;49[No. RR-9]), including a cochlear implant.

6. Influenza vaccine. *(Minimum age: 6 months for trivalent inactivated influenza vaccine [TIV]; 2 years for live, attenuated influenza vaccine [LAIV])*
 • Administer annually to children aged 6 months through 18 years.
 • For healthy nonpregnant persons (i.e., those who do not have underlying medical conditions that predispose them to influenza complications) aged 2 through 49 years, either LAIV or TIV may be used.
 • Children receiving TIV should receive 0.25 mL if aged 6 through 35 months or 0.5 mL if aged 3 years or older.
 • Administer 2 doses (separated by at least 4 weeks) to children aged younger than 9 years who are receiving influenza vaccine for the first time or who were vaccinated for the first time during the previous influenza season but only received 1 dose.

7. Measles, mumps, and rubella vaccine (MMR). *(Minimum age: 12 months)*
 • Administer the second dose at age 4 through 6 years. However, the second dose may be administered before age 4, provided at least 28 days have elapsed since the first dose.

8. Varicella vaccine. *(Minimum age: 12 months)*
 • Administer the second dose at age 4 through 6 years. However, the second dose may be administered before age 4, provided at least 3 months have elapsed since the first dose.
 • For children aged 12 months through 12 years the minimum interval between doses is 3 months. However, if the second dose was administered at least 28 days after the first dose, it can be accepted as valid.

9. Hepatitis A vaccine (HepA). *(Minimum age: 12 months)*
 • Administer to all children aged 1 year (i.e., aged 12 through 23 months). Administer 2 doses at least 6 months apart.
 • Children not fully vaccinated by age 2 years can be vaccinated at subsequent visits.
 • HepA also is recommended for children older than 1 year who live in areas where vaccination programs target older children or who are at increased risk of infection. See *MMWR* 2006;55(No. RR-7).

10. Meningococcal vaccine. *(Minimum age: 2 years for meningococcal conjugate vaccine [MCV] and for meningococcal polysaccharide vaccine [MPSV])*
 • Administer MCV to children aged 2 through 10 years with terminal complement component deficiency, anatomic or functional asplenia, and certain other high-risk groups. See *MMWR* 2005;54(No. RR-7).
 • Persons who received MPSV 3 or more years previously and who remain at increased risk for meningococcal disease should be revaccinated with MCV.

The Recommended Immunization Schedules for Persons Aged 0 Through 18 Years are approved by the Advisory Committee on Immunization Practices (www.cdc.gov/vaccines/recs/acip/), the American Academy of Pediatrics (http://www.aap.org), and the American Academy of Family Physicians (http://www.aafp.org).
DEPARTMENT OF HEALTH AND HUMAN SERVICES • CENTERS FOR DISEASE CONTROL AND PREVENTION

D.2 Recommended Immunization Schedule for Persons Aged 7 Through 18 Years—United States • 2009

For those who fall behind or start late, see the schedule below and the catch-up schedule

Vaccine ▼ Age ▶	7–10 years	11–12 years	13–18 years
Tetanus, Diphtheria, Pertussis[1]	see footnote 1	Tdap	Tdap
Human Papillomavirus[2]	see footnote 2	HPV (3 doses)	HPV Series
Meningococcal[3]	MCV	MCV	MCV
Influenza[4]	Influenza (Yearly)		
Pneumococcal[5]	PPSV		
Hepatitis A[6]	HepA Series		
Hepatitis B[7]	HepB Series		
Inactivated Poliovirus[8]	IPV Series		
Measles, Mumps, Rubella[9]	MMR Series		
Varicella[10]	Varicella Series		

Range of recommended ages

Catch-up immunization

Certain high-risk groups

This schedule indicates the recommended ages for routine administration of currently licensed vaccines, as of December 1, 2008, for children aged 7 through 18 years. Any dose not administered at the recommended age should be administered at a subsequent visit, when indicated and feasible. Licensed combination vaccines may be used whenever any component of the combination is indicated and other components are not contraindicated and if approved by the Food and Drug Administration for that dose of the series. Providers should consult the relevant Advisory Committee on Immunization Practices statement for detailed recommendations, including high-risk conditions: http://www.cdc.gov/vaccines/pubs/acip-list.htm. Clinically significant adverse events that follow immunization should be reported to the Vaccine Adverse Event Reporting System (VAERS). Guidance about how to obtain and complete a VAERS form is available at http://www.vaers.hhs.gov or by telephone, 800-822-7967.

1. Tetanus and diphtheria toxoids and acellular pertussis vaccine (Tdap). *(Minimum age: 10 years for BOOSTRIX® and 11 years for ADACEL®)*
- Administer at age 11 or 12 years for those who have completed the recommended childhood DTP/DTaP vaccination series and have not received a tetanus and diphtheria toxoid (Td) booster dose.
- Persons aged 13 through 18 years who have not received Tdap should receive a dose.
- A 5-year interval from the last Td dose is encouraged when Tdap is used as a booster dose; however, a shorter interval may be used if pertussis immunity is needed.

2. Human papillomavirus vaccine (HPV). *(Minimum age: 9 years)*
- Administer the first dose to females at age 11 or 12 years.
- Administer the second dose 2 months after the first dose and the third dose 6 months after the first dose (at least 24 weeks after the first dose).
- Administer the series to females at age 13 through 18 years if not previously vaccinated.

3. Meningococcal conjugate vaccine (MCV).
- Administer at age 11 or 12 years, or at age 13 through 18 years if not previously vaccinated.
- Administer to previously unvaccinated college freshmen living in a dormitory.
- MCV is recommended for children aged 2 through 10 years with terminal complement component deficiency, anatomic or functional asplenia, and certain other groups at high risk. See *MMWR* 2005;54(No. RR-7).
- Persons who received MPSV 5 or more years previously and remain at increased risk for meningococcal disease should be revaccinated with MCV.

4. Influenza vaccine.
- Administer annually to children aged 6 months through 18 years.
- For healthy nonpregnant persons (i.e., those who do not have underlying medical conditions that predispose them to influenza complications) aged 2 through 49 years, either LAIV or TIV may be used.
- Administer 2 doses (separated by at least 4 weeks) to children aged younger than 9 years who are receiving influenza vaccine for the first time or who were vaccinated for the first time during the previous influenza season but only received 1 dose.

5. Pneumococcal polysaccharide vaccine (PPSV).
- Administer to children with certain underlying medical conditions (see *MMWR* 1997;46[No. RR-8]), including a cochlear implant. A single revaccination should be administered to children with functional or anatomic asplenia or other immunocompromising conditions after 5 years.

6. Hepatitis A vaccine (HepA).
- Administer 2 doses at least 6 months apart.
- HepA is recommended for children older than 1 year who live in areas where vaccination programs target older children or who are at increased risk of infection. See *MMWR* 2006;55(No. RR-7).

7. Hepatitis B vaccine (HepB).
- Administer the 3-dose series to those not previously vaccinated.
- A 2-dose series (separated by at least 4 months) of adult formulation Recombivax HB® is licensed for children aged 11 through 15 years.

8. Inactivated poliovirus vaccine (IPV).
- For children who received an all-IPV or all-oral poliovirus (OPV) series, a fourth dose is not necessary if the third dose was administered at age 4 years or older.
- If both OPV and IPV were administered as part of a series, a total of 4 doses should be administered, regardless of the child's current age.

9. Measles, mumps, and rubella vaccine (MMR).
- If not previously vaccinated, administer 2 doses or the second dose for those who have received only 1 dose, with at least 28 days between doses.

10. Varicella vaccine.
- For persons aged 7 through 18 years without evidence of immunity (see *MMWR* 2007;56[No. RR-4]), administer 2 doses if not previously vaccinated or the second dose if they have received only 1 dose.
- For persons aged 7 through 12 years, the minimum interval between doses is 3 months. However, if the second dose was administered at least 28 days after the first dose, it can be accepted as valid.
- For persons aged 13 years and older, the minimum interval between doses is 28 days.

The Recommended Immunization Schedules for Persons Aged 0 Through 18 Years are approved by the Advisory Committee on Immunization Practices (www.cdc.gov/vaccines/recs/acip), the American Academy of Pediatrics (http://www.aap.org), and the American Academy of Family Physicians (http://www.aafp.org).
DEPARTMENT OF HEALTH AND HUMAN SERVICES • CENTERS FOR DISEASE CONTROL AND PREVENTION

D.3 CATCH-UP IMMUNIZATION SCHEDULE FOR PERSONS AGED 4 MONTHS THROUGH 18 YEARS WHO START LATE OR WHO ARE MORE THAN 1 MONTH BEHIND—UNITED STATES • 2009

The table below provides catch-up schedules and minimum intervals between doses for children whose vaccinations have been delayed. A vaccine series does not need to be restarted, regardless of the time that has elapsed between doses. Use the section appropriate for the child's age.

CATCH-UP SCHEDULE FOR PERSONS AGED 4 MONTHS THROUGH 6 YEARS

Vaccine	Minimum Age for Dose 1	Minimum Interval Between Doses			
		Dose 1 to Dose 2	Dose 2 to Dose 3	Dose 3 to Dose 4	Dose 4 to Dose 5
Hepatitis B[1]	Birth	4 weeks	8 weeks (and at least 16 weeks after first dose)		
Rotavirus[2]	6 wks	4 weeks	4 weeks[2]		
Diphtheria, Tetanus, Pertussis[3]	6 wks	4 weeks	4 weeks	6 months	6 months[3]
Haemophilus influenzae type b[4]	6 wks	4 weeks if first dose administered at younger than age 12 months / 8 weeks (as final dose) if first dose administered at age 12-14 months / No further doses needed if first dose administered at age 15 months or older	4 weeks[4] if current age is younger than 12 months / 8 weeks (as final dose)[4] if current age is 12 months or older and second dose administered at younger than age 15 months / No further doses needed if previous dose administered at age 15 months or older	8 weeks (as final dose) This dose only necessary for children aged 12 months through 59 months who received 3 doses before age 12 months	
Pneumococcal[5]	6 wks	4 weeks if first dose administered at younger than age 12 months / 8 weeks (as final dose for healthy children) if first dose administered at age 12 months or older or current age 24 through 59 months / No further doses needed for healthy children if first dose administered at age 24 months or older	4 weeks if current age is younger than 12 months / 8 weeks (as final dose for healthy children) if current age is 12 months or older / No further doses needed for healthy children if previous dose administered at age 24 months or older	8 weeks (as final dose) This dose only necessary for children aged 12 months through 59 months who received 3 doses before age 12 months or for high-risk children who received 3 doses at any age	
Inactivated Poliovirus[6]	6 wks	4 weeks	4 weeks	4 weeks[6]	
Measles, Mumps, Rubella[7]	12 mos	4 weeks			
Varicella[8]	12 mos	3 months			
Hepatitis A[9]	12 mos	6 months			

CATCH-UP SCHEDULE FOR PERSONS AGED 7 THROUGH 18 YEARS

Vaccine	Minimum Age for Dose 1	Dose 1 to Dose 2	Dose 2 to Dose 3	Dose 3 to Dose 4	
Tetanus, Diphtheria/ Tetanus, Diphtheria, Pertussis[10]	7 yrs[10]	4 weeks	4 weeks if first dose administered at younger than age 12 months / 6 months if first dose administered at age 12 months or older	6 months if first dose administered at younger than age 12 months	
Human Papillomavirus[11]	9 yrs	Routine dosing intervals are recommended[11]			
Hepatitis A[9]	12 mos	6 months			
Hepatitis B[1]	Birth	4 weeks	8 weeks (and at least 16 weeks after first dose)		
Inactivated Poliovirus[6]	6 wks	4 weeks	4 weeks	4 weeks[6]	
Measles, Mumps, Rubella[7]	12 mos	4 weeks			
Varicella[8]	12 mos	3 months if the person is younger than age 13 years / 4 weeks if the person is aged 13 years or older			

1. Hepatitis B vaccine (HepB).
- Administer the 3-dose series to those not previously vaccinated.
- A 2-dose series (separated by at least 4 months) of adult formulation Recombivax HB® is licensed for children aged 11 through 15 years.

2. Rotavirus vaccine (RV).
- The maximum age for the first dose is 14 weeks 6 days. Vaccination should not be initiated for infants aged 15 weeks or older (i.e., 15 weeks 0 days or older).
- Administer the final dose in the series by age 8 months 0 days.
- If Rotarix® was administered for the first and second doses, a third dose is not indicated.

3. Diphtheria and tetanus toxoids and acellular pertussis vaccine (DTaP).
- The fifth dose is not necessary if the fourth dose was administered at age 4 years or older.

4. Haemophilus influenzae type b conjugate vaccine (Hib).
- Hib vaccine is not generally recommended for persons aged 5 years or older. No efficacy data are available on which to base a recommendation concerning use of Hib vaccine for older children and adults. However, studies suggest good immunogenicity in persons who have sickle cell disease, leukemia, or HIV infection, or who have had a splenectomy; administering 1 dose of Hib vaccine to these persons is not contraindicated.
- If the first 2 doses were PRP-OMP (PedvaxHIB® or Comvax®), and administered at age 11 months or younger, the third (and final) dose should be administered at age 12 through 15 months and at least 8 weeks after the second dose.
- If the first dose was administered at age 7 through 11 months, administer 2 doses separated by 4 weeks and a final dose at age 12 through 15 months.

5. Pneumococcal vaccine.
- Administer 1 dose of pneumococcal conjugate vaccine (PCV) to all healthy children aged 24 through 59 months who have not received at least 1 dose of PCV on or after age 12 months.
- For children aged 24 through 59 months with underlying medical conditions, administer 1 dose of PCV if 3 doses were received previously or administer 2 doses of PCV at least 8 weeks apart if fewer than 3 doses were received previously.
- Administer pneumococcal polysaccharide vaccine (PPSV) to children aged 2 years or older with certain underlying medical conditions (see MMWR 2000;49[No. RR-9]), including a cochlear implant, at least 8 weeks after the last dose of PCV.

6. Inactivated poliovirus vaccine (IPV).
- For children who received an all-IPV or all-oral poliovirus (OPV) series, a fourth dose is not necessary if the third dose was administered at age 4 years or older.
- If both OPV and IPV were administered as part of a series, a total of 4 doses should be administered, regardless of the child's current age.

7. Measles, mumps, and rubella vaccine (MMR).
- Administer the second dose at age 4 through 6 years. However, the second dose may be administered before age 4, provided at least 28 days have elapsed since the first dose.
- If not previously vaccinated, administer 2 doses with at least 28 days between doses.

8. Varicella vaccine.
- Administer the second dose at age 4 through 6 years. However, the second dose may be administered before age 4, provided at least 3 months have elapsed since the first dose.
- For persons aged 12 months through 12 years, the minimum interval between doses is 3 months. However, if the second dose was administered at least 28 days after the first dose, it can be accepted as valid.
- For persons aged 13 years and older, the minimum interval between doses is 28 days.

9. Hepatitis A vaccine (HepA).
- HepA is recommended for children older than 1 year who live in areas where vaccination programs target older children or who are at increased risk of infection. See MMWR 2006;55[No. RR-7].

10. Tetanus and diphtheria toxoids vaccine (Td) and tetanus and diphtheria toxoids and acellular pertussis vaccine (Tdap).
- Doses of DTaP are counted as part of the Td/Tdap series.
- Tdap should be substituted for a single dose of Td in the catch-up series or as a booster for children aged 10 through 18 years; use Td for other doses.

11. Human papillomavirus vaccine (HPV).
- Administer the series to females at age 13 through 18 years if not previously vaccinated.
- Use recommended routine dosing intervals for series catch-up (i.e., the second and third doses should be administered at 2 and 6 months after the first dose). However, the minimum interval between the first and second doses is 4 weeks. The minimum interval between the second and third doses is 12 weeks, and the third dose should be given at least 24 weeks after the first dose.

Information about reporting reactions after immunization is available online at http://www.vaers.hhs.gov or by telephone, 800-822-7967. Suspected cases of vaccine-preventable diseases should be reported to the state or local health department. Additional information, including precautions and contraindications for immunization, is available from the National Center for Immunization and Respiratory Diseases at http://www.cdc.gov/vaccines or telephone, 800-CDC-INFO (800-232-4636).

DEPARTMENT OF HEALTH AND HUMAN SERVICES • CENTERS FOR DISEASE CONTROL AND PREVENTION

Appendixes

D.4 Summary of Recommendations for Childhood and Adolescent Immunization

Vaccine name and route	Schedule for routine vaccination and other guidelines (any vaccine can be given with another)	Schedule for catch-up vaccination and related issues	Contraindications and precautions (mild illness is not a contraindication)
Hepatitis B (HepB) *Give IM*	• Vaccinate all children age 0 through 18yrs. • Vaccinate all newborns with monovalent vaccine prior to hospital discharge. Give dose #2 at age 1–2m and the final dose at age 6–18m (the last dose in the infant series should not be given earlier than age 24wks). After the birth dose, the series may be completed using 2 doses of single-antigen vaccine or up to 3 doses of Comvax (ages 2m, 4m, 12–15m) or Pediarix (ages 2m, 4m, 6m), which may result in giving a total of 4 doses of hepatitis B vaccine. • **If mother is HBsAg-positive:** give the newborn HBIG + dose #1 within 12hrs of birth; complete series at age 6m or, if using Comvax, at age 12–15m. • **If mother's HBsAg status is unknown:** give the newborn dose #1 within 12hrs of birth. If mother is subsequently found to be HBsAg positive, give infant HBIG within 7d of birth and follow the schedule for infants born to HBsAg-positive mothers.	• Do not restart series, no matter how long since previous dose. • 3-dose series can be started at any age. • Minimum spacing between doses: 4wks between #1 and #2, 8wks between #2 and #3, and at least 16wks between #1 and #3 (e.g., 0-, 2-, 4m; 0-, 1-, 4m). **Special Notes on Hepatitis B Vaccine (HepB)** **Dosing of HepB:** Vaccine brands are interchangeable. For persons age 0 through 19yrs, give 0.5 mL of either Engerix-B or Recombivax HB. **Alternative dosing schedule for unvaccinated adolescents age 11 through 15yrs:** Give 2 doses Recombivax HB 1.0 mL (adult formulation) spaced 4–6m apart. (Engerix-B is not licensed for a 2-dose schedule.) **For preterm infants:** Consult ACIP hepatitis B recommendations (*MMWR* 2005; 54 [RR-16]).*	**Contraindication** Previous anaphylaxis to this vaccine or to any of its components. **Precaution** Moderate or severe acute illness.
DTaP, DT (Diphtheria, tetanus, acellular pertussis) *Give IM*	• Give to children at ages 2m, 4m, 6m, 15–18m, 4–6yrs. • May give dose #1 as early as age 6wks. • May give #4 as early as age 12m if 6m have elapsed since #3 and the child is unlikely to return at age 15–18m. • Do not give DTaP/DT to children age 7yrs and older. • If possible, use the same DTaP product for all doses.	• #2 and #3 may be given 4wks after previous dose. • #4 may be given 6m after #3. • If #4 is given before 4th birthday, wait at least 6m for #5 (age 4–6yrs). • If #4 is given after 4th birthday, #5 is not needed.	**Contraindications** • Previous anaphylaxis to this vaccine or to any of its components. • For DTaP/Tdap only: encephalopathy within 7d after DTP/DTaP. **Precautions** • Moderate or severe acute illness. • History of Arthus reaction following a prior dose of tetanus- and/or diphtheria-toxoid-containing vaccine, including MCV.
Td, Tdap (Tetanus, diphtheria, acellular pertussis) *Give IM*	• Give 1-time Tdap dose to adolescents age 11–12yrs if 5yrs have elapsed since last dose DTaP; then boost every 10yrs with Td. • Give 1-time dose of Tdap to all adolescents who have not received previous Tdap. Special efforts should be made to give Tdap to persons age 11yrs and older who are - in contact with infants younger than age 12m. - healthcare workers with direct patient contact. • In pregnancy, when indicated, give Td or Tdap in 2nd or 3rd trimester. If not administered during pregnancy, give Tdap in immediate postpartum period.	• If never vaccinated with tetanus- and diphtheria-containing vaccine: give Td dose #1 now, dose #2 4wks later, and dose #3 6m after #2, then give booster every 10yrs. A 1-time Tdap may be substituted for any dose in the series, preferably as dose #1. For persons who previously received a Td booster, an interval of 2yrs or less between Td and Tdap may be used.	• Guillain-Barré syndrome within 6wks after previous dose of tetanus toxoid-containing vaccine. • For DTaP only: Any of these events following a previous dose of DTP/DTaP: 1) temperature of 105°F (40.5°C) or higher within 48hrs; 2) continuous crying for 3hrs or more within 48hrs; 3) collapse or shock-like state within 48hrs; 4) convulsion with or without fever within 3d. • For DTaP/Tdap only: Unstable neurologic disorder. **Note:** Use of Td or Tdap is not contraindicated in pregnancy. At the provider's discretion, either vaccine may be administered during the 2nd or 3rd trimester.
Polio (IPV) *Give SC or IM*	• Give to children at ages 2m, 4m, 6–18m, 4–6yrs. • May give dose #1 as early as age 6wks. • Not routinely recommended for U.S. residents age 18yrs and older (except certain travelers).	• All doses should be separated by at least 4wks. • If dose #3 is given after 4th birthday, dose #4 is not needed.	**Contraindication** Previous anaphylaxis to this vaccine or to any of its components. **Precautions** • Moderate or severe acute illness. • Pregnancy.
Human papillomavirus (HPV) *Give IM*	• Give 3-dose series to girls at age 11–12yrs on a 0, 2, 6m schedule. (May be given as early as age 9yrs.) • Vaccinate all older girls and women (through age 26yrs) who were not previously vaccinated.	Minimum spacing between doses: 4wks between #1 and #2; 12 wks between #2 and #3. Overall, there must be at least 24wks between doses #1 and #3.	**Contraindication** Previous anaphylaxis to this vaccine or to any of its components. **Precautions** • Moderate or severe acute illness. • Pregnancy.

*This document was adapted from the recommendations of the Advisory Committee on Immunization Practices (ACIP). To obtain copies of the recommendations, call the CDC-INFO Contact Center at (800) 232-4636; visit CDC's website at www.cdc.gov/vaccines/pubs/ACIP-list.htm; or visit the Immunization Action Coalition (IAC) website at www.immunize.org/acip. This table is revised periodically. Visit IAC's website at www.immunize.org/childrules to make sure you have the most current version.

Technical content reviewed by the Centers for Disease Control and Prevention, November 2008.

www.immunize.org/catg.d/p2010.pdf • Item #P2010 (11/08)

Immunization Action Coalition • 1573 Selby Avenue • Saint Paul, MN 55104 • (651) 647-9009 • www.immunize.org • www.vaccineinformation.org • admin@immunize.org

Vaccine name and route	Schedule for routine vaccination and other guidelines (any vaccine can be given with another)	Schedule for catch-up vaccine administration and related issues	Contraindications and precautions (mild illness is not a contraindication)
Varicella (Var) (Chickenpox) *Give SC*	• Give dose #1 at age 12–15m. • Give dose #2 at age 4–6yrs. Dose #2 may be given earlier if at least 3m since dose #1. • Give a second dose to all older children and adolescents with history of only 1 dose. • MMRV may be used in children age 12m through 12yrs.	• If younger than age 13yrs, space dose #1 and #2 at least 3m apart. If age 13yrs or older, space at least 4wks apart. • May use as postexposure prophylaxis if given within 5d. • If Var and either MMR, LAIV, and/or yellow fever vaccine are not given on the same day, space them at least 28d apart.	**Contraindications** • Previous anaphylaxis to this vaccine or to any of its components. • Pregnancy or possibility of pregnancy within 4wks. • Children on high-dose immunosuppressive therapy or who are immunocompromised because of malignancy and primary or acquired cellular immunodeficiency, including HIV/AIDS (although vaccination may be considered if CD4+ T-lymphocyte percentages are either 15% or greater in children ages 1 through 8yrs or 200 cells/mL or greater in children age 9yrs or older). **Precautions** • Moderate or severe acute illness. • If blood, plasma, and/or immune globulin (IG or VZIG) were given in past 11m, see ACIP statement *General Recommendations on Immunization* regarding time to wait before vaccinating. **Note:** For patients with humoral immunodeficiency or leukemia, see ACIP recommendations*.
MMR (Measles, mumps, rubella) *Give SC*	• Give dose #1 at age 12–15m. • Give dose #2 at age 4–6yrs. Dose #2 may be given earlier if at least 4wks since dose #1. • Give a second dose to all older children and teens with history of only 1 dose. • MMRV may be used in children age 12m through 12yrs.	• If MMR and either Var, LAIV, and/or yellow fever vaccine are not given on the same day, space them at least 28d apart. • When using MMR for both doses, minimum interval is 4wks. • When using MMRV for both doses, minimum interval is 3m. • Within 72hrs of measles exposure, give 1 dose of MMR as postexposure prophylaxis to susceptible healthy children age 12m and older.	**Contraindications** • Previous anaphylaxis to this vaccine or to any of its components. • Pregnancy or possibility of pregnancy within 4wks. • Severe immunodeficiency (e.g., hematologic and solid tumors; receiving chemotherapy; congenital immunodeficiency; long-term immunosuppressive therapy, or severely symptomatic HIV). Note: HIV infection is NOT a contraindication to MMR for children who are not severely immunocompromised (consult ACIP MMR recommendations [*MMWR* 1998;47 [RR-8] for details*). **Precautions** • Moderate or severe acute illness. • If blood, plasma, or immune globulin given in past 11m, see ACIP statement *General Recommendations on Immunization* regarding time to wait before vaccinating. • History of thrombocytopenia or thrombocytopenic purpura. **Note:** MMR is not contraindicated if a TST (tuberculosis skin test) was recently applied. If TST and MMR are not given on same day, delay TST for at least 4wks after MMR.
Influenza Trivalent inactivated influenza vaccine (TIV) *Give IM* Live attenuated influenza vaccine (LAIV) *Give intranasally*	• Vaccinate all children and teens age 6m through 18yrs, as well as all household contacts of infants and children through age 59m (4yrs 11m). • Vaccinate persons age 19yrs and older who - have a risk factor (e.g., pregnancy, heart or lung disease, renal, hepatic, hematologic, or metabolic disorder [including diabetes], immunosuppression, or have a condition that compromises respiratory function or that can increase the risk of aspiration) or live in a chronic-care facility. - live or work with at-risk people as listed above. • All other persons who want to reduce the likelihood of becoming ill with influenza or of spreading it to others. • LAIV may be given to healthy, non-pregnant persons age 2–49yrs. • Give 2 doses to first-time vaccinees age 6m through 8yrs. • For TIV, give 0.25 mL dose to children age 6–35m and 0.5 mL dose if age 3yrs and older.	• Vaccinate all children and teens age 6m through 18yrs, as well as all household contacts of infants and children through age 59m (4yrs 11m). • Give 2 doses to first-time vaccinees age 6m through 8yrs, spaced 4wks apart.	**Contraindications** • Previous anaphylaxis to this vaccine, to any of its components, or to eggs. • For LAIV only: Pregnancy, asthma, reactive airways disease, or other chronic disorder of the pulmonary or cardiovascular systems; an underlying medical condition, including metabolic diseases such as diabetes, renal dysfunction, and hemoglobinopathies; known or suspected immune deficiency diseases or immunosuppressed states; for children younger than age 5yrs, possible reactive airways disease (e.g., recurrent wheezing or a wheezing episode within the past 12m). **Precautions** • Moderate or severe acute illness. • History of Guillain-Barré syndrome within 6wks of a previous influenza vaccination. **Note:** If LAIV and either MMR, Var, and/or yellow fever vaccine are not given on the same day, space them at least 28d apart.
Rotavirus (RV) *Give orally*	• Rotarix (RV1): give at age 2m, 4m • RotaTeq (RV5): give at age 2m, 4m, 6m • May give dose #1 as early as age 6wks. • Give dose #3 no later than age 8m 0 days.	• Do not begin series in infants older than age 15wks 0 days. • Intervals between doses may be as short as 4wks. • If prior vaccination included use of different or unknown brand(s), a total of 3 doses should be given.	**Contraindication** Previous anaphylaxis to this vaccine or to any of its components, including latex for RV1. **Precautions** • Moderate or severe acute illness. • Altered immunocompetence. • Moderate to severe acute gastroenteritis or chronic gastrointestinal disease. • History of intussusception.

continued

Appendixes

Vaccine name and route	Schedule for routine vaccination and other guidelines (any vaccine can be given with another)	Schedule for catch-up vaccination and related issues	Contraindications and precautions (mild illness is not a contraindication)
Hib (*Haemophilus influenzae type b*) *Give IM*	• ActHib (PRP-T); give at age 2m, 4m, 6m, 12–15m (booster dose). • PedvaxHIB or Comvax (containing PRP-OMP): give at age 2m, 4m, 12–15m (booster dose). • Dose #1 of Hib vaccine should not be given earlier than age 6wks. • The last dose (booster dose) is given no earlier than age 12m and a minimum of 8wks after the previous dose. • Hib vaccines are interchangeable; however, if different brands of Hib vaccines are administered for dose #1 and dose #2, a total of 3 doses are necessary to complete the primary series in infants. • Any Hib vaccine may be used for the booster dose. • Hib is not routinely given to children age 5yrs and older.	**All Hib vaccines:** • If #1 was given at 12–14m, give booster in 8wks. • Give only 1 dose to unvaccinated children from age 15 through 59m. **ActHib:** • #2 and #3 may be given 4wks after previous dose. • If #1 was given at age 7–11m, only 3 doses are needed; #2 is given 4–8wks after #1, then boost at age 12–15m (wait at least 8wks after dose #2). **PedvaxHIB and Comvax:** • #2 may be given 4wks after dose #1.	**Contraindications** • Previous anaphylaxis to this vaccine or to any of its components. • Age younger than 6wks. **Precaution** Moderate or severe acute illness.
Pneumo. conjugate (PCV) *Give IM*	• Give at ages 2m, 4m, 6m, 12–15m. • Dose #1 may be given as early as age 6wks. • Give 1 dose to unvaccinated healthy children age 24–59m. • For high-risk** children ages 24–59m, give 2 doses at least 8wks apart if previous vaccinations were fewer than 3 doses, or give 1 dose if previously received 3 doses. • PCV is not routinely given to children age 5yrs and older. ****High-risk:** Those with sickle cell disease; anatomic/functional asplenia; chronic cardiac, pulmonary, or renal disease; diabetes; cerebrospinal fluid leaks; HIV infection; immunosuppression; diseases associated with immunosuppressive and/or radiation therapy; or who have or will have a cochlear implant.	• For age 7–11m: If history of 0–2 doses, give additional doses 4wks apart with no more than 3 total doses by age 12m; then give booster 8wks later. • For age 12–23m: If 0–1 dose before age 12m, give 2 doses at least 8wks apart. If 2–3 doses before age 12m, give 1 dose at least 8wks after previous dose. • For age 24–59m: If patient has had no previous doses, or has a history of 1–3 doses given before age 12m but no booster dose, or has a history of only 1 dose given at age 12–23m, give 1 dose now.	**Contraindication** Previous anaphylaxis to this vaccine or to any of its components. **Precaution** Moderate or severe acute illness.
Pneumo. polysacch. (PPSV) *Give IM or SC*	• Give 1 dose at least 8wks after final dose of PCV to high-risk children age 2yrs and older. • For children who are immunocompromised or have sickle cell disease or functional or anatomic asplenia, give a 2nd dose of PPSV 5yrs after previous PPSV (consult ACIP PPSV recommendations at http://www.cdc.gov/vaccines/pubs/ACIP-list.htm*).		**Contraindication** Previous anaphylaxis to this vaccine or to any of its components. **Precaution** Moderate or severe acute illness.
Hepatitis A (HepA) *Give IM*	• Give 2 doses to all children at age 1yr (12–23m) spaced 6m apart. • Vaccinate all previously unvaccinated children and adolescents age 2 years and older who - Live in a state, county, or community with a routine vaccination program already in place for children age 2yrs and older. - Travel anywhere except U.S., W. Europe, N. Zealand, Australia, Canada, or Japan. - Wish to be protected from HAV infection. - Have chronic liver disease, clotting factor disorder, or are MSM adolescents. - Are injecting or non-injecting drug users.	• Minimum interval between doses is 6m. • Children who are not fully vaccinated by age 2yrs can be vaccinated at subsequent visits. • Consider routine vaccination of children age 2yrs and older in areas with no existing program. • Give 1 dose as postexposure prophylaxis to incompletely vaccinated children age 12m and older who have recently (during the past 2wks) been exposed to hepatitis A virus.	**Contraindication** Previous anaphylaxis to this vaccine or to any of its components. **Precautions** • Moderate or severe acute illness. • Pregnancy.
Meningococcal conjugate (MCV) *Give IM* **polysaccharide (MPSV)** *Give SC*	• Give 1-time dose of MCV to adolescents age 11 through 18yrs. • Vaccinate all college freshmen living in dorms who have not been vaccinated. • Vaccinate all children age 2yrs and older who have any of the following risk factors (MCV is preferable to MPSV): - Anatomic or functional asplenia, or terminal complement component deficiency. - Travel to or reside in countries in which meningococcal disease is hyperendemic or epidemic (e.g., the "meningitis belt" of Sub-Saharan Africa).	If previously vaccinated with MPSV and risk continues, give MCV 5yrs after MPSV.	**Contraindication** Previous anaphylaxis to this vaccine or to any of its components, including diphtheria toxoid (for MCV). **Precautions** • Moderate or severe acute illness. • For MCV only: history of Guillain-Barré syndrome (GBS).

D.5 Summary of Recommendations for Adult Immunization

Vaccine name and route	For whom vaccination is recommended	Schedule for vaccine administration (any vaccine can be given with another)	Contraindications and precautions (mild illness is not a contraindication)
Influenza Trivalent inactivated influenza vaccine (TIV) *Give IM* ___ Live attenuated influenza vaccine (LAIV) *Give intranasally*	• All persons who want to reduce the likelihood of becoming ill with influenza or of spreading it to others. • Persons age 50yrs and older. [TIV only] • Persons with medical problems (e.g., heart or lung disease, renal, hepatic, hematologic, or metabolic disorder [including diabetes], immunosuppression). [TIV only] • Persons with any condition that compromises respiratory function or the handling of respiratory secretions or that can increase the risk of aspiration (e.g., cognitive dysfunction, spinal cord injury, seizure disorder, or other neuromuscular disorder). [TIV only] • Persons living in chronic care facilities. [TIV only] • Persons who work or live with high-risk people. • Women who will be pregnant during the influenza season (December–spring). [If currently pregnant, TIV only] • All healthcare personnel and other persons who provide direct care to high-risk people. • Household contacts and out-of-home caregivers of children age 0–59m. • Travelers at risk for complications of influenza who go to areas where influenza activity exists or who may be among people from areas of the world where there is current influenza activity (e.g., on organized tours). [TIV only] • Students or other persons in institutional settings (e.g., residents of dormitories or correctional facilities). **Note:** LAIV may not be given to some of the persons listed to the left; see contraindications listed in far right column.	• Give 1 dose every year in the fall or winter. • Begin vaccination services as soon as vaccine is available and continue until the supply is depleted. • Continue to give vaccine to unvaccinated adults throughout the influenza season (including when influenza activity is present in the community) and at other times when the risk of influenza exists. • If 2 or more of the following live virus vaccines are to be given—LAIV, MMR, Var, and/or yellow fever vaccine—they should be given on the same day. If they are not, space them by at least 28d.	**Contraindications** • Previous anaphylactic reaction to this vaccine, to any of its components, or to eggs. • For LAIV only, age 50 years or older, pregnancy, asthma, reactive airway disease or other chronic disorder of the pulmonary or cardiovascular system; an underlying medical condition, including metabolic disease such as diabetes, renal dysfunction, and hemoglobinopathy; a known or suspected immune deficiency disease or immunosuppressed state. **Precautions** • Moderate or severe acute illness. • History of Guillain-Barré syndrome (GBS) within 6wks of previous influenza vaccination.

Pneumococcal polysaccharide (PPSV) *Give IM or SC*	• Persons age 65yrs and older.
	• Persons who have chronic illness or other risk factors, including chronic cardiac or pulmonary disease, chronic liver disease, alcoholism, diabetes, CSF leaks, cigarette smoking, as well as people living in special environments or social settings (including Alaska Natives and certain American Indian populations age 50 through 64 years if recommended by local public health authorities).
	• Those at highest risk of fatal pneumococcal infection, including persons who
	  - have anatomic asplenia, functional asplenia, or sickle cell disease
	  - have an immunocompromising condition, including HIV infection, leukemia, lymphoma, Hodgkin's disease, multiple myeloma, generalized malignancy, chronic renal failure, or nephrotic syndrome
	  - are receiving immunosuppressive chemotherapy (including corticosteroids)
	  - have received an organ or bone marrow transplant
	  - are candidates for or recipients of cochlear implants.
		• Give 1 dose if unvaccinated or if previous vaccination history is unknown.
		• Give a 1-time revaccination at least 5yrs after 1st dose to persons
		  - age 65yrs and older if the 1st dose was given prior to age 65yrs
		  - at highest risk of fatal pneumococcal infection or rapid antibody loss (see the 3rd bullet in the box to left for listings of persons at highest risk)
			Contraindication
			Previous anaphylactic reaction to this vaccine or to any of its components.
			Precaution
			Moderate or severe acute illness.

Zoster (shingles) (Zos) *Give SC*	• Persons age 60yrs and older.	• Give 1-time dose if unvaccinated, regardless of previous history of herpes zoster (shingles) or chickenpox.	**Contraindications** • Previous anaphylactic reaction to any component of zoster vaccine (e.g., gelatin & neomycin). • Primary cellular or acquired immunodeficiency. • Pregnancy. **Precaution** Moderate or severe acute illness.

*This document was adapted from the recommendations of the Advisory Committee on Immunization Practices (ACIP). To obtain copies of these recommendations, call the CDC-INFO Contact Center at (800) 232-4636; visit CDC's website at www.cdc.gov/vaccines/pubs/ACIP-list.htm; or visit the Immunization Action Coalition (IAC) website at www.immunize.org/acip. This table is revised periodically. Visit IAC's website at www.immuniz.org/adultrules to make sure you have the most current version.

Technical content reviewed by the Centers for Disease Control and Prevention, November 2008.

Immunization Action Coalition   •   1573 Selby Avenue   •   Saint Paul, MN 55104   •   (651) 647-9009   •   www.immunize.org   •   www.vaccineinformation.org

www.immunize.org/catg.d/p2011.pdf   •   Item #P2011 (11/08)

admin@immunize.org

continued

Appendixes

Vaccine name and route	For whom vaccination is recommended	Schedule for vaccine administration (any vaccine can be given with another)	Contraindications and precautions (mild illness is not a contraindication)
Hepatitis B (HepB) *Give IM* Brands may be used interchangeably.	• All persons through age 18yrs. • All adults wishing to be protected from hepatitis B virus infection. • High-risk persons, including household contacts and sex partners of HBsAg-positive persons; injecting drug users; sexually active persons not in a long-term, mutually monogamous relationship; men who have sex with men; persons with HIV; persons seeking evaluation or treatment for an STD; patients receiving hemodialysis and patients with renal disease that may result in dialysis; healthcare personnel and public safety workers who are exposed to blood; clients and staff of institutions for the developmentally disabled; inmates of long-term correctional facilities; and certain international travelers. • Persons with chronic liver disease. **Note:** Provide serologic screening for immigrants from endemic areas. If patient is chronically infected, assure appropriate disease management. Screen sex partners and household members; give HepB at the same visit if not already vaccinated.	• Give 3 doses on a 0, 1, 6m schedule. • Alternative timing options for vaccination include 0, 2, 4m and 0, 1, 4m. • There must be at least 4wks between doses #1 and #2, and at least 8wks between doses #2 and #3. Overall, there must be at least 16wks between doses #1 and #3. **Schedule for those who have fallen behind:** If the series is delayed between doses, DO NOT start the series over. Continue from where you left off.	**Contraindication** Previous anaphylactic reaction to this vaccine or to any of its components. **Precaution** Moderate or severe acute illness.
Hepatitis A (HepA) *Give IM* Brands may be used interchangeably.	• All persons wishing to be protected from hepatitis A virus (HAV) infection. • Persons who travel or work anywhere EXCEPT the U.S., Western Europe, New Zealand, Australia, Canada, and Japan. • Persons with chronic liver disease; injecting and non-injecting drug users; men who have sex with men; people with HAV in experimental lab settings (not routine medical laboratories); persons who receive clotting-factor concentrates; persons who work with HAV in experimental lab settings (not routine medical laboratories); food handlers when health authorities or private employers determine vaccination to be appropriate. • Unvaccinated adults age 40yrs or younger with recent (within 2 wks) exposure to HAV. For persons older than age 40yrs with recent (within 2 wks) exposure to HAV, immune globulin is preferred over HepA vaccine.	For Twinrix® (hepatitis A and B combination vaccine [GSK]) for patients age 18yrs and older only: give 3 doses on a 0, 1, 6m schedule. There must be at least 4wks between doses #1 and #2, and at least 5m between doses #2 and #3. An alternative schedule can also be used at 0, 7d, 21–30d, and a booster at 12m. • Give 2 doses. • The minimum interval between doses #1 and #2 is 6m. • If dose #2 is delayed, do not repeat dose #1. Just give dose #2.	**Contraindication** Previous anaphylactic reaction to this vaccine or to any of its components. **Precautions** • Moderate or severe acute illness. • Safety during pregnancy has not been determined, so benefits must be weighed against potential risk.
Td, Tdap (Tetanus, diphtheria, pertussis) *Give IM*	• All adults who lack written documentation of a primary series consisting of at least 3 doses of tetanus- and diphtheria-toxoid-containing vaccine. • A booster dose of tetanus- and diphtheria-toxoid-containing vaccine may be needed for wound management as early as 5yrs after receiving a previous dose, so consult ACIP recommendations.* • Using tetanus toxoid (TT) instead of Td or Tdap is not recommended. • In pregnancy, when indicated, give Td or Tdap in 2nd or 3rd trimester. If not administered during pregnancy, give Tdap in immediate postpartum period. **For Tdap only:** • All adults younger than age 65yrs who have not already received Tdap. • Adults in contact with infants younger than age 12m (e.g., parents, grandparents younger than age 65yrs, childcare providers, healthcare personnel) who have not received a dose of Tdap should be prioritized for vaccination. • Healthcare personnel who work in hospitals or ambulatory care settings and have direct patient contact and who have not received Tdap.	• For persons who are unvaccinated or behind, complete the primary series with Td (spaced at 0, 1–2m, 6–12m intervals). One-time dose of Tdap may be used for any dose if younger than age 65yrs. • Give Td booster every 10yrs after the primary series has been completed. For adults younger than age 65yrs, a 1-time dose of Tdap is recommended to replace the next Td. • Intervals of 2yrs or less between Td and Tdap may be used. **Note:** The two Tdap products are licensed for different age groups: Adacel™ (sanofi) for use in persons age 11–64yrs and Boostrix® (GSK) for use in persons age 10–18yrs.	**Contraindications** • Previous anaphylactic reaction to this vaccine or to any of its components. • For Tdap only, history of encephalopathy within 7d following DTP/DTaP. **Precautions** • Moderate or severe acute illness. • GBS within 6wks of receiving a previous dose of tetanus-toxoid-containing vaccine. • Unstable neurologic condition. • History of Arthus reaction following a previous dose of tetanus- and/or diphtheria-toxoid-containing vaccine, including MCV. **Note:** Use of Td/Tdap is not contraindicated in pregnancy. Either vaccine may be given during trimester #2 or #3 at the provider's discretion.
Polio (IPV) *Give IM or SC*	Not routinely recommended for U.S. residents age 18yrs and older. **Note:** Adults living in the U.S. who never received or completed a primary series of polio vaccine need not be vaccinated unless they intend to travel to areas where exposure to wild-type virus is likely (i.e., India, Pakistan, Afghanistan, and Nigeria). Previously vaccinated adults can receive 1 booster dose if traveling to polio endemic areas.	• Refer to ACIP recommendations* regarding unique situations, schedules, and dosing information.	**Contraindication** Previous anaphylactic or neurologic reaction to this vaccine or to any of its components. **Precautions** • Moderate or severe acute illness. • Pregnancy.

Vaccine name and route	For whom vaccination is recommended	Schedule for vaccine administration (any vaccine can be given with another)	Contraindications and precautions (mild illness is not a contraindication)
Varicella (Var) (Chickenpox) *Give SC*	• All adults without evidence of immunity. **Note:** Evidence of immunity is defined as written documentation of 2 doses of varicella vaccine; a history of varicella disease or herpes zoster (shingles) based on healthcare-provider diagnosis; laboratory evidence of immunity; laboratory confirmation of disease; and/or birth in the U.S. before 1980, with the exceptions that follow. Healthcare personnel (HCP) and pregnant women born in the U.S. before 1980 who do not meet any of the criteria above should be tested. If they are not immune, give the first dose of varicella vaccine immediately (HCP) or postpartum and before hospital discharge (pregnant women). Give the second dose 4–8 wks later. Routine post-vaccination testing is not recommended.	• Give 2 doses. • Dose #2 is given 4–8wks after dose #1. • If the second dose is delayed, do not repeat dose #1. Just give dose #2. • If 2 or more of the following live virus vaccines are to be given—LAIV, MMR, Var, and/or yellow fever vaccine—they should be given on the same day. If they are not, space them by at least 28d. • May use as postexposure prophylaxis if given within 5d.	**Contraindications** • Previous anaphylactic reaction to this vaccine or to any of its components. • Pregnancy or possibility of pregnancy within 4wks. • Persons on high-dose immunosuppressive therapy or who are immunocompromised because of malignancy and primary or acquired cellular immunodeficiency, including HIV/AIDS (although vaccination may be considered if CD4+ T-lymphocyte counts are greater than or equal to 200 cells/μL. See *MMWR* 2007;56,RR-4). **Precautions** • Moderate or severe acute illness. • If blood, plasma, and/or immune globulin (IG or VZIG) were given in past 11m, see ACIP statement *General Recommendations on Immunization* regarding time to wait before vaccinating.
Meningo-coccal Conjugate vaccine (MCV) *Give IM* Polysaccharide vaccine (MPSV) *Give SC*	• All persons age 11 through 18yrs. • College freshmen living in a dormitory. • Persons with anatomic or functional asplenia or with a terminal-complement component deficiency. • Persons who travel to or reside in countries in which meningococcal disease is hyperendemic or epidemic (e.g., the "meningitis belt" of Sub-Saharan Africa). • Microbiologists routinely exposed to isolates of *N. meningitidis*.	• Give 1 dose. • If previous vaccine was MPSV, revaccinate after 3yrs if risk continues. • Revaccination after MCV is not recommended. • MCV is preferred over MPSV for persons age ≥ 55yrs and younger, although MPSV is an acceptable alternative.	**Contraindication** Previous anaphylactic or neurologic reaction to this vaccine or to any of its components, including diphtheria toxoid (for MCV). **Precautions** • Moderate or severe acute illness. • For MCV only, history of Guillain-Barré syndrome (GBS).
MMR (Measles, mumps, rubella) *Give SC*	• Persons born in 1957 or later (especially those born outside the U.S.) should receive at least 1 dose of MMR if there is no serologic proof of immunity or documentation of a dose given on or after the first birthday. • Persons in high-risk groups, such as healthcare personnel (paid, unpaid, or volunteer), students entering college and other post–high school educational institutions, and international travelers, should receive a total of 2 doses. • Persons born before 1957 are usually considered immune, but proof of immunity (serology or vaccination) may be desirable for healthcare personnel. • Women of childbearing age who do not have acceptable evidence of rubella immunity or vaccination.	• Give 1 or 2 doses (see criteria in 1st and 2nd bullets in box to left). • If dose #2 is recommended, give it no sooner than 4wks after dose #1. • If a pregnant woman is found to be rubella susceptible, give 1 dose of MMR postpartum. • If 2 or more of the following live virus vaccines are to be given—LAIV, MMR, Var, and/or yellow fever vaccine—they should be given on the same day. If they are not, space them by at least 28d. • Within 72hrs of measles exposure, give 1 dose as postexposure prophylaxis to susceptible adults.	**Contraindications** • Previous anaphylactic reaction to this vaccine or to any of its components. • Pregnancy or possibility of pregnancy within 4wks. • Severe immunodeficiency (e.g., hematologic and solid tumors; receiving chemotherapy; congenital immunodeficiency; long-term immunosuppressive therapy; or severely symptomatic HIV). **Note:** HIV infection is NOT a contraindication to MMR for those who are not severely immunocompromised (i.e., CD4+ T-lymphocyte counts are greater than or equal to 200 cells/μL). **Precautions** • Moderate or severe acute illness. • If blood, plasma, and/or immune globulin were given in past 11m, see ACIP statement *General Recommendations on Immunization* regarding time to wait before vaccinating. • History of thrombocytopenia or thrombocytopenic purpura. **Note:** If TST (tuberculosis skin test) and MMR are both needed but not given on same day delay TST for 4–6wks after MMR.
Human papillomavirus (HPV) *Give IM*	All previously unvaccinated women through age 26yrs.	• Give 3 doses on a 0, 2, 6m schedule. • There must be at least 4wks between doses #1 and #2 and at least 12wks between doses #2 and #3. Overall, there must be at least 24wks between doses #1 and #3.	**Contraindication** Previous anaphylactic reaction to this vaccine or to any of its components. **Precautions** • Moderate or severe acute illness. • Data on vaccination in pregnancy are limited. Vaccination should be delayed until after completion of the pregnancy.

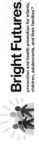

American Academy of Pediatrics
DEDICATED TO THE HEALTH OF ALL CHILDREN®

Recommendations for Preventive Pediatric Health Care

Bright Futures/American Academy of Pediatrics

Each child and family is unique; therefore, these **Recommendations for Preventive Pediatric Health Care** are designed for the care of children who are receiving competent parenting, have no manifestations of any important health problems, and are growing and developing in satisfactory fashion. **Additional visits may become necessary** if circumstances suggest variations from normal.

Developmental, psychosocial, and chronic disease issues for children and adolescents may require frequent counseling and treatment visits separate from preventive care visits.

These guidelines represent a consensus by the American Academy of Pediatrics (AAP) and Bright Futures. The AAP continues to emphasize the great importance of **continuity of care** in comprehensive health supervision and the need to avoid **fragmentation of care.**

The recommendations in this statement do not indicate an exclusive course of treatment or standard of medical care. Variations, taking into account individual circumstances, may be appropriate.

Copyright © 2008 by the American Academy of Pediatrics.

No part of this statement may be reproduced in any form or by any means without prior written permission from the American Academy of Pediatrics except for one copy for personal use.

Bright Futures.
prevention and health promotion for infants, children, adolescents, and their families™

AGE[1]	PRENATAL[2]	NEWBORN[3]	3–5 d[4]	By 1 mo	2 mo	4 mo	6 mo	9 mo	12 m	15 mo	18 mo	24 mo	30 mo	3 y	4 y	5 y	6 y	7 y	8 y	9 y	10 y	11 y	12 y	13 y	14 y	15 y	16 y	17 y	18 y	19 y	20 y	21 y
HISTORY Initial/Interval	●	●	●	●	●	●	●	●	●	●	●	●	●	●	●	●	●	●	●	●	●	●	●	●	●	●	●	●	●	●	●	●
MEASUREMENTS Length/Height and Weight		●	●	●	●	●	●	●	●	●	●	●	●	●	●	●	●	●	●	●	●	●	●	●	●	●	●	●	●	●	●	●
Head Circumference		●	●	●	●	●	●	●	●	●	●	●																				
Weight for Length		●	●	●	●	●	●	●	●	●	●																					
Body Mass Index[5]												●	●	●	●	●	●	●	●	●	●	●	●	●	●	●	●	●	●	●	●	●
Blood Pressure[5]		★	★	★	★	★	★	★	★	★	★	★	★	●	●	●	●	●	●	●	●	●	●	●	●	●	●	●	●	●	●	●
SENSORY SCREENING Vision[6]		★	★	★	★	★	★	★	★	★	★	★	★	●	●	●	●	★	●	★	●	★	●	★	★	●	★	★	●	★	★	★
Hearing[7]		●	★	★	★	★	★	★	★	★	★	★	★	★	●	●	●	★	●	★	●	★	★	★	★	★	★	★	★	★	★	★
DEVELOPMENTAL/BEHAVIORAL ASSESSMENT Developmental Screening[8]								●			●		●																			
Autism Screening[9]											●	●																				
Developmental Surveillance[8]		●	●	●	●	●	●		●	●		●		●	●	●	●	●	●	●	●	●	●	●	●	●	●	●	●	●	●	●
Psychosocial/Behavioral Assessment		●	●	●	●	●	●	●	●	●	●	●	●	●	●	●	●	●	●	●	●	●	●	●	●	●	●	●	●	●	●	●
Alcohol and Drug Use Assessment																						★	★	★	★	★	★	★	★	★	★	★
PHYSICAL EXAMINATION[10]		●	●	●	●	●	●	●	●	●	●	●	●	●	●	●	●	●	●	●	●	●	●	●	●	●	●	●	●	●	●	●
PROCEDURES[11] Newborn Metabolic/Hemoglobin Screening[12]		●	●—→	●																												
Immunization[13]		●	●	●	●	●	●	●	●	●	●	●	●	●	●	●	●	●	●	●	●	●	●	●	●	●	●	●	●	●	●	●
Hematocrit or Hemoglobin[14]						★			● or ★	★	★	★	★	★	★	★	★	★	★	★	★	★	★	★	★	★	★	★	★	★	★	★
Lead Screening[15]							★	★[16]	● or ★[21]		★	● or ★[21]		★	★	★	★															
Tuberculin Test[17]				★			★		★			★		★	★	★	★	★	★	★	★	★	★	★	★	★	★	★	★	★	★	★
Dyslipidemia Screening[18]												★			★		★		★	←→	★	←→				←→			↑			↓
STI Screening[19]																						★	★	★	★	★	★	★	★	★	★	★
Cervical Dysplasia Screening[20]																													★—→	★	★	★
ORAL HEALTH[21]							★	★	● or ★[21]		● or ★[21]	● or ★[21]	● or ★[21]	●[22]			●[22]															
ANTICIPATORY GUIDANCE[23]	●	●	●	●	●	●	●	●	●	●	●	●	●	●	●	●	●	●	●	●	●	●	●	●	●	●	●	●	●	●	●	●

1. If a child comes under care for the first time at any point on the schedule, or if any items are not accomplished at the suggested age, the schedule should be brought up to date at the earliest possible time.

2. A prenatal visit is recommended for parents who are at high risk, for first-time parents, and for those who request a conference. The prenatal visit should include anticipatory guidance, pertinent medical history, and a discussion of benefits of breastfeeding and planned method of feeding per AAP statement "The Prenatal Visit" (2001) [URL: http://aappolicy.aappublications.org/cgi/content/full/pediatrics;107/6/1456].

3. Every infant should have a newborn evaluation after birth, breastfeeding encouraged, and instruction and support offered.

4. Every infant should have an evaluation within 3 to 5 days of birth and within 48 to 72 hours after discharge from the hospital to include evaluation for feeding and jaundice. Breastfeeding infants should receive formal breastfeeding evaluation, encouragement, and instruction as recommended in AAP statement "Breastfeeding and the Use of Human Milk" (2005) [URL: http://aappolicy.aappublications.org/cgi/content/full/pediatrics;115/2/496]. For newborns discharged in less than 48 hours after delivery, the infant must be examined within 48 hours of discharge per AAP statement "Hospital Stay for Healthy Term Newborns" (2004) [URL: http://aappolicy.aappublications.org/cgi/content/full/pediatrics;113/5/1434].

5. Blood pressure measurement in infants and children with specific risk conditions should be performed at visits before age 3 years.

6. If the patient is uncooperative, rescreen within 6 months per the AAP statement "Eye Examination in Infants, Children, and Young Adults by Pediatricians" (2007) [URL: http://aappolicy.aappublications.org/cgi/content/full/pediatrics;111/4/902].

7. All newborns should be screened per the AAP statement "Year 2000 Position Statement: Principles and Guidelines for Early Hearing Detection and Intervention Programs" (2000) [URL: http://aappolicy.aappublications.org/cgi/content/full/pediatrics;106/4/798], Joint Committee on Infant Hearing, Year 2007 position statement: principles and guidelines for early hearing detection and intervention programs. Pediatrics; 2007;120:898–921.

8. AAP Council on Children With Disabilities, AAP Section on Developmental Behavioral Pediatrics, AAP Bright Futures Steering Committee, AAP Medical Home Initiatives for Children With Special Needs Project Advisory Committee. Identifying infants and young children with developmental disorders in the medical home: an algorithm for developmental surveillance and screening. Pediatrics. 2006;118:405–420 [URL: http://aappolicy.aappublications.org/cgi/content/full/pediatrics;118/1/405].

9. Gupta VB, Hyman SL, Johnson CP, et al. Identifying children with autism early? Pediatrics. 2007;119:152–153 [URL: http://pediatrics.aappublications.org/cgi/content/full/119/1/152].

10. At each visit, age-appropriate physical examination is essential, with infant totally unclothed, older child undressed and suitably draped.

11. These may be modified, depending on entry point into schedule and individual need.

12. Newborn metabolic and hemoglobinopathy screening should be done according to state law. Results should be reviewed at visits and appropriate retesting or referral done as needed.

13. Schedules per the Committee on Infectious Diseases, published annually in the January issue of Pediatrics. Every visit should be an opportunity to update and complete a child's immunizations.

14. See AAP Pediatric Nutrition Handbook, 5th Edition (2003) for a discussion of universal and selective screening options. See also Recommendations to prevent and control iron deficiency in the United States. MMWR. 1998;47(RR-3):1–36.

15. For children at risk of lead exposure, consult the AAP statement "Lead Exposure in Children: Prevention, Detection, and Management" (2005) [URL: http://aappolicy.aappublications.org/cgi/content/full/pediatrics;116/4/1036]. Additionally, screening should be done in accordance with state law where applicable.

16. Perform risk assessments or screens as appropriate, based on universal screening requirements for patients with Medicaid or high prevalence areas.

17. Tuberculosis testing per recommendations of the Committee on Infectious Diseases, published in the current edition of Red Book: Report of the Committee on Infectious Diseases. Testing should be done on recognition of high-risk factors.

18. "Third Report of the National Cholesterol Education Program (NCEP) Expert Panel on Detection, Evaluation, and Treatment of High Blood Cholesterol in Adults (Adult Treatment Panel III) Final Report" (2002) [URL: http://circ.ahajournals.org/cgi/content/full/106/25/3143] and "The Expert Committee Recommendations on the Assessment, Prevention, and Treatment of Child and Adolescent Overweight and Obesity," Supplement to Pediatrics. In press.

19. All sexually active patients should be screened for sexually transmitted infections (STIs).

20. All sexually active girls should have screening for cervical dysplasia as part of a pelvic examination beginning within 3 years of onset of sexual activity or age 21 (whichever comes first).

21. Referral to dental home, if available. Otherwise, administer oral health risk assessment. If the primary water source is deficient in fluoride, consider oral fluoride supplementation.

22. At the visits for 3 years and 6 years of age, it should be determined whether the patient has a dental home. If the patient does not have a dental home, a referral should be made to one. If the primary water source is deficient in fluoride, consider oral fluoride supplementation.

23. Refer to the specific guidance by age as listed in Bright Futures Guidelines. (Hagan JF, Shaw JS, Duncan PM, eds. Bright Futures: Guidelines for Health Supervision of Infants, Children, and Adolescents. 3rd ed. Elk Grove Village, IL: American Academy of Pediatrics; 2008.)

KEY

● = to be performed   ★ = risk assessment to be performed, with appropriate action to follow, if positive   ● = range during which a service may be provided, with the symbol indicating the preferred age   ←——→ = range during which a service may be provided

Appendix E

Guidelines for Practice

E.1 INFECTION CONTROL GUIDELINES FOR HOME CARE

The practice of Universal Precautions means that all blood and body fluids are treated as potentially infectious. Universal Precautions procedures are implemented to prevent exposure and infection of caregivers. It is an important practice because many infections are subclinical.

- Use extreme care when handling needles, scalpels, and razors to prevent injuries. Do not recap, bend, break, or remove the needle from a syringe before disposal. Discard needles and syringes in puncture-resistant containers made of plastic or metal and dispose of them in a local landfill.
- Barrier precautions—such as gloves, masks, eye covering, and gowns—should be worn when contact with blood and body fluids is expected. Gloves must be worn when in contact with body fluids, mucous membranes, and nonintact skin and when drawing blood. Masks and eye coverings are recommended when droplets or splashes of blood or other body fluids are expected. Gowns, aprons, or smocks should be worn to protect regular clothing from splashes of blood or body fluids.
- Handwashing is the single most important practice in preventing infections. Handwashing should be done before and after providing client care and before and after preparing food, eating, feeding, or using the bathroom.

- Soiled dressings and perineal pads should be placed inside polyethylene garbage bags using two bags, one inside the other as a liner.
- HIV is easily decontaminated by common disinfectants such as Lysol and is rapidly killed by household bleach. Surfaces can be disinfected with a solution of 1 part bleach to 10 parts water. A new solution must be prepared daily to retain its disinfectant properties. Bathrooms and kitchens can be safely shared with persons infected with HIV, but towels, razors, and toothbrushes should not be shared. Household cleaning can be done in a regular manner unless there are spills of blood or body fluids. If a spill occurs, wear gloves and decontaminate the area by flooding the spill with a disinfectant, then use paper towels to remove visible debris, and reapply the disinfectant.
- Kitchen counters, dishes, and laundry should be cleaned in warm water and detergent after use. Bathrooms may be cleaned with a household disinfectant.

E.2 ACCIDENT PREVENTION IN CHILDREN

Age	Development	Major Accidents	Anticipatory Guidance
Neonate to 1 month	Is unable to protect self; when on abdomen can lift and turn head; dependent, requires protection; little control over body and movements.	Motor vehicles	Use approved car seat. Do not hold infant in lap. Never leave infant in car unattended.
		Strangulation	Spacing between crib bars should be no more than $2^3/_8$ inches apart. Avoid tying anything, including pacifiers, around neck. Fasten mobiles securely.
		Suffocation and injuries	Crib mattress should fit firmly to sides. Do not use pillows; use bumper pads. Support infant's head when lifting, holding, or bathing.
		Burns, including sunburn	Avoid bathing near hot water faucets. Test water temperature before bath. Set home water temperature less than 120 °F to 130 °F. Avoid handling hot liquids, and do not smoke while handling infant. Keep out of direct sunlight, and use sunscreen. Use flame-resistant clothing and furniture. Have smoke detectors and fire extinguishers in the home. Develop a fire plan for the home.
2 to 3 months	Begins gross motor movements of wiggling, squirming, thrashing, rolling.	Falls	Never leave infant unattended (at any age) for any reason. Keep one hand on infant while giving care. Keep crib sides up. Use infant seat on floor or playpen.
4 to 5 months	Mouths objects; brings hands to mouth.	Aspiration and choking	Do not prop bottles (at any age). Burp well before putting infant in crib. Toys should be too large for infant to swallow, nonbreakable, and free of sharp edges, strings, and detachable parts. Keep diaper pins closed during changing. Keep small objects (e.g., buttons, coins) out of reach. Use only one-piece pacifiers with a large shield.
		Suffocation	Keep all plastic bags out of reach. Keep stuffed animals out of crib.
		Lead poisoning	Check toys and other objects for lead-free paint.
6 to 7 months	Sits without support; has a firm grasp; rolls and creeps.	Falls and falling objects	Use safety strap in stroller or high chair. Use sturdy high chair or feeding table. Keep doors to stairs and outside locked; use safety gates. Avoid use of hanging tablecloths. Remove knickknacks and breakables.
		Ingestion	Keep small objects, medicine, and plants out of reach. Have poison control number posted. Lock up medicine, cleaning agents, insecticides, etc. Keep trashcans out of reach or use locklids.
		Injuries and electric shock	Cover wall outlets. Place furniture so cords are inaccessible. Check furniture for sharp corners—pad or remove. Inspect toys for breakage. Keep sharp objects out of reach.

Age	Development	Major Accidents	Anticipatory Guidance
8 to 12 months	Pulls to stand; crawls, grabs; beginning to walk; enjoys exploring.	Burns	Crawl around on floor and investigate what child could reach or get into.
			Keep all hot food and drinks away from table edge; turn pot handles inward on stove.
			Keep matches and lighters out of reach.
			Keep kitchen closed up or gated.
			Never leave child unattended near fireplace or stove.
			Place guards around open hearths, registers, stoves, and fans.
			Do not iron when child is crawling nearby.
		Choking	Do not give child small hard foods, such as peanuts, raw vegetables, popcorn.
			Inspect toys for broken parts.
			Keep floors, counters, tables free of small objects.
		Motor vehicle accidents	Continue use of car seat.
		Poisoning	Keep doors locked.
			See previous discussion.
1 to 2 years	Walks up and down stairs; stoops and recovers; climbs; likes to take things apart.	Falls and injuries	Supervise children in most activities, especially up and down stairs, out of doors, and at playgrounds.
			Lock all windows; when opening, do so from top only.
			Remove any objects or furniture in front of window that child could use as a ladder.
			Permit climbing within child's capabilities.
			Remove bumper pads or toys in crib that child could use to climb on.
			Check toys, especially riding ones, for damage.
			Keep small, pointed, or sharp objects out of reach.
			Keep out of way of swings.
		Burns	Teach child meaning of hot.
			Avoid use of flowing clothing.
		Drowning	Continue to supervise bath/toilet use.
			Supervise all water sport activity (e.g., wading pools, swimming, boating); use floats and/or life jackets.
			Teach child to respect water and seek swimming lessons.
		Motor vehicle accidents	Continue to use appropriate car seat.
			Keep doors and windows locked.
			Do not permit child to hang out of windows.
			Hold onto child when crossing street or in parking lots.
			Do not permit child to ride toys near street.
		Poisoning and ingestion	Use childproof caps on medications.
			Do not regard medicine as candy.
			Do not give one child another's prescription.
2 to 4 years	More adventuresome and curious; explores body orifices; more independent, with limited cognition, imitates.	Falls and injuries	Teach child to be cautious around strange animals.
			Supervise play at playground.
			Keep small objects and foods (peanuts, beans) that can be inserted into orifices out of reach; check buttons on clothes and toys.
			Discontinue use of crib when height of crib rail is 75% of toddler's height.
			Keep stairs well-lighted and free of clutter.
			Give toys a safety check.
			Discourage running in house, and limit outdoor running to safe places.

Continued

Appendixes

Age	Development	Major Accidents	Anticipatory Guidance
			Teach child to respect street and cars.
			Teach child to stay away from and out of old appliances.
		Drowning	Continue to teach water safety.
			Supervise all water activities.
			Continue with swimming lessons.
		Motor vehicle accidents	See previous discussion.
	Play increases to include rougher games and bike riding. Cognition improving and can identify good and bad.	Burns	Teach child what to do if fire breaks out; hold household drills.
			Teach child to roll and smother clothes if they catch on fire.
			Teach child about danger of matches, lighters, stove.
			Recheck radiators, space heaters, fireplaces, and protective guards.
		Drowning	Continue swimming lessons.
			Use floats or lifejacket if child cannot swim.
			Swim only where supervision is available (parent or lifeguard).
		Motor vehicle accidents	Teach pedestrian safety, providing example for child.
			Do not permit playing in street.
			Use adult seatbelt if child is over 60–80 pounds.
		Falls, injuries	Make periodic checks on playground or play area used frequently.
			Check on child when out playing.
			Instruct child in safe use of toys; keep in good condition.
			Keep away from driveways and streets.
			If possible, provide fenced-in play area.
			Set a good example by using seatbelt, looking before crossing street, etc.
		Poisoning and ingestions	Do not become lax about keeping medication, etc., locked up.
			Teach child to respect harmful objects, and use a symbol to indicate "danger or harmful" to child.
			Routinely check house, basement, and garage for harmful substances within reach.
4 to 6 years	Continues to be curious, daring, and imitative; frequently plays out of sight.		Involve child in safety discussions.
			Continue previously described activities when using household tools and equipment.
School age	Increased motor coordination and cognitive ability; increased peer and group activity and involvement in sports; assumes more responsibility for self and well-being.	Motor vehicle and bicycle accidents	Involve child in safety discussion and planning.
			Assign safety responsibilities, such as checking bike.
			Teach child not to ride with strangers.
			Teach child how to contact the police and fire department and physician.
			Be certain child knows address and phone number.
			Discuss bicycle and pedestrian safety.
			Discuss bicycle riding rules:
			Always wear an approved bike helmet.
			Do not hitch a ride on moving vehicles.
			Do not ride on dark streets.
			Use headlight or reflector light at night; wear bright clothes.
			Do not dart from behind parked cars.
			Do not carry passengers on bicycle.
			Keep bike in good repair.

Age	Development	Major Accidents	Anticipatory Guidance
			Do not use the street as a playground.
			Use seatbelts.
		Injuries	Teach child to participate in sports safely using appropriate gear.
			Permit only supervised sport activities.
			Teach child proper use of household gadgets and equipment; supervise as necessary.
		Drowning	Teach the following swimming rules:
			Swim only where a lifeguard is present.
			Use buddy system.
			Know water depth before diving.
			Wear life jacket while boating or skiing or if nonswimmer.
			No horseplay or calling for help jokingly.
		Falls	See bicycle rules.
			Discuss climbing trees:
			Avoid slippery shoes.
			Avoid weak or dead branches.
			Keep a secure handhold.
		Burns	Continue household drills.
			Camp with supervision.
			Teach proper campfire and barbecue care.
			Use safe camping gear, including flame-retardant clothes.
Adolescence	Seeking identity and establishment of independence; subject to strong peer pressure; rejects unsought advice; has a need for physical activity; spends most of free time away from home.	Drowning	Most important to have cooperation of adolescent when discussing and implementing safety measures.
			See previous sections.
			Never too late to learn to swim.
			Enroll in lifesaving classes.
		Firearms accidents	Avoid having loaded guns in household.
			Learn safety handling if involved in sport hunting.
			Keep guns in locked closet and ammunition in separate locked area.
			Never assume gun is not loaded.
			Never point gun at another.
		Motor vehicle accidents	Take driver's education.
			Use seatbelts for self and passengers.
			Practice pedestrian safety.
			Do not drive under the influence of drugs or alcohol.
			Do not hitchhike or pick up hitchhikers.
		Alcohol, drugs, and tobacco	Discuss effects of substance use and abuse.
			Assist teen to identify other ways to achieve self-esteem, independence, and peer acceptance.

E.3 THE HEALTH INSURANCE PORTABILITY AND ACCOUNTABILITY ACT (HIPAA): WHAT DOES IT MEAN FOR PUBLIC HEALTH NURSES?

Public Health Nursing Practice—definition: the synthesis of nursing and public health theory applied to promoting and preserving the health of populations. The practice focuses on the community as a whole and on the effect of the community's health status (resources) on the health of individuals, families, and groups. The goal is to prevent disease and disability and promote and protect the health of the community as a whole.

EXPLANATION
- Federal privacy standards were created by the Department of Health and Human Services (HHS) to protect patients' medical records and other health information provided to health plans, doctors, hospitals, and other health care providers.
  - These standards took effect on April 14, 2003.
  - The standardization of electronic transactions, and the elimination of inefficient paper forms, will save the health care industry over $29 billion in the next 10 years.

PRIVACY RULE
- Protects the confidentiality of individually identifiable health information, whether it is on paper, in computers, or communicated orally.
  - Protected health information (PHI) is the name for this individually identifiable health information.
  - Limits the ways that health plans, pharmacies, hospitals, and other covered entities can use patients' personal medical information.

PATIENT PROTECTIONS
- Patients should be able to see, obtain copies of, and make corrections to their medical records.
- Patients should receive a notice from health care providers regarding how their personal medical information may be used by them and their rights under the privacy regulation. Patients can restrict this use.
- Limits have been set on how health care providers can use individually identifiable health information. Doctors, nurses, and other providers can share information needed to treat a patient. For purposes other than medical care, personal health information generally may not be used.
- Pharmacies, health plans, and other covered entities must obtain an individual's authorization before disclosing patient information for marketing purposes.

PUBLIC HEALTH SERVICES AND PHI
Overview: Although protection of health information is important, PHI is used for the public good by health officials to identify, monitor, and respond to disease, death, and disability among populations. Examples of ways PHI is used include public health surveillance, program evaluation, terrorism preparedness, outbreak investigations, direct health services, and public health research. Public health authorities have taken precautions in the past to protect the privacy of individuals and will continue to do so under HIPAA. The privacy rule, however, still permits PHI to be shared for important public health purposes.

PERMITTED PHI DISCLOSURES TO A PUBLIC HEALTH AUTHORITY WITHOUT AUTHORIZATION
- Reporting of disease, injury, and vital events
- Conducting public health surveillance, investigations, and interventions
- Reporting child abuse or neglect to a public health or other government authority legally authorized to receive such reports
- To a person subject to the jurisdiction of the Food and Drug Administration (FDA) concerning the quality, safety, or effectiveness of an FDA-related product or activity for which that person has responsibility
- To a person who may have been exposed to a communicable disease or may be at risk for contracting or spreading a disease or condition, when legally authorized to notify the person as necessary to conduct a public health intervention or investigation
- To an individual's employer, under certain circumstances and conditions, as needed for the employer to meet the requirements of the Occupational Safety and Health Administration, Mine Safety and Health Administration, or similar state law

HIPAA AND NURSING RESEARCH
Definitions
Covered entity: a health plan, a health care clearinghouse, or a health care provider who transmits any health information in electronic form.
Individually Identifiable Health Information (IIHI): information about an individual regarding his or her physical or mental health; the provision of health care; or the payment for the provision of health care; and which identifies the individual.
  - It is the covered entity's obligation not to disclose the information improperly when a researcher—seeks data that includes PHI.

A covered entity can disclose IIHI for research purposes under any of the following conditions:
1. The IIHI pertains only to deceased persons.
2. The IIHI can be examined for reviews preparatory to research if it is not removed from the covered entity.
3. Information that has been deidentified can be disclosed; this information is no longer considered IIHI and thus is not covered by HIPAA.
4. Data must be disclosed as part of a limited data set if the researcher has a data use agreement with the covered entity.
5. The researcher has a valid authorization from the research subject to disclose IIHI.
6. An IRB or Privacy board has waived the authorization requirement.

Creating Data
Researchers may also be creating IIHI. If the researcher is part of a covered entity, any PHI obtained by any means is covered by HIPAA, and the researcher and his or her institution are bound by HIPAA regulations. Most universities with nursing schools will be hybrid entities (i.e., some parts of the university are a covered entity and some are not). Researchers should check their institution's policies.

Disclosing Data

Nurse researchers should be aware that sharing data with colleagues and students may constitute disclosures of IIHI and they should conform to HIPAA regulations. In this case, the researcher is the holder of the IIHI and can disclose it only under appropriate conditions:

1. Patients agree to specific disclosures in the initial authorization.
2. Former patients sign an additional authorization.
3. An IRB or privacy board waives the need for authorization.
4. The holder allows the colleague to review the data to prepare a research protocol if the colleague takes no information away.
5. A holder enters the data in a limited data set and signs a data use agreement with the recipient.
6. A holder deidentifies the data and shares it freely.

From Olsen DP: HIPAA privacy regulations and nursing research, *Nurs Res* 52(5):344–348, 2003; U.S. Department of Health and Human Services: Fact sheet. Retrieved Jan 26, 2004, from www.hhs.gov/news/press/2002pres/hipaa.html; CDC: *HIPAA privacy rule and public health.* Retrieved Feb 12, 2004, from www.cdc.gov/mmwr/preview/mmwrhtml/su5201a1.htm.

E.4 LIVING WILL DIRECTIVE

Living Will Directive

My wishes regarding life-prolonging treatment and artificially provided nutrition and hydration to be provided to me if I no longer have decisional capacity, have a terminal condition, or become permanently unconscious have been indicated by checking and initialing the appropriate lines below. By checking and initialing the appropriate lines, I specifically:

Designate _____ as my health care surrogate(s) to make health care decisions for me in accordance with this directive when I no longer have decisional capacity. If _____ refuses or is not able to act for me, I designate _____ as my health care surrogate(s).

Any prior designation is revoked.

If I do not designate a surrogate, the following are my directions to my attending physician. If I have designated a surrogate, my surrogate shall comply with my wishes as indicated below:

_____ Direct that treatment be withheld or withdrawn, and that I be permitted to die naturally with only the administration of medication or the performance of any medical treatment deemed necessary to alleviate pain.

_____ DO NOT authorize that life-prolonging treatment be withheld or withdrawn.

_____ Authorize the withholding or withdrawal of artificially provided food, water, or other artificially provided nourishment or fluids.

_____ DO NOT authorize the withholding or withdrawal of artificially provided food, water, or other artificially provided nourishment or fluids.

_____ Authorize my surrogate, designated above, to withhold or withdraw artificially provided nourishment or fluids, or other treatment if the surrogate determines that withholding or withdrawing is in my best interest; but I do not mandate that withholding or withdrawing.

In the absence of my ability to give directions regarding the use of life-prolonging treatment and artificially provided nutrition and hydration, it is my intention that this directive shall be honored by my attending physician, my family, and any surrogate designated pursuant to this directive as the final expression of my legal right to refuse medical or surgical treatment and I accept the consequences of the refusal.

If I have been diagnosed as pregnant and that diagnosis is known to my attending physician, this directive shall have no force or effect during the course of my pregnancy.

I understand the full import of this directive and I am emotionally and mentally competent to make this directive.

Signed this _____ day of _____, 20____.

_____

Signature and address of the grantor.

If our joint presence, the grantor, who is of sound mind and eighteen years of age, or older, voluntarily dated and signed this writing or directed it to be dated and signed for the grantor.

_____

Signature and address of witness.

_____

Signature and address of witness.

OR

_____

_____ County

Before me, the undersigned authority, came the grantor who is of sound mind and eighteen (18) years of age, or older, and acknowledged that he voluntarily dated and signed this writing or directed it to be signed and dated as above.

Done this _____ day of _____, 20____.

_____

Signature of Notary Public or other.

_____

Date commission expires.

Execution of this document restricts withholding and withdrawing of some medical procedures. Consult State Revised Statutes or your attorney.

Screening Tools

F.1 SCREENING FOR COMMON ORTHOPEDIC PROBLEMS

Deformity

Congenital hip dislocation (CHD): Complete or partial displacement of femoral head out of the acetabulum.

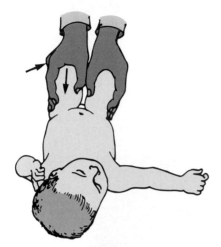

FIGURE F-1

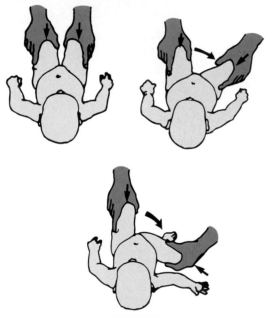

FIGURE F-2

Screening

Barlow's maneuver (for dislocation of femoral head): Flex hip to 90 degrees; grasp symphysis in front and sacrum in back with one hand; with other hand, apply lateral pressure to medial thigh with thumb and longitudinal pressure to knee with palm; abduct flexed hip. A positive sign is a sensation of abnormal movement. Reverse hands for examining other hip (Figure F-1).

Ortolani's maneuver (for reduction of femur): Abduct hip to 80 degrees, lifting proximal femur anteriorly with fingers placed on lateral thigh. A positive sign is a sensation of a jerk or snap with reduction into socket (Figure F-2).

Limited full abduction of hips: With child flat on back, abduct hips one at a time, then together. See Figure F-3 for degrees of hip abduction.

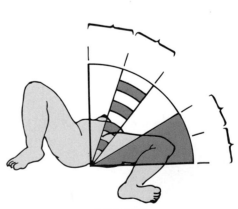

FIGURE F-3

Deformity

Metatarsus adductus (varus): Adduction or turning in of forefoot with high longitudinal arch and wide space between first and second toes. Commonly associated with tibial torsion.

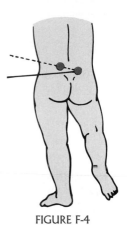

FIGURE F-4

Pes planus (flat feet): When child is weight bearing, longitudinal arch of foot appears flat on floor.
1. Pseudo flat feet: Very common until ages 2 to 3 years; created by plantar fat pad. Feet are flexible, exhibit hypermobility of joint, and have a low arch.
2. Rigid flat feet: Uncommon; created by tightness of heel cord or tarsal coalition (a cartilaginous fibrous or bony connection between bones).

Screening

Apparent shortening of femur:
1. Allis's sign: With child lying on back, pelvis flat, knees flexed, and feet planted firmly, observe knees. If one knee projects further anteriorly, the femur is longer; if one knee is higher, the tibia is longer.
2. With child on back, both legs are extended out with pressure on knees. Heels are matched and observed for equal or unequal length.
3. Trendelenburg's sign: With child standing on one leg, observe pelvis. When child stands on abnormal leg, the pelvis drops on the normal side (Figure F-4).

Test foot for flexibility, and elicit tonic foot reflexes. Rigidity is indicated by eversion or inversion when foot does not move beyond neutral position or does not respond to toe grasping or by dorsiflexing. Signs of metatarsus adductus are illustrated in Figure F-5.
1. Observe feet in weighted and unweighted position.
2. Stand child on toes. Arch disappears with weight bearing in flexible flat foot and reappears when on toes (Figure F-6).
3. Elicit dorsal and plantar flexion to rule out tight heel cord.
4. Elicit eversion and inversion flexion to rule out tarsal coalition.

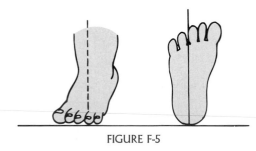

FIGURE F-5

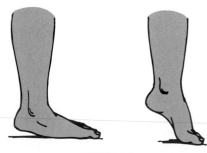

FIGURE F-6

Continued

Deformity

Genu valgum (knock knees): A deviant axis of thighs and calves of more than 10 to 15 degrees (normal from ages 2 to 6).

Genu varum (bowlegs): Deviant axis of thighs and calves, which is:
1. Physiological: Normal until ages 2 to 3 years; occurs with internal tibial torsion and genu valgum.
2. Pathological.

Screening

Same as for pseudo flat feet.

1. Observe axis of thighs and calves with child standing. Normally axes are parallel with 10 to 15 degrees deviance (Figure F-7).
2. Observe space between the knees from front to back. Normal spacing is 1½ inches.
3. Observe space between ankles from front and back. Normal spacing between medial malleoli at heel is 2 inches.
Same as for genu valgum.

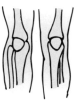 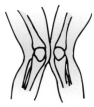 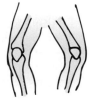

FIGURE F-7

Internal tibial torsion: Twisting or torsion of tibia usually accompanied by metatarsus adductus.

1. Examine legs for range of motion and flexibility of ankle, and elicit tonic foot reflexes.
2. Holding knee firmly with foot in neutral position, observe medial and lateral malleoli. The normal angle between them is approximately 15 to 20 degrees (Figure F-8).
3. Have child sit on examining table and draw a circle over the patellar and external malleoli. With patella facing forward, only anterior edge of malleolar circle should be seen (Figure F-9).

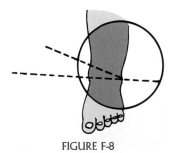

FIGURE F-8

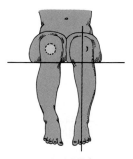

FIGURE F-9

Deformity

Scoliosis: S-shaped lateral curvature of spine with rotation of vertical bodies.

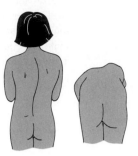

FIGURE F-10

Screening

Screening is implemented as follows:

1. Ask the child to bend forward in a 50% flexing position with shoulders drooping forward and arms and head dangling. Observe the spine from above the head and inspect for any lateral curvature or prominent projection of the rib cage on one side (Figure F-10).
2. While the child is standing erect with weight equal on both feet, observe for the following:
    a. Difference in levels of shoulders, scapula, and hips
    b. Differences in the size of the spaces between the arms and the trunk
    c. Prominence of either scapulae or hip
    d. A curve in the vertebral spinous process alignment
3. Ask the child to walk, and make observations discussed in No. 2 and observe for the presence of a waddle, limp, or tilt.

F.2 Vision and Hearing Screening Procedures

Method	Age	Procedure	Normal Response
Vision			
Following	Infancy	Shine light or hold bright object directly in front of infant's line of vision; move slowly from side to side.	Follow light or bright object up to 180 degrees.
Turn to light response	Infancy	Hold back of head to bright light source.	Eyes turn toward source of light.
Optokinetic drum	Infancy	Twirl drum with stripes slowly in front of infant's eyes.	Nystagmus occurs.
Hirschberg reflex (corneal light reflex)	Infancy through adolescence	Shine penlight into child's eyes; note where light reflex falls. For older children: have child focus and stare at a point 14 inches and then 20 inches away before shining light into eyes.	Light reflex falls in same position in eye.
Cover test	Toddler through adolescence	Have child focus on specified spot first 14 inches, then 20 inches away. While child is focusing, one eye is completely covered for 5 to 10 seconds. Cover is then removed and eye observed for movement. Procedure repeated for other eye.	No wandering or sharp jerky movement of eyes noted, indicating ability to focus.
Snellen E	Preschool	Child is instructed to point finger in direction that the E or table legs are pointing from a distance of 20 feet. Test each eye separately, then together. Test as far down on chart as child can go.	Visual acuity of 20/30–20/40.
Snellen alphabet	School age through adolescence	Child stands 20 feet from chart and reads letters. Each eye is tested separately and then together. Testing usually started at 20/30 or 20/40 line and child is allowed to test as far down chart as possible. Passing score consists of reading the majority of letters (or E's) on each line.	Visual acuity of 20/20.
Hearing			
Startle reflex	Newborn	Loud noise or bang made near infant's ears.	Jumps at noise, blinks, cries, or widens eyes.
Tracks sound	3–6 months	Make noise, call name, or sing.	Eyes shift toward sound; responds to mother's voice; coos to verbalization.

Continued

Method	Age	Procedure	Normal Response
Recognizes sound	6–8 months	As preceding, from out of line of vision.	Turns head toward sound; responds to name, babbles to verbalization.
Localization of sound	8–12 months	Call name, or use tuning fork or say words.	Localizes source of sound; turns head (and body at times) toward sound, repeats words.
Pure tone screening—play	Toddler to preschool	Demonstrate to child by putting headphones on and making believe you hear sound. As you say "I hear it," put a block in box or ring on holder. Put headphones on child and give block or ring to use. Sound a 50-dB tone at 1000 Hz and guide child's hand with block to box. When child can do this alone, begin screening. Set at 25 dB at 1000 Hz. If child responds, go to 2000, 4000, and 6000 Hz. Praise child and place new block in hand. Switch to other ear and test.	Should respond at 25 dB at any frequency.
Pure tone audiometry	School age through adolescence	Explain procedure to child. Place headphones on ears. Test one ear at a time in sequence as preceding (i.e., 25 dB at 1000, 2000, 4000, and 6000 Hz). Have child raise hand to indicate sound is heard.	Should respond at 25 dB at any frequency.
Tuning fork test	Some preschoolers; school age through adolescence		
Weber test		Strike tuning fork to make it vibrate, and place the stem in midline of scalp. Ask child if sound is same in both ears or louder in either ear.	Sound heard equally well in both ears.
Rinne test		Strike tuning fork until it vibrates, place stem on child's mastoid until the child no longer hears it. Then place vibrating fingers of fork 1 to 2 inches in front of concha. Ask child if he or she can still hear the sound.	Sound from fingers of fork vibrating in air should be heard when child can no longer hear sound with stem against mastoid (i.e., air conduction is greater than bone conduction).

F.3 TANNER STAGES OF PUBERTY

Both Sexes	**Pubic Hair**
Stage 1	Prepubescent: no pubic hair
Stage 2	Sparse growth along labia or at base of penis; long, slightly pigmented, downy
Stage 3	Darker, coarser, curly hair spreading sparsely over junction of the pubes
Stage 4	Dark, coarse, adult-like in texture but smaller area of distribution
Stage 5	Adult-like in quantity and distribution; spread to medial surface of thighs
Stage 6	Spread up linea alba

Boys	**Genitalia Development**
Stage 1	Prepubescent: no change from childhood
Stage 2	Scrotum and testes enlarge; scrotal skin reddened and thicker in texture
Stage 3	Penis elongates; further enlargement of scrotum and testes
Stage 4	Penis enlarges with increased size of glans; scrotal skin continues to darken
Stage 5	Genitalia adult-like in size, shape, and pigmentation

Girls	**Breast Development**
Stage 1	Prepubescent: elevation of papilla only
Stage 2	Development of breast bud; diameter of areola increases; papilla and breast form small mound
Stage 3	Enlargement of breast and areola with no separation of contours
Stage 4	Areola and papilla form secondary mound above the level of the breast
Stage 5	Mature stage: projection of papilla only, due to recession of the areola to the general contour of the breast

Assessment Tools

G.1 COMMUNITY-AS-PARTNER MODEL

The community-as-partner model was developed to illustrate public health nursing as a synthesis of public health and nursing. The model, originally titled the *community-as-client* model, has evolved to incorporate the philosophy that nurses work with communities as partners. This is congruent with what was learned about how communities (and people, for that matter) change and grow best, that is, by full involvement and self-empowerment, not by imposed programs and structures.

The model's "heart" is the assessment wheel (Figure G-1), which shows that the people actually are the community—the core elements. Without people there is no community, and it is the people (their demographics, values, beliefs, and history) that are of interest to the public health nurse. Surrounding the people, and integral with them, are the identified eight subsystems of a community. These subsystems (physical environment, education, safety and transportation, politics and government, health and social services, communication, economics, and recreation) both affect and are affected by the people. To understand this interaction, it is necessary to understand each subsystem; therefore, it is necessary to incorporate its assessment into the assessment of the people.

The "wheel" (actually the entire community, including the people and subsystems) is shown with broken lines between each subsystem to show that these are not discrete, but that all subsystems affect each other. Within the community are lines of resistance, those "strengths" that defend against stressors (e.g., a school-based program to prevent teen violence); identifying strengths in the community is as important as identifying "problems." Surrounding the community are lines of defense, depicted in the model as "flexible" and "normal" to indicate that there are two types of defense: one is the usual (normal) "health" of a community and the other is more dynamic (flexible) and changes more rapidly. Two illustrations may

assist in clarifying these lines. The flexible line of defense may be a temporary response to a stressor. For instance, an environmental stressor such as flash flooding or a major fire may call into play resources from within the community and from surrounding areas; these resources are considered the flexible lines of defense. The normal line of defense is the usual level of health a community has reached over time. Examples of normal lines of defense include the immunization rate, adequate housing, or access to Meals-on-Wheels for shut-ins; all of these contribute to the health of the community.

Stressors affect the community and may be from the community or from outside the community. Either way, the community's response to stressors is mitigated by its overall health state, that is, by the strength of its lines of resistance and defense. Knowing these strengths is one purpose of the community assessment. In the analysis phase of the nursing process, the nurse will weigh the stressor and the degree of reaction it causes in order to describe a community nursing diagnosis that, in turn, will give direction to goals and interventions. One method for stating the community nursing diagnosis is to state the "problem" as the degree of reaction (from which the goal is derived) and to state the "as related to" as stressors ("causes" that help define needed interventions). Using this method, an example of a community nursing diagnosis might be as follows: High rate of tuberculosis (the problem, the degree of reaction) related to poor hygiene and sanitation, crowded living conditions, poverty, and consumption of raw milk (stressors) as manifested by open garbage and poor ventilation; an average of 5.6 persons per household; and sale of raw milk for income (the "data" collected in your assessment).

Think for a moment how each subsystem contributes to the health of the community. The nurse can see how an inadequate infrastructure, such as lack of modern sewage treatment or unemployment, can affect the health of all of the citizens.

Many models exist to provide a framework for assessing a community. This systems model gives one other way to describe a community. Working with the community is a vital and challenging task for nurses. Using a model wherein the community is viewed as a partner will help formulate community-focused interventions and promote the health of the entire community.

Elizabeth T. Anderson, RN, FAAN, DrPH
Professor and Chair, Department of Community Health and Technology
University of Texas School of Nursing at Galveston
University of Texas Medical Branch
Galveston, Texas

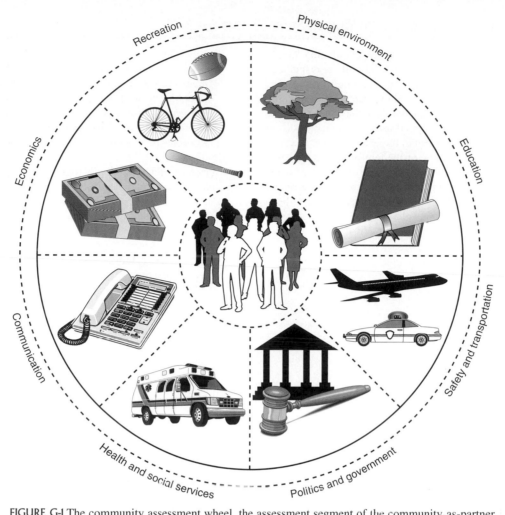

FIGURE G-I The community assessment wheel, the assessment segment of the community as-partner model. (From Anderson ET, McFarlane J: *Community-as-partner theory and practice in nursing,* ed 3, Philadelphia, 2000, Lippincott Williams & Wilkins.)

G.2 FRIEDMAN FAMILY ASSESSMENT MODEL (SHORT FORM)

Before using the following guidelines in completing family assessments, two words of caution. First, not all areas included below will be germane for each of the families visited. The guidelines are comprehensive and allow depth when probing is necessary. The student should not feel that every subarea needs to be covered when the broad area of inquiry poses no problems to the family or concern to the health worker. Second, by virtue of the interdependence of the family system, one will find unavoidable redundancy. For the sake of efficiency, the assessor should try not to repeat data, but to refer the reader back to sections where this information has already been described.

IDENTIFYING DATA

1. Family name
2. Address and phone
3. Family composition (see table)
4. Type of family form
5. Cultural (ethnic) background
6. Religious identification
7. Social class status
8. Family's recreational or leisure-time activities

DEVELOPMENTAL STAGE AND HISTORY OF FAMILY

9. Family's present developmental stage
10. Extent of developmental tasks fulfillment
11. Nuclear family history
12. History of family of origin of both parents

ENVIRONMENTAL DATA

13. Characteristics of home
14. Characteristics of neighborhood and larger community
15. Family's geographic mobility
16. Family's associations and transactions with community
17. Family's social support network (ecomap)

FAMILY STRUCTURE

18. Communication patterns
    Extent of functional and dysfunctional communication (types of recurring patterns)
    Extent of emotional (affective) messages and how expressed
    Characteristics of communication within family subsystems
    Extent of congruent and incongruent messages
    Types of dysfunctional communication processes seen in family
    Areas of open and closed communication
    Familial and external variables affecting communication
19. Power structure
    Power outcomes
    Decision-making process
    Power bases
    Variables affecting family power
    Overall family system and subsystem power
20. Role structure
    Formal role structure
    Informal role structure
    Analysis of role models (optional)
    Variables affecting role structure

21. Family values
    Compare the family to American or family's reference group values and/or identify important family values and their importance (priority) in family
    Congruence between the family's values and the family's reference group or wider community
    Congruence between the family's values and family member's values
    Variables influencing family values
    Values consciously or unconsciously held
    Presence of value conflicts in family
    Effect of the above values and value conflicts on health status of family

FAMILY FUNCTIONS

22. Affective function
    Family's need-response patterns
    Mutual nurturance, closeness, and identification
    Separateness and connectedness
23. Socialization function
    Family child-rearing practices
    Adaptability of child-rearing practices for family form and family's situation
    Who is (are) socializing agent(s) for child(ren)?
    Value of children in family
    Cultural beliefs that influence family's child-rearing patterns
    Social class influence on child-rearing patterns
    Estimation about whether family is at risk for child-rearing problems and, if so, indication of high-risk factors
    Adequacy of home environment for children's needs to play
24. Health care function
    Family's health beliefs, values, and behavior
    Family's definitions of health-illness and their level of knowledge
    Family's perceived health status and illness susceptibility
    Family's dietary practices
    Adequacy of family diet (recommended 24-hour food history record)
    Function of mealtimes and attitudes toward food and mealtimes
    Shopping (and its planning) practices
    Person(s) responsible for planning, shopping, and preparation of meals
    Sleep and rest habits
    Physical activity and recreation practices (not covered earlier)
    Family's drug habits
    Family's role in self-care practices
    Medically based preventive measures (physicals, eye and hearing tests, and immunizations)
    Dental health practices
    Family health history (both general and specific diseases—environmentally and genetically related)
    Health care services received
    Feelings and perceptions regarding health services
    Emergency health services
    Source of payments for health and other services
    Logistics of receiving care

FAMILY STRESS AND COPING

25. Short- and long-term familial stressors and strengths
26. Extent of family's ability to respond, based on objective appraisal of stress-producing situations
27. Coping strategies utilized (present/past)
    Differences in family members' ways of coping

Family's inner coping strategies
Family's external coping strategies
28. Dysfunctional adaptive strategies utilized (present/past; extent of usage)

Family Composition Form

Name (Last, First)	Gender	Relationship	Date and Place of Birth	Occupation	Education
1. (Father)					
2. (Mother)					
3. (Oldest child)					
4.					
5.					
6.					
7.					
8.					

From Friedman MM, Bowden VR, Jones EG: *Family nursing: research, theory, and practice,* ed 5, 2003. Electronically reproduced by permission of Pearson Education, Inc., Upper Saddle River, New Jersey.

G.3 COMPREHENSIVE OCCUPATIONAL AND ENVIRONMENTAL HEALTH HISTORY

WORK HISTORY

1. List your current and past longest held jobs, including the military:

Company	Dates Employed	Job Title	Known Exposures

2. Do you work full-time? NO ___ YES ___ How many hours per week? ___
3. Do you work part-time? NO ___ YES ___ How many hours per week? ___
4. Please describe any health problems or injuries that you have experienced in connection with your present or past jobs:

5. Have you ever had to change jobs due to health problems or injuries? YES ___ NO ___
   If yes, describe:

   Did any of your co-workers experience similar problems?

6. In what type of business do you currently work?

7. Describe your work (what you actually do).

8. Have you had any current or past exposure (through breathing or touching) to any of the following?

___ Acids	___ Chlorinated	___ Fiberglass	___ Noise (loud)	___ Styrene
___ Alcohols	naphthalenes	___ Halothane	___ PBBs	___ Talc
___ Alkalis	___ Chloroform	___ Heat (severe)	___ PCBs	___ TDI or MDI
___ Ammonia	___ Chloroprene	___ Isocyanates	___ Perchloroethylene	___ Toluene
___ Arsenic	___ Chromates	___ Ketones	___ Pesticides	___ Trichloroethylene
___ Asbestos	___ Coal dust	___ Lead	___ Phenol	___ Trinitrotoluene
___ Benzene	___ Cold (severe)	___ Manganese	___ Phosgene	___ Vibration
___ Beryllium	___ Dichlorobenzene	___ Mercury	___ Radiation	___ Vinyl chloride
___ Cadmium	___ Ethylene	___ Methylene	___ Rock dust	___ Welding fumes
___ Carbon	dibromide	chloride	___ Silica powder	___ X-rays
tetrachloride	___ Ethylene dichloride	___ Nickel	___ Solvents	

9. Did you receive any safety training about these agents? YES ___ NO ___
   Explain.

10. Are you involved in any work processes such as grinding, welding, soldering, or polishing that create dust, mists, or fumes? YES ___ NO ___
    If yes, describe.

11. Did you use any of the following personal protective equipment when exposed?
    ___ Boots ___ Coveralls ___ Earplugs/earmuffs ___ Glasses/goggles ___ Gloves ___ Respirator
    ___ Safety shoes ___ Shield ___ Sleeves ___ Welding mask

12. Is your work environmental generally clean? YES ___ NO ___
    If no, describe.

13. What ventilation systems are used in your workplace?

14. Do they seem to work? Are you aware of any chemical odors in your environment?
    If so, explain.

15. Where do you eat, smoke, and take your breaks when you are on the job?

16. Do you use a uniform or have clothing that you wear only to work? YES ___ NO ___

17. How is your work clothing laundered (at home, by employer, etc.)?

18. How often do you wash your hands at work, and how do you wash them (running water, special soaps, etc.)?

19. Do you shower before leaving the worksite? YES ___ NO ___

20. Do you have any physical symptoms associated with work? YES ___ NO ___
    If yes, describe.

21. Are other workers similarly affected? YES ___ NO ___

HOME EXPOSURES

1. Which of the following do you have in your home?
   ___ Air conditioner ___ Air purifier ___ Central heating (gas or oil?) ___ Fireplace ___ Electric stove
   ___ Wood stove
2. In approximately what year was your home built? _____
3. Have there been any recent renovations? YES ___ NO ___
   If yes, describe.

4. Have you recently installed new carpet, bought new furniture, or refinished existing furniture? YES ___ NO ___
   If yes, explain.

5. Do you use pesticides around your home or garden? YES ___ NO ___
   If yes, describe.

6. What household cleaners do you use? (List most common and any new products you use.)

7. List all hobbies done at your home.

8. Are any of the agents listed earlier for work exposures encountered in hobbies or recreational activities? YES ___ NO ___

9. Is any special protective equipment or ventilation used during hobbies? YES ___ NO ___
   Explain.

10. What are the occupations of other household members?

11. Do other household members have contact with any form of chemicals at work or during leisure activities? YES ___ NO ___
    If yes, explain.

12. Is anyone else in your home environment having symptoms similar to yours? YES ___ NO ___
    If yes, explain.

COMMUNITY EXPOSURES

1. Are any of the following located in your community?
   ___ Industrial plant ___ Landfill ___ Major source of air pollution ___ Toxic spill ___ Waste site ___ Other
2. What is your source of drinking water?
   ___ Private well ___ Public water source ___ Other
3. Are neighbors experiencing any health problems similar to yours? YES ___ NO ___
   If yes, explain.

KEY OCCUPATIONAL AND ENVIRONMENTAL HEALTH QUESTIONS TO BE ASKED WITH ALL HISTORIES

1. What are your current and past longest-held jobs?

2. Have you been exposed to any radiation or chemical liquids, dusts, mists, or fumes? YES ___ NO ___
3. Is there any relationship between current symptoms and activities at work or at home? YES ___ NO ___

Modified from Pope AM, Snyder MA, Mood LH, editors: *Nursing, health, and environment: strengthening the relationship to improve the public's health,* Washington, DC, 1995, National Academy Press.

G.4 OMAHA SYSTEM PROBLEM CLASSIFICATION SCHEME WITH CASE STUDY APPLICATION

DOMAINS AND PROBLEMS OF THE OMAHA SYSTEM PROBLEM CLASSIFICATION SCHEME

Environmental Domain

Material resources and physical surroundings both inside and outside the living area, neighborhood, and broader community:

    Income
    Sanitation
    Residence
    Neighborhood/workplace safety

Psychosocial Domain

Patterns of behavior, emotion, communication, relationships, and development:

    Communication with community resources
    Social contact
    Role change
    Interpersonal relationship
    Spirituality
    Grief
    Mental health
    Sexuality
    Caretaking/parenting
    Neglect
    Abuse
    Growth and development

Physiological Domain

Functions and processes that maintain life:

    Hearing
    Vision
    Speech and language
    Oral health
    Cognition
    Pain
    Consciousness
    Skin
    Neuromusculoskeletal function
    Respiration
    Circulation
    Digestion-hydration
    Bowel function
    Urinary function
    Reproductive function
    Pregnancy
    Postpartum
    Communicable/infectious condition

Health-related Behaviors Domain

Patterns of activity that maintain or promote wellness, promote recovery, and decrease the risk of disease:

    Nutrition
    Sleep and rest patterns
    Physical activity
    Personal care
    Substance use
    Family planning
    Health care supervision
    Medication regimen

CATEGORIES OF THE OMAHA SYSTEM INTERVENTION SCHEME

Teaching, Guidance, and Counseling

Activities designed to provide information and materials, encourage action and responsibility for self-care and coping, and assist the individual, family, or community to make decisions and solve problems.

Treatments and Procedures

Technical activities such as wound care, specimen collection, resistive exercises, and medication prescriptions that are designed to prevent, decrease, or alleviate signs and symptoms for the individual, family, or community.

Case Management

Activities such as coordination, advocacy, and referral that facilitate service delivery; promote assertiveness; guide the individual, family, or community toward the use of appropriate community resources; and improve communication among health and human service providers.

Surveillance

Activities such as detection, measurement, critical analysis, and monitoring intended to identify the individual, family, or community's status in relation to a given condition or phenomenon.

TARGETS OF THE OMAHA SYSTEM INTERVENTION SCHEME

- Anatomy/physiology
- Anger management
- Behavior modification
- Bladder care
- Bonding/attachment
- Bowel care
- Cardiac care
- Caretaking/parenting skills
- Cast care
- Communication
- Community outreach worker services
- Continuity of care
- Coping skills
- Day care/respite
- Dietary management
- Discipline
- Dressing change/wound care
- Durable medical equipment
- Education
- Employment
- End-of-life care
- Environment
- Exercises
- Family planning care
- Feeding procedures
- Finances
- Gait training
- Genetics
- Growth/development care
- Home

- Homemaking/housekeeping
- Infection precautions
- Interaction
- Interpreter/translator services
- Laboratory findings
- Legal system
- Medical/dental care
- Medication action/side effects
- Medication administration
- Medication coordination/ordering
- Medication prescription
- Medication set-up
- Mobility/transfers
- Nursing care
- Nutritionist care
- Occupational therapy care
- Ostomy care
- Other community resources
- Paraprofessional/aide care
- Personal hygiene
- Physical therapy care
- Positioning
- Recreational therapy care

- Relaxation/breathing techniques
- Respiratory care
- Respiratory therapy care
- Rest/sleep
- Safety
- Screening procedures
- Sickness/injury care
- Signs/symptoms–mental/emotional
- Signs/symptoms–physical
- Skin care
- Social work/counseling care
- Specimen collection
- Speech and language pathology care
- Spiritual care
- Stimulation/nurturance
- Stress management
- Substance use cessation
- Supplies
- Support group
- Support system
- Transportation
- Wellness
- Other

Omaha System Problem Rating Scale for Outcomes

Concept	1	2	3	4	5
Knowledge: Ability of the client to remember and interpret information	No knowledge	Minimal knowledge	Basic knowledge	Adequate knowledge	Superior knowledge
Behavior: Observable responses, actions, or activities of the client fitting the occasion or purpose	Not appropriate behavior	Rarely appropriate behavior	Inconsistently appropriate behavior	Usually appropriate behavior	Consistently appropriate behavior
Status: Condition of the client in relation to the objective and subjective defining characteristics	Extreme signs/symptoms	Severe signs/symptoms	Moderate signs/symptoms	Minimal signs/symptoms	No signs/symptoms

CASE STUDY
MARTHA P.: OLDER WOMAN LIVING IN A DETERIORATING HOME

Joan B. Castleman, RN, MS, Clinical Associate Professor
College of Nursing, University of Florida
Gainesville, Florida

Information Obtained During the First Visit/Encounter

Martha P. was a 93-year-old woman who lived by herself in a deteriorating house. She had kyphosis and arthritis that contributed to her unsteady gait. Martha rarely used her cane in her house, but steadied herself by holding onto furniture.

When a student nurse arrived, Martha was shivering under a thin blanket. Boxes filled with old papers were stacked along the walls. The student nurse asked Martha if she had wood for the stove that heated the house. She replied that she ran out of wood yesterday. "I don't know what I'm going to do, but I'm not leaving this house."

She reported that people from a church had brought the last load of wood. The student asked permission to contact Concerned Neighbors, a volunteer organization that could provide firewood. Martha was pleased. The student expressed concern that the boxes of paper, especially those near the stove, were a fire hazard. "Those boxes have been there for years, and I use them to light the stove." When the student asked if she could help Martha move the four boxes near the stove to the other wall, she grudgingly agreed.

The student nurse noted that Martha was wearing a "Lifeline necklace," a fall alert system, and asked about her history of falls. Martha described how she moved around her home and fell in the bathroom last week when she was trying to take a sponge bath. She pushed the button, and "two nice gentlemen from the fire department came to pick me up." The student and Martha walked around her house. They talked about where she fell in the past, how fortunate she was not to have injuries, and ways to decrease her risk of falling in the future. Martha was willing to have a personal care assistant visit weekly to help her with a bath and shampoo as long there was no charge. Before leaving, the student took Martha's vital signs and blood pressure, and noted that they were within normal limits. The student called Concerned Neighbors and arranged for firewood to be delivered that day; the student also telephoned a local health assistance organization to schedule a home health aide to provide personal care for the next week. Although Martha sounded grumpy, she asked the student to return.

APPLICATION OF THE OMAHA SYSTEM

Domain: Environmental
    Problem: Residence (High Priority)
    Problem Classification Scheme
    Modifiers: Individual and actual
    Signs/symptoms of actual:
Inadequate heating/cooling
Cluttered living space
Unsafe storage of dangerous objects/substances
    Intervention Scheme
    Category: Teaching, guidance, and counseling
    Targets and client-specific information:
Safety (moved boxes away from stove; Martha unwilling to dispose of papers)
    Category: Case management
    Targets and client-specific information:
Other community resource (referred to Concerned Neighbors; arranged delivery of firewood)
    Category: Surveillance
    Targets and client-specific information:
Housing (needed wood)
    Problem Rating Scale for Outcomes
    Knowledge: 2—minimal knowledge (not aware/unwilling to recognize fire hazards)
    Behavior: 2—rarely appropriate behavior (unable/unwilling to make changes)
    Status: 2—severe signs/symptoms (residence was livable but needed changes)
Domain: Physiological
    Problem: Neuromusculoskeletal Function (High Priority)
Problem Classification Scheme
    Modifiers: Individual and actual
    Signs/symptoms of actual:
Limited range of motion
Decreased balance
Gait/ambulation disturbance
    Intervention Scheme
    Category: Teaching, guidance, and counseling
    Targets and client-specific information:
Mobility/transfers (ways to decrease risk of falling, absence of injuries, continue wearing " Lifeline necklace")
    Category: Surveillance
    Targets and client-specific information:

Mobility/transfers (how, when falls occurred)
Signs/symptoms—physical (falls/injuries; vital signs, blood pressure)
    Problem Rating Scale for Outcomes
    Knowledge: 2—minimal knowledge (knew few options to decrease falls)
    Behavior: 2—rarely appropriate behavior (had not used cane in the house; did wear and use the "Lifeline necklace")
    Status: 3—moderate signs/symptoms (activities restricted, fell last week)
Domain: Health-Related Behaviors
    Problem: Personal Care (High Priority)
Problem Classification Scheme
    Modifiers: Individual and actual
    Signs/symptoms of actual:
Difficulty with bathing
Difficulty shampooing/combing hair
    Intervention Scheme
    Category: Teaching, guidance, and counseling
    Targets and client-specific information:
Personal hygiene (needed help with bathing, shampoo)
    Category: Case management
    Targets and client-specific information:
Paraprofessional/aide care (referred to health assistance organization for home health aide)
    Problem Rating Scale for Outcomes
    Knowledge: 3—basic knowledge (knew she needed to bathe, but was not aware of assistance)
    Behavior: 3—inconsistently appropriate behavior (tried to take a sponge bath)
    Status: 3—moderate signs/symptoms (cannot bathe safely without help)

This case illustrates use of the Omaha System with a client in the home. Talk with your classmates and other colleagues about how this form of documenting care would help guide your practice as a home care nurse, ensuring the highest quality possible and client safety.

From Martin K: *The Omaha System: a key to practice, documentation, and information management,* St. Louis, Mo, 2005, Elsevier.

Appendix H

Essential Elements of Public Health Nursing

H.1 EXAMPLES OF PUBLIC HEALTH NURSING ROLES AND IMPLEMENTING PUBLIC HEALTH FUNCTIONS

This document is intended to clearly present the role of public health nurses in Virginia as members of the multidisciplinary public health team in a changing health care environment. The following matrices present the role of public health nursing in Virginia. The following definitions were used to develop these matrices.

Essential Element is taken from the National Association of City and County Health Officials' (NACCHO) Document "Blueprint for a Healthy Community." The following public health essential elements are used as a framework to present the role of public health nursing in Virginia:

- Conducting Community Assessments
- Preventing and Controlling Epidemics
- Providing a Safe and Healthy Environment
- Measuring Performance, Effectiveness, and Outcomes of Health Services

- Promoting Healthy Lifestyles
- Providing Targeted Outreach and Forming Partnerships
- Providing Personal Health Care Services
- Conducting Research and Innovation
- Mobilizing the Community for Action

Public Health Function is defined as a broad public health activity needed to ensure a strong, flexible, accountable public health structure. It may require a multidisciplinary team to carry out.

Public Health Nurse Role is the activity the public health nurse is responsible for, either alone or as a member of a team, to accomplish the stated public health function. This can be the public health nurse at the local level or at the state level.

State Role is what public health nurses need from the state level to do their jobs (e.g., policy, aggregate data, training). This refers to any Central Office program or staff, not just nurses.

A process was implemented that would involve all public health nurses in Virginia. Although this lengthened the timeline to completion, it will ensure that the final document represents a consensus developed through creative open dialogue.

From National Association of City and County Health Officials: *Blueprint for a healthy community: a guide for local health departments,* Washington, DC, 1994, the Association.

ESSENTIAL ELEMENT 1: Conduct Community Assessment: Systematically collect, assemble, analyze, and make available health-related data for the purpose of identifying and responding to community and state level public health concerns and conducting epidemiologic and other population-based studies.

Public Health Function	PHN Roles	State Roles
Develop frameworks, methodologies, and tools for standardizing data collection and analysis and reporting across all jurisdictions and providers.	• Provide, review, and comment on proposed methodologies and tools for data collection. • Field test tools and methods.	• Collaborate with professional organizations and academic and governmental institutions to develop and test tools and methods. • Provide educational opportunities in areas of and use of tools. • Work with local level agencies to standardize definitions, data collected, etc. across jurisdictions and among all stakeholders (schools, community-based organizations, and private providers).
Collect and analyze data.	• Collaborate with the community to identify population-based needs and gaps in service. • Analyze data and needs, knowledge, attitudes, and practices of specific populations. • Identify patterns of diseases; illness and injury and develop or stimulate development of programs to respond to identified trends.	• Provide aggregated data to the local level in a timely and accurate manner. • Provide census tract-level aggregated data to the local level. • Provide national and state comparisons to be used with local data to obtain trends and assist localities in documenting need, progress, etc. to attain standard outcomes.

ESSENTIAL ELEMENT 2: Preventing and Controlling Epidemics: Monitoring disease trends and investigating and containing diseases and injuries.

Public Health Function	PHN Roles	State Roles
Develop programs that prevent, contain, and control the transmission of diseases and danger of injuries (including violence).	• Provide community-wide preventive measures in the form of health education and mobilization of community resources. • Ensure isolation/containment measures when necessary. • Ensure adequate preventive immunizations. • Implement programs that control the transmission of diseases and danger of injuries during disasters.	• Work with local jurisdictions to develop tools such as videos, PSAs, and/or posters that local jurisdictions can use. • Work with local jurisdictions to develop disaster plans for the control of the transmission of diseases and danger of injuries during disasters. • Facilitate state level partnerships that promote health, healthy lifestyles, and wellness (individual and family).
Develop regulatory guidelines for the prevention of targeted diseases.	• Implement regulatory measures. • Implement OSHA Guidelines for Blood Borne Pathogens and the Prevention of the Transmission of TB in Health Care Settings.	• In partnership with localities, develop regulatory guidelines. • Serve as a clearinghouse or source of information.

ESSENTIAL ELEMENT 3: Providing a Safe and Healthy Environment: Maintaining clean and safe air, water, food, and facilities both in the community and the home environment.

Public Health Function	PHN Roles	State Roles
Develop methods/tools for the collection and analysis of health-related data (occurrence of mortality and morbidity relating to both communicable and chronic diseases, injury registries, sentinel event establishment, environmental quality, etc.).	• Provide reporting guidelines and consultation regarding disease prevention, diagnosis, treatment, and follow-up of cases/contacts to physicians and institutions (emergency department, university and secondary school student health, prisons, industries, etc.). • Conduct/participate in community needs assessments to determine customer/provider knowledge deficits and perceptions of need.	• Develop standard methodology and tools for the collection and analysis of health-related data. • Provide training in the area of data collection and analysis. • Evaluate activities and outcomes of interactions. • Work in partnership with localities to develop programs based on data analysis needs.

ESSENTIAL ELEMENT 3: Providing a Safe and Healthy Environment—cont'd

Public Health Function	PHN Roles	State Roles
	• Provide education to individuals, providers, targeted populations, etc., in response to knowledge deficits, disease outbreaks, toxic waste emissions, etc. • Provide individual follow-up/case management of communicable diseases that are transmitted by air, water, food and fomites (TB, hepatitis A, salmonella, and staphylococcus, etc.).	
Develop programs that promote a safe environment in the home.	• Provide childhood lead poisoning screenings and follow-up. • Teach clients to inspect homes for safety violations and toxic substances and to practice safe behaviors; assist families to access/use available resources/safety devices. • Assess/teach regarding safe food selection, preparation, and storage. • Train/supervise volunteers/auxiliary personnel in the performance of the above tasks. • Teach families that all men, women, and children have a right to a safe environment free of physical and mental abuse.	• Provide consultation and technical assistance to state and local organizations regarding laws and regulations that protect health and ensure safety. • In partnership with localities, develop and evaluate educational programs.
Develop programs that promote a safe environment in the workplace.	• Provide consultation in the implementation of OSHA regulations relating to occupational exposure to diseases. • Provide educational programs related to healthy lifestyles (smoking cessation, back protection, etc). • Ensure provision of screenings for individuals to determine baselines and the occurrence of infectious diseases and preventable deterioration of health and function: hearing, back soundness, lung capacity, RMS indicators, PPDs, etc. • Assist in policy/practice development to address the prevention of the above. • Provide immunizations.	• Monitor and assist localities to implement prevention activities. • Assist localities in developing and evaluating educational programs. • Monitor outcomes of screening activities and evaluate interventions.
Develop programs that promote a safe environment in the school setting.	• Provide consultations on the implementation of OSHA regulations relating to occupational exposure to diseases. • Provide educational programs related to healthy lifestyles (smoking cessation, etc.). • Ensure provision of screenings for students to determine baselines and the occurrence of infectious disease and preventable deterioration of health and function. • Assist in policy/practice development to address prevention of the above. • Provide immunizations.	• Develop guidelines that ensure accountability in meeting standards set forth. • Ensure that policy is developed to protect children in the school environment. • Monitor the immunization status of children and provide immunizations during outbreaks and evaluate activities.
Develop programs that promote a safe environment in the community.	• Identify population clusters exhibiting an unhealthy environment; provide consultation/group education regarding preventive measures.	• In times of disaster, facilitate the availability of resources across jurisdictions. • Have a statewide plan.

Appendixes

ESSENTIAL ELEMENT 3: Providing a Safe and Healthy Environment—cont'd

Public Health Function	PHN Roles	State Roles
	• Participate in the development of local disaster plans to ensure provision of safe water, food, air, and facilities. • Respond in time of natural disasters such as floods, tornadoes, and hurricanes. • Participate in developing plans for shelter management during disasters, especially "Special Needs" shelters that may require nursing staff.	• Ensure that localities have developed plans to protect the public in time of national and/or other disasters. • Coordinate efforts statewide. • Assist localities in responding. • Evaluate efforts.
Develop and issue standards that guide regulations, mandate, policy, and program development.	• Survey worksites, schools, institutions, etc. for compliance to regulations that protect health and ensure safety.	• Develop a systematic evaluation tool for the collection of data to measure trends.
Develop protocols to ensure accountability of all health care providers, public and private.	• Provide technical assistance, i.e., interpretation, implementation, and evaluation processes.	• Assist localities in developing standards to mandate accountability.
Provide inservice to all providers of health care services.	• Share and implement knowledge gained in inservices.	• Provide consultation/technical assistance to localities.

ESSENTIAL ELEMENT 4: Measuring Performance, Effectiveness, and Outcomes of Health Services: Monitoring health care providers and the health care system to identify gaps in service, deteriorating health status indicators, effectiveness of interventions, and the accessibility and quality of personal and population-wide health services.

Public Health Function	PHN Roles	State Roles
Promote competency in public health issues throughout the health delivery system.	• Provide educational and technical assistance in areas such as case management and appropriate treatment and control of communicable diseases to the community.	• Develop appropriate regulatory, educational, and technical assistance programs. • Provide technical assistance and training to local health departments for local forecasting and interpretation of data.
Collect data.	• Participate in data collection with a target population. • Ensure that the data collection system supports the objectives of programs serving the community by participating in the design and operation of data collection systems. • Collect data via surveys, polls, interviews, and focus groups that will enable assessment of the community's perception of health status and understanding how the system works and how to obtain needed service.	• Work with localities (health districts, private providers, other state and local agencies) to develop standard data elements and definitions across jurisdictions and among all stakeholders, especially for consistency in coding of population-based data. • Identify data collection and analytic issues related to monitoring the impact of health system changes such as costs and benefits of record linkage, strategies for ensuring confidentiality, and strategies for analyzing trends in health within a broader social and economic context. • Advocate for uniform data collection from all managed care plans so that outcomes and health trends can be analyzed and tracked and sentinel events reported.
Analyze data to ensure the accurate diagnosis of health status, identification of threats to health, and assessment of health service needs.	• Participate in a systematic approach to convert data into information that will identify gaps in service at the local and state level and will lead to action. • Monitor health status indicators to identify emerging problems and facilitate community-wide responses to identified problems. • Facilitate data analysis as part of a local collaborative effort.	• Develop a systematic, integrated statewide approach to converting data into information that directs action. • Ensure that resources to analyze data, such as hardware and software, are available at the local level. • Work with localities (health districts, private providers, other state and local agencies) to address issues related to variable access to technology, confidentiality issues.

ESSENTIAL ELEMENT 4: Measuring Performance, Effectiveness, and Outcomes of Health Services—cont'd

Public Health Function	PHN Roles	State Roles
		• Educate and train currently employed public health nurses in areas of epidemiology and population-based services.
Monitor health status indicators for the entire population and for specific population groups and/or geographic areas.	• Identify target populations that may be at risk for public health problems such as communicable diseases and unidentified and untreated chronic diseases. • Conduct surveys or observe targeted populations such as preschools, child care centers, and high-risk census tracks to identify health status. • Monitor health care utilization of vulnerable populations at the local and regional level.	• Develop methodology for identification, measurement, and analysis of key indicators of health care utilization of vulnerable populations
Monitor and assess availability, cost-effectiveness, and outcomes of personal and population-based health services.	• Identify gaps in services (e.g., a neighborhood with deteriorating immunization rates may indicate a lack of available primary care services). • Ensure that all receive the same quality of care, including comprehensive preventive services. • Monitor the impact of health system reforms on vulnerable populations. • Evaluate the effectiveness and outcomes of care. • Plan interventions based on the health of the overall population, not just for those in the health care system. • Identify interventions that are effective and replicable.	• Develop analyses that demonstrate the cost effectiveness of investment in public health services. • Develop protocols and technical assistance for ensuring accountability of Medicaid-managed care plans and other government-funded plans for service delivery and overall health status of their covered populations. • Identify standard theoretical, methodological, and measurement issues that are specific to population subgroups for monitoring the impact of health system changes on vulnerable populations.
Disseminate information.	• Disseminate information to the public on community health status, including how to access and use the services appropriately. • Disseminate information to other health care providers regarding gaps in services or deteriorating health status indicators.	• Ensure a mechanism for public accountability of performance and outcomes through public dissemination of information and, in particular, ensure that underservice, a risk inherent in capitated plans, is measurable through available data. • Ensure that information is provided to communities, local health departments, managed care plans, and other appropriate state agencies.

ESSENTIAL ELEMENT 5: Promoting Healthy Lifestyles: Providing health education to individuals, families, and communities.

Public Health Function	PHN Roles	State Roles
Promote informed decision making of residents about things that influence their health on a daily basis.	• Exert influence through contact with individuals and community groups. • Accept and issue challenges concerning healthy lifestyles to all contacts. • Reinforce and reward positive informed decisions made for healthy lifestyles.	• Develop and monitor standards to determine changes in behavior.

ESSENTIAL ELEMENT 5: Promoting Healthy Lifestyles—cont'd

Public Health Function	PHN Roles	State Roles
Promote effective use of media to encourage both personal and community responsibility for informed decision making.	• Be a resource for the community. • Gather data and address findings as appropriate. • Work with community groups to promote accurate information for healthy lifestyles through the media. • Utilize current information and other agencies' resources to maximize information accessible to the public.	• Assist localities to provide current information to community organizations and other state organizations. • Serve as a resource for localities and work with media.
Develop a public awareness/marketing campaign to demonstrate the importance of public health to overall health improvement and its proper place in the health delivery system.	• Provide education to special groups, e.g., local politicians, school boards, PTAs, churches, civic groups, and news media, regarding the benefits of preventive health.	• Develop training activities to assist localities in marketing.
Develop public information and education systems/programs through partnerships.	• Provide educational sessions/programs to the public regarding the components of healthy lifestyles. • Access grants/other funding sources to promote healthy lifestyle decisions (e.g., cervical and breast cancer prevention; bike helmets, hypertension). • Provide/promote teaching for individuals and families at every opportunity (home, clinic, community settings).	• Assist localities in developing and evaluating educational programs. • Assist localities in funding. • Hold regional/state training sessions. • Evaluate outcomes and plan ongoing educational systems/programs.

ESSENTIAL ELEMENT 6: Providing Targeted Outreach and Forming Partnerships: Ensuring access to services, including those that lead to self-sufficiency, for all vulnerable populations and ensuring the development of culturally appropriate care.

Public Health Function	PHN Roles	State Roles
Ensure accessibility to health services that will improve morbidity, decrease mortality, and improve health status outcomes.	• Provide family-centered case management services for high-risk and hard-to-reach populations that focus on linking families with needed services. • Improve access to care by forming partnerships with appropriate community individuals and entities. • Increase the influence of cultural diversity on system design and on access to care, as well as on individual services rendered. • Ensure that translation services are available for the non-English-speaking populations. • Participate in ongoing community assessment to identify areas of concern and needs for rules. • Provide outreach services that focus on preventing epidemics and the spread of disease, such as tuberculosis and sexually transmitted diseases.	• Provide funds in cooperation with the locality. • Ensure policy development that includes case management and is culturally sensitive. • Provide adequate ongoing continuing education for the staff (especially in areas common to all localities). • Participate in state-level contract development to ensure that contracts with health plans require and include incentives for health plans to offer and deliver preventive health services in the minimum benefits package. • Educate financing officials about the roles of public health both in performing core public health services and in ensuring access to personal health services.

ESSENTIAL ELEMENT 7: Providing Personal Health Care Services: Provide targeted direct services to high-risk populations.

Public Health Function	PHN Roles	State Roles
Provide direct services for specific diseases that threaten the health of the community and develop programs that prevent, contain, and control the transmission of infectious diseases.	Plan, develop, implement, and evaluate: • Sexually transmitted disease services • Communicable disease services • HIV/AIDS services • Tuberculosis control services • Develop and implement guidelines for the prevention of the above targeted disease.	• Establish standards/criteria for personal health care. • Work with local health departments to assist in developing infrastructure and management techniques to facilitate record-keeping and appropriate financial monitoring and tracking systems, which enable local health departments to enter into contractual arrangements for preventive health and primary care services.
Provide health services, including preventive health services, to high-risk and vulnerable populations (e.g., the uninsured working poor), and in geographic areas in which primary health care services are not readily accessible or available in a privatized setting.	• Provide coordination, follow-up, referral, and case management as indicated. • Integrate supportive services, such as counseling, social work, and nutrition, into primary care services. • Assess the existing community medical capacity for referral and follow-up.	• Continue to work at the state and local level to build primary and preventive health services capacity, particularly in traditionally underserved areas, to ensure availability to providers and primary care sites essential to primary care access.

ESSENTIAL ELEMENT 8: Conducting Research and Innovation: Discovering and applying improved health care delivery mechanisms and clinical interventions.

Public Health Function	PHN Roles	State Roles
Ensure ongoing prevention research relating to biomedical and behavioral aspects of health promotion and prevention of disease and injury.	• Develop outcome measures. • Identify research priorities for target communities and develop and conduct scientific and operations research for health promotion and disease/injury prevention.	• Provide training in the area of measuring program effectiveness.
Implement pilot or demonstration projects.	• Develop and implement linkages with academic centers, ensuring that clients and populations who participate in research projects benefit as a result of the research.	• Support evaluations and research that demonstrate the benefits of public health, as well as the consequences of failure to support public health interventions.

ESSENTIAL ELEMENT 9: Mobilizing the Community for Action: Providing leadership and initiating collaboration.

Public Health Function	PHN Roles	State Roles
Provide leadership to stimulate the development of networks or partnerships that will ensure the availability of comprehensive primary health care services to all regardless of the ability to pay.	• Advocate for improved health. • Disseminate health information. • Build coalitions. • Make recommendations for policy implementation or revision.	• Facilitate the establishment and enhancement of statewide high-quality, needed health services. • Administer quality improvement programs.
Initiate collaboration with other community organizations to ensure the leadership role in resolving a public health issue.	• Facilitate resources that manage environmental risk and maintain and improve community health. • Provide information for a community group working on impacting policy at the local, state, or federal level. • Use results of community health assessments to stimulate the community to develop a plan to respond to identified gaps in service.	• Uses information-gathering techniques of assessment to assist policy/legislature activities to develop needed health services and functions that require statewide action or standards. • Recommend programs to carry out policies.

Appendixes

H.2 AMERICAN NURSES ASSOCIATION STANDARDS OF CARE OF PUBLIC HEALTH NURSING PRACTICE

Standard 1. Assessment: The public health nurse collects comprehensive data pertinent to the health status of populations.

Standard 2. Population Diagnosis and Priorities: The public health nurse analyzes the assessment data to determine the population diagnoses and priorities.

Standard 3. Outcomes Identification: The public health nurse identifies expected outcomes for a plan that is based on population diagnoses and priorities.

Standard 4. Planning: The public health nurse develops a plan that reflects best practices by identifying strategies, action plans, and alternatives to attain expected outcomes.

Standard 5. Implementation: The public health nurse implements the identified plan by partnering with others.

Standard 5A. Coordination: The public health nurse coordinates programs, services, and other activities to implement the identified plan.

Standard 5B. Health Education and Health Promotion: The public health nurse employs multiple strategies to promote health, prevent disease, and ensure a safe environment for populations.

Standard 5C. Consultation: The public health nurse provides consultation to various community groups and officials to facilitate the implementation of programs and services.

Standard 5D. Regulatory Activities: The public health nurse identifies, interprets, and implements public health laws, regulations, and policies.

Standard 6. Evaluation: The public health nurse evaluates the health status of the population.

From American Nurses Association: *Public health nursing: Scope and standards of practice*, Silver Spring, Md, 2007, ANA.

H.3 QUAD COUNCIL PUBLIC HEALTH NURSING CORE COMPETENCIES AND SKILL LEVELS

The Quad Council of Public Health Nursing Organizations is an alliance of the four national nursing organizations that address public health nursing issues: the Association of Community Health Nurse Educators (ACHNE), the American Nurses Association's Congress on Nursing Practice and Economics (ANA), the American Public Health Association—Public Health Nursing Section (APHA), and the Association of State and Territorial Directors of Nursing (ASTDN). In 2000, prompted in part by work on educating the public health workforce being done under the leadership of the Centers for Disease Control and Prevention (CDC), the Quad Council began the development of a set of national public health nursing competencies.

The approach utilized by the Quad Council was to start with the Council on Linkages between Academia and Public Health Practice (COL) "Core Competencies for Public Health Professionals" and to determine their application to two levels of public health nursing practice: the staff nurse/generalist role and the manager/specialist/consultant role.

The "Quad Council PHN Competencies" document is designed for use with other documents. It complements the "Definition of Public Health Nursing" adopted by the APHA's Public Health Nursing Section in 1996 and the *Scope and Standards of Public Health Nursing* (Quad Council, 2000). Differentiating PHN competencies at the generalist and specialist levels will help clarify the PHN specialty for both the discipline of nursing and the profession of public health. In addition, the ability to identify PHN competencies should facilitate collaboration among public health nurses and other public health professionals in education, practice, and research to improve the public's health.

In developing the competencies, the Quad Council members concurred that the generalist level would reflect preparation at the baccalaureate level.

Further, the specialist level competencies described in this document reflect preparation at the master's level in public health nursing and/or public health.

The Quad Council determined that although the Council on Linkages competencies were developed with the understanding that public health practice is population focused and public health nursing is also population focused, one of the unique contributions of public health nurses is the ability to apply these principles at the individual and family level *within the context of population-focused practice.*

These competencies can be found through the WebLinks on this book's Evolve website at http://evolve.elsevier.com/stanhope/foundations.

H.4 Minnesota Department of Health Public Health Interventions Wheel

Public Health Interventions

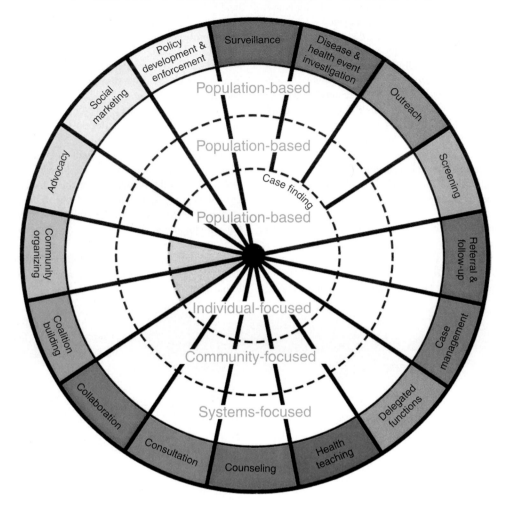

March 2001

Minnesota Department of Health
Division of Community Health Services
Public Health Nursing Section

Minnesota Department of Health Public Health Intervention Wheel. (From Section of Public Health Nursing, Minnesota Department of Health: *Public Health Interventions,* 2001, available at www.health. state.mn.us/divs/chs/phn/.)

DEFINITION OF POPULATION-BASED PRACTICE
Population-Based Practice
1. **Focuses on entire populations**
   A **population** is a collection of individuals who have one or more personal or environmental characteristics in common.[1]
   A **population-of-interest** is a population essentially healthy but who could improve factors that promote or protect health.

A **population-at-risk** is a population with a common identified risk factor or risk exposure that poses a threat to health. Population-based practice always begins with identifying everyone who is in the population-of-interest or the population-at-risk. It is not limited to only those who seek service or who are poor or otherwise vulnerable.

2. **Grounded in an assessment of the population's health status**
   Population-based practice reflects the priorities of the community. Community priorities are determined through an assessment of the population's health status and a prioritization process.

---

[1]Williams, CA, Highriter ME: Community health nursing: population focus and evaluation, *Public Health Rev* 7(3–4):197–221, 1978.

3. Considers the broad determinants of health

Population-based practice focuses on the entire range of factors that determine health rather than just personal health risks or disease. Health determinants include income and social status, social support networks, education, employment and working conditions, biology and genetic endowment, physical environment, personal health practices and coping skills, and health services.

4. Emphasizes all levels of prevention

Prevention is anticipatory action taken to prevent the occurrence of an event or to minimize its effect after it has occurred.[2] Not every event is preventable, but every event does have a preventable component. Primary prevention promotes health or keeps problems from occurring; secondary prevention detects and treats problems early; tertiary prevention keeps existing problems from getting worse. Whenever possible, population-based practice emphasize primary prevention.

5. Intervenes with communities, systems, individuals, and families

Population-based practice intervenes with communities, with the systems involving the health of communities, and/or with the individuals and families that comprise communities. Community-focused practice changes community norms, attitudes, awareness, practices, and behaviors. Systems-focused practice changes organizations, policies, laws, and power structures of the systems that affect health. Individual/family-focused practice changes knowledge, attitudes, beliefs, values, practices, and behaviors of individuals (identified as belonging to a population), alone or as part of a family, class, or group. Interventions at each level of practice contribute to the overall goal of improving population health status.

[2]Turnock, B: *Public Health: What It Is and How It Works*, Gaithersburg, Md, 2008, Jones & Bartlett.

PUBLIC HEALTH INTERVENTIONS WITH DEFINITIONS

Public Health Intervention	Definition
Surveillance	Describes and monitors health events through ongoing and systematic collection, analysis, and interpretation of health data for the purpose of planning, implementing, and evaluating public health interventions. (Modified from MMWR, 1988.)
Disease and other health event investigation	Systematically gathers and analyzes data regarding threats to the health of populations, ascertains the source of the threat, identifies cases and others at risk, and determines control measures.
Outreach	Locates populations-of-interest or populations-at-risk and provides information about the nature of the concern, what can be done about it, and how services can be obtained.
Screening	Identifies individuals with unrecognized health risk factors or asymptomatic disease conditions in populations.
Case finding	Locates individuals and families with identified risk factors and connects them with resources.
Referral and follow-up	Assists individuals, families, groups, organizations, and/or communities to identify and access necessary resources in order to prevent or resolve problems or concerns.
Case management	Optimizes self care capabilities of individuals and families and the capacity of systems and communities to coordinate and provide services.
Delegated functions	Directs care tasks that a registered professional nurse carries out under the authority of a health care practitioner as allowed by law. Delegated functions also include any direct care tasks that a registered professional nurse entrusts to other appropriate personnel to perform.
Health teaching	Communicates facts, ideas, and skills that change knowledge, attitudes, values, beliefs, behaviors, and practices of individuals, families, systems, and/or communities.
Counseling	Establishes an interpersonal relationship with a community, a system, family, or individual intended to increase or enhance their capacity for self-care and coping. Counseling engages the community, a system, family, or individual at an emotional level.
Consultation	Seeks information and generates optional solutions to perceived problems or issues through interactive problem solving with a community, system, family, or individual. The community, system, family, or individual selects and acts on the option best meeting the circumstances.
Collaboration	Commits two or more persons or organizations to achieve a common goal through enhancing the capacity of one or more of the members to promote and protect health. (Modified from Henneman EA, Lee J, Cohen J: Collaboration: a concept analysis, *J Advan Nurs* 21:103–109, 1995.)
Coalition building	Promotes and develops alliances among organizations or constituencies for a common purpose. It builds linkages, solves problems, and/or enhances local leadership to address health concerns.
Community organizing	Helps community groups to identify common problems or goals, mobilize resources, and develop and implement strategies for reaching the goals they collectively have set. (Modified from Minkler M, editor: *Community Organizing and Community Building for Health*, New Brunswick, NJ, 1997, Rutgers University Press.)
Advocacy	Pleads someone's cause or acts on someone's behalf, with a focus on developing the community, system, individual, or family's capacity to plead their own cause or act on their own behalf.

Public Health Intervention	Definition
Social marketing	Utilizes commercial marketing principles and technologies for programs designed to influence the knowledge, attitudes, values, beliefs, behaviors, and practices of the population-of-interest.
Policy development	Places health issues on decision-makers' agendas, acquires a plan of resolution, and determines needed resources. Policy development results in laws, rules and regulation, ordinances, and policies.
Policy enforcement	Compels others to comply with the laws, rules, regulations, ordinances, and policies created in conjunction with policy development.

THREE LEVELS OF PUBLIC HEALTH PRACTICE

Public health interventions are population-based if they consider all levels of practice. This concept is represented by the three inner rings of the model. The inner rings of the model are labeled community-focused, systems-focused, and individual/family-focused.

A population-based approach considers intervening at all possible levels of practice. Interventions may be directed at the entire population within a community, the systems that affect the health of those populations, and/or the individuals and families within those populations known to be at risk.

Levels	Definition
Population-based **community-focused** practice	Changes community norms, community attitudes, community awareness, community practices, and community behaviors. They are directed toward entire populations within the community or occasionally toward target groups within those populations. Community-focused practice is measured in terms of what proportion of the population actually changes.
Population-based **systems-focused** practice	Changes organizations, policies, laws, and power structures. The focus is not directly on individuals and communities but on the systems that affect health. Changing systems is often a more effective and long-lasting way to affect population health than requiring change from every individual in a community.
Population-based **individual-focused** practice	Changes knowledge, attitudes, beliefs, practices, and behaviors of individuals. This practice level is directed at individuals, alone or as part of a family, class, or group. Individuals receive services because they are identified as belonging to a population-at-risk.

(From Section of Public Health Nursing, Minnesota Department of Health: Public Health Interventions, 2001, available at www.health.state.mn.us/divs/chs/phn/.)

Answers to Clinical Application Questions

CHAPTER 1

C and G are population focused, looking at the needs of their subpopulation and planning programs to meet their needs. A, B, D, and F are likely to be practicing nursing in the community if their focus is health protection, health promotion, and disease prevention of the individuals and/or families in their subpopulations. B and D are more likely to be practicing community-based nursing, caring for clients who are ill. E is neither community based nor community health.

CHAPTER 2

A. It is easier to use a population-focused approach to solving these problems. If a nurse can show through a community needs assessment that these are problems for a large number of people in the community and are putting the community at risk for increased health problems, more costly health care, and less social and economic growth, it might be possible to convince policymakers to establish programs directed at these problems. With limited health care dollars, the emphasis is on the greatest good for the greatest number.

B. An historical approach will build understanding of the public policy elements limiting care of various populations. This involves exploring what attempts have been made in the past to innovate or reform services for these populations, determining what has limited these attempts, and identifying examples of programs or policies that have been successful.

CHAPTER 3

The correct answer is D. The nurse's responsibility is to educate clients about appropriate health care resources in their community and to allow families to choose care based on their own unique needs and preferences.

CHAPTER 4

A.1. Ann's job entailed monitoring federal money and supervising funded programs within her division.

A.2. The federal government had allocated considerable money to the state agency to subsidize pediatric primary care programs.

A.3. The pediatric primary care programs had never been formally evaluated.

A.4. The director of the state agency was using considerable federal money targeted for the pediatric primary care program in his district to supplement home health care services for indigent homebound elderly persons.

B.1. The first ethical issue involved the inappropriate allocation of federal funds.

B.2. The second ethical issue involved a statewide lack of accountability regarding the use of federal funds.

B.3. The third ethical issue involved the conflict that occurs when two equally indigent populations need primary care services but inadequate money is available to subsidize both.

C.1. Ann developed new policies for the allocation of funds. For any agency within the state to receive funding from the Division of Primary Care, the agency had to follow the new policies.

C.2. Ann also initiated a task force to develop specific procedures for the policies she developed. The procedures and their implementation were reviewed by the task force monthly. The task force comprised representatives from the federal government and all the state-funded primary care programs. The task force became a safety net for anyone misappropriating federal funds, thus ensuring accountability.

C.3. Periodic unannounced site visits to all agencies within the state were made by peer administrators from the 20 districts in the State Health Department.

C.4. Regarding the pediatric primary care program in his district, the director for the state agency would receive funds only if he submitted specified monthly reports to Ann about the pediatric program's performance.

C.5. The director for the state agency and his staff were given help regarding how to interpret the policies and follow the procedures.

C.6. As a result of Ann's initiatives, the director for the state agency followed the new guidelines, which ensured that the pediatric primary care program received all of the money the program was due. In addition, he sought new funding to assist indigent homebound elderly persons with chronic illnesses in his district.

CHAPTER 5

The correct answer is C. Ms. Johnson was serving as a cultural broker between the patient and the professional health care system and facilitated effective communication. She provided an opportunity for clarification of any misinformation regarding cancer treatment. Ms. Johnson also facilitated open communication with the father and his family.

CHAPTER 6

Answers to the first case scenario:

A. You would include in your assessment a Denver Developmental Screening Test (Denver II) on Billy to determine the neurological effects of the lead on his growth and development, an assessment of the population to find the total child population younger than 6 years who may benefit from screening, and a community assessment to find the number of older homes in the community that may have lead-based paint.

B. Prevention strategies would include assisting the parents in enrolling Billy in Head Start to stimulate his development because of his altered growth and development state, a blood level screening program for children younger than 6 years in the community to determine other children who may need to be referred for treatment, and a community-wide lead poisoning prevention program that includes educational materials about where lead is found in home environments and how to test for it. The nurse can target parent group leaders, local newspapers, and the school system to distribute educational materials.

Answers to the second case scenario:

Possible responses to the problem are (1) short-term: alternate drinking water (bottled), and (2) long-term: extension of water lines from a nearby municipality, monitoring and clean-up of the contaminated groundwater (including testing other wells), testing children for lead poisoning, and informing the community of the risks and remedies.

CHAPTER 7

A plan of action to influence the health department about its decision to close the prenatal clinic would include the following:

1. Review the state register in the law library to see if regulations for the block grants had been finalized.
2. Check state health statistics, including vital statistics providing the current infant and maternity mortality rates in the state, and compare these with national statistics.
3. Review the literature for research that would show the relationships between prenatal care, normal deliveries, and complications of pregnancy and delivery.

4. After the discussion, hold a group meeting with the state nurses association to create answers. The next step is to have the groups contact their local senators and representatives to ask for a meeting to discuss the issue.
5. Contact the legal aid society to find a lawyer interested in consulting with them in preparing written and oral testimony.
6. Present the testimony to the state health department during the process of preparing the regulations for the block grants.

CHAPTER 8

A. Agencies are reimbursed for visits either by private insurance or Medicare or by clients through self-pay.
B. The payment for the visit is determined by using a cost basis or a charge basis. A cost basis reflects the actual cost to the agency to deliver the service. A charge basis reflects the cost plus additional monies charged for the visit, which may include indigent care visits or profit to be paid to stockholders if the agency is a for-profit agency.
C. Nursing care costs, although they may be known, are usually not used alone to determine the costs of a visit. The visit cost includes money for lights, water, supplies, secretarial and administrative salaries and benefits, and salaries and benefits for nurses.
D. There is rationing in all of health care. Home health visits are rationed by the criteria set by the federal government for Medicare clients, such as a limited number of visits per year, and by private insurance, which also limits the number of visits per year. The individual client who must pay out of pocket sets his or her own limits and self-rations the amount he or she may be willing to pay for home health visits.
E. Improved health outcomes, reduced cost of care, and economic growth because of increased productivity of workers.

CHAPTER 9

The correct answer is D. There is controversy about prostate cancer screening, and the experts disagree. The American Cancer Society recommends that prostate cancer screening be offered only after men are informed of their risk and benefits. Age recommendations for screening are 45 years and older in African-American men and 50 years and older in white men. Prostate cancer screening should be offered to men who have 10 years or more of life expectancy left.

Population risks include incontinence and impotence for some but not all forms of treatment for prostate cancer. Individual risks for Rob are increased because of his family history of prostate cancer, as well as personal lifestyle habits of smoking and consumption of a high-fat diet. It is believed that hereditary cancer is more aggressive than regular cancer.

Population benefits include increased survival rates when prostate cancer is detected in the early stages rather than the advanced stages, 100% versus 31%. Personal benefits may include decreased psychological stress from fear of dying from prostate cancer, especially with a family history of a father dying from prostate cancer.

Two loci have been identified for hereditary prostate cancer: one on chromosome 1 and one on chromosome X. However, additional research is needed before the gene is available for cancer susceptibility testing in high-risk men. A high risk for cancer susceptibility testing is usually defined as having several family members with cancer and/or an earlier age of onset than normal for the cancer. Cancer susceptibility testing is not appropriate for all persons; it is appropriate only for persons in the high-risk group. Genetic testing is new, and there are many misconceptions. Nurses are often some of the first health professionals who come into contact with at-risk persons and/or who are asked questions by the public. Therefore it is critical that nurses know and understand the basic concepts of cancer susceptibility testing. In addition, nurses need to know referral sources that include genetic counselors for additional genetic information.

CHAPTER 10

A. All four choices
B. EBP in nursing takes into account the best evidence from research findings and evidence from community knowledge and experience to make decisions that promote the health of the community in a culturally appropriate manner.

CHAPTER 11

The correct answer is C. This community health education need will require in-depth planning to meet the needs of the community. If Kristi works with the local health department and presents both a community forum and informational brochures, she can reach more of the target audience either in person or through the literature.

CHAPTER 12

The correct answer is B. A high level of community motivation is critical for any community-focused intervention and will help ensure active community involvement in the planning process and commitment to the intervention itself.

CHAPTER 13

The correct sequence is C, B, A, D. The first piece of information (C) is essential to understanding the level, amount, and nature of services the client is eligible to receive. The client must be informed, her needs assessed, and her options discussed (B). Family care options must be understood to formulate resource possibilities for the client (A). Arrangement for a facility site visit may or may not be essential but may be preferred (D).

CHAPTER 14

The correct answer is A. Sharing her feelings with a trained professional who is familiar with the devastating circumstances in which Paula is involved will be most helpful. Although calling home might be comforting, family members

with no experience in disaster work would not be able to fully appreciate the stress that Paula is experiencing.

CHAPTER 15

1. The pandemic may come in waves and exposure to flu could last for months.
2. It is important for families and businesses to be prepared.
3. There will be disruption in services, including hospitals, banks, schools, and post offices.
4. People may not be able to go to work; thus there may be a possible loss of income.
5. There may not be any transportation.
6. Support systems for individuals and families need to be developed.

CHAPTER 16

Eva would include all the steps in planning her project. She contacted the pastor of the church who was planning to open the soup kitchen to discuss the issue (formulation and assessment). She found him very receptive to the idea of developing a solution to the health care needs of the homeless. In her assessment, Eva found that no other health services were available to the homeless in the community. She looked at national data to estimate the needs and size of the population. She talked with the faculty to discuss potential solutions to the problem. She talked to members of the homeless population to obtain their perceptions of their needs.

On completing her assessment, Eva conceptualized the solutions. Several solutions were possible: work with the health department, attempt to provide better care through the local medical center, or open a clinic on site at the soup kitchen where most of the people gathered so that transportation would not be a problem.

After considering the solutions, Eva detailed the plan looking at the resources needed for opening a clinic at the soup kitchen. She considered supplies, equipment, facilities, and acceptability to the clients. She also considered the time involved, the activities required to implement a program, and funding sources.

In evaluating the possibilities, Eva considered the cost, the client and community benefits, and acceptability to clients, self, faculty, and the church. Although it would have been easier for her to choose to work with the health department or the medical center, she knew that the solution most acceptable to the clients would be to have a clinic located at the soup kitchen. The clinic would be more accessible, transportation would not be needed, and health services through the clinic could possibly prevent more costly hospital and emergency care (value).

Eva presented her plan to the faculty and the church. She convinced them that it would not be a costly endeavor. She had found nurses in the community who volunteered to help, she had contacted a carpenter who would donate his time to build an examining room in the back of the soup kitchen, and she had met with community physicians who had promised to provide equipment. The client assessment indicated that a first-aid and health assessment clinic was what was needed most. With approval from all (implementation), Eva began the clinic in 1981, seeing 25 to 35 clients a week, 1 hour per day for 5 days per week.

Eva evaluated the relevance of the program via the needs assessment process. She tracked the progress of the program by keeping records of her activities. She kept track of the resources in relation to the number of persons served (efficiency) and used these data to convince the church and the college of nursing to fund the ongoing clinic operation after she graduated. A summative evaluation of the clinic was completed by the faculty at the end of 4 years. The program's impact was outstanding. The clinic had grown. The client demand was high; most of the health problems could be handled at the clinic, which eliminated the cost burden to the community for more expensive health care; and it was highly acceptable to the clients (effectiveness). This clinic began as a service to 25 people for 1 hour per day. Today this clinic is open all day, 5 days per week, has more than 900 clients per year, and provides for more than 5000 client visits per year. The success of this clinic shows the effect that one nursing student can have on a community.

CHAPTER 17

A. Outcomes of parenting education should provide evidence that behavior change has occurred because of the educational intervention. Oscar might use the outcome measure of episodes of praising children. He could construct a questionnaire for clients of the nurses who attended classes on teaching parenting skills and for clients of nurses who had not attended classes as a control group. A possible question for the client questionnaire would be the following: Each week, how many times do you praise your child/children for doing something well? A. 0; B. 1; C. 2; D. 3; E. 4 or more.

B. An increase in this measure over time would indicate that the nurses had provided quality instruction that had improved the praising behavior in the parent. The differences in responses between the clients of the nurses who were taught parenting skills and those who received no instruction could be statistically analyzed for significant differences.

CHAPTER 18

A. No. The idealized version never existed. There have always been stressors that presented challenges for families. Although not as prominent in the past, differing family structures have always existed within U.S. society.

B. According to a report from the National Commission on Children, people are both discouraged and encouraged about the status of America's families. The contradictions in this report indicate a disparity between people's perceptions of their own families (healthy) and the perception of families outside their own (unhealthy or dysfunctional).

C. There are liberal people in our society who believe the definition of family should include two-parent, single-parent, remarried, gay, adoptive, foster, and many other

alternative family forms. That is, families are what people define them to be and the government, with its health and economic sanctions, should be supportive of all family groups. However, there are conservative people who believe that the definition of families should remain limited to blood, legal, and adoptive guidelines.

D. How we ourselves define family will influence how we live, how we provide nursing care to families, and what health and welfare programs we are willing to support in the society.

CHAPTER 19

A. A home visit. This would allow for a more extensive assessment of the family within the four models of health: clinical, role-performance, adaptive, and eudaemonistic. The nurse would phone the home to make an appointment for a home visit.

B. At the first home visit, it would be determined whether Amy and her mother were interested in continuing nursing service. During her visit with Amy and her mother, the nurse would add to her assessment by exploring with them what they saw as problems and concerns. This is consistent with an approach focused on empowerment.

C. Schedule a second visit to include Amy's boyfriend and father. During the second visit, additional areas related to the clinical health of the family, in terms of acute or chronic conditions, would be assessed using a family genogram.

D. Yes, negotiate a contract to continue visiting with Amy, but the visits would need to occur at school during a study period. The focus would be on prenatal teaching for the nurse, with Amy agreeing to attend a group for pregnant students offered at the school. Visits also would be arranged with Amy's mother to discuss her concerns. These approaches reflected acknowledgment of the family's abilities to be actively and competently involved in resolving problems they had identified. Over time, the contract would be modified and expanded to include well-child supervision during the year following the birth of a healthy baby boy.

CHAPTER 20

A. The correct answers are numbers 3, 4, and 5. First, the nurse completed a physical examination and administered the Mini-Mental Status Examination short form (to assess cognitive function) and found that Mrs. Eldridge had eight errors.

The medications, an antihypertensive and a diuretic, were verified with the physician and the pharmacist. One pill bottle did not have a label, and the pharmacist said the unknown medication was probably a sleeping pill because its description fit one that had been prescribed. The pharmacist said that the sleeping pill prescription was old and had not been refilled in some time.

A meeting was arranged with the son at the health department after a neighbor agreed to stay with Mrs. Eldridge. After the nurse revealed what had been observed, the son was both shocked and saddened. He went on to say that he had an uneasy feeling about his mother for the past couple of weeks but that he "just couldn't put a finger on what was going on." Because of Mrs. Eldridge's obvious cognitive impairment, the nurse asked for validation of what information she had been able to obtain. She learned that Mrs. Eldridge had been hypertensive for several years and had always been faithful about taking her medications, keeping appointments, and eating a healthy diet. He went on to say that he had been dreading the day when he would have to look for a nursing home for his mother for an extended stay.

Mrs. Eldridge's son and the nurse met again 2 weeks later at Mrs. Eldridge's home. The home and Mrs. Eldridge were clean, and Mrs. Eldridge apologized for not remembering the first meeting. It appeared that the sleeping pill, which she had taken to help with the sad feeling and insomnia that accompanied the anniversary of her husband's death, had caused Mrs. Eldridge's intellectual impairment. Mrs. Eldridge and her son had a frank discussion about her living arrangements, and both agreed she would stay in her apartment. Mrs. Eldridge also wished that should her health deteriorate to a point that all hope for recovery was lost, she be allowed to die a peaceful death. The nurse suggested that both mother and son discuss this issue and come to an agreement on the advance directive measure; both agreed.

B. The following factors make this situation difficult:
— Mrs. Eldridge lives alone.
— Mrs. Eldridge demonstrates problems with memory and self-care.
— The nurse must balance Mrs. Eldridge's autonomy with the need to intervene for her safety.

CHAPTER 21

A. Check Ms. Green for proteinuria (because of her pitting edema and complaints of a mild headache). Contact the health department and arrange for her to be seen soon by the nurse practitioner to determine what medication she needs, what dietary restrictions and additions she needs, what intervals of work and rest will help her, and whether she needs any meals brought to her or she needs to get some meals from a local shelter.

B. Ms. Green is likely approaching preeclampsia. She may be on the brink of an emergence of her psychotic illness. Her nutrition may be inadequate, with too much salt and fat. Her psychotropic medicine needs to be regulated and taken regularly. Find out if she needs help to pay for the medicine and the vitamins. Investigate whether she can really take care of this infant. Determine if the father is a source of financial and emotional support.

CHAPTER 22

A. Nursing roles include coordination, referred, case management.

B. Liz might coordinate obtaining nutritious food for Ethyl by arranging for Meals-On-Wheels to deliver a hot meal daily and extra meals for the weekend to be delivered on Friday.

C.1. Because Ethyl is alone a lot, the Meals-On-Wheels driver can be taught to observe any unusual or out-of-the-ordinary behaviors. Should anything be noticed, the driver should call the Coordinating Assessment and Monitoring (CAM) Agency in the hospital emergency department.

C.2. Liz might also arrange through the Senior Center for their van to take Ethyl into town weekly to shop and/or visit the physician.

C.3. Liz can also arrange for Ethyl's sister, Suzanna, to call Ethyl each day to check on her.

D.1. After the episode in which Ethyl was found in her yard, Liz coordinated with her neighbor to organize a rotating system among other neighbors so that one person went by to see Ethyl daily.

D.2. A remote monitoring system was put into Ethyl's home so she can call the CAM whenever she does not feel "up to par."

D.3. The most significant outcome achieved by Liz's case management would be to arrange sufficient basic services to allow Ethyl to remain at home. These include the following:
• Coordinating food (both Meals-On-Wheels and grocery shopping)
• Organizing a team of people to regularly check on Ethyl both to determine her health status and also to provide stimulation and socialization
• Arranging transportation to obtain regular health care
• Ensuring that Ethyl knows how to use technology to communicate with others in her circle of support as well as health care providers (e.g., a portable cellular phone or a remote paging systems)

CHAPTER 23

1. Develop a separate young fathers program, and recruit a male program leader.
2. Develop a school-based childcare center for students and teachers, and use the center as a service learning opportunity for teen program participants.
3. Design a presentation on violence—both intimate partner violence and child violence.
4. Recruit volunteer adult mentors to work closely with individual teens throughout their pregnancy.

CHAPTER 24

A. Consider Mr. Jones' readiness for change, educational needs regarding health effects of smoking, and risks to family members from sidestream smoke.

B. Consider support groups such as AA for Mr. Jones and Alanon for Anne and how this could be helpful. Is it realistic for Anne to stop her grandfather from drinking if he doesn't want to? What else would be helpful to know about his drinking (e.g., where he drinks, what his behavior is like when he is drinking, health risks related to drinking, effects of his drinking on her children), and how would this affect the interventions?

C. Is there evidence of Anne's concern about her children's health as a place to begin? If Anne is not ready to stop "cold turkey," what steps can she begin to take toward the ultimate goal of stopping? What local resources are available?

D. Consider Anne's knowledge of good parenting skills. Consider counseling needs—what stressors are Anne and her children dealing with in their family and environment? How does age affect the potential interventions? Which child is at greater risk? Consider school resources, day care possibilities, and community resources for recreational activities.

E. Consider what the local neighborhood can do to help and what community resources are available. Which community leaders might be helpful? Could Ms. Doe facilitate a meeting between the local neighbors and law enforcement to help establish helpful communication and relationships? What prevention and treatment programs are available and at what cost? Are legislators aware of the cost benefits of drug treatment compared with law enforcement?

CHAPTER 25

A. The nurse needs to listen carefully to the pain and anguish the daughter felt about hitting her mother. She can convey a nonjudgmental attitude and help the daughter and mother explore ways in which both of their needs could be more effectively met. She can provide information and resources to allow the daughter some respite from constant caretaking and a way to continue her own activities.

B.1. Assess the situation: Mrs. Smith felt stiff and seemed to have more joint pain from her arthritis in the mornings. With further assessment it became clear that by late afternoon her joints were more flexible and less painful.

B.2. Discuss options with the family: When nurse, daughter, and client discussed their options, they decided that Mary would wash only her mother's anal area in the morning and put clean pads under her if indicated. Total hygienic care would be done in the late afternoon.

B.3. Teach alternative approaches: Mrs. Jones demonstrated to Mary alternative ways to move, turn, and wash her mother to minimize the strain on her arthritic joints and to incorporate some effective exercise into the bath.

B.4. Make appropriate referrals and coordinate services: On two mornings each week, a home health care aide was engaged to stay with Mrs. Smith. Mary could then do family shopping and errands and participate in activities in which she had previously been involved.

C. Mrs. Jones will need to monitor the situation carefully for any further signs of abuse. Any further instance of violence must be discussed with the daughter and immediately reported. In a subsequent visit, the nurse evaluated the effectiveness of her teaching and learned that Mary and her mother were working much more cooperatively on Mrs. Smith's care.

CHAPTER 26

A. The best answer is the third one. Trusted leaders provide an entry point into the community; they can help develop a plan that is best suited to meet perceived and actual needs.

B. The best answer is the first one. Trust in public health programs must be developed before a crisis situation occurs. The assistance of community leaders at the time of crisis is extremely helpful, but will be more effective if word of mouth has already established that public health officials are not associated with immigration. An appeal for the safety of friends and family may sometimes be more effective than emphasizing the threat to the individual.

C. The best answer is probably a combination of all four choices and may depend on the literacy level of the community. Some immigrant groups are largely illiterate in their own language.

D. All of these options have possibilities, but the best answer is the second one since community leaders know best how to reach their members in a culturally appropriate manner. However, state-produced materials, if culturally and linguistically appropriate, are very helpful because they are already developed. An ongoing relationship with community representatives is necessary because disease control messages often need to be developed and delivered quickly.

CHAPTER 27

A. Questions the nurse asks Yvonne seek information about past injection drug use and sexual partners. The nurse evaluates Yvonne's comfort in sharing the information with Phil as she explores what she believes Phil's response might be. The nurse offers to role-play the situation of Yvonne telling Phil about the possibility of his infection, risks, and the importance of testing for the HIV antibody. Rather than contacting other previous sexual and drug-using partners herself, Yvonne requests that the health department staff contact them about being tested for possible infection. She gives the nurse the names and addresses of two additional drug-using partners.

B. The most immediate concerns for Yvonne are the need to seek ongoing care to monitor the HIV infection and to decide whether to continue the pregnancy. The nurse asks Yvonne whether she has a primary health care provider. The information given includes providing Yvonne with a list of providers and counseling her about the importance of establishing an ongoing relationship with a primary health care provider for follow-up of the HIV infection. She tells Yvonne that important information about her health may be identified that will help determine her ability to carry and deliver the baby if she chooses to continue the pregnancy. Other important information includes the implications of the test results, such as how they may affect the infant's and mother's health.

C. The nurse explains that transmission to the fetus is possible during the pregnancy and she may have a greater chance of progressing from asymptomatic infection to symptomatic HIV disease but that medications would be given to try to prevent this. The nurse explores possibilities with Yvonne about the decision regarding her ability to physically, emotionally, and financially cope with rearing a child that possibly may be ill. Family members and other potential resources are assessed. The need for Yvonne to tell health care providers or blood handlers about the HIV infection is reviewed. The nurse schedules a second appointment for follow-up counseling 1 week after the initial test results are given. She also gives Yvonne the telephone number of the local AIDS support group and arranges to make a home visit to her in 2 days.

D. At the follow-up home and clinic visits, specific information is given regarding infection control in the home and safer sexual relations. The nurse ensures that Yvonne is taking steps toward receiving prenatal care and medical care for the HIV infection. The nurse reviews information about how to maintain health and avoid stressors and contracts with Yvonne to initiate home visits to provide reinforcement of adequate prenatal nutrition and teaching and to assess Yvonne's physical health as the pregnancy progresses.

CHAPTER 28

The correct answer is C. The team was organized to develop the case definition, plan the interview questions and sampling, and organize the specimen collection. Interviews were used to determine characteristics of the illness and to attempt to identify the source by dietary recall and living arrangements. The dietary recall was focused on the food consumed during the three meals before illness onset. While the interviews were being conducted, an environmental investigation concentrated on food preparation, service, and storage, along with housekeeping procedures. The administrative staff of the retirement community kept a daily log documenting all interventions implemented to determine what effect the measures undertaken to stop the spread of illness may have actually had on controlling the spread of illness.

It was initially thought that the infectious agent was a "Norwalk-like" virus, classified under the heading of human caliciviruses (HCV). Specimen testing, however, confirmed the presence of a virus strain similar to the Mexican virus, also an HCV but classified in a genogroup different from the Norwalk virus. Clinically, symptoms are indistinguishable. Fecal–oral spread through food contamination, close person-to-person contact, and possible respiratory spread were hypothesized for this highly contagious virus.

Much is to be learned about the transmission from persons who are asymptomatic. A majority of the residents of the facility became ill even after the institutional precautions were implemented, such as closing the dining room and limiting contacts among residents, encouraging disinfection of common areas of the retirement community, and emphasizing

personal hygiene and glove use by staff. Ill staff members were told to stay home until at least 2 days after their symptoms subsided. Handwashing by the staff was emphasized using antibacterial soap and drying with paper towels. The use of disposable items was encouraged when possible. The recent increase in gastrointestinal illness in older populations in the state highlights the fragile state of health of many of the residents. As a result of this investigation, recommendations for control measures during outbreaks of gastroenteritis in institutions became incorporated into a checklist for long-term care facilities. This increases the level of awareness of the importance of strict adherence to hygienic practices in institutional settings.

CHAPTER 29

Regardless of the earliest beginnings, the following elements are needed to shape the path:
- Discussions
- Questions
- Eliciting statements of healthy and unhealthy events in the lives of the members
- Surveying the physical, social, emotional, and spiritual environmental conditions of the faith community

Formation of a broadly representative wellness committee will help to plan the formal and informal assessment methods and careful documentation of activities and communication.

Building on strengths of the congregation, gathering information on leaders and valued activities in the congregation, and becoming informed regarding lines of authority and communication help provide a foundation for the service. The best answer is D: "Assessing the needs of the congregational members through a survey." This increases interest and involvement of the members. Results assist in bringing a possible goal into focus. If the majority of the congregation is older than 55 years, it would be helpful to assess areas such as the need for retirement planning, the current health status and adequacy of health financing options, involvement in caregiving for parents as well as adult children, the need for involvement in meaningful volunteer activities, and the ability to holistically engage in activities appropriate for the life stage. Assessment would also include the impact of the group older than age 55 on the remainder of the congregation and the surrounding community. Information regarding resources within the church and geopolitical community is helpful.

Organizing and implementing a health fair to address identified needs often is beneficial in the following ways:
- Creating awareness of health needs
- Providing information to act on identified health concerns
- Increasing the visibility of the value of health and faith connections
- Promoting interest for additional congregational members to become involved in the parish nurse and health ministry program

The greater the involvement by the members, the greater the ownership of the program by the total faith community.

Evaluation of the activity will yield information regarding which areas or activities should be continued or reinforced, which need to change focus, and which should be omitted.

In addition to the group and population activities, the parish nurse meets regularly with the pastoral staff and coordinates with other committee chairs. Together, they identify individuals requiring further assessment or support; become aware of issues that need to be clarified, supported, or addressed; and determine individuals, groups, or issues that have not yet become a part of the parish nurse or congregational wellness program. Home visits, phone calls, and visits to hospitals or community agencies are also part of the parish nurse's weekly activities. Agendas might include advocacy and interpretation with a health care provider, monitoring dementia progress, supporting a new mother embarking on a "new" career at home, leading a support group, therapeutic touch, prayer, and visualization.

CHAPTER 30

A. The following strategies help develop trust:
   — Respect the family's customs and space and use sensitivity regarding the timing of questions.
   — Be flexible and keep promises; this is even more important in the home.
   — Give the family a time range when making an appointment to allow for delays at other homes and for traffic.
   — Provide the client and family information about the referral, the purpose of the visit, what services are available, and how to contact the agency.
   — Deal first with the issue that is uppermost on the client's mind, not what is first on the nurse's agenda. This strategy will decrease client anxiety and improve the ability to understand and focus on what the nurse needs to tell them.
B. The assessment in the home environment should include the following:
   — Take a detailed history.
   — Do a physical assessment.
   — Walk through the important parts of the house (bedroom, bathroom, kitchen, hallways) to obtain baseline data for forming the plan of care.
   — Listen to clients to get the most important clues to health status and effective teaching strategies.
   — Begin to complete the necessary forms to ensure that the information is obtained. Some clients will not be able to complete all the forms and provide the required information on the first visit because of pain or fatigue. Focus on the essentials and complete the rest of the forms on a second visit.

C. Client contact must include the following:
   — Set short-term and long-term goals with clients.
   — Have a plan for every visit to progress toward the goals.
   — Inform clients and families that home health services are time limited and that they need to learn to provide their own care.
   — Set limits, model expected behaviors, and write in the behaviors of the client.
   — Develop principles to facilitate and encourage self-care.
   — Plan for modifying care to allow as much independence as possible.
   — Write plans to teach the client rather than do for the client.
D. Learning style is assessed by understanding adult learning principles and asking the client about the characteristics that indicate the preferred learning style.

CHAPTER 31

The correct answer is A. Use this opportunity to show how school nurses respond to the primary, secondary, and tertiary prevention health needs of children and families.

CHAPTER 32

The correct answer is D. This is an example of how the epidemiologic triad can be used to assess clients and plan nursing care. It illustrates the usefulness of approaching occupational health problems with an epidemiologic perspective.

Index

Index